Magnetic Resonance Imaging in Orthopaedics & Sports Medicine

Magnetic Resonance Imaging in Orthopaedics & Sports Medicine

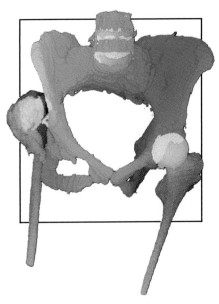

David W. Stoller, M.D.

Director
California Advanced Imaging
San Francisco, California

Assistant Clinical Professor of Radiology
University of California at San Francisco
San Francisco, California

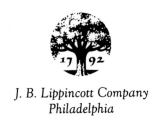

J. B. Lippincott Company
Philadelphia

Acquisitions Editor: Charles McCormick, Jr.
Sponsoring Editor: Kimberley Cox
Project Editor: Molly E. Dickmeyer
Indexer: Sandi Schroeder
Designer: Doug Smock
Production Manager: Caren Erlichman
Production Coordinator: David T. Murphy, Jr.
Compositor: Tapsco, Inc.
Prepress: Jay's Publishers Services, Inc.
Printer/Binder: Arcata Graphics/Kingsport

6   5   4   3   2

Library of Congress Cataloging-in-Publication Data

Stoller, David W.
  Magnetic resonance imaging in orthopaedics and sports medicine/ David W. Stoller.
    p.   cm.
  Includes bibliographical references and index.
  ISBN 0-397-51144-2
  1. Orthopedics—Diagnosis.   2. Magnetic resonance imaging.
  3. Sports—Accidents and injuries—Diagnosis.   I. Title.
  [DNLM: 1. Athletic Injuries.   2. Magnetic Resonance Imaging.
  3. Orthopedics.   QT 260 S875m]
  RD734.5.M33S75 1993
  617.5'807548—dc20
  DNLM/DLC
  for Library of Congress   *92-49358*
                                                                  CIP

The authors and publisher have exerted every effort to ensure that drug selection and dosage set forth in this text are in accord with current recommendations and practice at the time of publication. However, in view of ongoing research, changes in government regulations, and the constant flow of information relating to drug therapy and drug reactions, the reader is urged to check the package insert for each drug for any change in indications and dosage and for added warnings and precautions. This is particularly important when the recommended agent is a new or infrequently employed drug.

All of the color anatomy figures that appear in this book are reproduced with permission from Gosling's Human Anatomy, *2nd edition, J. A. Gosling, P. F. Harris, J. R. Humpherson, I. Whitmore, P. L. T. Willan, eds., published by Gower Medical Publishing, London, 1990.*

Many of the black and white images that appear in this book have been previously published in Magnetic Resonance Imaging in Orthopaedics and Rheumatology, *D. W. Stoller, et al, published by J. B. Lippincott Company, Philadelphia, 1989.*

To my lovely wife, Marcia, for her extraordinary love and support, and to both of our families, for understanding and accommodating the sacrifices of personal time

Contributors

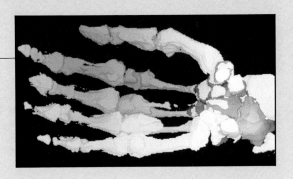

Lesley J. Anderson, M.D.
Orthopaedic Surgeon
California Pacific Medical Center
San Francisco, California

Gordon A. Brody, M.D.
Chief, Hand Surgery
Grant Orthopaedic Institute
Columbus, Ohio

W. Dilworth Cannon, Jr., M.D.
Professor of Clinical Orthopaedics
   and Director of Sports Medicine
University of California at San Francisco
San Francisco, California

Richard H. Griffey, Ph.D.
Director of Magnetic Resonance Imaging Education
Baylor University Medical Center
Dallas, Texas

Steven E. Harms, M.D.
Medical Director
Magnetic Resonance Imaging Department
Baylor University Medical Center
Dallas, Texas

Thomas R. Lindquist, Ph.D.
President
Lindquist and Associates Systems and Software
Eden Prairie, Minnesota

William J. Maloney, M.D.
Assistant Clinical Professor
Stanford University
Palo Alto, California

Attending Orthopaedic Surgeon
Palo Alto Medical Clinic
Palo Alto, California

Bruce A. Porter, M.D.
Medical Director
First Hill Diagnostic Imaging Center
Seattle, Washington

Frank G. Shellock, Ph.D.
Director of Research, Development and
   Advanced Applications
Tower Imaging
Los Angeles, California

Assistant Professor of Radiological Sciences
UCLA School of Medicine
Los Angeles, California

Terri M. Steinkirchner, M.D.
Staff Pathologist
Department of Pathology
Walnut Creek Kaiser Medical Center
Walnut Creek, California

David W. Stoller, M.D.
Director
California Advanced Imaging
San Francisco, California

Assistant Clinical Professor of Radiology
University of California at San Francisco
San Francisco, California

Eugene M. Wolf, M.D.
Department of Orthopaedics
California Pacific Medical Center
San Francisco, California

Foreword

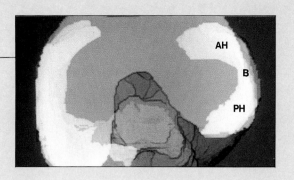

Magnetic resonance imaging is the most significant diagnostic test performed on orthopaedic and sports medicine patients. Frequently, it is the definitive examination, providing invaluable information to help the surgeon not only to understand the underlying pathology but also to make the critical decision regarding surgical intervention. In 1985, when MR imaging of the knee first became available, the clinical decision-making process was rarely influenced by its results, the direction of treatment being determined by the physical examination and arthrogram. With the advent of improved and sophisticated equipment, today MR imaging is indispensable in the work-up of patients with knee disorders and is fast approaching the same state of excellence for shoulder maladies. It is especially important to the professional athlete who depends on quick, accurate diagnoses to support treatment programs and to provide him or her with information that will help determine their return to play.

The accuracy of MR imaging for detection of meniscal and anterior cruciate ligament tears has risen to over 90%. In the shoulder, the diagnosis of subtle labral tears and abnormal capsular attachments, including SLAP lesions, now is made possible by these imaging techniques, thereby avoiding invasive techniques and radiation exposure. Occasionally, when further information is sought from diagnostic MR imaging, the use of intraarticular or intravenous gadolinium provides surface topographic details as well as information on vascular patterns within tissues. But the orthopaedist and radiologist should also be aware of the limitations of MR imaging, such as in the evaluation of the knee after partial meniscectomy or after meniscal repair, instances in which a grade III signal may persist despite clinical and arthroscopic evidence of satisfactory healing.

The present compendium of musculoskeletal MR imaging is all encompassing: from the shoulder to the foot and ankle, and from bone marrow imaging to bone and soft tissue tumors. *Magnetic Resonance Imaging in Orthopaedics and Sports Medicine* is composed of over 1100 pages and over 2500 images. The beginning section provides a valuable introduction into the physics and science of MR imaging for the nonradiologist. Chapter 2, on three-dimensional MR rendering techniques, provides some interesting clinical and research concepts on volumetric analysis of internal structures, such as the menisci. Preoperative MR imaging sizing for allograft surgery is also possible. The kinematics of meniscal motion during flexion and extension as determined by MR imaging has helped to better understand knee biomechanics.

Dr. Stoller's text should become a key reference source for the libraries of both radiologists and orthopaedists. It is extremely readable, and its ample illustrations help clarify points made in the text. *Magnetic Resonance Imaging in Orthopaedics and Sports Medicine* is the most comprehensive work to date on musculoskeletal imaging and should remain a classic for years to come.

W. DILWORTH CANNON, JR., M.D.
Professor of Clinical Orthopaedics
Director of Sports Medicine
Department of Orthopaedic Surgery
University of California at San Francisco

Preface

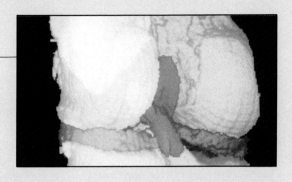

The indications and applications of MR imaging in the fields of orthopaedics and sports medicine have shown exponential growth and refinement since its initial clinical introduction in 1983. With the development of advanced systems hardware, work stations, phased array coils, and advanced software programs including fast-imaging techniques and high resolution imaging options (*e.g.,* 512 acquisition matrices, volume acquisition, and reformation) MR continues to both replace and complement CT in the evaluation of disorders affecting the axial and appendicular skeleton.

Magnetic Resonance Imaging in Orthopaedics and Sports Medicine was written to replace my 1989 textbook, *Magnetic Resonance Imaging in Orthopaedics and Rheumatology.* Significant advances in the understanding and application of MR imaging in the wrist, shoulder, knee, and hip have been incorporated with the assistance of orthopaedic contributors. Separate chapters on marrow disorders, tumors, kinematic imaging, and three-dimensional rendering techniques are included. Because the quality of magnetic resonance studies is related to an accurate correlation with gross anatomy and surgical findings, detailed multiplanar MR normal anatomy sections have been incorporated into the appendicular joint chapters, as have relevant gross surgical dissection color images. Arthroscopic and histologic photographs have been included to support anatomic and pathologic findings.

Magnetic Resonance Imaging in Orthopaedics and Sports Medicine is a complete and current reference that addresses the growing need of radiologists, orthopaedic surgeons, and sports medicine physicians to understand and incorporate new clinical applications of bone and joint imaging into their practices.

DAVID W. STOLLER, M.D.

Acknowledgments

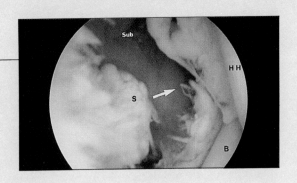

I appreciate and acknowledge the following individuals for their contributions:

J. A. Gosling, M.D., M.B., Ch.B., P. F. Harris, M.D., M.B., Ch.B., M.Sc., J. R. Humpherson, M.B., Ch.B., I. Whitmore, M.D., M.B., B.S., L.R.C.P., M.R.C.S., and P. L. T. Willan, M.B., Ch.B., F.R.C.S., for providing superior quality gross anatomic color plates from their text, *Human Anatomy*, second edition, Gower Medical Publishing.

Robert Ashley and the Squibb Diagnostics Group, for their encouragement and assistance.

Jay Miller, Bob Edmeyer, Kuldip Ahluwalia, Bill Kennedy, and Hans Grillmeyer of General Electric, for their ongoing support of my interest in MR basic science, clinical research, and MR education.

The industrious technologist staff at California Advanced Imaging: Carolin Elmquist, Carol Greene, and Michael Wehry.

JoAnn Alonzo of California Advanced Imaging, for her invaluable contributions and encouragement throughout the dispatch of the manuscript.

Wendy Jovero, for typing the first draft of the manuscript.

Katherine Pitcoff, who served as my West Coast editor, for tirelessly preparing manuscript for presentation to J. B. Lippincott.

Charles McCormick, Medical Editor at J. B. Lippincott, for his efforts and appreciation of the necessary quality required to bring this textbook to fruition. Charles' foresight and independent character enabled him to orchestrate this project to completion despite varied opinions and recommendations of others in his field.

Peter Fairfield and the staff of Gamma Photographic Laboratories in San Francisco, for photography of text images with unmatched professional quality, produced in record-breaking time.

John V. Crues III, M.D., for Figures 5–123, 12–7, 12–8, 12–9, 12–10, 13–6, 13–98, and 13–107.

Jerrold H. Mink, M.D., for Figure 13–81.

Sheila Moore, M.D., for Figures 3–59, 3–80, 12–14, 12–55, 13–73, and 13–100.

David Seidenwurm, M.D., for Figures 13–32, 13–39, 13–40, 13–68, 13–76, and 13–110.

Jeremy McCreary, M.D., for Figure 8–67.

John Hunter, M.D., for Figure 13–31.

Neil Chafetz, M.D., for Figure 4–111.

Barbara Griffiths, M.D., for Figure 4–32.

Michael Schneider, M.D., for Figure 4–272.

Bob Princenthal, for Figure 5–48.

Harry K. Genant, M.D., for Figures 3–34, 11–34, 11–77, 11–113, 13–19, 13–44, and 13–46.

Clyde A. Helms, M.D., for Figure 9–5.

Russell Fritz, M.D., for Figure 6–34.

Frank Shellock, Ph.D., for Figures 10–9, 10–13, 10–35, 10–38, and 10–42, from *MRI of the Musculoskeletal System. A Teaching File,* Raven Press.

Phillip Brody, M.D., for Figure 12–21.

David Rubenstein, M.D., for Figure 8–90.

Jacque Anderson, M.D., of Royal North Shore Hospital, Sydney, Australia, for Figures 5–72 and 5–99.

James Glick, M.D., for the arthroscopic photographs in Chapter 3.

Contents

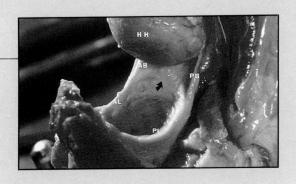

Magnetic Resonance Imaging in Orthopaedics & Sports Medicine

CHAPTER 1

Richard H. Griffey
Steven E. Harms

Generation and Manipulation of Magnetic Resonance Images

Magnetic resonance (MR) imaging, which uses nonionizing radiation and has no demonstrated adverse effects, has rapidly evolved into an accepted modality for medical imaging of disease processes in soft tissues. Magnetic resonance images provide a digital representation of tissue characteristics related to spatial location and can be obtained in any tissue plane. This chapter provides an overview of MR fundamentals and addresses the factors that affect the differences in appearance (*i.e.,* contrast) among tissues in MR imaging. The current generation of advanced MR techniques is presented, including magnetic resonance angiography (MRA), magnetic resonance spectroscopy (MRS), and an introduction to three-dimensional (3D) MR imaging (see Chap. 2). More detailed discussions on the fundamentals of MR can be found in other sources.[1-5]

The appearance of an MR image is a function of the chemical composition of the various types of tissue. For example, soft tissues are composed of approximately 70% water and 10% to 15% adipose, which generate all the MR signal. At the atomic level, water and adipose are composed of hydrogen, oxygen, carbon, and phosphorus atoms. The hydrogen atom contains a proton and an orbiting electron. Understanding how an MR image is produced begins with a knowledge of magnetic fields and how these atomic components of water and fat interact with such fields.

FUNDAMENTALS OF MAGNETISM

A familiar example of magnetism is an ordinary compass needle. Like any magnet, the compass needle has a north pole and a south pole—a reflection of the dipolar nature of magnetism. The compass needle has a weak internal magnetic field called a magnetic moment. The earth also has an internal magnetic field, which is stronger than the magnetic field of the compass needle. In the presence of the strong magnetic field from the earth, the weak magnetic moment of the compass needle aligns with the stronger magnetic field and the needle points north. It is possible to introduce another magnetic field, such as a bar magnet, which has a magnetic field comparable in strength to the earth's magnetic field, and to twist the compass needle out of alignment with the earth's magnetic field. When the bar magnet is removed, the compass needle returns to the normal condition of pointing north in the same direction as the earth's magnetic field.

The magnetic fields associated with MR are less intuitive, but follow these same principles. A spinning, charged particle produces a local magnetic field. The proton has a positive charge and spins like a top about its internal axis, as shown in Figure 1–1. The local magnetic field of the proton is called the magnetic dipole moment, and causes the proton to behave like a tiny, weak bar magnet or a weak compass needle. In the absence of any external forces, the magnetic moments of protons in tissue are oriented randomly, as shown in Figure 1–2A. If the ensemble of protons are placed in a strong, static magnetic field (B_0), their magnetic dipoles align with and against the strong field (Fig. 1–2B). The distribution of alignments are nearly evenly divided due to the effects of thermal energy. The magnetic moments aligned with the main field are canceled by neighbors aligned against the main field. Slightly more than one-half of the magnetic moments align parallel with the B_0 field, however, because it takes less energy for the small magnetic moments to align with the stronger main magnetic field.

The MR signal is generated from extra magnetic moments that are aligned parallel with B_0. At a magnetic field strength of 1.5 tesla (T), used in many clinical scanners, only approximately 8 of 2,000,000 proton magnetic moments aligned with B_0 do not have a corresponding proton magnetic moment aligned against B_0. This slight excess of protons in the lower energy state, whose individual magnetic moments add up, create the net magnetization vector. The alignment of the magnetic moments, which occurs when the protons are placed in the B_0 field, causes the patient to acquire a slight magnetization. This process is reversible, because the magnetic moments lose alignment when the person is removed from the strong static magnetic field.

Magnetic resonance sensitivity increases as a function of magnetic field strength, because more energy is required for magnetic moments to align against the main magnetic field with increasing field strength, and a higher percentage of magnetic moments adopt the low-energy state aligned with the main B_0 field. Magnetic resonance images have low signal-to-noise ratio (SNR) compared with that of computed tomography or x-ray, because this net magnetization vector is detected from such a small percentage of the protons in the tissue.

PRECESSION AND RESONANCE

Precession and resonance are physical phenomena central to understanding MR. Both result from the interaction of an object with a force. Common examples of precession include the movement of the earth and planets around the sun, the swing of a pendulum, and the rotation of a spinning top. In these cases, the precessional motion results from the effect of an orienting gravitational field on the motion of the object. The precessional motion of the magnetic dipole moment induced by the force of a strong magnetic field is analogous.

Resonance involves the exchange of energy between two systems. A familiar example of resonance is the vibration of two tuning forks. When energy is applied to a single tuning fork (*i.e.,* when it is struck), it resonates at a characteristic frequency. The vibration of the air produced by the first tuning fork induces resonance in a second nearby tuning fork and causes the second fork to vibrate as well. The interaction of the precessing magnetic moments with a second perturbing magnetic field is another example of resonance. In each of these examples, the motion of the object has a periodic return to the same physical location, resulting from its inherent energy (*i.e.,* momentum) or applied energy. Resonance and precession can be measured in units of numbers of cycles per period of time. A common unit of this type is cycles per second, or hertz (Hz). This unit can be scaled by a multiplier, for example, 1 million, to produce units of millions of cycles per second, or megahertz (MHz).

Precession

When a person is placed in a strong magnetic field, alignment of the magnetic moments of the protons in water and fat generates a net magnetization in the tissue. The aligned magnetic moments also precess about the main magnetic field. This precession of the magnetic moments about the main magnetic field is a cyclic process with a characteristic frequency (Fig. 1–3). A good analogy is the precession of a spinning top about the gravitational field of the earth. As the top spins, the pull of gravity is balanced by centrifugal force and the top begins to precess. As the protons spin, the attraction of the main magnetic field is balanced by centrifugal force, and the proton and its magnetic moment begin to precess. For protons in tissue, the relationship between the magnetic field strength B_0 and the precessional frequency μ is given by the Larmor equation

$$nu = gamma \times B_0$$

where gamma is a physical constant (*i.e.,* 42.58 MHz/T) for the proton. Other MR-sensitive nuclei such as phosphorus-31 have lower values for gamma and precess at lower frequencies.

Resonance

The net magnetism produced by precessing magnetic moments in tissue is small and cannot be measured directly with any accuracy. Instead, it is detected indirectly with a second perturbing magnetic field (B_1). A compass needle and two magnets provide a model for this process. When a compass needle is placed in a strong magnetic field (B_0), the needle aligns with the lines of magnetic flux (Fig. 1–4A). If a second perturbing magnetic field (B_1, from a second bar magnet) is placed perpendicular to the aligned compass needle, the needle realigns in a new position (Fig. 1–4B). When the B_1 field is removed, the compass needle begins to oscillate about B_0 (Fig. 1–4C). The resonant frequency of oscillation is governed by the strength of the aligning field (B_0), whereas the amplitude of the oscillation is determined by the strength of the perturbing field (B_1).

An analogous sequence of events is used to induce resonance in MR studies of tissue. The patient is placed in a strong magnetic field (B_0) to align the magnetic moments of water and fat protons in the tissue. Next, a perturbing magnetic field (B_1) is applied through a short (*i.e.,* 1 to 3 msec) pulse of a radiofrequency (RF) wave at the Larmor frequency. Radiofrequency waves have inherent perpendicular oscillating electric and magnetic field components. Therefore, a pulse of a 63.86 MHz RF wave briefly creates a magnetic field that oscillates at 63.86 MHz. The magnetic moments resonate and begin to precess about this perturbing B_1 magnetic field, and the net magnetization in tissue is realigned about a new axis away from equilibrium (Fig. 1–5). This realignment of the net magnetization vector at a new position introduces phase coherence to the individual magnetic moments in a plane perpendicular to the direction of the B_0 magnetic field. After the RF pulse is turned off and the perturbing mag-

netic field B_1 is removed, the displaced individual magnetic moments begin to precess coherently about the B_0 field at the characteristic frequency nu given by the Larmor equation.

The resonance of the bulk magnetic moment from tissue is detected as a very small (μA) current induced in an RF antenna tuned to the Larmor frequency and located perpendicular to the B_0 field. Both the antenna used to perturb the magnetic moments and the antenna used to detect their precession must be tuned to the Larmor frequency and located perpendicular to the B_0 field.

This detection process is similar to the generation of electricity by a dynamo in a power station. In the dynamo shown in Figure 1–6, the moving water turns a turbine attached to a bar magnet. The turbine and magnet rotate at a fixed frequency and produce a magnetic field that oscillates at the same frequency (*e.g.,* the turbine and magnet rotate at 60 Hz and produce a magnetic field that oscillates at 60 Hz). If the bar magnet is near a coil of wire, the oscillating magnetic field generates electric current in the coil of wire. The electric current varies from positive to negative at a resonant frequency of 60 Hz as the bar magnet swings around near the coil of wire. This alternating current then can be stored.

Similarly, after excitation, the protons in tissue behave like tiny bar magnets rotating at the Larmor frequency. When a coil of wire (*i.e.,* the MR antenna) is located near the tissue, the rotating magnetic field caused by precession of the net magnetic moment from the tissue generates a current that resonates at the Larmor frequency in the wire of the MR antenna. The amplitude of the detected signal in an MR scan is related to the size of the net magnetic moment per volume of tissue and the duration and amplitude of the applied perturbing magnetic field (B_1). The voltage induced in the antenna is digitized and stored in an MR imaging computer as a function of time.

Energy Levels

This process can also be described in quantum mechanical terms as a probability function for inducing a transition between two energy levels that correspond to the states where the magnetic moment is aligned with and against the main magnetic field. This quantum mechanical description of resonance is equally valid, but is based on a mathematical description that is difficult to visualize.

Rotating Frame of Reference

A reexamination of the precession of the net magnetization vector in tissue, as seen in Figure 1–3, shows that after excitation the precession of the bulk magnetic moment traces out a circular path. If the observer's perspective is redefined, instead of viewing this precession from the side, it is viewed looking down the direction of the static magnetic field B_0, which will be defined as the Z axis in this new coordinate system. This is illustrated in Figure 1–7A, where the intensity of the net magnetization vector is projected onto a plane that contains the X and Y axes. The vector precesses at the Larmor frequency, perhaps in a counterclockwise direction (*i.e.,* an arbitrary choice), and it can now be seen that the precession of the magnetization is a 3D process with an associated amplitude (*i.e.,* length) and phase (*i.e.,* relative position in the X,Y plane). These attributes can be visualized by plotting the relative position of the net magnetization vector in the X,Y plane *versus* time. The result (Fig. 1–7B) is a sine or cosine wave that resonates at the Larmor frequency. As the net magnetization vector precesses, the change in apparent position is reflected as a change in the phase of the projected vector in the X,Y plane.

If the observer also is precessing counterclockwise at the Larmor frequency, the net magnetization vector appears to be stationary. This is called the rotating frame of reference, and is commonly used in descriptions of MR scans to aid in the visualization of the effects that RF pulses, magnetic field gradient pulses, and relaxation processes have on the net magnetization vector.

Changes in the phase and Larmor frequency of a net magnetization vector relative to the position of the observer at a fixed frequency and phase can be detected. If the observer is diligent and continuously records the position of the precessing vectors, those vectors will appear to move away from the fixed reference point at some relative frequency (Fig. 1–8). However, imagine that the observer is sleepy and only opens his or her eye periodically for a brief instant to perform a measurement and recording. In this case, the precessing vectors don't appear to move continually, but adopt a new relative position in the X,Y plane each time the observer makes a measurement. The new position is recorded as phase information relative to the position of the observer. If enough observations are performed, the frequency of the precessing vectors can be determined indirectly by measuring the rate of change in the phase of the vectors and by converting this rate of change into frequency information (see Fig. 1–8).

The two methods—direct measurement of frequency and indirect determination of frequency from phase changes—yield an identical result. Every MR signal has a frequency and a phase; thus, changes in either of these two attributes can be measured via phase encoding or frequency encoding and converted into frequency information to produce a two-dimensional (2D) MR image.

MAKING A MAGNETIC RESONANCE IMAGE

The generation of an MR image inherently is a four-dimensional problem that involves three spatial coordinates (*i.e.,* X, Y, Z) and one contrast dimension that reflects the signal intensity within each volume element (*i.e.,* voxel) of tissue. The spatial origin of the signal must be defined with suitable resolution in three orthogonal planes, whereas the signal intensity in the contrast dimension must be above the level of the background noise. In practice, the resolution in one spatial dimension (*i.e.,* slice dimension) may be compressed to one point to save time, producing a 2D image of a single slice. This method for generating a 2D slice-selective image is the basis for the following discussion. The benefits of true 3D volume imaging are presented later in this chapter.

Equipment

The following equipment is required to produce an MR image:

- a large homogeneous static magnetic field (B_0) to align the tissue magnetization
- magnetic field gradient coils, which produce linear variations in the effective magnetic field as a function of spatial position in X, Y, and Z
- an RF antenna, or RF coil, to produce a perturbing magnetic field (B_1) and to measure the MR signal
- a computer to store time domain data on frequency and phase and to convert this data to frequency information through the mathematical function called three-dimensional Fourier transform (3DFT; Fig. 1–9)
- a method to display the images through appropriate media such as film or a computer workstation.

Magnetic Field Gradient

In a perfectly homogeneous static magnetic field, all the magnetic moments for each proton of water or fat would precess at the same Larmor frequency. However, the strength of the magnetic field can be made to vary throughout the magnet in a linear and predictable fashion, using the magnetic field gradient coils. All MR scanners have magnetic field gradient coils that introduce a linear change in the magnetic field B_0 oriented along three orthogonal directions:

1. Left to right across the bore of the magnet
2. Up and down in the bore of the magnet
3. Along the length of the bore of the magnet (X, Y, and Z axes in the rotating frame coordinate system).

At the exact center of the gradient coil, the linear change in magnetic field strength for all three directions is zero. This location, where each of the gradient coils induce no change in magnetic field strength, is called the isocenter of the magnet. At this point, magnetic moments always precess at the normal frequency governed by the strength of the main magnetic field. Away from isocenter, the strength of the main static magnetic field B_0 is altered by the gradient coils.

The precessional frequency of the magnetization depends on the effective strength of the total magnetic field, as calculated from the Larmor equation. Therefore, the precessional frequencies can be made to vary as a function of spatial position by applying a magnetic field gradient in the X, Y, or Z direction.

This concept of magnetic field gradient, central to all MR processes, is illustrated in Figure 1–10. If a 10-cm long container filled with water is placed in the bore of a 1.5 T magnet, all the protons will resonate at a frequency of 63.876000 MHz. However, in the presence of a magnetic field gradient with a strength of 10 mT/m (1 gauss/cm) applied along the Z axis (*i.e.*, the length of the magnet bore), the water protons resonate over a range of frequencies determined by the following equation:

$$(10 \text{ cm long}) \times (0.1 \text{ mT/m}) \times (42.58 \text{ MHz/T}) = 42{,}580 \text{ Hz}.$$

Since the strength of the magnetic field gradient is linear as a function of position along Z, the resonant frequency is directly related to the spatial position. We use this relationship to generate MR images.

Two-Dimensional Magnetic Resonance Imaging

The generation of a 2D MR image requires three steps:

1. Selection of a slice of tissue for study in a first dimension (*i.e.*, slice direction)
2. Definition of the spatial position in a second dimension by measuring the rate of change in the phase of the MR signal produced by varying the amplitude of a magnetic field gradient pulse (*i.e.*, phase-encoding direction)
3. Definition of the spatial position in the third dimension by detecting the signals in the presence of a magnetic field gradient (*i.e.*, read-out direction).

Slice Selection

As shown in Figure 1–10, in the presence of a 1 gauss/cm magnetic field gradient, the water protons in the 10-cm dish resonate over a frequency range of 42,580 Hz ($\pm 21{,}290$ Hz), with a frequency of 63.876000 MHz at the gradient isocenter. If the RF pulse used to generate the perturbing magnetic field at 63.876000 MHz has a bandwidth of only 2129 Hz, the signal from a 5-mm section of the dish centered about the isocenter can be excited selectively when the magnetic field gradient is turned

on. If the frequency of the slice-selective pulse is varied, for example, to 63.878129 MHz (+2129 Hz), a 5-mm slice can be generated at a location 5 mm to the left (*i.e.*, high-frequency side) of the slice at isocenter. In this fashion, 20 contiguous 5-mm thick MR images of the entire object could be generated using frequency-selective RF pulses to excite each slice.

Phase and Phase Encoding

As shown earlier, precessing magnetization has an amplitude and a relative position in the X,Y plane. In the presence of a magnetic field gradient perpendicular to the direction of the slice gradient, the magnetization vectors in different spatial locations experience different effective magnetic field strengths as a linear function of their position and, as governed by the Larmor equation, resonate at different frequencies. This condition leads to dephasing of the magnetization vectors in different parts of the slice plane. The amount of dephasing that the net magnetization vector experiences is a function of the position in the gradient (Fig. 1–11), the strength of the applied gradient, and the length of time that the gradient pulse is on.

When the field gradient pulse is turned off, the vectors experience only the B_0 magnetic field, and then resonate at their original frequencies. However, the vectors remember the amount of dephasing they received during the time the field gradient pulse was applied (*i.e.*, phase-encoding time). The strength of the applied field gradient pulse can be varied many times, and the amount of dephasing that occurs with each variation can be measured for magnetization in all parts of the slice plane. The rates of change in the phase of the magnetization for proximate regions of tissue are small, and a large number (128 to 256) of phase-encoding steps are required to produce adequate resolution in the time domain. These rates are converted into frequency information via 3DFT and finally into the exact spatial location from the known strength and duration of the phase-encoding gradient pulse.

Read-Out Dimension and Frequency Encoding

As shown in Figure 1–10, the relative spatial position of an object can be estimated from the resonant frequency in the presence of a magnetic field gradient. However, the resonant frequency is determined indirectly. The MR signal is measured and stored as amplitude (*i.e.*, voltage) *versus* time information while the read-out field gradient is applied. The spatial resolution in this dimension is determined by the number of points that are sampled and the frequency bandwidth. The strength of the read-out gradient and the bandwidth determine the field of

(text continues on page 12)

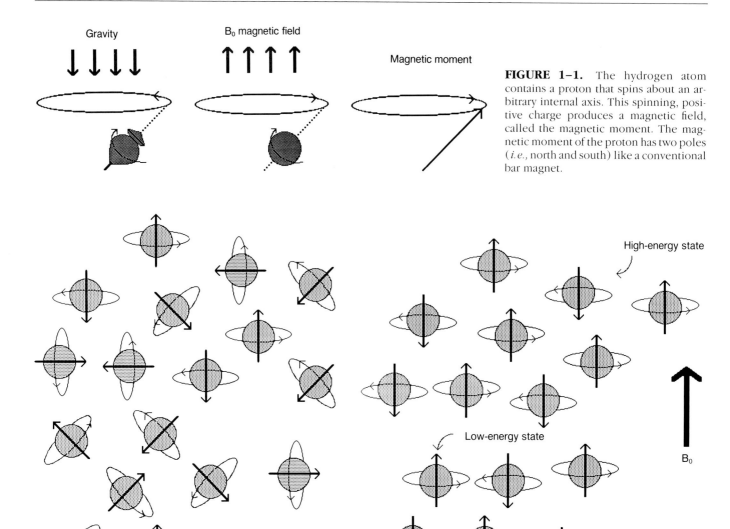

FIGURE 1–1. The hydrogen atom contains a proton that spins about an arbitrary internal axis. This spinning, positive charge produces a magnetic field, called the magnetic moment. The magnetic moment of the proton has two poles (*i.e.,* north and south) like a conventional bar magnet.

FIGURE 1–2. (**A**) A collection of protons at thermal equilibrium in the absence of a strong magnetic field. The magnetic moments produced by the spinning of the nucleus are oriented randomly. (**B**) The same collection of protons at thermal equilibrium in the presence of a strong magnetic field. The magnetic moments are aligned with or against the magnetic field B_0.

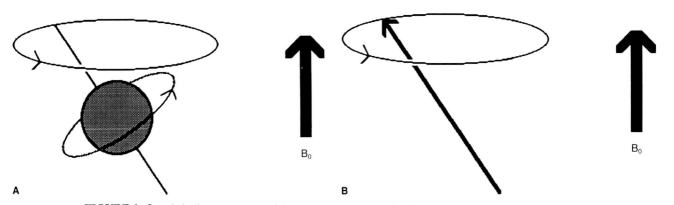

FIGURE 1–3. (**A**) The precession of the spinning proton and (**B**) the magnetic moment of the proton in the presence of a strong external magnetic field.

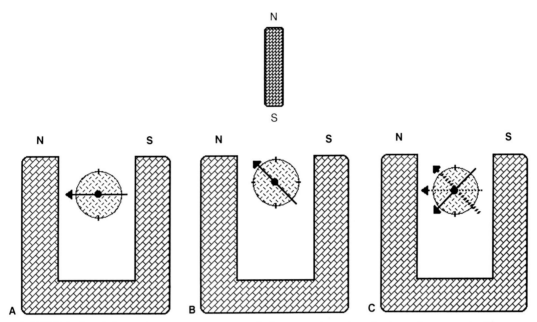

FIGURE 1–4. (**A**) Positioning a compass needle between the poles of a strong bar magnet will cause it to orient itself toward the north pole of the magnet. (**B**) Reorientation of the compass needle is caused by a second perturbing magnetic field. (**C**) Induction of precession in the compass needle occurs when the second perturbing magnetic field is removed.

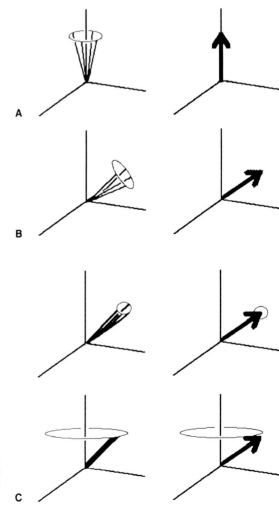

FIGURE 1–5. Note the effects of the perturbing B_1 magnetic field on the bulk magnetization vector (**A**) at the start of the B_1 pulse; (**B**) at the end of the B_1 pulse; (**C**) some time after the pulse as the individual magnetic moments precess at their Larmor frequencies.

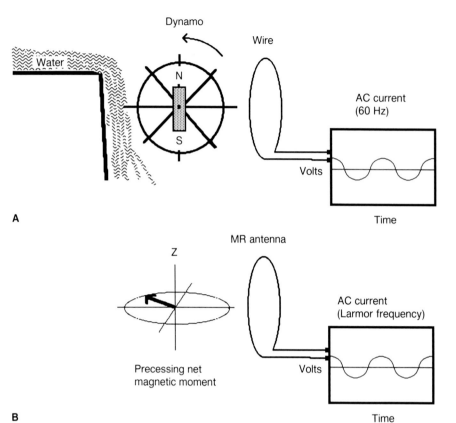

FIGURE 1–6. The dynamo model for detection of the MR signal. (**A**) A model dynamo produces current in a loop of wire through the circular motion of the bar magnet induced by the flow of water over the paddle wheels. (**B**) A model magnetic moment produces current in a loop of wire (*i.e.,* MR antenna) through precession at the Larmor frequency. The effect is analogous to the model dynamo, although the model magnetic moment rotates in a plane perpendicular to the plane of the dynamo's bar magnet.

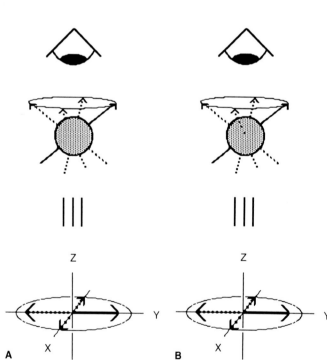

FIGURE 1–7. A view of a precessing magnetization vector after perturbation (**A**) from along the Z axis (*i.e.,* along the axis of the strong magnetic field), and the corresponding model of precession in the rotating frame of reference (**B**) continuously monitored from along the Y axis. The amplitude of the magnetization vector is zero when viewed head-on, and has maximum and minimum values when viewed from the side.

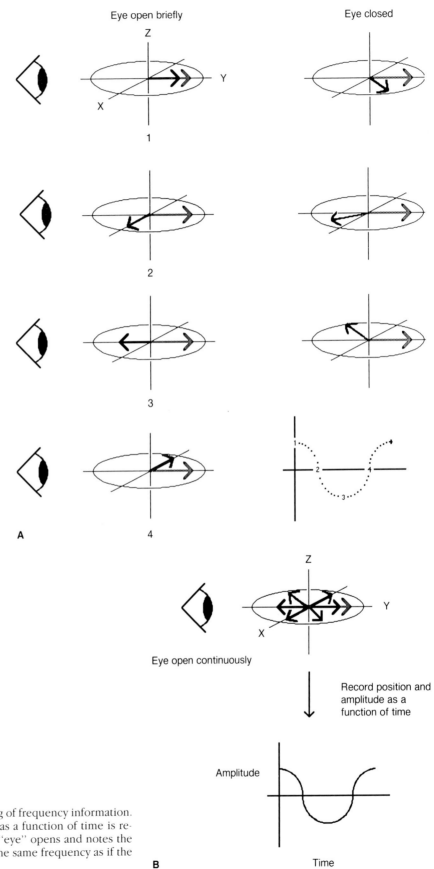

FIGURE 1–8. A model for the phase encoding of frequency information. (**A**) The amplitude of the magnetization vector as a function of time is recorded in the lower right corner each time the "eye" opens and notes the position. (**B**) This periodic sampling measures the same frequency as if the eye had been open the entire time.

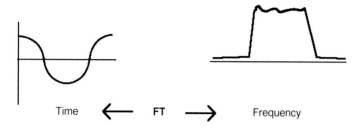

Time ⟵ FT ⟶ Frequency

FIGURE 1-9. The 3D Fourier transform converts time to frequency information. Hence, signals measured in the time domain can be converted into frequency information used to produce MR images.

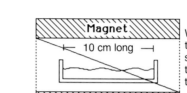

$v = 63.867$ MHz

A ⟵ B_0

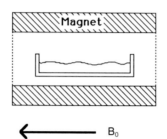

When the magnetic field gradient is turned on, the effective magnetic field strength is altered by an amount equal to ΔB_0 from one end of the magnet to the other.

FIGURE 1-10. (**A**) When a 10-cm long tub of water is placed in a homogeneous static magnetic field B_0, all the water protons precess at a single frequency, nu. (**B**) In the presence of a magnetic-field gradient ΔB_0 with a strength of 1 gauss/cm applied along the Z axis, the water magnetization resonates over a frequency range of 63.888–63.846 MHz as a function of the spatial position in the magnetic-field gradient. (**C**) In the presence of a magnetic-field gradient with a strength of 1 gauss/cm, the water magnetization in the central 1-cm region resonates over a frequency range of 4257 Hz. If a radio-frequency pulse with a bandwidth of 4257 Hz is used as the perturbing B_1 magnetic field, only the water magnetization in the 1-cm region will be excited.

B

$B_0 + \Delta B_0$ $B_0 - \Delta B_0$

$v = 63.888$ MHz $v = 63.846$ MHz

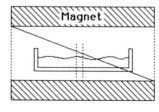

C

>1 cm, $\Delta v = 4257$ Hz

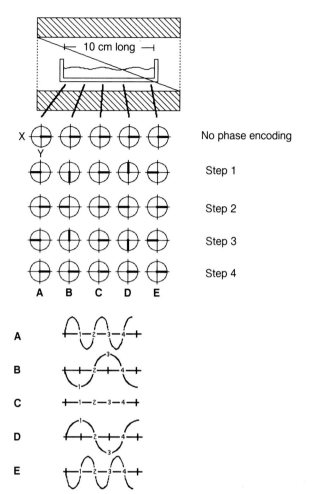

FIGURE 1–11. The phase-encoding process. In the presence of a magnetic-field gradient pulse, the magnetic moments temporarily precess at faster or slower speeds. This produces a shift in the phase of the detected signal. The change in phase is shown for five locations, labeled A–E, following four different magnetic-field gradient pulses, numbered 1–4. The resulting phase maps for A–E are shown (*bottom*).

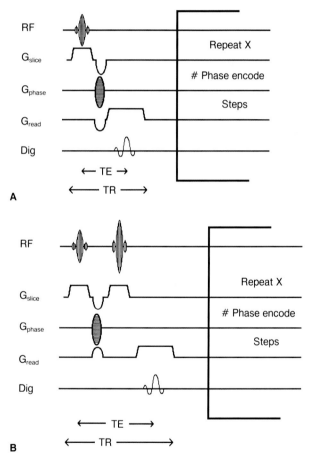

FIGURE 1–12. Timing diagrams for (**A**) a gradient-echo pulse sequence and (**B**) a spin-echo pulse sequence. Time is increasing from left to right for each of the radiofrequency (RF) and gradient pulse waveforms. (Dig, analog/digital converter; G_{phase}, phase-encoding gradient; G_{read}, read-out or frequency gradient; G_{slice}, slice-encoding gradient.)

view (FOV). If the frequency bandwidth in the read-out dimension is 16,000 Hz, 512 points will have to be sampled to be able to distinguish signals that differ by 30 Hz.

The read-out bandwidth also affects the SNR in an image. The amount of noise stored by the computer is proportional to the bandwidth. A four-fold decrease in the read-out bandwidth reduces the noise by a factor of four, with a two-fold improvement in image SNR. This variable bandwidth strategy is used on many commercial MR units to improve the SNR in images acquired at long echo times (TE).

Three-Dimensional Magnetic Resonance Imaging

Conventional 2D imaging often sacrifices resolution and complete coverage in the slice dimension for speed. These trade-offs probably are acceptable in studies of the brain and body in which the organs are large and homogeneous. However, in regions that contain fine structures, such as the knee, the volume averaging, lack of contiguous slices, and thicker slices associated with 2D MR imaging can obscure pathology. Three-dimensional MR imaging can be used to generate a set of contiguous images having nearly isotropic voxels, which provide high-resolution detail of fine pathologic processes. In addition, images corresponding to any plane of tissue can be generated and viewed from a 3D data set. Hence, it is not necessary to spend time obtaining separate sets of images in all three conventional image planes. This added flexibility is advantageous for following pathologic processes such as damage to ligaments or cartilage that do not track through a single image plane.

To date, the clinical use of 3D MR imaging has been restricted because of limitations in the performance of computers and gradients available on MR instruments. For example, a 16-bit, $128 \times 128 \times 256$ point 3D data set requires 8 megabytes of computer memory. Storage, 3DFT, and reformatting of 3D data sets can be time-consuming on conventional MR imaging computers, making dedicated image processing workstations necessary for viewing 3D images. However, the usefulness and diagnostic importance of 3D MR imaging has spawned a new generation of MR imaging hardware to provide users with the required capabilities.

The steps involved in producing a 3D MR image are very similar to the steps used to make a 2D image. A thick slab 3D image can be produced by exciting a large (8 to 20 cm) slice, followed by phase encoding using stepped gradient pulses in both the slice-encoding and phase-encoding dimensions. This method is used when a limited number of slice-encoding steps are to be used. A volume 3D image can be produced by performing the initial excitation with a nonselective pulse, followed by application of a large number (128 or more) of encoding

steps in the slice and phase dimensions. The data sets may be interpolated in one or more dimensions to yield true isotropic 3D images.

Image Generation

An MR image is produced through the following steps:

1. Excite a slice of magnetization in the presence of a magnetic field gradient in one direction.
2. Encode spatial position in the second direction (a third direction for 3D) by measuring the rate of change in the phase of the signals caused by a series of pulsed field gradients of differing amplitudes (*i.e.,* phase encoding).
3. Encode spatial position in the third direction by indirectly measuring the resonant frequency in the presence of a magnetic field gradient (*i.e.,* frequency read-out).

These steps must be performed in the proper order for the image to be generated properly.

The series of RF and gradient events for producing an MR image can be drawn schematically as a function of time. Such pulse timing diagrams for a gradient-echo sequence and a spin-echo sequence are shown in Figure 1–12. The gradient-echo sequence begins with the selection of a slice of tissue by applying a narrow-band RF pulse with the shape of a sine function [sine(x)/x] in the presence of a magnetic field gradient. The phase error introduced by the magnetic field gradient during the slice selection process is reversed when a magnetic field gradient pulse of the opposite sign and one-half the area is applied after the slice-selection process. Next, the appropriate phase-encoding magnetic field gradient pulse is applied. This is often concomitant with the slice refocusing gradient pulse and a dephasing gradient pulse— whose area is equal to one-half of the area of the read-out gradient pulse—applied along the read-out direction during the signal acquisition period. Finally, the signal is detected in the presence of the read-out magnetic field gradient. A full echo generally is stored during the digitization period, although this is not required.

The data are stored in the MR imaging computer as voltage amplitude *versus* time. The computer performs a 3DFT to convert the time data from the read-out dimension and the rate of change of the signal phase from the phase-encoding dimension into frequency information. Frequency differences are proportional to the distance from the isocenter in a calibrated magnetic field gradient, and the frequency information directly corresponds to the spatial location in both directions. The resulting MR image has a resolution of 1 point in the slice direction. In the image plane, however, the resolution is represented by the following:

$$\frac{FOV}{\begin{array}{c} number\ of \\ phase\text{-}encoding\ steps \end{array}} \times \frac{FOV}{\begin{array}{c} number\ of\ points\ stored \\ during\ read\text{-}out \end{array}}.$$

Therefore, greater resolution for smaller structures can be achieved only by increasing the number of phase-encoding steps and the time required to make the image or by decreasing the FOV to alter the size of the voxels in the image. Each voxel contains signal intensity corresponding to the voltage measured during data acquisition. The enhancement or attenuation of this signal intensity using known variables produces contrast in the MR image.

PARAMETERS AFFECTING THE APPEARANCE OF MAGNETIC RESONANCE IMAGES

The appearance of an MR image is determined by many parameters. In general, these parameters can be divided into two classes:

1. Those that have a fixed value governed by the physics of MR
2. Those that can be modified by the user to alter the appearance of the image.

The goal of any MR study is to generate images of tissue anatomy in which the contrast-to-noise ratio (CNR) is sufficient to allow identification of the disease process. This is accomplished by varying the user-defined parameters to maximize differences in the values of intrinsic parameters and to emphasize differences in signal intensity between voxels containing normal and pathologic tissues.

Intrinsic Parameters

Intrinsic parameters are tissue-dependent and not under operator control. Examples of intrinsic parameters are the density of water and fat within tissue, blood flow, and the rates of relaxation of the magnetic moments back to equilibrium after perturbation. Some intrinsic parameters are invariant among all tissues (*e.g.,* the strength of the magnetic field).

Proton Density

A common pathologic condition is the accumulation of edematous fluid around a tumor. The edema has a higher proportion of water than surrounding normal tissue, and hence a higher density of protons per unit volume. This increase in density of protons per unit volume can be observed using MR imaging methods that emphasize or attenuate the signal intensity in voxels based on the proton density. Typically, proton-density–weighted MR images are obtained using the shortest possible TE and a repetition time (TR) that allows full T1 relaxation of all magnetic moments back to equilibrium.

Relaxation Times

After it is excited, the MR signal cannot be detected forever. It decays as the result of two different types of relaxation processes:

1. The return of the bulk magnetic moment to thermal equilibrium.
2. The loss of phase coherence in the net magnetization as a result of interactions with other magnetic moments in the tissue.

The rate at which these processes return the net magnetization to equilibrium is critical, because the MR experiment must be repeated for each phase-encoding step, and the amount of magnetization available for study depends on how many of the magnetic moments are realigned with the main magnetic field.

T2 and T2* Relaxation Times. After excitation, the MR signal present in the X,Y plane decays exponentially to zero over time. The time required for 63% of the signal to disappear irreversibly is called the T2 relaxation time or the transverse or spin–spin relaxation time (Fig. 1–13). This decay is caused by the many processes that produce a loss of phase coherence in the MR signal. After the RF pulse, all the magnetic moments initially precess with identical phases. However, variations in the effective magnetic field strength cause the magnetic moments to precess at different frequencies for short periods of time. This results in the dephasing of the vector bundle in the X,Y plane illustrated in Figure 1–13 and a decrease in the signal available for detection. Variations in the local magnetic field strength can be produced by binding to macromolecules, interactions with magnetic dipoles of other nuclei such as oxygen, and vibration of chemical bonds.

The T2* and T2 relaxation processes originate from inhomogeneities in the strength of the main magnetic field (T2*), or close interactions with other magnetic dipoles (T2). After the initial RF pulse, the individual magnetic moments precess in phase at frequencies determined by the local magnetic field strength. For a variety of reasons, however, including differences in tissue composition, the main magnetic field B_0 is not homogeneous. As the magnetic moments traverse regions of altered magnetic field strength, they momentarily precess at higher and lower frequencies, causing dephasing of the net magnetization vector and T2* relaxation. This inhomogeneity in the main magnetic field varies slowly. Hence, the dephasing can be reversed by application of a second RF pulse with an amplitude of π radians (*i.e.,* 180°), which flips the magnetic moments in the X,Y plane and produces a reversal of the dephasing due to static magnetic field inhomogeneity.

The RF pulse can be applied many times, and multiple echoes can be formed and acquired as shown in Figure 1–14. Eventually, the signal amplitude decays as a function of the true T2 relaxation time, which is a function of irreversible dephasing caused by random, short duration interactions of the individual magnetic moments with neighboring magnetic moments.

T1 Relaxation Time. The T1 relaxation time (*i.e.,* spin–lattice or longitudinal relaxation time) is the time required to restore 63% of the equilibrium population of magnetic moments aligned with the B_0 magnetic field following the excitation pulse. T1 relaxation is an exponential process (Fig. 1–15). In the classic picture, T1 relaxation processes involve the transfer of energy from the excited individual magnetic moments to the surrounding lattice of magnetic moments in other molecules. This transfer of energy from the magnetic moments to the lattice restores the equilibrium alignment of the magnetic moments with the main magnetic field. An example of a T1 relaxation process would be the transfer of energy from an excited magnetic dipole of an individual spin to the large and small effective magnetic dipoles of groups of spins on neighboring molecules. Unlike T2 relaxation, this T1 relaxation occurs only through oscillations of local magnetic moments that occur at the Larmor frequency. These local magnetic moments originate from tumbling macromolecules and other magnetic constituents of the lattice that couple to the relaxing magnetic moment.

The T1 relaxation time for any material varies as a function of magnetic field strength, since more variations occur in the local effective magnetic field strength at lower Larmor frequencies. Therefore, T1 relaxation times tend to decrease with decreasing magnetic field strengths. At all Larmor frequencies, few paths exist to produce T1 relaxation, and the T1 relaxation time is always longer than or equal to the T2 relaxation time. Figure 1–15 contains a pictorial representation of T1 relaxation and a graph showing the exponential recovery of aligned magnetization as a function of time after the initial RF pulse.

Extrinsic Parameters

Many types of operator-controlled parameters can alter image appearance. These include timing events, such as TR, TE, and, in inversion recovery studies, the spin-inversion time. Other parameters that affect image appearance are slice thickness, digital resolution, and FOV. Image appearance can also be changed by applying more than one RF pulse prior to data collection.

TR and TE

Typically, 128 or 256 phase-encoding steps are required in an MR acquisition. The TR is the amount of time between consecutive phase-encoding steps, and the TE is the time between the initial perturbing RF pulse and the center of the acquisition period. TR is generally longer than TE, except for some steady-state fast-scan methods such as contrast-enhanced fast acquisition in steady state (CE-FAST) or fast imaging with steady-state precession (FISP).

Slice Thickness, Field of View, and Resolution

All MR images suffer from volume averaging effects to some degree. This is most serious in the slice direction, where the effective voxel size is often 3 or 5 mm deep. Thinner slices can be obtained with 3D sequences at the expense of longer acquisition times. The size of the FOV can be modified to prevent wrap-around artifacts and to increase the in-plane resolution for a fixed number of data points. When the resolution in a spatial dimension is doubled for a fixed total acquisition time, only one-half as much signal is detected in each voxel and the SNR in the image is decreased by a factor of 2. Scanning for twice as long does not provide twice the signal, because the SNR only increases with the square root of the number of averages (n).

Pulse Tip Angle

When the second perturbing magnetic field B_1 is applied, the individual magnetic moments precess about the new effective magnetic field. Hence, their final position is a function of the strength and duration of the perturbing field B_1. As illustrated in the rotating frame diagram of Figure 1–4, the maximum signal is detected when the B_1 magnetic field produces a displacement of $\pi/2$ radians (*i.e.,* 90°) away from the Z axis, and the bulk magnetization vector is placed in the X,Y plane. The geometric angle between the position of the net magnetization vector and the Z axis is called the pulse tip angle. The pulse tip angle can strongly affect the contrast in an image. An example of this relationship is shown in Figure 1–16.

Signal-to-Noise Ratio and Scan Time

As discussed in the preceding sections, the SNR in an MR image is a function of many things. Invariant parameters such as the magnetic field strength influence the SNR, as do the intrinsic parameters unique to tissues such as proton density [N(H)] and T1, T2*, and T2 relaxation times. The extrinsic operator-controlled parameters that affect the SNR are the following:

- TE
- TR
- flip angle
- FOV and sampling bandwidth in each spatial dimension (FOV_x and FOV_y, where x = read-out and y = phase-encode directions)
- slice thickness (Δz)

- n
- number of points sampled in each spatial dimension (#x and #y)
- image noise level (N).

With a fixed field strength, flip angle, and noise level, the SNR can be calculated according to the following formula:

$$SNR \frac{f(\text{intrinsic}) \bullet f(\text{extrinsic})}{N}.$$

The function for the dependence of the signal strength on the intrinsic parameters in an spin-echo pulse sequence is given as the following equation:

$$f(\text{intrinsic}) \approx N(\text{H}) \bullet (1 - e^{-(\text{TR/T1})}) \bullet (e^{-(\text{TE/T2})}).$$

The TR is linked to T1, such that only variations in TR affect the amount of T1 weighting, or signal attenuation, in an MR image. Similarly, TE is linked to T2, and variations in the extrinsic parameter TE affect the amount of T2 weighting (*i.e.,* signal attenuation) in an image. Both T1- and T2-weighted images have lower SNRs than proton density images because contrast is produced by attenuating one signal component. These relationships between TR/T1 and TE/T2 form the basis for the following discussion of image appearance.

For any given combination of invariant and intrinsic parameters with TR and TE, the equation for the signal strength as a function of the remaining extrinsic parameters is given as the following:

$$f(\text{extrinsic}) \approx \Delta z \bullet (\sqrt{n}) \bullet \frac{\text{FOV}_x}{\#x} \bullet \frac{\text{FOV}_y}{\#y}.$$

This relationship has no impact on the contrast in an image, but does have several other important consequences. For example, a two-fold magnification (*i.e.,* fixed-matrix size but reducing the FOV by one-half) reduces the SNR per voxel in the image by a factor of 4. A two-fold increase in resolution (*i.e.,* doubling the matrix size in both the phase-encoding and read-out dimensions for a fixed FOV) reduces the SNR by $2\sqrt{2}$ but doubles the scan time (TS), because the TS is increased to sample twice as many phase-encode steps. Sampling for twice as long (*i.e.,* n twice as large) increases the SNR by a maximum of only $\sqrt{2}$.

The total TS for a 2D or 3D image can be defined from TR, #y, #z, and n as the following equation:

$$TS = TR \bullet \#y \bullet n \bullet \#z.$$

It follows from this equation that increasing the number of n, the number of phase-encode steps (#y and #z; #z = 1 for a 2D image), or TR, increases the time required to complete the scan. In spin-echo imaging, signal averaging is the only way to improve the SNR without altering image resolution. The situation is more complex in fast scans, where the SNR is a function of the TR,

type of pulse, and flip angle. If the TS is held constant, an improvement in SNR can be realized only by increasing the slice thickness, increasing the FOV, or decreasing the resolution.

Contrast-to-Noise Ratio

The ability to differentiate among tissues is limited by both the inherent SNR level and the difference in signal strength (*i.e.,* contrast) between adjacent voxels. For example, if the signal strength in voxel 1 is defined as S1 and in an adjacent voxel as S2, and N in the image is uniformly distributed (*i.e.,* no artifacts are present), then the CNR is given as the following equation:

$$CNR \approx \frac{|S1 - S2|}{N}.$$

This equation suggests that the contrast in an MR image can be improved by reducing the noise level or by manipulating the differential attenuation of signal in normal *versus* pathologic tissues using the extrinsic parameters. Strategies for manipulating image contrast are discussed in the next section.

MANIPULATING EXTRINSIC PARAMETERS TO VARY IMAGE CONTRAST

Echo Formation

The discussion of production of an MR image thus far has been concerned with excitation of a slice, followed by generation of a gradient echo that is detected during application of a read-out gradient and contains phase information on spatial position in the phase-encoding dimension. Two methods commonly are used to form the echo:

1. Refocusing of the read-out gradient to form a gradient echo
2. Simultaneous formation of a gradient echo and an RF echo using gradient reversal and an additional RF pulse.

The characteristics of the detected signal are influenced strongly by the method used to generate the echo.

Gradient Echoes

The gradient-echo method collects the residual free induction decay (FID) signal still present after the initial excitation pulse. The FID disappears to zero at a time, designated T2*, that is shorter than the natural T2 relaxation time. At very short TEs, the signal attenuation from T2 and T2* are approximately equivalent, and gradient-echo images provide an accurate representation of tissue signal intensity. However, at TEs longer than 10 msec, the signal intensity in gradient-echo images is attenuated strongly by T2*.

Spin Echoes

Nearly 40 years ago, Hahn demonstrated that the FID signal could be regenerated by applying a second RF pulse.[5] This second pulse reverses and refocuses the dephasing of the magnetization produced by long-lived magnetic field inhomogeneities (*i.e.,* T2* relaxation) and forms an echo at a time equal to the interval between the two RF pulses. When the amplitude of the second RF pulse produces an inversion of the signal in the X,Y plane, the echo formed during the digitization period is called a spin echo. The second pulse has an optimum amplitude of π radians (180°) to produce the maximum intensity of the spin echo. The signal intensity decays with time as an exponential function of the T2 relaxation time, not the T2* relaxation time (see Fig. 1–14).

It can be seen, therefore, that the contrast in an image generated from a gradient echo differs significantly from that of an image generated from a spin echo. The contrast in a gradient-echo image can be varied using "pre-pulses" to invert the magnetization prior to the fast scan, by increasing (or decreasing) the repetition and TEs, and by selecting from among the different types of gradient echo that can be acquired.

Spin-echo imaging methods collect the data after application of a 180° pulse to refocus T2*-induced dephasing. The contrast in spin-echo images is a function of the T1 and T2 relaxation times and the TR and TE, with no contribution from T2*.

T1-Weighted Magnetic Resonance Imaging and TR

All MR images are T1-weighted to some degree, since the net magnetization is not restored to 100% until a period equal to 7 • (T1 relaxation time) after the initial excitation. The T1 relaxation times for water and fat in the body range from 100 to 2000 msec. At a TR value of 500 msec and a TE of 15 msec, the primary source of signal attenuation in an spin-echo image is the progressive saturation of the magnetic moments by the repetitive slice selection pulses. This is demonstrated in Figure 1–17 for sagittal images from a knee obtained with a 3-mm slice thickness. The signal from fat is bright, whereas image intensities from areas of muscle and fluid in a meniscal cyst are lower. At longer TR values, the amount of signal attenuation due to incomplete T1 relaxation is reduced, and the images move toward a proton density appearance. T1-weighted images also can be produced using a preliminary inversion-recovery pulse and delay time. However, this method requires a sufficiently long TR interval to ensure that the magnetization has returned to equilibrium prior to the next inversion pulse.

Proton Density Weighting

Images where the contrast is governed by the relative concentration of water in the tissue can be generated using long repetition (TR > 2 sec) times and short TEs (TE < 20 msec). These images are called proton-density–weighted images, and they have high SNR, because the signal intensity is only slightly attenuated by T1 or T2 relaxation processes. Proton-density–weighted images provide improved anatomic detail, because the high SNR of these images can be used to visualize fine structure. They are usually obtained in conjunction with a long-echo T2-weighted image and are useful for interpretation of areas of high signal intensity observed on the T2-weighted scan in which anatomic detail is obscured. A proton-density–weighted image of a knee with a meniscal cyst is presented in Figure 1–18.

T2 Weighting and TE

Fluids and edema can be emphasized on MR images by using long TE times because they have longer T2 relaxation times than normal tissues. At long TEs, the exponential signal decay due to T2 relaxation attenuates the signal from fluid and edema more slowly than signal from fat, muscle, or normal connective tissues. Therefore, fluid and edema appear bright on T2-weighted MR images acquired using long TE times and long TR times. For example, in a T2-weighted sagittal image from the same knee, the synovial fluid and region of cyst appear bright in the image, whereas regions of muscle appear dark (Fig. 1–19).

Two-Dimensional *versus* Three-Dimensional Imaging

As noted earlier, true volume 3D MR imaging allows reconstruction of any image plane from the 3D data set. This is particularly useful for following small structures such as nerves, blood vessels, and cartilage. Pseudo-3D data sets can be produced from 2D studies that have been acquired radially or by contiguous slices, but this method suffers from signal attenuation where slices intersect or overlap. In addition, the resolution in the slice dimension is low and fine structures can be obscured. An example of a T1-weighted coronal image reformatted from a series of 32 contiguous sagittal slices is presented in Figure 1–20. The in-plane resolution is very low in the slice direction and the features appear smeared.

The corresponding coronal image generated from a sagittal 3D image data set is shown in Figure 1–21. Acquisition of data from a volume using nearly isotropic voxel sizes in each dimension permits observation of multiple planes without any reduction in diagnostic quality. This approach to imaging is most useful in situations in which multiple image planes or views along nonorthogonal planes are required, since image planes are calculated off-line on an image workstation. This method reduces total magnet time because patient preparation time used for positioning and slice definition is decreased. Finally, repeat studies are not required to sample multiple contiguous thin slices.

Manipulation of Contrast in Fast Scans

Most fast-scan techniques use small RF tip angles and gradient refocusing to acquire a gradient echo. In any fast-scan method the image contrast is a mixture of T1 and T2* weighting, with some dependence on the flip angle. As already noted, T2* relaxation proceeds more rapidly than conventional T2 relaxation, and fast-scan sequences are more sensitive to the effects of magnetic field inhomogeneities and signal drop-out at air–tissue interfaces. Fast-scan images can appear similar to either T1- or T2-weighted spin-echo scans depending on the choice of TR, TE, type of magnetization spoiling, type of echo that is acquired, and type of RF pulse.

The simplest fast-scan technique for acquiring a gradient echo is outlined in Figure 1–12A. These conventional fast, low-angle shot (FLASH) images are like T1-weighted spin-echo images because of the saturating effects of the repetitive low-angle RF pulses and large amplitude spoiler gradients.[6] Such FLASH or spoiled gradient recalled acquisition in the steady state (GRASS) images usually suffer from low SNR, and several excitations must be added together to produce images with acceptable SNR. A GRASS image obtained from a knee using a 45° flip angle and 8 averages is presented in Figure 1–22. The amount of magnetization available for imaging during the next phase-encoding step is increased as TR is increased, and multiplanar gradient-echo images have less T1 weighting and more T2* weighting.[7]

Pure proton density gradient-echo images can be obtained using the 3D fast adiabatic trajectory in the steady state (FATS) technique with adiabatic RF pulses and a short TE of 2.8 msec.[8] Fast-scan methods such as CE-FAST, sagittal, 3D, steady-state free precession (SSFP), and PSIF—which store a high-order echo generated by combinations of RF and gradient pulses—tend to be strongly T2*-weighted because the effective TE is two to three times that of the TR.[9] These types of fast-scan images are useful for demonstrating fluid, which has very high intensity relative to other soft tissues. Unfortunately, these images are not truly T2-weighted, and lesions that would be hyperintense on T2-weighted spin-echo images such as bone bruises and tumors may not be seen on SSFP and CE-FAST scans.

An example of a 3D SSFP image from a knee containing a meniscal cyst is presented in Figure 1–23. The regions of fluid appear to have very high intensity, but the SNR for other tissues is very low.

A combination of two RF pulses applied in rapid succession is called a composite pulse. Composite pulses are used in field echo aquisition with a short TR and echo reduction (FASTER) to achieve better SNR, improved T1 weighting, and fewer artifacts.[10] The second RF pulse is used to convert nonresonant magnetization into transverse magnetization, which contributes to the steady-state coherence. A FASTER image of a knee is presented in Figure 1–24.

Fat Suppression

In many cases, detection of a pathologic process is hindered by the presence of a large signal from neighboring adipose tissue. In such cases, the suppression of the fat signal offers improved conspicuity and sensitivity. The signal from fat can be suppressed in a number of ways, such as inversion recovery techniques (*e.g.*, short TI inversion recovery, or STIR), in which an inversion time where signal from fat is nullified; preliminary saturation of the magnetic moments from fat; selective excitation of the signal from water; and chopper methods in which the phase of the fat and water signals are altered.[11] In 2D MR imaging, all these methods have benefits and drawbacks. In 3D imaging, selective excitation of the signal from water using adiabatic techniques is possible, because no slice selection gradient is required.[12] These fat-suppressed 3D images have high SNRs without errors associated with 2D methods. An example of a fat-suppressed 3D fast adiabatic trajectory in a steady state (FATS) image of the knee is provided in Figure 1–25. The signal from bone and adipose have been suppressed by a factor of >150. The slice thickness of 1.25 mm allows excellent visualization of fine detail in the region of pathology in this image.

Kinematic Studies

Multiple MR images can be obtained at various defined stations of joint movement and displayed in rapid succession to provide a kinematic display that resembles joint motion. These techniques have been effectively used for the temporomandibular joint, knee, wrist, and ankle. The amount of imaging time spent at each station is critical because multiple stations are needed for the kinematic display. A reasonable TS per station is approximately 80 seconds, and the number of stations needed is approximately 6 to 12. Fast scans or short TR spin-echo sequences can be used. Kinematic MR imaging is discussed in detail in Chapter 10.

FUTURE APPLICATIONS OF MAGNETIC RESONANCE IMAGING

Conventional MR imaging is already established in clinical practice for visualization of soft tissue and pathology,

(text continues on page 22)

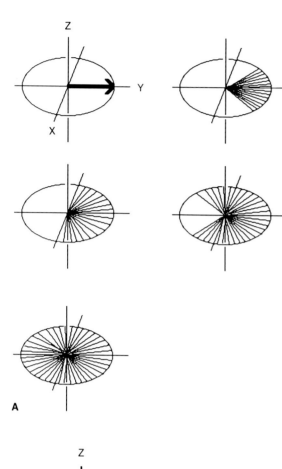

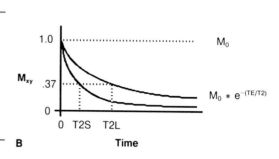

FIGURE 1–13. Evolution of transverse magnetization produced by T2 relaxation processes. (**A**) Immediately following the radiofrequency pulse, the transverse magnetization has maximum phase coherence. The magnetization continually loses phase coherence due to changes in the precession frequency caused by variations in the local magnetic-field strength, and dephases as a function of time. (**B**) A graph of the decay of the transverse magnetization M_{xy} as a function of TE from a starting value of M_0 shows two decay rates: a short T2 relaxation time (T2S) and a long T2 relaxation time (T2L).

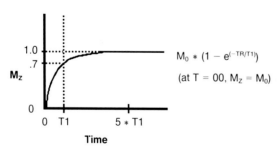

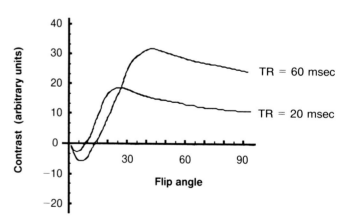

FIGURE 1–14. Evolution of transverse magnetization as a function of time in a spin-echo sequence with four echoes. Following the initial slice pulse, sequential application of 180° pulses produces refocussing of T2* dephasing due to magnetic-field inhomogeneities and balanced magnetic-field gradient pulses. The maximum amplitude of each echo decays over a time T2, which is the time period for irreversible dephasing of transverse magnetization.

FIGURE 1–15. Contrast depends on the magnitude of the initial pulse, as seen for two tissues with a T1 of 500, 800 msec. Restoration of longitudinal magnetization occurs as a function of time following a single $\pi/2$ radiofrequency (RF) pulse. After the $\pi/2$ RF pulse, the longitudinal magnetization is zero. The magnetization continues to precess at the Larmor frequency until it has returned to its equilibrium position with a longitudinal component M_0. The amount of longitudinal magnetization is restored as an exponential function of time.

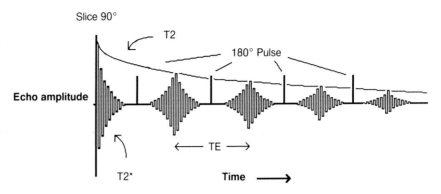

FIGURE 1–16. Tissue contrast depends on the magnitude of the initial radiofrequency (RF) pulse for a model system of two tissues with different T1 longitudinal relaxation times. As the flip angle of the RF pulse increases, the contrast between the two tissues becomes strongly dependent on the TR used between pulses. However, there is a flip angle that produces the optimum contrast for the given T1 values of 500 and 800 msec (*e.g.,* values for white matter and gray matter in the brain).

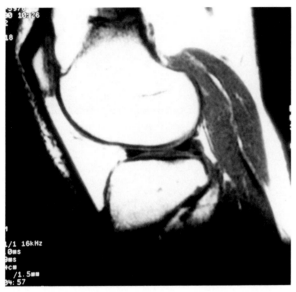

FIGURE 1–17. A T1-weighted sagittal image from the knee of a patient with a meniscal cyst. A TR of 500 msec and a TE of 15 msec have been employed using a 3-mm slice thickness and a 16-cm field of view with 256 points. The meniscus is very hypointense, the cyst and articular cartilage are hypointense, the muscle has moderate intensity, and the fat is hyperintense.

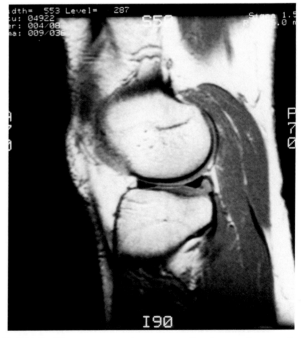

FIGURE 1–18. A proton-density–weighted sagittal image from the knee of a patient with a meniscal cyst. A TR of 2000 msec and a TE of 15 msec have been employed using a 3-mm slice thickness and a 16-cm field of view with 256 points. Less contrast among tissues is seen as compared with the T1-weighted image.

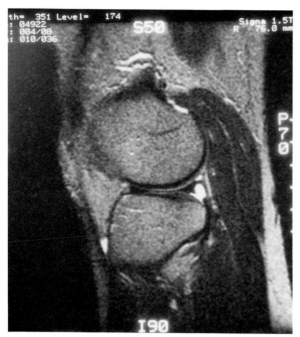

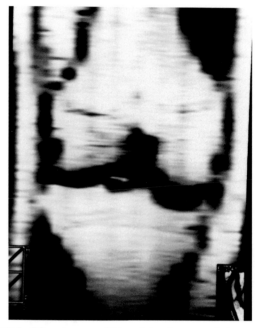

FIGURE 1–19. A T2-weighted sagittal image from the knee of a patient with a meniscal cyst. A TR of 2000 msec and a TE of 80 msec have been employed using a 3-mm slice thickness and a 16-cm field of view with 256 points. The meniscus remains hypointense, whereas the cyst is hyperintense. Fat displays moderate intensity, and muscle is hypointense. This image suffers from a significant deficit in signal-to-noise ratio compared with that found on the T1-weighted and proton-density–weighted images.

FIGURE 1–20. A coronal T1-weighted image of a knee was generated from a series of 32 contiguous sagittal 2D spin-echo images. The in-plane resolution is 32 × 128 points. A TR of 500 msec and a TE of 15 msec were used. Two-dimensional slices with the thinnest commercially available section thickness are inadequate for multiplanar reformations.

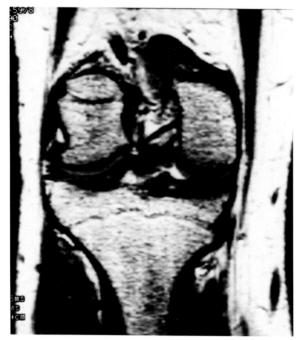

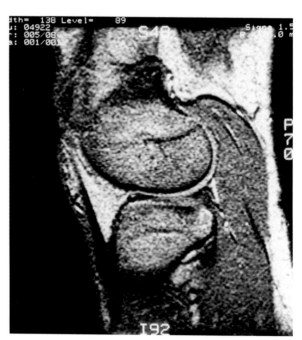

FIGURE 1–21. A coronal T1-weighted image of a knee was generated from a sagittal 3D field-echo acquisition with a short TR and echo reduction (FASTER) data set. The in-plane resolution is 128 × 128 points. A TR of 18 msec and a TE of 3.2 msec were used. Reformations using thin-slice 3D data produce images that have image quality nearly identical to images of the original acquisition plane.

FIGURE 1–22. A sagittal spoiled gradient recalled acquisition in the steady state (GRASS) image of a knee was generated using a TR of 33 msec and a TE of 5.6 msec with a total of four averages using a 5-mm slice thickness, a 16-cm field of view, and 256 data points. This image has similar contrast to the T1-weighted spin-echo image, but suffers from poor signal-to-noise ratio.

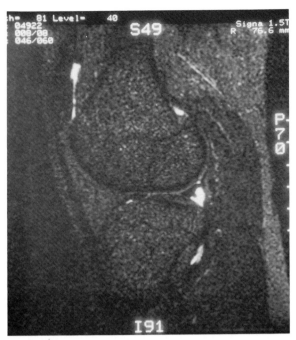

FIGURE 1–23. A sagittal 3D steady-state free precession (SSFP) of a knee with a meniscal cyst. A TR of 33 msec and a TE of 9.0 msec were used. The effective TE was 66–99 msec. A total of two averages have been used with a 1.25-mm slice thickness, a 16-cm field of view, and 128 × 128 × 256 data points. Note the high intensity fluid signal that allows easy identification of the cyst. Normal tissues are difficult to identify due to decreased signal-to-noise ratio caused by T2* losses.

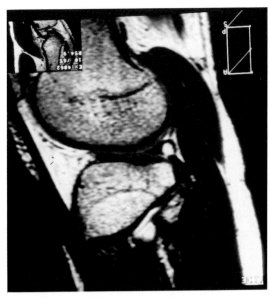

FIGURE 1–24. The field-echo acquisition with a short TR and echo reduction (FASTER) image shows T1-weighted contrast similar to the T1-weighted spin-echo (see Fig. 1–17) and T1-weighted, spoiled gradient recalled acquisition in the steady state (GRASS) images, except that fluids are hyperintense due to the presence of long T2 species in the steady-state signal. If hyperintense fluid is not desirable, radiofrequency spoiling can be used with the FASTER sequence to make fluids appear hypointense.

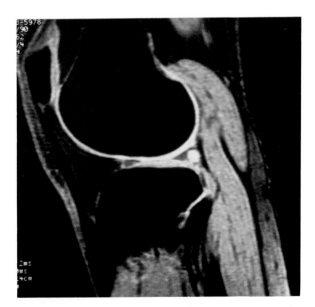

FIGURE 1–25. A 3D fast adiabatic trajectory in the steady state (FATS) image of a knee with a meniscal cyst. A TR of 18 msec, a TE of 2.8 msec, and a slice thickness of 1.25 mm have been employed. One average was obtained for a 128 × 128 × 256 data matrix and a 16-cm field of view. Bone marrow is hypointense due to fat suppression. Note the reversal in contrast between fat and muscle when compared with the proton-density–weighted and T1-weighted scans (see Figs 1–18, 1–20, and 1–21). Fluid and cartilage are hyperintense.

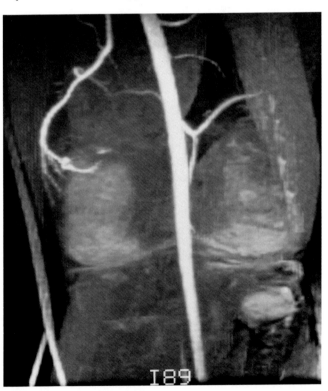

FIGURE 1–26. A maximum pixel ray casting of a 3D fast adiabatic trajectory in the steady state (FATS) image of a knee with an osteosarcoma. The reformatted image was generated using a standard ray-casting method on a Sun 3-260 workstation with a TAAC board (Sun Macrosystems, Mountain View, CA). The FATS sequence can produce high-quality basis and angiographic images in the same scan. Even though this sequence is nonselective and proton density weighted, high signal intensity is produced from vessels due to the acquisition of signal from frequency-shifted spins.

and several new MR techniques are moving toward clinical acceptance. The image quality available in fast-scanning techniques is improving rapidly, and real-time MR imaging is now possible using echo planar imaging or "turbo" gradient-echo techniques. Magnetic resonance angiographic images are also dramatically improved, and MRA is now approved by the Food and Drug Administration. Magnetic resonance spectroscopy generates information on tissue metabolism and has been used to study energetics and disease conditions in patients. Current research into the slow movement of water and blood (*i.e.,* diffusion and perfusion) shows great promise for evaluation of hydrodynamics in the extracellular, interstitial, and intracellular spaces of tissue.[13]

Magnetic Resonance Angiography

The signal from flowing blood can be observed selectively using MRA techniques. This is accomplished using 2D and 3D time-of-flight (TOF) methods in which the signal from blood is refreshed by inflow, and phase–contrast difference methods in which moving spins acquire a phase shift relative to stationary spins.[14,15] Different techniques can be used to enhance the signal from arterial and venous structures relative to static tissue. In TOF methods, thin 2D or thick 3D slabs can be excited to saturate the signal from static spins. When thick slabs are used, the signal from blood flowing slowly within the slab also can be saturated. Therefore, SNR for venous structures is superior with 2D TOF MRA compared with that found with 3D methods.

Time-of-flight methods use computational postprocessing tools to find the pixels with the maximum signal intensity after conventional fast-scan data has been obtained. In fast scans, blood that flows into the slice has the highest signal strength, and the reconstructed data sets yield images in which the vessels are enhanced compared with that found in normal tissue. The maximum pixel images can be enhanced by suppression of the signal from fat and by administration of gadolinium contrast agents to enhance the signal from blood.

The 3D FATS technique has been used to simultaneously produce both high quality vascular images and multiple anatomic slices in a single scan.[16] This method uses TOF and improved capture of off-resonance flowing spins to enhance the SNR from vessels. The use of maximum pixel intensity ray tracing on a workstation generates the vascular images. An example of the high quality vascular and multiple anatomic slices produced by this integrated approach is shown in Figure 1–26.

Magnetic Resonance Spectroscopy

Information on tissue metabolism and energetics can be obtained with MRS. The protons and phosphorus atoms in metabolites such as lactate, creatine, phosphocreatine, and adenosine triphosphate have unique magnetic environments that can be observed using MRS. The effective magnetic fields differ by only parts per million, and are small compared with the strength of the magnetic field gradients used to make MR images. In MRS, therefore, the MR signal is detected in the absence of read-out gradients to provide high-resolution information on the distribution of frequencies induced by chemical differences. Levels of inorganic phosphate, phosphocreatine, and adenosine triphosphate can be estimated using phosphorus MR.[17] Spatial localization to specific volumes of tissue is achieved using slice-selective gradients, phase encoding, or both.[18] With proton MRS, it is possible to detect anaerobic metabolism by means of the production of lactic acid.[19] Although MRS is a powerful tool for research studies of tissue biochemistry, clinical applications still are being developed.

Quicker Scanning Methods

A number of new techniques for obtaining MR images in real time have been developed. Echo planar imaging methods produce a low-resolution MR image in 30 to 60 msec from a single excitation pulse.[20,21] The amplitude of the read-out gradient is reversed rapidly for each of 32 to 64 phase-encoding steps applied after the single RF excitation. The image contrast is a complex function of T2* (or T2 for echo-planar) and T1, and the SNR generally is low. In most fast-scan imaging methods, the major limitation on the duration of TE is the magic TE of 4.4 msec required at 1.5 T to generate in-phase images. At multiples of this TE, the signals from water and fat are in phase because the phase evolution due to the difference in chemical shift is equal to 2π radians. The images have more signal intensity than fast scans performed using a TE of 2.2, 6.6, or 11 msec, because the signals from fat and water do not cancel each other. As already discussed, the contrast in fast-scan methods can be altered in a variety of ways to generate T1-weighted, proton-density–weighted, T2-weighted, or other types of images.

REFERENCES

1. Stark DD, Bradley WG, eds. Magnetic resonance imaging. St. Louis: CV Mosby, 1988.
2. Mink JH, Reicher MA, Crues JV III, eds. Magnetic resonance imaging of the knee. New York: Raven Press, 1987.
3. Wehrli FW, Shaw D, Kneeland JB, eds. Biomedical magnetic resonance imaging: principles, methodology, and applications. New York: VCH Publishers, 1988.
4. Matwiyoff NA. Magnetic resonance workbook. New York: Raven Press, 1989.
5. Hahn EL. Spin echoes. Phys Rev 1950;80:580.
6. Haase A. Applications to T1, T2, and chemical-shift imaging. Magn Reson Med 1990;13(1):77. Snapshot FLASH MRI.

7. Reischer MA, Lufkin RB, Smith S, et al. AJR 1986;147:363.

8. Harms SE, Flamig DP, Griffey RH. New MR pulse sequence: fat-suppressed steady state. Radiology 1990;270:177.

9. Gyngell ML. The application of steady-state free precession in rapid 2DFT NMR imaging: FAST and CE-FAST sequences. Magn Reson Imaging 1988;6:415.

10. Harms SE, Flamig DP, Fisher CF, Fulmer JM. New method for fast MR imaging of the knee. Radiology 1989;173:743.

11. Vinitski S, Mitchell DG, Szumowski J, Burk DL Jr, Rifkin MD. Variable flip angle imaging and fat suppression in combined gradient and spin-echo (GREASE) techniques. Magn Reson Imaging 1990;8:131.

12. Harms SE, Flamig DP, Griffey RH. Clinical applications of a new fat suppressed, steady state pulse sequence for high resolution 3D applications. In: Book of abstracts. vol. 1. New York: Society of Magnetic Resonance in Medicine, 1990:187.

13. LeBihan D, Breton E, Lallemand D, Grenier P, Cabanis E, Laval-Jeantet M. MR imaging of intravoxel incoherent motors: application to diffusion and perfusion in neurologic disorders. Radiology 1986;161:401.

14. Nishimura DG. Time-of-flight MR angiography. Magn Reson Med 1990:14(2):194.

15. Steinberg FL, Yucel EK, Dumoulin CL, Souza SP. Peripheral vascular and abdominal applications of MR flow imaging techniques. Magn Reson Med 1990;14(2):315.

16. Harms SE, Flamig DP, Siemers PT, Glastad KA, Pierce B. Zero scan time vascular MR imaging. Radiology 1990;144:177.

17. Luyten PR, Bruntink G, Sloff FM, et al. Broadband proton decoupling in human 31P NMR spectroscopy. NMR Biomed 1989;1(4):177.

18. Van Vaals JJ, Bergman AH, den Boef JH, et al. A single-shot method for water suppressed localization and editing of spectra, images, and spectroscopic images. Magn Reson Med 1990;16:451.

19. Griffey RH. Tumor characterization using unconventional MR modalities. Invest Radiol 1990;24(12):985.

20. Mansfield P. Multi-planar image formation using NMR spin echoes. J Physiol Chem 1977;10:L55.

21. Farzaneh F, Riederer SJ, Pelc NJ. Analysis of T2 limitations and off-resonance effects on spatial resolution and artifacts in echo-planar imaging. Magn Reson Med 1990;14(1):123.

CHAPTER 2

Thomas R. Lindquist

Three-Dimensional Magnetic Resonance Rendering Techniques

Although radiologists are skilled at interpreting original cross-sectional images, situations exist in which the complexity of an anatomic region, or the need to improve communication with other physicians, warrants computer-based medical three-dimensional (3D) imaging. Three-dimensional rendering is a technique for producing images that ideally approach the clarity and style of a medical artist's illustration. In a medical illustration, the artist has the freedom to select what to depict, what vantage point to use, how to shade and color structures of interest, and how to use cutaway views or transparency to best effect. In producing computer-based 3D images, computer algorithms do much of the work as the individual user makes decisions to guide the process.

Unlike a typical computer graphics task, which renders images from precise geometrical descriptions of idealized objects, medical 3D rendering must faithfully extract and represent clinical features of interest that lie embedded within millions of original image data points, such as those generated by a magnetic resonance (MR) scanner. Despite formidable challenges, technical advances have already reached a point at which clinically useful 3D renderings from MR data are being obtained. This chapter reviews some of the methods for 3D processing using a commercially available computerized workstation.

For readers interested in technical details, the surface-rendering algorithms used within this workstation have roots that can be found in Artzy and colleagues.[1] However, in its handling of multiple surfaces and volumes, the approach taken here is substantially different from other volume-rendering approaches (*e.g.,* Levoy's).[2] Surveys of the overall field of 3D medical image rendering algorithms can be found in Tiede and colleagues[3] and in Stytz and colleagues.[4]

TWO-DIMENSIONAL IMAGES AND THREE-DIMENSIONAL VOLUMES

Three-dimensional processing begins with the acquisition of a set of two-dimensional (2D) cross-sectional images. These may come from a 3D or volume acquisition on the MR scanner, or from any acquisition in which a sufficient number of thin original image slices can capture the anatomic structure of interest at the required detail in all three dimensions.

Image Quality

The quality of a three-dimensionally rendered image depends to a great extent on the quality and coverage of the original cross-sectional 2D images from which it is derived. If the original 2D images have poor spatial resolution, so will the resultant 3D image. If gaps in coverage exist between the original slices, the small structures that lie in these gaps will not be seen in the 3D image. Similarly, if the original images represent a relatively thick slab of anatomy, small details in the slice-to-slice direction will be lost, even if each original image seems sharp in its own plane. In addition, inconsistencies in the original images, caused by poor signal-to-noise ratio (SNR) or drop-offs in sensitivity, generally also appear in the 3D image. In fact, the inconsistency is probably accentuated in the 3D image, because numerical consistency in the image data is usually more critical to a 3D processing algorithm than to a human observer of a 2D image. The human eye easily accommodates gradual drop-offs in brightness across an image, whereas a simple threshold-based classification algorithm responds incorrectly when the inherent contrast of a structure (compared with its surroundings) is less than the nonuniformities caused by the imaging technique.

Acquisition Parameters

When 3D processing of images from an acquisition is anticipated, the choice of acquisition parameters (*e.g.,* coils, slice selections, pulse sequences) should not only ensure adequate in-plane spatial resolution and SNR for the tissues of interest, but should also provide sufficient self-consistency and sufficient sampling, both within each image and from image to image. If high spatial resolution is to be maintained in all three dimensions, the acquired image set should have a large number of thin, contiguous slices, as is the case when a 3D volume acquisition is performed.

It should be noted that the methods described in this chapter allow for and can exploit multiple acquisitions from the same patient. For example, one pulse sequence that yields T1-weighted images may be performed to make a particular tissue visibly brighter than or darker than its surroundings. A second pulse sequence that yields T2-weighted images may be performed to enhance the contrast of a different tissue. As long as the two original image sets have the same geometric locations, they may be used jointly to produce combined 3D renderings that show the two (or more) tissues at once, each derived from its most favorable acquisition.

Data Processing

After the original images have been acquired, they may be electronically transmitted from the MR scanner to a workstation computer equipped with a suitable direct link. If a direct link is not installed, the MR scanner may save the images on an archive tape, which can then be brought to the workstation computer for input.

Figure 2–1 summarizes how the acquired data is then used as input for 3D processing. The user first selects a set of original 2D cross-sectional MR images and then defines, using tools created for the medical imaging workstation, one or more 3D volumes, each representing an anatomic structure of interest. The resultant volumes are then used for interactive rendering or for batch high-resolution rendering. The final rendered images may represent single or multiple anatomic structures and may optionally make use of color or transparency to best depict the features of clinical interest.

SEGMENTATION

The most useful 3D renderings usually include only those anatomic structures that are most relevant to the case at hand. Rendering more structures tends to cover up or obfuscate the area to be examined. This leads to the need for segmentation, or the extraction of a desired structure (*i.e.,* the one that is to be seen in the renderings) from other structures in the same original image set. In a few cases, segmentation may be defined entirely by the image data itself (*e.g.,* when all pixels of a particular brightness are selected). More typically, however, segmentation is determined by geometric constraints (*e.g.,* disarticulation boundaries imposed by a user) or by connectivity requirements. Methods for segmentation are discussed later in the chapter.

It should be noted that segmentation in no way precludes examining multiple anatomic structures. Rather, it provides entirely separate representations for each structure of interest, giving the user a set of building blocks, any combination of which can be collectively rendered.

Preprocessing

The segmentation of data may be facilitated by performing one of a variety of automatic preprocessing algorithms prior to segmentation. One such algorithm is a smoothing filter, which reduces the noise of the original image set. Although this operation also results in a small loss in spatial resolution, the gain in smoothness of tissue values makes this type of preprocessing warranted, unless the highest possible spatial resolution is needed.

Another preprocessing algorithm, specifically developed for MR, performs an autonormalization function; that is, the algorithm derives sensitivity correction information from the original image set itself and applies that correction information to the original images. This process yields images with significantly improved consistency in brightness and contrast.

Segmentation Tools

Generating Binary Volumes

Segmentation is the processing step that generates a 3D binary volume from the original, or preprocessed, image set. The binary volume represents a particular anatomic structure of interest to the user (*e.g.,* the meniscus in a knee study). The binary volume contains one bit of information for each location (*i.e.,* voxel) in 3D space, defining whether or not that voxel is in or out of the structure of interest.

Two independent criteria must both be satisfied for a given voxel to be considered in the structure of interest.

1. The brightness at the voxel's location, as seen in the original images, must be within a specified range of values selected by the user for that tissue. The user determines the range by viewing the original image and interactively adjusting the range of brightness. Pixels with values in the range are given a distinctive color to indicate which will be included in the resultant binary volume.
2. The voxel's location must lie within a geometric volume of interest and any disarticulation boundaries established by the user. The user defines these boundaries by means of various manual and automatic boundary-drawing tools.

As an example of segmentation, Figure 2–2 illustrates three stages in the generation of a meniscal volume from an axial knee study. The left image shows one original image, as acquired from an MR scanner. The middle image shows the effect of preprocessing by means of a smoothing filter to improve SNR, even though this results in a slight loss in spatial resolution. The third image shows the results of selecting a threshold range of pixel values—those in the user-selected range for the meniscus are medium gray—and defining disarticulation boundaries—in white—to further limit what will be present in the binary volume and hence in the final 3D renderings. In this case, the disarticulation contour was drawn automatically by the workstation computer in response to a single point placed by the user in the interior of the meniscus. In this example, the binary volume being defined will contain only the meniscus, because other tissue that is in the same range of brightness (*i.e.,* pixel value) is not included within the disarticulation contour defined here.

Disarticulation Methods

Disarticulation methods warrant discussion in some detail. The automatic-boundary–generating method, as noted previously in the chapter, is able to generate, with some limitations, the boundary between the in-threshold–range pixels and those that are outside the threshold range. This can be done provided that there are few, if any, pixels along the boundary that are in the currently defined in-threshold range yet not a part of the desired tissue. Automatic boundary generation cannot be used when abutting tissues have nearly the same brightness for the pulse sequence that was used or when there is partial volume averaging of abutting tissues.

When fully automatic methods cannot be used, the user can hand-trace the desired disarticulation contour with the workstation computer's mouse. Alternatively, automatically generated contours may be edited by the user by manually tracing over the portion to be changed.

It is necessary for the user to ensure that disarticulation contours are properly set on each original slice that contains any anatomic structure to be included in a particular binary volume. To assist in this, computer tools allow the replication of disarticulation contours through a number of adjacent slices. For automatically generated contours, the workstation computer uses the geometric center of an existing contour to begin generating a contour on the next slice.

After the threshold range has been selected and any required disarticulation contours have been defined, the binary volume representing the desired anatomic structure is computed. The procedure used here may be repeated for as many different binary volumes as the user may eventually wish to render.

Intermediate Three-Dimensional Data

Thus far, the concept of segmentation leading to binary volumes has been described in some detail. A binary volume is one of several intermediate 3D data structures that may be used in a workstation. Although these data structures cannot be directly viewed as 2D images, they are important in terms of their information content and their effect on the final images.

Processing Binary Volumes

As already discussed, a binary volume is a concise and useful representation of the results of segmentation. It may, for example, be used as input for a program that interactively rotates, cuts, measures, renders, and displays such volumes. It may also be used as input to a 3D surface-extraction program that generates yet another intermediate data structure called a voxel surface.

The spatial resolution content of a binary volume is fundamentally limited by the spatial resolution of the original slices from which it was built and by the center-to-center distance of the original slices. To retain even this much spatial resolution, there must be at least as

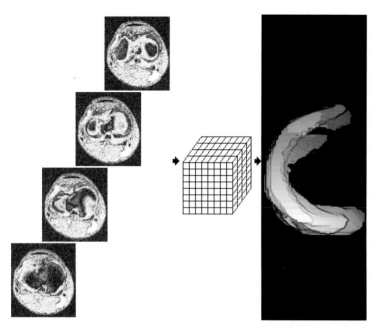

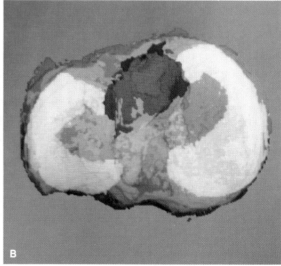

FIGURE 2–1. Original MR images (*left*) are acquired and processed into one or more 3D volumes (*middle*), which are subsequently used to render the final images (*right*).

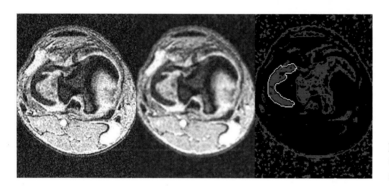

FIGURE 2–2. Original image (*left*), after preprocessing (*middle*), and after segmentation operations to extract meniscus (*right*).

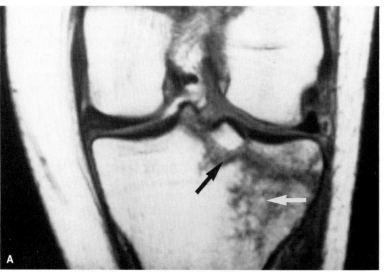

FIGURE 2–3. (**A**) A 3D MR T1-weighted coronal image of a lateral tibial plateau fracture (*black arrow*) involving the anterior intercondyloid fossa and tibial spine. Adjacent marrow hemorrhage (*white arrow*) is identified by diffuse low signal intensity. (**B**) The corresponding axial 3D rendering generated from 0.7-mm axial 3D Fourier transform images demonstrates anterior tibial plateau avulsion (*dark green*) separate from marrow edema (*light gray*) and meniscal cartilages (*transparent yellow*).

many volume elements (*i.e.,* voxels) as there were total pixels in all the original slices. In practice, because the slice-to-slice distance is usually considerably larger than the original pixel size, volumes are usually computed using some form of interpolation in at least the slice-to-slice direction. The interpolation computation not only does slice-to-slice pixel value interpolation but also derives new disarticulation contours at the interpolated slice positions. Typically, a volume is built with voxels that are approximately cubic; that is, the voxel size in the slice-to-slice direction is chosen to be as small as its size in the original image plane. This yields a binary volume which, when rendered, looks less blocky, although the resolution is not improved.

It should be noted that volumes other than binary volumes may also be generated. Such volumes may contain the full resolution pixel values of the original image data (*e.g.,* 12 bits per voxel instead of 1) and are useful for volume rendering.

Voxel Surfaces

When a large number of high-resolution surface renderings are to be made, a surface representation such as the voxel surface data structure becomes useful. As its name implies, a voxel surface contains information on only those voxels that lie on the surface of a binary volume. A voxel surface can be generated by means of a 3D boundary detection program applied to an existing binary volume. In addition, if the user has placed a "seed point" on some desired anatomic point that can be selected on any original image, the boundary detection algorithm limits itself to generating only those surface elements that are connected to the user-specified seed point. This may be useful for excluding unwanted anatomic structures or noise.

RENDERING OF SURFACES

The algorithms used in surface rendering normally perform hidden surface removal; that is, for each pixel in the rendered image, only the projected element of that surface closest to the viewer is retained. The rendered brightness of a surface element is normally modeled after the diffuse reflection of light from a surface. The brightest surface elements are those closest to the viewer and tipped most favorably to reflect light to the viewer, as with "miner's lamp illumination." If the selected rendering parameters make brightness decrease rapidly with the tipping angle, the surface takes on a somewhat specular appearance.

Using the segmentation methods just described, the most natural-looking surface renderings are obtained when disarticulations do not actually cut through in-

threshold regions. The best mathematical estimates of actual surface orientation come from the image pixels that are immediately exterior to the in-threshold pixels; thus, these neighboring pixels should not be eliminated unless necessary. The rightmost images of Figures 2–1 and 2–3B are examples of surface renderings.

RENDERING OF VOLUMES

Volume rendering techniques have been developed as an alternative to the surface rendering method. In volume rendering, rays are mathematically projected through the entire volume, not just its surface elements. In addition, the full resolution (*e.g.,* 12 bits per voxel) of the original slice data may be retained and used during the projection process. Color assignments may be made to different ranges in the values of the voxels. Opacity assignments may also be made to different structures.

In one type of volume rendering, opacities are assigned only to voxel surfaces. In certain other systems, all voxels have opacity, and gradients in the voxel values may be computed during the volume rendering to give surfacelike renderings. In either case, volume-rendering methods can produce quasiradiographic images, in which the brightness of a pixel in the final rendered image is related to the summed voxel values along a ray. Unlike actual radiographs, these images can be derived from any multislice modality, such as MR. These images can be generated with or without disarticulations and at any desired pose.

There is another method of generating 2D images from volumes that is based on a maximum or minimum intensity projection algorithm. Such images are useful mainly in portraying vasculature, from original bright blood or dark blood images acquired using a suitable magnetic resonance angiographic (MRA) technique. There is no segmentation or true 3D representation of different tissues in this method; therefore, its application is limited primarily to MRA.

CO-RENDERING

In many cases, it is desirable to view one anatomic structure in the context of several nearby structures. Software is available that allows such co-rendering, up to a limit of eight objects, any of which may be of either a surface or volumetric type. Arbitrary or standardized colors and brightnesses may be assigned to each object. In addition, any desired opacity can be assigned to any surface.

The final images are based on a rendering model in which the rendered simulated light from a deeper object is partially absorbed when passing through any intervening surface. The final color of any pixel is the net effect of all the brightnesses and attenuations that occur along the ray that passes through that pixel.

IMAGE PRESENTATION

Since its introduction a few years ago, the laser imager has proven to be a high-quality hard copy device that is well suited to multiformat presentation of gray-scale images from digital modalities such as MR. Many 3D images, however, benefit from the addition of color or motion, making it desirable to have some sort of supplemental output available such as color hard copy, a remote color display system, or videotaping. This may be achieved by ancillary devices and systems (*e.g.,* a color laser imager), which obtain color images from the primary workstation either digitally or by video.

For "true" 3D viewing, rendered images can be computed at poses that are at roughly 5° to 10° rotational increments about an axis vertical to the observer. Any two consecutive images then form a stereo pair. Stereo pairs can be displayed or filmed using a side-by-side format and viewed directly by persons who can do crossed-eye stereo viewing. Another approach is to use ancillary equipment with a special display and glasses. Although the 3D effect of stereo-pair viewing can be rather dramatic, its contribution to the clinical interpretation of the rendered images is questionable.

As technology continues to evolve, the use of low-cost remote workstations for interactive 3D operations is becoming feasible. In the not-too-distant future, media delivered from the radiology department to surgeons, radiation treatment planners, and other referring physicians could well include electronically transmitted data files with 3D volumes, which can then be interactively reviewed, analyzed, and discussed using a desktop computer.

REFERENCES

1. Artzy E, Frieder G, Herman GT. The theory, design, implementation, and evaluation of a three-dimensional surface detection algorithm. Comput Graphics Image Process 1981;15:1.
2. Levoy M. Display of surfaces from volume data. IEEE Comput Graphics Appl 1988;8(3):29.
3. Tiede U, et al. Investigation of medical 3D-rendering algorithms. IEEE Comput Graphics Appl 1990;10(2):41.
4. Stytz MR, Frieder G, Frieder O. Three-dimensional medical imaging: algorithms and computer systems. ACM Computing Surveys 1991; 23(4):421.

CHAPTER 3

David W. Stoller
William J. Maloney

The Hip

The hip (*i.e.,* the acetabulum, femoral articulation, and supporting soft tissue, muscle, and cartilage structures) is a functionally and structurally complex joint. Disease processes involving the hip joint include trauma, osteonecrosis, arthritis, infection, and neoplasia, conditions that are frequently not detected by conventional radiographic techniques until they have reached an advanced clinical stage. The various imaging modalities have different strengths and weaknesses in facilitating diagnosis: plain films are limited in assessment of soft tissues and articular structures; contrast arthrography is useful in evaluation of the joint spaces and for sampling of synovial fluid in cases of infection; and computed tomography (CT), by reformatting axial scans with sufficient bone detail to generate sagittal and coronal images, provides a multiplanar three-dimensional (3D) perspective on hip disease.[1]

Magnetic resonance (MR) imaging has also been successfully used to evaluate pathologic processes in the hip.[2,3] The excellent spatial and contrast resolution provided by MR facilitates early detection and evaluation of femoral head osteonecrosis, definition of hyaline articular cartilage in arthritis, identification of joint effusions, and characterization of osseous and soft tissue tumors about the hip. With direct, noninvasive MR imaging of bone marrow, fractures and infiltrative diseases can be identified earlier than with radiographic studies. In addition, the cartilaginous epiphysis in an infant or a child, which is not yet visible on routine radiographs, can be demonstrated on MR images. The use of surface coils in MR of the hip allows more anatatomic details of the hip joint capsule and acetabular labrum to be seen.

IMAGING PROTOCOLS FOR THE HIP

With the body coil, which is used in most MR examinations of the hip, and with a large (32–40-cm) field of view (FOV), both hips are seen and can be compared (Fig. 3–1).

T1-weighted images can be acquired in axial, sagittal, or coronal planes with repetition time (TR) values of 500 to 600 msec and echo time (TE) values of 20 msec or less (Fig. 3–2). Examinations are performed with a 192 × 256 or 256 × 256 acquisition matrix using 1 or 2 excitations (NEX). Thin (3–5 mm) sections are obtained either contiguously or with a minimal interslice gap. Three-millimeter sections are preferred in pediatric patients or when precise assessments are required to image articular cartilage surfaces and the labrum. Three-dimensional Fourier transform (3DFT) volume images allow acquisition of slices to 1 mm in thickness (Fig. 3–3).

Conventional T2-weighted images, acquired in the axial imaging plane with a TR of 2000 msec and TE of 20 and 80 msec, are useful in the evaluation of arthritis, infection, and neoplasia. Coronal T2*-weighted and short TI inversion recovery (STIR) sequences are useful in identifying hip effusions, bone marrow pathology, osseous trauma, and muscle hemorrhage and edema (Fig. 3–4).[4-6]

When imaging a single hip in the sagittal plane, smaller FOVs (24 cm) should be used to obtain high spatial resolution (Fig. 3–5). Signal-to-noise ratio may be a limiting factor, however. With a shoulder surface coil placed anterolateral to the hip joint, FOVs as small as 18 cm and 20 cm can be used (Fig. 3–6). These images are obtained with T1-weighted or T2*-weighted contrast to display capsular and ligamentous anatomy. This technique is particularly useful in separating femoral head from acetabular articular cartilage and for demonstrating intraarticular loose bodies.[7]

ANATOMY OF THE HIP

Gross Anatomy

The femoral head represents a multiaxial, synovial ball-and-socket joint (Fig. 3–7). The acetabulum provides bony coverage of 40% of the femoral head (Fig. 3–8). The dense fibrocartilaginous labrum of the acetabulum increases the depth of the acetabulum (Fig. 3–9). The acetabular fossa contains the ligamentum teres and fat pad or pulvinar. The innominate bone, or hip bone, includes the ilium, ischium, and pubic bones. At birth, the triradiate or Y cartilage, located at the center of the acetabulum, separates the ilium, ischium, and pubis.[8,9] The fovea capitis, a small depression on the medial femoral head, is the site of attachment of the ligamentum teres originating in the acetabular fossa (Fig. 3–10). The transverse acetabular ligament bridges the notch at the inferolateral acetabulum and, together with the acetabular labrum, forms a complete ring around the acetabulum. The femoral head, covered by articular cartilage, forms two-thirds of a sphere proximal to its transition into the femoral neck. There is no articular cartilage surface over the fovea capitis. The femoral head articular cartilage surface measures 3 mm in its thickest regions posteriorly and superiorly, thinning to 0.5 mm along its peripheral and inferior margins.

The inelastic fibrous capsule of the hip joint is reinforced by the iliofemoral, pubofemoral, and ischiofemoral ligaments (Figs. 3–11 and 3–12). The iliofemoral ligament, or ligament of Bigelow, is the strongest and thickest of the capsular ligaments and has an inverted Y shape anteriorly. The pubofemoral and ischiofemoral ligaments are less substantial. Deep circular fibers from the ischiofemoral ligament form the zona orbicularis. Twisting and shortening of the capsule limits full hip extension. The main hip abductors, the gluteus minimis and gluteus medius, insert on the greater trochanter. The iliopsoas tendon, a major hip flexor, passes anterior to the hip joint and attaches to the lesser trochanter.

The calcar femorale represents weight-bearing bone radiating from the inferomedial femoral cortex toward the greater tuberosity. Weight-bearing stress trabeculae form the boundaries of Ward's triangle in the femoral neck and head. On conventional radiography, Ward's triangle appears as a region of decreased bone density distal to the intersection of femoral neck weight-bearing trabeculae. The secondary ossification centers of the femoral head, the greater and lesser trochanters, appear at 4 to 7 months of fetal development. In the adult, the mean femoral neck shaft angle is 125° and femoral anteversion averages 14°. The neck shaft and femoral anteversion angles decrease during skeletal maturation.

The intertrochanteric line between the greater and lesser trochanters of the femur is the attachment site of the iliofemoral ligament; therefore, it can be seen that 95% of the femoral neck is intracapsular.

The medial and lateral circumflex arteries provide most of the blood supply to the femoral head and proximal femur through anastomotic rings at the base of the femoral neck and head. The lateral part of this extracapsular arterial ring provides most of the blood supply to the femoral head. The obturator artery provides a variable vascular supply to the femoral head through the ligamentum teres.

Normal Magnetic Resonance Appearance of the Hip

Axial Images

The axial plane displays the relationship between the femoral head and the acetabulum with supporting musculature on cross-sectional gross images (Fig. 3–13) and MR scans (Fig. 3–14). Axial images made at the level of the acetabular roof may show a partial volume effect with the femoral head. Signal intensity inhomogeneity within the acetabulum is secondary to a greater distribution of red (*i.e.,* hematopoietic) marrow stores. The hip musculature demonstrates intermediate signal intensity on T1-weighted images. The gluteal muscles—the gluteus medius laterally, the gluteus minimis deep, and the gluteus maximus posteriorly—can be differentiated from one another by high signal intensity fat along fascial divisions. The tensor fasciae latae muscle is seen anterior to the gluteus medius and is bordered anteriorly by subcutaneous fat. The iliopsoas muscle group is anterior to the femoral head in a twelve-o'clock position. The sartorius muscle is the most anterior, and the rectus femoris is positioned between the more lateral tensor fasciae latae and the medial iliopsoas. The obturator internus muscle is visualized medial to the anterior and posterior acetabular columns.

The sciatic nerve, located directly posterior to the posterior column of the acetabulum, is visualized with intermediate signal intensity. The external iliac vessels, which are of low signal intensity, are medial to the iliopsoas muscle and anterior to the anterior acetabular column. The low signal intensity tendon of the rectus femoris blends with the low signal intensity cortex of the anterior inferior iliac spine. The reflected head of the rectus femoris tendon is lateral to the iliofemoral ligament and follows the contours of the lateral acetabulum. At the level of the femoral head, the more distal femoral artery and vein are visualized. The femoral head articular cartilage demonstrates intermediate signal intensity, and the anterior and posterior fibrocartilaginous acetabular labrum may also be identified at this level. The acetabular labrum is triangular, with the apex oriented laterally.

At the level of the greater trochanter and femoral neck, the obturator internus is identified medial to the pubis and ischium. The iliofemoral ligament is of low signal intensity and blends with the dark (*i.e.,* low signal intensity) cortex of the anterior femoral neck. The sciatic nerve, lateral to the ischial tuberosity, is encased in fat between the quadratus femoris muscle anteriorly and the gluteus maximus muscle posteriorly. The iliotibial tract can be seen peripherally as a thin, low signal intensity band surrounded by high signal intensity fat on the medial and lateral surfaces. The low signal intensity obturator vessels are encased in high signal intensity fat and can be identified posterolateral to the pubic bone, between the pectineus and obturator internus muscles. The adductor muscles anteromedially, the obturator externus and the quadratus femoris muscles medially, the ischial tuberosity attachment of the long head of the biceps femoris, and the semitendinosus tendons posteriorly, can be visualized at the level of the proximal femur. The ischiofemoral ligament is also identified anterior to the quadratus femoris, medial to the ischium, and applied to the posterior hip capsule. The sacrotuberous ligament is seen posteromedial to the ischium.

Sagittal Images

The gluteus medius muscle and the tendon attachment to the greater trochanter are demonstrated on lateral sagittal images (Fig. 3–15). The tendon of the obturator externus is anterior and inferior to the greater trochanter. The piriformis tendon is situated between the iliofemoral ligament anteriorly and the gluteus medius tendon posteriorly. On lateral sagittal images, the ilium, the anterior inferior iliac spine, the acetabular roof, and the femoral head are visualized on the same sagittal section. The iliofemoral ligament extends inferiorly directly anterior to the anterior acetabular labrum. The iliopsoas muscle and tendon course obliquely anterior to the iliofemoral ligament anterior to the femoral head. The ischiofemoral ligament is closely applied to the posterior femoral head surface, anterior to the inferior gemellus muscle and obturator internus tendon. The femoral physeal scar is seen as a horizontal band of low signal intensity, in an anterior to posterior orientation. In the sagittal plane, the intermediate signal intensity hyaline articular cartilage of the femoral head and acetabulum can be separately defined, and the posterior gluteal and anterior rectus femoris muscles are displayed in the long axis.

Distally, the vastus musculature is imaged anterior to the proximal femoral diaphysis and the biceps femoris is viewed posteriorly. The sciatic nerve can be followed longitudinally between the anterior quadratus femoris and the posterior gluteus maximus. The low signal intensity attachment of the sartorius to the anterosuperior iliac spine is shown anteriorly on sagittal images. The low signal intensity iliopsoas tendon spans the hip joint anteriorly, crossing to its insertion on the lesser trochanter. The adductor muscle group is displayed inferior to and medial to the iliopsoas tendon and the pectineus muscle.

(text continues on page 57)

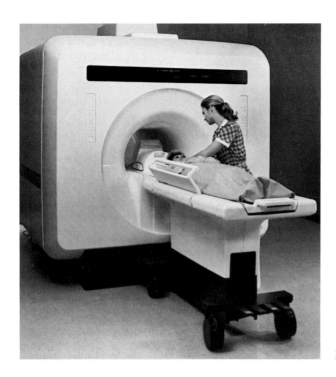

FIGURE 3–1. Body coil for MR imaging of the hip.

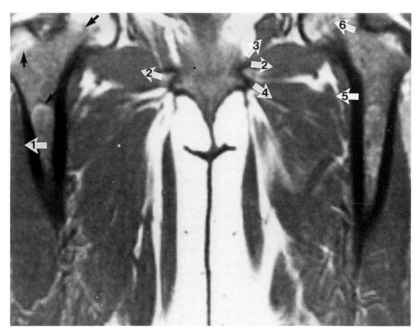

FIGURE 3–2. A T1-weighted coronal image through the hips shows the vastus lateralis muscle (1), obturator externus muscle (2), obturator internus muscle (3), adductor magnus muscle (4), iliopsoas muscle (5), and femoral head (6). Normal red marrow (low signal intensity) and yellow marrow (bright signal intensity) inhomogeneity (*black arrows*) is present. (TR, 600 msec; TE, 20 msec.)

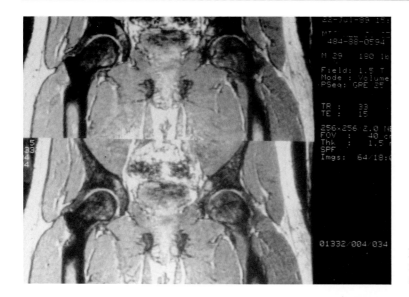

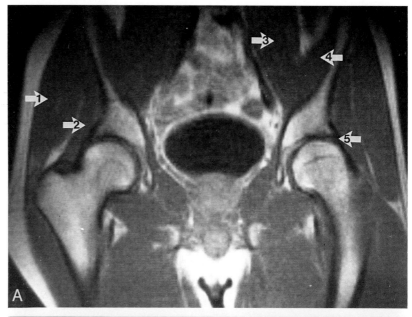

FIGURE 3–3. Three-dimensional Fourier transform coronal 5-mm images through the hips. (TR, 33 msec; TE, 15 msec; flip angle, 25°.)

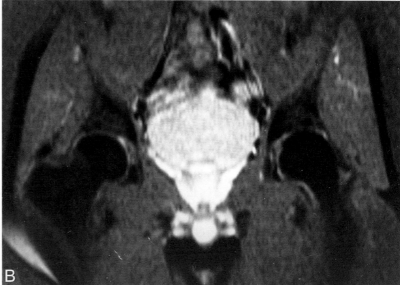

FIGURE 3–4. Coronal image through the mid-hips. (**A**) T1-weighted image shows the gluteus medius muscle (1), gluteus minimus muscle (2), psoas muscle (3), iliacus (4), and labrum (5). (TR, 600 msec; TE, 20 msec.) (**B**) The corresponding short TI inversion recovery image demonstrates a dark signal from areas of null fat signal intensity. (TR, 1400 msec; TI, 125 msec; TE, 40 msec.)

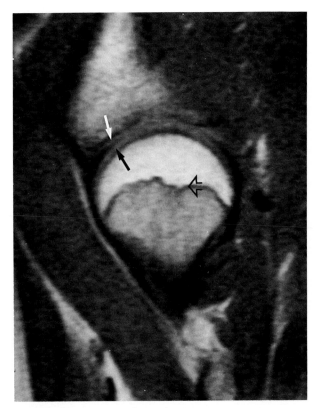

FIGURE 3–5. T1-weighted sagittal image of the femoral head in a 12-year-old child shows separation of hyaline articular cartilage in the acetabulum (*white arrow*) and femoral head (*black arrow*). The open physis, represented by low signal intensity, is transversely oriented (*open arrow*). (TR, 600 msec; TE, 20 msec.)

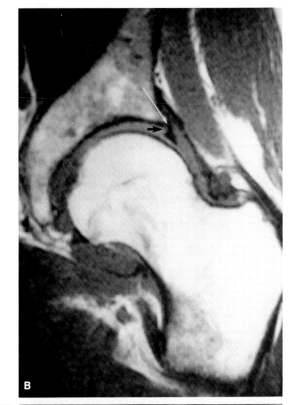

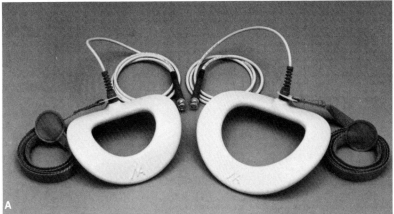

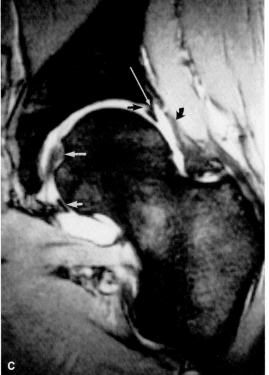

FIGURE 3–6. Capsular anatomy. (**A**) Shoulder surface coils are used to image the hip joint. (**B**) A T1-weighted coronal image obtained with the surface coil displays low signal intensity labrum (*white arrow*) and intermediate signal intensity articular cartilage (*black arrow*). The lateral extent of the articular cartilage should not be mistaken for a partial labral tear. (TR, 500 msec; TE, 20 msec.) (**C**) A coronal T2*-weighted image obtained with the surface coil identifies capsular structures in contrast to the bright signal intensity joint fluid. The acetabular labrum (*long white arrow*) and cartilage (*straight black arrow*), ligamentum teres (*medium white arrow*), transverse ligament (*short white arrow*), and iliofemoral ligament (*curved black arrow*) are noted. (TR, 400 msec; TE, 15 msec; flip angle, 20°.)

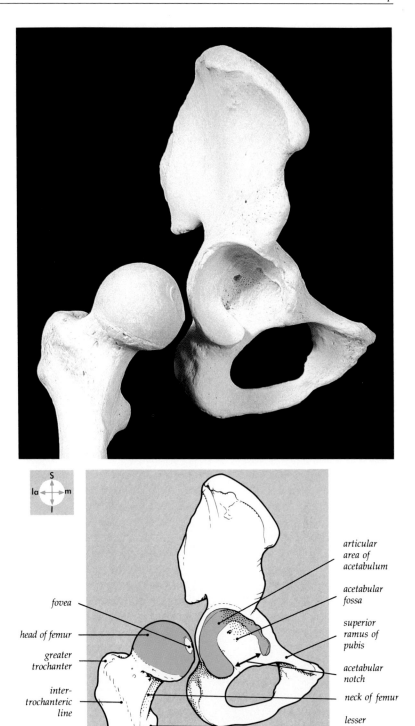

FIGURE 3-7. Articular surfaces of the hip joint are comprised of the acetabulum of the hip bone and the head of the femur.

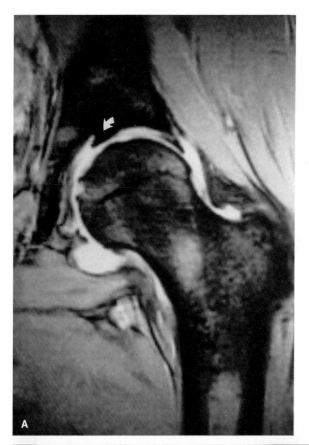

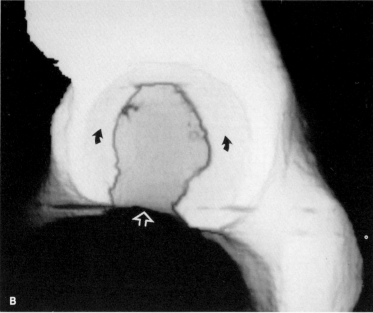

FIGURE 3–8. A normal cortical articular ridge of the acetabulum (*arrow*) is seen on (**A**) T2*-weighted coronal and (**B**) 3D CT images. This bony ridge should not be mistaken for osseous pathology. The acetabular notch (*open arrow*) is shown on 3D CT rendering. (**A**: TR, 400 msec; TE, 20 msec; flip angle, 25°.)

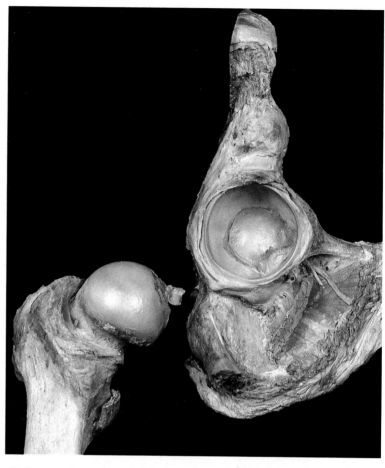

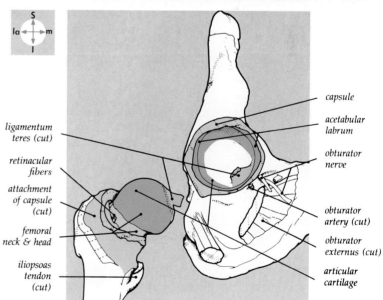

capsule

acetabular
labrum

obturator
nerve

obturator
artery (cut)

obturator
externus (cut)

articular
cartilage

ligamentum
teres (cut)

retinacular
fibers

attachment
of capsule
(cut)

femoral
neck & head

iliopsoas
tendon
(cut)

FIGURE 3–9. Internal features are revealed by disarticulation of the joint after cutting the ligamentum teres and joint capsule.

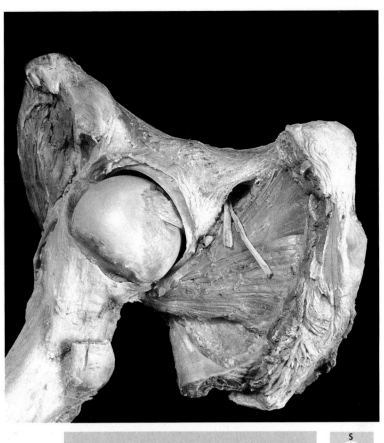

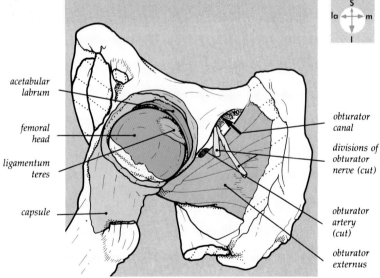

acetabular labrum

femoral head

ligamentum teres

capsule

obturator canal

divisions of obturator nerve (cut)

obturator artery (cut)

obturator externus

FIGURE 3–10. The joint capsule has been opened anteriorly and reflected to show the interior of the joint. The femur has been abducted and externally rotated.

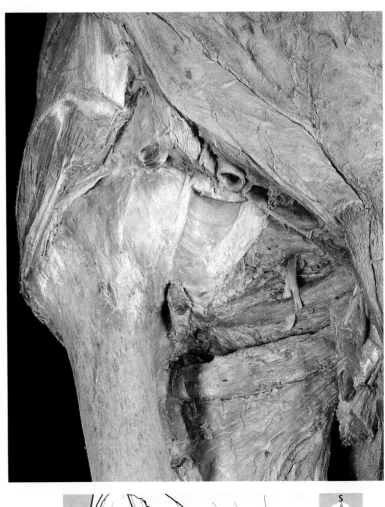

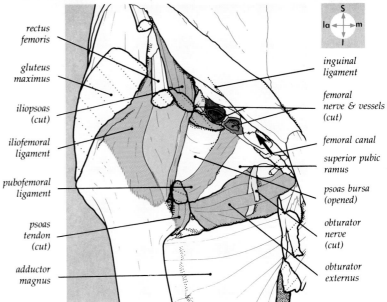

rectus
femoris

gluteus
maximus

iliopsoas
(cut)

iliofemoral
ligament

pubofemoral
ligament

psoas
tendon
(cut)

adductor
magnus

inguinal
ligament

femoral
nerve & vessels
(cut)

femoral canal

superior pubic
ramus

psoas bursa
(opened)

obturator
nerve
(cut)

obturator
externus

FIGURE 3–11. Anterior surface of the joint capsule,
associated ligaments, and adjacent structures.

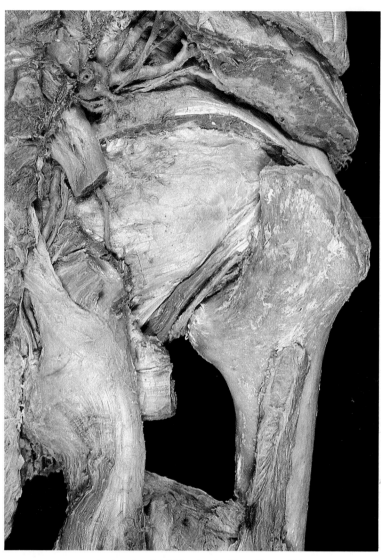

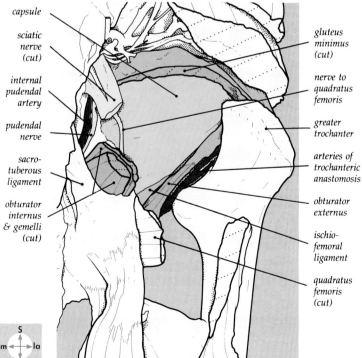

capsule

sciatic
nerve
(cut)

internal
pudendal
artery

pudendal
nerve

sacro-
tuberous
ligament

obturator
internus
& gemelli
(cut)

gluteus
minimus
(cut)

nerve to
quadratus
femoris

greater
trochanter

arteries of
trochanteric
anastomosis

obturator
externus

ischio-
femoral
ligament

quadratus
femoris
(cut)

FIGURE 3–12. Posterior surface of the joint capsule and the ischiofemoral ligament.

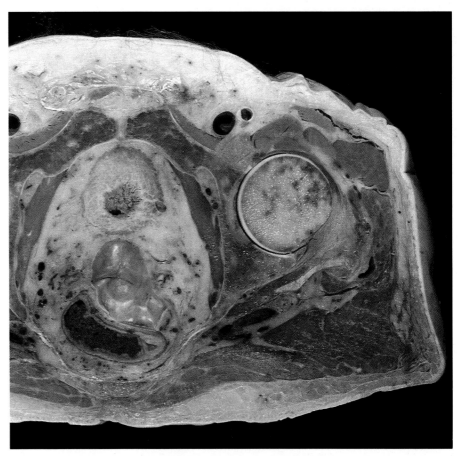

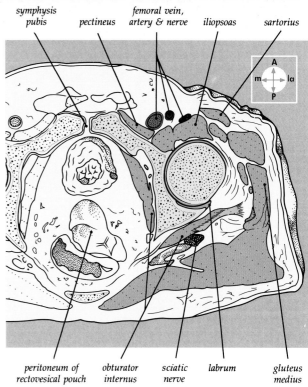

FIGURE 3–13. A transverse section through the hip joint shows its anatomic relations.

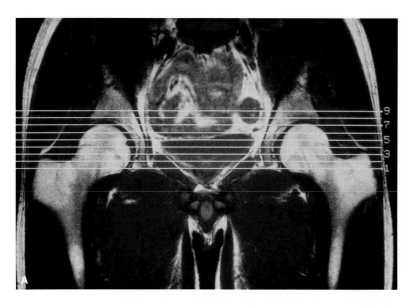

FIGURE 3–14. Normal axial MR anatomy. (**A**) This coronal localizer was used to graphically prescribe axial T1-weighted image locations from (**B**) superior to (**J**) inferior.

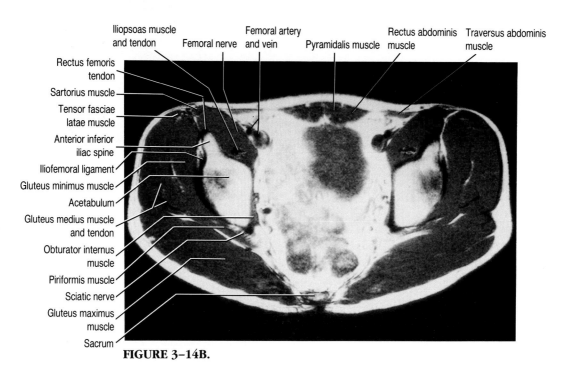

FIGURE 3–14B.

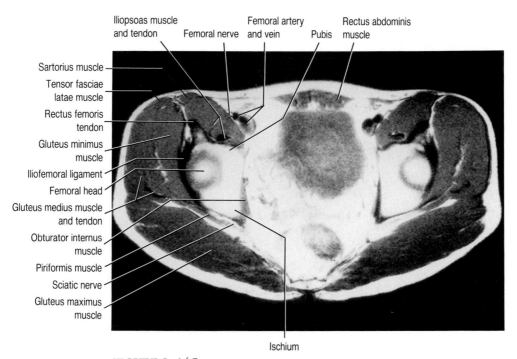

Iliopsoas muscle and tendon   Femoral nerve   Femoral artery and vein   Pubis   Rectus abdominis muscle

Sartorius muscle

Tensor fasciae latae muscle

Rectus femoris tendon

Gluteus minimus muscle

Iliofemoral ligament

Femoral head

Gluteus medius muscle and tendon

Obturator internus muscle

Piriformis muscle

Sciatic nerve

Gluteus maximus muscle

Ischium

FIGURE 3–14C.

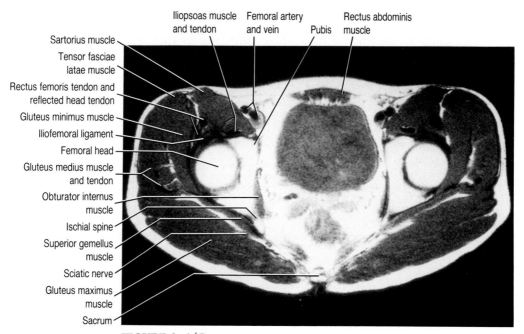

Iliopsoas muscle and tendon   Femoral artery and vein   Pubis   Rectus abdominis muscle

Sartorius muscle

Tensor fasciae latae muscle

Rectus femoris tendon and reflected head tendon

Gluteus minimus muscle

Iliofemoral ligament

Femoral head

Gluteus medius muscle and tendon

Obturator internus muscle

Ischial spine

Superior gemellus muscle

Sciatic nerve

Gluteus maximus muscle

Sacrum

FIGURE 3–14D.

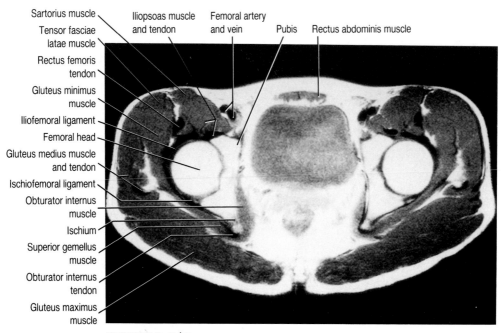

Sartorius muscle
Tensor fasciae latae muscle
Rectus femoris tendon
Gluteus minimus muscle
Iliofemoral ligament
Femoral head
Gluteus medius muscle and tendon
Ischiofemoral ligament
Obturator internus muscle
Ischium
Superior gemellus muscle
Obturator internus tendon
Gluteus maximus muscle

Iliopsoas muscle and tendon
Femoral artery and vein
Pubis
Rectus abdominis muscle

FIGURE 3–14E.

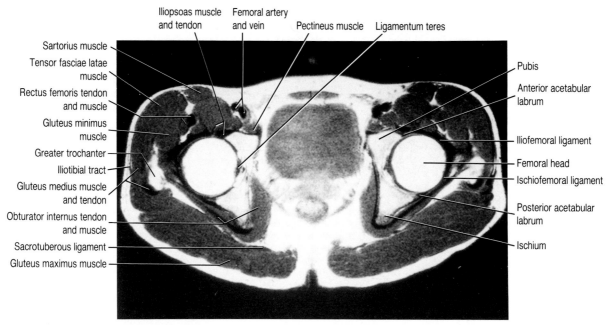

Iliopsoas muscle and tendon
Femoral artery and vein
Pectineus muscle
Ligamentum teres

Sartorius muscle
Tensor fasciae latae muscle
Rectus femoris tendon and muscle
Gluteus minimus muscle
Greater trochanter
Iliotibial tract
Gluteus medius muscle and tendon
Obturator internus tendon and muscle
Sacrotuberous ligament
Gluteus maximus muscle

Pubis
Anterior acetabular labrum
Iliofemoral ligament
Femoral head
Ischiofemoral ligament
Posterior acetabular labrum
Ischium

FIGURE 3–14F.

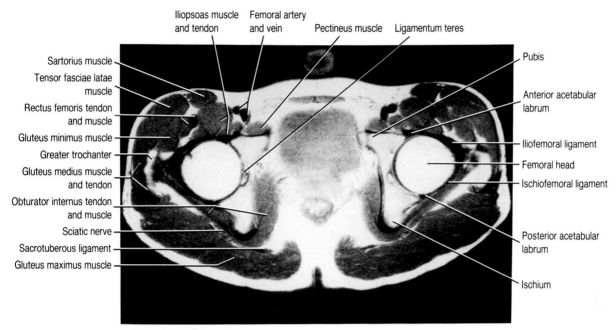

Iliopsoas muscle and tendon
Femoral artery and vein
Pectineus muscle
Ligamentum teres

Sartorius muscle
Tensor fasciae latae muscle
Rectus femoris tendon and muscle
Gluteus minimus muscle
Greater trochanter
Gluteus medius muscle and tendon
Obturator internus tendon and muscle
Sciatic nerve
Sacrotuberous ligament
Gluteus maximus muscle

Pubis
Anterior acetabular labrum
Iliofemoral ligament
Femoral head
Ischiofemoral ligament
Posterior acetabular labrum
Ischium

FIGURE 3–14G.

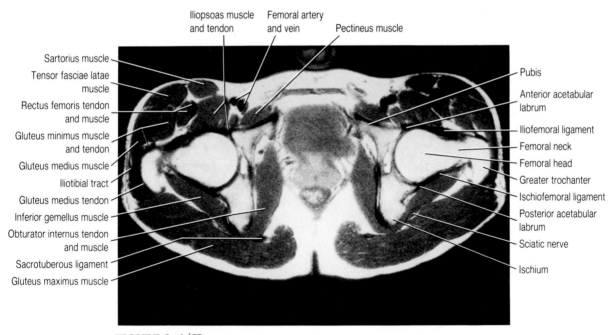

Iliopsoas muscle and tendon
Femoral artery and vein
Pectineus muscle

Sartorius muscle
Tensor fasciae latae muscle
Rectus femoris tendon and muscle
Gluteus minimus muscle and tendon
Gluteus medius muscle
Iliotibial tract
Gluteus medius tendon
Inferior gemellus muscle
Obturator internus tendon and muscle
Sacrotuberous ligament
Gluteus maximus muscle

Pubis
Anterior acetabular labrum
Iliofemoral ligament
Femoral neck
Femoral head
Greater trochanter
Ischiofemoral ligament
Posterior acetabular labrum
Sciatic nerve
Ischium

FIGURE 3–14H.

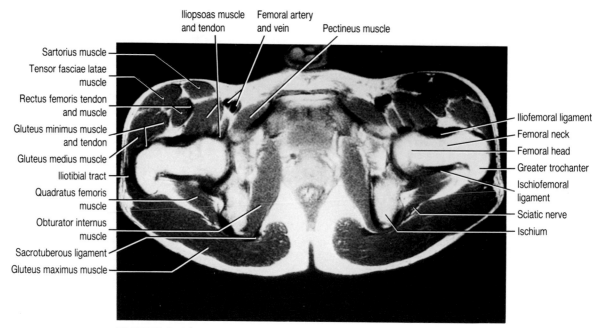

FIGURE 3–14I.

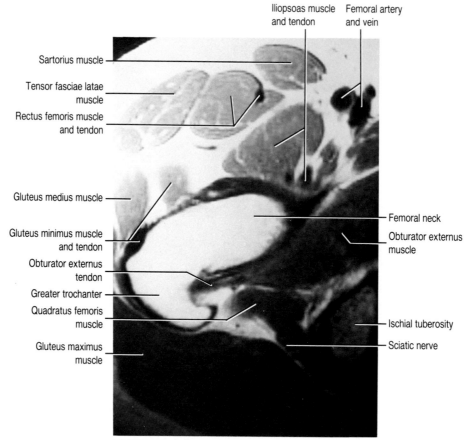

FIGURE 3–14J.

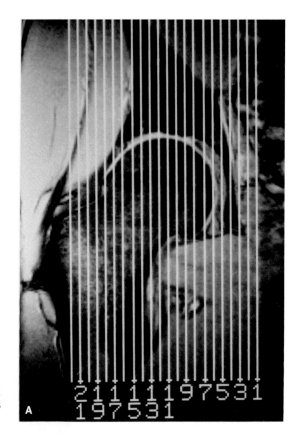

FIGURE 3–15. Normal sagittal MR anatomy. (**A**) This T2*-weighted coronal localizer was used to graphically prescribe sagittal T1-weighted image locations from (**B**) medial to (**O**) lateral.

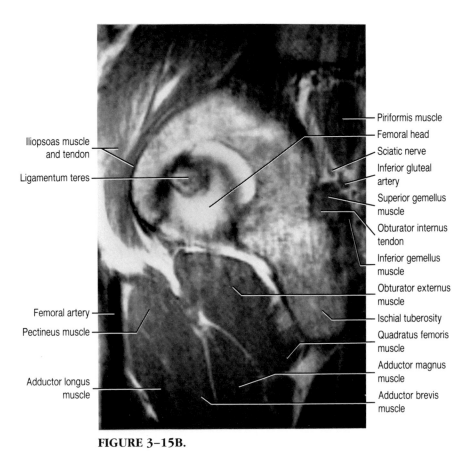

Iliopsoas muscle and tendon

Ligamentum teres

Femoral artery

Pectineus muscle

Adductor longus muscle

Piriformis muscle

Femoral head

Sciatic nerve

Inferior gluteal artery

Superior gemellus muscle

Obturator internus tendon

Inferior gemellus muscle

Obturator externus muscle

Ischial tuberosity

Quadratus femoris muscle

Adductor magnus muscle

Adductor brevis muscle

FIGURE 3–15B.

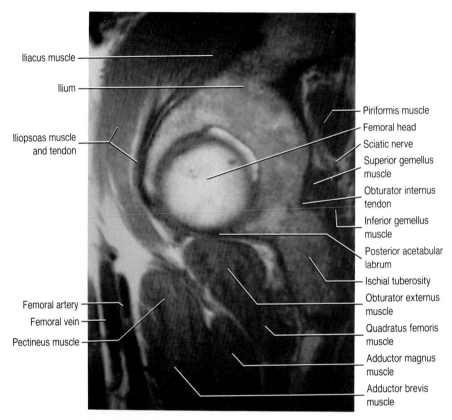

Iliacus muscle

Ilium

Iliopsoas muscle
and tendon

Femoral artery

Femoral vein

Pectineus muscle

Piriformis muscle

Femoral head

Sciatic nerve

Superior gemellus
muscle

Obturator internus
tendon

Inferior gemellus
muscle

Posterior acetabular
labrum

Ischial tuberosity

Obturator externus
muscle

Quadratus femoris
muscle

Adductor magnus
muscle

Adductor brevis
muscle

FIGURE 3–15C.

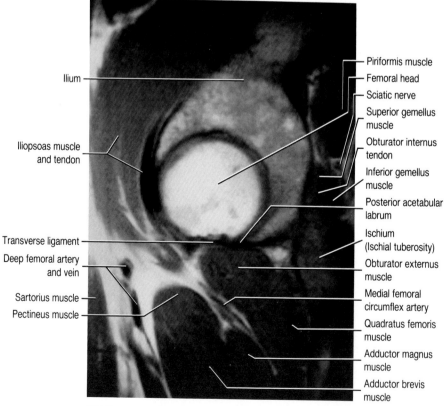

Ilium

Iliopsoas muscle
and tendon

Transverse ligament

Deep femoral artery
and vein

Sartorius muscle

Pectineus muscle

Piriformis muscle

Femoral head

Sciatic nerve

Superior gemellus
muscle

Obturator internus
tendon

Inferior gemellus
muscle

Posterior acetabular
labrum

Ischium
(Ischial tuberosity)

Obturator externus
muscle

Medial femoral
circumflex artery

Quadratus femoris
muscle

Adductor magnus
muscle

Adductor brevis
muscle

FIGURE 3–15D.

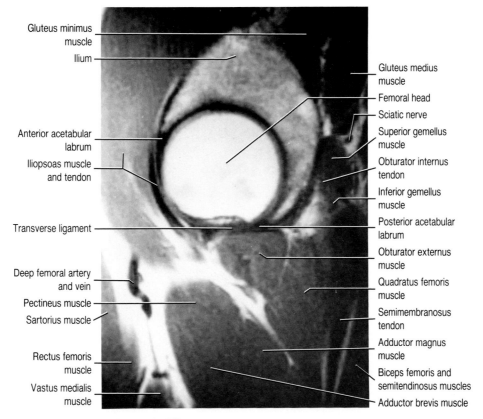

Gluteus minimus muscle

Ilium

Anterior acetabular labrum

Iliopsoas muscle and tendon

Transverse ligament

Deep femoral artery and vein

Pectineus muscle

Sartorius muscle

Rectus femoris muscle

Vastus medialis muscle

Gluteus medius muscle

Femoral head

Sciatic nerve

Superior gemellus muscle

Obturator internus tendon

Inferior gemellus muscle

Posterior acetabular labrum

Obturator externus muscle

Quadratus femoris muscle

Semimembranosus tendon

Adductor magnus muscle

Biceps femoris and semitendinosus muscles

Adductor brevis muscle

FIGURE 3–15E.

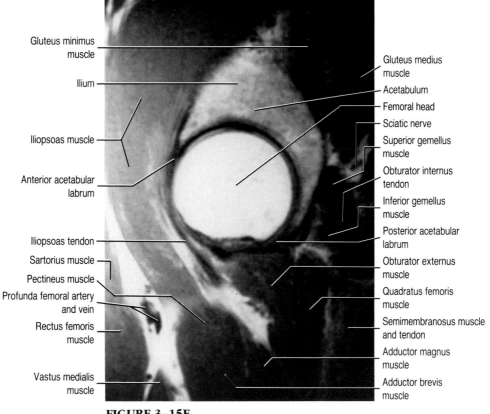

Gluteus minimus muscle

Ilium

Iliopsoas muscle

Anterior acetabular labrum

Iliopsoas tendon

Sartorius muscle

Pectineus muscle

Profunda femoral artery and vein

Rectus femoris muscle

Vastus medialis muscle

Gluteus medius muscle

Acetabulum

Femoral head

Sciatic nerve

Superior gemellus muscle

Obturator internus tendon

Inferior gemellus muscle

Posterior acetabular labrum

Obturator externus muscle

Quadratus femoris muscle

Semimembranosus muscle and tendon

Adductor magnus muscle

Adductor brevis muscle

FIGURE 3–15F.

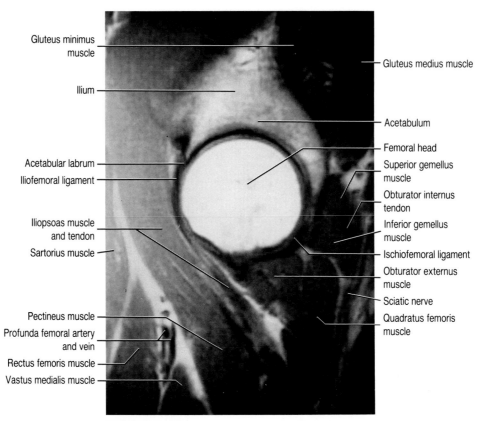

Gluteus minimus muscle

Ilium

Acetabular labrum

Iliofemoral ligament

Iliopsoas muscle and tendon

Sartorius muscle

Pectineus muscle

Profunda femoral artery and vein

Rectus femoris muscle

Vastus medialis muscle

Gluteus medius muscle

Acetabulum

Femoral head

Superior gemellus muscle

Obturator internus tendon

Inferior gemellus muscle

Ischiofemoral ligament

Obturator externus muscle

Sciatic nerve

Quadratus femoris muscle

FIGURE 3–15G.

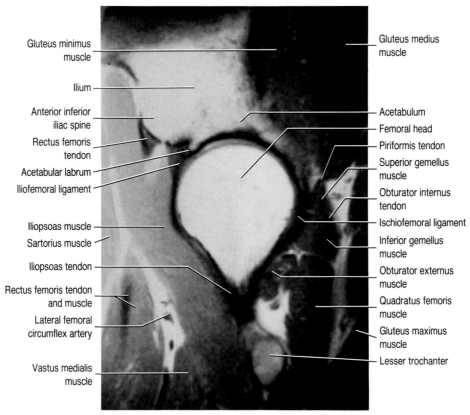

Gluteus minimus muscle

Ilium

Anterior inferior iliac spine

Rectus femoris tendon

Acetabular labrum

Iliofemoral ligament

Iliopsoas muscle

Sartorius muscle

Iliopsoas tendon

Rectus femoris tendon and muscle

Lateral femoral circumflex artery

Vastus medialis muscle

Gluteus medius muscle

Acetabulum

Femoral head

Piriformis tendon

Superior gemellus muscle

Obturator internus tendon

Ischiofemoral ligament

Inferior gemellus muscle

Obturator externus muscle

Quadratus femoris muscle

Gluteus maximus muscle

Lesser trochanter

FIGURE 3–15H.

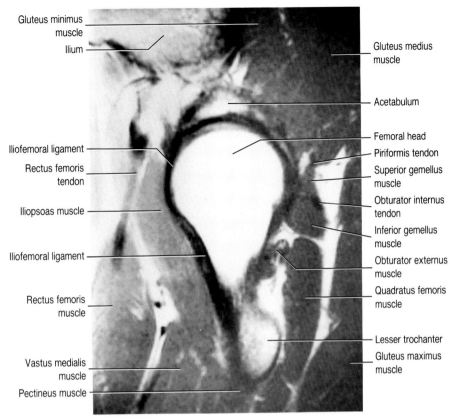

Gluteus minimus
muscle

Ilium

Iliofemoral ligament

Rectus femoris
tendon

Iliopsoas muscle

Iliofemoral ligament

Rectus femoris
muscle

Vastus medialis
muscle

Pectineus muscle

Gluteus medius
muscle

Acetabulum

Femoral head

Piriformis tendon

Superior gemellus
muscle

Obturator internus
tendon

Inferior gemellus
muscle

Obturator externus
muscle

Quadratus femoris
muscle

Lesser trochanter

Gluteus maximus
muscle

FIGURE 3–15I.

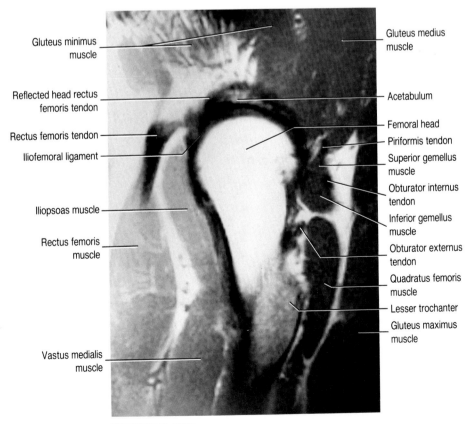

Gluteus minimus
muscle

Reflected head rectus
femoris tendon

Rectus femoris tendon

Iliofemoral ligament

Iliopsoas muscle

Rectus femoris
muscle

Vastus medialis
muscle

Gluteus medius
muscle

Acetabulum

Femoral head

Piriformis tendon

Superior gemellus
muscle

Obturator internus
tendon

Inferior gemellus
muscle

Obturator externus
tendon

Quadratus femoris
muscle

Lesser trochanter

Gluteus maximus
muscle

FIGURE 3–15J.

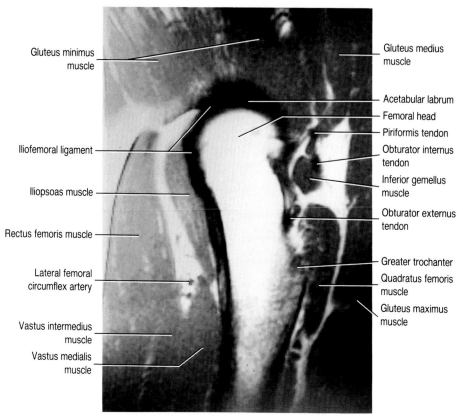

Gluteus minimus muscle

Iliofemoral ligament

Iliopsoas muscle

Rectus femoris muscle

Lateral femoral circumflex artery

Vastus intermedius muscle

Vastus medialis muscle

Gluteus medius muscle

Acetabular labrum

Femoral head

Piriformis tendon

Obturator internus tendon

Inferior gemellus muscle

Obturator externus tendon

Greater trochanter

Quadratus femoris muscle

Gluteus maximus muscle

FIGURE 3–15K.

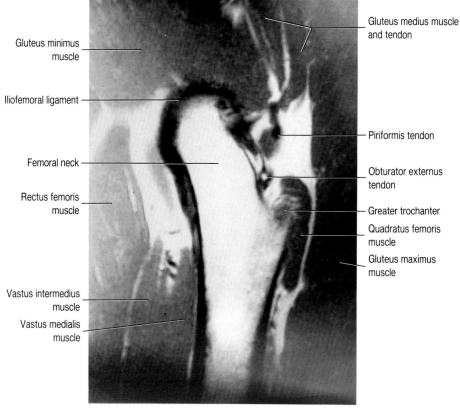

Gluteus minimus muscle

Iliofemoral ligament

Femoral neck

Rectus femoris muscle

Vastus intermedius muscle

Vastus medialis muscle

Gluteus medius muscle and tendon

Piriformis tendon

Obturator externus tendon

Greater trochanter

Quadratus femoris muscle

Gluteus maximus muscle

FIGURE 3–15L.

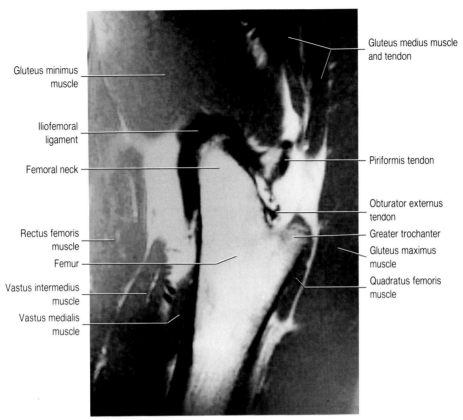

Gluteus minimus muscle

Iliofemoral ligament

Femoral neck

Rectus femoris muscle

Femur

Vastus intermedius muscle

Vastus medialis muscle

Gluteus medius muscle and tendon

Piriformis tendon

Obturator externus tendon

Greater trochanter

Gluteus maximus muscle

Quadratus femoris muscle

FIGURE 3–15M.

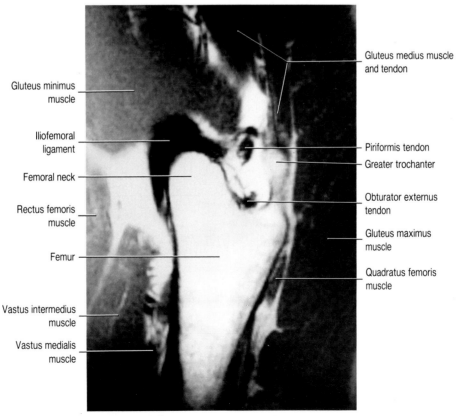

Gluteus minimus muscle

Iliofemoral ligament

Femoral neck

Rectus femoris muscle

Femur

Vastus intermedius muscle

Vastus medialis muscle

Gluteus medius muscle and tendon

Piriformis tendon

Greater trochanter

Obturator externus tendon

Gluteus maximus muscle

Quadratus femoris muscle

FIGURE 3–15N.

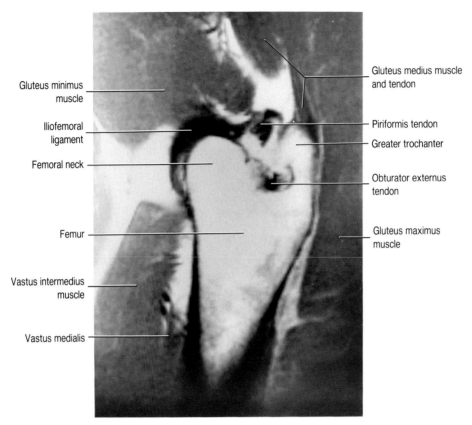

Gluteus minimus muscle

Iliofemoral ligament

Femoral neck

Femur

Vastus intermedius muscle

Vastus medialis

Gluteus medius muscle and tendon

Piriformis tendon

Greater trochanter

Obturator externus tendon

Gluteus maximus muscle

FIGURE 3–15O.

On medial sagittal images the acetabulum encompasses 75% of the femoral head, and the low signal intensity transverse acetabular ligament bridges the uncovered anterior inferior gap. On extreme medial images through the hip joint, the ligamentum teres may be seen within the acetabular fossa. At this level, the ischial tuberosity can be seen posterior and inferior to the acetabular fossa.

Coronal Images

The coronal plane is used in the evaluation of the acetabular labrum, the hip joint space, and the subchondral acetabular and femoral marrow as seen on coronal gross (Fig. 3–16) and MR sections (Fig. 3–17). Acetabular and femoral head articular cartilage may be more difficult to separate on coronal images than on sagittal images. The fibrocartilaginous limbus (or acetabular labrum), is visualized as a low signal intensity triangle interposed between the superolateral aspect of the femoral head and the inferolateral aspect of the acetabulum. The joint capsule is visualized as a low signal intensity structure circumscribing the femoral neck. In the presence of fluid, the capsule distends and the lateral and medial margins become convex. Anterior coronal images demonstrate the iliac crest in continuity with the acetabulum. A defect in the articular cartilage of the femoral head can be seen medially at the ligamentum teres insertion site. The reflected head of the rectus femoris is shown lateral to the proximal portion of the iliofemoral ligament.

Anteriorly, the iliopsoas muscle and tendon are in a seven-o'clock position relative to the femoral head. The low signal intensity iliofemoral ligament is present on the lateral aspect of the femoral neck near the greater trochanter. The superior acetabular labrum is located deep to the proximal portion of the iliofemoral ligament along the lateral inferior margin of the acetabulum. The orbicular zone may be identified as a small outpouching on the medial aspect of the junction of the femoral head and neck. The intraarticular femoral fat pad is located between the medial femoral head and the acetabulum and displays increased signal intensity on T1-weighted images. The obturator externus muscle crosses the femoral neck on posterior coronal images. Inhomogeneity of marrow signal intensity in the acetabulum, ilium, and ischium is a normal finding on T1-weighted images. This represents normal red and yellow marrow inhomogeneity.

PATHOLOGY OF THE HIP

Avascular Necrosis

Avascular necrosis (AVN) of bone most commonly involves the femoral head. It is usually caused by trauma, typically occurring after a displaced femoral neck fracture and less frequently after a fracture–dislocation of the hip. Necrosis results when the vascular supply to the femoral head is disrupted at the time of injury. Nontraumatic AVN occurs in a younger population and is commonly bilateral.[10] Although its etiology is not well understood, a popular theory suggests a vascular etiology secondary to fat embolism leading to inflammation and focal intravascular coagulation.[11] Nontraumatic AVN is associated with several clinical conditions such as alcoholism, hypercortisolism, Gaucher's disease, obesity, hemoglobinopathies, pancreatitis, and dysbaric phenomena (Fig. 3–18). In a significant number of cases, none of the known risk factors can be identified, and the disease is considered idiopathic.[12-14]

Diagnosis

Early diagnosis is important in improving the chances of saving the femoral head, because all prophylactic treatment procedures (discussed later in the chapter) are more successful in the initial stages of AVN. This becomes an issue when evaluating an asymptomatic hip in a patient with nontraumatic AVN on the contralateral side (Fig. 3–19). In addition to MR imaging, nuclear scintigraphy with technetium-labeled phosphate analogues such as methylene diphosphonate (*i.e.,* ^{99m}TC-MDP), has been used for the early detection of osteonecrosis.[15] During the acute phase of the disease, decreased uptake of bone tracer is associated with vascular compromise. Increased radiopharmaceutical accumulation occurs with chronic vascular stasis in repair and in revascularization. Blood flow (*i.e.,* dynamic) scanning has been used to assess regional blood flow. The specificity of marrow scanning with technetium sulfur colloid (^{99m}TC-sulfur colloid) is variable and depends on the underlying disease status and the pattern of marrow distribution.

Magnetic Resonance Imaging. In detection of AVN of the hip, MR imaging has been reported to be more sensitive than CT or radionuclide bone scintigraphy.[16,17] In differentiating AVN from non-AVN disease of the femoral head, MR imaging has been reported to have a specificity of 98% and a sensitivity of 97%.[18] Magnetic resonance imaging is also effective in assessing joint effusions, marrow conversion, edema, and articular cartilage congruity, none of which is possible with bone scintigraphy, standard radiographs, or CT.

Evaluation of patients with osteonecrosis can be accomplished with a T1-weighted axial localizer and either a T1- or T2-weighted spin-echo coronal sequence. Imaging in the sagittal plane may be helpful in defining early changes of cortical flattening associated with subchondral collapse (see Fig. 3–19). Short TI inversion recovery pulse sequences, which negate yellow marrow-fat signal, provide excellent contrast for the detection of marrow replacement, fluid, and necrotic tissue (Fig. 3–

20). Premature fatty marrow conversion associated with osteonecrosis can be detected using chemical-shift imaging techniques. On fat-selective and water-selective images, fatty and hematopoietic marrow and distribution of water within the ischemic focus can be differentiated. Gradient-echo coronal images, although not as sensitive for fluid within reparative tissue and necrosis, demonstrate associated hip joint effusions, subchondral fluid, and changes in articular cartilage contours (Figs. 3–21 to 3–23). When compared with coronal images acquired with a body coil, sagittal images acquired with a surface coil and a small FOV may provide superior anteroposterior (AP) and superoinferior localization of AVN by demonstrating joint-space narrowing, articular cartilage fracture, and the double-line sign (Fig. 3–24).[19] The characteristic double-line sign can be observed in up to 80% of lesions and cannot be attributed to a chemical-shift artifact or misrepresentation (Fig. 3–25). On T2-weighted images it is visualized as an inner border of high signal intensity, paralleling the low signal intensity periphery.

Staging

There are a number of staging systems for AVN,[11,20–23] but the most popular is that of Ficat and Arlet,[21] modified to include preclinical and preradiologic stages of the disease.[20] The modification is important because the disease can be present in the absence of clinical and radiologic signs.

In stage 0 disease, diagnosed on the basis of scintigraphic or MR imaging when a painful contralateral hip is being evaluated, no clinical or radiographic changes are found (Fig. 3–26).

In stage I and stage II disease, the joint line remains normal and the femoral head is spherical. In stage I disease, the trabeculae appear normal or slightly porotic and progress to diffuse porosis and sclerosis in stage II. Pathologic specimens in these early stages show viable bone on necrotic bone with marrow spaces infiltrated by mononuclear cells and histiocytes; this explains the radiographic changes. In stage II disease, a shell of reactive bone delimits the area of infarct. Within this area, the trabeculae and marrow spaces are acellular.

The onset of stage III disease is marked by the loss of the spherical shape of the femoral head. The AP radiograph may appear normal, but the lateral view often reveals a crescent sign, or radiolucency, under the subchondral bone, which represents a fracture between the subchondral bone and the underlying femoral head. The necrotic area becomes radiodense as a result of mineral deposition in the marrow spaces. The joint space remains preserved or may actually increase.

In stage IV disease, the femoral head undergoes further collapse, leading to articular cartilage destruction and joint-space narrowing (Fig. 3–27). Segmental collapse and subchondral fracture may result in pain and disability. This is often the stage at which the patient presents for evaluation, although patients may present prior to this stage. The etiology of pain in these patients has been attributed to increased intraosseous pressure and microfracture.

The specificity of radiographic staging of osteonecrosis is improved by the use of CT, which is also helpful in defining the associated sclerotic arc, detecting acetabular dome and femoral head contour changes, assessing the joint space, and evaluating the extent of femoral head involvement.[24] Disruption of the normal pattern of bony trabeculae has been observed in osteonecrosis of the femoral head.[25] Clumping and fusion of peripheral aspects of the femoral head asterisk may be identified prior to conventional radiographic sclerosis or subchondral fracture. These CT changes do not, however, reflect the early vascular marrow histologic processes in osteonecrosis.

Magnetic Resonance Staging. Mitchell and colleagues have described an MR classification system for AVN based on qualitative assessment of alterations in the central region of MR signal intensity in the osteonecrotic focus.[15,26]

In MR class A disease, the osteonecrotic lesion demonstrates signal characteristics analogous to fat: a central region of high signal intensity on short TR/TE settings (T1-weighted) and intermediate signal intensity on long TR/TE settings (T2-weighted) (Figs. 3–28 and 3–29). Class B hips demonstrate the signal characteristics of blood or hemorrhage: high signal intensity on both short and long TR/TE sequences (Fig. 3–30). Hips identified as class C demonstrate the signal properties of fluid: low signal intensity on short TR/TE sequences and high signal intensity on long TR/TE sequences (Fig. 3–31). Class D hips exhibit the signal characteristics of fibrous tissue—low signal intensity on short and long TR/TE sequences (Fig. 3–32). In all four classes, there is a peripheral band of low signal intensity that outlines the central focus of AVN. This border is most visible on T1-weighted images of class A and B hips, where the central focus of necrosis is bright in signal intensity, and on T2-weighted images of class C hips. Manipulation of TR/TE pulse parameters does not affect the low signal intensity border.

Treatment

The aim of treatment is to save the femoral head, not replace it, because most patients with nontraumatic AVN are relatively young. Unfortunately, surprisingly little is written about the natural history of the disease. Some clinicians still recommend restricted activity and protected weight bearing as initial therapy, and Steinberg and colleagues have published a retrospective study of 48 patients treated nonoperatively.[27] Their results indicate

(text continues on page 77)

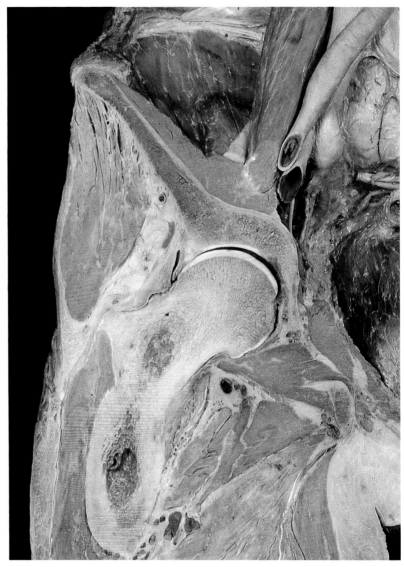

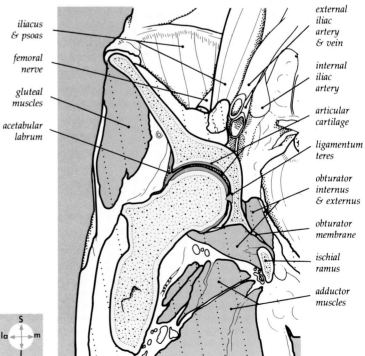

iliacus
& psoas

femoral
nerve

gluteal
muscles

acetabular
labrum

external
iliac
artery
& vein

internal
iliac
artery

articular
cartilage

ligamentum
teres

obturator
internus
& externus

obturator
membrane

ischial
ramus

adductor
muscles

S
la ← → m
I

FIGURE 3–16. A coronal section through the hip joint
shows its anatomic relations.

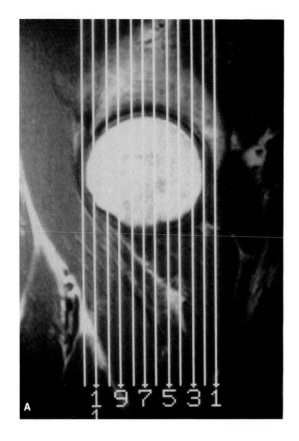

FIGURE 3–17. Normal coronal MR anatomy. (**A**) This sagittal localizer was used to graphically prescribe coronal T1-weighted image location from (**B**) anterior to (**L**) posterior.

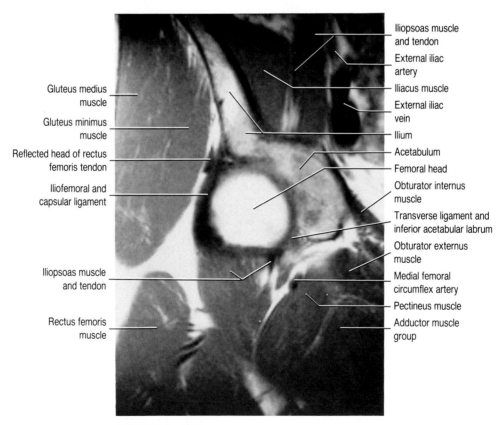

Gluteus medius muscle

Gluteus minimus muscle

Reflected head of rectus femoris tendon

Iliofemoral and capsular ligament

Iliopsoas muscle and tendon

Rectus femoris muscle

Iliopsoas muscle and tendon

External iliac artery

Iliacus muscle

External iliac vein

Ilium

Acetabulum

Femoral head

Obturator internus muscle

Transverse ligament and inferior acetabular labrum

Obturator externus muscle

Medial femoral circumflex artery

Pectineus muscle

Adductor muscle group

FIGURE 3–17B.

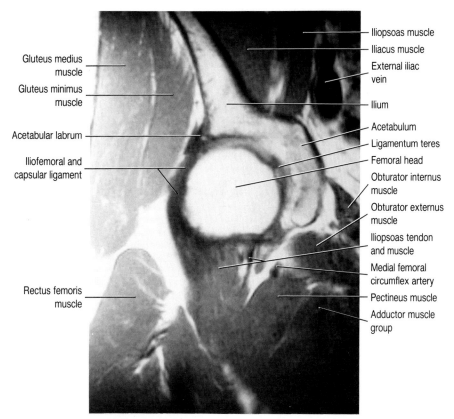

Gluteus medius muscle

Gluteus minimus muscle

Acetabular labrum

Iliofemoral and capsular ligament

Rectus femoris muscle

Iliopsoas muscle

Iliacus muscle

External iliac vein

Ilium

Acetabulum

Ligamentum teres

Femoral head

Obturator internus muscle

Obturator externus muscle

Iliopsoas tendon and muscle

Medial femoral circumflex artery

Pectineus muscle

Adductor muscle group

FIGURE 3–17C.

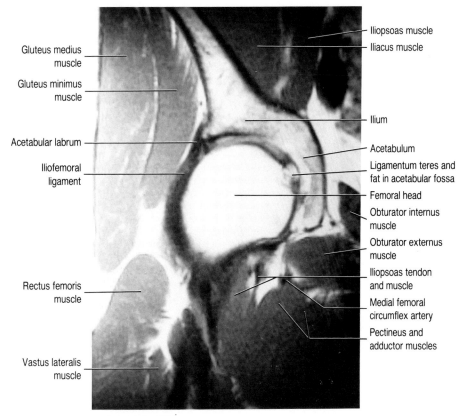

Gluteus medius muscle

Gluteus minimus muscle

Acetabular labrum

Iliofemoral ligament

Rectus femoris muscle

Vastus lateralis muscle

Iliopsoas muscle

Iliacus muscle

Ilium

Acetabulum

Ligamentum teres and fat in acetabular fossa

Femoral head

Obturator internus muscle

Obturator externus muscle

Iliopsoas tendon and muscle

Medial femoral circumflex artery

Pectineus and adductor muscles

FIGURE 3–17D.

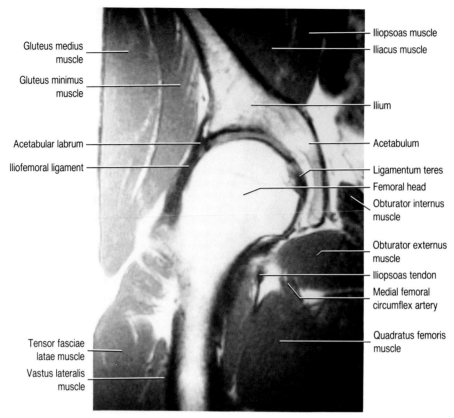

Gluteus medius muscle

Gluteus minimus muscle

Acetabular labrum

Iliofemoral ligament

Tensor fasciae latae muscle

Vastus lateralis muscle

Iliopsoas muscle

Iliacus muscle

Ilium

Acetabulum

Ligamentum teres

Femoral head

Obturator internus muscle

Obturator externus muscle

Iliopsoas tendon

Medial femoral circumflex artery

Quadratus femoris muscle

FIGURE 3–17E.

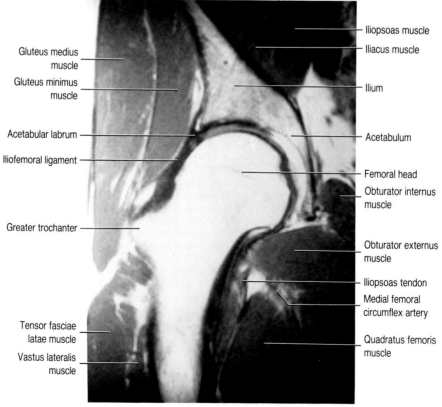

Gluteus medius muscle

Gluteus minimus muscle

Acetabular labrum

Iliofemoral ligament

Greater trochanter

Tensor fasciae latae muscle

Vastus lateralis muscle

Iliopsoas muscle

Iliacus muscle

Ilium

Acetabulum

Femoral head

Obturator internus muscle

Obturator externus muscle

Iliopsoas tendon

Medial femoral circumflex artery

Quadratus femoris muscle

FIGURE 3–17F.

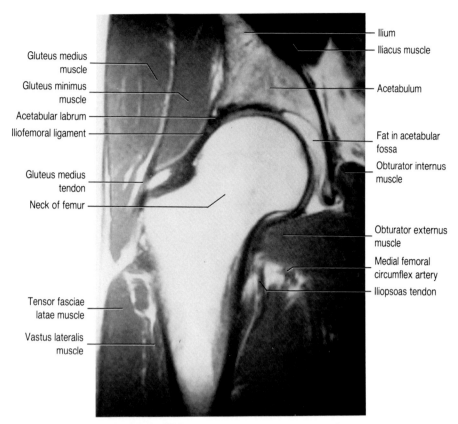

Gluteus medius muscle

Gluteus minimus muscle

Acetabular labrum

Iliofemoral ligament

Gluteus medius tendon

Neck of femur

Tensor fasciae latae muscle

Vastus lateralis muscle

Ilium

Iliacus muscle

Acetabulum

Fat in acetabular fossa

Obturator internus muscle

Obturator externus muscle

Medial femoral circumflex artery

Iliopsoas tendon

FIGURE 3–17G.

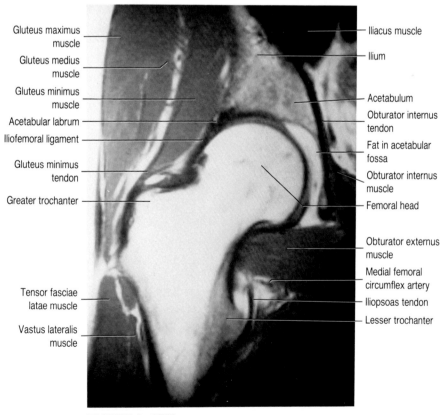

Gluteus maximus muscle

Gluteus medius muscle

Gluteus minimus muscle

Acetabular labrum

Iliofemoral ligament

Gluteus minimus tendon

Greater trochanter

Tensor fasciae latae muscle

Vastus lateralis muscle

Iliacus muscle

Ilium

Acetabulum

Obturator internus tendon

Fat in acetabular fossa

Obturator internus muscle

Femoral head

Obturator externus muscle

Medial femoral circumflex artery

Iliopsoas tendon

Lesser trochanter

FIGURE 3–17H.

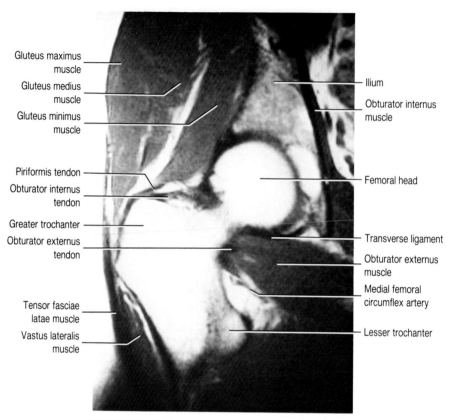

Gluteus maximus muscle

Gluteus medius muscle

Gluteus minimus muscle

Piriformis tendon

Obturator internus tendon

Greater trochanter

Obturator externus tendon

Tensor fasciae latae muscle

Vastus lateralis muscle

Ilium

Obturator internus muscle

Femoral head

Transverse ligament

Obturator externus muscle

Medial femoral circumflex artery

Lesser trochanter

FIGURE 3–17I.

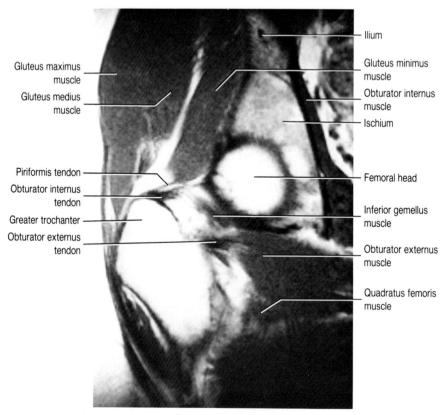

Gluteus maximus muscle

Gluteus medius muscle

Piriformis tendon

Obturator internus tendon

Greater trochanter

Obturator externus tendon

Ilium

Gluteus minimus muscle

Obturator internus muscle

Ischium

Femoral head

Inferior gemellus muscle

Obturator externus muscle

Quadratus femoris muscle

FIGURE 3–17J.

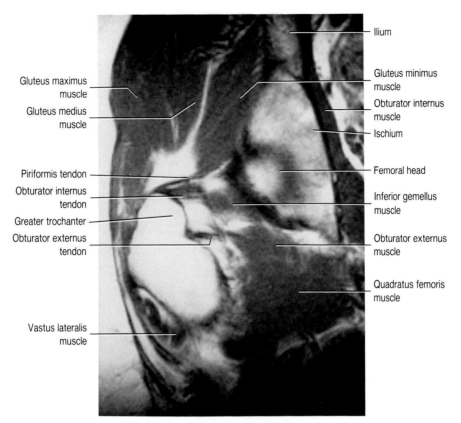

Gluteus maximus muscle

Gluteus medius muscle

Piriformis tendon

Obturator internus tendon

Greater trochanter

Obturator externus tendon

Vastus lateralis muscle

Ilium

Gluteus minimus muscle

Obturator internus muscle

Ischium

Femoral head

Inferior gemellus muscle

Obturator externus muscle

Quadratus femoris muscle

FIGURE 3–17K.

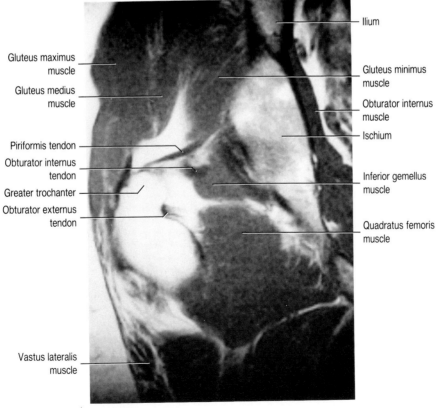

Gluteus maximus muscle

Gluteus medius muscle

Piriformis tendon

Obturator internus tendon

Greater trochanter

Obturator externus tendon

Vastus lateralis muscle

Ilium

Gluteus minimus muscle

Obturator internus muscle

Ischium

Inferior gemellus muscle

Quadratus femoris muscle

FIGURE 3–17L.

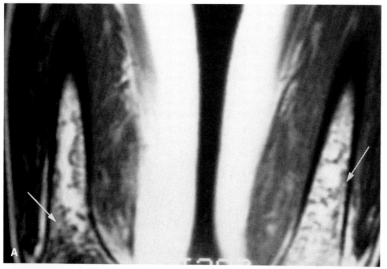

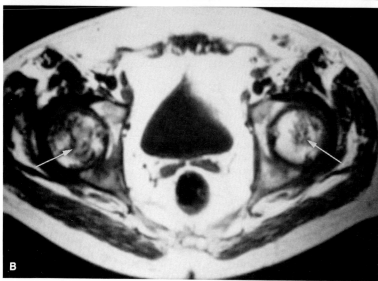

FIGURE 3–18. Diffuse osteonecrosis (*arrows*) demonstrates low signal intensity. Serpiginous areas can be seen on (**A**) T1-weighted coronal and (**B**) axial images in a patient with history of ethanol abuse. (TR, 600 msec; TE, 20 msec.)

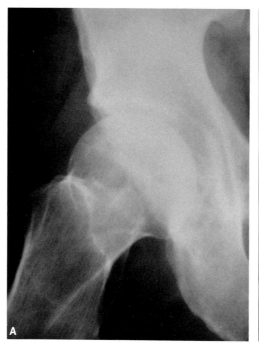

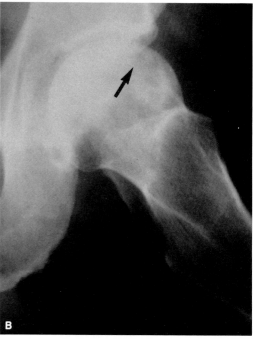

FIGURE 3–19.

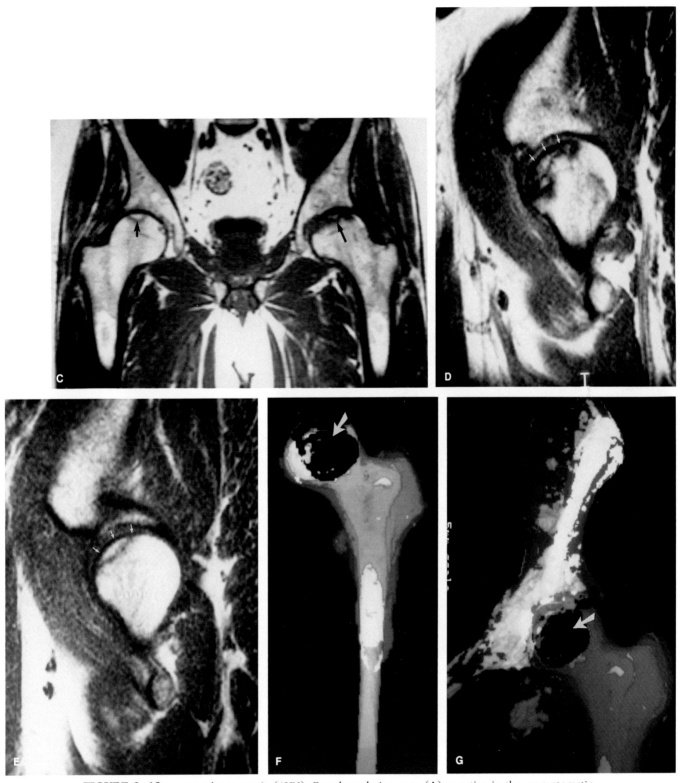

FIGURE 3–19. Avascular necrosis (AVN). Frog-lateral views are (**A**) negative in the asymptomatic right hip and (**B**) show patchy sclerosis of the left femoral head (*arrow*) in the symptomatic left hip. (**C**) The coronal T1-weighted image demonstrates AVN with greater than 30% involvement in the left femoral head (*long arrow*) and less than 10% involvement of the right femoral head (*short arrow*). (**D**) Sagittal T1-weighted images more accurately depict early subchondral collapse with flattening (*arrows*) of the left femoral head, but (**E**) show normal spherical morphology of the right femoral head (*arrows*). Three-dimensional MR rendering and mapping of the left femoral head AVN (*arrows*) (**F**) with and (**G**) without the femur disarticulated.

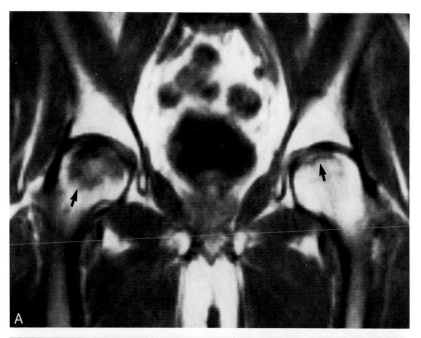

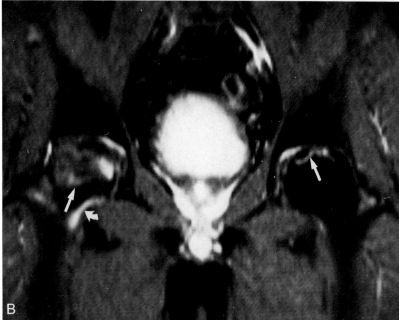

FIGURE 3–20. Avascular necrosis (AVN). (**A**) On a T1-weighted image, bilateral osteonecrosis of the hips demonstrates low signal intensity (*arrows*). (TR, 600 msec; TE, 20 msec.) (**B**) On a short TI inversion recovery image, AVN (*straight arrows*) and associated joint effusion (*curved arrow*) demonstrate bright signal intensity. (TR, 1400 msec; TI, 125 msec; TE, 40 msec.)

FIGURE 3–21. Avascular necrosis (AVN). (**A**) A T1-weighted coronal image demonstrates a low signal intensity focus of AVN (*large arrow*). The apparent cortical outline is shown (*small arrows*). (**B**) The T2*-weighted coronal image identifies a subchondral fracture (*arrows*) with fluid signal intensity in the necrotic interface.

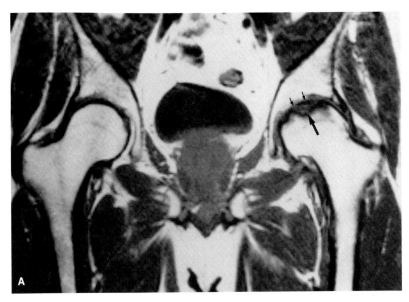

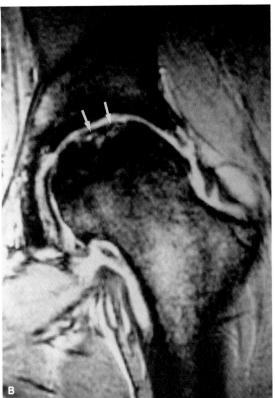

FIGURE 3–22. Avascular necrosis. Subchondral fluid in the osteonecrotic focus (*open arrows*) demonstrates (**A**) low signal intensity on a coronal T1-weighted image and (**B**) bright signal intensity on a T2*-weighted image.

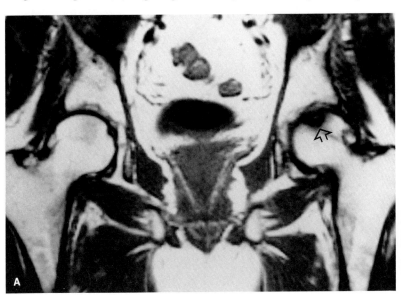

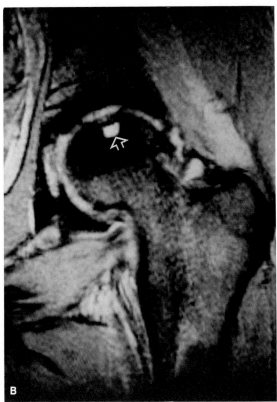

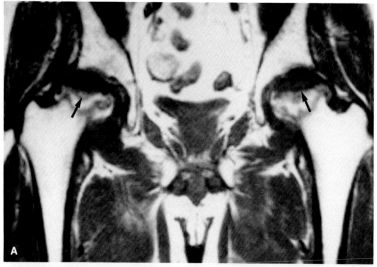

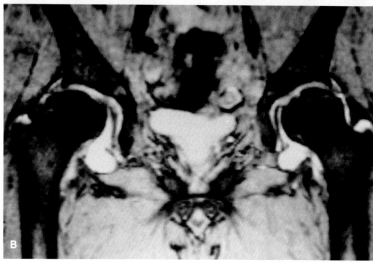

FIGURE 3–23. Bilateral avascular necrosis. (**A**) Superior delineation of the necrotic focus (*arrows*) is seen on a T1-weighted coronal image, and (**B**) spherical morphology of left femoral head is displayed on a T2*-weighted image. The right femoral head shows remodeling and flattening of its superior articular surface.

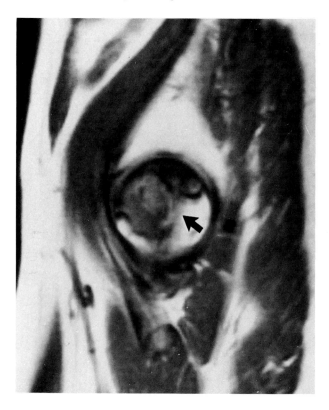

FIGURE 3–24. Femoral head osteonecrosis demonstrates low signal intensity on a T1-weighted sagittal image (*arrow*). The sagittal imaging plane displays anterior-to-posterior relationships in determining the extent of femoral head involvement. (TR, 600 msec; TE, 20 msec.)

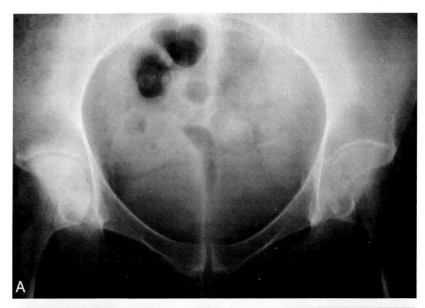

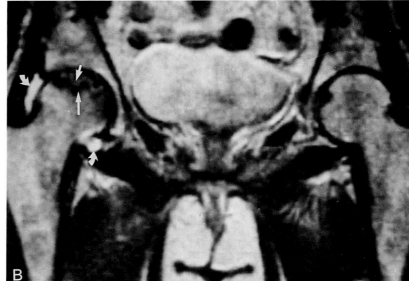

FIGURE 3–25. (**A**) An anteroposterior radiograph in a patient with right hip pain is unremarkable. (**B**) A T2-weighted coronal image displays right femoral head osteonecrosis with the characteristic double-line sign. Low signal intensity periphery (*long straight arrow*) and high signal intensity inner border (*short straight arrow*) are differentiated. Bright signal intensity hip effusion is also shown (*curved arrows*). (TR, 2000 msec; TE 60 msec.)

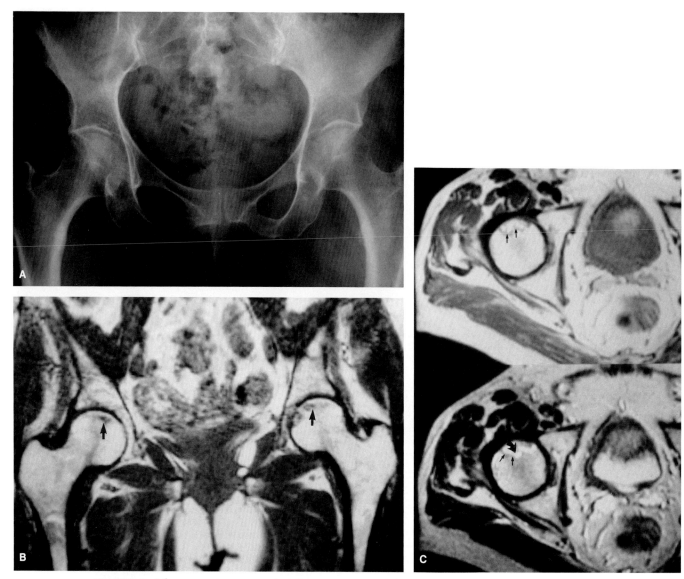

FIGURE 3–26. Avascular necrosis (AVN) in Ficat stage 0. (**A**) An anteroposterior radiograph is negative in a patient presenting with unilateral hip pain. (**B**) A T1-weighted coronal image displays stage 0 disease with bilateral AVN (*arrows*) demonstrating central fat signal intensity. (TR, 600 msec; TE, 20 msec.) (**C**) On a T2-weighted coronal image, the double-line sign with a low signal intensity peripheral border (*straight arrows*) and a high signal intensity inner band (*curved arrow*) is seen. (TR, 2000 msec; TE, 20, 80 msec.)

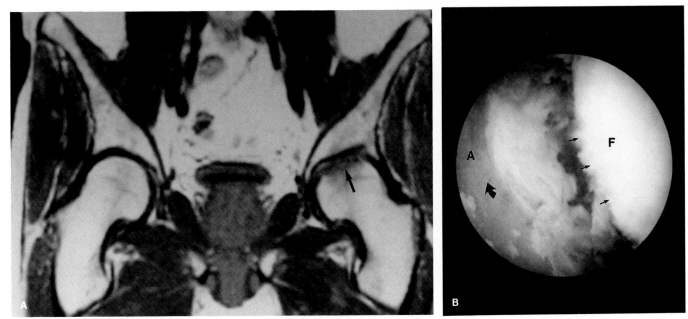

FIGURE 3–27. Avascular necrosis in Ficat stage IV. (**A**) A T1-weighted coronal image demonstrates left femoral head osteonecrosis (*arrow*) with associated flattening of the superior surface of the femoral head and joint-space narrowing. (TR, 600 msec; TE, 20 msec.) (**B**) At arthroscopy degenerative changes of the femoral head (*small arrows*) and denuded acetabular articular cartilage (*curved arrow*) associated with secondary narrowing of the hip joint are seen. (A, acetabulum; F, femur.)

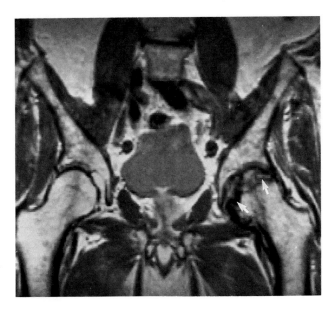

FIGURE 3–28. Osteonecrosis of the left femoral head demonstrates a central focus of high signal intensity (*arrows*) on a T1-weighted coronal image. (TR, 600 msec; TE, 20 msec.)

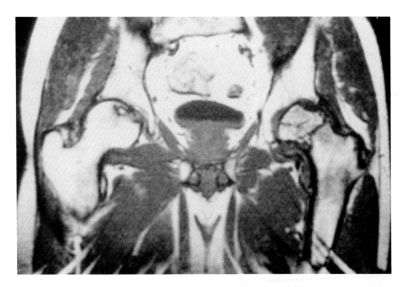

FIGURE 3–29. Avascular necrosis (AVN), class A. Bilateral AVN demonstrates fat marrow signal intensity. The sclerotic interface of the left femoral head involvement mimics a femoral neck fracture. (TR, 600 msec; TE, 20 msec.)

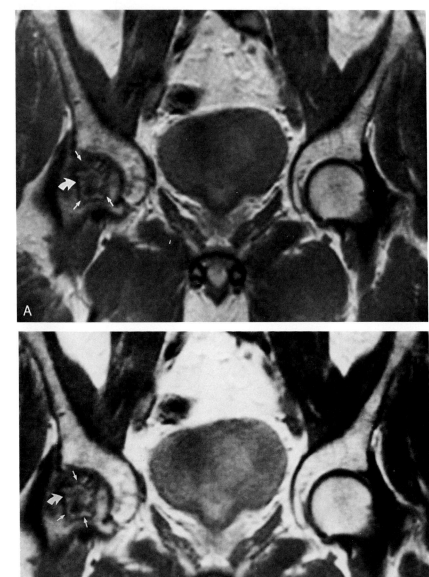

FIGURE 3–30. Right femoral head osteonecrosis (*straight arrows*) demonstrates intermediate to high signal intensity on (**A**) T1-weighted and (**B**) T2-intermediate–weighted images. The lesion is demarcated by a peripheral rim of low signal intensity (*curved arrows*).

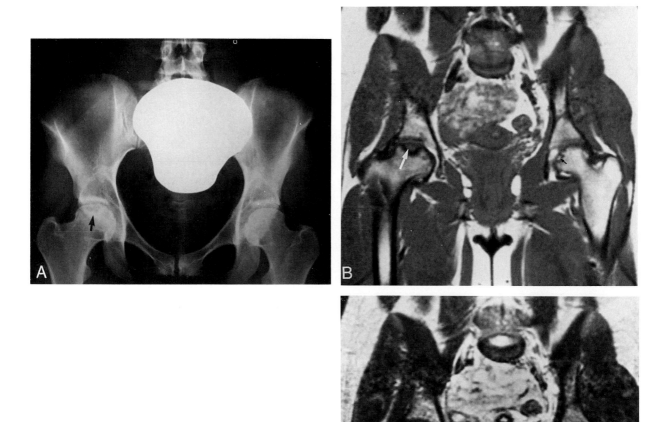

FIGURE 3–31. Bilateral avascular necrosis (AVN), class C. (**A**) An anteroposterior radiograph shows a focus of osteonecrosis with a sclerotic border (*arrow*) seen in the right femoral head. The left femoral head is without visible defect. The focus of osteonecrosis (*large arrows*) demonstrates (**B**) low to intermediate signal intensity on the corresponding intermediate-weighted image and (**C**) high signal intensity characteristic of class C AVN on a T2-weighted image. An associated focus of AVN is seen in the contralateral hip (*small arrows*).

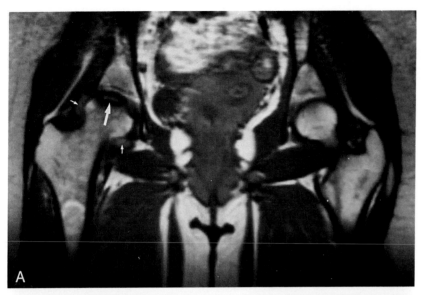

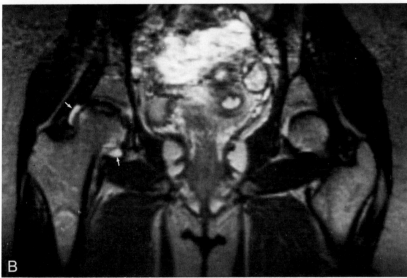

FIGURE 3–32. Osteonecrosis, class D. Right femoral head osteonecrosis with low signal intensity focus (*large arrow*) on (**A**) T1-weighted and (**B**) T2-weighted images. Associated capsular effusion demonstrates an increased signal intensity on the T1-weighted image (*small arrows*). (**A**: TR, 800 msec; TE, 20 msec; **B**: TR, 2000 msec; TE, 60 msec.)

that limiting weight bearing had no beneficial effect on the outcome, and disease was progressive in 92% of patients. A subsequent study showed disease progression in over 80% of patients regardless of the stage of disease at presentation, and progression of the disease in all patients who presented with some collapse of the femoral head.[10]

Many clinicians recommend early surgical intervention because of the high rate of progression with nonoperative treatment. Conservative or prophylactic procedures include core decompression with or without bone grafts,[10,20,28–33] osteotomy,[13,34] and electrical stimulation.[32,35,36] Core decompression is the most commonly used procedure in this group. The rationale in core decompression is to alleviate the elevated intraosseous pressure, permitting neovascularization (Fig. 3–33). Success rates reported in the literature vary dramatically— from 40% to 90% depending on the criteria used to grade results. Cancellous, cortical, muscle pedicle, and microvascular bone grafts have been used with core depression. The use of a cortical graft for necrotic bone was first described by Phemister,[37] and the procedure was later modified by Bonfiglio.[28] Urbaniak first used a vascularized fibular graft after coring of the femoral head.[38]

A variety of proximal femoral osteotomies have been used with variable results.[14,32] The principle underlying osteotomy involves redirecting stresses from structurally compromised trabeculae, and this procedure is most successful in cases in which limited femoral head involvement exists. In addition, patients who remain on corticosteroids or who have persistent metabolic bone disease do not benefit greatly from osteotomy. Pulsed electromagnetic fields and implantable direct current stimulators have also been used in the treatment of AVN, with variable results.[32,35,36]

After the femoral head has collapsed, the success of prophylactic procedures diminishes significantly. The chance of saving the femoral head is small, and most patients go on to require femoral head replacement. In general, total hip replacement is more reliable than a bipolar endoprosthesis.[39] Hip fusion is also an alternative in young patients with unilateral disease, especially the heavy, active male.

Clinical and Pathologic Correlation

Symptoms of patients with AVN correlate with MR classification and are least severe in class A hips and most severe in class D hips. MR signal intensity, therefore, can be seen to follow a chronologic progression from acute (*i.e.,* class A) to chronic (*i.e.,* class D) osteonecrosis.

When compared with conventional radiographic staging, 50% of radiographic stage 1 and 83% of stage 2 lesions imaged with fatlike central signal intensity were classified as MR class A. Class A lesions were infrequent in more advanced radiographic stages.

Magnetic resonance findings can also be correlated with histologic changes (Fig. 3–34). The central region of high signal intensity corresponds to necrosis of bone and marrow, prior to the development of capillary and mesenchymal ingrowth.[40] The low signal intensity peripheral band corresponds to a sclerotic margin of reactive tissue at the interface between necrotic and viable bone. Low signal intensity on T1-weighted images and intermediate-to-high signal intensity on T2-weighted images can be attributed to the high water content of mesenchymal tissue and thickened trabecular bone. The double-line sign is thought to represent a hyperemic or inflammatory response causing granulation tissue inside the reactive bone interface.[15] In areas of proposed vascular engorgement and inflammation, decreased signal intensity on T2-weighted images has been associated with successful core decompression treatments (see Fig. 3–33).[15]

Beltran and colleagues have correlated collapse of the femoral head after core decompression with the extent or percentage of involvement of AVN as determined preoperatively by MR imaging.[41] When less than 25% of the weight-bearing surface was involved, femoral head collapse did not occur after core decompression. With 25% to 50% involvement, femoral head collapse occurred in 43% of hips. With greater than 50% involvement, femoral head collapse occurred in 87% of hips. Mean time to collapse was 6.7 months after diagnosis and treatment. Therefore, if a large area or volume of the femoral head is involved, subchondral collapse may occur with core decompression despite the absence of subchondral fracture on conventional films.

In one case of osteonecrosis in Legg–Calvé–Perthes disease, return of yellow marrow signal intensity was recorded 8 months following a varus osteotomy. Joint effusions of low signal intensity on T1-weighted images and of high signal intensity on T2-weighted images are commonly associated with more advanced stages of AVN (Fig. 3–35).[42] It is not known whether the presence or absence of a joint effusion is of prognostic significance for the course and treatment of the disease.

A second pattern of MR signal intensity, diffuse low signal intensity on T1-weighted images with isointense or increased signal intensity on T2-weighted images, has been described by Turner and colleagues.[43] The area of diffuse low signal intensity on T1-weighted images extends from the femoral head and neck into the intertrochanteric area. Although no focal findings were identified initially, AVN was subsequently demonstrated by core biopsy and focal MR morphologic patterns specific for osteonecrosis. The diffuse pattern of low signal intensity in and adjacent to the femoral head was shown to be transient in five of six patients, and may represent bone marrow edema preceding focal anterosuperior femoral head osteonecrosis. When increased uptake on corresponding radionuclide bone scans also occurs, careful observation may be required to differentiate diffuse MR patterns of early osteonecrosis from transient osteoporosis of the hip. Bone marrow edema may represent a secondary phenomenon associated with the development of osteonecrosis, since these changes have also been reported in the acetabular bone prior to the development of sclerosis and granulation tissue at the interface surrounding devitalized or necrotic bone (Figs. 3–36 and 3–37).

Value of Magnetic Resonance Imaging

One of the most important contributions of MR imaging to the detection of AVN is identification of the osteonecrotic lesion in patients with normal bone scintigraphy and conventional radiographs.[44] Observation of focal MR abnormalities subsequent to the presentation of diffuse bone marrow edema has been reported as early as 6 to 8 weeks from the time of detection. The demonstration of marrow necrosis and acellular lacunas can differentiate osteonecrosis in its early stages from transient osteoporosis of the hip. The finding of symptomatic hip joint effusion prior to any alteration in marrow signal intensity may correspond to an elevation of intraosseous intramedullary pressures. Genez and colleagues has also confirmed that histologic findings of osteonecrosis may be present in the absence of abnormal MR findings in the early stage of the disease.[45] Positive MR findings for focal areas of osteonecrosis have been reported with negative radionuclide scans and normal CT findings.[46] Thus, asymptomatic persons at risk for AVN can be evaluated with MR imaging, and disease can be detected before changes are found with plain film radiographs, CT, or bone scintigraphy.

Chronologic or temporal staging and assessment of the percentage of marrow involvement offers the physician additional information and may facilitate the choice of therapeutic modality prior to reactive bone changes including subchondral fracture, collapse, and fragmentation. In the later stages (*i.e.,* stages 3 and 4) of osteonecrosis, core decompression is frequently used to palliate pain without altering disease progression.

A 3D MR rendering can be used to evaluate the volume of osteonecrotic involvement of the femoral head relative to its cross-sectional area (see Fig. 3–19). This technique can be useful in differentiating and separating the necrotic zone of involvement and in identifying its location in the femoral head and its relationship to the weight-bearing surface. Information from quantitative assessment of femoral head volume may assist in the decision to perform a core decompression or a rotational osteotomy.

Three-dimensional rendering is also best suited for display of osteonecrotic involvement of the anterior superior femoral head. Disarticulation of the femur and femoral head from the acetabulum may facilitate superior surface viewing of the femoral head and the associated necrotic focus (see Fig. 3–19). Separate disarticulation and composite volume rendering can be performed with associated joint effusions. Volume transmission enables viewing of the femoral head through the acetabulum using various degrees of pelvic rotation in horizontal and vertical planes.

Legg–Calvé–Perthes Disease

Legg–Calvé–Perthes disease is a childhood hip disorder that results in infarction of the bony epiphysis of the femoral head. Although the etiology is unclear, certain risk factors have been identified, including gender (*i.e.,* boys are affected four times more often than girls), socioeconomic class (*i.e.,* high incidence in low socioeconomic classes and children with low birth weight), and inguinal hernia and genitourinary anomalies in children.[47,48]

Legg–Calvé–Perthes disease is a dynamic condition, and the physical examination depends on the stage of the disease at the time of presentation. Early in the disease, the physical findings are similar to those of irritable hip syndrome. The child often has a limp with groin, thigh, or knee pain. The most common age group is 4 to 9 years. Children who present with knee pain must be carefully examined for hip pathology. As the disease progresses, a flexion and adduction contracture may develop, and lateral overgrowth of the femoral head cartilage may cause loss of abduction. Attempts at abduction lead to hinging and possible subluxation of the femoral head. Eventually, the hip may only move in the flexion–extension plane.

Diagnosis

A diagnosis of Legg–Calvé–Perthes disease is usually made from radiographs. Signs include widening of the inferomedial joint space, epiphyseal sclerosis, a subchondral fracture line, and a small epiphysis. Plain film radiograph findings may be negative early in the course of the disease, and scintigraphy and MR imaging may provide additional information.

Staging

The most commonly used classification systems for Legg–Calvé–Perthes disease are based on radiographic estimates of the amount of femoral head involvement. Catterall has defined four groups,[49] and Salter has described two groups based on such estimates.[50] In Catterall's classification,[49] group I represents involvement of the anterior aspect of the epiphysis without a metaphysical reaction, sequestrum, or subchondral fracture line. Group II shows more extensive or severe involvement of the anterior aspect of the epiphysis, with preservation of the medial and lateral segments. A sequestrum is pres-

(text continues on page 82)

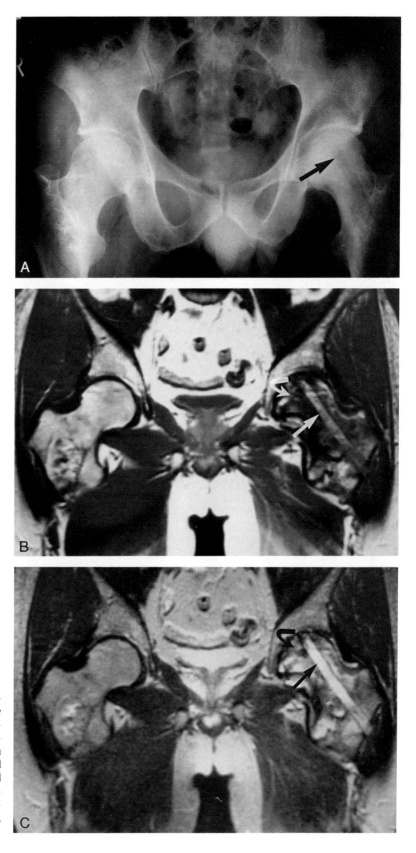

FIGURE 3–33. Core decompression. (**A**) An antero-posterior radiograph allows identification of the core decompression tract for osteonecrosis (*arrow*). Unsuccessful core decompression for left femoral head osteonecrosis (*curved arrows*) with diffuse vascular edema is seen with (**B**) low signal intensity on a T1-weighted image and (**C**) high signal intensity on a T2-weighted image. The core tract (*straight arrows*) displays increased signal intensity from fluid contents on the T2-weighted image. (**B**: TR, 600 msec; TE, 20 msec; **C**: TR, 2000 msec; TE, 60 msec.)

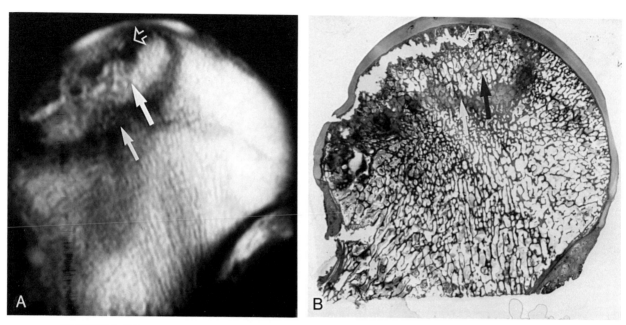

FIGURE 3–34. Osteonecrosis. (**A**) A T1-weighted coronal image demonstrates high signal intensity cortical necrosis (*large arrow*), low signal intensity sclerotic peripheral interface between necrosis and viable marrow (*small arrow*), and low signal intensity subchondral fracture (*open arrow*). (TR, 600 msec; TE, 20 msec.) (**B**) A macroslide of a gross specimen shows corresponding subchondral collapse (*open arrow*), reactive periphery (*white arrow*), and cortical necrosis (*black arrow*).

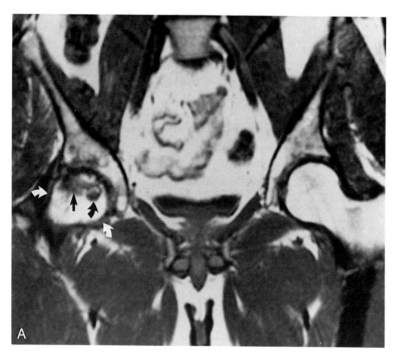

FIGURE 3–35. Advanced osteonecrosis with low signal intensity central cortical focus (*straight arrows*) on (**A**) T1-weighted and (**B**) T2-weighted images. Associated joint-space narrowing, degenerative cyst (*curved black arrows*), and effusion (*curved white arrows*) are indicated. Cyst and hip effusion demonstrate low signal intensity on T1-weighted sequences and high signal intensity on T2-weighted sequences. (**A**: TR, 800 msec; TE, 20 msec; **B**: TR, 1500 msec; TE 80 msec.)

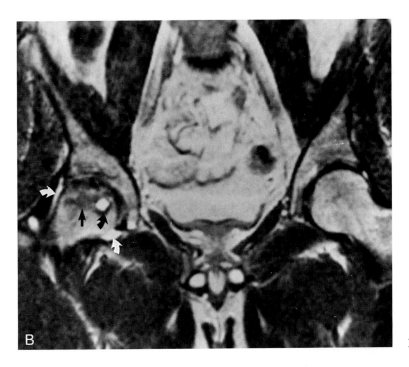

FIGURE 3–35. *(Continued)*

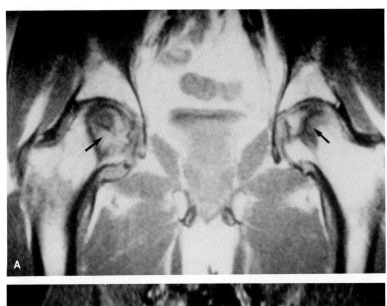

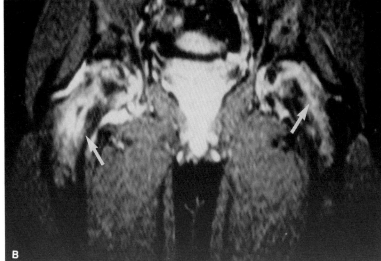

FIGURE 3–36. Avascular necrosis. Bilateral class A necrosis (*arrows*) on (**A**) coronal T1-weighted and (**B**) short TI inversion recovery (STIR) images. Femoral neck edema or hyperemia (*arrows*) is best demonstrated on STIR images. (**A**: TR, 600 msec; TE, 20 msec; **B**: TR, 1400 msec; TI, 125 msec; TE, 40 msec.)

ent, as is a metaphyseal reaction anterolaterally. A subchondral fracture line is present; the line does not extend to the apex of the femoral epiphysis. In group III, the entire epiphysis is dense. There is a diffuse metaphyseal reaction with femoral neck widening. A subchondral fracture line is visualized posteriorly. Group IV disease is characterized by involvement of the entire femoral head, with flattening, mushrooming, and eventual collapse. There is an extensive metaphyseal reaction and associated posterior remodeling. In Catterall's grouping of Legg–Calvé–Perthes disease, it should be possible to separate group I cases without sequestrum or metaphyseal lesion from cases of groups II and III with viable bone posteriorly and medially and from group IV cases, in which the entire epiphysis is involved, with collapse and loss of epiphyseal height. The more advanced the stage at the time of presentation, the poorer the prognosis. It is important to understand that the disease is progressive, and final radiographic staging may take up to 9 months. Green and colleagues have correlated the amount of epiphyseal extrusion with prognosis: when more than 20% of the epiphysis is extruded laterally, the prognosis is poor; when more than 50% of the femoral head is also involved, only 8% have good results.[51] Pathologically, the early stages of the disease are characterized by overgrowth of the articular cartilage medially and laterally.[52,53] Infarction within the femoral head can lead to trabecular fracture and decreased epiphyseal height.

On radiographic examination, increased bony tissue density is found in the area of infarction, which represents appositional new bone and calcification of necrotic marrow. Revascularization occurs through creeping substitution of necrotic bone with fibrocartilage, causing the fragmented appearance seen on plain film radiographs during this phase of the disease. The thickened articular cartilage is repaired from subchondral bone and from within the abnormal cartilage anteriorly and laterally. Unossified cartilage that streams down from the growth plate can lead to metaphyseal cysts. In the late stages, the fibrocartilage is reossified. The last area to heal is superior and anterior.

Treatment

It is important to determine prognosis at the time of presentation, because more than 50% of patients with Legg–Calvé–Perthes disease do well with no treatment. The younger the child at the time of presentation, the better the prognosis. Children who present after 8 years of age do poorly. Generally girls do not do as well and may have a more severe form of the disease. The earlier the stage of the disease at the time of presentation, the better the prognosis. Cattarall has identified clinical and radiographic "head at risks" signs that he correlated with

the chance of developing significant femoral head deformity.[49] Clinically, progressive loss of movement, adduction contracture, flexion with abduction, and obesity all are poor prognostic signs. Radiographically, both epiphyseal and metaphyseal signs are associated with a prognosis, although some are controversial. The epiphyseal signs are calcification lateral to the epiphysis and a lytic area laterally (*i.e.,* Gage's sign). In the metaphysis, Catterall identifies horizontal inclination of the growth plate and diffuse metaphyseal reaction as risk signs. Two or more of these signs correlate with a poor prognosis.[49] Lateral subluxation of the femoral head is also associated with a poor outcome.

The decision whether to treat a particular patient is sometimes a difficult one. Catterall recommends definitive treatment for all "at-risk" cases, for groups II and III disease in patients older than 7 years of age, and for group IV cases in which serious deformity has not occurred.[49] Group I cases and group II and III cases that are not "at risk" can be observed. Arthrography may be helpful in determining incongruity of the femoral head. After healing is established radiographically, treatment is not required because the femoral head will not deteriorate further. Radiographic signs of healing are an increase in height and size of viable bone on the medial side of the epiphysis and an increase in height and quality of new bone formed laterally.

The principles of treatment involve restoration of hip motion and decreasing the forces across the hip joint. To accomplish this, the femoral hip must be positioned within the acetabulum. This can be achieved with physical therapy and bracing or femoral osteotomy. Neither treatment modality is clearly superior, and both have advantages and disadvantages. In the long term, approximately 86% of patients develop osteoarthritis, but most are able to function relatively well until the fifth or sixth decade of life.[54]

Magnetic Resonance Imaging

Magnetic resonance imaging has been used to identify both morphologic and signal characteristics of the femoral epiphysis in the early stages of radiographically negative disease (Fig. 3–38) and in more advanced disease (Fig. 3–39). In addition to low signal intensity within the epiphyseal marrow center on T1- and T2-weighted images, associated findings include an intraarticular effusion and a small, laterally displaced ossification nucleus.[55,56]

Revascularization of the necrotic portion of the femoral epiphysis has been shown in a case of Legg–Calvé–Perthes disease treated with varus osteotomy. The initial low signal intensity focus was replaced with high signal intensity marrow fat. Coxa plana and coxa magna can occur with later remodeling (Fig. 3–40). Before the diffuse loss of signal intensity of the ossific nucleus is observed, low signal intensity irregularity occurs along the periphery of the fat-containing ossific nucleus and, in one case, a linear area of low signal intensity traversed the femoral ossification center (see Fig. 3–38). These changes correlate with positive bone scintigraphy in stage 1 disease.

T2*-weighted images are useful in evaluating the thickness of the articular cartilage that is visualized with an increased signal intensity. Coronal or sagittal images may be used to display both acetabular and femoral head cartilage surfaces. Measurements of acetabular and femoral head articular cartilage show an increased thickness in affected hips.

Loss of containment of the femoral head in the acetabulum was identified in a majority of cases studied by Rush and colleagues, who found hypertrophy of the synovium within the iliopsoas recess of the hip capsule in 7 of 20 cases.[56a] This was visualized as a frondlike structure adjacent to the inferomedial joint space.

Ranner and colleagues, in a study of 13 patients with Legg–Calvé–Perthes disease among 45 patients presenting with acute hip pain, demonstrated that MR imaging showed equal sensitivity to isotope bone scans and more precise localization of involvement than conventional radiography.[57] Although revascularization of the necrotic focus may be more accurately determined with nuclear scintigraphy, MR imaging is preferable for evaluating the position, form, and size of the femoral head and surrounding soft tissues. Bone marrow edema, detected on MR scans in pediatric patients with symptomatic hips, has been shown to resolve without AVN.

Slipped Capital Femoral Epiphysis

Slipped capital femoral epiphysis (SCFE) is a childhood disorder of the hip characterized by posterior inferior displacement of the proximal femoral epiphysis. Although the precise etiology is unknown, present theories indicate that obesity, trauma, and hormonal abnormalities play roles in development of the disease.[58] Mechanically, a vertical growth plate and retroversion of the femoral neck appear to be risk factors.[59] Histologically, the slip occurs through the zone of hypertrophy in the growth plate. Agamanolis and colleagues demonstrated a generalized chondrocyte degeneration throughout the growth plate suggesting a primary pathology.[60]

The child usually presents with pain and a limp. The pain can often be located only in the thigh or knee; thus the diagnosis is frequently missed. It is important to remember that knee pain in the child can be secondary to hip disease. On physical examination, there is frequently limitation of motion, especially internal rotation and abduction. As the examiner flexes the hip, it moves into external rotation and the patient often holds the leg externally rotated when standing.

Diagnosis

Initial evaluation should include both AP and frog lateral radiographs. Since the major direction of the slip is usually posterior, it is often most easily noted on a frog lateral view. Both hips should be evaluated, because slips are bilateral in 20% to 25% of cases.

Classification

Slipped capital femoral epiphysis can be classified either according to the duration of symptoms or the degree of slippage. Acute slips may be diagnosed in patients who have had symptoms for less than 3 weeks, and in whom no chronic radiographic changes are found. Symptoms lasting 3 weeks or longer indicate a chronic slip, and chronic radiographic changes include resorption of the superior femoral neck and new bone formation on the inferior femoral neck. An acute on chronic slip has chronic symptoms and radiographic changes with an acute progression of the slip. Slips are also classified as mild, moderate, or severe based on the amount of slippage.

Treatment

The goal of treatment of SCFE is to stabilize the femoral capital epiphysis leading to early fusion of the growth plate. For mild to moderate slips, the most common procedure is pinning *in situ*. Many types of hardware have been used, such as a variety of multiple pin techniques and single screws. With severe slips, some authors advocate a gentle closed reduction, open reduction, or cuneiform osteotomy.[61] The complication rate is high with internal fixation.[62] Chondrolysis can occur and has been attributed to pin penetration. Unrecognized pin penetration is a major problem. Avascular necrosis, another serious complication of treatment in SCFE, may follow closed reduction, open reduction, osteotomy, or vascular damage from internal fixation. It is important to remember that this is an iatrogenic complication. Bone graft epiphysiodesis has gained popularity in some centers because of the high complication rate with internal fixation.[63] In the long term, the biomechanical abnormality that results predisposes the patient to degenerative arthritis.[64]

Magnetic Resonance Imaging

Although MR imaging has played a limited role in the evaluation of SCFE, it has the ability to identify the morphology of the articular cartilage epiphysis prior to the development of bright signal intensity fat within the femoral ossification center.[57] The widened growth plate and epiphyseal slippage are clearly demonstrated on MR images (Fig. 3–41). Magnetic resonance imaging may also be useful in identifying associated osteonecrosis—reported in up to 15% of children—prior to its appearance on conventional radiographs.[65] Associated incongruity of the joint surfaces and changes in the articular cartilage covering of the femoral head and acetabulum are best seen on coronal and axial plane images. The relationship of the femoral epiphysis to its containment within the acetabulum is best displayed on axial images showing anterior and posterior position relative to the acetabulum.

Congenital Dysplasia of the Hip

In congenital dysplasia (*i.e.,* dislocation) of the hip (CDH), also known as infantile hip dysplasia, the left hip is affected in 40% to 60% of cases and bilateral involvement occurs in 20%. Infants at risk for CDH include those with a positive family history; breach presentation; torticollis; scoliosis; metatarsus adductus; and structural abnormalities such as underdevelopment of the anterior capsule, ligament of Bigelow, or rectus muscle.

Classification

Dunn and associates have classified CDH according to the configuration of the acetabulum and the limbus.[66] A type 1 hip is characterized by positional instability. In types 2 and 3, the hip is subluxed and dislocated, respectively. In dislocation of the femoral epiphysis, the femoral head is uncovered by the cartilaginous acetabulum and displaced superolaterally. The hourglass configuration of the joint capsule is caused by compression between the limbus and the ligamentum teres. Constriction by the iliopsoas tendon may block attempts at reduction. Most cases of CDH present with a type 1 hip and positional instability. Failed hip reduction may be secondary to thickening of the ligamentum teres, an infolded or blunted limbus, and severe deformity of the acetabulum or femoral head.

Diagnosis

Ortolani's and Barlow's tests are used in the early postnatal period to assess the dislocated and dislocatable hip, respectively. In Ortolani's test, abduction at 90° flexion with anterior pressure directs a dislocated femoral head into the acetabulum. In Barlow's test, an unstable femoral head can be dislocated by application of posterior pressure in adduction.

Radiographic diagnosis of CDH is more accurate than either of the above-mentioned clinical tests. Conventional

radiographic assessment of the ossific nucleus relative to Hilgenreiner's line demonstrates its location in the lower medial quadrant. Shenton's line, connecting the medial border of the femoral metaphysis and the superior border of the obturator foramen, should form a smooth uninterrupted arc in the normal or nonsubluxed or dislocated hip. The acetabular index (*i.e.,* the slope of the ossified acetabular roof), which is 27° to 30° at birth, is an unreliable measurement in newborns and changes with rotation of the pelvis. A 45° bilateral abduction and internal rotation view or Van Rosen view may prematurely reduce the positionally unstable hip.

Ultrasonography has been used to evaluate the cartilaginous femoral head prior to the appearance of the ossific nucleus in children up to 1 year of age. This technique, however, may also be used in older children. Osseous dysplasia of the acetabular rim and coverage of the acetabular roof can be assessed. Computed tomography has had limited use because of the association of ionizing radiation. This technique, however, may have applications in patients in plaster or with equivocal conventional radiographs.

Magnetic Resonance Imaging

Magnetic resonance imaging has been successfully used in the evaluation of congenital hip dysplasia and dislocation (Fig. 3–42).[64] The femoral epiphyseal articular cartilage displays intermediate signal intensity on T1-weighted images, and bright signal intensity on gradient-echo images. T1-weighted coronal and axial images display the exact position of the intermediate signal intensity cartilaginous femoral head. This is important when the position of the femoral head is uncertain on conventional radiographs and when serial follow-up examinations, in and out of plaster casts, are required, eliminating the need to repeatedly expose the child to ionizing radiation. T2-weighted images are helpful when evaluating complications associated with CDH, such as ischemic necrosis and associated effusions, which are not effectively detected with ultrasound or conventional radiography. Three-dimensional MR rendering is useful in displaying complex femoral head and acetabular spatial relationships as well as associated dysplasia (Fig. 3–43).[67]

With MR imaging, the etiology of CDH and failure to achieve adequate reduction can be determined without the use of invasive arthrography.[68] However, an hourglass configuration of the acetabulum or an inverted, hypertrophied limbus must be excluded. With inversion, the intermediate signal intensity limbus is often seen in the lateral aspect of the joint, with increased fat (*i.e.,* high signal intensity on T1-weighted images) noted medially. An interposed iliopsoas tendon crossing the joint space prevents reduction of the femoral head in the acetabulum and may create an hourglass configuration of the joint capsule. Whereas supralateral subluxation or dislocation is identified on coronal MR images, the axial plane best demonstrates AP relationships and dysplasia of the acetabular wall (Fig. 3–44).

Magnetic resonance imaging is also useful in the long-term follow-up and postoperative evaluation of patients with CDH (Fig. 3–45). There is no artifact from plaster or fiberglass abduction spica casts, allowing for noninvasive evaluations of the femoral head. Adult sequelae of CDH may require reconstruction of the acetabulum using a shelf procedure to redirect, reposition, and augment the hip socket (Fig. 3–46).

Miscellaneous Pediatric Hip Conditions

Multiple epiphyseal dysplasia is an autosomal dominant condition involving the epiphyseal chondrocytes of the growth plate with resultant joint incongruity and premature degenerative arthritis. MR imaging demonstrates irregularity of the femoral head and articular and cortical surfaces (Fig. 3–47). Joint-space narrowing and secondary degenerative joint disease are present by the third or fourth decade of life.

Proximal focal femoral deficiency is a term used to describe the unilateral lack of or shortening of the proximal segments of the femur. The radiographic classification system (classes A–D) is based on the presence or absence of a femoral head or acetabular dysplasia and on the shape of the femoral segment.[69] We have used MR to evaluate severe pseudoarthrosis and subtrochanteric varus deformity (Fig. 3–48). On MR examination, fibrous and osseous connections between the femoral head and shaft can be differentiated.

Diaphyseal sclerosis, or Engelmann's disease, is characterized by long bone sclerosis involving both endosteal and cortical surfaces with relative sparing of the epiphysis and metaphysis. Bilateral symmetry and varying degrees of pain are usually associated with this condition. Although MR is not indicated as the initial study of choice, its use allows the assessment of low signal intensity cortical thickening without the ionizing radiation (Fig. 3–49).

Hip Pain in the Athlete

Overuse Syndromes

The most common cause of hip pain in the athlete is secondary to overuse resulting in tendinitis, bursitis, or muscle strain. Runners are most prone to these types of injuries, which are often associated with repetitive drills or a change in the intensity or duration of a workout schedule. Muscle edema involving the adductor muscle groups has been demonstrated without tears in marathon and ultramarathon runners (Fig. 3–50). The antagonist muscle groups are most susceptible to injury. Although the injury can occur anywhere within the muscle, the origin or insertion of the muscle is most likely to be affected. In the adductors, the resulting tendinitis and periostitis cause the so-called pulled groin. Similarly, the pulled hamstring usually is a result of periostitis/tendinitis at the ischial tuberosity where the hamstring muscles originate.

In evaluating the athlete with hip pain, a careful history is critical. The physician needs a detailed account of the training habits of the athlete and any recent modifications to that regimen. On physical examination, pain can often be elicited with deep palpation in the area of the musculotendinous junction or the muscle itself. In addition, pain with resistive muscle contraction can localize the traumatized muscle group.

Muscle Strains. Muscle strains can be graded using a system similar to the that used for ligament injuries. A grade 1 strain may simply result in a muscle spasm or cramp. In grade 2 strains, which result from true overuse, discomfort occurs during sporting activity or training but usually resolves with rest. The grade 3 strain is a true muscle tear that can occur within the muscle, at the muscle-tendon junction, or at the origin or insertion of the muscle.

Muscle tears and avulsions demonstrate high signal intensity on T2-weighted images in areas of edema or hemorrhage.[70-72] Magnetic resonance axial imaging is useful for the demonstration of associated muscle retraction and atrophy, which will have high signal intensity on T1-weighted images. Coronal or sagittal images provide a longitudinal display of the entire muscle group on a single image. A comparison with the contralateral extremity is important in evaluating relative symmetry of muscle groups. Magnetic resonance in a grade 1 muscle strain shows edema and or hemorrhage with preservation of muscle morphology (Fig. 3–51). In a grade 2 muscle strain or tear, hemorrhage with tearing and disruption of up to 50% of muscle fibers occurs (Figs. 3–52 and 3–53). Subacute hemorrhage, of bright signal intensity on T1-weighted images, is commonly seen in grade 2 injuries (Fig. 3–54). There is complete tearing with or without muscle retraction in grade 3 muscle tears (Fig. 3–55).

Treatment of a grade 2 strain centers on identifying the offending activity. The injury usually responds to cutting back or altering the training schedule. Cycling or swimming can be temporarily substituted for running to maintain aerobic conditioning. Physiotherapy is initially beneficial to aid in decreasing muscle spasm and then to regain flexibility and strength. Grade 3 strains are more difficult to treat and usually require a period of 6 to 8

(text continues on page 98)

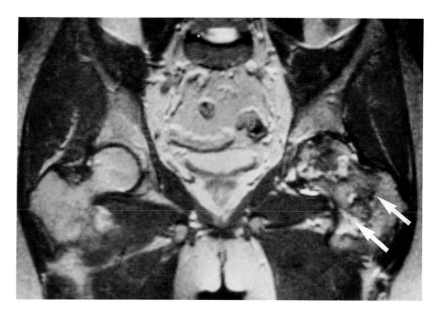

FIGURE 3–37. A T2-weighted coronal image showing a diffuse pattern of osteonecrosis in the femoral head and neck (*arrows*) with a high signal intensity area of marrow edema. (TR, 2000 msec; TE, 60 msec.)

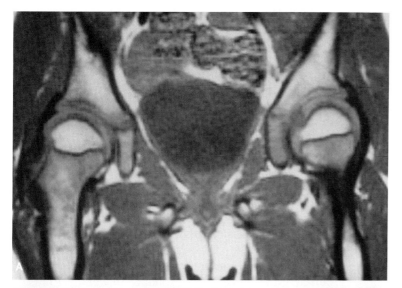

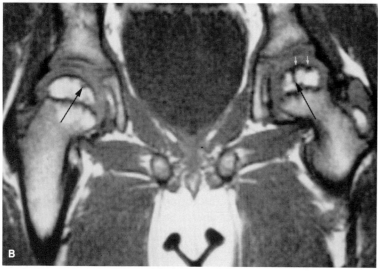

FIGURE 3–38. T1-weighted coronal images in Legg–Calvé–Perthes disease. (**A**) Normal femoral head capital epiphyses. (**B**) The earliest MR presentation of Legg–Calvé–Perthes disease shows peripheral irregularity of marrow-fat–containing epiphyseal ossification center (*white arrows*). Low signal intensity foci or linear segments are seen within the right and left ossification centers (*black arrows*). No subarticular collapse is present, and conventional radiographs are normal. (TR, 500 msec; TE, 20 msec.)

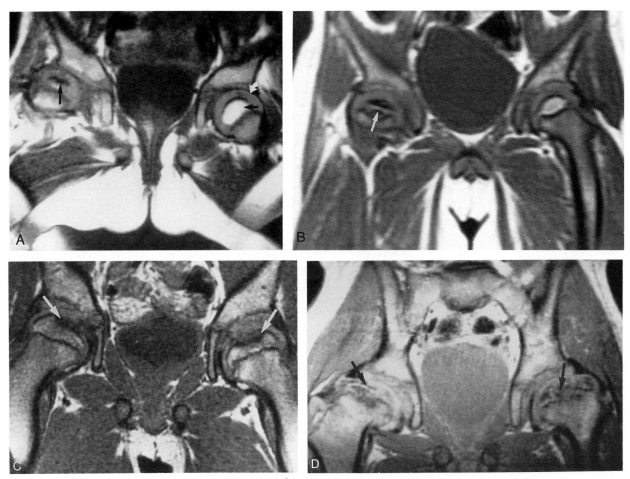

FIGURE 3–39.   Coronal T1-weighted images show the spectrum of Legg–Calvé–Perthes disease from (**A**, **B**) early to (**C**, **D**) late advanced involvement. (**A**) Small, laterally displaced ossific nucleus with loss of yellow marrow signal intensity (*long black arrow*) is present early in the disease. Normal contralateral epiphyseal cartilage (*curved arrow*) and high signal intensity marrow (*short black arrow*) are seen. (**B**) Complete loss of right femoral epiphyseal marrow signal intensity (*arrow*) occurs as the disease progresses. (**C**) Bilateral low signal intensity osteonecrosis foci in the femoral epiphysis (*arrows*) becomes apparent later in the disease. Articular cartilage is thinner in the older child. (**D**) Advanced remodeling in Legg–Calvé–Perthes disease with coxa plana and coxa magna of the femoral heads (*arrows*) is indicative of late advanced involvement. (TR, 600 msec; TE, 20 msec.)

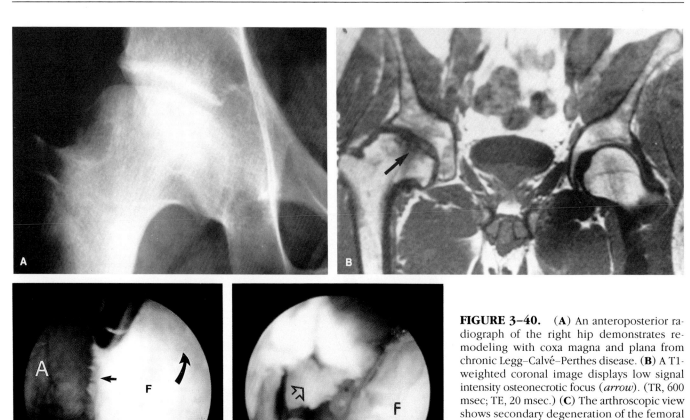

FIGURE 3–40. (**A**) An anteroposterior radiograph of the right hip demonstrates remodeling with coxa magna and plana from chronic Legg–Calvé–Perthes disease. (**B**) A T1-weighted coronal image displays low signal intensity osteonecrotic focus (*arrow*). (TR, 600 msec; TE, 20 msec.) (**C**) The arthroscopic view shows secondary degeneration of the femoral head (F) articular cartilage (*straight arrow*). The transition from white articular cartilage to exposed yellow bone (*curved arrow*) is shown. (**D**) Arthroscopy also reveals intraarticular cartilage debris (*open arrow*). (A, acetabulum.)

FIGURE 3–41. Slipped capital femoral epiphysis. (**A**) An anteroposterior radiograph shows varus deformity (*arrow*). (**B**) T1-weighted coronal and (**C**) axial images demonstrate fracture and varus deformity (*arrows*). Epiphyseal marrow signal intensity is preserved. (TR, 500 sec; TE, 30 msec.)

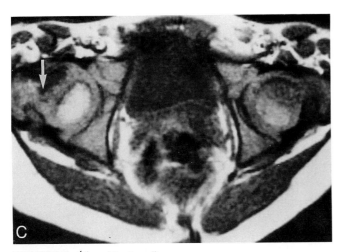

FIGURE 3–41. *(Continued)*

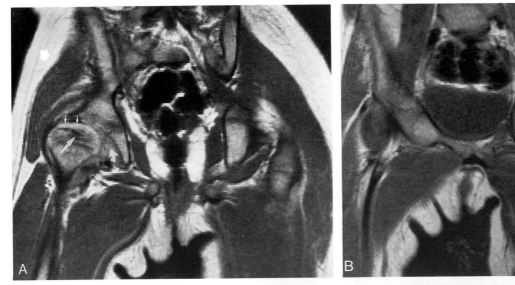

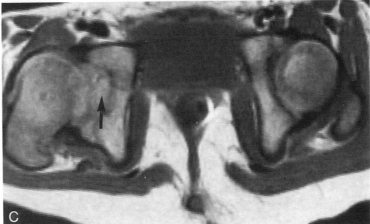

FIGURE 3–42. T1-weighted images showing congenital dislocation of the hip. (**A**) Superolateral subluxation of the right femoral head and interposed soft tissue (*curved arrow*) is seen within the acetabulum. Osteonecrosis (*large straight arrow*) and flattening of the cartilaginous epiphysis (*small straight arrows*) are also present. (**B**) A normal left hip is shown for comparison. Note the intact intermediate signal intensity articular cartilage (*curved arrow*) and bright signal intensity yellow marrow epiphyseal center (*straight arrow*). (**C**) An axial image shows interposed cartilage (*arrow*) that resulted in lateral subluxation. Normal anteroposterior relationships are maintained. (TR, 600 msec; TE, 20 msec.)

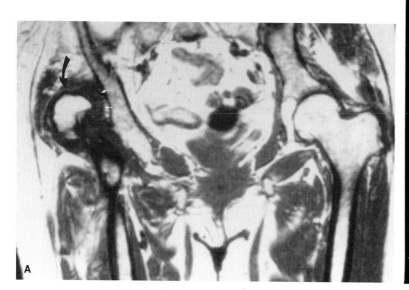

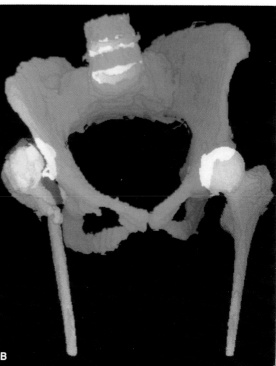

FIGURE 3–43. (**A**) A T1-weighted coronal image of congenital dysplasia of the hip (CDH). Severe acetabular dysplasia and deformity of the femoral head (*curved black arrow*) is shown in an adult patient with untreated congenital dysplasia of the hip. The pseudocapsule is outlined (*white arrows*). (TR, 500 msec; TE, 20 msec.) (**B**) Three-dimensional MR rendering of CDH. (Blue, pelvis and spine; orange, femur; red, capsule.)

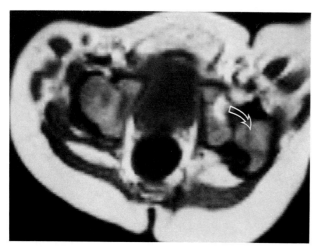

FIGURE 3–44. This T1-weighted axial image demonstrates left posterior dislocation (*arrow*) in congenital dislocation of the hip. Associated acetabular dysplasia is shown. (TR, 600 msec; TE, 20 msec.)

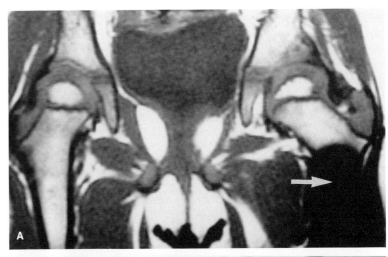

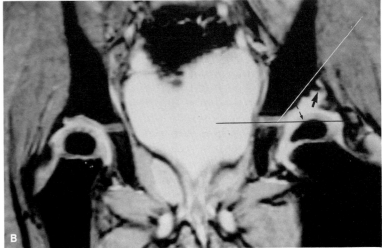

FIGURE 3-45. Coronal (**A**) T1-weighted and (**B**) T2*-weighted images in congenital dysplasia of the hip treated with varus osteotomy (*white arrow*). The acetabulum is shallow, and the labrum is inverted (*black arrows*). The acetabular index formed by Hilgenreiner's or the Y-line through the triradiate cartilage and tangent through acetabular roof is abnormal (>30°). (**A**: TR, 500 msec; TE, 20 msec; **B**: TR, 400; TE, 20 msec; flip angle, 25°.)

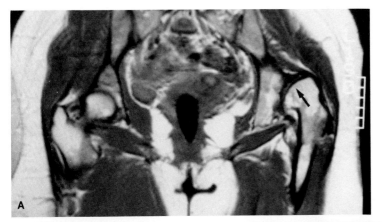

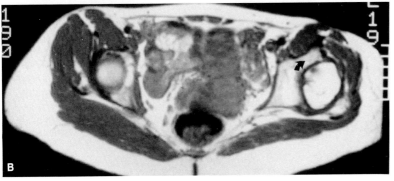

FIGURE 3-46. (**A**) Coronal and (**B**) axial T1-weighted images in an adult patient with chronic congenital dysplasia of the hip deformities of the acetabulum (*curved arrow*) and remodeling of the femoral head (*straight arrow*). (TR, 500 msec; TE, 15 msec.)

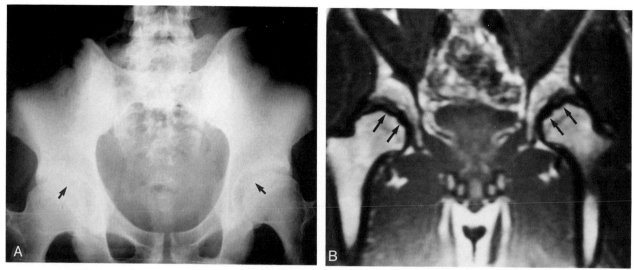

FIGURE 3–47. (**A**) An anteroposterior radiograph and (**B**) a T1-weighted coronal image show multiple epiphyseal dysplasia and bilateral irregularity of the femoral head (*arrows*). (TR, 800 msec; TE, 20 msec.)

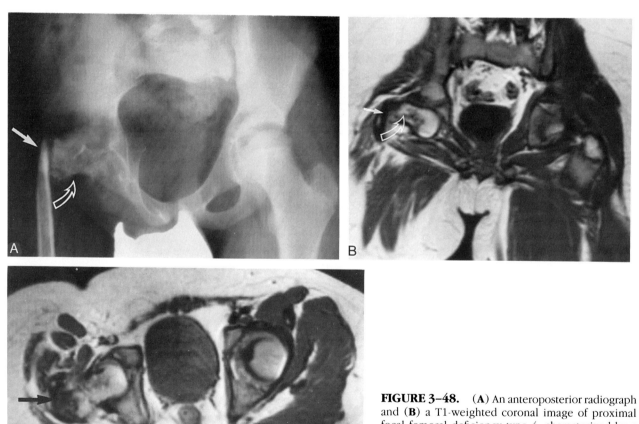

FIGURE 3–48. (**A**) An anteroposterior radiograph and (**B**) a T1-weighted coronal image of proximal focal femoral deficiency type 4, characterized by a short, sharply tapered dysgenic femoral shaft (*straight arrow*) and resultant coxa vara deformity (*curved open arrow*). (**C**) A T1-weighted axial image demonstrates a region of low signal intensity pseudarthrosis (*arrow*) bridging the femoral head and neck to the ossified diaphysis. (TR, 600 msec; TE, 20 msec.)

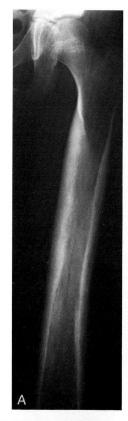

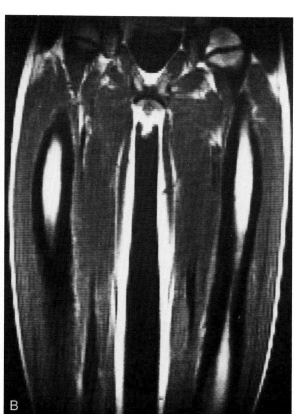

FIGURE 3–49. (**A**) An anteroposterior radiograph of the femur shows diaphyseal sclerosis characteristic of Englemann's disease. (**B**) The corresponding T1-weighted coronal MR image demonstrates low signal intensity cortical thickening. (TR, 500 msec; TE, 40 msec.)

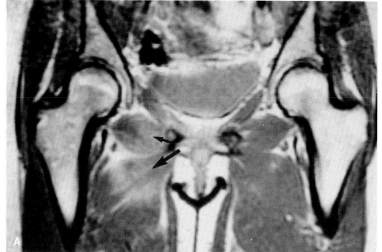

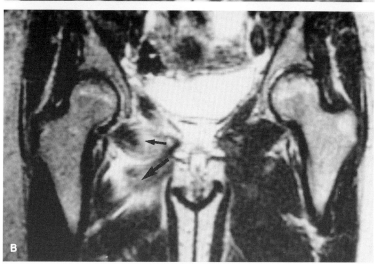

FIGURE 3–50. After a 100-mile run, an ultramarathon runner presented with a grade 1 muscle strain. Coronal (**A**) intermediate-weighted and (**B**) T2-weighted images display increased signal intensity edema and hemorrhage involving the obturator externus (*small arrow*) and adductor brevis muscles (*large arrow*). Normal muscle size and morphology were preserved. (TR, 2000 msec; TE, 20, 80 msec.)

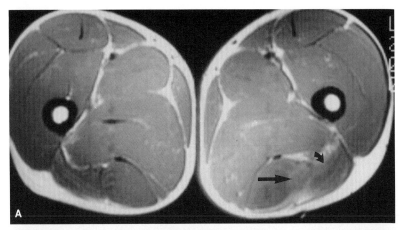

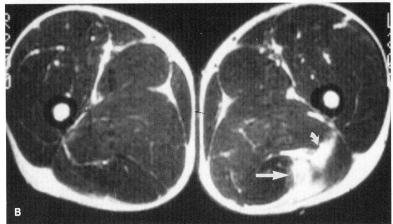

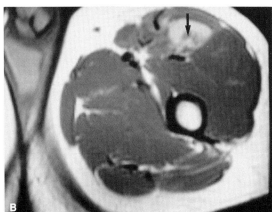

FIGURE 3–51. A grade 1 muscle strain caused edema and hemorrhage in the lateral aspect of the semitendinosus muscle (*straight arrow*) and medial aspect of the biceps femoris muscle (*curved arrow*) in a professional sprinter who presented with acute thigh pain. (**A**) Normal muscle morphology is shown on an intermediate-weighted image, whereas (**B**) edema and hemorrhage are demonstrated on the T2-weighted image. (TR, 2000; TE, 20, 80 msec.)

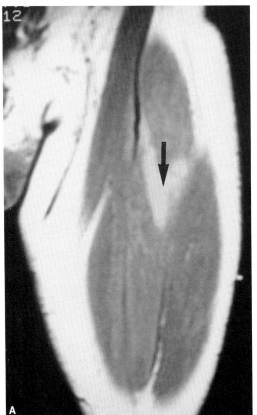

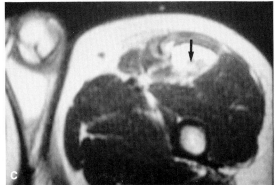

FIGURE 3–52.

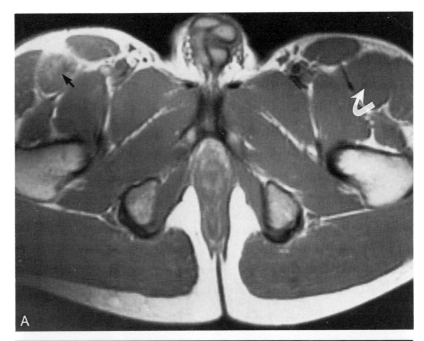

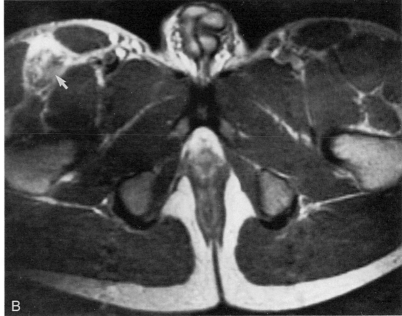

FIGURE 3–53. A grade 2 muscle tear of the right rectus femoris muscle with atrophy and edema (*arrows*) is shown on (**A**) intermediate-weighted and (**B**) T2-weighted axial images. Edematous muscle fibers display increased signal intensity on the T2-weighted image. A normally sized left rectus femoris muscle is shown for comparison (*curved arrow*). (TR, 2000 msec; TE, 20, 80 msec.)

◄ **FIGURE 3–52.** Focal hemorrhage and disruption of approximately 50% of the rectus femoris muscle fibers (*arrows*) are present on (**A**) intermediate-weighted coronal and (**B**) axial and (**C**) T2-weighted axial images of a grade 2 muscle strain. Loss of normal muscle morphology with discontinuity of muscle fibers can be seen on both the intermediate- and the T2-weighted images. (TR, 2000 msec; TE, 20, 80 msec.)

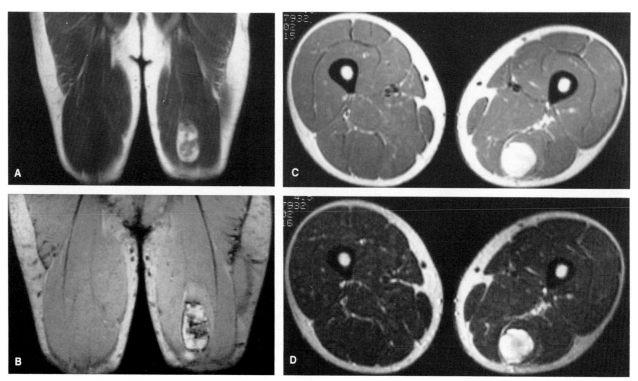

FIGURE 3-54. A grade 2 semitendinosus muscle tear is indicated by hemorrhage seen on coronal (**A**) T1-weighted and (**B**) T2*-weighted images. A subacute hemorrhage, of bright intensity on the T1-weighted image, shows focal areas of hemosiderin on the T2*-weighted image. (**A:** TR, 600 msec; TE, 20 msec; **B:** TR, 500 msec; TE, 20 msec; flip angle, 25°.) Axial (**C**) intermediate-weighted and (**D**) T2-weighted images show semitendinosus hemorrhage involving disruption of approximately 50% of the muscle fibers. (**C, D:** TR, 2000 msec; TE, 20, 80 msec.)

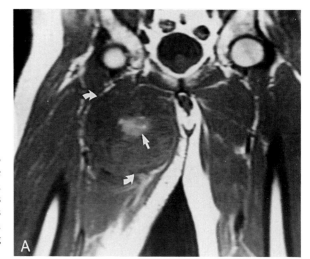

FIGURE 3-55. (**A**) A T1-weighted image displays a complete grade 3 rupture of the adductor magnus muscle (*curved arrow*) with central subacute hemorrhagic component demonstrating bright signal intensity. (TR, 600 msec; TE, 20 msec.) Axial (**B**) intermediate-weighted and (**C**) T2-weighted images demonstrate increasing signal intensity within the edematous muscle fibers (*curved arrows*). The central hemorrhagic component (*straight arrow*) seen on the intermediate-weighted scan becomes isointense with surrounding edema on T2-weighted image. (**B, C:** TR, 2000 msec; TE, 20, 80 msec.)

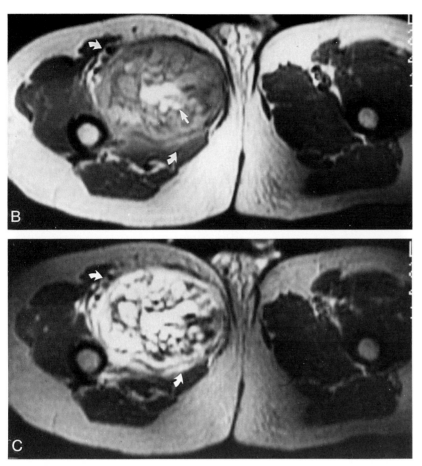

FIGURE 3-55. *(Continued)*

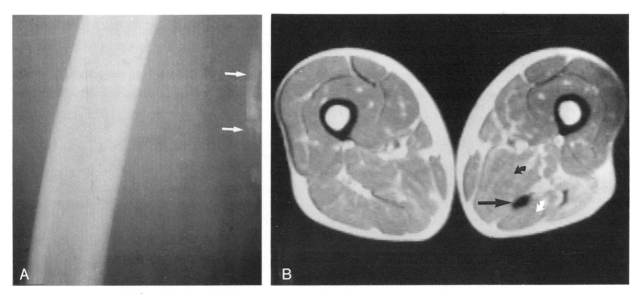

FIGURE 3-56. (**A**) A lateral radiograph of the thigh shows myositis ossificans demonstrating linear calcification (*arrows*). (**B**) A T1-weighted axial image shows low signal intensity calcific deposition (*straight arrow*) in the fascial plane between the semitendinosus muscle (*curved white arrow*) and the semimembranosus muscle (*curved black arrow*). (TR, 800 msec; TE, 20 msec.)

weeks of rest. Return to full activity is allowed when pain has resolved and muscle strength has returned. This can be effectively judged by using Cybex testing.

Although conventional radiography should remain the initial diagnostic examination for excluding post-traumatic myositis ossificans, MR scans have imaged small areas of calcification or ossification as signal void, or low signal intensity on T1- and T2-weighted images (Fig. 3–56).

Intramuscular hemorrhage may occur spontaneously or with minimal trauma in patients on anticoagulants (Fig. 3–57). On MR examination of a diabetic patient, intramuscular hemosiderin deposits in sites of insulin injections have been identified (Fig. 3–58).

Muscle and soft tissue inflammation may appear similar to a grade 1 muscle strain; however, the grade 1 strain is usually more diffuse and invades more than one muscle group. Acute fasciitis was detected in a 3-year-old boy as a diffuse increase in signal intensity conforming to the involved muscle group (Fig. 3–59). Corresponding gallium scintigraphy and CT were negative in this case. Soft tissue edema in infection demonstrates low signal intensity on T1-weighted images and increased signal intensity on T2-weighted images. If soft tissue infection is suspected, MR evaluation may be the examination of choice.

Bursitis. Two main bursal groups can become inflamed and cause hip pain in the athlete:

1. The trochanteric bursa, which is actually three discrete bursae
2. The deep gluteal or ischiogluteal bursa.

In addition, the iliopsoas bursa, which lies deep to the iliopsoas muscle, can less frequently cause hip pain.

The trochanteric bursa becomes inflamed with repetitive irritation of the tensor fascia latae sliding over the greater trochanter (Fig. 3–60). This condition is common in runners and participants in racquet sports, causing pain in the lateral aspect of the thigh. Inflammation of the deep gluteal bursa causes pain deep in the buttock and can be confused with referred pain from the lower back. In both cases, it is important to differentiate between bursitis and lumbar disease. Treatment consists of activity modification, physical therapy, and nonsteroidal antiinflammatory medications. Occasionally, local steroid injection and, less commonly, surgical intervention play a role.

Iliopsoas bursitis may be accompanied by a snapping sensation caused by the psoas tendon passing over the iliopectineal eminence on the pubis. Treatment is initially conservative, but if pain and snapping persist, the prominence on the iliopectineal eminence can be resected along with a partial release of the iliopsoas tendon.

Axial MR images with T2 weighting have been useful in demonstrating iliopsoas bursal collections adjacent to the iliopsoas tendon in patients presenting with clicking of the hip during range-of-motion activities with internal and external rotation (Fig. 3–61). Identification of bursal fluid correlates with snapping or clicking of the hip on clinical examination. Bursal fluid should not be mistaken for a malignant soft tissue neoplasm such as synovial sarcoma, which has similar imaging characteristics (*i.e.,* low signal intensity on T1-weighted images and bright signal intensity on T2-weighted images).

Avulsion Fracture

Three bony structures in the hip region are prone to avulsion injury:

1. The anterior superior iliac spines
2. The anterior inferior iliac spines
3. The ischial tuberosity.

These injuries most frequently occur in adolescents or young adults participating in athletics and are becoming more common. It is important to evaluate the contralateral side as well as the injured side in these injuries because they occur through secondary centers of ossification and because what appears to be a fracture may simply be an anatomic variant. Axial T2-weighted, T2*-weighted, or STIR images are usually necessary to identify areas of edema or hemorrhage associated with these fractures. When imaging with fat marrow signal, which is bright on T1-weighted images, or cortical signal intensity, which demonstrates low signal intensity on T1-weighted images, avulsed bone appears dark on either gradient-echo or STIR images and may be indistinguishable from adjacent tendons or ligaments on these pulse sequences. MR evaluation of avulsion fractures should follow an initial evaluation with conventional film radiography or bone scintigraphy. The anterior superior iliac spine is injured secondary to overpull of the sartorius muscle. This occurs with the hip in extension and the knee flexed, and thus can be seen in kicking athletes such as soccer players.

Avulsion of the anterior inferior iliac spine is less common than injury to the anterior superior iliac spine and occurs as a result of overpull of the straight head of the rectus (Fig. 3–62). The mechanism of injury and the type of athlete at risk are similar in both injuries, and both are treated in the same manner. A few days of bed rest for pain relief, followed by protected weight bearing until comfort is achieved, is adequate.[73]

Avulsion fracture of the ischial tuberosity results from overpull of the hamstring muscles. This occurs with the hip flexed and the knee in extension. During physical examination this maneuver elicits pain as does rectal examination. Gymnasts are prone to this injury and Milch described seeing it in a dancer doing splits.[74] Treatment is a short period of bed rest followed by protected weight bearing. Although the fracture invariably heals, exuberant callus formation can occur causing chronic pain.[75] Excision may be required for pain relief and has been confused with malignancy, leading to biopsy.

Heterotopic Ossification

Heterotopic ossification occurs secondary to trauma or surgery, or in patients who have sustained burns or paralysis. Patients with ankylosing spondylitis and diffuse idiopathic skeletal hyperostosis are also at risk for heterotopic bone formation. Large areas of bone marrow containing mature heterotopic ossification demonstrate fat marrow signal intensity on T1-weighted images (Fig. 3–63). Capsular trauma may produce bone formations that resemble an avulsion-type injury (Figs. 3–64 and 3–65).

Fractures of the Femur and Acetabulum

Fractures about the hip may be associated with significant morbidity, especially when diagnosis and treatment are delayed.[76-78] Femoral fractures are classified as either intra- or extracapsular. Intracapsular femoral neck fractures are subcapital, transcervical, or basicervical in location. The incidence of post-traumatic osteonecrosis increases as the fracture site nears the femoral head, culminating in a 30% incidence for fractures in closest proximity to the femoral head. The less common capital fracture is an intracapsular fracture of the femoral head. Extracapsular fractures are intertrochanteric or subtrochanteric.

Stress fractures of the hip most frequently involve the femoral neck. They occur in two patient populations:

1. The young adult, in whom stress fractures result from overuse and repeated stress to normal bone (*e.g.,* military recruits and runners)
2. Osteoporotic women, in whom the fractures are more appropriately termed insufficiency fractures, and may occur with normal activity or a seemingly insignificant increase in activity.[79,80]

Patients usually present with pain aggravated by weight bearing, and passive movement is often painful, especially rotation. Radiographs are often normal, and symptoms can be subtle. A careful history and a high index of suspicion are necessary to avoid missing the injury.

Classification and Treatment

Blickenstaff and Morris classified stress fractures into three types.[81,82] In type I fractures, plain radiographs reveal endosteal or periosteal callus without a definite fracture line; and in type II fractures, a fracture line is clearly seen. Type III fractures are displaced. Treatment may be based on the fracture type. For type I fractures, some physicians recommend bed rest until the patient is pain-free, followed by progressive weight bearing. DeLee, however, recommends prophylactic pinning for type I fractures, especially if the callus is on the lateral or tension side of the femoral neck.[82a] Type 2 and 3 fractures are treated with internal fixation. The complication rate with internal fixation of type 3 fractures is high and includes nonunion, malunion, and aseptic necrosis.

Diagnosis and Magnetic Resonance Imaging

In general, fractures of the acetabulum are best assessed with thin section CT and subsequent image reformation and 3D rendering (Fig. 3–66). Magnetic resonance imaging in direct coronal, sagittal, and axial orthogonal planes is helpful in the evaluation of the acetabular columns and subchondral marrow. The lateral aspect of the acetabulum is formed by the anterior and posterior columns with the intervening superior dome of the acetabulum. Anterior column fractures are associated with external rotation of the femoral head, and posterior column fractures are associated with internal rotation of the femoral head.[83] Retained fragments within the hip joint are usually seen on axial T1- and T2-weighted images. Disarticulation of the femoral head on 3D CT renderings can be used to identify size, morphology, and number of osseous fragments. The association of AVN (18%) in posterior fractures can also be evaluated with MR.

Capital fractures are often radiographically occult, especially when the spherical morphology of the femoral head is maintained or when an area of impacted trabecular (*i.e.,* subchondral) bone is involved (Figs. 3–67 and 3–68). Axial and sagittal images may provide better delineation of fracture morphology than coronal plane images (Fig. 3–69).

With fractures of the proximal femur—including femoral neck stress fractures—radiographic signs of cortical disruption may be subtle, especially if there is either an incomplete or complete fracture without displacement of the medial trabeculae (Figs. 3–70 and 3–71).[84,85] Magnetic resonance imaging is particularly useful in identifying nondisplaced femoral neck fractures that require surgical treatment but are not detected on routine radiography (Fig. 3–72). Although bone scintigraphy is also sensitive to fractures, it is nonspecific. With MR imaging, it is possible to demonstrate the morphology of the fracture segment not identifiable on bone scans. Three-dimensional CT or MR rendering can display varus or valgus deformities and postoperative screw placement (Fig. 3–73). In displaced fractures, complicating osteonecrosis can be excluded on an MR image, and viability of the femoral head can be assessed (Figs. 3–74 through 3–76).

(text continues on page 115)

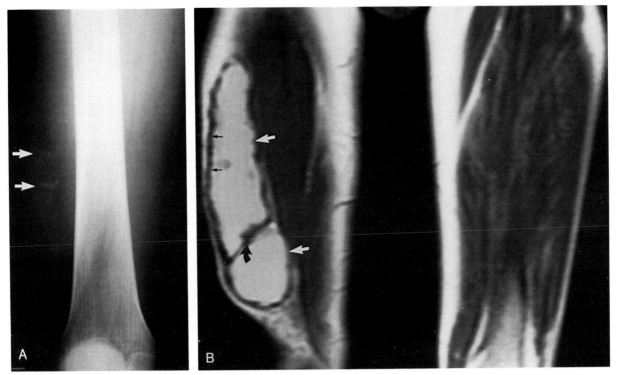

FIGURE 3–57. (**A**) An anterior thigh hemorrhage shows focal soft-tissue calcific deposition (*arrows*) in an anteroposterior radiograph. (**B**) A T1-weighted coronal image displays a high signal intensity subacute hemorrhage in the region of the vastus lateralis muscle (*white arrows*). The low signal intensity hemosiderin periphery (*small black arrows*) and internal septations (*curved arrow*) are shown. (TR, 800 msec; TE, 20 msec.)

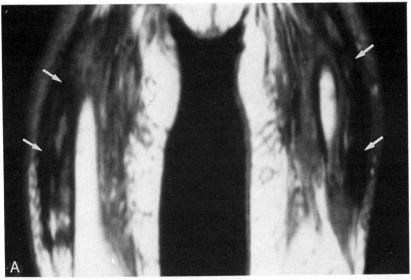

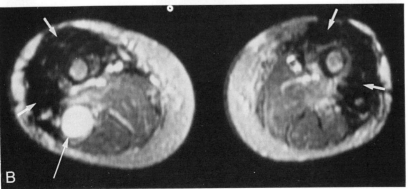

FIGURE 3–58. Chronic intramuscular hemorrhage was caused by repeated injections of insulin in this diabetic patient. Low signal intensity paramagnetic hemosiderin deposition (*short arrows*) in vastus lateralis and intermedius muscles can be seen on (**A**) T1-weighted coronal and (**B**) axial images. High signal intensity focal subacute hemorrhage is shown within the long head of the biceps femoris muscle (*long arrow*) on the axial image. (TR, 600 msec; TE, 20 msec.)

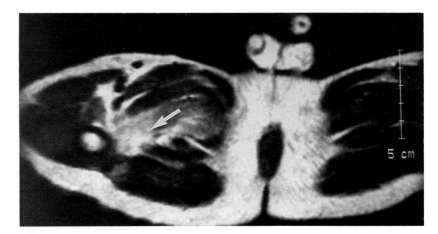

FIGURE 3-59. High signal intensity edema (*arrow*) along the muscle fascial plane is seen on this T2-weighted axial image in a 3 year old boy with acute fasciitis. (TR, 200 msec; TE, 60 msec.)

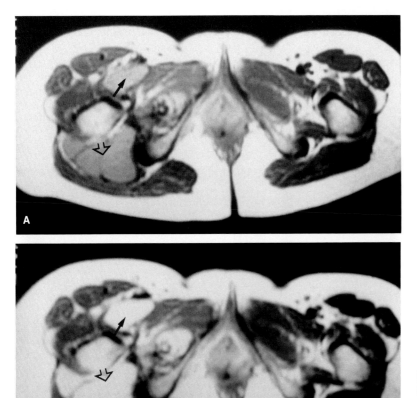

FIGURE 3-60. Trochanteric bursitis. Axial (**A**) intermediate-weighted and (**B**) T2-weighted images display inflammation with synovial fluid distention in the trochanteric and ischiotrochanteric bursa in a patient with rheumatoid arthritis (*open arrow*). There is associated involvement of the iliopsoas bursa (*black arrow*). No hip effusion is present. (TR, 200 msec; TE, 20, 80 msec.)

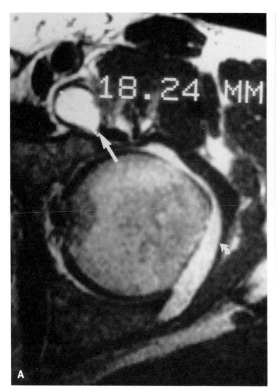

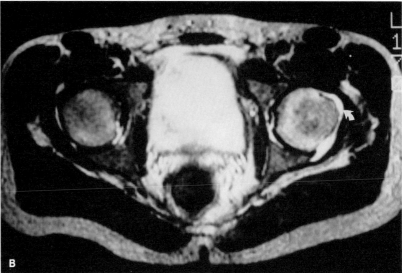

FIGURE 3–61. T2-weighted images of iliopsoas bursitis. (**A**) High signal intensity iliopsoas bursal distention can be seen medial to the iliopsoas tendon (*arrow*). Associated joint effusion is indicated (*curved arrow*). (**B**) Three months later, complete resolution of bursal fluid with no interval change in joint effusion (*curved arrow*) has taken place. The initial complaint of bursitis with hip clicking in internal and external rotation was also resolved.

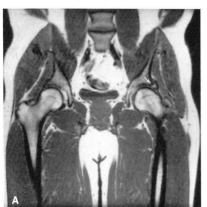

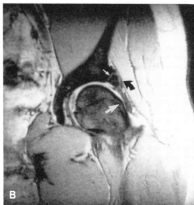

FIGURE 3–62. This old acetabular margin anterior inferior iliac spine avulsion fracture (*small white arrow*) is shown at the attachment of the reflected head of the rectus femoris (*curved black arrow*) on (**A**) a T1-weighted image obtained with a body coil and on (**B**) a T2*-weighted image obtained with a surface coil. Remodeling of the opposing surface of the femoral head has taken place (*large white arrow*). (**A**: TR 600 msec; TE, 20 msec; **B**: TR, 400 msec; TE, 20 msec; flip angle, 25°.)

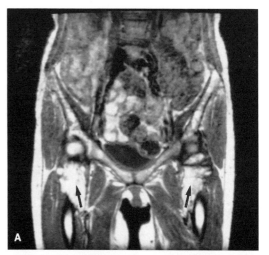

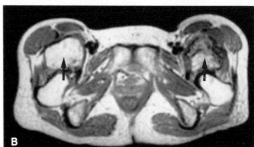

FIGURE 3–63. (**A**) T1-weighted coronal and (**B**) axial images of massive mature heterotopic bone (*arrows*) located anterior to the hip joints and extending to the level of the lesser trochanters in a patient with Guillain–Barré paralysis. (TR, 600 msec; TE, 20 msec.)

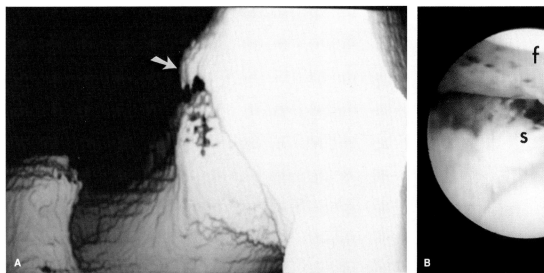
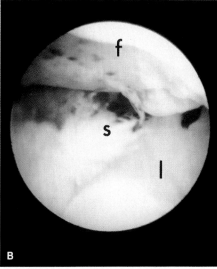

FIGURE 3-64. (**A**) Three-dimensional CT rendering of posterior capsule trauma (*arrow*) with heterotopic ossification shown in posterior view of the left hip. (**B**) An arthroscopic view shows the hyperplastic synovium (S) located deep to the capsular ossification. (F, femur; L, labrum.)

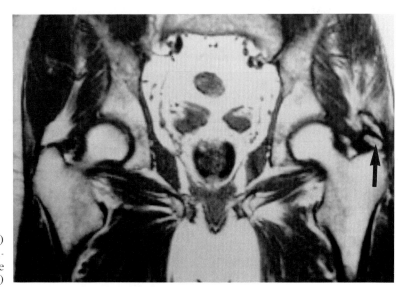

FIGURE 3-65. Heterotopic bone formation (*arrow*) occurred after capsular trauma to the left hip. On T1-weighted coronal image, mature ossifications demonstrate fat marrow signal intensity. (TR, 600 msec; TE, 20 msec.)

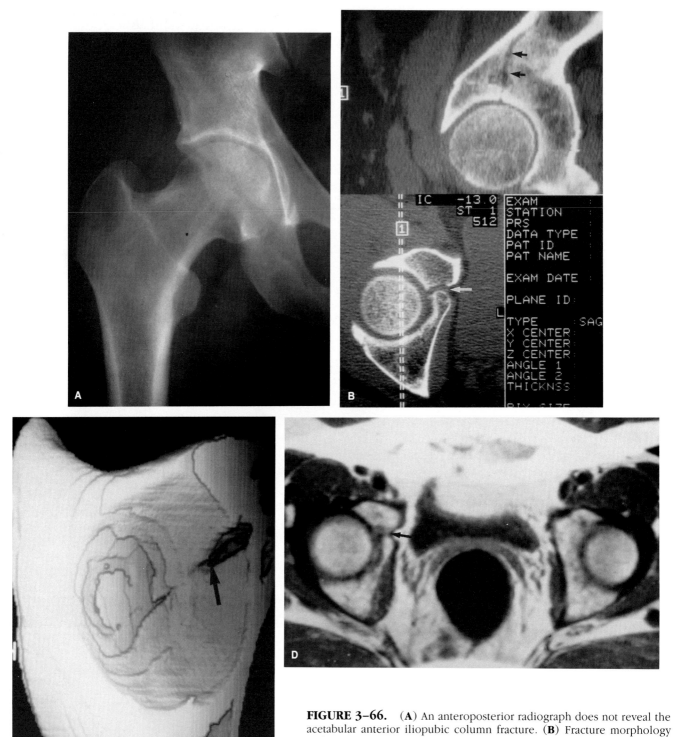

FIGURE 3–66. (**A**) An anteroposterior radiograph does not reveal the acetabular anterior iliopubic column fracture. (**B**) Fracture morphology and extent are optimally displayed on 2D axial (*white arrow*) and reformatted (*black arrows*) CT scans. (**C**) Three-dimensional CT rendering allows identification of the anterior column fracture (*arrow*) with disarticulated femur. (**D**) The corresponding axial T1-weighted image also displays the low signal intensity anterior column fracture (*arrow*). (TR, 600 msec; TE, 20 msec.)

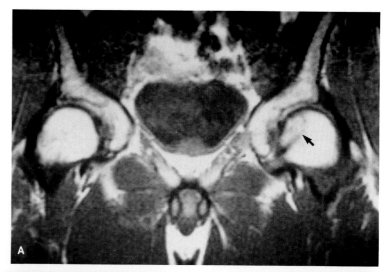

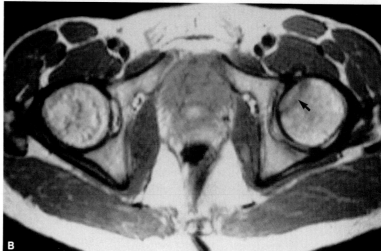

FIGURE 3–67. This radiographically occult chronic capital fracture (*arrows*) was diagnosed 4 months post-trauma. (**A**) The T1-weighted coronal and (**B**) axial images demonstrate the fracture as a nondisplaced linear area of decreased signal intensity. (TR, 600 msec; TE, 200 msec.)

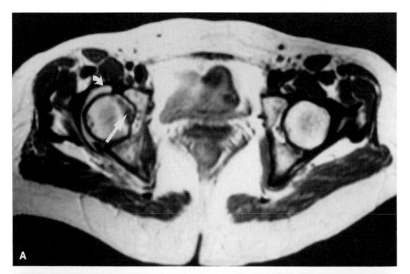

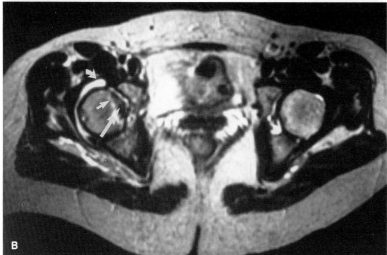

FIGURE 3–68. On axial (**A**) intermediate-weighted and (**B**) T2-weighted images, a capital (*i.e.,* femoral head) impaction fracture is displayed with a wide band of low signal intensity (*large arrows*), peripheral hemorrhage (*small arrow*), and associated effusion (*curved arrows*). A wide band instead of a thin linear segment is consistent with a larger area of trabecular microfracture. (TR, 2000 msec; TE, 20, 80 msec.)

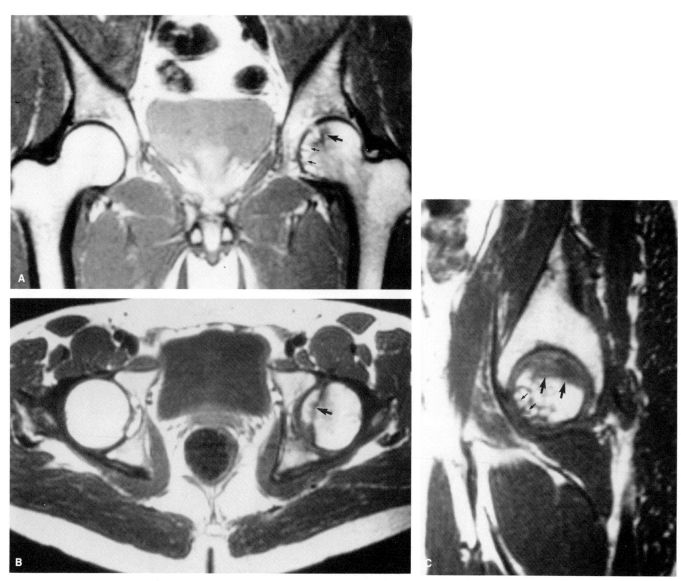

FIGURE 3–69. (**A**) A radiographically occult capital fracture (*large arrow*) is shown with associated bright signal intensity marrow hemorrhage (*small arrows*) on a T1-weighted coronal image. (**B**) The T1-weighted axial image also reveals the fracture (*arrow*). (**C**) The T1-weighted sagittal image accurately depicts the linear area of decreased signal intensity at the fracture site (*arrows*). (TR, 500 msec; TE, 20 msec.)

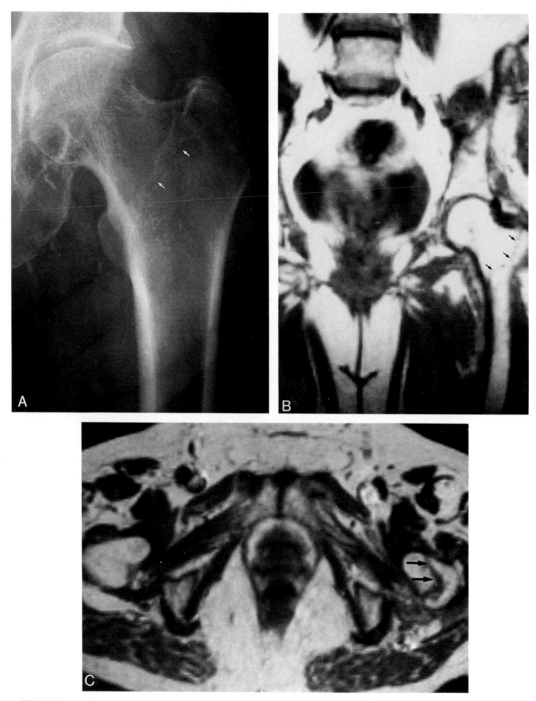

FIGURE 3–70. (**A**) This nondisplaced intertrochanteric femoral fracture was missed on the initial anteroposterior radiograph (*arrows*). The corresponding (**B**) T1-weighted coronal and (**C**) axial images demonstrate low signal intensity at the fracture segment (*arrows*). (**B, C**: TR, 1000 msec; TE, 40 msec.)

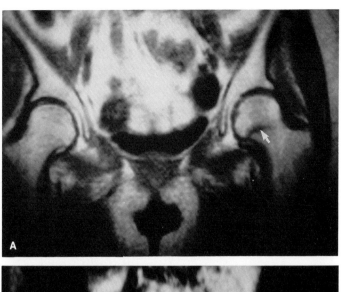

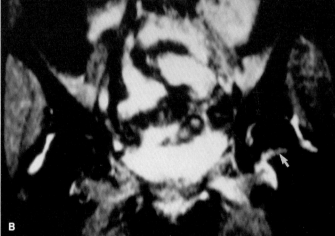

FIGURE 3–71. This femoral neck stress fracture (*arrows*) extends to the cortex of the medial femoral neck. Linear fracture morphology is (**A**) low in signal intensity on a T1-weighted image and (**B**) high in signal intensity on short TI inversion recovery image. (**A**: TR, 500 msec; TE, 20 msec; **B**: TR, 1400 msec; TI, 125 msec; TE, 40 msec.)

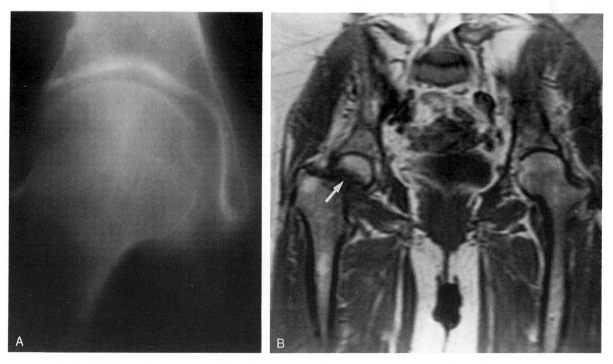

FIGURE 3–72. (**A**) This nondisplaced femoral neck fracture was missed on plain film tomography. (**B**) The fracture was detected as a low signal intensity segment (*arrow*) on a T1-weighted coronal image. The patient's fracture was subsequently pinned at surgery. (TR, 800 msec; TE, 20 msec.)

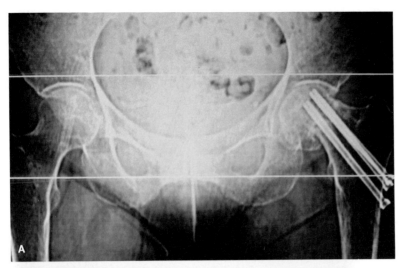

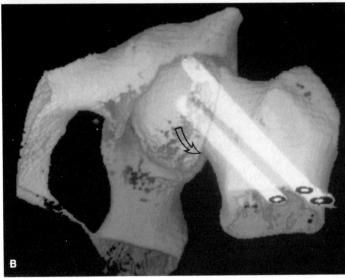

FIGURE 3–73. (**A**) An anteroposterior radiograph shows a left subcapital fracture with three titanium cortical screws. (**B**) A 3D CT image best displays the varus deformity (*curved open arrow*) and spatial placement of the titanium screws relative to the femoral neck and fracture.

FIGURE 3–74. (**A**) This anteroposterior radiograph demonstrates a right femoral neck fracture in varus deformation. (**B**) The T1-weighted coronal image displays a linear cervical neck fracture (*straight solid arrow*) and low signal intensity proximal femoral marrow edema (*open arrow*). Mild asymmetry in the femoral head marrow signal intensity is observed at this stage (*curved solid arrow*). (TR, 600 msec; TE, 20 msec.)

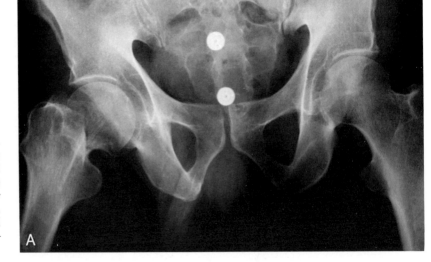

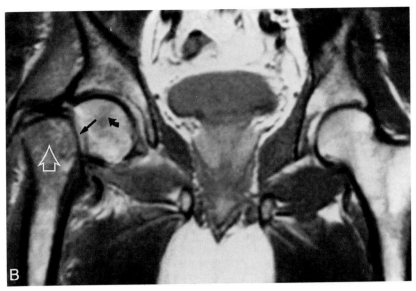

FIGURE 3–74. *(Continued)*

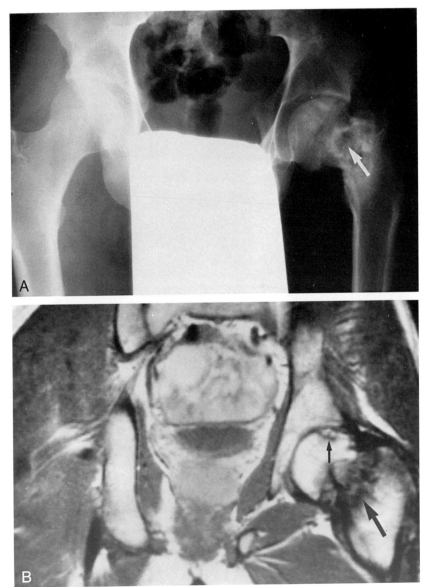

FIGURE 3–75. (**A**) An anteroposterior radiograph shows an untreated left femoral neck fracture (*arrow*). (**B**) The corresponding T1-weighted coronal image demonstrates the low signal intensity sclerotic fracture site (*large arrow*) and associated focus of femoral head osteonecrosis (*small arrow*). (TR, 800 msec; TE, 20 msec.)

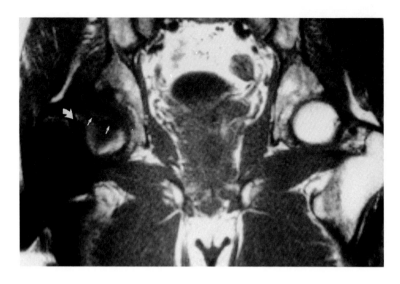

FIGURE 3–76. Osteonecrosis has developed as a complication of this midcervical femoral neck fracture after operative fixation. The metallic artifact does not preclude identification of the fracture site (*curved arrow*) or the osteonecrosis (*straight arrows*) on a T1-weighted coronal image. (TR, 500 msec; TE, 20 msec.)

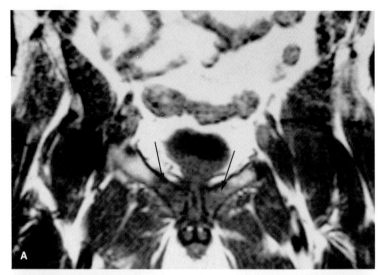

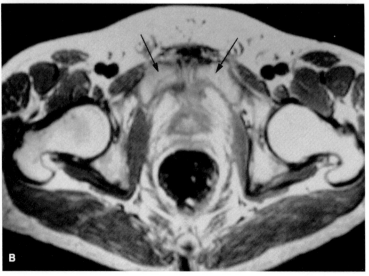

FIGURE 3–77. Bilateral superior pubic rami stress fractures (*arrows*) occurred in an ultramarathon runner. Diffuse trabecular marrow edema and hemorrhage are seen at (**A**) low signal intensity on a T1-weighted coronal image and (**B**) with increased signal intensity on axial intermediate-weighted and (**C**) T2-weighted images (**A**: TR, 600 msec; TE, 20 msec; **B**, **C**: TR, 2000 msec; TE, 20, 80 msec.)

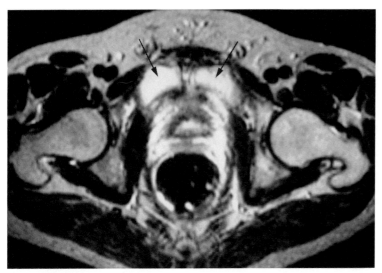

FIGURE 3–77. *(Continued)*

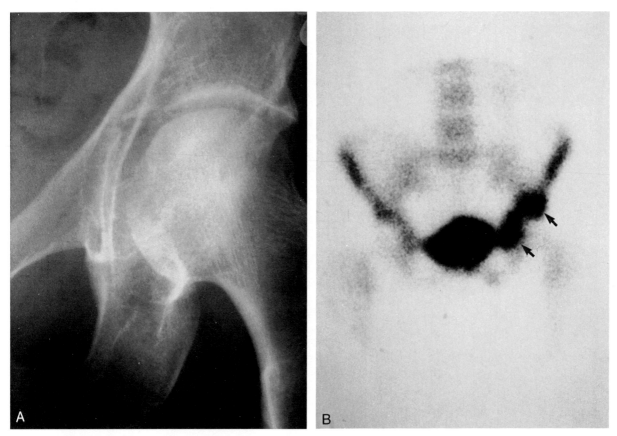

FIGURE 3–78. (**A**) An anteroposterior radiograph in a patient with primary biliary cirrhosis and hip pain is negative for acetabular stress fracture. (**B**) A ^{99m}TC-MDP bone scan shows uptake indicative of fracture in the left supraacetabular area (*arrows*). (**C**) A T1-weighted coronal image displays diffuse low signal intensity marrow edema in the left acetabular roof (*arrows*). (TR, 1000 msec; TE, 40 msec.) (**D**) Thin section CT shows multiple sites of cortical disruption, revealing the anterior column stress fracture (*arrows*). *(continued)*

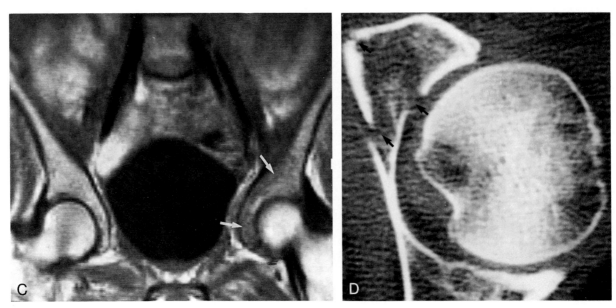

FIGURE 3–78. *(Continued)*

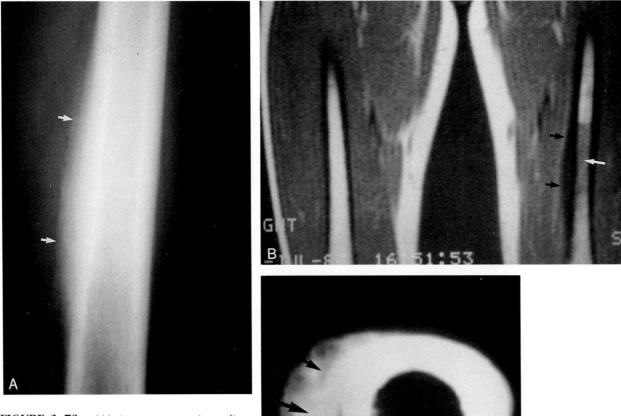

FIGURE 3–79. (**A**) An anteroposterior radiograph shows thickened periosteal reaction in the medial femoral shaft in response to a stress fracture (*arrows*). (**B**) The corresponding T1-weighted coronal image demonstrates thickened medial cortex (*black arrows*) and marrow edema (*white arrow*) as low signal intensity. (TR, 1000 msec; TE, 20 msec.) (**C**) Axial CT allows identification of the stress fracture (*small arrows*) and the adjacent periosteal reaction (*large arrows*).

T1-weighted images provide the best contrast for the low signal intensity fracture segment in contrast to adjacent bright signal intensity marrow fat. STIR images have shown greater sensitivity than gradient-echo techniques in displaying associated hemorrhage and edema at the fracture site.

The differential diagnosis of fatigue and insufficiency stress fractures may be difficult, and both infection and neoplasia need to be ruled out.[86] Stress fractures about the acetabulum, ilium, pubis, and femur may be associated with extensive edema, which demonstrates low signal intensity on T1-weighted images and high signal intensity on T2-weighted, T2*-weighted, or STIR images when there is no identifiable fracture segment (Fig. 3-77). Thin section, high resolution CT may be necessary to achieve the precise cortical detail needed to display subtle cortical discontinuities (Figs. 3-78 and 3-79).

Magnetic resonance imaging affords direct visualization of cartilage prior to the appearance of ossification centers, which facilitates the identification of physeal fractures (Fig. 3-80). In complex hemipelvis fracture–dislocations, MR or CT can be used to assess interruptions of both the anterior and posterior pelvic ring segments and sacroiliac joint separation (Fig. 3-81).

Dislocations

Dislocation of the femoral head is usually associated with a fracture of the acetabulum, the femoral head, or both. Anterior dislocations are less frequent than posterior dislocations, and are most commonly identified anteroinferiorly.[86,87] Anterior cortical fractures of the femoral head and fractures of the acetabular rim are associated with posterior dislocations.[88,89]

Chronic arthritis and AVN may complicate dislocations and fractures of the hip, and MR imaging is helpful in their early identification. In one case of posterior fracture–dislocation of the hip, MR imaging revealed an impacted femoral head fracture (low signal intensity on T1-weighted images), an acetabular rim fracture (high signal intensity hemorrhage), and multiple intraarticular fragments that were subsequently removed through an arthroscope (Fig. 3-82). At a 6-month follow-up, MR imaging showed the development of osteonecrosis at the initial site of fracture. Thus, it may be difficult to predict the subsequent development of osteonecrosis in a patient sustaining a low signal intensity compression fracture of the femoral head.

Axial MR images may be used to follow the course of the sciatic nerve, which is injured in 8% to 19% of posterior hip dislocations. Treatment of fracture–dislocations involves reduction of the hip and treatment of the associated fracture. Open surgery is required to debride osteochondral fragments. Immediate reduction of dislocation may decrease the incidence of AVN, although this practice is controversial.

Labral Tears

By performing the MR examination with a surface coil placed over the hip joint, it is possible to resolve the anatomic detail of the acetabular labrum (Fig. 3-83).[2] The normal labrum, triangular in cross section, is seen on coronal planar images as a low signal intensity triangle located between the lateral acetabulum and the femoral head (Fig. 3-84). Labral tears present with symptoms of pain, decreased range of motion, and clicking. Neither conventional radiographs nor arthrography are satisfactory for accurate identification of labral defects, but experience with MR evaluation of labral tears shows promise. In several patients with persistent pain and clicking with hip flexion and rotation, increased signal intensity or disruption of the labrum could be identified on T2*-weighted images using 18- to 20-cm FOVs (Fig. 3-85). Labral tears were subsequently confirmed at hip arthroscopy. Extension of acetabular articular cartilage along the medial aspect of the fibrous labrum should not be mistaken for a partial labral tear or detachment (see Fig. 3-84).

Arthritis

Joint Effusions

The volume of joint fluid in the normal hip is small, and it does not generate sufficient signal for detection. Joint effusions, however, demonstrate low signal intensity on T1-weighted images and increased signal intensity on T2-weighted images.[90] On coronal images, small collections of joint fluid first accumulate superiorly in the recess border by the labrum of the acetabulum and inferomedially by the transverse ligament. With larger effusions, the medial and lateral joint capsule is distended and has convex margins. Joint effusions are also easily identified on axial and sagittal images (Fig. 3-86).

Osteoarthritis

Osteoarthritis is by far the most common form of articular cartilage degeneration. In general, incidence increases with age, and, although the etiology remains unclear, two mechanical theories predominate:

1. Excessive stress on normal tissue
2. Abnormal response to normal forces.

In addition, the biologic response resulting in inflammation undoubtedly contributes to cartilage degeneration. Most osteoarthritis in the hip is thought to be secondary to an underlying condition such as an old SCFE, dysplasia, Legg–Calvé–Perthes disease in childhood, or anatomic variants such as an intraacetabular labrum.

Diagnosis and Treatment. The diagnosis of osteoarthritis is made by radiographic evaluation. Classically, there is loss of the joint space and sclerosis of the subchondral bone. Other changes include osteophyte and cyst formation.

The first line of treatment involves activity modification support (*e.g.,* a cane) and nonsteroidal antiinflammatory medications. When these modalities are no longer effective, surgery may be considered. The most common surgical procedure performed is total joint replacement, but osteotomies and arthrodesis remain viable options in appropriately selected patients.

Magnetic Resonance Imaging. T1- and T2*-weighted images of the hip have been used to detect the early changes of osteoarthritis (Figs. 3–87 and 3–88).[91] Articular cartilage attenuation is best demonstrated on either sagittal or coronal images, but separation of acetabular and femoral head articular cartilage is better displayed in the sagittal plane. Stress-thickened trabeculae can be seen with low signal intensity on T1- and T2-weighted images before there is evidence of subchondral sclerosis on conventional radiographs. Small subchondral cystic lesions can be identified on MR scans before superior joint-space narrowing, lateral acetabular and femoral head osteophytes, and medial femoral buttressing occur. Herniation pits of the femoral neck are not part of the spectrum of osteoarthritis of the hip and are considered incidental findings on conventional radiographs. These pits are related to mechanical or pressure effects of the anterior hip capsule on the proximal femoral neck.[91a] These small cortical defects or cavities (<1 cm in diameter), located in the anterior superior aspect of the lateral femoral neck, are defined by a low signal intensity sclerotic border and display either the low signal intensity of fibrous tissue or the high signal intensity of fluid on T2-weighted images. Synovium-filled degenerative cysts about the hip are identified with low signal intensity on T1-weighted images and with uniform high signal intensity on T2-weighted or T2*-weighted images (Fig. 3–89). These cysts may be present within the subchondral bone of the acetabulum and are referred to as Egger's cysts (Fig. 3–90).[92] Osteoarthritis may also be associated with or superimposed on osteonecrosis of the femoral head. In osteonecrosis, there is greater involvement of the femoral head prior to joint-space narrowing and reciprocal changes within the acetabulum.

Synovial Chondromatosis and Loose Bodies

The hip is commonly involved in synovial chondromatosis (*i.e.,* osteochondromatosis), a monarticular synovium-based cartilage metaplasia.[93] Development of intraarticular loose bodies may result in destruction of hyaline articular cartilage and progress to osteoarthritis. On T2-weighted MR imaging, the multiple, ossified loose bodies in synovial chondromatosis are seen as foci of intermediate signal intensity, bathed in the surrounding joint effusion that is bright in signal intensity. These nodules may demonstrate the high signal intensity characteristics of fatty marrow on T1- and T2-weighted images (Fig. 3–91).

Surface coil imaging of the hips has improved the identification of intraarticular loose bodies, which may be missed on images acquired with body coils and larger FOVs. On axial images, interruption of the low signal intensity space between the femoral head and the acetabulum is interposed with cartilaginous or osteocartilaginous tissue (Fig. 3–92). A cartilaginous loose body demonstrates low-to-intermediate signal intensity and is not detectable on corresponding radiographs (Fig. 3–93). The haversian fat pad or pulvinar in the acetabular fossa should not be confused with a loose body when viewing a T2*-weighted contrast image (Fig. 3–94).

Rheumatoid Arthritis

Rheumatoid arthritis is a systemic disease that most frequently affects the small joints of the hands and feet. The etiology remains unknown, but the disorder is associated with HLA-DR4 and has been classified as an autoimmune disease. Although articular cartilage contains immune complexes in this disease, these complexes have not been shown to stimulate inflammatory reactions in peripheral blood lymphocyte or monocytes.[94] An infectious etiology has also been postulated.

Diagnosis. The criteria for the diagnosis of rheumatoid arthritis were established in 1958 and modified in 1987.[94a] These criteria include the following:

- morning stiffness
- arthritis of three or more joints
- arthritis of the hand joints
- symmetric arthritis
- rheumatoid nodules
- serum rheumatoid factor
- radiographic changes.

Although rheumatoid factor is estimated to be positive in approximately 75% of rheumatoid arthritis cases, a positive rheumatoid factor alone is not sufficient for a diagnosis of rheumatoid arthritis. Conversely, the diagnosis can be made in a patient who tests negative for rheumatoid factor.

(text continues on page 127)

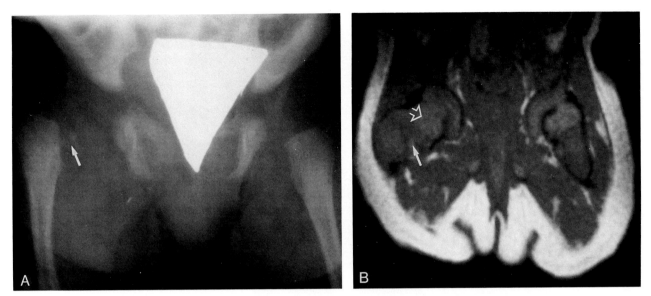

FIGURE 3–80. (**A**) An anteroposterior radiograph shows a physeal fracture (*arrow*) simulating congenital dislocation of the right hip. (**B**) The corresponding T1-weighted coronal image allows identification of the fracture site (*solid arrow*) and the normally seated cartilaginous epiphyseal center (*open arrow*). (TR, 500 msec; TE, 30 msec.)

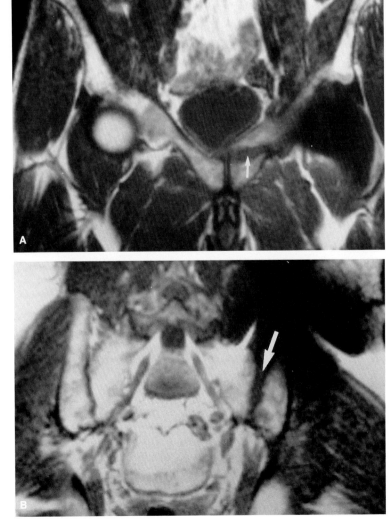

FIGURE 3–81. Malgaigne fracture. Coronal T1-weighted images show (**A**) a superior left pubic ramus fracture (*arrow*) and (**B**) a separation of the ipsilateral sacroiliac joint (*arrow*). The extent of sacroiliac involvement was not initially recognized on conventional radiographs. Low signal intensity metallic artifact can be seen overlying the left hip and sacroiliac joint. (TR, 600 msec; TE, 20 msec.)

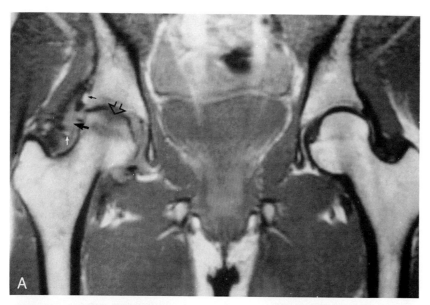

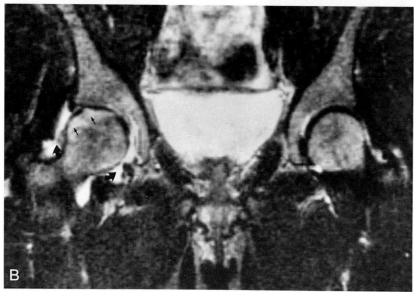

FIGURE 3–82. Posterior hip dislocation occurred after reduction in this patient. (**A**) A T1-weighted coronal image demonstrates femoral head compression fracture (*open arrow*), acetabular rim fracture (*small black arrow*), joint effusion (*large black arrow*), and intraarticular loose bodies (*white arrow*). (TR, 100 msec; TE, 20 msec.) (**B**) The corresponding T2-weighted coronal image displays high signal intensity capsular effusion (*curved arrows*) and edema in the area of the compression fracture (*straight arrows*). (TR, 2000 msec; TE, 60 msec.) (**C**) Hip arthroscopy allows identification of the acetabular fracture (Ac), loose body (LB) and femoral head (FH). (A, anterior, P, posterior). (**D**) A follow-up radiograph taken at 6 months postinjury shows the sclerotic focus within the femoral head (*large arrow*). The site of the old acetabular rim fracture is marked (*small arrow*). The corresponding coronal (**E**) T1-weighted and (**F**) T2-weighted images demonstrate the interval progression of osteonecrosis at 6 months postinjury (*arrows*). (**E**: TR, 600 msec; TE, 20 msec; **F**: TR, 2000 msec; TE, 60 msec.)

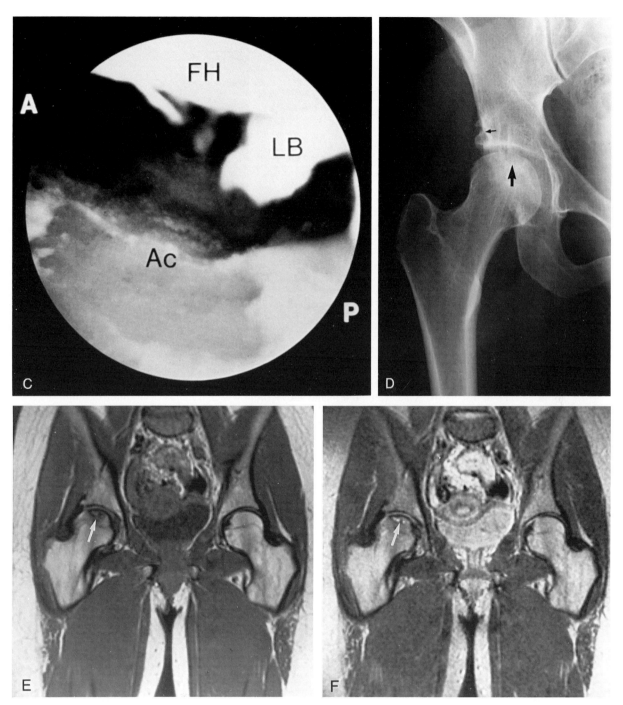

FIGURE 3–82. *(Continued)*

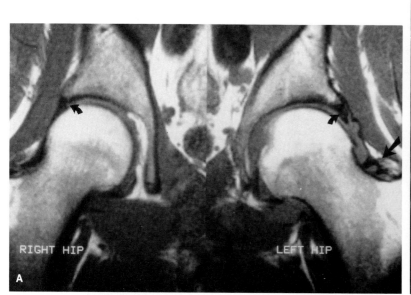

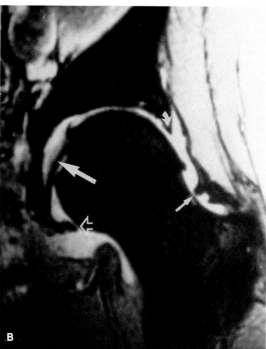

FIGURE 3–83. Normal labral anatomy. (**A**) A T1-weighted coronal image shows the low signal intensity triangular-shaped acetabular labrum (*curved arrow*) and the iliofemoral ligament (*straight arrow*). (TR, 600 msec; TE, 20 msec.) (**B**) A T2*-weighted image shows the low signal intensity labrum extending from the lateral acetabulum (*curved arrow*), the iliofemoral ligament (*small straight arrow*), the ligamentum teres (*large straight arrow*), and the transverse ligament (*open arrow*). (TR, 400 msec; TE, 20 msec; flip angle, 25°.)

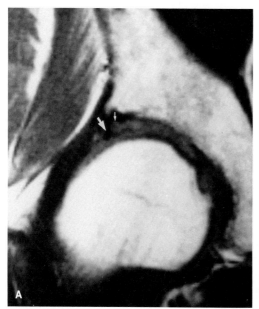

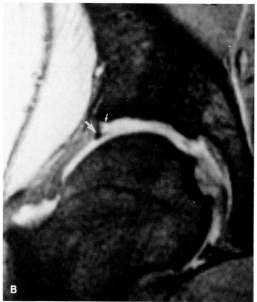

FIGURE 3–84. The normal acetabular labrum appears as a low signal intensity focus (*large arrows*) on (**A**) T1-weighted and (**B**) T2*-weighted images. The adjacent articular cartilage (*small arrows*) appears bright on a T2*-weighted image and should not be mistaken for a tear. (**A**: TR, 600 msec; TE, 20 msec; **B**: TR, 400 msec; TE, 20 msec; flip angle, 25°.)

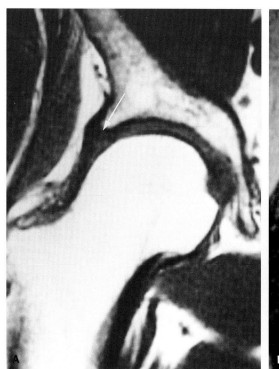

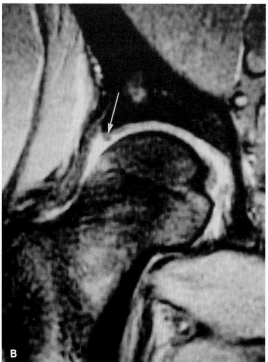

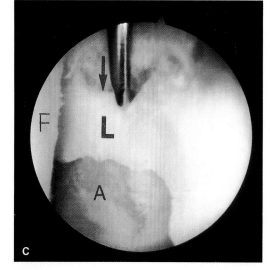

FIGURE 3–85. Coronal (**A**) T1-weighted and (**B**) T2*-weighted images show a blunted and torn acetabular labrum with absence of normal low signal intensity triangular morphology (*arrows*). (**A**: TR, 600 msec; TE, 20 msec; **B**: TR, 400 msec; TE, 20 msec; flip angle, 25°.) (**C**) An arthroscopic view of the labral tear (*arrow*) shows degenerative acetabular articular cartilage in transition from white hyaline cartilage to yellow exposed bone surfaces (F, femoral head; A, acetabulum; L, labrum.)

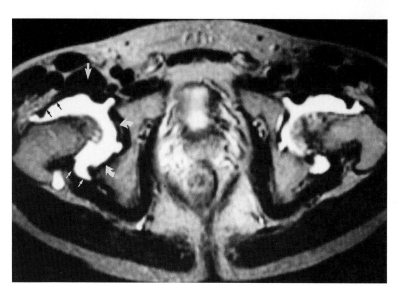

FIGURE 3–86. Distribution of joint effusion at the level of the femoral neck is shown on a T2-weighted axial image. The iliopsoas muscle (*large white arrow*), iliofemoral ligament (*small black arrows*), ischiofemoral (*small white arrows*), and acetabular cortical ridge (*curved arrows*) are identified. (TR, 2000 msec; TE, 80 msec.)

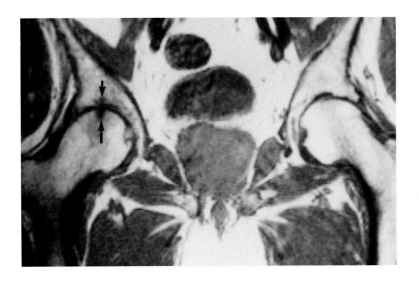

FIGURE 3–87. A T1-weighted coronal image of osteoarthritis reveals superior joint-space narrowing, loss of articular cartilage, and subchondral sclerosis in the opposing surfaces of the femoral head (*large arrow*) and acetabulum (*small arrow*). (TR, 600 msec; TE, 20 msec.)

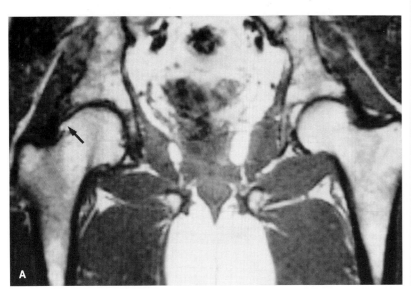

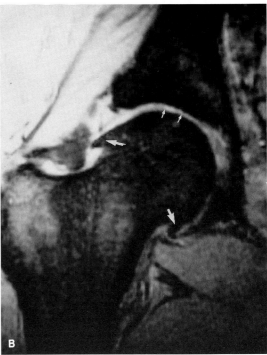

FIGURE 3–88. In osteoarthritis, coronal (**A**) T1-weighted and (**B**) T2*-weighted surface coil images demonstrate superior joint-space narrowing with attenuated articular cartilage (*small arrows*) and subcapital osteophytes (*large arrows*). (**A**: TR, 500 msec; TE, 20 msec; **B**: TR, 400 msec; TE, 20 msec; flip angle, 25°.)

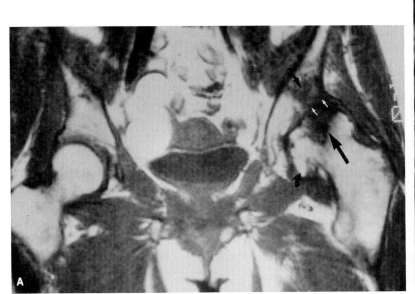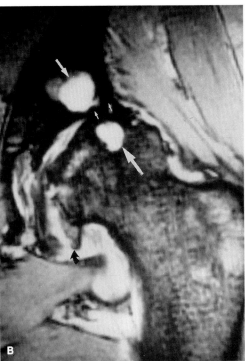

FIGURE 3–89. In osteoarthritis, coronal (**A**) T1-weighted and (**B**) T2*-weighted surface coil images display the advanced changes of osteoarthritis with acetabular and femoral head subchondral cysts (*black arrows*), sclerosis, medial subcapital osteophyte (*curved arrow*), and denuded articular cartilage (*white arrows*). Characteristic superior joint-space narrowing is present. (**A**: TR, 600 msec; TE, 20 msec; **B**: TR, 400 msec; TE, 20 msec; flip angle, 25°.)

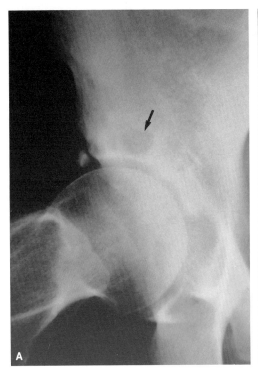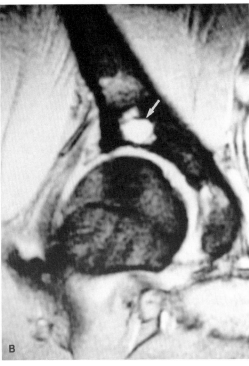

FIGURE 3–90. (**A**) An anteroposterior radiograph and (**B**) a T2*-weighted coronal image show the subchondral, synovial filled cyst of the acetabulum (*i.e.,* Egger's cyst; *arrows*) which is an early sign of osteoarthritis. Synovial fluid contents demonstrate bright signal intensity on a T2*-weighted image. (TR, 400 msec; TE, 20 msec; flip angle, 25°.)

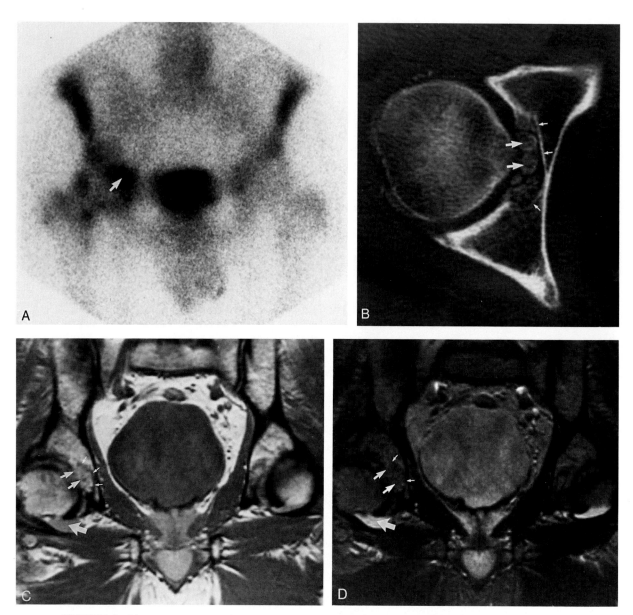

FIGURE 3–91. Synovial chondromatosis (*i.e., osteochondromatosis*). (**A**) A ⁹⁹ᵐTC-MDP bone scan shows uptake of bone tracer in the right hip (*arrow*). (**B**) An axial CT scan reveals multiple intraarticular loose bodies (*large arrows*) contained within the acetabular convexity (*small arrows*). The corresponding coronal (**C**) T1-weighted and (**D**) T2-weighted images demonstrate marrow signal intensity in the synovium-based free fragment (*medium arrows*). The inner wall of the acetabulum is demarcated (*small arrows*). Joint effusion (*large arrows*) generates increased signal intensity with T2 weighting.

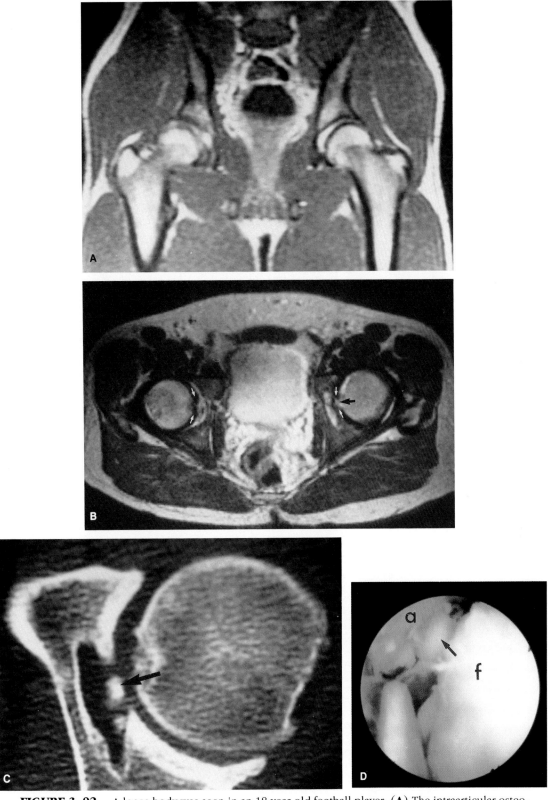

FIGURE 3–92. A loose body was seen in an 18-year-old football player. (**A**) The intraarticular osteo-chondral fragment was not seen on the T1-weighted image. (TR, 600 msec; TE, 20 msec.) (**B**) On the T2-weighted axial image, an intraarticular loose body (*black arrow*) blocks the normal low signal intensity left hip joint space (*white arrows*). (TR, 2000 msec; TE, 80 msec.) (**C**) Cortical detail of the osteochondral fragment (*arrow*) is shown on an 1.5-mm axial CT scan. (**D**) The corresponding arthroscopic view allows identification of the position of the loose body (*arrow*) between the acetabulum (a) and femoral head (f).

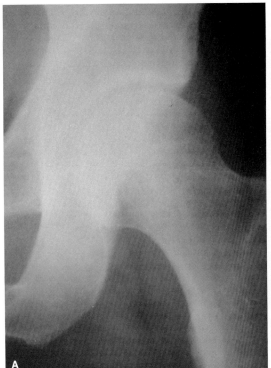

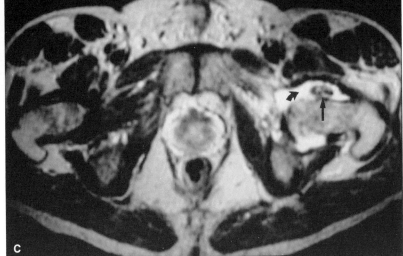

FIGURE 3–93. (**A**) An anteroposterior radiograph of the left hip is negative for a cartilaginous loose body. The intermediate signal intensity cartilaginous intraarticular fragment (*straight arrow*) is revealed within the anterior joint capsule anterior to the femoral neck on (**B**) intermediate-weighted and (**C**) T2-weighted axial images. The corticated low signal intensity peripheral rim cannot be seen. Associated joint effusion demonstrates high signal intensity on the T2-weighted axial image (*curved arrow*). (TR, 2000 msec; TE, 20, 80 msec.)

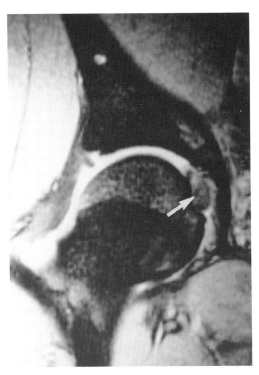

FIGURE 3–94. On a T2*-weighted coronal image, the normal low signal intensity fat pad in the acetabular fossa (*arrow*) mimics an intraarticular loose body. (TR, 400 msec; TE, 20 msec; flip angle, 25°.)

Approximately 50% of patients with rheumatoid arthritis have radiographic evidence of hip disease, although early in the course of the disease plain film radiographs may be negative.[95,96] Radiographic changes in the hip are usually bilateral, although unilateral lesions have been described and may confuse the initial diagnosis.[97] The earliest radiographic findings are symmetric loss of joint space reflecting cartilage loss and periarticular osteopenia. With complete loss of joint space, bony erosion can occur and result in protrusio acetabuli. Protrusio acetabuli may also be associated with steroid therapy.

Treatment. Drug therapy has been useful in decreasing symptoms of rheumatoid arthritis, but has not been proven to alter the natural history of the disease. When drug therapy fails to control the synovitis, synovectomy is an option. When radiographic evidence of significant joint destruction is found, synovectomy is less likely to be beneficial. The role of synovectomy in the hip is not established. When medical management fails to control symptoms in the hip, total hip replacement provides good pain relief.

Magnetic Resonance Imaging. Magnetic resonance examination of the hip joint in patients with juvenile rheumatoid (*i.e.*, chronic) arthritis demonstrates irregularities of the femoral capital epiphysis and growth plate, as well as osseous erosions that may be underestimated on conventional radiographs (Fig. 3–95).[98,99] Thinning of the hyaline articular cartilage can be identified on coronal and sagittal images before radiographic evidence of joint-space narrowing occurs (Fig. 3–96). Synovial hypertrophy, seen as low to intermediate signal intensity, is not a common finding. Rheumatoid arthritis patients on corticosteroid therapy who are at risk for osteonecrosis can be evaluated with MR imaging during acute episodes of pain (Fig. 3–97). Hip protrusio secondary to rheumatoid arthritis is more common than idiopathic protrusio acetabuli (Fig. 3–98).

Ankylosing Spondylitis

Ankylosing spondylitis is an autoimmune disorder associated with HLA-B27. Although not diagnostic, approximately 90% of Caucasian patients with ankylosing spondylitis are HLA-B27–positive. Unlike rheumatoid arthritis, which predominantly affects small joints, ankylosing spondylitis involves the spine and larger joints. The hip is frequently involved and may be the site of initial involvement. Overall, 17% to 35% of patients with ankylosing spondylitis have hip disease.[100] Hip disease is most commonly found in patients with adolescent onset of disease. The role of MR imaging in ankylosing spondylitis has not been defined, and initial evaluation with conventional radiography is the standard for diagnostic evaluation.

Pigmented Villonodular Synovitis

Pigmented villonodular synovitis (PVNS) results from an abnormal proliferation of synovial cells. The etiology is unknown. Although similar lesions can be induced experimentally in animals by repeated intraarticular injections of blood, patients usually deny significant trauma in the clinical situation. Histologically, a hyperplastic layer of synovial cells with large numbers of histiocytes and giant cells can contain hemosiderin, which causes the pigmentation.

The disease usually presents in the third to fifth decade of life, with clinical complaints of joint pain aggravated by activity. Although the knee is the joint most commonly affected, the hip joint may also be involved. The diagnosis can be difficult, and delay in diagnosis is common. In a study by Chung and Janes, the delay in diagnosis ranged from 2.5 to 11 years after the onset of symptoms.[101]

Early in the disease, radiographs are often negative. Lateral, multiple cystic areas can be seen in the acetabulum and femoral head and neck. Unlike the cysts in osteoarthritis, cysts in ankylosing spondylitis are often located away from the areas of maximum weight bearing. Arthrography can be very helpful diagnostically. On aspiration, blood-stained yellow joint fluid is noted. The arthrogram usually demonstrates a large joint space with many irregularities.

The presence of hemosiderin in a hemorrhagic effusion or in PVNS of the hip can be detected with high sensitivity with MR using T1-weighted and T2*-weighted images (Fig. 3–99).[2,102] It may be difficult, however, to differentiate hemorrhagic effusion or hemorrhagic synovium from the repeated bouts of hemosiderin deposition that occur in PVNS. The MR characteristics of PVNS reflect the proportions of hemorrhage, hemosiderin, fibrous tissue, inflamed synovium, and effusion. Thus, low-to-intermediate increased signal intensity areas may be defined on T2-weighted, T2*-weighted, or STIR images (Fig. 3–100).

Synovectomy is the treatment of choice. Radiation is now used sparingly and reserved for recurrent lesions or incomplete resections.[103] Eventually, articular cartilage damage may necessitate a salvage procedure. Arthrodesis or total joint replacement are viable alternatives, depending on the patient.

Amyloid Hip

Patients on long-term hemodialysis are at risk for an osteoarthropathy that has been reported to affect the hand, wrist, and less commonly, the spine.[2,104] Large cystic erosions have also been observed in the hip. These lesions are thought to represent a spectrum of amyloid (*i.e.*, β-microglobulin) deposition occurring in synovium, tendons, and cysts. In a chronic hemodialysis patient with amyloid of the hips, MR examination reveals intermediate

(text continues on page 134)

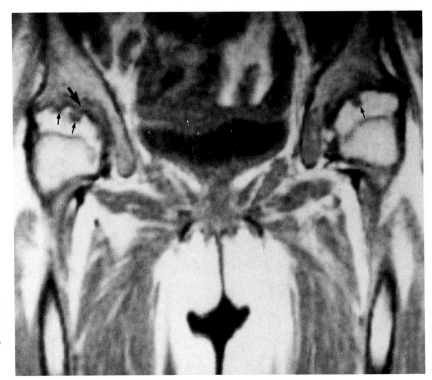

FIGURE 3–95. A T1-weighted coronal image of the hips showing low signal intensity subchondral cysts (*small arrows*) and denuded intermediate signal intensity hyaline articular cartilage (*large arrow*) is characteristic of juvenile chronic arthritis. (TR, 800 msec; TE, 20 msec.)

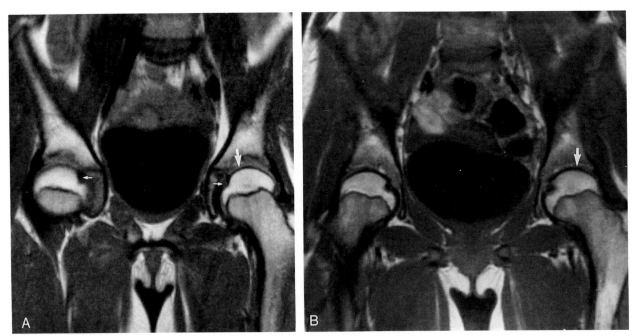

FIGURE 3–96. Early juvenile chronic arthritis. (**A**) T1-weighted coronal images of normal, age-matched control hips in a 9-year-old child with intact, intermediate signal intensity articular cartilage (*large arrow*). Normal low signal intensity fovea are present (*small arrows*). (**B**) A T1-weighted coronal image shows attenuated articular cartilage in the early stages of juvenile rheumatoid arthritis (*arrow*). (TR, 600 msec; TE, 20 msec.)

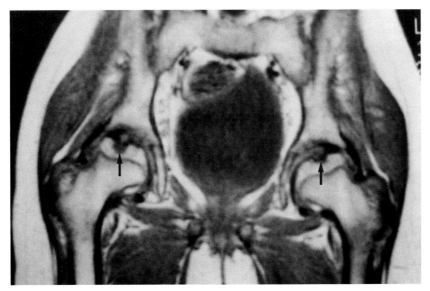

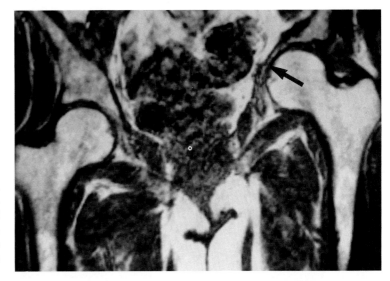

FIGURE 3–97. This T1-weighted image shows bilateral osteonecrosis in a juvenile rheumatoid arthritis patient who is on steroid therapy. Necrotic foci demonstrate low signal intensity on the weight-bearing surface (*arrows*). (TR, 600 msec; TE, 20 msec.)

FIGURE 3–98. A T1-weighted coronal image of idiopathic protrusio acetabuli shows gross medial convex protrusion of acetabular wall into pelvis (*arrow*) with medial position of the acetabular line relative to the ilioischial line. No history of rheumatoid arthritis, ankylosing spondylitis, osteoarthritis, or infection were noted. (TR, 500 msec; TE, 20 msec.)

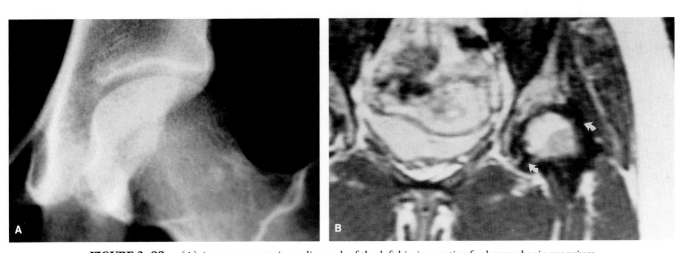

FIGURE 3–99. (**A**) An anteroposterior radiograph of the left hip is negative for hemorrhagic synovium. (**B**) On the T1-weighted image, low signal intensity hemosiderin and thickened synovium (*curved arrows*) are seen. (TR, 600 msec; TE, 20 msec.) Arthroscopy shows (**C**) hemorrhagic synovium (*arrow*) and (**D**) a detached sheet of acetabular cartilage (*arrow*).

(continued)

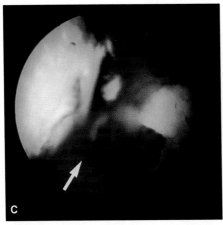

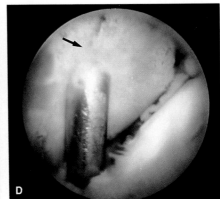

FIGURE 3–99. *(Continued)*

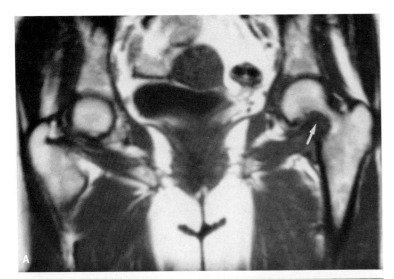

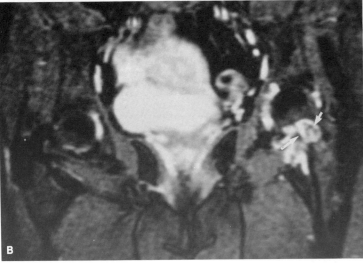

FIGURE 3–100. Pigmented villonodular synovitis presents as cystic erosion (*large arrow*) of the medial femoral neck on (**A**) T1-weighted and (**B**) short TI inversion recovery (STIR) coronal images. Central low signal intensity hemosiderin deposits (*small arrow*) are demonstrated on the STIR image. Synovial inflammation, hemorrhage, and capsular effusion also contribute to signal heterogeneity.

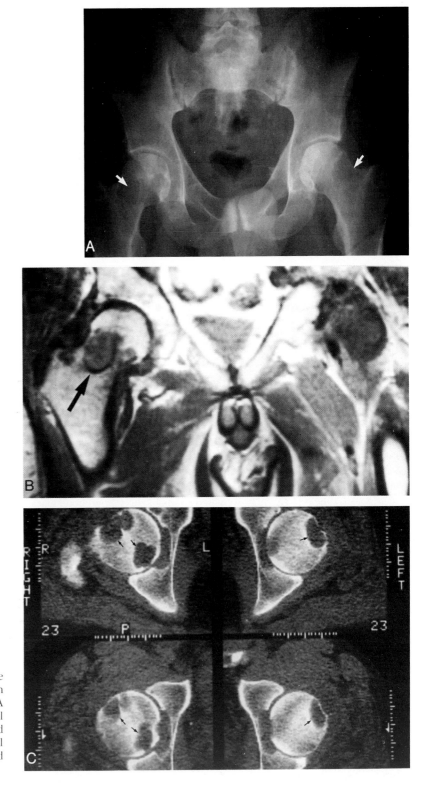

FIGURE 3–101. (**A**) Large cystic erosions of the femoral neck as seen on an anteroposterior radiograph in a patient on chronic renal dialysis (*arrows*). (**B**) A T1-weighted coronal image shows intermediate signal intensity amyloid deposits in the femoral head and neck (*arrow*). (TR, 600 msec; TE, 20 msec.) (**C**) Axial CT shows multiple cystic erosions of the femoral head (*arrows*).

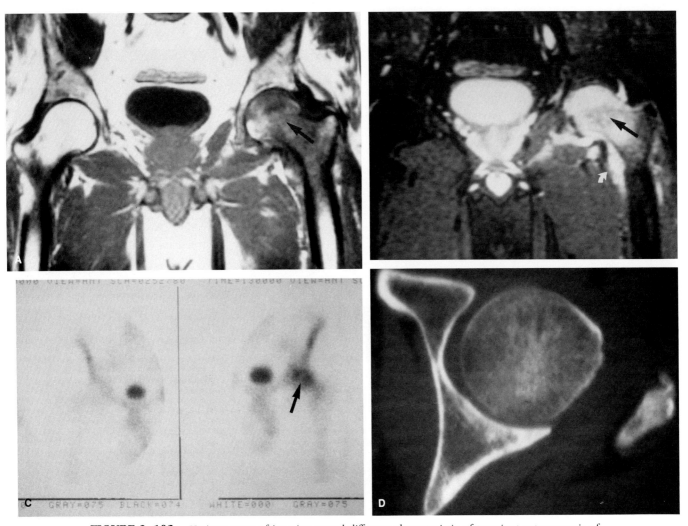

FIGURE 3–102. Various types of imaging reveal different characteristic of transient osteoporosis of the hip. (**A**) A T1-weighted coronal image shows bone marrow edema with diffuse low signal intensity within the left femoral head and neck (*arrow*). (TR, 600 msec; TE, 20 msec.) (**B**) A coronal short TI inversion recovery image displays the increased signal intensity of marrow (*straight arrow*) and associated effusion (*curved arrow*). (TR, 2000 msec; TI, 160 msec; TE, 43 msec.) (**C**) The ⁹⁹ᵐTC-MDP bone scan shows uptake in the left femoral head (*arrow*). (**D**) An axial CT scan demonstrates demineralization of trabecular bone.

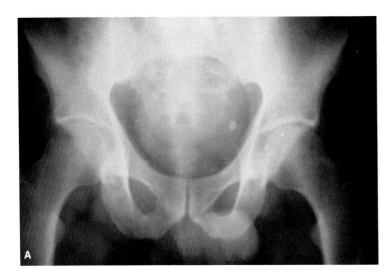

FIGURE 3–103. The appearance of transient osteoporosis of the hips is similar to that of avascular necrosis in imaging. (**A**) On an anteroposterior radiograph of the pelvis, subtle demineralization of right femoral head can be seen. (**B**) A ⁹⁹ᵐTC-MDP bone scan shows increased uptake (*arrow*) in the right femoral head and neck. (**C**) On a T1-weighted coronal image, low signal intensity alteration of fat marrow (*curved arrow*) is seen diffusely throughout right femoral head and neck. A small area of decreased signal in the left femoral head may represent the initial focus of osteonecrosis (*straight arrow*). However, patient's symptoms resolved within 4 months. (TR, 600 msec; TE, 20 msec.) (**D**) A coronal short TI inversion recovery image demonstrates high signal intensity marrow hyperemia (*curved arrow*). An associated joint effusion is present (*straight arrows*), and no osteonecrosis developed on follow up examination. (TR, 2000 msec; TI, 160 msec; TE, 43 msec.)

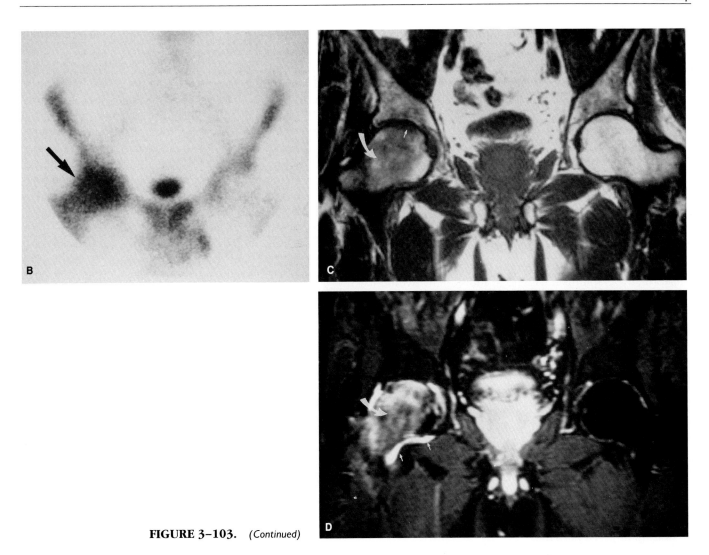

FIGURE 3–103. *(Continued)*

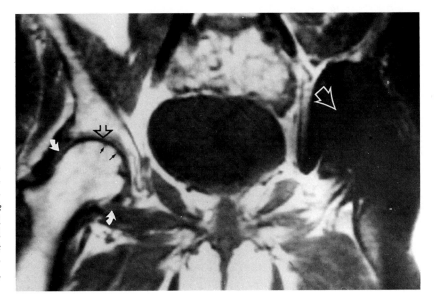

FIGURE 3–104. A T1-weighted image in degenerative osteoarthritis of the right hip shows superior joint-space narrowing, attenuated intermediate signal intensity articular cartilage (*open black arrow*), and small low signal intensity subchondral cysts (*straight arrows*). Signal void from the total hip prosthesis occurred (*open white arrow*). There is minimal joint effusion, which demonstrates intermediate signal intensity (*curved arrows*). (TR, 600 msec; TE, 20 msec.)

signal intensity masses in the femoral head and neck on T1-weighted images (Fig. 3–101). Only minimal increase in signal intensity occurs on T2-weighted images. Magnetic resonance examination also reveals an associated soft tissue component not noticeable on plain radiographs.

Miscellaneous Disorders of the Hip

Gaucher's Disease

Gaucher's disease is a rare hereditary disorder of lipid metabolism resulting in an accumulation of glucocerebroside in the reticuloendothelial system. The adult chronic non-neuropathic form can present at any age. In this form, hypersplenism with bone and skin involvement is present. The femur is the most common bone involved, and the hip joint is the most common symptomatic joint. Histologic sections demonstrate foamy histiocytes in marrow biopsies. Clinically, patients present with bone pain, and the picture can be confused with osteomyelitis. It is not uncommon for patients with Gaucher's disease to present with a low-grade fever as well as an elevated sedimentation rate and white blood cell count. In addition, on physical examination, erythema in the hip or thigh region may be found. Actual infection is rare and usually iatrogenic. Avascular necrosis of the femoral head is a common complication in these patients and often necessitates joint replacement, the results of which are not reliable. A thick, fibrous membrane often forms at the bone–cement interface and may lead to early aseptic loosening in these patients.

In addition to the usefulness of MR imaging in identifying complicating AVN of the femoral head, marrow changes seen in Gaucher's disease of the pelvis and femur can be characterized by coarse inhomogeneity of marrow on T1-weighted images and increased signal intensity on STIR fat-suppression images.

Transient Osteoporosis of the Hip

Transient osteoporosis of the hip is a rare disorder that was originally described in women in the third trimester of pregnancy.[105] Since then, it also has been described in both men and nonpregnant women.[106,107] The cause is unknown, but its similarity to reflex sympathetic dystrophy suggests a neurogenic origin.[106] The disease may be bilateral in men, but in women the left hip is almost exclusively involved. The disease is self-limited, but may take months to resolve. The patients presents with hip pain and limp in the absence of infection or trauma. On physical examination, hip motion is limited, and passive range of motion is painful. Treatment, which can include steroids, nonsteroidal anti-inflammatory drugs, and nonweight bearing or partial weight bearing, is provided on the basis of symptoms, and recovery can be expected.

Transient osteoporosis of the hip must be differentiated from tuberculosis, stress fracture, AVN, malignancy, synovial chondromatosis, and PVS. The laboratory evaluation is unremarkable except for intermittent elevation in the sedimentation rate. Radiographs reveal osteopenia around the hip joint, but these changes may lag 3 to 6 weeks behind the development of groin pain. Radiographic changes frequently develop after positive findings are made on bone scintigraphy, which shows intense homogeneous uptake within the femoral head and the neck. Although demineralization is present in the active phase of the disease, the radiographic picture eventually returns to normal. The pain resolves, and motion is restored.

Magnetic resonance imaging has been used to characterize a low signal intensity pattern in transient osteoporosis of the hip on T1-weighted images and uniform increased signal intensity on T2-weighted or STIR images (Fig. 3–102). Associated joint effusions are commonly seen on T2-weighted and STIR images.[108,109] Resolution of clinical and magnetic resonance abnormalities have been reported within 6 to 10 months. Histopathologic evidence of increased bone turnover and a mild inflammatory reaction are found on biopsy. The signal intensity changes in transient osteoporosis of the hip are thus thought to be related to an increased amount of free water. Extension of marrow involvement to the epiphysis and lack of soft tissue involvement are characteristic on MR imaging. The MR findings in preosteonecrosis marrow edema, reflex sympathetic dystrophy, and regional migratory osteoporosis may be similar to those described for transient osteoporosis of the hip (Fig. 3–103).

Joint Prostheses

Metallic total joint prostheses or arthroplasties generate sufficient low signal intensity artifact to prevent an accurate determination of component loosening or infection (Fig. 3–104).[110,111] Proximal and medial migration of the prosthesis into the pelvis, however, which complicates prosthetic revision and replacement, can be assessed by MR imaging. In such instances, proximity to neurovascular structures can be assessed without invasive angiography.

REFERENCES

1. Fishman EK, et al. Multiplanar (MPR) imaging of the hip. Radiographics 1986;6:7.
2. Stoller DW, Genant HK. Magnetic resonance imaging of the knee and hip. Arthritis Rheum 1990;33(3):441.
3. Pitt MJ, Lund PJ, Speer DP. Imaging of the pelvis and hip. Orthop Clin North Am 1990;21(3):545.

4. Porter BA, et al. Low field STIR imaging of avascular necrosis, marrow edema, and infarction. Radiology 1987;165:83.

5. Gillepsy T III, et al. Magnetic resonance imaging of osteonecrosis. Radiol Clin North Am 1986;24:193.

6. Berquist TH, ed. Imaging of orthopedic trauma and surgery. Philadelphia: WB Saunders, 1986:181.

7. Wrazidlo W, Schneider S, et al. Imaging of the hip joint hyaline cartilage with MR tomography using a gradient echo sequence with fat-water phase coherence. ROFO 1990;152(1):56.

8. Johnson ND, Wood BP, et al. MR imaging anatomy of the infant hip. AJR 1989;153(1):127.

9. Bos CF, et al. A correlative study of MR images and cryo-sections of the neonatal hip. Surg Radiol Anat 1990;12(1):43.

10. Steinberg MA. Management of avascular necrosis of the femoral head—an overview. In: Bassett FH, ed. Instructional Course Lectures, 1988;37:41.

11. Jones JP. Fat embolism and osteonecrosis. Orthop Clin North Am 1985;16:595.

12. Cruess RL. Osteonecrosis of bone: current concepts as to etiology and pathogenesis. Clin Orthop 1986;208:30.

13. Gotschalk F. Indications and results of intertrochanteric osteotomy in osteonecrosis of the femoral head. Clin Orthop 1989;249:219.

14. Jacobs B. Epidemiology of traumatic and nontraumatic osteonecrosis. Clin Orthop 1978;130:51.

15. Mitchell DG, et al. Femoral head avascular necrosis: correlation of MR imaging, radiographic staging, radionuclide imaging and clinical findings. Radiology 1987;162:709.

16. Beltran J, et al. Femoral head avascular necrosis: MR imaging with clinical-pathologic and radionuclide correlation. Radiology 1988;166:215.

17. Mitchell MD, et al. Avascular necrosis of the hip: comparison on MR, CT and scintigraphy. AJR 1986;147:67.

18. Glickstein MR, et al. Avascular necrosis versus other diseases of the hip: sensitivity of MR imaging. Radiology 1988;169(1):213.

19. Shuman WP, et al. MR imaging of avascular necrosis of the femoral head: value of small-field-of-view sagittal surface-coil images. AJR 1988;150:1073.

20. Ficat R. Treatment of avascular necrosis of the femoral head in the hip. Proceedings of the 11th Open Scientific Meeting of the Hip Society. St. Louis: CV Mosby, 1983;279.

21. Ficat RP, Arlet J. Necrosis of the femoral head. In: Hungerford DS, ed: Ischemia and necrosis of the bone. Baltimore: Williams & Williams, 1980.

22. Jones JP. Osteonecrosis. In: McCarthy DJ, ed. Arthritis and allied conditions. 10th ed. Philadelphia: Lea & Febiger, 1985:1356.

23. Springfield DS, Enneking WF. Idiopathic aseptic necrosis. In: Bones and joints. Baltimore: Williams & Williams, 1976:61.

24. Fishman EK, et al. Multiplanar (MPR) imaging of the hip. RadioGraphics 1986;6:7.

25. Dee R, et al. Ischemic necrosis of the femoral head. In: Dee R, ed. Principles of orthopaedic practice. vol 2. New York: McGraw-Hill, 1989:1357.

26. Markisz JA, et al. Segmental patterns of avascular necrosis of the femoral heads: early detection with MR imaging. Radiology 1987;162:717.

27. Steinberg MD, Hayken GD, Steinberg DR. The conservative management of avascular necrosis of the femoral head. In: Arlet J, Ficat RP, Hungerford DS, eds. Bone circulation. Baltimore: Williams & Wilkins, 1984:334.

28. Bonfiglio M, Voke E. Aseptic necrosis of the femoral head and nonunion of the femoral neck. J Bone Joint Surg [Am] 1968;50:48.

29. Camp JF, Colwell CW. Core decompression of the femoral head for osteonecrosis. J Bone Joint Surg [Am] 1986;68:1213.

30. Hungerford DS. Bone marrow pressure, venography, and core decompression in ischemic necrosis of the femoral head. In: Proceedings of the Seventh Open Scientific Meeting of the Hip Society. St. Louis: CV Mosby, 1979:218.

31. Marcus ND, Enneking WF, Massam RA. The silent hip in idiopathic aseptic necrosis: treatment by bone grafting. J Bone Joint Surg [Am] 1973;55:1351.

32. Steinberg MD, Brighton CT, et al. Osteonecrosis of the femoral head: results of core decompression and grafting with and without electrical stimulation. Clin Orthop 1989;249:199.

33. Stulberg BN, Bauer TW, Belhobek GH. Making core decompression work. Clin Orthop 1990;261:186.

34. Sugioka YU, Kaysuki T, Hotokebuchi T. Transtrochanteric rotational osteotomy of the femoral head for treatment of osteonecrosis. Clin Orthop 1982;169:115.

35. Aaron RK, Lennox D, Bunce GE, Ebert T. The conservative treatment of osteonecrosis of the femoral head. Clin Orthop 1989;249:209.

36. Steinberg MD. Early results in the treatment of avascular necrosis of the femoral head with electrical stimulation. Orthop Clin North Am 1984;15:163.

37. Phemister DB. Treatment of the necrotic head of the femur in adults. J Bone Joint Surg 1949;31A:55.

38. Urbaniak J, Nunley JA, Goldner RD, et al. Treatment of avascular necrosis of the femoral head by vascularized graft. Presented at 8th Combined Meeting of Orthopedic Associations of the English Speaking World. Washington DC: May 3–8, 1987.

39. Cabanela MD. Bipolar versus total hip arthroplasty for avascular necrosis of the femoral head: a comparison. Clin Orthop 1990;261:59.

40. Lang P, et al. 2.0 T MR imaging of the femoral head in avascular necrosis: histologic correlation (abstr). Sixth Annual Meeting and Exhibition of the Society of Magnetic Resonance in Medicine. New York City: August 17, 1987.

41. Beltran J, et al. Core decompression for avascular necrosis of the femoral head: correlation between long-term results and preoperative MR staging. Radiology 1990;175:533.

42. Mankey M, et al. Comparison of magnetic resonance imaging and bone scan in the early detection of osteonecrosis of the femoral head. Presented to the Academy of Orthopedic Surgeons. January, 1987.

43. Turner DA, et al. Femoral capital osteonecrosis: MR finding of diffuse marrow abnormalities without focal lesions. Radiology 1989;171:135.

44. Stulberg BN, et al. Multimodality approach to osteonecrosis of the femoral head. Clin Orthop 1989;240:181.

45. Genez BM, et al. Early osteonecrosis of the femoral head: detection in high-risk patients with MR imaging. Radiology 1988;168:521.

46. Coleman BG, et al. Radiographically negative avascular necrosis: detection with MR imaging. Radiology 1988;168:525.

47. Wynee-Davies R, Gormley J. The etiology of Perthes disease. J Bone Joint Surg [Br] 1978;60:6.

48. Catterall A, Lloyd-Roberts GC, Wynne-Davies R. Association of Perthes disease with congenital anomalies of the genitourinary tract and inguinal region. Lancet 1971;1:996.

49. Catterall A. The natural history of Perthes disease. J Bone Joint Surg [Br] 1971;53:37.

50. Salter RB, Thompson, GH. Legg-Calvé-Perthes disease: the prognostic significance of the subchondral fracture and a two-group classification of the femoral head involvement. J Bone Joint Surg [Br] 1978;60:6.

51. Green NE, Beauchamp RD, Griffin PD. Epiphyseal extrusion as a prognostic index in Legg-Calvé-Perthes disease. J Bone Joint Surg [Am] 1981;63:900.

52. Cattarall A, Pringle H, Byers, PD, et al. A review of the morphology of Perthes disease. J Bone Joint Surg [Br] 1982;64:269.

53. Dolman CL, Bell HM. The pathology of Legg-Calvé-Perthes syndrome. J Bone Joint Surg [Am] 1973;55:184.

54. Weinstein SL. Legg-Calvé-Perthes disease: results of long-term follow-up. In: The Proceedings of the 13th Open Scientific Meeting of the Hip Society. St Louis: CV Mosby, 1985:28.

55. Easton EJ Jr, et al. Magnetic resonance imaging and scintigraphy in Legg-Perthes's disease: diagnosis, treatment and prognosis. Radiology 1987;165:35.

56. Heuck A, et al. Magnetic resonance imaging in the evaluation of Legg-Perthes' disease. Radiology 1987;165:83.

56a. Rush BH, Bramson RT, Odgen JA. Legg-Calvé-Perthes disease: detection of cartilagenous and synovial changes with MR imaging. Radiology 1988;167:473.

57. Ranner G. Magnetic resonance imaging in children with acute hip pain. Pediatr Radiol 1989;20(1):67.

58. Wilcox PG, Weiner DS, Leighley D. Maturation factors in slipped capital femoral epiphysis. J Pediatr Orthop 1988;8:196.

59. Gelberman RH, Cohen MS, Shaw BA, et al. The association of femoral retroversion with slipped capital femoral epiphysis. J Bone Joint Surg [Am] 1986;68:1000.

60. Agamanolis DP, Weiner DS, Lloyd JK. Slipped capital femoral epiphysis: a pathological study. II. An ultrasound study of 23 cases. J Pediatr Orthop 1985;5:47.

61. Crawford AH. The role of osteotomy in the treatment of slipped capital femoral epiphysis. In: Barr JS, ed. Instruction Course Lectures. vol 38. Las Vegas: American Academy of Orthopaedic Surgeons, 1989:273.

62. Swiontkowski MF. Slipped capital femoral epiphysis. Complications relative to internal fixation. Orthopaedics 1983;6:705.

63. Wiener DS. Bone graft epiphysiodesis in the treatment of slipped capital femoral epiphysis. In: Barr JS, ed. Instruction Course Lectures. vol 38. Las Vegas: American Academy of Orthopaedic Surgeons, 1989:63.

64. Stuhlberg SD, Cordell LD, et al. Unrecognized childhood hip disease: a major cause of idiopathic osteoarthritis of the hip. In: The hip: proceedings of the Hip Society. St Louis: CV Mosby, 1975:212.

65. Johnson ND, et al. Complex infantile and congenital hip dislocation: assessment with MR imaging. Radiology 1988;168(1):151.

66. Dunn PM. The anatomy and pathology of congenital dislocation of the hip. Clin Orthop 1976;119:23.

67. Lang P, et al. Three-dimensional digital displays in congenital dislocation of the hip: preliminary experience. J Pediatr Orthop 1989;9(5):532.

68. Lang P, et al. Three-dimensional CT and MR imaging in congenital dislocation of the hip: technical considerations. Radiology 1987;165:279.

69. Hillman JS, et al. Proximal femoral focal deficiency: radiologic analysis of 49 cases. Radiology 1987;165:769.

70. Ehman RI, Berquist TH. Magnetic resonance imaging of musculoskeletal trauma. Radiol Clin North Am 1986;24:291.

71. Fisher MK, et al. MRI of the normal and pathological musculoskeletal system. Magn Reson Imaging 1986;4:491.

72. Doons GC, et al. MR imaging of intramuscular hemorrhage. J Comput Assist Tomogr 1985;9:908.

73. Cleaves EN. Fracture avulsion of the anterior superior iliac spine of the ilium. J Bone Joint Surg [Am] 1938;20:490.

74. Milch H. Avulsion fracture of the tuberosity of the ischium. J Bone Joint Surg [Am] 1926;8:832.

75. Rogge EA, Romano RL. Avulsion of the ischial apophysis. J Bone Joint Surg [Am] 1956;38:442.

76. Tile M, Kellam J, Joyce M. Fractures of the acetabulum, classification, management protocol and results of treatment. J Bone Joint Surg [Br] 1985;67:173.

77. Fairclough J, et al. Bone scanning for suspected hip fractures. Radiology 1987;164:886.

78. Griffiths HJ, et al. Computed tomography in the management of acetabular fractures. Radiology 1985;154:567.

79. Devas M. Stress fractures. New York: Churchill-Livingston, 1975.

80. Gilbert RS, Johnson HA. Stress fractures in military recruits: a review of twelve years' experience. Milit Med 1966;131:716.

81. Blickenstaff LD, Morris JM. Fatigue fracture of the femoral neck. J Bone Joint Surg [Am] 1966;48:1031.

82. Morris JM, Blickenstaff LD. Fatigue fractures. Springfield, IL: Charles C Thomas, 1967.

82a. DeLee JC. Dislocations and fracture-dislocations of the hip. In: Rockwood CA Jr, Green DP, eds. Fractures and dislocations. 2nd ed. Philadelphia: JB Lippincott, 1984:1287.

83. Tile M. Fractures of the acetabulum. In: Steinberg ME, ed. The hip and its disorders. Philadelphia: WB Saunders, 1991:201.

84. Deutsch AL, et al. Occult fractures of the proximal femur: MR imaging. Radiology 1989;170(1,pt1):113.

85. Berger PE, et al. MRI demonstration of radiographically occult fractures: what have we been missing? RadioGraphics 1989;9(3):407.

86. Stafford SA, et al. MRI in stress fracture. AJR 1986;147:553.

87. Berquist TH, Coventry MB. The pelvis and hips. In: Berquist TH, ed. Imaging of orthopaedic trauma and surgery. Philadelphia: WB Saunders, 1986:181.

88. Richardson P, et al. CT detection of cortical fracture of the femoral head associated with posterior hip dislocation. AJR 1990;155:93.

89. Tehranzadah J, et al. Osteochondral impaction of the femoral head associated with hip dislocation: CT study in 35 patients. AJR 1990;155:1049.

90. Mitchell DG, et al. MRI of joint fluid in the normal and ischemic hip. AJR 1986;146:1215.

91. Li KC, et al. MRI in osteoarthritis of the hip: gradations of severity. Magn Reson Imaging 1988;6(3):229.

91a. Mokes SR, Volger JB, Spritzer CE, et al. Herniation pits of the femoral neck: appearance at MR imaging. Radiology 1989;172:231.

92. Haller J, et al. Juxtaacetabular ganglionic (or synovial) cysts: CT and MR features. J Comput Assist Tomogr 1989;13(6):976.

93. Szypryt P, et al. Synovial chondromatosis of the hip joint presenting as a pathological fracture. Br J Radiol 1986;59:399.

94. Schurman DJ, Palathumpat MC, et al. Biochemistry and antigenicity of osteoarthritic and rheumatoid cartilage. J Orthop Res 1986;4:255.

94a. Arnett FC, Edworthy SM, et al. The American Rheumatism Association 1987 revised criteria for the clarification of rheumatoid arthritis. Arthritis Rheum 1988;31:315.

95. Duthie R, Harris C. A radiographic and clinical survey of hip joints in seropositive rheumatoid arthritis. Acta Orthop Scand 1969;40:346.

96. Glick EN, Mason RM, Wely WG. Rheumatoid arthritis affecting the hip joint. Ann Rheum Dis 1963;22:416.

97. Resnick D, Williams D, Weisman MH, Slaughter L. Rheumatoid arthritis and pseudo-rheumatoid arthritis in calcium pyrophosphate crystal deposition disease. Radiology 1981;140:615.

98. Stoller DW. MRI in juvenile (chronic) arthritis. Charleston, SC: Presented to Association of University Radiologists, March 22, 1987.

99. Senac MO Jr, et al. MR imaging in juvenile rheumatoid arthritis. AJR 1988;150(4):873.

100. Wilkinson M, Bywaters EGL. Clinical features and course of ankylosing spondylitis as seen in a follow-up of 222 hospital referred cases. Ann Rheum Dis 17:209, 1958.

101. Chung SMK, Janes JM. Diffuse pigmented villonodular synovitis of the hip joint. J Bone Joint Surg [Am] 1965;47:293.

102. Jelinek JS, et al. Imaging of pigmented villonodular synovitis with emphasis on MR imaging. AJR 1989;152(2):337.

103. McMaster PE. Pigmented villonodular synovitis with invasion of bone. J Bone Joint Surg [Am] 1960;42:1170.

104. Brancaccio D, et al. Amyloid arthropathy in patients on regular dialysis: a newly discovered disease. Radiology 1987;65(P): 335.

105. Curtiss PH, Kincaid WE. Transitory demineralization of the hip in pregnancy. J Bone Joint Surg [Am] 1959;41:1327.

106. Lequesne M. Transient osteoporosis of the hip. A nontraumatic variety of Sudeck's atrophy. Ann Rheum Dis 1968;27:463.

107. Pantazopoulos T, Exarchou E, Hartofilikidis-Garofalidis G. Idiopathic transient osteoporosis of the hip. J Bone Joint Surg [Am] 1973;55:315.

108. Bloem JL. Transient osteoporosis of the hip: MR imaging. Radiology 1988;167(3):753.

109. Kerr R. Transient osteoporosis of the hip. Orthopaedics 1990; 13(4):485.

110. Feldman F, et al. MR imaging of soft-tissue reaction to prostheses. Radiology 1987;165(P):84.

111. Laakman RW, et al. MR imaging in patients with metallic implants. Radiology 1985;157:711.

CHAPTER 4

David W. Stoller
W. Dilworth Cannon, Jr.
Lesley J. Anderson

The Knee

Significant advances have been made in magnetic resonance (MR) imaging of the knee since its initial application in the evaluation of the meniscus, and routine examinations now encompass a wide spectrum of internal knee derangements and articular disorders.[1-4] A noninvasive modality, MR imaging has virtually replaced conventional arthrography in the evaluation of the menisci and the cruciate ligaments. Knee arthrography is presently performed to evaluate loosening of total joint arthroplasty and to document communication with an atypical popliteal cyst when not seen on MR imaging.

Radial imaging and three-dimensional (3D) volume techniques have demonstrated the versatility of MR imaging in the evaluation of meniscal tears (Fig. 4–1). Images of meniscal tears have also been reformatted in a curved, sagittal technique, allowing the C-shaped meniscus to be unraveled in the sagittal plane (Fig. 4–2). With MR imaging, the anatomic and pathologic definition of soft tissue, ligaments, and cartilage is superior to that seen with computed tomography (CT). Due to the multiplanar and thin section capabilities of MR imaging, combined with the ability to evaluate subchondral bone and marrow, MR imaging is now being recommended instead of CT for the evaluation of tibial plateau fractures of the knee.

The introduction of kinematic MR techniques provides a new perspective on assessing the biomechanics of the patellofemoral joint and the normal function of ligamentous structures of the knee (Fig. 4–3). Fast-scan techniques, including 3D Fourier transform (FT) volume imaging with submillimeter capability can be acquired with as many as 120 images through the knee joint in a single acquisition. These images can be reformatted retrospectively in any orthogonal or oblique plane (Fig. 4–4).

Magnetic resonance imaging is unique in its ability to evaluate the internal structure as well as the surface of the meniscus.[5] With conventional arthrography, intraarticular injection of contrast permits visualization of the surface anatomy, but does not allow delineation of fibro-cartilage structure or subchondral bone. Intravenous gadolinium contrast (Gd-DTPA) MR imaging has been used to enhance areas of pannus in images of inflammatory arthritis. More precise evaluation of articular cartilage surfaces and meniscal repairs may be facilitated by the intraarticular administration of gadolinium.

IMAGING PROTOCOLS FOR THE KNEE

A routine MR examination with imaging in the axial, sagittal, and coronal planes can be performed in less than 10 minutes of acquisition time. Magnetic resonance stress testing of ligamentous structures (*e.g.,* MR anterior drawer test; varus and valgus stress test) may increase the accuracy of joint evaluations. Manipulation of the knee joint—necessary to perform an arthrogram—is not required in MR studies. This is particularly important in patients who have sustained trauma with associated joint effusions and who cannot tolerate physical examination without anesthesia. Three-dimensional rendering techniques permit disarticulation of specified areas of pathology, generating surface, and volume detail (Fig. 4–5). The soft-tissue discrimination possible with MR imaging differentiates cortex, marrow, ligaments, tendons, muscle, synovium, and vascular and cartilage elements; this is not possible with conventional radiographic techniques.[6,7]

Routine Protocols

A circumferential extremity coil provides uniform signal-to-noise ratio (SNR) across the knee, without the posterior to anterior signal drop-off observed in imaging with planar surface coils (Fig. 4–6). In the evaluation of internal knee derangements, routine protocols include T1-weighted images in the axial, sagittal, and coronal planes. T2*-weighted two-dimensional (2D) or 3DFT gradient-echo sagittal images replace or complement routine T1-weighted sagittal images in evaluation of the meniscus and cruciate ligaments. Although less sensitive to the spectrum of meniscal degenerations, a conventional T2-weighted spin-echo protocol can be obtained in the sagittal plane. T2*-weighted axial images are used to assess articular cartilage in the patellofemoral joint in the evaluation of chondromalacia. T1-weighted images with a repetition time (TR) of 400 to 600 milliseconds (msec) and an echo time (TE) of 15 to 20 msec are obtained with an acquisition matrix of 256 × 256, a field of view (FOV) of 14 to 16 cm, and 1 NEX (number of excitations). Gradient-echo images are acquired at an acquisition matrix of 128, 192, or 256. TI can be reduced by obtaining 3D volume acquisitions with 64 or 128 images and an acquisition matrix of 192. A 16-cm FOV provides adequate imaging of the quadriceps patellar mechanism in the sagittal plane. In pediatric patients, the FOV should be 12 cm or less to increase spatial resolution.

Imaging Planes

The axial acquisition through the patellofemoral joint is used as an initial localizer for subsequent sagittal and coronal plane images. Meniscal and cruciate pathology is primarily evaluated on sagittal plane images, whereas the medial and lateral collateral ligaments (MCL; LCL) are displayed on coronal plane images. The MCL and LCL can be routinely identified on 1-mm 3DFT sagittal images. Cruciate anatomy and pathology is secondarily evaluated in the coronal and axial imaging planes. Meniscal lesions should be secondarily evaluated in the coronal plane.

Patient Positioning

Imaging studies are performed with the patient in the supine position and the knee placed in 10° to 15° of external rotation to realign the anterior cruciate ligament (ACL) parallel with the sagittal imaging plane. The rotation of the knee does not need to be changed for imaging in either the axial or the coronal planes. The ACL can be seen on 1- to 3-mm 3DFT sagittal images without external rotation of the leg.

Slice Thickness

Axial, sagittal, and coronal plane images are obtained in 5-mm sections without an interslice gap. Thinner sections (*i.e.,* 3 mm) do not increase the accuracy of detecting meniscal pathology. In pediatric patients, however, 3-mm slices allow optimum medial-to-lateral joint coverage in the sagittal plane and anterior-to-posterior coverage

in the coronal plane. In cases of inadequate imaging of the ACL, 3-mm oblique sagittal images can be obtained through the ACL, which is identified on the axial localizer, to optimize the display of its femoral and tibial attachments.[8] Short TRs (*i.e.,* 300 to 400 msec) minimize the TI for this additional sequence. Three-dimensional FT volume protocols using a 1- to 2-mm slice thickness, however, obviate the need for oblique cruciate imaging.

T2, T2*, and Short TI Inversion Recovery Protocols: Application and Techniques

Acute trauma, arthritis, infection, and neoplasia require T2- or T2*-weighted images. Conventional T2-weighted images are generated with a TR of 2000 msec; a TE of 20, 80 msec; a 256 × 192 on 128 acquisition matrix, and 1 NEX. The introduction of fast spin-echo techniques may increase the routine application of long TR/TE protocols with significant reduction in TI. Effective T2 or T2* contrast can be obtained with refocused 2DFT gradient-echo images with a flip angle of less than 90°, TR of 400 to 600 msec, TE of 15 msec, flip angle of 20°, and an acquisition matrix that is 256 × 192. Imaging time can be reduced by using 3DFT gradient-echo volumetric imaging, which can also reduce slice thickness to 0.7 mm. Three-dimensional FT images are acquired with a TR of 55 msec, TE of 15 msec, and flip angle of 10°. These images can be reformatted without loss of spatial resolution.[9]

T2*-weighted radial images of the knee, which can be obtained simultaneously with coronal or sagittal images, demonstrate meniscocapsular anatomy and have been used to evaluate peripheral meniscal tears. T2 or T2* contrast is helpful in highlighting ligamentous edema in collateral ligaments in the coronal imaging plane or cruciate ligaments in the sagittal imaging plane. Sagittal images provide the most information in early synovial reactions and cartilage erosions, as seen in patients with degenerative or inflammatory arthritis. Posterior femoral condylar defects, however, are best displayed on posterior coronal images. Trabecular bone contusions and fractures are identified with greater sensitivity on short TI inversion recovery (STIR) images than on T2- or T2*-weighted scans.

For STIR protocols, we typically use a TR of 1400 to 2000 msec, a TE of 43 msec, and a TI of 140 to 160 msec. Neoplastic lesions, both benign and malignant, require either T1- and T2- or T1- and T2*-weighted images in the axial plane to demonstrate compartment and neurovascular anatomy. T2*-weighted fast-scan sagittal or coronal images delineate the proximal and distal extent of tumor in one image. Fat-suppression or ChemSat pro-

(text continues on page 146)

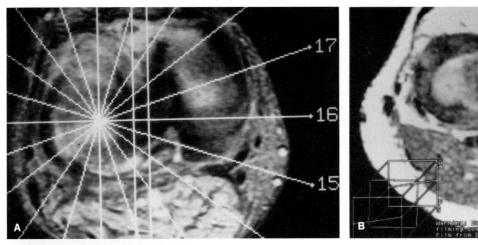

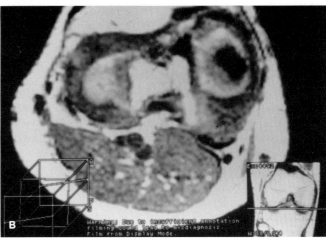

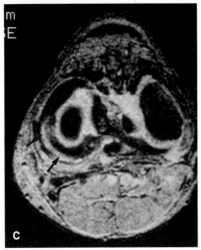

FIGURE 4–1. (**A**) A Localizer indicates radial and sagittal prescription locations. (**B**) This retrospectively formatted 3D Fourier transform (FT) 1-mm axial image was made in the plane of the menisci. (**C**) A direct 0.7-mm 3DFT T2*-weighted image shows a high signal intensity longitudinal tear of the medial meniscus (*arrow*).

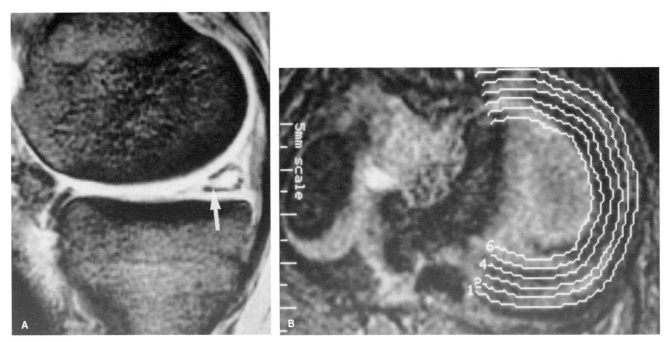

FIGURE 4–2.

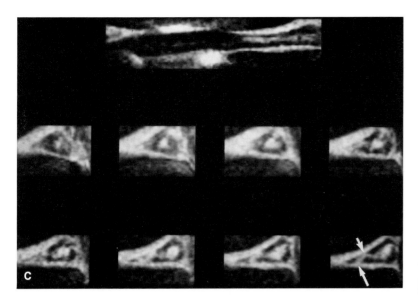

FIGURE 4-2. *(Continued)*

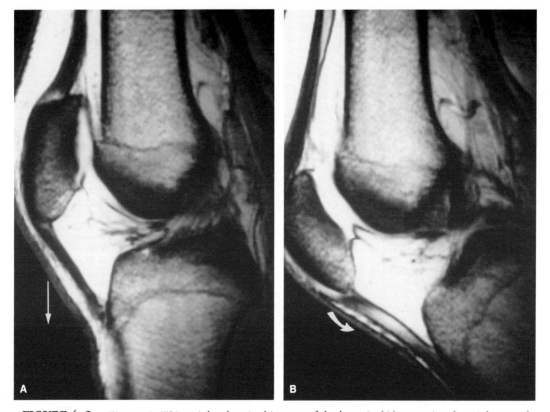

FIGURE 4-3. Kinematic T2*-weighted sagittal images of the knee in (**A**) extension (*straight arrow*) and (**B**) partial knee flexion (*curved arrow*).

FIGURE 4-2. (**A**) A T2*-weighted sagittal image shows a high signal intensity posterior horn medial meniscal tear (*arrow*). (**B**) A 3DFT axial image shows curved sagittal prescriptions designated along parallel meniscal contour lines. (**C**) The corresponding curved sagittal image artificially elongates the meniscal fibrocartilage and tear (*top*). More precise superior (*small arrow*) and inferior (*large arrow*) tear morphology is shown in sections obtained perpendicular to the curved sagittal reformatted image (*middle, bottom*).

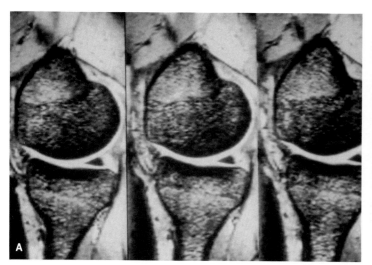

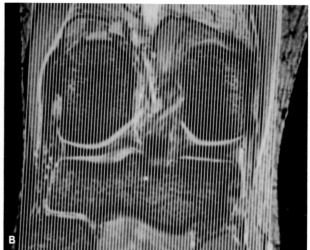

FIGURE 4–4. (**A**) These 0.6-mm sagittal reformatted images were generated from (**B**) a coronal 1-mm 3D Fourier transform volume scan.

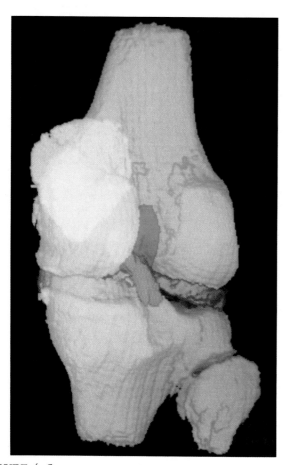

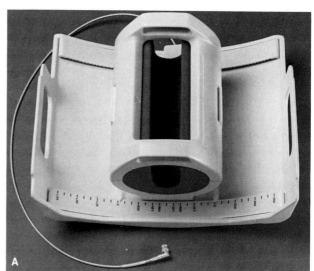

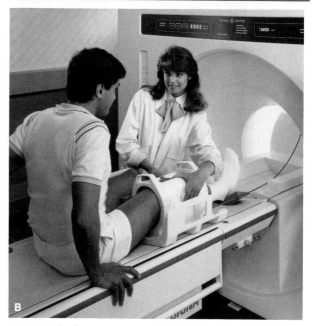

FIGURE 4–5. A 3D MR rendering in a posterior oblique projection shows the anterior cruciate ligament (dark blue), the posterior cruciate ligament (green), and the meniscal structures (yellow).

FIGURE 4–6.

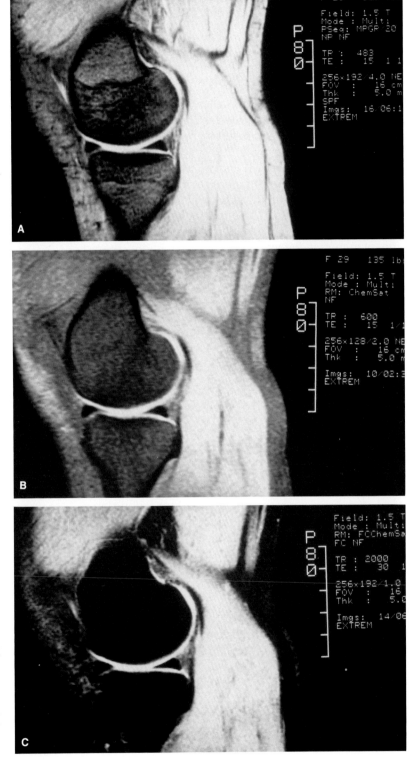

FIGURE 4–7. A comparison of (**A**) T2*-weighted contrast with (**B, C**) fat-saturation protocols. Although marrow fat is of low signal intensity in all images, only the ChemSat images show low signal intensity from all fat-containing tissues (*i.e.,* subcutaneous fat). Note that the longer the TR and TE of the protocol, the greater the degree of fat saturation. ChemSat is used to apply a frequency-selective presaturation pulse to fat before the excitation pulse, destroying the longitudinal magnetization of fat.

FIGURE 4–6. (**A**) A circumferential transmit-and-receive surface coil used in imaging the knee. (**B**) The coil as it is positioned on the patient.

tocols can be used to eliminate fat signal intensity, although T1 and T2 contrast are not additive as on STIR images (Fig. 4–7).

Artifacts and Photography

Popliteal artery pulsation artifacts can be minimized by exchanging the phase- and frequency-encoded directions in the sagittal imaging plane.[10]

Although high-contrast, narrow window-width photography has been used to emphasize or highlight internal signal intensities within the fibrocartilaginous meniscus, we have not found this to be routinely necessary (Fig. 4–8). Gradient-echo images adequately display the spectrum of meniscal degenerations and tear without contrast adjustment.

NORMAL GROSS AND MAGNETIC RESONANCE ANATOMY OF THE KNEE

Axial Images

Axial joint dissection displays the osseous relationships among the patella, femur, and tibia (Fig. 4–9). Circumferential surface anatomy of the menisci and attachments of the cruciate and collateral ligaments is shown with disarticulation of the femur from the tibia (Fig. 4–10). Axial plane images have an important role in routine knee evaluation (Fig. 4–11). Medial and lateral patellar facets and articular cartilage, because of their oblique orientation, are most accurately demonstrated on axial images through the patellofemoral joint. Patellofemoral disease (*i.e.,* chondromalacia) may be over- or underestimated on sagittal images alone. One-millimeter 3DFT axial images have been used to define circumferential meniscal tear patterns and to create 3D composite images using a workstation. Axial plane images are also used as localizers to determine sagittal and coronal coverage when short TR (*i.e.,* 600 msec) sequences are used. Sagittal reformations from axial 3DFT volume acquisitions can be used to display cross-sectional meniscal anatomy. Although the axial plane can be used to display meniscal structure, routine axial images at 5 mm are not sensitive (sections are too thick) to meniscal pathology. Sagittal images, which section the meniscus perpendicular to its surface, provide the best demonstration of internal meniscal anatomy and pathology.

The tibial plateau surface is seen on inferior axial images through the knee joint. The posterior cruciate insertion is displayed on the posterior tibial surface and demonstrates low signal intensity on cross section. The popliteus muscle is seen posterior to the tibia at the level of the superior tibiofibular joint. At the midjoint level, the medial and lateral menisci are seen with uniform low signal intensity. The medial meniscus has an open C-shaped configuration with a narrow anterior horn and wider posterior horn. The lateral meniscus has a more circular shape and consistent width. Three-millimeter or thinner sections will display both menisci on axial images.

The transverse ligament of the knee is seen as a band of low signal intensity connecting the anterior horn to the lateral and medial menisci. It can be identified where it traverses Hoffa's infrapatellar fat pad, which, in contrast to the ligament, demonstrates bright signal intensity.

The semimembranosus and semitendinosus tendons are seen as circular structures of low signal intensity located lateral to the medial head of the gastrocnemius muscle and posterior to the medial tibial plateau. The semimembranosus tendon appears larger than the semitendinosus tendon. The sartorius muscle is elliptical and the gracilis tendon is circular. These muscles are located more medial and posterior than the semimembranosus and semitendinosus, and are in line with the MCL, which crosses the peripheral joint line. Proximal to its insertion on the fibular head, the biceps femoris tendon is positioned anterolateral to the lateral head of the gastrocnemius muscle. The popliteal artery is found anterior to the popliteal vein, anterior to and between the two heads of the gastrocnemius muscle. The popliteal artery is located posterior to the posterior horn of the lateral meniscus and is potentially at risk for injury during meniscectomy.

In cross section, the low signal intensity lateral or fibular collateral ligament may be surrounded by high signal intensity fat. The ACL and posterior cruciate ligament (PCL) insertions can be seen within the intercondylar notch. The ACL can be identified superior to the joint line, 15° to 20° off-axis, in an anteromedial orientation.[11] The PCL is circular in cross section. The origin of the ACL can be seen on the medial aspect of the lateral femoral condyle and the PCL can be seen on the lateral aspect of the medial femoral condyle.

Hoffa's infrapatellar fat pad is bordered by the low signal intensity iliotibial band laterally, the medial retinaculum medially, and the thick patellar tendon anteriorly. The common peroneal nerve is located lateral to the plantaris muscle, demonstrates low-to-intermediate signal intensity, and is encased in fat. At the level of the femoral condyles, the tibial nerve is located posterior to the popliteal vein and demonstrates intermediate signal intensity.

The larger lateral patellar facet and the oblique medial patellar facet are also seen in the axial plane. The thick articular cartilage surfaces of the patella are shown at intermediate signal intensity on T1- and T2-weighted images and at increased signal intensity—but less than surrounding fluid—on T2*-weighted images. Both the medial and lateral patellar retinacular attachments are seen at the level of the patellofemoral joint and are of low signal intensity. Medial and lateral reflections of the suprapatellar bursa should not be mistaken for retinacular attachments or plicae.

Sagittal Images

Sagittal plane dissection displays the components of the medial (Fig. 4–12) and lateral (Fig. 4–13) collateral ligaments and adjacent capsule. The patellofemoral compartment, quadriceps, and patellar tendon are demonstrated on midsagittal gross anatomy (Fig. 4–14). The ACL and PCL are best displayed on sagittal images (Figs. 4–15 and 4–16). The lateral or fibular collateral ligament and the biceps femoris tendon may also be seen in peripheral sagittal sections. Images in the sagittal plane are key in evaluating meniscal anatomy for both degenerations and tears. The MCL is usually not defined in the sagittal plane unless thin section 3DFT volume images are acquired. Complex meniscal and bucket-handle tears may require examination of coronal images to identify displaced meniscal tissue or fragments.

On medial sagittal images, the low signal intensity semimembranosus tendon and intermediate signal muscle are seen posteriorly. The vastus medialis muscle makes up the bulk of the musculature anterior to the medial femoral condyle. On T1-weighted images, fatty (*i.e.,* yellow) marrow demonstrates bright signal intensity, whereas adjacent cortical bone demonstrates uniform low signal intensity. Femoral and tibial hyaline articular cartilage can be seen at intermediate signal intensity on T1- and conventional T2-weighted images, and with bright signal intensity on T2*-weighted images. Anterolateral femoral articular cartilage is particularly thick and is frequently the site of early erosions or attenuation in osteoarthritis. The tibial cortex appears thicker than the femoral cortical bone because of a chemical-shift artifact.

The medial meniscus, which is composed of fibrocartilage, demonstrates uniform low signal intensity. The body of the medial meniscus has a continuous or bowtie shape on at least one or two consecutive sagittal images taken in 5-mm sections. In medial compartment images approaching the intercondylar notch, the separate anterior and posterior horns of the medial meniscus can be seen. The meniscal horns appear as opposing triangles on a minimum of two to three consecutive sagittal images. The posterior horn of the medial meniscus is larger than the opposing anterior horn. The medial head of the gastrocnemius muscle sweeps posteriorly from its origin along the distal femur. A small band of high signal intensity fat representing the bursa is seen between the posterior horn of the medial meniscus and the low signal intensity posterior capsule.

When viewing sagittal images in the medial to lateral direction, the PCL is seen before the ACL comes into view. The thick, uniform, low signal intensity PCL arcs from its anterolateral origin on the medial femoral condyle to its insertion on the posterior inferior tibial surface. With partial knee flexion, the convex curve of the PCL becomes taut. The anterior and posterior meniscofemoral ligaments (*i.e.,* the ligaments of Humphrey and Wrisberg, respectively) are seen individually or together on either side of the PCL.

In the lateral portion of the intercondylar notch, the ACL extends obliquely from its semicircular origin on the posteromedial lateral femoral condyle to its insertion, which starts 15 mm from the anterior border of the tibial articular surface (between the tibial spines). On average, it is 30 mm in length through the anterior intercondylar area.[12,13] The ACL is composed of two functional bands of fibers (*i.e.,* anteromedial and posterolateral); however, these bands are not differentiated on sagittal images. Independent of partial voluming with the lateral femoral condyle, anterior cruciate fibers may display a minimally higher signal intensity than the PCL. The ACL is normally seen on at least one sagittal image when the knee is properly positioned in 10° to 15° of external rotation and 5-mm–thick sections are used. With 1-mm 3DFT protocols, however, the ACL can be seen on several sagittal images. Fiber bundle striations of the ACL are prominent at femoral and tibial attachments, especially when oblique sagittal images are performed to display attachment sites.

Portions of both cruciate ligaments may be observed on the same sagittal section. Excessive external rotation of the knee causes elongation of the anterior to posterior dimensions of the femoral condyles.

On midsagittal sections, the quadriceps and patellar tendons, which demonstrate low signal intensity, are seen at their anterior attachments to the superior and inferior patellar poles, respectively. Hoffa's infrapatellar fat pad is directly posterior to the patellar tendon and demonstrates bright signal intensity. The posterior patellar articular cartilage displays a smooth convex arc on sections through the medial and lateral patellar facets. In the absence of joint fluid, the collapsed patellar bursa is not seen proximal to the superior pole of the patella.

On intercondylar sagittal sections, the popliteal vessels are seen in the long axis, with the artery anterior and the vein posterior.

The conjoined insertion of the LCL and the biceps femoris tendon on the fibular head can be identified on extreme lateral sagittal sections. The lateral head of the gastrocnemius muscle is seen posterior to the fibula and follows an inferior course from the distal lateral femoral condyle behind the popliteus muscle. The low signal intensity popliteus tendon and its intermittent signal intensity sheath are seen in their expected anatomic loca-

(text continues on page 175)

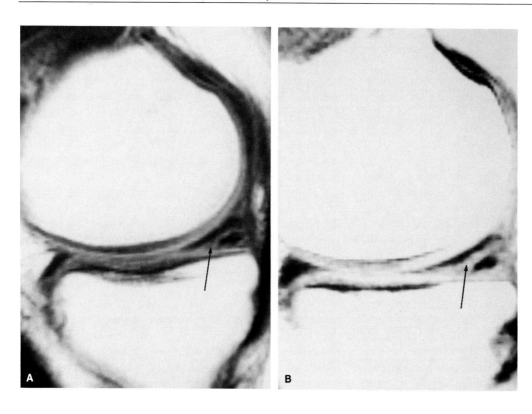

FIGURE 4–8. (**A**) A grade 3 signal intensity MR image shows a posterior horn medial meniscal tear (*arrow*). (**B**) The tear (*arrow*) is also shown with high contrast photography.

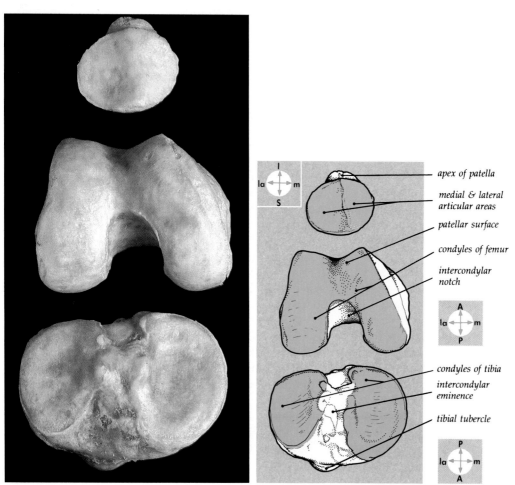

apex of patella

medial & lateral articular areas

patellar surface

condyles of femur

intercondylar notch

condyles of tibia

intercondylar eminence

tibial tubercle

FIGURE 4–9. The articular surfaces of the patella, femur, and tibia.

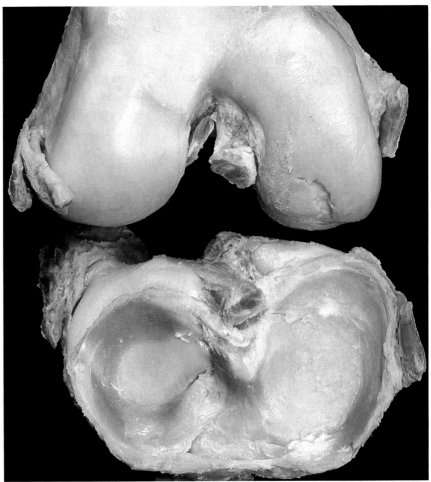

FIGURE 4–10. The attachments of the cruciate ligaments and the shape and attachments of the menisci. Cutting the cruciate and collateral ligaments allows the femur to be separated from the tibia.

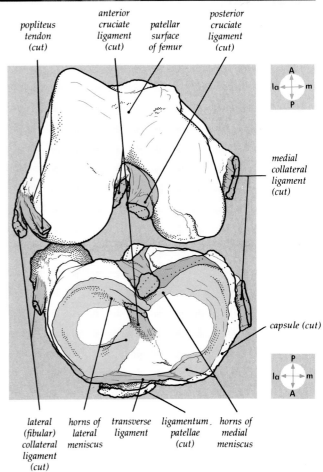

popliteus
tendon
(cut)

anterior
cruciate
ligament
(cut)

patellar
surface
of femur

posterior
cruciate
ligament
(cut)

medial
collateral
ligament
(cut)

capsule (cut)

lateral
(fibular)
collateral
ligament
(cut)

horns of
lateral
meniscus

transverse
ligament

ligamentum
patellae
(cut)

horns of
medial
meniscus

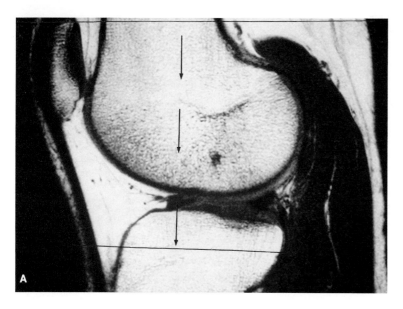

FIGURE 4-11. Normal axial MR anatomy. (**A**) This T1-weighted sagittal localizer was used to graphically prescribe image locations from (**B**) superior to (**N**) inferior.

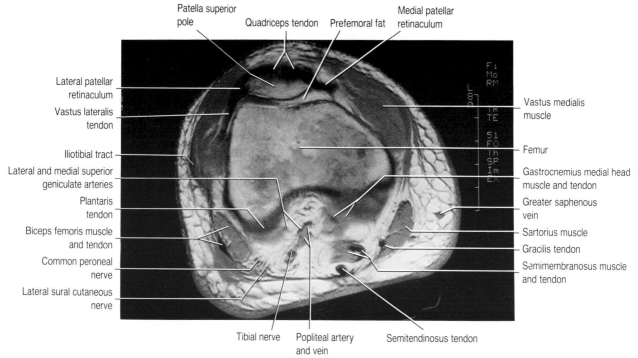

Patella superior pole

Quadriceps tendon

Prefemoral fat

Medial patellar retinaculum

Lateral patellar retinaculum

Vastus lateralis tendon

Iliotibial tract

Lateral and medial superior geniculate arteries

Plantaris tendon

Biceps femoris muscle and tendon

Common peroneal nerve

Lateral sural cutaneous nerve

Vastus medialis muscle

Femur

Gastrocnemius medial head muscle and tendon

Greater saphenous vein

Sartorius muscle

Gracilis tendon

Semimembranosus muscle and tendon

Tibial nerve

Popliteal artery and vein

Semitendinosus tendon

FIGURE 4-11B.

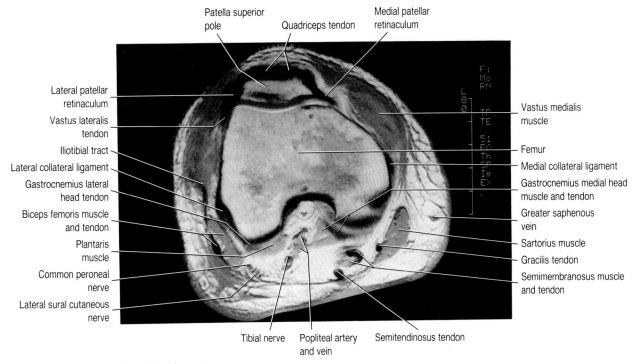

Patella superior pole
Quadriceps tendon
Medial patellar retinaculum
Lateral patellar retinaculum
Vastus lateralis tendon
Iliotibial tract
Lateral collateral ligament
Gastrocnemius lateral head tendon
Biceps femoris muscle and tendon
Plantaris muscle
Common peroneal nerve
Lateral sural cutaneous nerve
Vastus medialis muscle
Femur
Medial collateral ligament
Gastrocnemius medial head muscle and tendon
Greater saphenous vein
Sartorius muscle
Gracilis tendon
Semimembranosus muscle and tendon
Tibial nerve
Popliteal artery and vein
Semitendinosus tendon

FIGURE 4–11C.

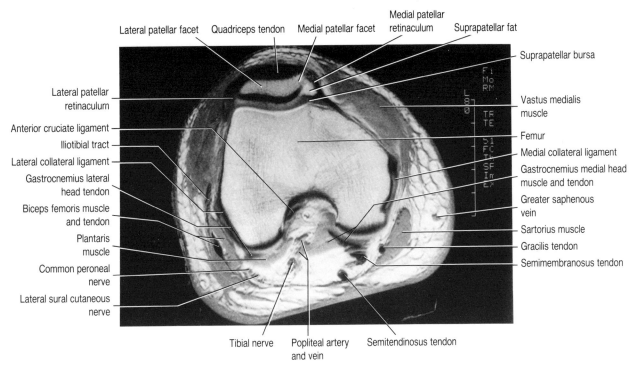

Lateral patellar facet
Quadriceps tendon
Medial patellar facet
Medial patellar retinaculum
Suprapatellar fat
Lateral patellar retinaculum
Anterior cruciate ligament
Iliotibial tract
Lateral collateral ligament
Gastrocnemius lateral head tendon
Biceps femoris muscle and tendon
Plantaris muscle
Common peroneal nerve
Lateral sural cutaneous nerve
Suprapatellar bursa
Vastus medialis muscle
Femur
Medial collateral ligament
Gastrocnemius medial head muscle and tendon
Greater saphenous vein
Sartorius muscle
Gracilis tendon
Semimembranosus tendon
Tibial nerve
Popliteal artery and vein
Semitendinosus tendon

FIGURE 4–11D.

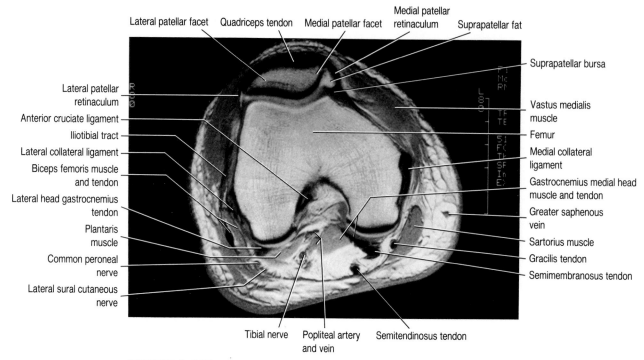

Lateral patellar facet Quadriceps tendon Medial patellar facet Medial patellar retinaculum Suprapatellar fat

Suprapatellar bursa

Lateral patellar retinaculum

Vastus medialis muscle

Anterior cruciate ligament

Femur

Iliotibial tract

Medial collateral ligament

Lateral collateral ligament

Biceps femoris muscle and tendon

Gastrocnemius medial head muscle and tendon

Lateral head gastrocnemius tendon

Greater saphenous vein

Plantaris muscle

Sartorius muscle

Common peroneal nerve

Gracilis tendon

Semimembranosus tendon

Lateral sural cutaneous nerve

Tibial nerve Popliteal artery and vein Semitendinosus tendon

FIGURE 4–11E.

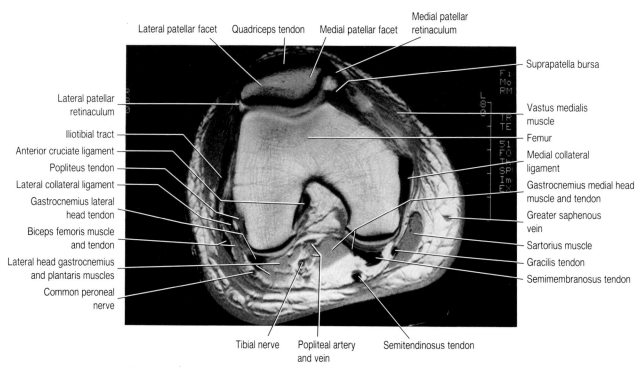

Lateral patellar facet Quadriceps tendon Medial patellar facet Medial patellar retinaculum

Suprapatella bursa

Lateral patellar retinaculum

Vastus medialis muscle

Iliotibial tract

Femur

Anterior cruciate ligament

Medial collateral ligament

Popliteus tendon

Lateral collateral ligament

Gastrocnemius medial head muscle and tendon

Gastrocnemius lateral head tendon

Greater saphenous vein

Biceps femoris muscle and tendon

Sartorius muscle

Lateral head gastrocnemius and plantaris muscles

Gracilis tendon

Common peroneal nerve

Semimembranosus tendon

Tibial nerve Popliteal artery and vein Semitendinosus tendon

FIGURE 4–11F.

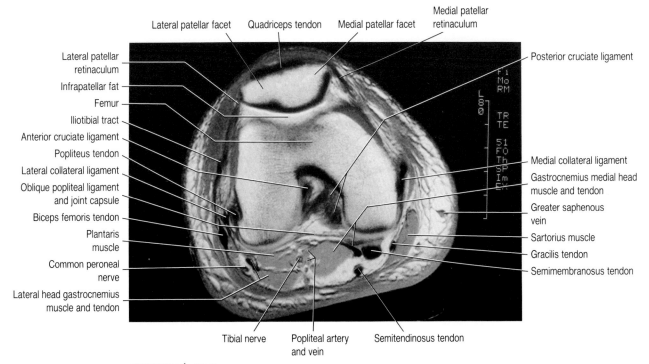

Lateral patellar facet   Quadriceps tendon   Medial patellar facet   Medial patellar retinaculum

Lateral patellar retinaculum
Infrapatellar fat
Femur
Iliotibial tract
Anterior cruciate ligament
Popliteus tendon
Lateral collateral ligament
Oblique popliteal ligament and joint capsule
Biceps femoris tendon
Plantaris muscle
Common peroneal nerve
Lateral head gastrocnemius muscle and tendon

Posterior cruciate ligament
Medial collateral ligament
Gastrocnemius medial head muscle and tendon
Greater saphenous vein
Sartorius muscle
Gracilis tendon
Semimembranosus tendon

Tibial nerve   Popliteal artery and vein   Semitendinosus tendon

FIGURE 4–11G.

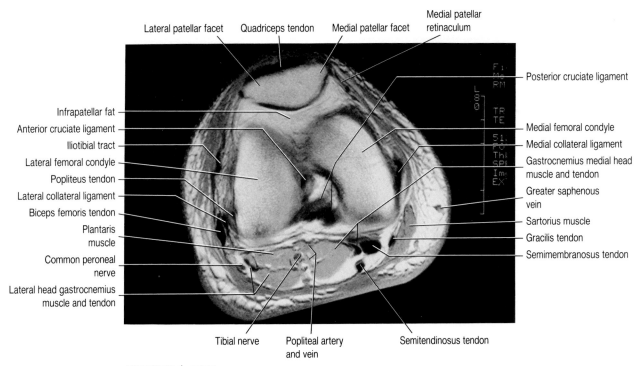

Lateral patellar facet   Quadriceps tendon   Medial patellar facet   Medial patellar retinaculum

Infrapatellar fat
Anterior cruciate ligament
Iliotibial tract
Lateral femoral condyle
Popliteus tendon
Lateral collateral ligament
Biceps femoris tendon
Plantaris muscle
Common peroneal nerve
Lateral head gastrocnemius muscle and tendon

Posterior cruciate ligament
Medial femoral condyle
Medial collateral ligament
Gastrocnemius medial head muscle and tendon
Greater saphenous vein
Sartorius muscle
Gracilis tendon
Semimembranosus tendon

Tibial nerve   Popliteal artery and vein   Semitendinosus tendon

FIGURE 4–11H.

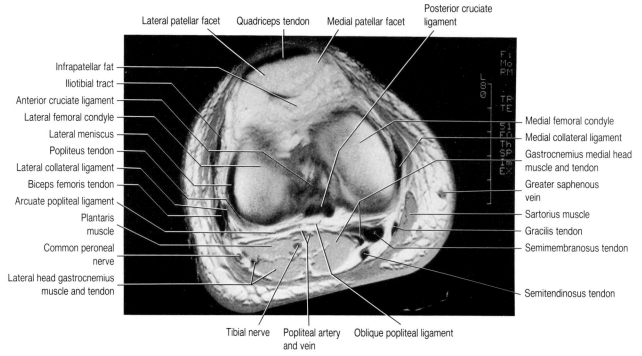

Lateral patellar facet — Quadriceps tendon — Medial patellar facet — Posterior cruciate ligament

Infrapatellar fat
Iliotibial tract
Anterior cruciate ligament
Lateral femoral condyle
Lateral meniscus
Popliteus tendon
Lateral collateral ligament
Biceps femoris tendon
Arcuate popliteal ligament
Plantaris muscle
Common peroneal nerve
Lateral head gastrocnemius muscle and tendon

Medial femoral condyle
Medial collateral ligament
Gastrocnemius medial head muscle and tendon
Greater saphenous vein
Sartorius muscle
Gracilis tendon
Semimembranosus tendon
Semitendinosus tendon

Tibial nerve — Popliteal artery and vein — Oblique popliteal ligament

FIGURE 4–11I.

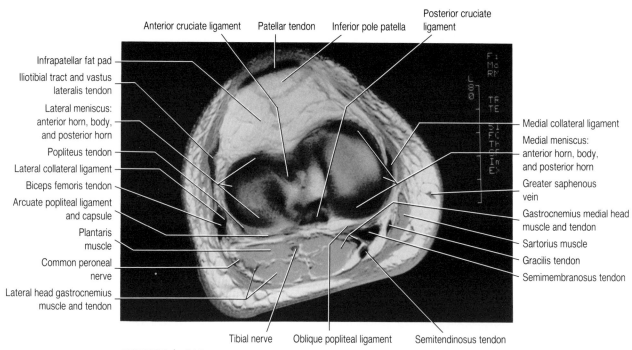

Anterior cruciate ligament — Patellar tendon — Inferior pole patella — Posterior cruciate ligament

Infrapatellar fat pad
Iliotibial tract and vastus lateralis tendon
Lateral meniscus: anterior horn, body, and posterior horn
Popliteus tendon
Lateral collateral ligament
Biceps femoris tendon
Arcuate popliteal ligament and capsule
Plantaris muscle
Common peroneal nerve
Lateral head gastrocnemius muscle and tendon

Medial collateral ligament
Medial meniscus: anterior horn, body, and posterior horn
Greater saphenous vein
Gastrocnemius medial head muscle and tendon
Sartorius muscle
Gracilis tendon
Semimembranosus tendon

Tibial nerve — Oblique popliteal ligament — Semitendinosus tendon

FIGURE 4–11J.

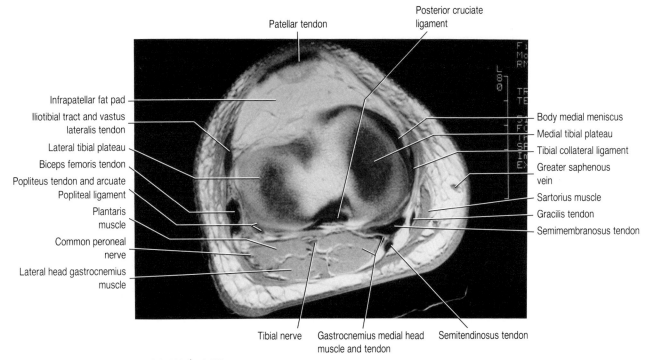

Patellar tendon

Posterior cruciate ligament

Infrapatellar fat pad

Iliotibial tract and vastus lateralis tendon

Lateral tibial plateau

Biceps femoris tendon

Popliteus tendon and arcuate Popliteal ligament

Plantaris muscle

Common peroneal nerve

Lateral head gastrocnemius muscle

Body medial meniscus

Medial tibial plateau

Tibial collateral ligament

Greater saphenous vein

Sartorius muscle

Gracilis tendon

Semimembranosus tendon

Tibial nerve

Gastrocnemius medial head muscle and tendon

Semitendinosus tendon

FIGURE 4–11K.

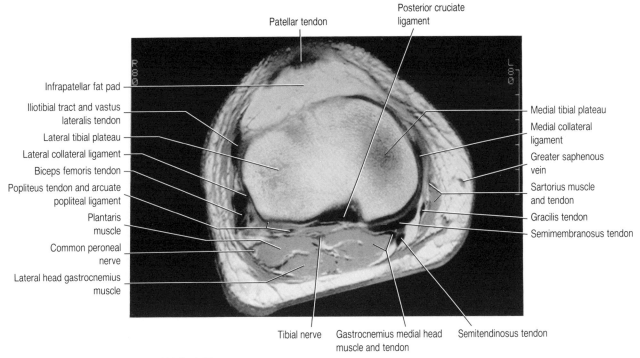

Patellar tendon

Posterior cruciate ligament

Infrapatellar fat pad

Iliotibial tract and vastus lateralis tendon

Lateral tibial plateau

Lateral collateral ligament

Biceps femoris tendon

Popliteus tendon and arcuate popliteal ligament

Plantaris muscle

Common peroneal nerve

Lateral head gastrocnemius muscle

Medial tibial plateau

Medial collateral ligament

Greater saphenous vein

Sartorius muscle and tendon

Gracilis tendon

Semimembranosus tendon

Tibial nerve

Gastrocnemius medial head muscle and tendon

Semitendinosus tendon

FIGURE 4–11L.

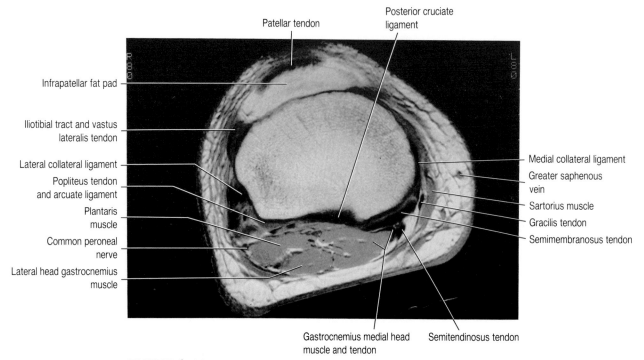

Patellar tendon

Posterior cruciate ligament

Infrapatellar fat pad

Iliotibial tract and vastus lateralis tendon

Lateral collateral ligament

Popliteus tendon and arcuate ligament

Plantaris muscle

Common peroneal nerve

Lateral head gastrocnemius muscle

Medial collateral ligament

Greater saphenous vein

Sartorius muscle

Gracilis tendon

Semimembranosus tendon

Gastrocnemius medial head muscle and tendon

Semitendinosus tendon

FIGURE 4–11M.

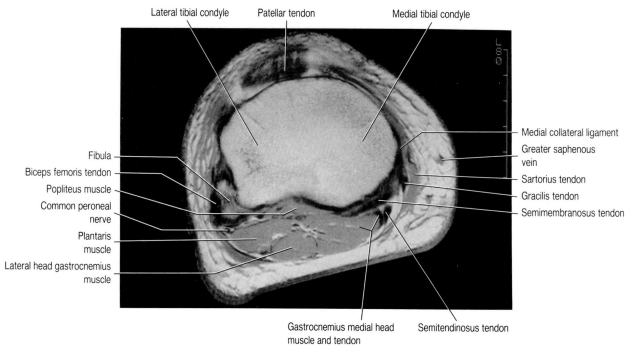

Lateral tibial condyle

Patellar tendon

Medial tibial condyle

Fibula

Biceps femoris tendon

Popliteus muscle

Common peroneal nerve

Plantaris muscle

Lateral head gastrocnemius muscle

Medial collateral ligament

Greater saphenous vein

Sartorius tendon

Gracilis tendon

Semimembranosus tendon

Gastrocnemius medial head muscle and tendon

Semitendinosus tendon

FIGURE 4–11N.

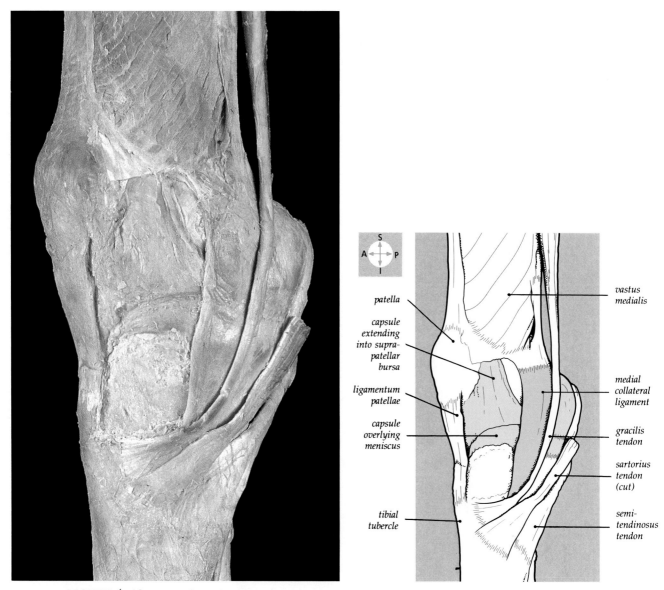

FIGURE 4–12. Superficial dissection from the medial aspect reveals the medial collateral ligament, capsule, and insertions of the sartorius, gracilis, and semitendinosus tendons.

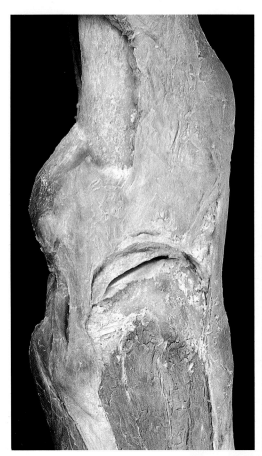

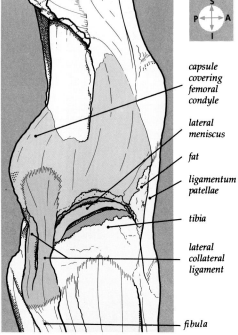

capsule
covering
femoral
condyle

lateral
meniscus

fat

ligamentum
patellae

tibia

lateral
collateral
ligament

fibula

FIGURE 4–13. Dissection from the lateral aspect shows the lateral collateral ligament and the meniscus, which are revealed by removing part of the capsule.

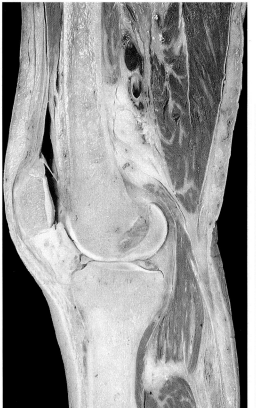

FIGURE 4–14.

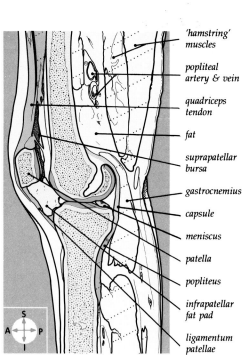

'hamstring'
muscles

popliteal
artery & vein

quadriceps
tendon

fat

suprapatellar
bursa

gastrocnemius

capsule

meniscus

patella

popliteus

infrapatellar
fat pad

ligamentum
patellae

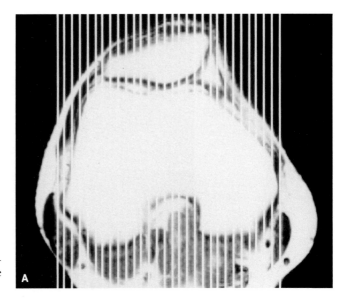

FIGURE 4–15. Normal sagittal MR anatomy of the medial compartment. (**A**) This T1-weighted localizer was used to prescribe image locations (**B**) through (**P**).

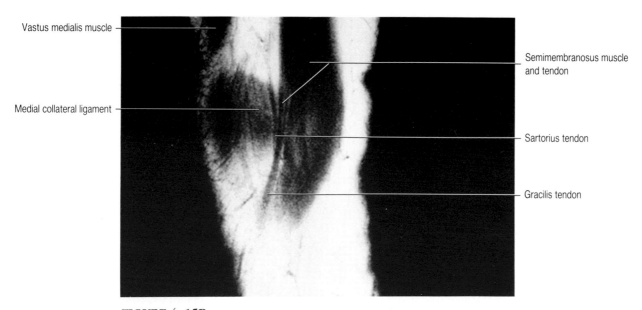

Vastus medialis muscle

Medial collateral ligament

Semimembranosus muscle and tendon

Sartorius tendon

Gracilis tendon

FIGURE 4–15B.

◄ **FIGURE 4–14.** A sagittal section through the knee joint shows the articular surfaces and suprapatellar pouch.

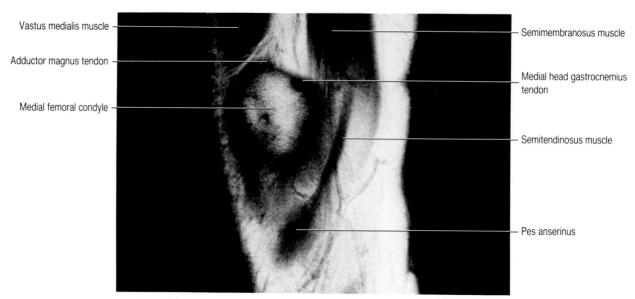

Vastus medialis muscle

Adductor magnus tendon

Medial femoral condyle

Semimembranosus muscle

Medial head gastrocnemius tendon

Semitendinosus muscle

Pes anserinus

FIGURE 4–15C.

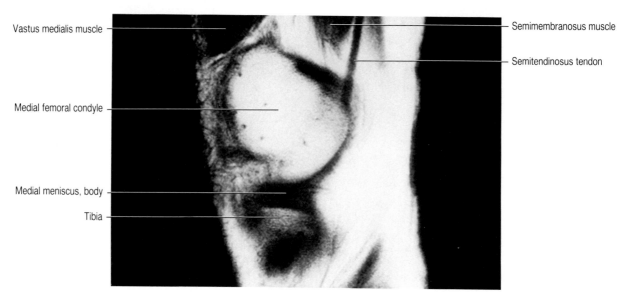

Vastus medialis muscle

Medial femoral condyle

Medial meniscus, body

Tibia

Semimembranosus muscle

Semitendinosus tendon

FIGURE 4–15D.

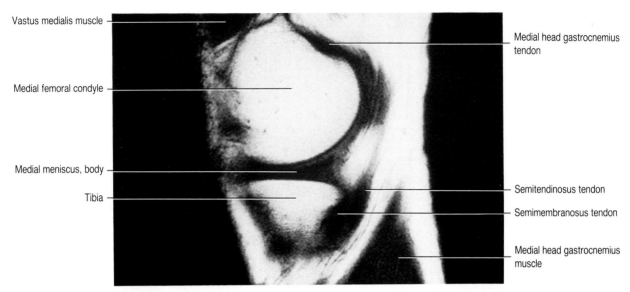

Vastus medialis muscle

Medial femoral condyle

Medial meniscus, body

Tibia

Medial head gastrocnemius tendon

Semitendinosus tendon

Semimembranosus tendon

Medial head gastrocnemius muscle

FIGURE 4–15E.

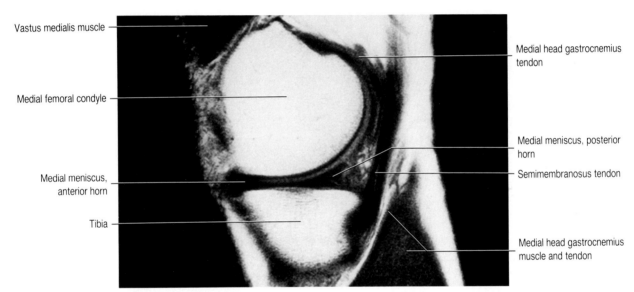

Vastus medialis muscle

Medial femoral condyle

Medial meniscus, anterior horn

Tibia

Medial head gastrocnemius tendon

Medial meniscus, posterior horn

Semimembranosus tendon

Medial head gastrocnemius muscle and tendon

FIGURE 4–15F.

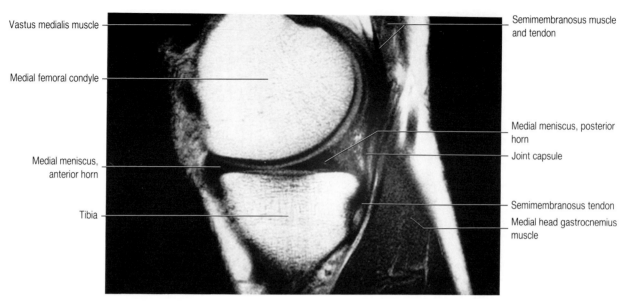

Vastus medialis muscle

Medial femoral condyle

Medial meniscus, anterior horn

Tibia

Semimembranosus muscle and tendon

Medial meniscus, posterior horn

Joint capsule

Semimembranosus tendon

Medial head gastrocnemius muscle

FIGURE 4–15G.

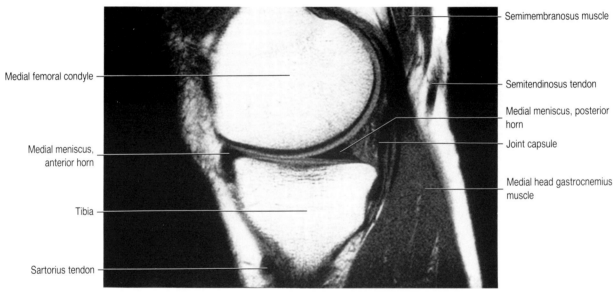

Medial femoral condyle

Medial meniscus, anterior horn

Tibia

Sartorius tendon

Semimembranosus muscle

Semitendinosus tendon

Medial meniscus, posterior horn

Joint capsule

Medial head gastrocnemius muscle

FIGURE 4–15H.

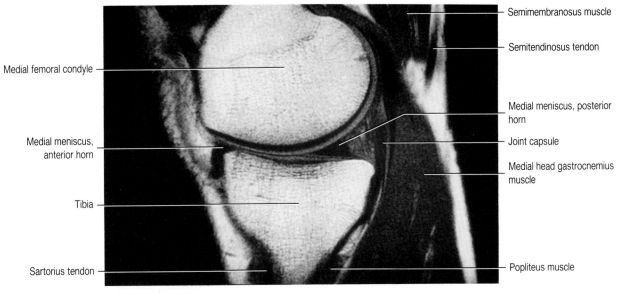

Medial femoral condyle

Medial meniscus, anterior horn

Tibia

Sartorius tendon

Semimembranosus muscle

Semitendinosus tendon

Medial meniscus, posterior horn

Joint capsule

Medial head gastrocnemius muscle

Popliteus muscle

FIGURE 4–15I.

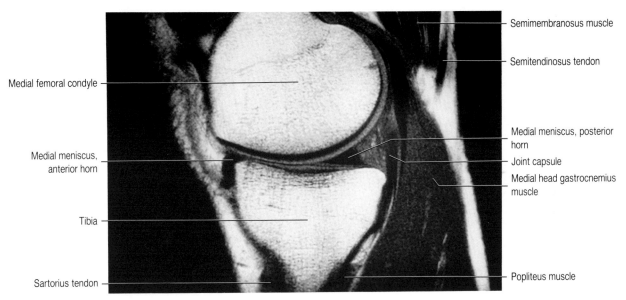

Medial femoral condyle

Medial meniscus, anterior horn

Tibia

Sartorius tendon

Semimembranosus muscle

Semitendinosus tendon

Medial meniscus, posterior horn

Joint capsule

Medial head gastrocnemius muscle

Popliteus muscle

FIGURE 4–15J.

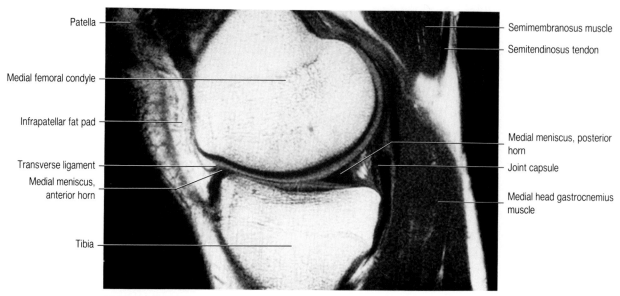

Patella

Medial femoral condyle

Infrapatellar fat pad

Transverse ligament

Medial meniscus, anterior horn

Tibia

Semimembranosus muscle

Semitendinosus tendon

Medial meniscus, posterior horn

Joint capsule

Medial head gastrocnemius muscle

FIGURE 4–15K.

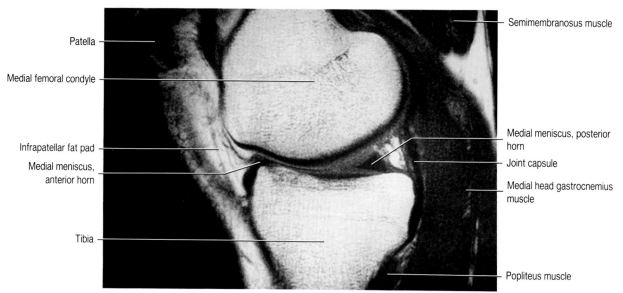

Patella

Medial femoral condyle

Infrapatellar fat pad

Medial meniscus, anterior horn

Tibia

Semimembranosus muscle

Medial meniscus, posterior horn

Joint capsule

Medial head gastrocnemius muscle

Popliteus muscle

FIGURE 4–15L.

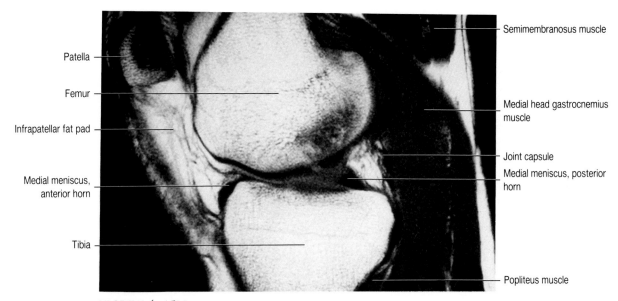

Patella

Femur

Infrapatellar fat pad

Medial meniscus, anterior horn

Tibia

Semimembranosus muscle

Medial head gastrocnemius muscle

Joint capsule

Medial meniscus, posterior horn

Popliteus muscle

FIGURE 4–15M.

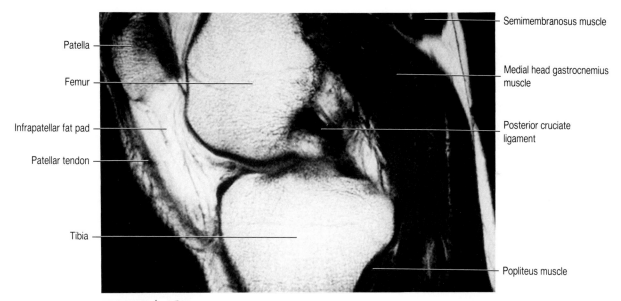

Patella

Femur

Infrapatellar fat pad

Patellar tendon

Tibia

Semimembranosus muscle

Medial head gastrocnemius muscle

Posterior cruciate ligament

Popliteus muscle

FIGURE 4–15N.

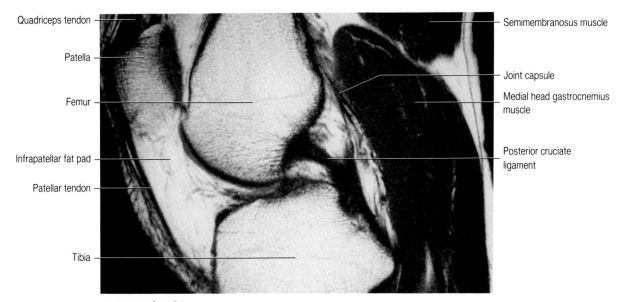

Quadriceps tendon
Patella
Femur
Infrapatellar fat pad
Patellar tendon
Tibia

Semimembranosus muscle
Joint capsule
Medial head gastrocnemius muscle
Posterior cruciate ligament

FIGURE 4–15O.

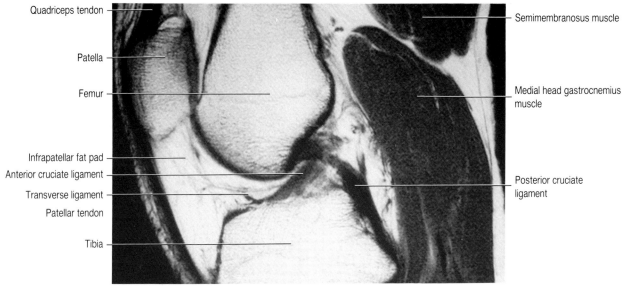

Quadriceps tendon
Patella
Femur
Infrapatellar fat pad
Anterior cruciate ligament
Transverse ligament
Patellar tendon
Tibia

Semimembranosus muscle
Medial head gastrocnemius muscle
Posterior cruciate ligament

FIGURE 4–15P.

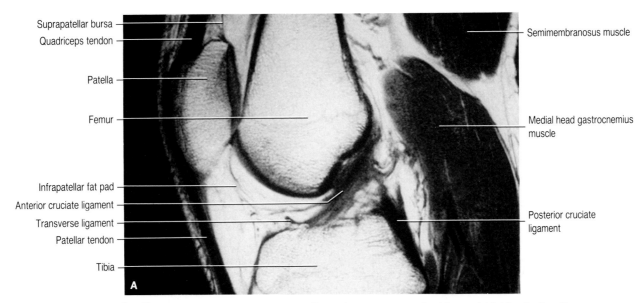

Suprapatellar bursa

Quadriceps tendon

Patella

Femur

Infrapatellar fat pad

Anterior cruciate ligament

Transverse ligament

Patellar tendon

Tibia

Semimembranosus muscle

Medial head gastrocnemius muscle

Posterior cruciate ligament

FIGURE 4–16. Normal sagittal MR anatomy of lateral compartment. See Figure 4-15*A* for the localizer that was used to prescribe image locations (**A**) through (**P**).

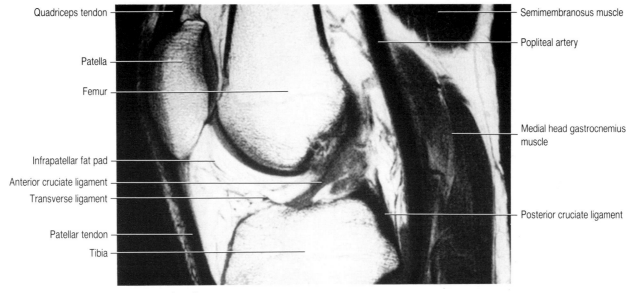

Quadriceps tendon

Patella

Femur

Infrapatellar fat pad

Anterior cruciate ligament

Transverse ligament

Patellar tendon

Tibia

Semimembranosus muscle

Popliteal artery

Medial head gastrocnemius muscle

Posterior cruciate ligament

FIGURE 4–16B.

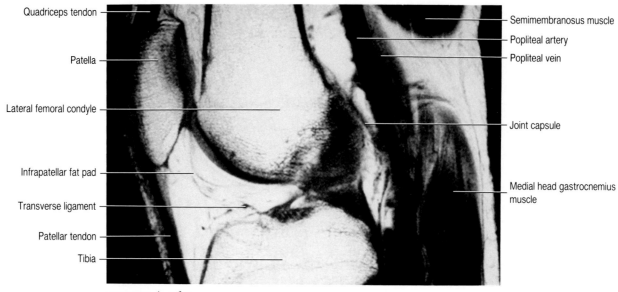

Quadriceps tendon

Patella

Lateral femoral condyle

Infrapatellar fat pad

Transverse ligament

Patellar tendon

Tibia

Semimembranosus muscle

Popliteal artery

Popliteal vein

Joint capsule

Medial head gastrocnemius muscle

FIGURE 4–16C.

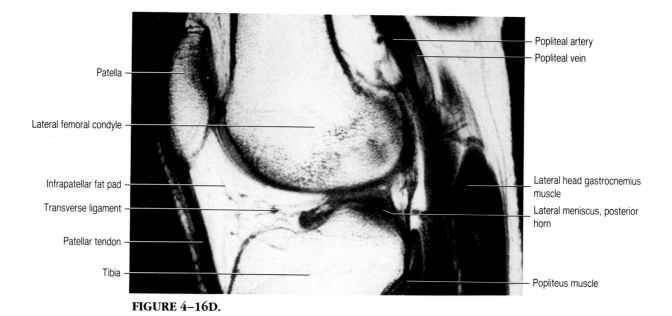

Patella

Lateral femoral condyle

Infrapatellar fat pad

Transverse ligament

Patellar tendon

Tibia

Popliteal artery

Popliteal vein

Lateral head gastrocnemius muscle

Lateral meniscus, posterior horn

Popliteus muscle

FIGURE 4–16D.

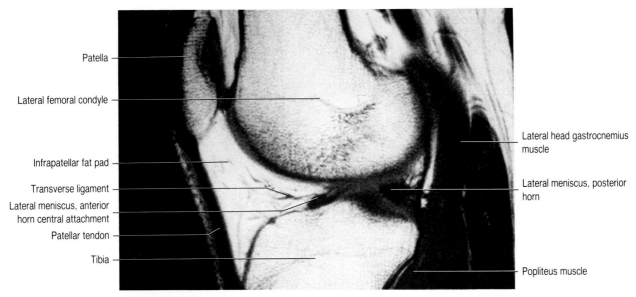

Patella

Lateral femoral condyle

Infrapatellar fat pad

Transverse ligament
Lateral meniscus, anterior
horn central attachment
Patellar tendon

Tibia

Lateral head gastrocnemius
muscle

Lateral meniscus, posterior
horn

Popliteus muscle

FIGURE 4–16E.

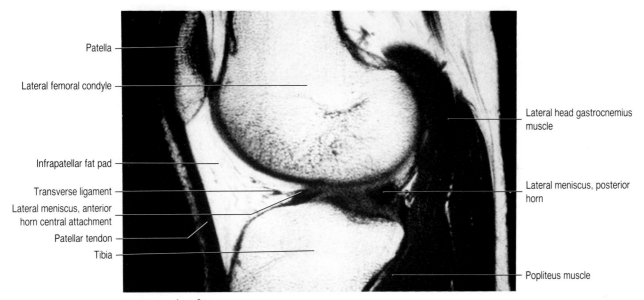

Patella

Lateral femoral condyle

Infrapatellar fat pad

Transverse ligament
Lateral meniscus, anterior
horn central attachment
Patellar tendon
Tibia

Lateral head gastrocnemius
muscle

Lateral meniscus, posterior
horn

Popliteus muscle

FIGURE 4–16F.

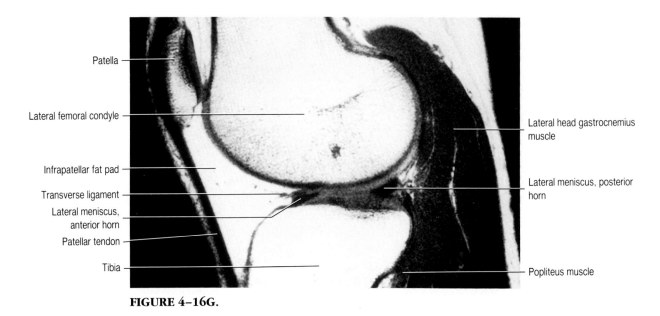

Patella

Lateral femoral condyle

Infrapatellar fat pad

Transverse ligament

Lateral meniscus, anterior horn

Patellar tendon

Tibia

Lateral head gastrocnemius muscle

Lateral meniscus, posterior horn

Popliteus muscle

FIGURE 4–16G.

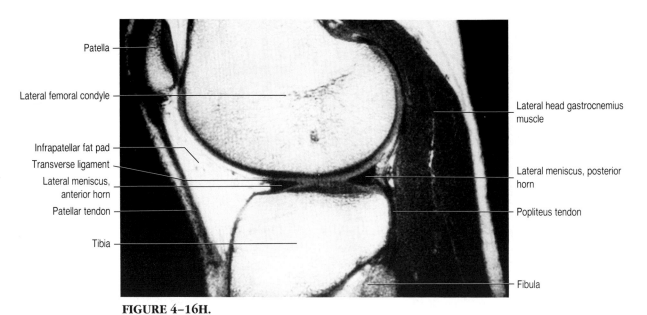

Patella

Lateral femoral condyle

Infrapatellar fat pad

Transverse ligament

Lateral meniscus, anterior horn

Patellar tendon

Tibia

Lateral head gastrocnemius muscle

Lateral meniscus, posterior horn

Popliteus tendon

Fibula

FIGURE 4–16H.

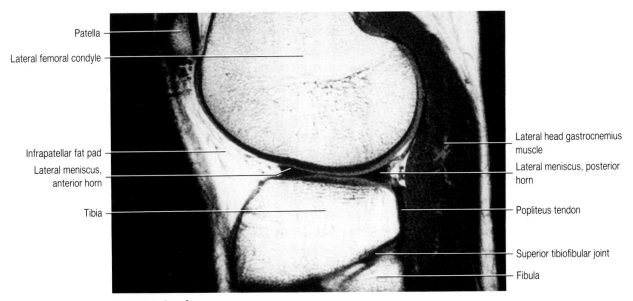

Patella

Lateral femoral condyle

Infrapatellar fat pad

Lateral meniscus, anterior horn

Tibia

Lateral head gastrocnemius muscle

Lateral meniscus, posterior horn

Popliteus tendon

Superior tibiofibular joint

Fibula

FIGURE 4–16I.

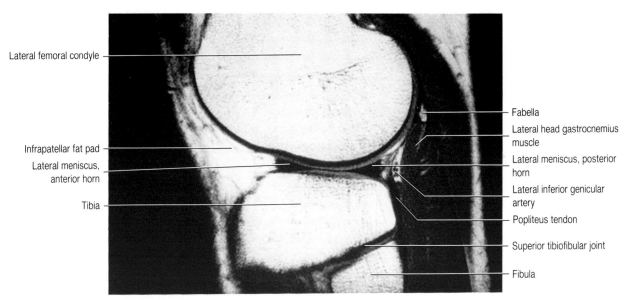

Lateral femoral condyle

Infrapatellar fat pad

Lateral meniscus, anterior horn

Tibia

Fabella

Lateral head gastrocnemius muscle

Lateral meniscus, posterior horn

Lateral inferior genicular artery

Popliteus tendon

Superior tibiofibular joint

Fibula

FIGURE 4–16J.

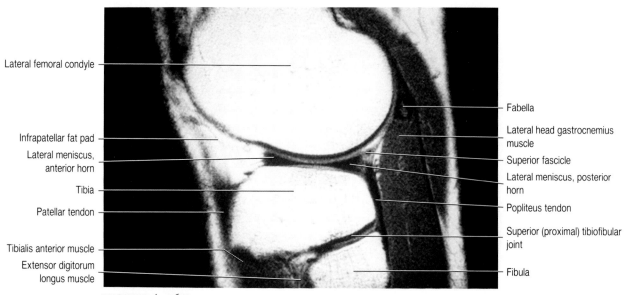

Lateral femoral condyle

Infrapatellar fat pad

Lateral meniscus, anterior horn

Tibia

Patellar tendon

Tibialis anterior muscle

Extensor digitorum longus muscle

Fabella

Lateral head gastrocnemius muscle

Superior fascicle

Lateral meniscus, posterior horn

Popliteus tendon

Superior (proximal) tibiofibular joint

Fibula

FIGURE 4–16K.

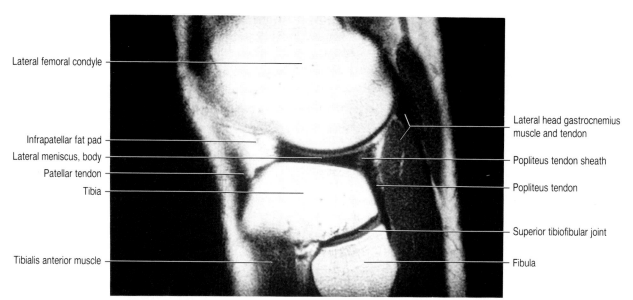

Lateral femoral condyle

Infrapatellar fat pad

Lateral meniscus, body

Patellar tendon

Tibia

Tibialis anterior muscle

Lateral head gastrocnemius muscle and tendon

Popliteus tendon sheath

Popliteus tendon

Superior tibiofibular joint

Fibula

FIGURE 4–16L.

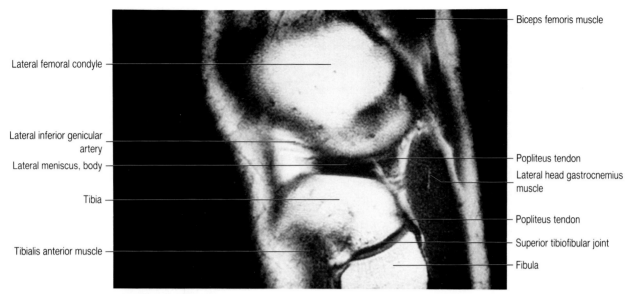

Biceps femoris muscle

Lateral femoral condyle

Lateral inferior genicular artery

Lateral meniscus, body

Tibia

Tibialis anterior muscle

Popliteus tendon

Lateral head gastrocnemius muscle

Popliteus tendon

Superior tibiofibular joint

Fibula

FIGURE 4–16M.

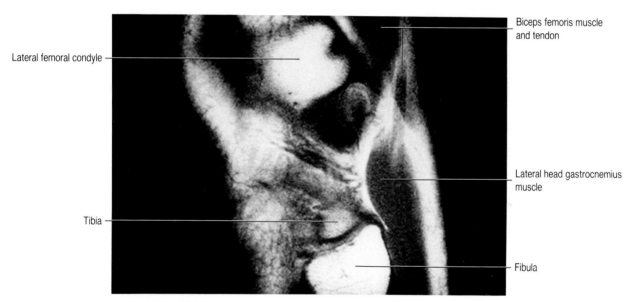

Biceps femoris muscle and tendon

Lateral femoral condyle

Lateral head gastrocnemius muscle

Tibia

Fibula

FIGURE 4–16N.

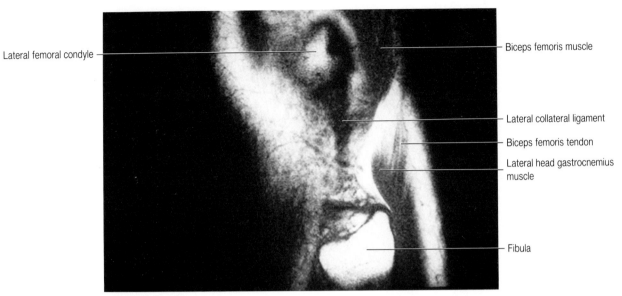

Lateral femoral condyle

Biceps femoris muscle

Lateral collateral ligament

Biceps femoris tendon

Lateral head gastrocnemius muscle

Fibula

FIGURE 4–16O.

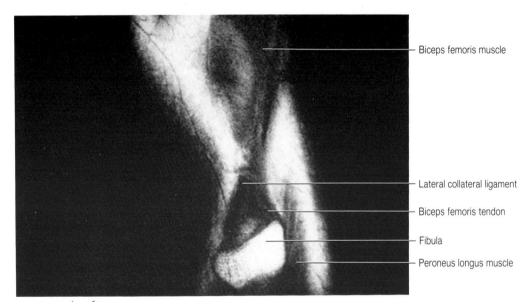

Biceps femoris muscle

Lateral collateral ligament

Biceps femoris tendon

Fibula

Peroneus longus muscle

FIGURE 4–16P.

tions between the capsule and the periphery of the lateral meniscus. Separate synovium-lined fascicles, or struts, of the meniscus allow intraarticular passage of the popliteus tendon. In its middle one-third (*i.e.,* body), the C-shaped lateral meniscus also demonstrates a bow-tie shape. On more medial sections through the lateral compartment, the separate triangular shapes of the anterior and posterior horns, which are oriented toward each other and nearly symmetric in size and shape, can be distinguished. The MCL is not routinely defined on 3- or 5-mm sagittal images.

Coronal Images

Coronal anatomic dissection from posterior to anterior demonstrates the posterior capsule (Fig. 4–17), the popliteus tendon (Fig. 4–18), the cruciate ligaments and menisci (Fig. 4–19), the collateral ligaments (Figs. 4–20 and 4–21), and the extensor mechanism (see Fig. 4–21). Coronal plane images (Fig. 4–22) are most frequently used to identify collateral ligament anatomy. They are also best for displaying the posterior femoral condyles—the sites of early articular erosions. The cruciate ligaments, although displayed to best advantage in the sagittal plane, can also be identified on coronal images. The oblique popliteal ligament and the arcuate popliteal ligament define the posterior capsule.

The low signal intensity popliteal vessels are also identified on posterior coronal images. The fibular collateral ligament is seen as a low signal intensity cord stretching from its insertion on the fibular head to the lateral epicondyle of the femur. It is separated from the lateral meniscus by the thickness of the popliteus tendon.

Anterior to the PCL, the meniscofemoral ligament is known as the ligament of Humphrey; posteriorly it is called the ligament of Wrisberg. Posteriorly, at the level of the femoral condyles, the meniscofemoral ligaments of Wrisberg and Humphrey may be observed as thin, low–spin-density bands extending from the posterior horn of the lateral meniscus to the lateral surface of the medial femoral condyle. The ligament of Humphrey is variable in size when identified. Either branch of the meniscofemoral ligament may be identified on one-third of sagittal images. The coexistence of both branches of the meniscofemoral ligament is seen in only 3% of examinations.[14]

The functional location of the anteromedial and posterolateral bands of the ACL may be discerned on anterior and posterior coronal images, respectively. The PCL is circular and of uniform low signal intensity on anterior and midcoronal sections. On posterior coronal images, the triangular attachment to the posterior cruciate can be differentiated as it fans out from the lateral aspect of the medial femoral condyle. The MCL is identified on mid-

coronal sections, anterior to sections in which the femoral condyles appear to fuse together with the distal metaphysis. The tibial or medial collateral ligament is seen as a band of low signal intensity extending from its femoral epicondylar attachment to the medial tibial condyle. It consists of superficial and deep layers attached to the periphery of the medial meniscus.

The femoral and tibial attachments of the uninjured or intact MCL demonstrate uniform dark signal intensity, indistinguishable from underlying cortical bone. From the plane of the posterior femoral condyles, the MCL is seen on at least two to three coronal images when acquired with 5-mm sections and no interslice gap. A line of intermediate signal intensity separating the medial meniscus from the deep layer of the MCL represents a small bursa. The body and the anterior and posterior horns of the medial and lateral menisci are seen as distinct segments, and not as opposing triangles as on sagittal images. On posterior coronal images, the planar section is parallel with the posterior curve of the C-shaped menisci, and the posterior horn may be displayed as a continuous band of low signal intensity.

Midcoronal sections demonstrate the anterior tibial spine, whereas anterior images are marked by the high signal intensity of Hoffa's infrapatellar fat pad anterior to the lateral knee compartment. Anteriorly, the iliotibial band blends with the lateral patellar retinaculum, and the vastus medialis is in continuity with its medial retinacular patellar attachment. The low signal intensity fibers of the quadriceps and patellar tendons can be identified on the most anterior sections in the same plane as the patella.

MENISCI

Imaging Protocols

T1-weighted or intermediate-weighted (*i.e.,* proton-density–weighted) images were initially described as optimal techniques for detecting meniscal lesions, which are sensitive to the T1 shortening of imbibed synovial fluid in tears and mucinous degenerations.[15,16] Techniques such as gradient-echo T2*-weighted 2DFT or 3DFT images, however, are sensitive to both the spectrum of grade 1 and 2 degenerations and grade 3 meniscal tears.[17] The technique of 3D field echo acquisition with a short TR and echo reduction (FASTER) which produces isotropic voxels without significant loss of image quality, is especially promising.[18] This technique displays fluid with increased signal intensity on T1-weighted contrast images and is as effective in identifying meniscal tears as conventional T2-weighted images. The rate of false-positives in detection of meniscal tears is lower with 3DFT GRASS sequences than with conventional 2D spin-echo sequences (TR, 2000 msec; TE, 20, 80 msec).[19] The first echo of a conventional T2-weighted pulse sequence produces intermediate contrast images for the identification of meniscal lesions, and the second echo identifies soft tissue and osseous pathology.

Acquisitions at 1 NEX without an interslice gap limits the SNR with these long TR and TE protocols. T1- or T2*-weighted images offer the advantage of reducing scanning time, providing thin contiguous slices, and allowing 3D reformatting in any plane.[9] Radial images, which show the meniscus perpendicular to orthogonal sagittal views, acquired with gradient-echo contrast can be used to evaluate peripheral meniscal tears and equivocal grade 2 or 3 lesions. This technique is also sensitive in identifying the meniscocapsular junction (Fig. 4–23). Contrast enhancement with intraarticular gadolinium may prove useful in identifying poor healing or retear of a primary meniscal repair. Simultaneous acquisition of radial and coronal or sagittal images is possible with multisection gradient-echo contrast (Fig. 4–24). Steady-state free procession images, where TR is shorter than T2, display heavily weighed T2 contrast; it may not be possible to detect grade 1 and 2 degenerations on these scans. However, this technique is sensitive to small amounts of fluid in meniscal tears or cysts.

Normal Magnetic Resonance Anatomy of the Menisci

The C-shaped fibrocartilaginous menisci or semilunar cartilages are attached to the condylar surface of the tibia and provide added mechanical stability to femorotibial gliding (Figs. 4–25 and 4–26). The meniscus protects the joint articular cartilage by acting as a buffer between femoral and tibial surfaces with loading. The meniscus provides joint lubrication and increases joint stability by providing congruity between femoral and tibial articular surfaces. The proximal or superior meniscal surface is smooth and concave, producing greater contact with the femoral condyles. Tibial attachments to the meniscus are made through the meniscofemoral and meniscotibial or coronary ligaments of the joint capsule. Except for the peripheral 10% to 25% of the meniscus, which is supplied by the perimeniscal capillary plexus, the adult meniscus is relatively avascular.[20,21] In the pediatric knee, the vascularity of the meniscus is already restricted to the peripheral one-third, whereas the inner two-thirds of the meniscus remain relatively avascular.[22]

Intact menisci demonstrate uniform low signal intensity on T1-, T2-, and T2*-weighted images. They are triangular in cross section and have an outer convex curve, and the apex is directed toward the intercondylar notch. The meniscus is arbitrarily divided into thirds—the anterior horn, the body, and the posterior horn (Fig. 4–27).

The microstructure of the meniscus is organized so that the collagen bundles form two distinct zones, the circumferential and the transverse (Fig. 4–28).[23] The circumferential fibers or bundles are found in the peripheral one-third of the meniscus. The transverse collagen fibers bridge the circumferential zone of the meniscus peripherally to the free edge of the meniscus. On cross section, the transverse zone of the meniscus is divided into superior and inferior leaves by the middle perforating collagen bundle (Fig. 4–29). Middle perforating collagen fibers normally cannot be distinguished from adjacent meniscal tissue on images. Secondary vertical collagen fibers, which function as secondary stabilizers, may be present within the transverse zone. The middle perforating bundle may demarcate the shear plane of the meniscus. In internal degenerations or tears, the middle-perforating collagen bundle corresponds to the location of the predominantly horizontal signal intensity.

The meniscocapsular junction is peripheral to the circumferential zone. The function of the circumferential collagen fibers is to resist longitudinal loading (*i.e.,* hoop stresses).[24] The menisci provide the following functions:

- transmit axial and torsional forces across the joint
- cushion mechanical loading
- limit compressive displacement
- distribute synovial fluid
- increase surface area for femoral condylar motion
- prevent synovial impingement.[25]

The stabilizing effect and vascularization of the peripheral one-third of the meniscus is the reason for attempts to preserve this tissue in partial meniscectomies. However, its preservation may not protect the joint from degenerative changes.[20,26]

Lateral Meniscus and the Screw-Home Mechanism

The lateral meniscus forms a tight C-shape and accommodates the popliteus tendon posteriorly (Fig. 4–30). It is separated from the lateral collateral (*i.e.,* extracapsular) ligament and has posterior horn attachments to the PCL and medial femoral condyle through the ligaments of Wrisberg and Humphrey. The more mobile lateral meniscus covers two-thirds of the tibial articular surface.[5] The popliteal recess allows passage of the popliteus tendon through a 1-cm hiatus in the posterolateral attachment of the lateral meniscus. The superior fascicle is seen medial to the inferior fascicle as the popliteus tendon penetrates the meniscocapsular junction. The function of the popliteal tendon attachments to the lateral meniscus is to pull the lateral meniscus posterior with knee flexion. Whereas the popliteus muscle can effectively rotate the tibia with the knee in extension, this unlocking of the knee from full extension is the reverse of the screw home mechanism of the knee. The screw home mechanism functions to lock the knee in extension with internal rotation of the femur relative to the tibia.[27,28]

Medial Meniscus

The medial meniscus has a wide posterior horn, narrows anteriorly, and has a more open C-shaped configuration than the circular lateral meniscus (Fig. 4–31). The less mobile medial meniscus attachment to the deep layer of the MCL and capsule render the medial meniscus more susceptible to injury. A small intermediate signal intensity bursa separates the posterior horn of the medial meniscus from the joint capsule.

Meniscal Degenerations and Tears

Pathogenesis

The rotation of the femur against a fixed tibia during flexion and extension places the menisci at risk for injury.[29] Tears involving the medial meniscus usually start on the inferior surface of the posterior horn. The lateral meniscus is more prone to transverse or oblique tears. Associated hemorrhage and tearing of the peripheral meniscal attachments contribute to the pain perceived in meniscal tears. Sequelae of complete meniscectomy include degenerative joint disease as well as increased instability, especially in the anterior cruciate-deficient knee.[24,26,30,31] These changes are less likely to occur with partial meniscectomy and are minimized with primary meniscal healing.

Magnetic Resonance of Meniscal Degenerations and Tears

Magnetic Resonance Accuracy. Compared with that of arthroscopy, the sensitivity of MR imaging to meniscal tears has been reported to be between 80% and 100%.[6,17,32–36] In a series by Mink and colleagues, 600 menisci were studied with an accuracy rate of 92%.[37] There were 9 false-negatives and 18 false-positives. With fast 3D MR imaging, there is a 95% concurrence between MR imaging and arthroscopy in detection of meniscal tears, and a 100% correlation with meniscal degenerations.[38] Li and colleagues studied 459 menisci and reported an arthroscopic correlation of 93%.[11] In excluding tears on normal MR examination of the meniscus, the negative predictive value of MR imaging approaches 100%. In a large multicenter series of 1014 patients, the MR imaging accuracy of diagnosis was 89% for the medial meniscus and 88% for the lateral meniscus.[39] The varia-

tions in detection rates compared with arthroscopy may be due to the following factors:

- learning curve on the part of the radiologist in interpreting MR signal intensities
- the experience of several different arthroscopists participating in the correlative studies
- false interpretation of areas of fibrillation or fraying as meniscal tears
- inability of arthroscopy to detect intrasubstance degenerative cleavage tears
- obstructed arthroscopic visualization of the posterior horn of the medial meniscus by the medial femoral condyle
- difficulty in accurately imaging the periphery of the meniscus at the meniscocapsular junction
- variability in performing examinations with different MR imagers and surface coils at a variety of field strengths.

Magnetic Resonance Appearance. The intact meniscus demonstrates homogeneous low signal intensity, regardless of the pulse sequence. Degenerations and tears of the meniscus demonstrate increased signal intensity, which is attributed to imbibed synovial fluid.[15] As synovial fluid diffuses through the meniscus, areas of degeneration and tears trap water molecules onto surface boundary layers, increasing the local spin density. This interaction of synovial fluid with large macromolecules in the meniscus slows the rotation rates of protons and shortens T1 and T2 values.[15] This explains the sensitivity of T1-weighted and intermediate-weighted (*i.e.,* proton-density–weighted) images in revealing meniscal degenerations and tears. Increased signal intensity in synovial fluid gaps has been confirmed in surgically induced tears in animal models.[40] On MR studies performed after arthrography, increased signal intensity may be observed on T2-weighted images. This change is related to the actions of joint fluid and a hyperosmolar contrast agent that draws fluid into meniscal separations. This creates a motional narrowing effect (*i.e.,* free water molecules in motion) allowing more mobile protons to be imaged separately from unbound water molecules.[41] In the absence of a joint effusion, meniscal degenerations and tears may actually decrease in signal intensity on T2-weighted images. On T2*-weighted refocused images, however, intrasubstance degenerations and tears generate increased signal intensities.[16] Therefore, gradient-echo sequences are extremely sensitive to the spectrum of meniscal degenerations and tears.

To understand the significance of increased signal intensity in meniscal abnormalities, an MR grading system has been developed and correlated with a pathologic (*i.e.,* histologic) model (Fig. 4–32). Areas of degeneration are shown with increased signal intensity in a spectrum of patterns or grades that are based on the signal distribution relative to an articular surface exclusive of the peripheral capsular margin of the meniscus, which is considered nonarticular.

In MR grade 1, a nonarticular focal or globular intrasubstance increased signal intensity is seen (Fig. 4–33). Histologically, grade 1 signal intensity correlates with foci of early mucinous degeneration and chondrocyte-deficient or hypocellular regions that are pale-staining on hematoxylin and eosin preparations. The terms mucinous, myxoid, and hyaline degeneration can be used interchangeably to describe the accumulation or increased production of mucopolysaccharide ground substance in stressed or strained areas of the meniscal fibrocartilage.[42,43] These changes usually occur in response to mechanical loading and degeneration. Grade 1 signal intensity may be observed in asymptomatic athletes and normal volunteers and is not clinically significant (Fig. 4–34).

In MR grade 2, a horizontal, linear intrasubstance increased signal intensity usually extends from the capsular periphery of the meniscus, but does not involve an articular surface (Fig. 4–35). Areas and bands of mucinous degeneration are more extensive in MR grade 2 than in MR grade 1 (Fig. 4–36). Although no distinct cleavage plane or tear is observed in grade 2 menisci, microscopic clefting and collagen fragmentation has been recorded in hypocellular regions of the fibrocartilaginous matrix. The middle perforating collagen bundle, a structure not ordinarily seen on MR images, sends out fibers that horizontally divide the meniscus into superior and inferior leaves.[44] The low–spin-density meniscus and middle-perforating collagen fibers cannot be differentiated in the normal knee because they both demonstrate low signal intensity. The middle-perforating collagen bundle creates a neutral or buffer plane for the superior femoral and inferior tibial frictional forces and is a site for preferential accumulation of mucinous ground substance that displays grade 2 signal intensity. This also represents the shear plane of the meniscus and is the site of horizontal degenerative tears of the meniscus.

Although patients with grade 2 menisci may or may not present with symptomatic knee pain, these lesions are prone to symptomatic grade 3 tears, especially in the posterior horns of the medial meniscus, the most common location of grade 2 signal intensity tears (Fig. 4–37).[45] The presence of mucinous degeneration is thus thought to represent potential structural weakening within collagen fibers. In the immature meniscus, vascular ingrowth that has been primarily reabsorbed cannot fully explain the finding of grade 2 signal intensity in young children without associated fibrocartilaginous degenerations.[22] In the adult, however, the finding of increased signal intensity distinctly correlates with areas of mucinous degeneration. T2*-weighted images frequently demonstrate the extent of intrasubstance degeneration more accurately than corresponding T1-weighted sagittal images (Fig. 4–38).

Postexercise studies have shown increased signal intensity in meniscal degenerations without alterations in morphology or grade of signal intensity.[46] In a separate prospective study of asymptomatic football players over a 1-year period, progression of grades of meniscal degenerations were recorded.[47] These preliminary findings, however, cannot be used to predict the temporal occurrence of meniscal tears from preexisting areas of intrasubstance degenerations.

A meniscus is considered MR grade 3 when the area of increased signal intensity communicates or extends to at least one articular surface (Fig. 4–39). Fibrocartilaginous separation or tears have been found in all menisci with grade 3 signal intensity. In 5% to 6% of grade 3 menisci, these disruptions represent what has been referred to in the orthopaedic literature as confined intrasubstance cleavage tears (Fig. 4–40).[48] Diagnosis of these closed meniscal tears requires surgical probing during arthroscopy and might be missed altogether on arthrographic examination. These disruptions also partly explain the 6% false-positive interpretations of grade 3 signal intensity when correlated with arthroscopy. A similar rate of false-negative correlations with arthroscopy may relate to spurious interpretation of areas of fraying or fibrillation as meniscal tears. Even without joint locking, the resultant edema and inflammation created by confined horizontal cleavage tears may be responsible for the clinical presentation of acute knee pain. Meniscal tears frequently occur adjacent to areas of intrasubstance degeneration (Fig. 4–41).

In addition to observing increased signal intensity within tears, the morphology (*i.e.,* size and shape) of the meniscus should be assessed when evaluating meniscal lesions (Figs. 4–42 and 4–43). The normal meniscus measures 3 to 5 mm in height. The medial meniscus varies in width from 6 mm at the anterior horn to 12 mm at the posterior horn. The lateral meniscus is consistent in width at 10 mm.[49]

Regenerative chondrocytes and synovial development, apparently attempts at meniscal repair, have been documented along the tear–meniscus interface (Fig. 4–44).[15] In fact, arthroscopic rasping is performed to induce a neovascular response by abrading synovium and creating a blood supply. Synovial ingrowth in degenerative tears is thought to contribute to the development of acute and chronic pain (Fig. 4–45). Hyperplasia of the synovium may also form, secondary to joint debris in degenerative osteoarthritis, and is arthroscopically resected. Peripheral perimeniscal capillary ingrowth may be seen perforating areas of degeneration and fibrocartilaginous separation, supporting the preferential healing in this location (Fig. 4–46).

(text continues on page 207)

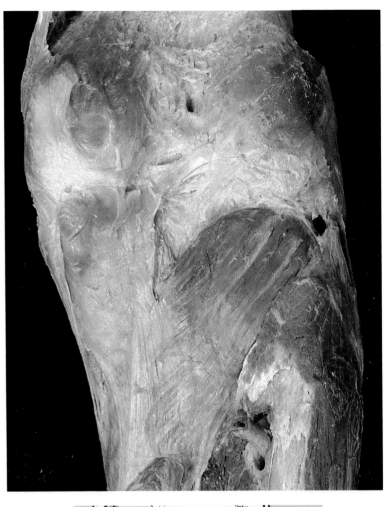

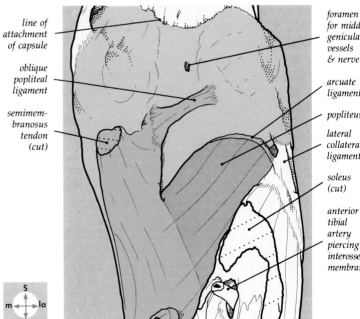

line of
attachment
of capsule

oblique
popliteal
ligament

semimem-
branosus
tendon
(cut)

foramen
for middle
genicular
vessels
& nerve

arcuate
ligament

popliteus

lateral
collateral
ligament

soleus
(cut)

anterior
tibial
artery
piercing
interosseous
membrane

FIGURE 4–17. Superficial dissection from the posterior aspect reveals the capsule, semimembranosus insertion, oblique popliteal ligament, popliteus and arcuate ligament.

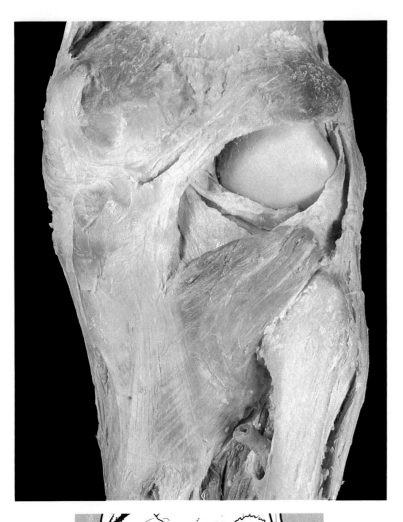

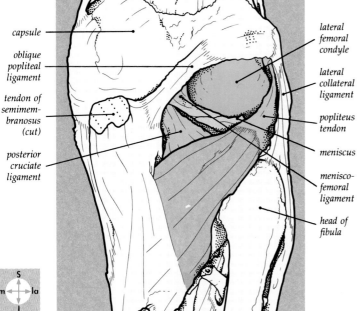

capsule

oblique
popliteal
ligament

tendon of
semimem-
branosus
(cut)

posterior
cruciate
ligament

lateral
femoral
condyle

lateral
collateral
ligament

popliteus
tendon

meniscus

menisco-
femoral
ligament

head of
fibula

FIGURE 4–18. The posterior part of the capsule has been removed to reveal the meniscofemoral and posterior cruciate ligaments and the popliteus tendon.

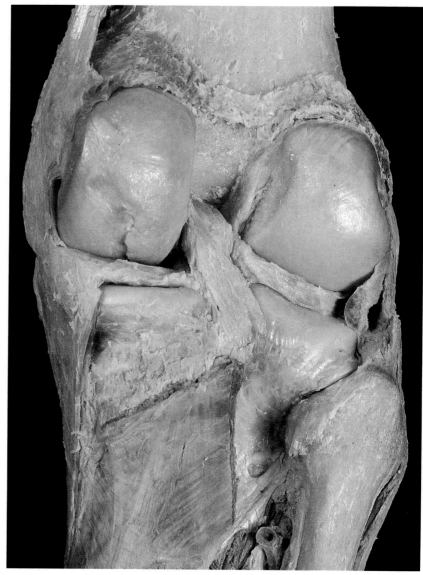

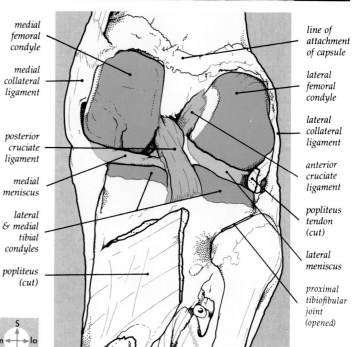

medial
femoral
condyle

medial
collateral
ligament

posterior
cruciate
ligament

medial
meniscus

lateral
& medial
tibial
condyles

popliteus
(cut)

line of
attachment
of capsule

lateral
femoral
condyle

lateral
collateral
ligament

anterior
cruciate
ligament

popliteus
tendon
(cut)

lateral
meniscus

proximal
tibiofibular
joint
(opened)

FIGURE 4–19. The posterior part of the capsule has been removed to reveal the anterior and posterior cruciate ligaments and menisci.

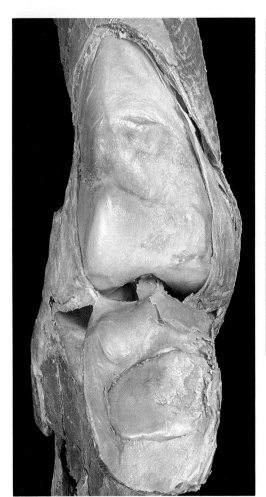

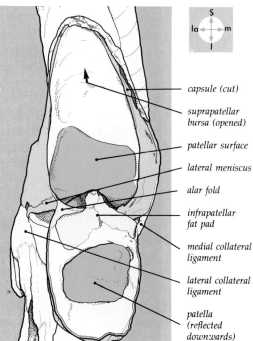

capsule (cut)

suprapatellar
bursa (opened)

patellar surface

lateral meniscus

alar fold

infrapatellar
fat pad

medial collateral
ligament

lateral collateral
ligament

patella
(reflected
downwards)

FIGURE 4–20. The interior of the joint and the suprapatellar pouch are exposed by opening the capsule anteriorly and reflecting the patella downward.

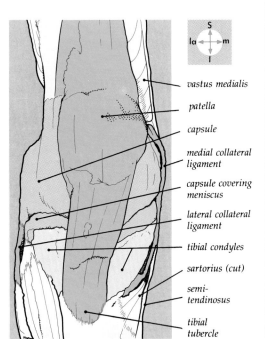

vastus medialis

patella

capsule

medial collateral
ligament

capsule covering
meniscus

lateral collateral
ligament

tibial condyles

sartorius (cut)

semi-
tendinosus

tibial
tubercle

FIGURE 4–21. Superficial dissection from the anterior aspect shows the ligamentum patellae, capsule, and medial and lateral collateral ligaments.

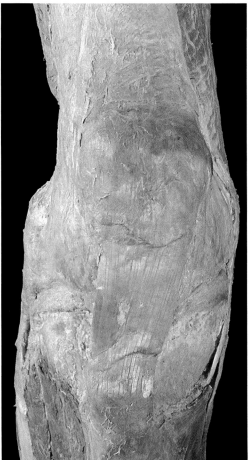

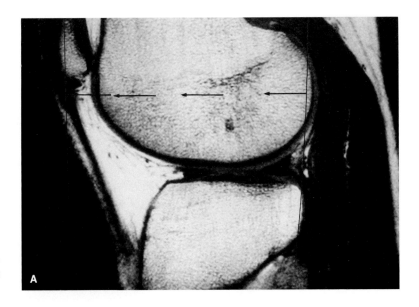

FIGURE 4–22. Normal coronal MR anatomy. (**A**) This T1-weighted sagittal localizer was used to prescribe image locations from (**B**) posterior to (**X**) anterior.

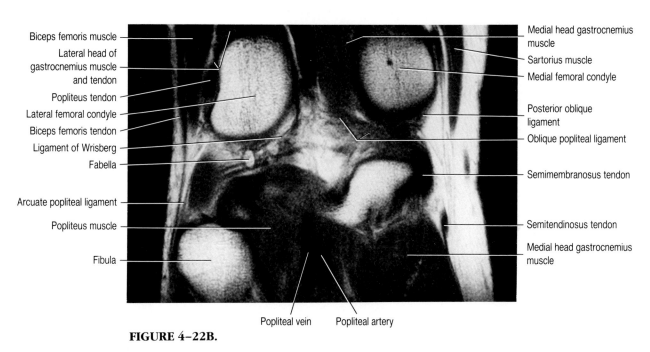

Biceps femoris muscle

Lateral head of gastrocnemius muscle and tendon

Popliteus tendon

Lateral femoral condyle

Biceps femoris tendon

Ligament of Wrisberg

Fabella

Arcuate popliteal ligament

Popliteus muscle

Fibula

Medial head gastrocnemius muscle

Sartorius muscle

Medial femoral condyle

Posterior oblique ligament

Oblique popliteal ligament

Semimembranosus tendon

Semitendinosus tendon

Medial head gastrocnemius muscle

Popliteal vein   Popliteal artery

FIGURE 4–22B.

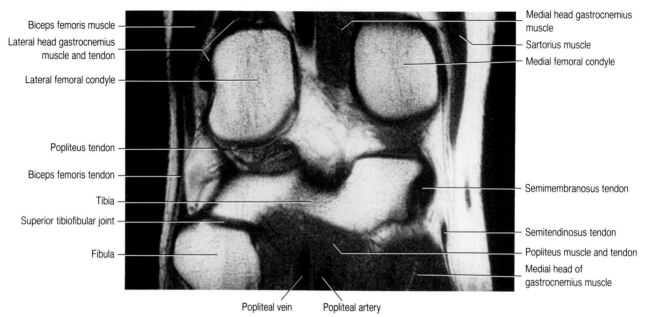

Biceps femoris muscle

Lateral head gastrocnemius muscle and tendon

Lateral femoral condyle

Popliteus tendon

Biceps femoris tendon

Tibia

Superior tibiofibular joint

Fibula

Medial head gastrocnemius muscle

Sartorius muscle

Medial femoral condyle

Semimembranosus tendon

Semitendinosus tendon

Popliteus muscle and tendon

Medial head of gastrocnemius muscle

Popliteal vein   Popliteal artery

FIGURE 4–22C.

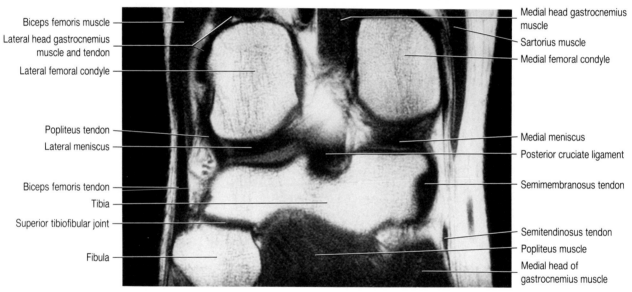

Biceps femoris muscle

Lateral head gastrocnemius muscle and tendon

Lateral femoral condyle

Popliteus tendon

Lateral meniscus

Biceps femoris tendon

Tibia

Superior tibiofibular joint

Fibula

Medial head gastrocnemius muscle

Sartorius muscle

Medial femoral condyle

Medial meniscus

Posterior cruciate ligament

Semimembranosus tendon

Semitendinosus tendon

Popliteus muscle

Medial head of gastrocnemius muscle

FIGURE 4–22D.

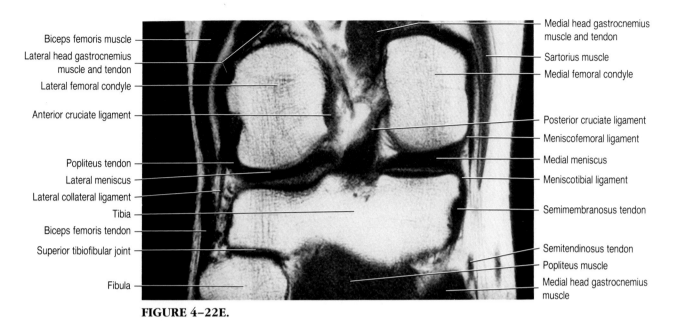

Biceps femoris muscle

Lateral head gastrocnemius
muscle and tendon

Lateral femoral condyle

Anterior cruciate ligament

Popliteus tendon
Lateral meniscus
Lateral collateral ligament
Tibia
Biceps femoris tendon
Superior tibiofibular joint

Fibula

Medial head gastrocnemius
muscle and tendon

Sartorius muscle
Medial femoral condyle

Posterior cruciate ligament
Meniscofemoral ligament
Medial meniscus
Meniscotibial ligament

Semimembranosus tendon

Semitendinosus tendon
Popliteus muscle
Medial head gastrocnemius
muscle

FIGURE 4–22E.

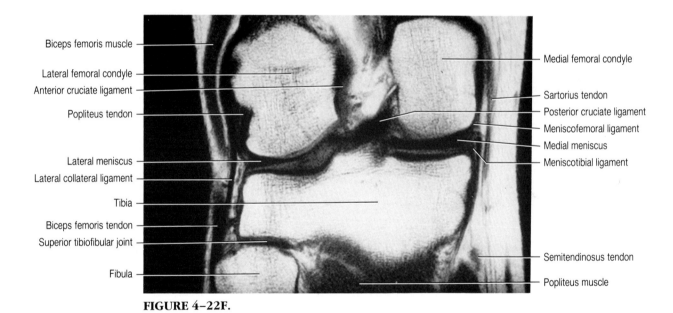

Biceps femoris muscle

Lateral femoral condyle
Anterior cruciate ligament

Popliteus tendon

Lateral meniscus
Lateral collateral ligament
Tibia
Biceps femoris tendon
Superior tibiofibular joint

Fibula

Medial femoral condyle

Sartorius tendon
Posterior cruciate ligament
Meniscofemoral ligament
Medial meniscus
Meniscotibial ligament

Semitendinosus tendon

Popliteus muscle

FIGURE 4–22F.

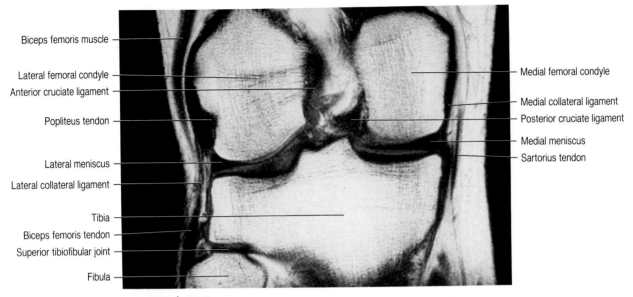

Biceps femoris muscle

Lateral femoral condyle
Anterior cruciate ligament

Popliteus tendon

Lateral meniscus

Lateral collateral ligament

Tibia
Biceps femoris tendon
Superior tibiofibular joint

Fibula

Medial femoral condyle

Medial collateral ligament
Posterior cruciate ligament
Medial meniscus
Sartorius tendon

FIGURE 4–22G.

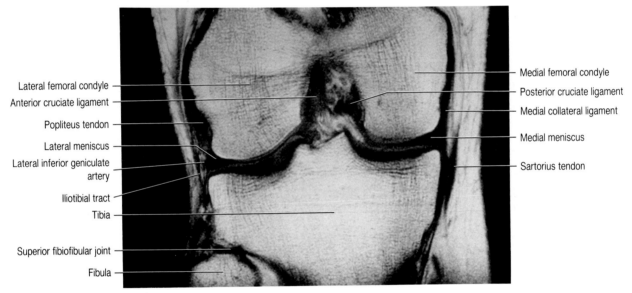

Lateral femoral condyle
Anterior cruciate ligament

Popliteus tendon

Lateral meniscus
Lateral inferior geniculate
artery

Iliotibial tract

Tibia

Superior fibiofibular joint

Fibula

Medial femoral condyle
Posterior cruciate ligament
Medial collateral ligament
Medial meniscus
Sartorius tendon

FIGURE 4–22H.

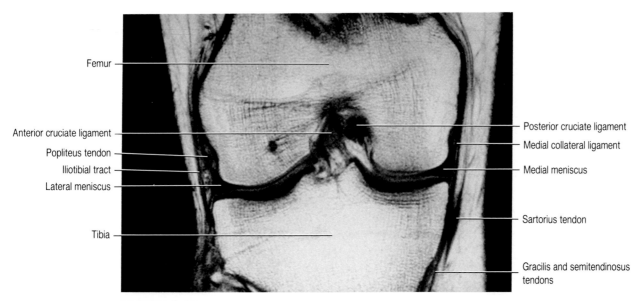

Femur

Anterior cruciate ligament
Popliteus tendon
Iliotibial tract
Lateral meniscus

Tibia

Posterior cruciate ligament
Medial collateral ligament

Medial meniscus

Sartorius tendon

Gracilis and semitendinosus tendons

FIGURE 4–22I.

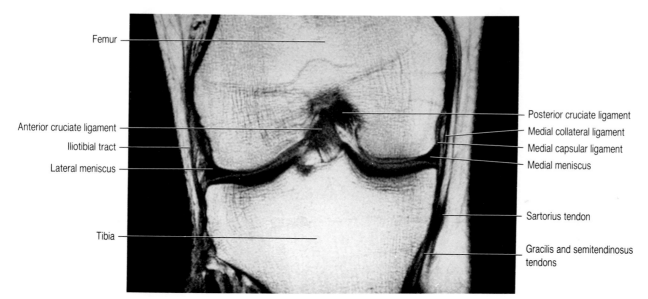

Femur

Anterior cruciate ligament
Iliotibial tract
Lateral meniscus

Tibia

Posterior cruciate ligament
Medial collateral ligament
Medial capsular ligament
Medial meniscus

Sartorius tendon

Gracilis and semitendinosus tendons

FIGURE 4–22J.

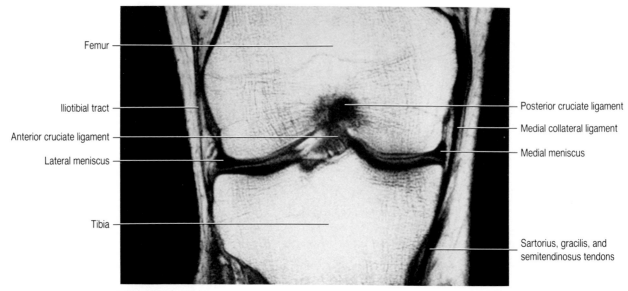

Femur

Iliotibial tract

Anterior cruciate ligament

Lateral meniscus

Tibia

Posterior cruciate ligament

Medial collateral ligament

Medial meniscus

Sartorius, gracilis, and semitendinosus tendons

FIGURE 4–22K.

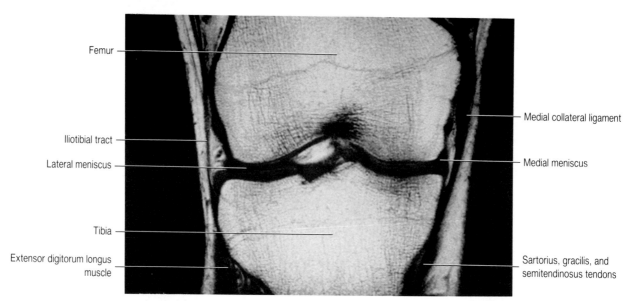

Femur

Iliotibial tract

Lateral meniscus

Tibia

Extensor digitorum longus muscle

Medial collateral ligament

Medial meniscus

Sartorius, gracilis, and semitendinosus tendons

FIGURE 4–22L.

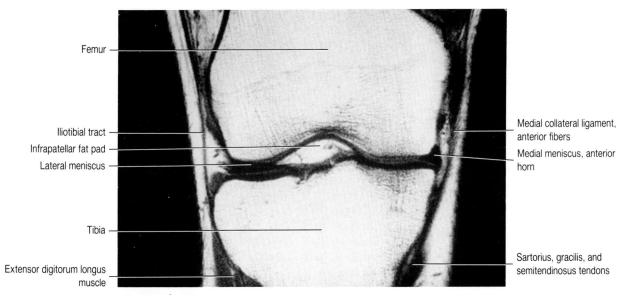

Femur

Iliotibial tract
Infrapatellar fat pad
Lateral meniscus

Tibia

Extensor digitorum longus
muscle

Medial collateral ligament,
anterior fibers

Medial meniscus, anterior
horn

Sartorius, gracilis, and
semitendinosus tendons

FIGURE 4–22M.

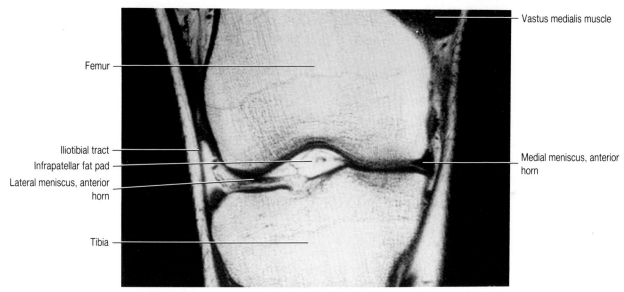

Vastus medialis muscle

Femur

Iliotibial tract
Infrapatellar fat pad
Lateral meniscus, anterior
horn

Tibia

Medial meniscus, anterior
horn

FIGURE 4–22N.

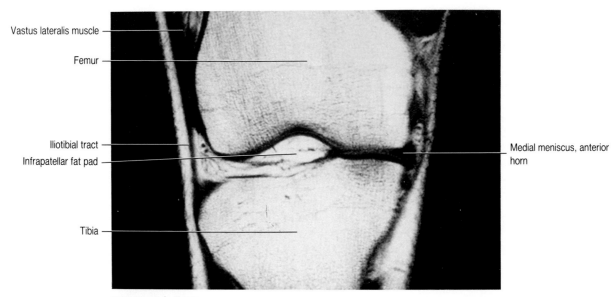

Vastus lateralis muscle

Femur

Iliotibial tract

Infrapatellar fat pad

Tibia

Medial meniscus, anterior horn

FIGURE 4–22O.

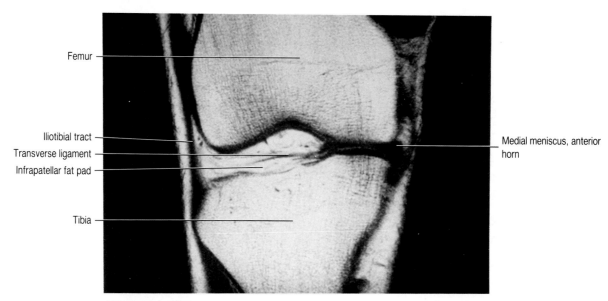

Femur

Iliotibial tract

Transverse ligament

Infrapatellar fat pad

Tibia

Medial meniscus, anterior horn

FIGURE 4–22P.

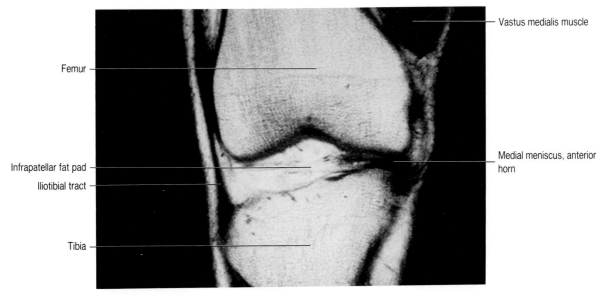

Vastus medialis muscle

Femur

Medial meniscus, anterior horn

Infrapatellar fat pad

Iliotibial tract

Tibia

FIGURE 4–22Q.

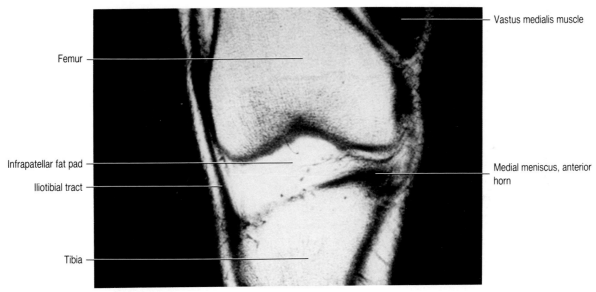

Vastus medialis muscle

Femur

Medial meniscus, anterior horn

Infrapatellar fat pad

Iliotibial tract

Tibia

FIGURE 4–22R.

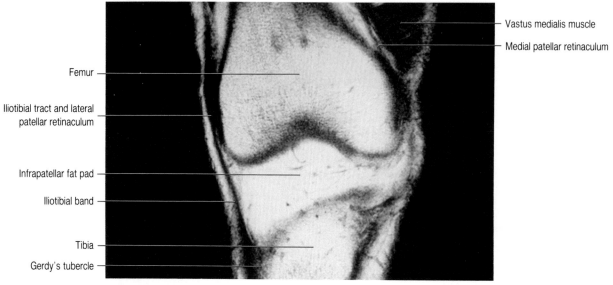

Vastus medialis muscle

Medial patellar retinaculum

Femur

Iliotibial tract and lateral patellar retinaculum

Infrapatellar fat pad

Iliotibial band

Tibia

Gerdy's tubercle

FIGURE 4–22S.

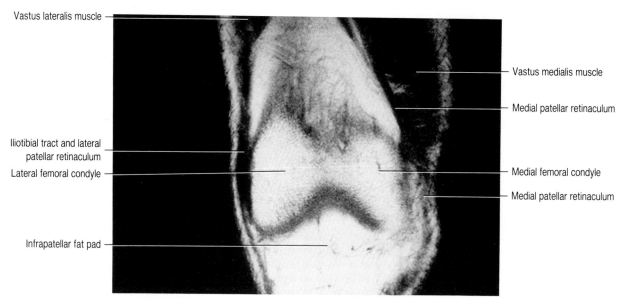

Vastus lateralis muscle

Iliotibial tract and lateral patellar retinaculum

Lateral femoral condyle

Infrapatellar fat pad

Vastus medialis muscle

Medial patellar retinaculum

Medial femoral condyle

Medial patellar retinaculum

FIGURE 4–22T.

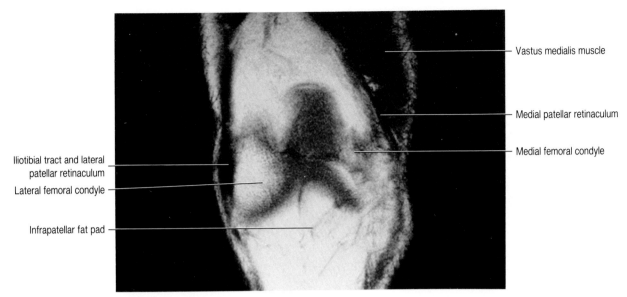

Vastus medialis muscle

Medial patellar retinaculum

Medial femoral condyle

Iliotibial tract and lateral
patellar retinaculum

Lateral femoral condyle

Infrapatellar fat pad

FIGURE 4–22U.

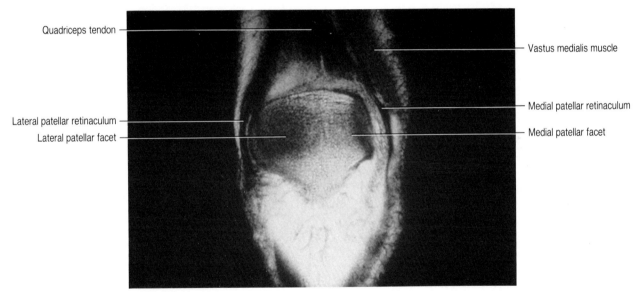

Quadriceps tendon

Vastus medialis muscle

Medial patellar retinaculum

Medial patellar facet

Lateral patellar retinaculum

Lateral patellar facet

FIGURE 4–22V.

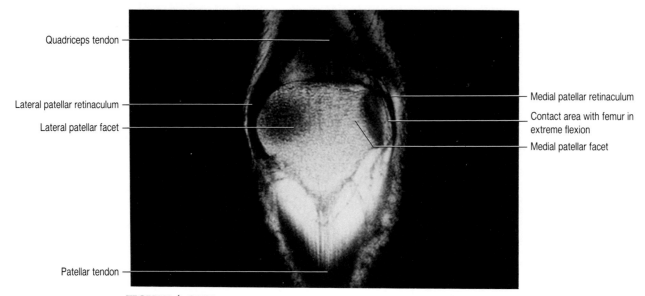

FIGURE 4–22W.

Quadriceps tendon

Lateral patellar retinaculum

Lateral patellar facet

Medial patellar retinaculum

Contact area with femur in extreme flexion

Medial patellar facet

Patellar tendon

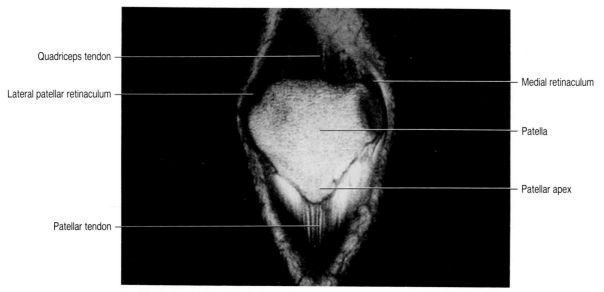

FIGURE 4–22X.

Quadriceps tendon

Lateral patellar retinaculum

Medial retinaculum

Patella

Patellar apex

Patellar tendon

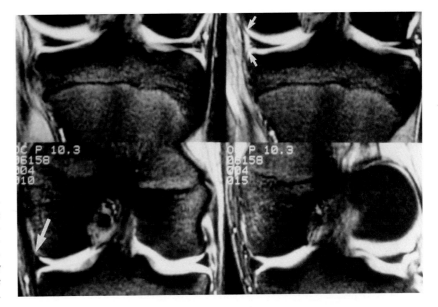

FIGURE 4–23. These T2*-weighted radial images progress from the posterior (*top left*) to the anterior (*bottom right*) horn of the medial meniscus. Normal meniscofemoral and meniscotibial attachments (*small arrows*) of the deep medial capsular layer (*i.e.,* ligament) are present. The closely applied meniscal attachment to the capsule and the medial collateral ligament is shown (*large arrow*).

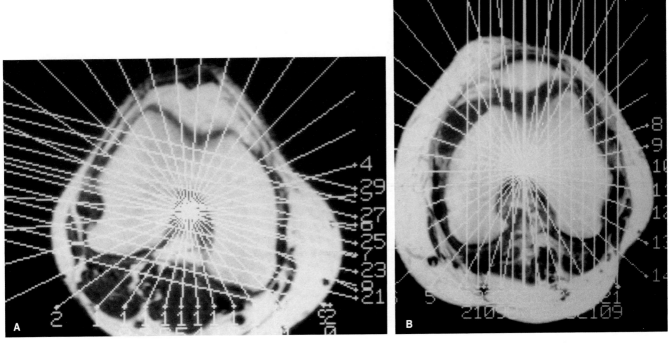

FIGURE 4–24. Normal MR anatomy. These T1-weighted axial localizers were used to prescribe simultaneous (**A**) radial–coronal and (**B**) radial–sagittal images.

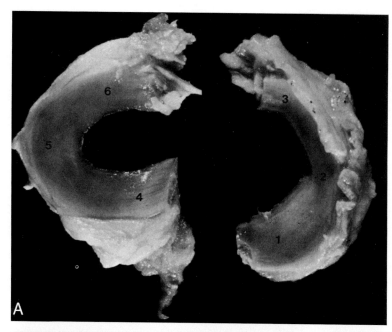

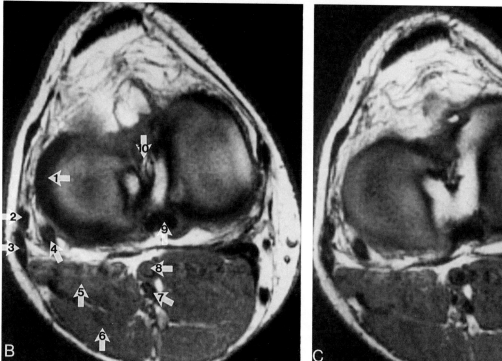

FIGURE 4–25. Axial anatomy of the menisci. (**A**) Gross anatomy of the lateral meniscus (*left*) and medial meniscus (*right*). The larger posterior horn of the medial meniscus is evident. (1, posterior horn of medial meniscus; 2, body of meniscus; 3, anterior horn of medial meniscus; 4, posterior horn of lateral meniscus; 5, body of lateral meniscus; 6, anterior horn of lateral meniscus.) (**B**) An axial image made in the plane of the lateral meniscus. (1, lateral meniscus; 2, fibular collateral ligament; 3, biceps femoris tendon; 4, popliteus tendon; 5, plantaris muscle; 6, lateral head of gastrocnemius muscle; 7, popliteal vein; 8, popliteal artery; 9, posterior cruciate ligament; 10, anterior cruciate ligament.) (**C**) An axial image made in the plane of the medial meniscus. (1, anterior horn of medial meniscus; 2, medial tibial collateral ligament; 3, posterior horn of medial meniscus; 4, gracilis tendon; 5, semimembranosus tendon; 6, semitendinosus tendon.)

FIGURE 4–26. Normal anatomy of the meniscus. (**A**) Line 1 of the gross specimen of the lateral meniscus represents the sagittal plane of section through the body of the lateral meniscus. Line 2 represents the sagittal plane of section through the anterior and body of the lateral meniscus. (**B**) The corresponding gross sagittal sections (1 and 2) are seen through the posterior horns (*curved black arrows*) and anterior and posterior horns (*straight white arrows*) of the lateral meniscus. The periphery or body of the meniscus has a continuous bow-tie appearance. The anterior and posterior horns are oriented as opposing triangles of fibrocartilage. (**C, D**) The corresponding sagittal plane images (1 and 2) demonstrate the low signal intensity body (*curved black arrows*) and anterior and posterior horns (*straight white arrows*) of the lateral meniscus.

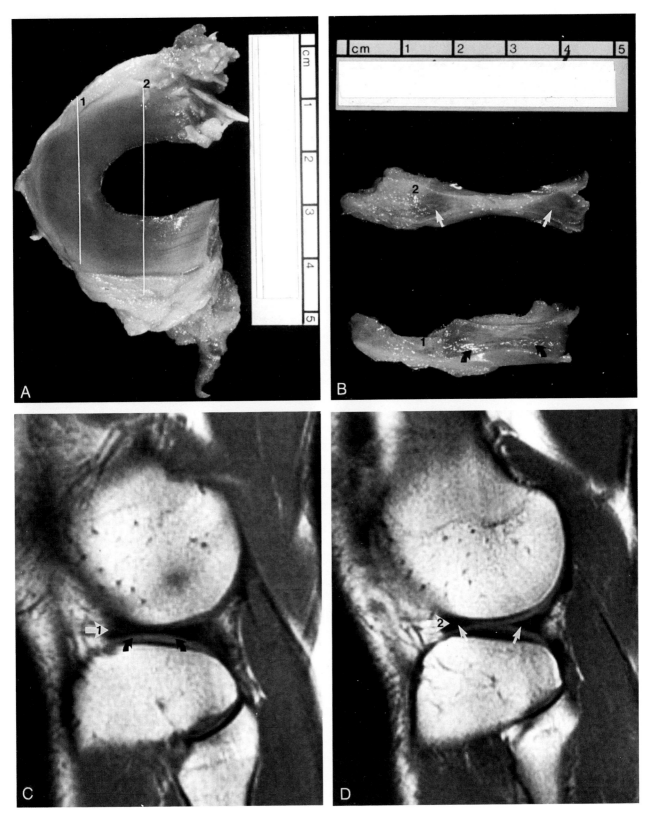

FIGURE 4–26.

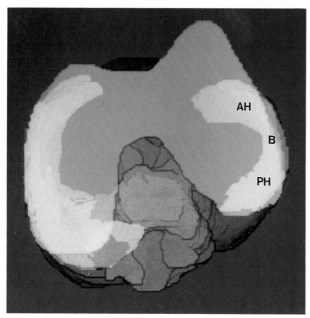

FIGURE 4–27. This 3D MR image rendering demonstrates the division of the lateral meniscus into the anterior horn (AH), body (B) and posterior horn (PH). A posterior tibial fracture, seen from above, is represented by the salmon-colored area.

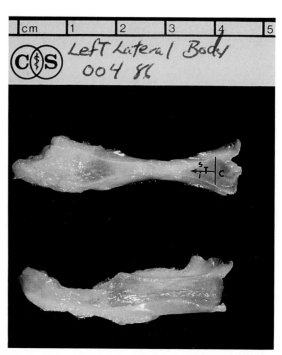

FIGURE 4–28. The circumferential (C) and transverse (T) zones of the meniscus. The middle perforating collagen bundle (*arrow*) divides the transverse zone into superior (s) and inferior (i) leaves.

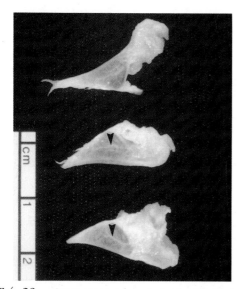

FIGURE 4–29. Gross meniscal sections identify the location of the middle perforating collagen bundle and the site of preferential horizontal mucinous degeneration (*arrowheads*).

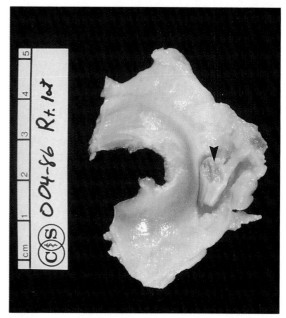

FIGURE 4–30. Gross anatomy of the lateral meniscus and associated popliteus tendon (*arrowhead*).

FIGURE 4–33. (**A**) A T1-weighted sagittal image shows grade 1 signal intensity (*arrow*) in the posterior horn of the lateral meniscus. (**B**) On a cut gross section, a focus of meniscal degeneration (*arrow*) can be seen. (**C**) The corresponding photomicrograph shows hypocellularity with decreased numbers of chondrocytes (*black arrow*) in pale-staining areas (*white arrow*). (H & E stain.)

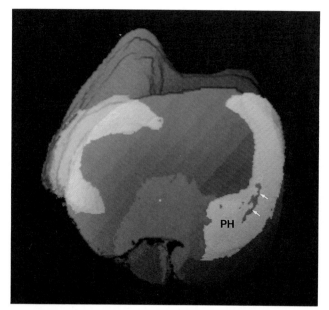

FIGURE 4–31. Normal posterior horn morphology of the medial meniscus (PH). A longitudinal tear pattern is shown (*arrows*). A posterior tibial fracture fragment can be seen from below when looking toward the femur.

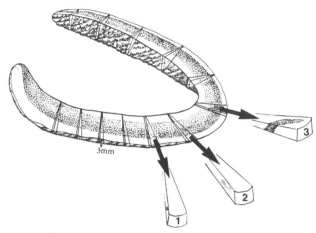

FIGURE 4–32. Representative grades of meniscal degeneration (grades 1 and 2) and tear (grade 3) are shown in relation to the gross meniscus.

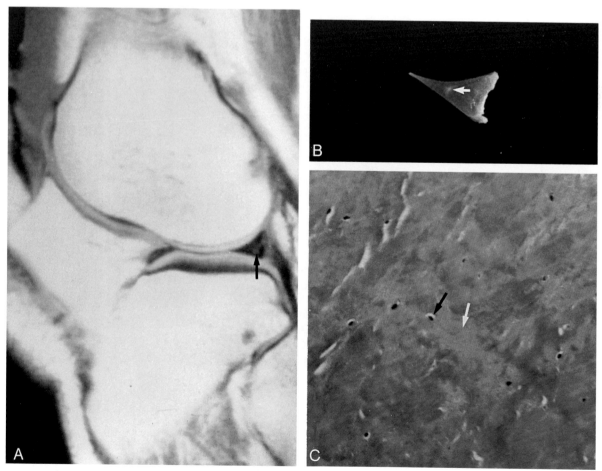

FIGURE 4–33.

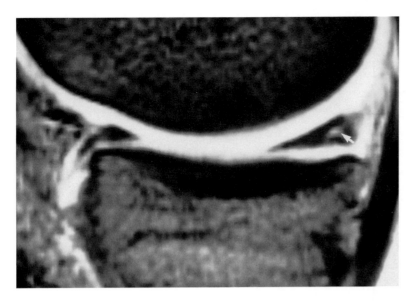

FIGURE 4–34. A T2*-weighted sagittal image shows grade 1 signal intensity (*arrow*) in the posterior horn of the medial meniscus in an athlete without medial compartment pain.

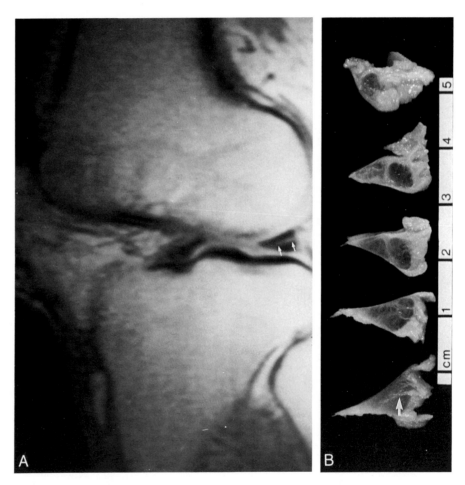

FIGURE 4–35. (**A**) A T1-weighted sagittal image demonstrates grade 2 signal intensity in the posterior horn of the lateral meniscus (*arrows*). (**B**) The corresponding gross section demonstrates linear mucinous meniscal degeneration (*arrow*). (**C**) The histologic correlation shows a focus of mucinous degeneration within the meniscal fibrocartilage (*arrows*).

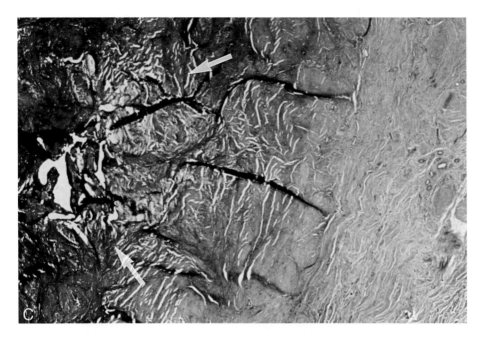

FIGURE 4-35. (Continued)

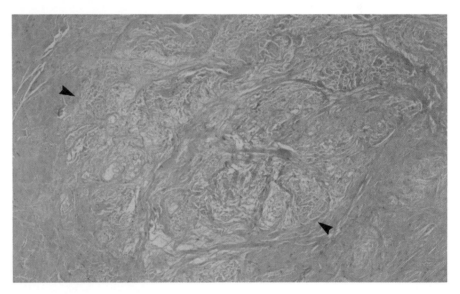

FIGURE 4-36. The region of mucinous degeneration (*arrowheads*) corresponds to grade 2 meniscal intrasubstance degeneration. (H & E stain.)

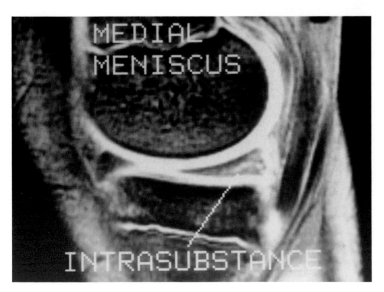

FIGURE 4-37. High grade 2 signal intensity is seen in the posterior horn of the medial meniscus on this T2*-weighted sagittal image.

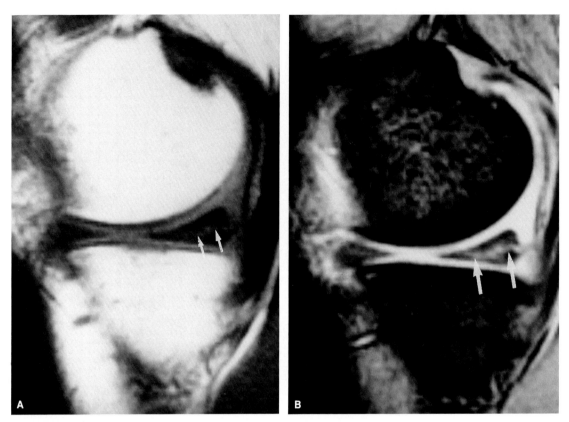

FIGURE 4–38. Prominent grade 2 signal intensity (*arrows*) is seen in the posterior horn of the medial meniscus on (**A**) T1-weighted and (**B**) T2*-weighted sagittal images. No surface extension of this intrasubstance degeneration has occurred.

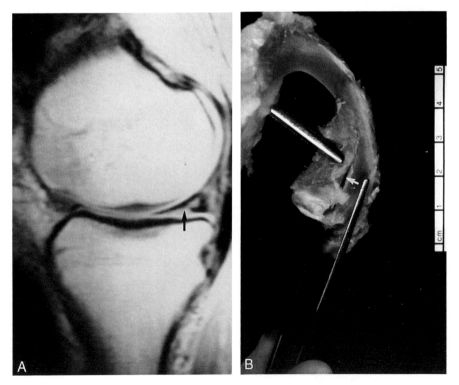

FIGURE 4–39. (**A**) A T1-weighted image shows grade 3 signal intensity extending to the inferior articular surface in the posterior horn of a medial meniscus flap tear (*arrow*). (**B**) On a gross specimen of the medial meniscus, a corresponding inferior surface tear (*arrow*) is revealed with probing. (**C**) Cut gross sagittal sections demonstrate the orientation of the inferior surface flap tear (*arrows*). (**D**) A photomicrograph of a grade 3 meniscal tear shows complete fibrocartilaginous separation (*large arrows*) with regenerative chondrocytes along the free edge of the torn meniscus (*small arrows*).

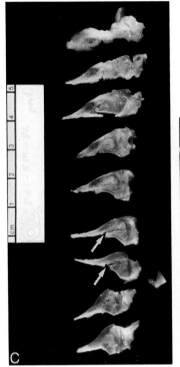

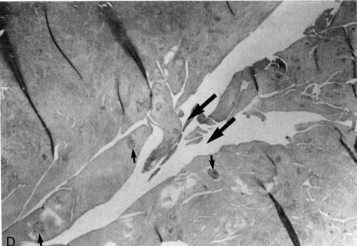

FIGURE 4–39. *(Continued)*

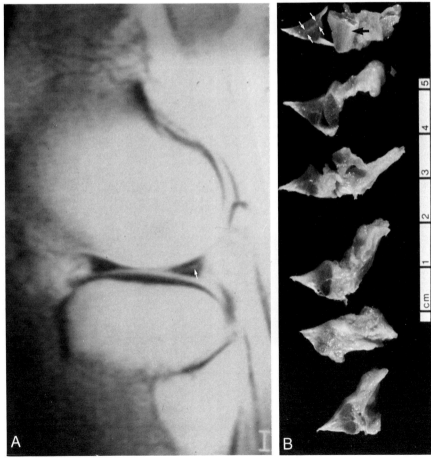

FIGURE 4–40. Closed meniscal tear. (**A**) On a T1-weighted sagittal image, a horizontal intrasubstance cleavage tear has grade 3 signal intensity (*white arrow*). (**B**) The sagittal gross section shows degeneration approaching the inferior surface of the meniscus without a visible surface tear (*white arrows*). The popliteus tendon is indicated (*black arrow*). (**C**) The corresponding photomicrograph demonstrates confined fibrocartilaginous separation (*arrows*). *(continued)*

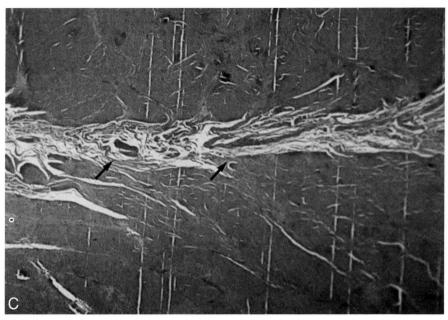

FIGURE 4-40. *(Continued)*

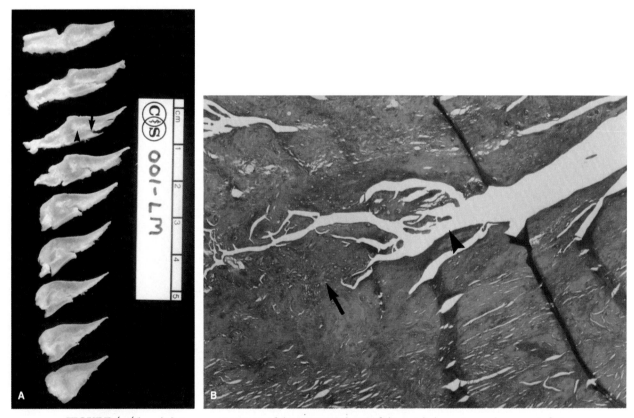

FIGURE 4-41. (**A**) A gross specimen of the posterior horn of the medial meniscus shows an inferior surface tear (*arrow*) adjacent to an area of intrasubstance degeneration (*arrowhead*). (**B**) The corresponding photomicrograph demonstrates a fibrocartilaginous tear (*arrowhead*) and surrounding (blue) mucinous degeneration (*arrow*). (Alcian blue stain.)

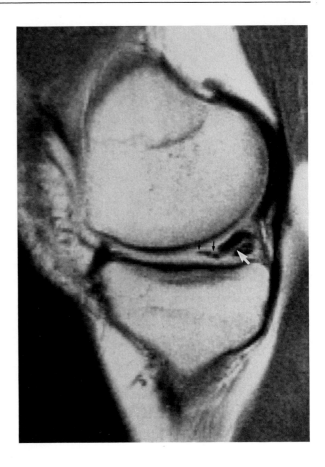

FIGURE 4–42. Intermediate-weighted sagittal images are used to demonstrate a grade 3 flap tear of the posterior horn of the medial meniscus (*white arrow*) with a truncated meniscal apex (*black arrows*).

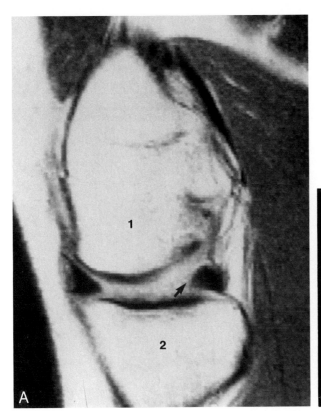

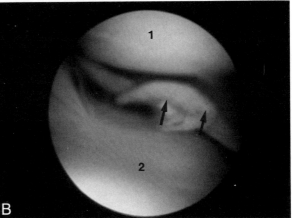

FIGURE 4–43. This torn medial meniscus shows abnormal morphology. (**A**) The T1-weighted sagittal image shows a blunted and foreshortened apex of the posterior horn of the medial meniscus (*arrow*). (1, femur; 2, tibia.) (**B**) The arthroscopic view demonstrates a complete flap tear (*arrows*) that extends to the truncated medial meniscus. (1, femur; 2, tibia.)

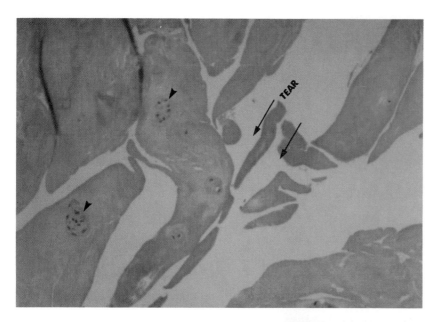

FIGURE 4-44. A high-power photomicrograph shows large regenerative chondrocytes (*arrowheads*) at the tear site (*long arrows*). (H & E stain.)

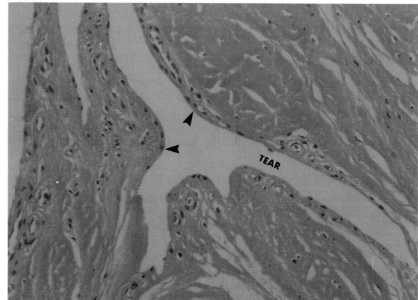

FIGURE 4-45. Peripheral synovial ingrowth into the meniscal tear cleavage plane can be seen in a photomicrograph. (H & E stain.)

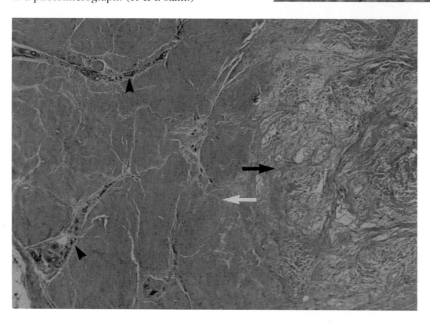

FIGURE 4-46. A perimeniscal capillary ingrowth (*arrowheads*) is directed toward an area of mucinous degeneration (*black arrow*). Normal adjacent meniscal tissue is shown (*white arrow*).

Acute traumatic tears have less predictable orientations and smaller areas of associated mucinous degeneration as sites for structural weakening than degenerative horizontal cleavage or flap tears (Fig. 4–47).[50] Grade 3 signal intensity is most frequent in the posterior horn of the medial meniscus, a finding supported by the observations of increased stress and strain generated on the undersurface of the meniscus with femorotibial rotations. Magnetic resonance makes a significant contribution in imaging this frequently injured site. The accuracy of arthroscopy in identifying inferior surface tears of the posteromedial meniscus is reported to be as low at 45% to 69%.[51,52] Furthermore, arthrographic and arthroscopic surface evaluations are insensitive to grade 1 and 2 intrasubstance degenerations as precursors to the formation of a defined meniscal tear. Magnetic resonance additionally detects multiple meniscal tears that may be overlooked on arthrography.

Three-Dimensional Rendering and Classification of Meniscal Tears

Cross-Sectional Patterns: Vertical and Horizontal Tears. The present system of classifying meniscal tears as grade 3 signal intensity relative to a meniscal articular surface does not accurately describe the anatomy of various horizontal and vertical tear patterns as identified during arthroscopic surgery of the knee.[53] Using the cross-sectional anatomy of the meniscus as demonstrated in sagittal images, meniscal tears can be classified into two primary tear planes, vertical or horizontal (Fig. 4–48). However, because most meniscal tears are not exclusively perpendicular or parallel with the tibial plateau surface, tears classified as either vertical (Fig. 4–49) or horizontal (Fig. 4–50) may have secondary tear patterns (*i.e.,* horizontal or vertical, respectively). For example, most horizontal tears have a secondary vertical vector association, with extension of the tear to the inferior surface of the meniscus (see Fig. 4–50).

An accurate description of the morphology and location of a tear is particularly useful in making the choice between primary meniscal repair and partial meniscectomy. We have developed a technique for displaying meniscal anatomy and pathology with 3D composite images spatially disarticulated from the knee joint, processed from 3DFT T2*-weighted images. With this technique, rotation of the meniscus and internal tear patterns are displayed.

Circumferential or Surface Patterns: Longitudinal, Transverse, and Oblique Tears. As viewed from the surface of the meniscus at arthroscopy, and relative to its circumference, three basic tear patterns are found:

1. Longitudinal
2. Transverse or radial
3. Oblique (Fig. 4–51).[23]

Vertical tears extend to the meniscal surface as either longitudinal, transverse, or oblique tears. Horizontal tears are either longitudinal or oblique, unless they remain in the plane of the middle perforating collagen bundle and extend to the meniscal apex as degenerative cleavage tears with approximately equally sized superior and inferior leaves (Fig. 4–52). Although horizontal tears have been referred to as fish-mouth tears, the description is imprecise. Horizontal tears are most frequently associated with meniscal cysts, and treatment of the underlying meniscal tear leads to involution of the meniscal cyst (Fig. 4–53). Complex tears display multiple combinations of vertical and horizontal tear patterns (Fig. 4–54).

Longitudinal Tears. A tear seen from the surface of the meniscus as longitudinal may be either vertical or horizontal on sagittal images (Figs. 4–55 and 4–56). Internal probing of a longitudinal surface tear during arthroscopy confirms these findings. Peripheral vertical tears are successfully treated with primary meniscal repair, whereas horizontal tears that extend into avascular fibrocartilage are treated with partial meniscectomy. The peripheral extension of the MR meniscal signal to the stable rim of the meniscus may assist the arthroscopist in performing a partial meniscectomy, but may not be appreciated at arthroscopy. This corresponds to the normal grade 3 appearance in postmeniscectomy MR images.

Bucket-Handle Tears. A displaced longitudinal tear of the meniscus, usually the medial meniscus, is called a bucket-handle tear because the separated central fragment resembles the handle of a bucket (Fig. 4–57).[15] The remaining larger peripheral section of the meniscus is the bucket. A bucket-handle tear effectively reduces the width of the meniscus, and peripheral sagittal images fail to demonstrate the normal bow-tie configuration in the body of the meniscus. The remaining anterior and posterior horns are often hypoplastic or truncated, with or without increased internal signal intensity. In the normal medial meniscus without tear, the posterior horn is wider and taller than the anterior horn. Foreshortening of the posterior horn of the medial meniscus without history of previous partial meniscectomy is associated with bucket-handle morphology. A displaced medial meniscal fragment can frequently be identified within the intercondylar notch on coronal images (Figs. 4–58 and 4–59).[54]

The medial displaced fragment of a bucket-handle tear is displayed on sagittal images as a low signal intensity band parallel and anterior to the PCL, but we have found this to be an uncommon presentation (Fig. 4–60).[55] In complex bucket-handle tears, 3DFT axial images show the relationship of the displaced tear to the remaining meniscus in a single section (Fig. 4–61). The lateral meniscus may also be the site of bucket-handle tears in which the body of the lateral meniscus is displaced into the intercondylar notch (Fig. 4–62).

Patients with bucket-handle tears may present with a locked knee or lack full extension. Single or multiple flaps of meniscal tissue may be generated. Bucket-handle tears may start as longitudinal tears with a primary horizontal tear pattern. A displaced vertical component subsequently generates a bucket-handle morphology. More commonly, bucket-handle tears are displaced vertical, longitudinal tears.

Transverse or Radial Tears. A transverse or radial tear is, by definition, a vertical tear perpendicular to the free edge of the meniscus (Fig. 4–63). No horizontal vector or flap degeneration is present in radial tears. On sagittal images, the only evidence of a radial tear may be increased signal intensity on one or two peripheral sections, since the sagittal plane sections the meniscus perpendicular to this tear pattern (Fig. 4–64). The middle one-third of the lateral meniscus is a common location for radial tears, probably because of its more circular shape and decreased radius of curvature, increased mobility because the posterior horn is pulled posteriorly in flexion, and excessive loading during valgus stress.[49,56,57]

Oblique Tears. An oblique tear, which represents a composite of a longitudinal and transverse or radial tear, starts on the free edge of the meniscus and curves obliquely into the meniscal fibrocartilage (Fig. 4–65). These tears are often referred to as flap or parrot-beak tears. A parrot-beak tear usually describes an oblique tear pattern with a smaller horizontal component. On cross-sectional images, oblique tears may display either a primary vertical or horizontal tear pattern (Fig. 4–66). From sagittal sections, without thin section axial images or a 3D composite image of the meniscus, it is difficult to differentiate between oblique and longitudinal tear morphology. However, when grade 3 signal intensity is seen to extend to the superior and inferior surface of the meniscus on separate sagittal images, oblique morphology may be inferred (Fig. 4–67). Oblique tears may generate an anterior- or posterior-based flap of meniscus.[23] Oblique tears are treated with arthroscopic resection of the flap and contouring of meniscal tissue to a stable rim through the remaining horizontal component (Fig. 4–68).[56]

Discoid Menisci

A discoid meniscus is a dysplastic meniscus that has lost its normal or semilunar shape and has a broad disklike configuration.[58-60] Lateral discoid menisci are more common than medial discoid menisci, and the degree of enlargement varies from mild hypertrophy to a bulky slab of fibrocartilage. It has been postulated that an abnormal posterior horn attachment, involving the inferior fascicle, contributes to the development of discoid growth.

Discoid menisci are susceptible to tears and cysts, and young patients often present with symptoms of torn cartilage (Fig. 4–69). Pain, clicking, and locking are common presenting clinical findings in children.[23,61] Treatment of the unstable inner segment of a discoid meniscus requires saucerization or resection (partial meniscectomy) to a stable rim. The ligament-of-Wrisberg–type discoid lateral meniscus is prone to medial displacement into the intercondylar notch and is best treated with total meniscectomy.[24,62]

Plain film radiographs of discoid menisci may demonstrate widening of the involved compartment, and arthrography demonstrates an elongated meniscus (Fig. 4–70).[24] On MR images, a discoid meniscus has a continuous or bow-tie appearance on three or more consecutive sagittal images (Fig. 4–71).[6,63] Demonstration of the anterior and posterior horns is limited to one or two sagittal sections adjacent to the intercondylar notch. Central tapering, seen in the normal meniscus on sagittal images, is lost in discoid fibrocartilage. The increased inferior-to-superior dimensions of the meniscus can be appreciated on both coronal and sagittal MR images. A discoid meniscus may be as much as 2 mm higher than the opposite meniscus.[63] Grade 2 signal intensity in a discoid meniscus may correlate with intrameniscal cavitation or cysts, and many orthopaedic surgeons recommend meniscectomy for the symptomatic discoid meniscus even without grade 3 signal intensity. In the presence of an effusion, the enlarged meniscus is outlined with high signal intensity fluid on T2- and T2*-weighted images. Coronal images show the extension of the meniscal apex into the intercondylar notch.

Pitfalls in Interpreting Meniscal Tears

Knowledge of the more common pitfalls encountered in MR imaging of the meniscus helps to maintain high specificity and accuracy of diagnostic interpretations of meniscal tears.[64-67]

Grade 2 *versus* Grade 3 Signal Intensity. In a small percentage of cases (less than 5% in our experience), it may be difficult to distinguish articular surface extension of signal intensity. In such cases, evaluation of the morphology of the meniscus as well as the degree and thickness of increased signal intensity may facilitate a more accurate interpretation. Weakening or decreased signal intensity of a grade 3 lesion as it approaches an articular surface, for example, favors the diagnosis of an intrasubstance cleavage tear that, at arthroscopy, might require surgical probing for detection. In the presence of a joint effusion, the grade 3 signal, which becomes more conspicuous on conventional T2 weighting, corresponds to a disrupted meniscal surface that facilitates the influx of free water molecules (*i.e.*, T2 prolongation; Fig. 4–72).

Radial imaging may be helpful in patients with peripheral signal intensity or when grade 2 and grade 3 signal intensity cannot be differentiated (Figs. 4–73 and

(text continues on page 227)

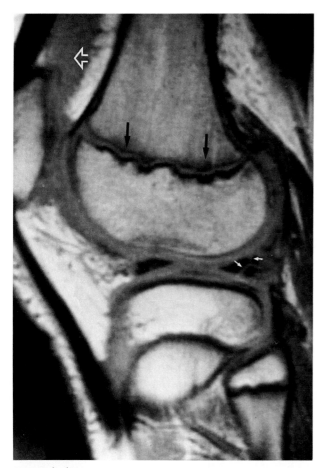

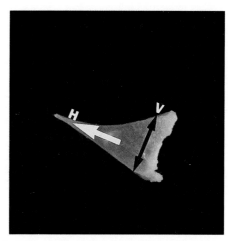

FIGURE 4–48. Idealized directions of horizontal (H, *white arrow*) and vertical (V, *black arrows*) tear patterns in a gross cross section of the meniscus.

FIGURE 4–47. A traumatic meniscal tear in a 12-year-old child. This complex tear of the posterior horn of the lateral meniscus communicates with both the superior and inferior articular surfaces (*white arrows*). A physeal scar (*black arrows*) and associated joint effusion (*open arrow*) are indicated.

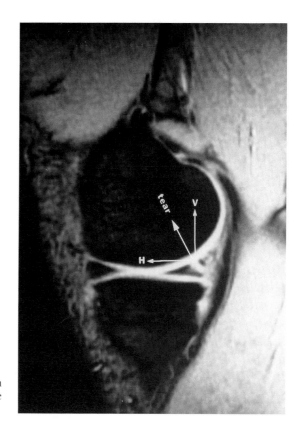

FIGURE 4–49. The vertical primary tear pattern (tear) is shown with both vertical (V) and horizontal (H) vector components. The tear is directed more than 45° from the horizontal component.

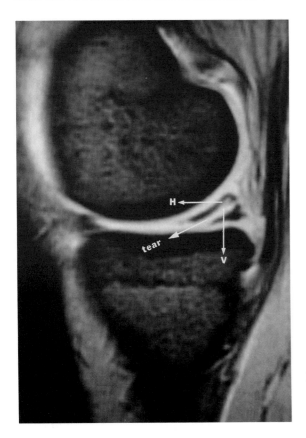

FIGURE 4–50. A horizontal primary tear pattern (tear) has both horizontal (H) and vertical (V) vector components. The direction of the tear is close to but less than 45° from the horizontal, indicating almost equal contributions from the horizontal and vertical vectors.

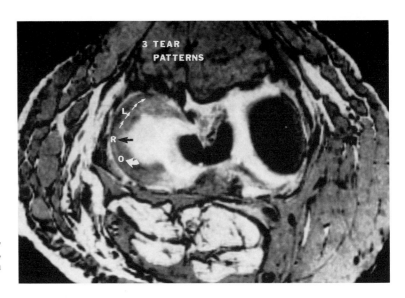

FIGURE 4–51. Longitudinal (L, *straight white arrows*), transverse or radial (R, *black arrow*), and oblique (O, *curved white arrow*) tear patterns are shown as seen from the surface of the lateral meniscus.

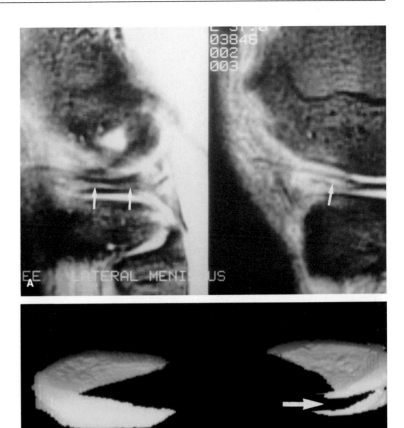

FIGURE 4–52. (**A**) A T2*-weighted sagittal image shows a horizontal tear (*arrows*) of the body (*left*) and anterior horn (*right*) of the lateral meniscus parallel with the tibial surface. (**B**) A 3D MR rendering displays a horizontal tear pattern (*arrow*) dividing the meniscus into superior and inferior leaves (*i.e.,* halves). Although most meniscal tears have horizontal components, a pure cleavage tear parallel with the tibial articular surface and extending to the apex is less common.

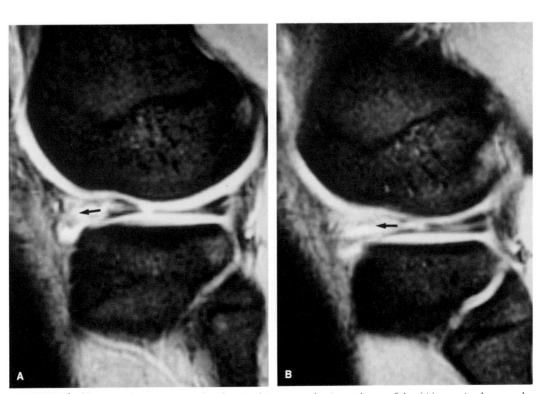

FIGURE 4–53. On these T2*-weighted sagittal images, a horizontal tear of the (**A**) anterior horn and (**B**) body of the lateral meniscus decompresses into an anterolateral meniscal cyst (*arrows*).

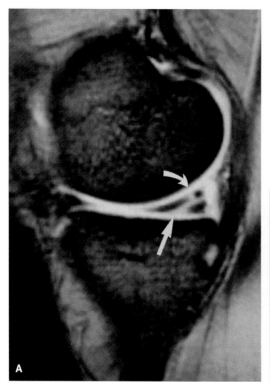

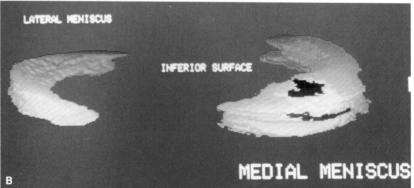

FIGURE 4–54. (**A**) A T2*-weighted image displays a complex tear pattern with superior (*curved arrow*) and inferior (*straight arrow*) meniscal tear extension. (**B**) A 3D MR rendering shows both vertical and horizontal components (*red*) in this complex oblique tear pattern.

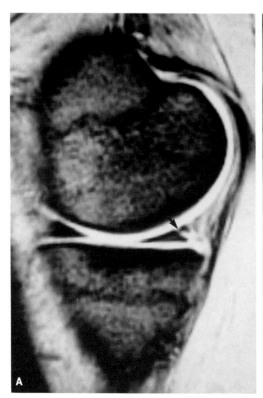

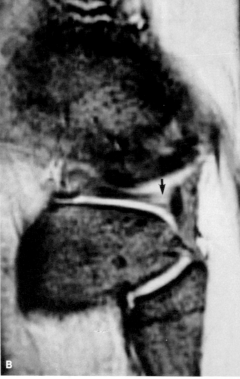

FIGURE 4–55. A longitudinal tear with the primary vertical tear pattern can be seen on meniscal cross section in the sagittal plane. Peripheral (*i.e.,* outer one-third of the meniscus) vertical tears of the posterior horn of the (**A**) medial and (**B**) lateral meniscus can be seen on T2*-weighted sagittal images. (**C**) The corresponding 3D MR rendering demonstrates superior surface extension of the medial meniscus (M), the longitudinal tear (*straight arrow*), and the peripheral location of the tear (*curved arrow*) of the lateral meniscus (L).

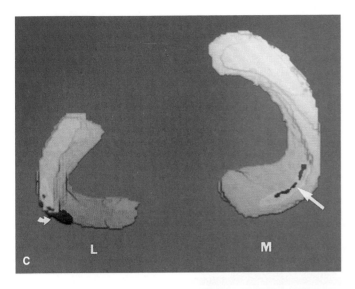

FIGURE 4-55. *(Continued)*

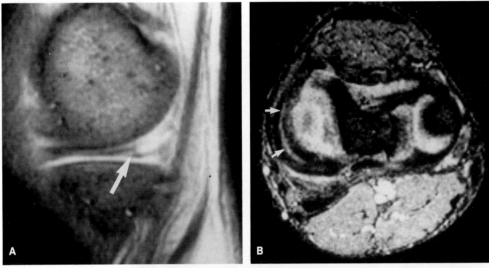

FIGURE 4-56. A longitudinal tear with a primary horizontal tear pattern as seen on meniscal cross section in the sagittal plane. (**A**) A T2*-weighted sagittal image shows a tear (*arrow*) of the posterior horn of the medial meniscus with primary horizontal morphology. (**B**) A 0.7-mm 3D Fourier transform axial image shows a longitudinal tear pattern (*arrows*). A 3D MR rendering displays an (**C**) inferior surface longitudinal tear (*arrows*) with (**D**) an intact superior meniscal surface. (**E**) Two months after MR study, arthroscopic examination revealed a displaced longitudinal tear (*all arrows*) with a bucket-handle morphology. (F, femur.) (**F**) A partial meniscectomy with remaining horizontal cleavage component (*arrows*) was performed after resection of the displaced bucket-handle fibrocartilage. Longitudinal tears can have either vertical or horizontal components. (F, femoral condyle; T, tibia.) *(continued)*

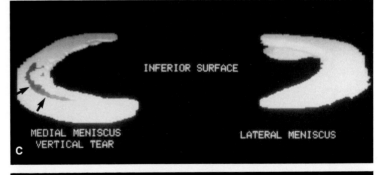

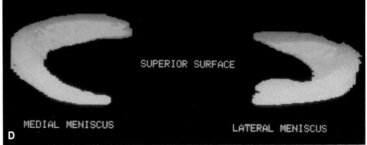

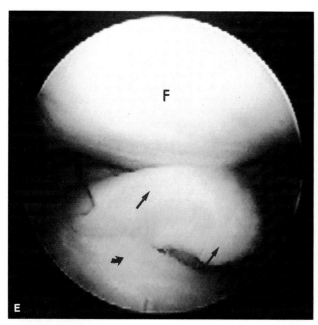

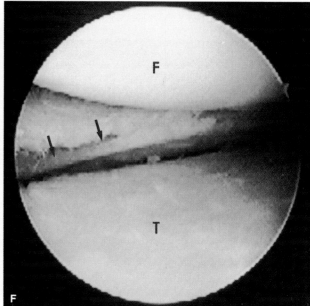

FIGURE 4–56. *(Continued)*

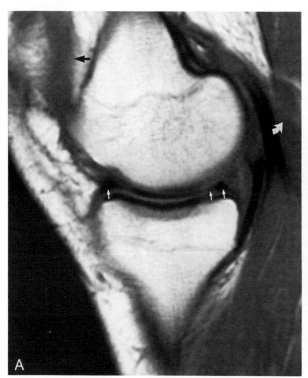

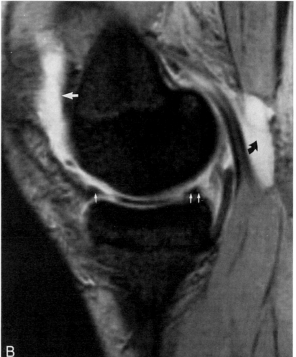

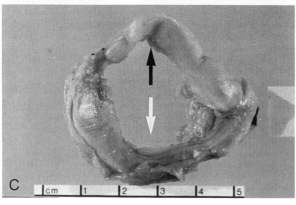

FIGURE 4–57. A bucket-handle tear with foreshortened anterior (*single small white arrows*) and posterior (*double small white arrows*) horns. Suprapatellar fluid (*large black arrows*) and a popliteal cyst (*curved arrows*) demonstrate (**A**) low signal intensity on T1-weighted sagittal image and (**B**) high signal intensity on T2*-weighted sagittal image. (**C**) A gross specimen demonstrates a displaced longitudinal bucket-handle tear (*black arrow*) from the medial meniscus (*white arrow*).

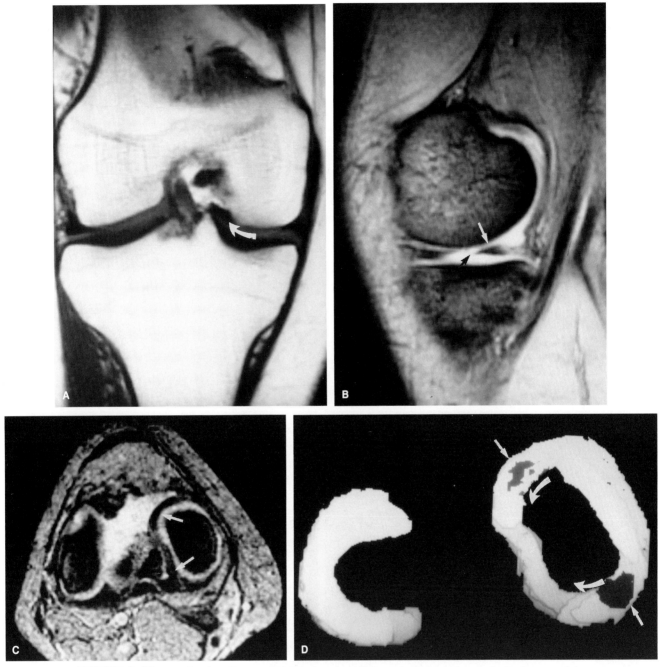

FIGURE 4–58. Bucket-handle tear. (**A**) Displaced medial meniscal tissue is seen in the intercondylar notch on a T1-weighted coronal image (*curved arrow*). (**B**) The T2*-weighted sagittal image shows a tear (*black arrow*) with foreshortening of the posterior horn of the medial meniscus (*white arrow*). (**C**) A 0.7-mm 3D Fourier transform T2*-weighted axial image reveals an intercondylar displaced meniscal tissue fragment (*arrows*). (**D**) A 3D MR rendering shows the bucket-handle tear pattern (*curved arrow*) with anterior and posterior tear points (*straight arrows*).

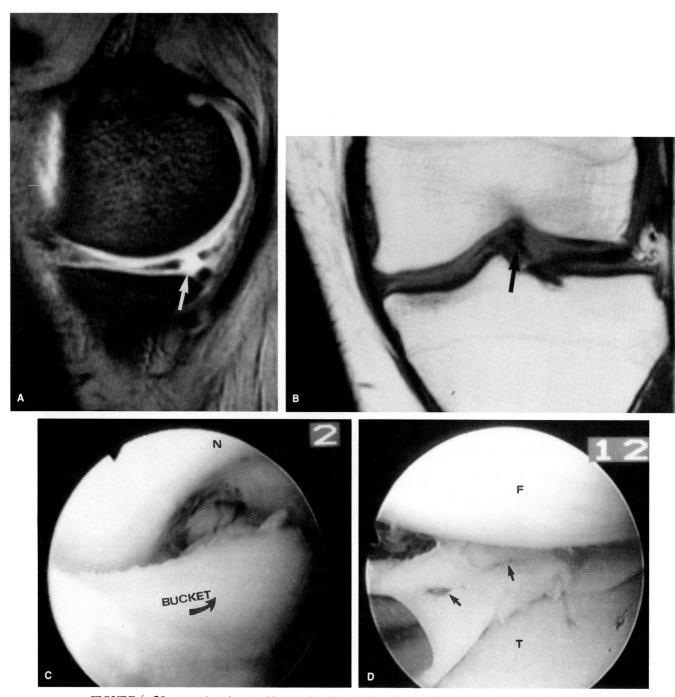

FIGURE 4–59. Displaced vertical longitudinal bucket-handle tear. (**A**) A T2*-weighted sagittal image displays a peripheral one-third vertical tear of the posterior horn of the medial meniscus (*arrow*). (**B**) On a T1-weighted coronal image, the bucket fragment (BUCKET) in intercondylar notch (*arrow*) demonstrates low signal intensity. (**C**) The arthroscopic photograph allows identification of the intercondylar notch (N) and bucket-handle fragment (*curved arrow*). (**D**) Another arthroscopic photograph shows primary arthroscopic repair approximating the separated meniscal fragments. Suture points are indicated (*arrows*). (F, femoral condyle; T, tibia.)

FIGURE 4–61. (**A**) A T1-weighted coronal image shows displaced meniscal tissue in the intercondylar notch (*curved arrow*). (**B**) Three-dimensional Fourier transform T2*-weighted axial images show bucket-handle morphology (*white arrow*) and tear points (*black arrow*).

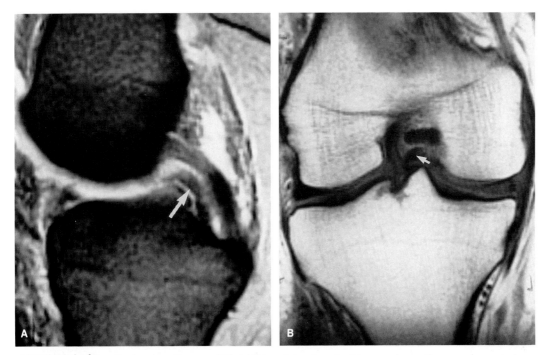

FIGURE 4–60. Bucket-handle tear. (**A**) A T2*-weighted sagittal image shows the pseudo-posterior-cruciate-ligament created by the displaced bucket-handle tear of the medial meniscus (*arrow*). (**B**) The corresponding T1-weighted coronal image allows identification of the displaced bucket meniscal fragment in the intercondylar notch (*arrow*).

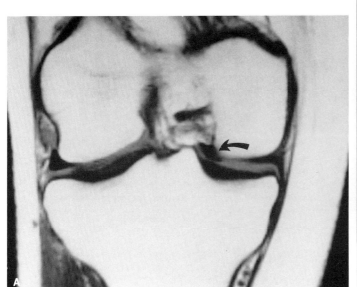

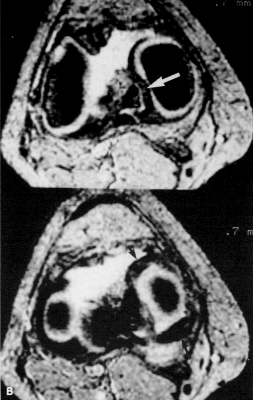

FIGURE 4–61.

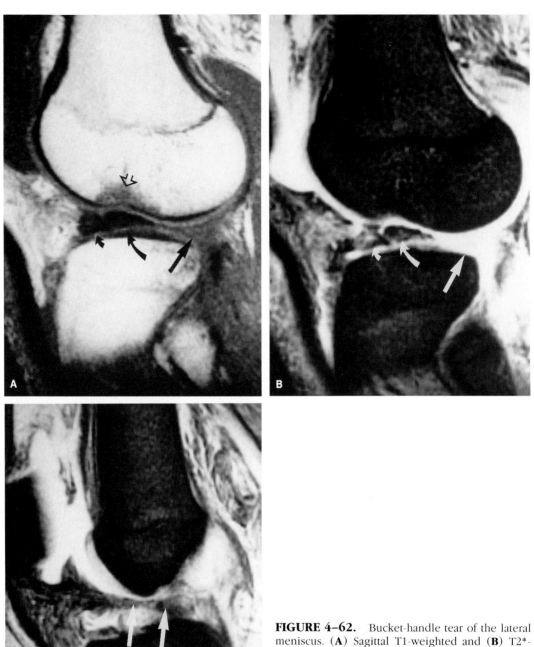

FIGURE 4–62. Bucket-handle tear of the lateral meniscus. (**A**) Sagittal T1-weighted and (**B**) T2*-weighted images show an anteriorly displaced posterior horn of the lateral meniscus (*large curved arrows*) adjacent to the anterior horn (*small curved arrows*). Note the absence of meniscal tissue in the expected location—the posterior horn of the lateral meniscus (*solid straight arrows*). Lateral femoral condylar bone contusion is seen on the T1-weighted sagittal image (*open arrow*). (**C**) A midsagittal T2*-weighted image shows the displaced portion of the body of the meniscus in the intercondylar notch (*arrows*).

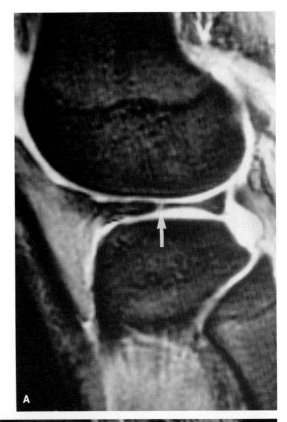

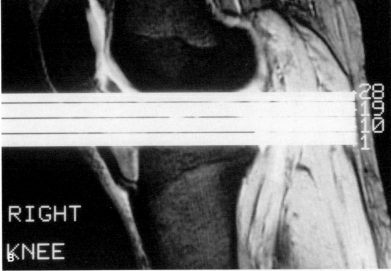

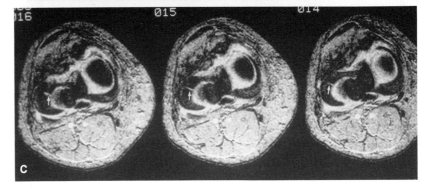

FIGURE 4–63. (**A**) A transverse or radial tear with grade 3 signal intensity is seen in the anterior horn–body junction of the lateral meniscus on a T2*-weighted sagittal image. (**B**) A T2*-weighted sagittal localizer is used to prescribe locations for 3D Fourier transform volume axial images through the meniscus. (**C**) The corresponding 0.7-mm axial images show the radial tear (*arrow*) of the free edge of the lateral meniscus in three separate images.

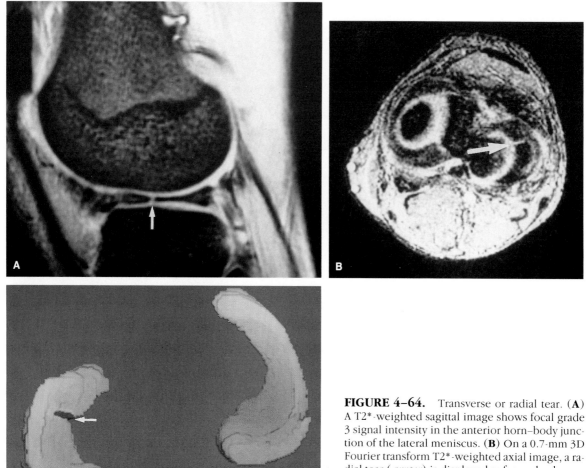

FIGURE 4–64. Transverse or radial tear. (**A**) A T2*-weighted sagittal image shows focal grade 3 signal intensity in the anterior horn–body junction of the lateral meniscus. (**B**) On a 0.7-mm 3D Fourier transform T2*-weighted axial image, a radial tear (*arrow*) is displayed as free-edge hyperintensity perpendicular to the concave edge of the meniscus. (**C**) The corresponding 3D MR rendering reveals the free-edge radial tear (*arrow*).

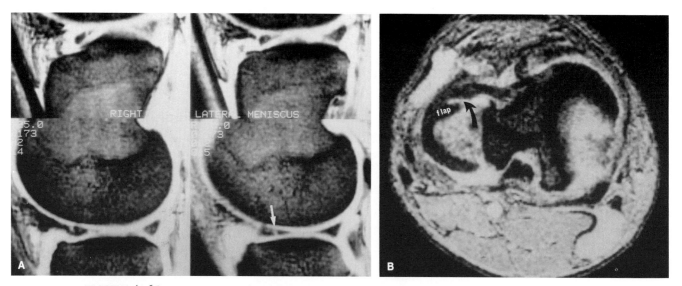

FIGURE 4–65. Oblique tear. (**A**) A T2*-weighted cross-sectional sagittal image shows a vertical tear that involves the anterior horn of the lateral meniscus (*arrow*). (**B**) A 0.7-mm 3D Fourier transform T2*-weighted axial image reveals an oblique tear pattern (*arrow*) with flap as seen from the circumferential surface of the meniscus (*arrow*). This surface tear pattern could not be easily identified from sagittal images alone.

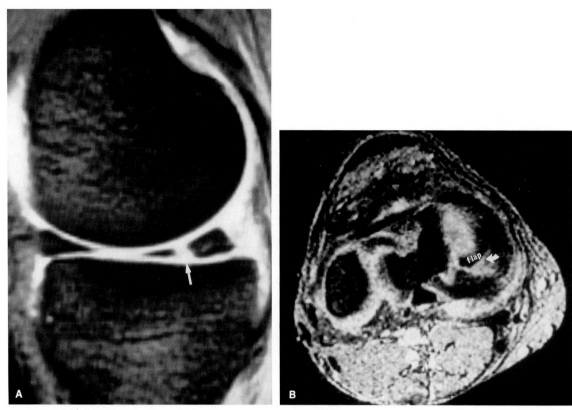

FIGURE 4–66. Vertical oblique or flap tear. (**A**) A T2*-weighted sagittal image shows a vertical tear (*arrow*) dividing the posterior horn of the medial meniscus. (**B**) The corresponding 0.7-mm 3D Fourier transform T2*-weighted axial image reveals flap tear morphology and allows identification of the oblique tear site (*curved arrow*).

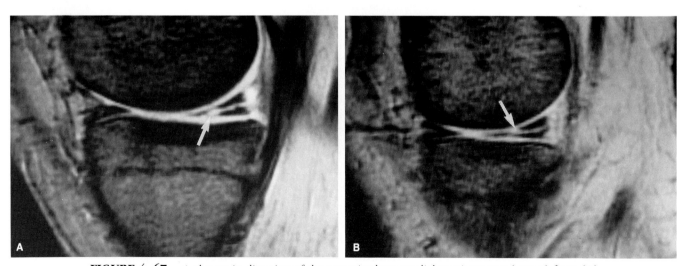

FIGURE 4–67. A change in direction of the posterior horn medial meniscus tear (*arrow*) from (**A**) the inferior surface to (**B**) the superior surface is frequently seen in oblique or flap tear morphology on T2*-weighted sagittal images.

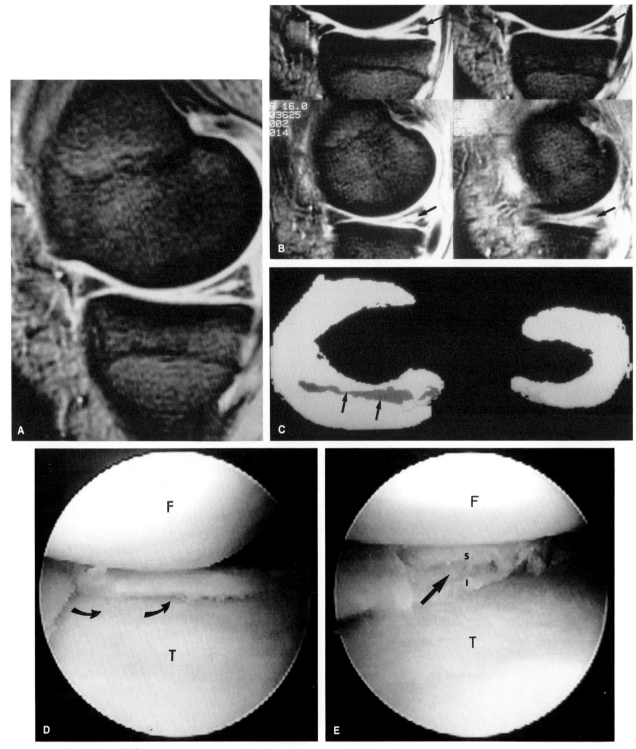

FIGURE 4–68. Oblique tear. Grade 3 signal intensity tear of the posterior horn of the medial meniscus is shown on (**A**) a single T2*-weighted sagittal image and (**B**) on a series of T2*-weighted sagittal images from the meniscal body to the posterior horn. Without observing a change in the direction of grade 3 signal intensity from the inferior to the superior surface of the meniscus, it is difficult to differentiate an oblique from a longitudinal tear. (**C**) Three-dimensional MR rendering demonstrates an oblique or flap tear pattern (*arrows*) as it appears from the inferior surface. (**D**) An arthroscopic photograph presents a flap tear with displacement of the meniscal flap toward the intercondylar area (*curved arrows*). (F, femur; T, tibia.) (**E**) Another arthroscopic photograph shows a stable meniscal rim, postmeniscal contouring, and flat excision with residual horizontal components (*arrow*) between stable superior (S) and inferior (I) meniscal leaves. (F, femur; T, tibia.)

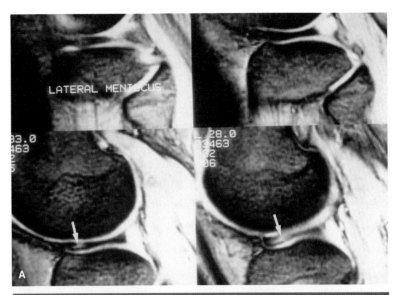

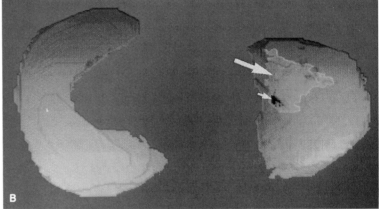

FIGURE 4-69. (**A**) A discoid lateral meniscus with slablike fibrocartilage morphology of the separate anterior and posterior horns is seen on consecutive T2*-weighted sagittal images. A superior surface tear is demonstrated (*arrow*) with associated intrasubstance degeneration. (**B**) Three-dimensional MR rendering shows intrasubstance degeneration (orange) and a superior surface tear (red).

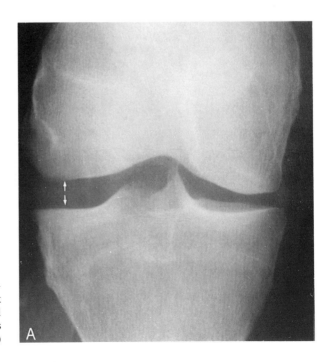

FIGURE 4-70. Discoid lateral meniscus. (**A**) An anterposterior radiograph reveals a widened lateral joint compartment (*arrows*). The thick slab of lateral meniscal fibrocartilage is seen as a continuous low signal intensity band in corresponding (**B**) coronal and (**C**) sagittal images (*arrows*). (continued)

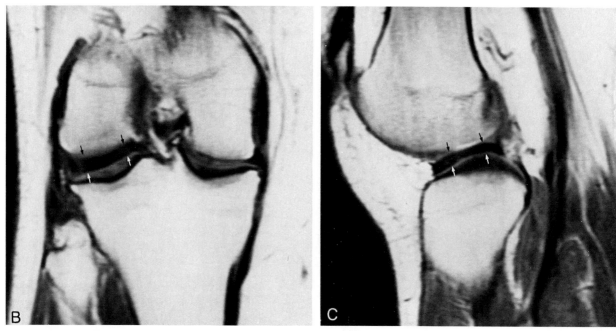

FIGURE 4–70. *(Continued)*

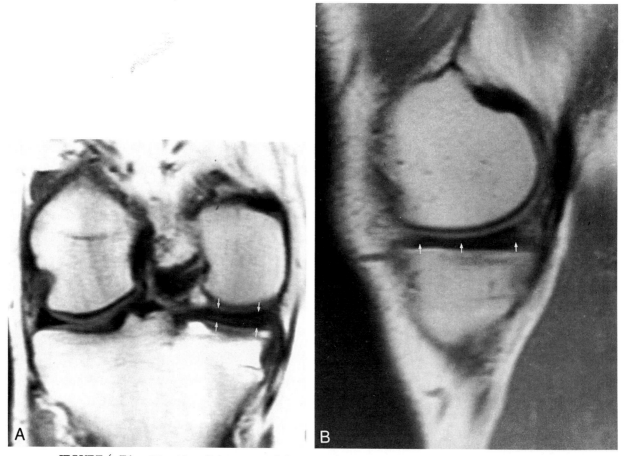

FIGURE 4–71. Discoid medial meniscus. (**A**) A coronal image demonstrates a dysplastic hypertrophied band of medial meniscal tissue (*arrows*). A discoid medial meniscus is rare. A continuous low signal intensity bow-tie appearance (*arrows*) is seen on multiple sagittal images from (**B**) the periphery toward (**C**) the intercondylar notch.

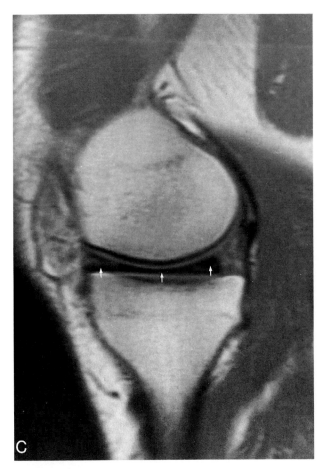

FIGURE 4–71. *(Continued)*

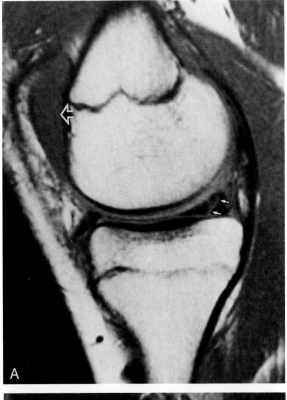

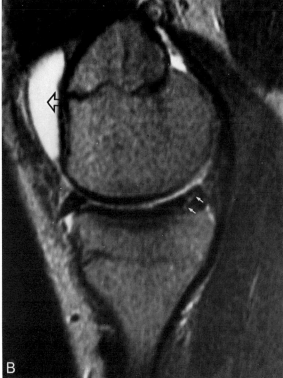

FIGURE 4–72. A posterior horn medial meniscus tear (*small arrows*) is seen on (**A**) T1-weighted and (**B**) T2-weighted images. The tear demonstrates increased signal intensity on the T2-weighted image.

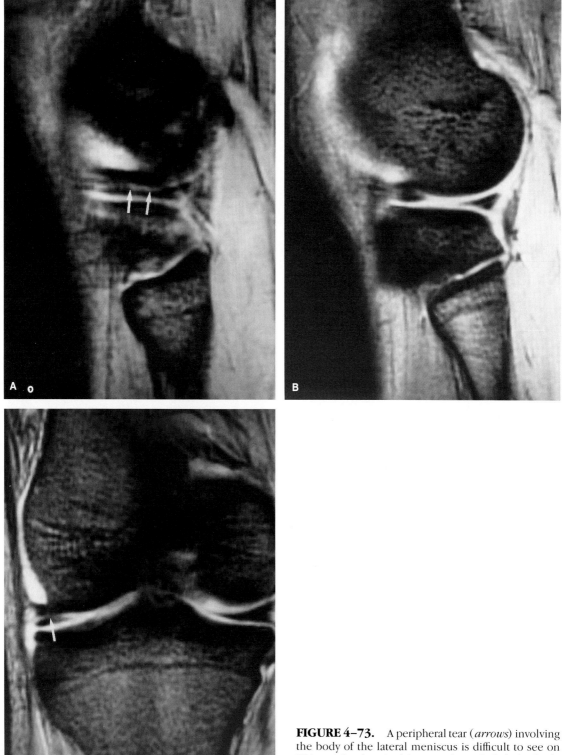

FIGURE 4–73. A peripheral tear (*arrows*) involving the body of the lateral meniscus is difficult to see on T2*-weighted sagittal images through (**A**) the body and (**B**) the posterior horn of the lateral meniscus. (**C**) On the corresponding radial T2*-weighted image through the body of the lateral meniscus, a grade 3 signal intensity tear (*arrow*) is easily identified.

4–74). By providing a view perpendicular to that seen on orthogonal sagittal images, extension to the superior or inferior surface of the meniscus can be more easily determined.

A less common pitfall involves a truncation artifact, which may mimic a meniscal tear when a 128 × 128 matrix with a 128-pixel phase-encoded axis is oriented in the superoinferior direction.[68] These artifacts are minimized when a 192 or 256 × 256 matrix is used.

Transverse Ligament. The transverse ligament of the knee, which connects the anterior horns of the medial and lateral menisci, can simulate an oblique tear adjacent to the anterior horn of the lateral meniscus (Fig. 4–75). The transverse ligament originates anterolateral to the central rhomboid attachment of the lateral meniscus. The central rhomboid attachment of the anterior horn of the lateral meniscus may normally demonstrate linear increased signal intensity. On sagittal or axial images, the transverse ligament can be identified coursing between the tibial attachment of the ACL and Hoffa's infrapatellar fat pad to its insertion on the anterior superior aspect of the anterior horn of the medial meniscus (Fig. 4–76).

The transverse ligament varies in diameter and is absent in 40% of gross specimens. In 30% of MR examinations, the fat that surrounds the low signal intensity ligament mimics grade 3 signal intensity (see Fig. 4–75). In less than 5% of cases, the medial extent of the transverse ligament may simulate a tear adjacent to the anterior horn of the medial meniscus (Fig. 4–77). Three-dimensional FT axial images, 1 mm or less, have been most successful in demonstrating the entire course of the transverse ligament as a low signal intensity band traversing Hoffa's infrapatellar fat pad. Two-dimensional axial images show the course of the transverse ligament less reliably (75%). On serial sagittal images, the round transverse ligament may be traced from the anterior horn of the lateral meniscus to the anterior horn of the medial meniscus. Isolated tears of the anterior horn of the lateral meniscus are rare, but can be easily differentiated from the transverse ligament pseudotear.

Rarely, a prominent branch vessel from the lateral inferior geniculate artery will produce a second pseudotear in this location (Fig. 4–78). In the presence of a joint effusion, increased signal intensity may be present in the interface between the transverse ligament and the anterior horn of the lateral meniscus, especially on T2- or T2*-weighted images (Fig. 4–79).

Fibrillation. Fibrillation or fraying on the concave free edge of the meniscus facing the intercondylar notch is seen as increased signal intensity restricted to the apex of the meniscus and does not represent meniscal tearing (Figs. 4–80 and 4–81). However, truncation or foreshortening of the meniscus is abnormal morphology and indicates a meniscal tear. A macerated meniscus imbibes synovial fluid throughout its substance and demonstrates a diffuse increase in signal intensity (multiple grade 3 tears) (Fig. 4–82).

Popliteus Tendon. In the posterior horn of the lateral meniscus, the popliteus tendon sheath may be mistaken for grade 3 signal and be falsely interpreted as a tear (Fig. 4–83). The popliteus tendon sheath is intermediate in signal intensity on T1- and T2-weighted images and courses in an oblique anterosuperior-to-posteroinferior direction, anterior to the low signal intensity popliteus tendon (Fig. 4–84). In the presence of a joint effusion, fluid in the popliteus sheath can be seen with bright signal intensity on T2- or T2*-weighted images (Fig. 4–85). In addition, the superior and inferior fascicles of the posterior horn of the lateral meniscus are best displayed on T2-weighted images in the presence of a small effusion (Fig. 4–86). A fascicle tear should not be confused with the normal superior and inferior meniscocapsular defects, which allow passage of the popliteus tendon through the popliteus hiatus (Fig. 4–87). The course of the popliteus muscle and tendon can be followed on serial posterior coronal images (Fig. 4–88). The thickness of the popliteus tendon sheath is variable and may be identified as a thin line or a thick band. A true peripheral lateral meniscal tear usually presents with a different obliquity than that described for the popliteus tendon sheath (Fig. 4–89). A vertical tear of the posterior horn of the lateral meniscus, however, may parallel the popliteus tendon sheath; in such cases, the popliteus tendon should be used as a landmark for the location of the peripheral edge of the meniscus (Fig. 4–90).

Partial Volume Imaging. The concave peripheral meniscal edge may produce the appearance of grade 2 signal intensity on peripheral sagittal images through the body of the meniscus.[66] This appearance is more commonly seen in the medial meniscus and is caused by partial volume imaging of fat and neurovascular structures lying in the concavity of the meniscus. Corresponding coronal thin section sagittal or radial images, however, display an intact meniscal structure.

Meniscofemoral Ligaments. Laterally, the meniscofemoral ligament consists of the ligament of Humphrey, which extends anterior to the PCL, and a posterior branch of the ligament of Wrisberg, seen posterior to the PCL (Figs. 4–91 and 4–92). Usually, one branch of the meniscofemoral ligament predominates. The ligament of Humphrey can be best seen on sagittal images, whereas the ligament of Wrisberg is best shown on posterior coronal images. The ligament of Humphrey can, however, be identified on coronal images (Fig. 4–93). Meniscal insertion of the meniscofemoral ligament may mimic the appearance of a vertical tear in the posterior horn of the lateral meniscus (Fig. 4–94).[67] This pseudotear can be seen extending obliquely from the superior meniscal surface directed posteriorly and inferiorly toward the inferior meniscal surface. A less common pattern is a vertical line parallel with the periphery of the meniscus. The medial capsular layer consists of meniscofemoral and meniscotibial or coronary ligament attachments, which may infrequently produce vertical signal intensity at the periphery of the posterior horn of the medial meniscus on sagittal images (Fig. 4–95).

Pseudo-Bucket-Handle Tear. Separate portions of the posterior horn may be mistaken for a bucket-handle tear because posterior coronal images traverse both the body and the posterior horn of the lateral meniscus, especially with the knee positioned in external rotation. This appearance is not usually encountered on posterior coronal images through the medial meniscus.

Pseudohypertrophy of the Anterior Horn. Complex meniscal tears may present with a unique MR appearance. In the lateral meniscus, the posterior horn may not be seen; it may be flipped anteriorly, occupying the space adjacent to the anterior horn (Figs. 4–96 and 4–97), creating pseudohypertrophy of the anterior horn fibrocartilage. This pattern is commonly seen in bucket-handle tears of the lateral meniscus.

Pseudo–Loose Body. Normal intercondylar notch fat signal intensity may be mistaken for a loose body on T2*-weighted coronal or sagittal images. This pitfall is not a problem when T1-weighted images are correlated with corresponding T2*-weighted images (Fig. 4–98).

Lax Meniscus Sign. Sometimes a lax or redundant folding of the superior and inferior surfaces of the medial meniscal contours is present without an associated fibrocartilage tear (Fig. 4–99). This finding is usually associated with some degree of joint effusion.

Vacuum Phenomenon. The magnetic susceptibility of normal amounts of intraarticular gas may produce a low signal intensity void or blooming artifact on gradient-echo images (Fig. 4–100). This artifact may be mistaken for a meniscal tear or articular cartilage injury.

Treatment of Meniscal Tears

The decision to perform a partial meniscectomy depends on the morphology of the tear and its extension to the free edge of the meniscus.[56] Horizontal tears should not be treated with primary meniscal repair. In displaced longitudinal vertical or bucket-handle tears, a partial meniscectomy is performed in which the displaced por-

tion of the meniscus is reduced with a probe prior to resection and the meniscus is then trimmed until stable tissue is exposed. A horizontal component is often present in the meniscal rim. Radial tears greater than 5 mm are usually symptomatic and resected at arthroscopy. Although usually associated with horizontal tears, meniscal cysts may be associated with deep radial tears. Partial meniscectomy with removal of the flap is performed in oblique tears. Stability of the remaining portion of the meniscus can be tested with a probe at arthroscopy and varies as a function of the horizontal or vertical components of the tear. In horizontal cleavage tears, the superior and inferior leaves are usually resected to an inferior stable rim of the meniscus. A 3-mm flap may be left.

Meniscal Transplantation. Meniscal transplantation, developed by Garret and associates, is used to delay the development of degenerative disease after meniscectomy.[69] In this procedure, age- and size-matched allograft menisci are sutured to a resected meniscal rim. The anterior and posterior meniscal horn meniscotibial attachments are preserved so that they can function as firm anchors for the generation of hoop stresses. This technique is indicated in young patients who have undergone total meniscectomy and who are likely to develop degenerative arthrosis by middle age. Degenerative arthrosis develops more rapidly when the lateral meniscus is removed than when the medial meniscus is removed.

Meniscal transplantation also contributes to stability in ACL-deficient knees with absent medial meniscal fibrocartilage. It may also contribute to preservation of joint function as part of a three- stage reconstruction, which includes repair of the meniscus, the ACL, and an associated osteochondral lesion.

Magnetic resonance is presently used to evaluate the integrity of the transplanted allograft, to determine proper sizing, and to follow peripheral healing at the suture site. Persistent grade 3 signal intensity may be seen after meniscal transplantation, during the process of peripheral revascularization (Fig. 4–101).

Postoperative Appearance of Menisci

It is difficult to identify tears in meniscal remnants after a partial meniscectomy (Fig. 4–102). Even in the absence of a retear, the meniscal remnant may demonstrate residual grade 3 signal intensity. There may also be residual signal intensity if one or both leaves of a cleavage component or a tear are removed. Correlation with the original tear pattern and knowledge of the arthroscopic procedure performed are necessary to accurately interpret MR findings. Postoperative meniscal fragments adjacent to the site of a meniscectomy may be identified on MR examination; however, the clinical significance of this finding relative to the patient's symptoms requires further investigation. A sharp surgical truncation of the apex of the meniscus with foreshortening is often seen after partial meniscectomy (Fig. 4–103). The meniscal tissue, however, may be contoured so that the remnant is identified with obvious blunting (Figs. 4–103 and 4–104). No meniscal tissue is seen after a total meniscectomy (Fig. 4–105).

Smith and colleagues have divided the MR characteristics of partial meniscectomies into three groups.[70] Group 1 menisci demonstrate near-normal length but no osteoarthritis. Group 2 menisci are significantly shortened, also without osteoarthritis (see Fig. 4–104). Group 3 menisci may be any length, but they demonstrate development of osteoarthritis (Fig. 4–106). Contour irregularities in group 2 menisci simulated meniscal fragmentation in 40% of segments studied; therefore, no rigid criteria for diagnosis of tears in meniscal segments with partial meniscectomy contour irregularities have been established (Fig. 4–107). Regenerated meniscal tissue (*i.e.,* rim) is composed of fibrous tissue, is smaller than normal, and demonstrates low to intermediate signal intensity on T1-, T2-, or T2*-weighted images.

Primary meniscal repairs may show grade 1, grade 2, or persistent grade 3 signal intensities on MR images (Fig. 4–108).[71] With second-look arthroscopy, it has been shown that a healed meniscal repair may demonstrate grade 3 signal intensity, making postoperative characterization of primary repairs difficult (Fig. 4–109). Intra-articular gadolinium may be helpful in identifying imbibed synovial fluid in menisci that are retorn after primary repair (Fig. 4–110).

Miscellaneous Meniscal Pathology

Meniscal Cysts

Meniscal cysts are collections of mucinous or synovial fluid traceable to the joint line (Figs. 4–111 and 4–112). These cysts may develop in response to trauma or degeneration and are associated with meniscectomy.[72,73] Meniscal cysts are more common laterally (ratio of lateral-to-medial occurrence is 7:1), and they often present at the middle third of the peripheral margin of the meniscus. Horizontal meniscal tears frequently communicate with meniscal cysts, with decompression of synovial fluid (see Fig. 4–112).[74] Meniscal cysts are uniformly low in signal intensity on T1-weighted images and increase in signal intensity on T2- or T2*-weighted images. Loculations may be seen in complex meniscal cysts, usually in those far removed from the site of origin (meniscal tear; Fig. 4–113). Medial meniscal cysts have been identified, extending from the posterior horn and dissecting peripherally to present in a more anterior location (Fig. 4–114).

Chondrocalcinosis

In chondrocalcinosis, meniscal calcifications are usually identified with conventional radiographic techniques. In five patients with calcium pyrophosphate disease (CPPD), MR studies using high contrast settings for photography revealed focal, low signal intensity calcification separate from adjacent low signal intensity meniscus. On T2*-weighted images, local susceptibility artifacts are seen around the foci of calcium pyrophosphate deposition, making them easier to identify (Fig. 4–115). Due to local magnetic susceptibility, however, CPPD crystals in either the meniscus or articular cartilage may dampen the signal intensity for meniscal degenerations and tears, falsely producing grade 2 signal intensity in a patient with grade 3 signal intensity on corresponding T1-weighted images. This limits the usefulness of gradient-echo imaging in the evaluation of degenerative menisci. Dicalcium phosphate dihydrate, hydroxyapatite, and calcium oxalate are also responsible for cartilaginous calcifications.[24] A meniscal ossicle is larger and occurs as an isolated focus in asymptomatic patients without history of antecedent trauma (Fig. 4–116).

Meniscocapsular Separations

Meniscocapsular separations or tears usually involve the less mobile medial meniscus (Fig. 4–117).[64] The thick medial one-third of the joint capsule or medial capsular ligament is divided into meniscofemoral and meniscotibial components.[75] These fibers are separated from the superficial fibers of the MCL by an interposed bursa and can best be seen on radial images through the medial compartment of the knee. The meniscocapsular junction is poorly seen on routine orthogonal coronal images. The posterior horn of the medial meniscus, fixed to the tibia by meniscotibial or coronary ligaments, is especially susceptible to tear at its capsular attachment. Even in the absence of grade 3 signal intensity through the meniscus, a separation at the meniscocapsular junction may have clinical significance in patient management if associated with pain.

Meniscocapsular tears less than 1 cm may heal without surgical intervention, because these tears occur through the vascularized periphery of the meniscus, adjacent to the perimeniscal capillary plexus.[49] Minor repair of these lesions also has a high success rate because of their peripheral location.

On sagittal MR images, the tibial plateau articular cartilage should be covered by the posterior horn of the medial meniscus without an exposed articular cartilage surface. Displacement of the posterior horn of the medial meniscus by 5 mm or more, uncovered tibial articular cartilage, or fluid interposed between the peripheral edge of the meniscus and capsule are suggestive of peripheral detachment.[49] However, quantitative measurement of meniscal displacement may be unreliable (Fig. 4–118). In addition, the meniscus may have fluid within the superior and inferior capsular recesses without intervention of the meniscocapsular junction (Fig. 4–119). Medial collateral ligament tears may be associated with meniscocapsular tears; in these patients, radial imaging may be used to supplement routine coronal and sagittal images. A complete peripheral detachment of the posterior horn is seen as a free-floating meniscus, especially if it is associated with a MCL tear (Figs. 4–120 and 4–121).

CRUCIATE LIGAMENTS

Anterior Cruciate Ligament

Functional Anatomy of the Anterior Cruciate Ligament

The cruciate ligaments are intracapsular and extrasynovial. The ACL is attached to the posteromedial aspect of the lateral femoral condyle anteriorly and extends inferior and medial to the anterior tibial intercondylar area for insertion between the anterior attachments of the menisci.[75] The ACL is 11 mm wide and 31 to 38 mm long.[12] It is composed of two functional fiber bundles that usually do not exist as distinct structures on gross examination.[76,77] The longer anteromedial bundle (AMB) tightens with knee flexion, whereas the shorter posterolateral bundle (PLB), which represents the bulk of the ACL, tightens with knee extension.[25] In flexion, the anteromedial fibers twist or spiral over the posterolateral fibers.[57] The ACL prevents anterior translation of the tibia and resists posterior translation of the femur.

Mechanism of Injury of the Anterior Cruciate Ligament

Anterior cruciate ligament failure can occur during external rotation and abduction with hyperextension, direct forward displacement of the tibia, or internal rotation with the knee in full extension.[29] With varus or valgus stress, the ACL is injured after collateral ligament failure. Forced valgus in external rotation is the most common mechanism of injury and causes disruption of the MCL.[12,78,79] Isolated ACL injuries are less common, but can occur with pivoting in deceleration, which causes forced internal rotation of the femur. In skiers, a forceful quadriceps contraction with passive anterior force applied through the forward movement of the ski boot may also cause isolated ACL injuries.[12] Catching and fixation of the ski tips is another mechanism of ACL injury in downhill skiers. Football clipping injuries with direct posterior trauma to the flexed knee usually produce both ACL and posterior capsular injury.

Associated Intraarticular Pathology

In acute isolated ACL injuries, 41% to 68% are associated with meniscal tears.[12,80,81] When this association occurs, the prognosis for meniscal repairs performed in conjunction with ACL reconstruction is improved.[82] Associated meniscal pathology is reported in between 85% to 91% of chronic ACL-deficient knees.[83] Injury to the meniscus and articular cartilage, especially in the medial compartment of the knee, is associated with episodes of anterior tibial subluxation.[12] Articular cartilage lesions, including erosions and chondral fractures of both medial and lateral compartments, have been observed in 23% of acute injuries and 54% of chronic injuries.[81]

Clinical Assessment of Anterior Cruciate Ligament Injury

Acute ACL tears are associated with acute hemarthrosis (75%) and an audible pop (34%) at the time of injury.[12,24] The ACL is the primary stabilizer for anterior tibial displacement; it can resist loads up to 400 N under maximum loading.[12] The AMB of the ACL must be disrupted before a positive anterior drawer sign performed in 90° of knee flexion is demonstrated with anterior tibial translation. The anterior drawer sign, however, usually requires associated disruption of the medial capsule.[84] A positive Lachman's sign (*i.e.,* an anterior drawer test performed between full extension and 15° of flexion) and a positive pivot shift test performed at 70° of flexion with valgus stress and internal rotation during knee extension may be seen in patients with isolated PLB rupture without an anterior drawer sign and with intact anteromedial fibers. In isolated tears of the ACL, the classic anterior drawer sign may give a false-negative result because the medial tibial plateau and meniscus abut the convex surface of the medial femoral condyle in flexion, which limits anterior tibial translation. These isolated tears are best identified with Lachman's test.[29]

In chronic tears, adhesions or attachments to the PCL result in increased laxity on clinical testing. Partial tears of the ACL are present in 24% to 39% of ACL injuries. When the knee is subjected to 20-pound anterior load testing, ACL ligament disruption is associated with anterior tibial translation or subluxation 3 mm greater in the involved knee than in the uninvolved knee. A grade I ACL represents interligamentous injury without a change in ligament length. In a grade II ACL, there is interligamentous injury and an increase in ligament length. A grade III ACL represents complete ligamentous disruption.

On arthrography, the ACL can be only indirectly assessed by observing air and contrast along the reflected synovial surface. Direct visualization of ligamentous fibers is not possible.

(text continues on page 254)

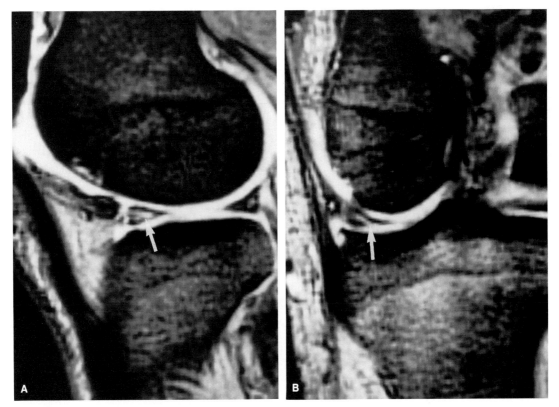

FIGURE 4–74. Grade 2 *versus* grade 3 signal intensity. (**A**) A T2*-weighted sagittal image shows what is presumed to be grade 2 signal intensity without clearly defined inferior surface extension in the anterior horn of the lateral meniscus (*arrow*). (**B**) The corresponding T2*-weighted radial image shows clearly defined grade 3 signal intensity that extends to the inferior lateral meniscal surface (*arrow*).

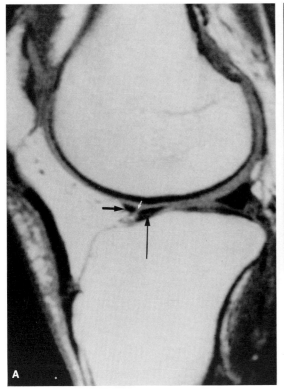

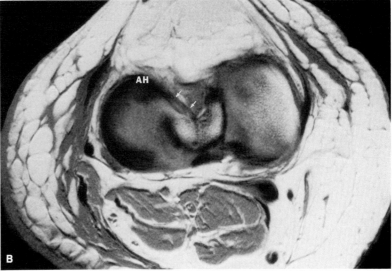

FIGURE 4–75. (**A**) A T1-weighted sagittal image of the transverse ligament of the knee shows an oblique pseudotear, created by fat (*white arrow*) associated with the low signal intensity transverse ligament of the knee (*short black arrow*). Normal signal intensity is identified in the central rhomboid attachment of the anterior horn of the lateral meniscus (*long black arrow*). (**B**) A T1-weighted axial image shows central rhomboid attachment (*small arrows*) of the anterior horn (AH) of the lateral meniscus.

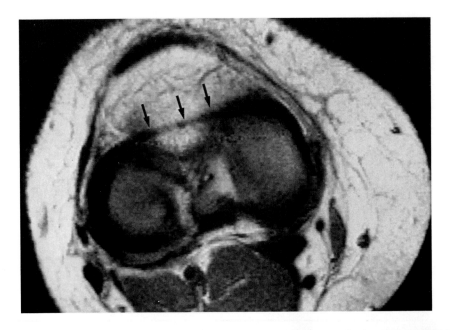

FIGURE 4–76. The low signal intensity transverse ligament of the knee is shown connecting the anterior horns of the medial and lateral meniscus (*arrows*) on a T1-weighted axial image. The ligament is surrounded by high signal intensity fat in Hoffa's infrapatellar fat pad.

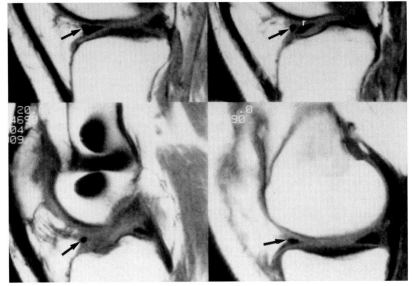

FIGURE 4–77. A T1-weighted sagittal image shows the transverse ligament (*arrows*) of the knee producing a pseudotear adjacent to the anterior horn of the lateral meniscus and the medial meniscus as it courses directly posterior to Hoffa's infrapatellar fat pad. Note the characteristic oblique line of intermediate signal intensity between the transverse ligament and lateral meniscus. The anterior horn of the lateral meniscus assumes a more rhomboid (r) shape at the site of its central ligamentous attachment to the tibia.

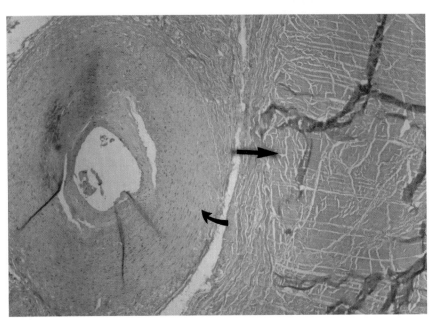

FIGURE 4–78. A photomicrograph shows proximity of the lateral inferior geniculate artery (*curved arrow*) to lateral meniscus (*straight arrow*). (H & E stain.)

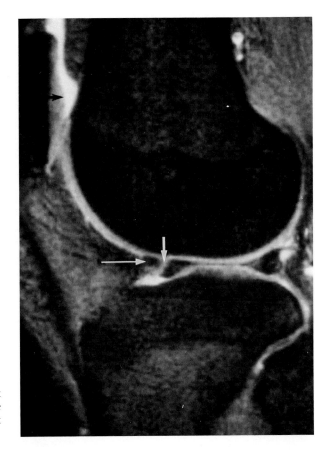

FIGURE 4–79. A T2*-weighted image shows the transverse ligament of the knee (*long white arrow*) separated from the anterior horn of the lateral meniscus by high signal intensity fluid (*small white arrow*). Bright signal intensity suprapatellar effusion is also seen (*small black arrow*).

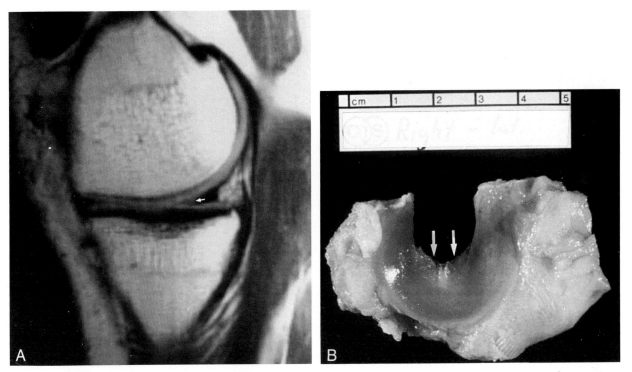

FIGURE 4–80. (**A**) Increased signal intensity restricted to the apex of the meniscus represents degenerative fibrillation or fraying (*arrows*). (**B**) The gross specimen shows a meniscus with fibrillation along concave free edge (*arrows*).

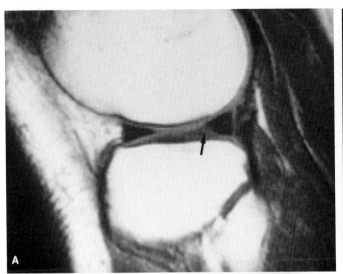

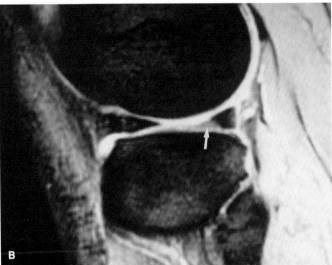

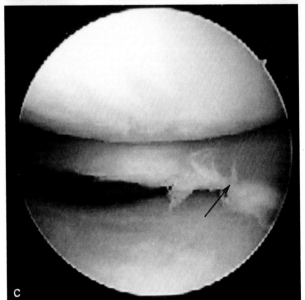

FIGURE 4–81. Free-edge fibrillation of the posterior horn of the lateral meniscus with an increased signal intensity apex is seen on (**A**) T1-weighted and (**B**) T2*-weighted sagittal images. (**C**) The arthroscopic view also shows lateral meniscal fibrillation.

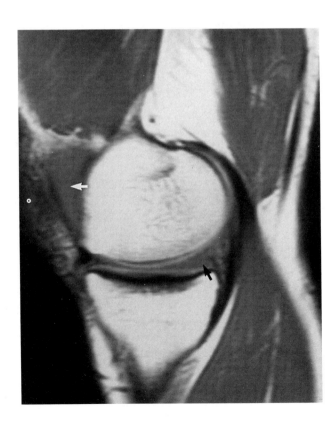

FIGURE 4–82. Increased signal intensity from imbibed synovial fluid in the macerated posterior horn of the medial meniscus (*black arrow*) is shown on this T2-weighted sagittal image. Adjacent joint effusion (*white arrow*) is indicated. T2-weighted sagittal image.

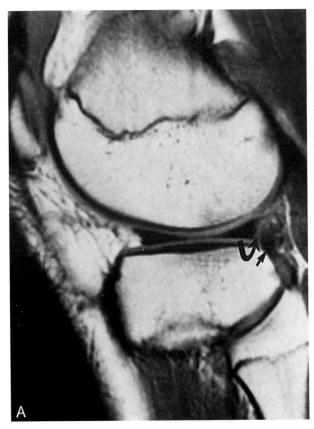

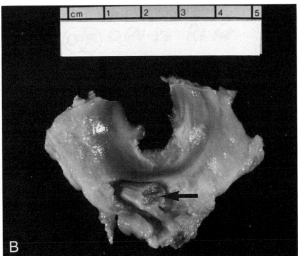

FIGURE 4–83. Popliteus tendon and sheath. (**A**) On a T1-weighted sagittal image, the popliteus tendon sheath demonstrates intermediate signal intensity (*curved arrow*) and the popliteus tendon (*straight arrow*) demonstrates low signal intensity. (**B**) The corresponding gross specimen shows the course of the popliteus tendon (*arrow*) along the posterior horn of the lateral meniscus.

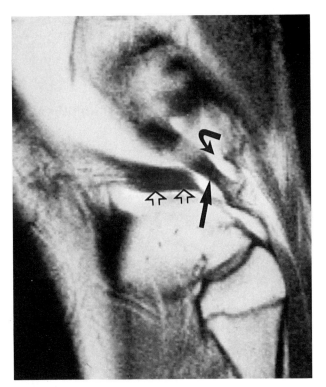

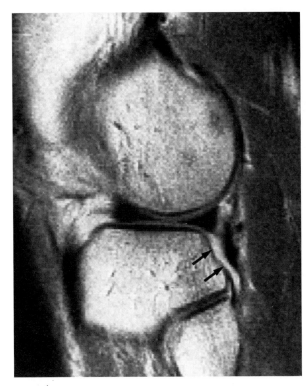

FIGURE 4–84. A T2-weighted peripheral sagittal image allows identification of the oblique course of the popliteus tendon (*straight arrow*) to its superior attachment along the lateral femoral condyle. The adjacent body of the lateral meniscus (*open arrows*) and high signal intensity synovial effusion (*curved arrow*) are shown.

FIGURE 4–85. A T2-weighted sagittal image shows high signal intensity fluid distending the popliteus tendon sheath (*arrows*).

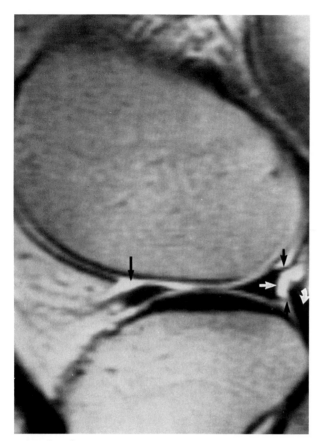

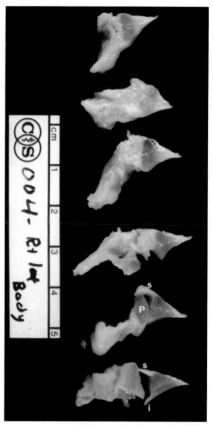

FIGURE 4–86. A T2-weighted sagittal image demonstrates high signal intensity joint fluid reflected over the lateral meniscus (*large black arrow*) and contained within the popliteus sheath (*straight white arrow*). Lateral meniscal struts (*small black arrows*) and the popliteus tendon (*curved white arrow*) are also seen.

FIGURE 4–87. A gross anatomic specimen allows the location of the superior (s) and inferior (i) fascicles. The popliteus tendon (P) passes normally through defects in the inferior and superior fascicles.

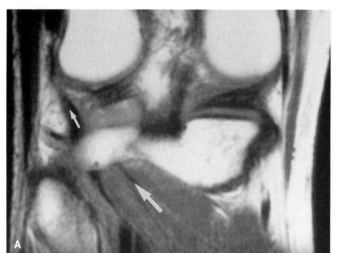

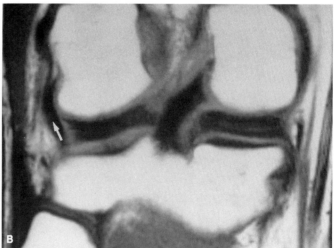

FIGURE 4–88. The normal course of the popliteus tendon (*white arrows*) through the popliteus hiatus is shown from (**A**) posterior through (**C**) anterior. The lateral collateral ligament (*black arrows*) is lateral to the popliteus tendon.

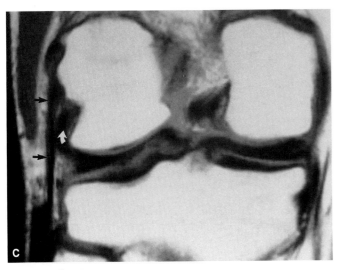

FIGURE 4–88. *(Continued)*

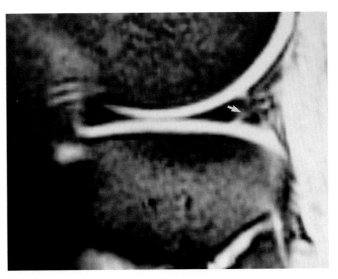

FIGURE 4–89. A tear of the posterior inferior corner of the lateral meniscus is revealed on a T2*-weighted sagittal image. The oblique direction of the tear is opposite to the expected course of the popliteus tendon (*arrow*).

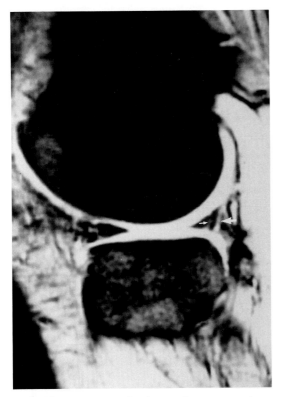

FIGURE 4–90. A T2*-weighted sagittal image reveals a vertical tear (*small arrow*) of the posterior horn of the lateral meniscus parallel with the popliteus tendon sheath (*large arrows*).

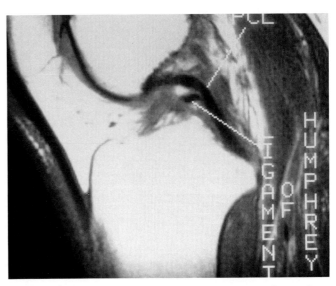

FIGURE 4–91. The low signal intensity ligament of Humphrey is prominent on a T1-weighted sagittal image.

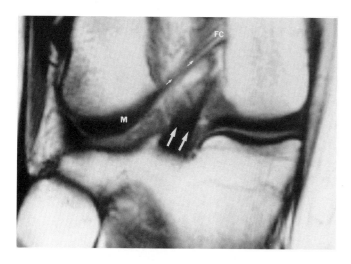

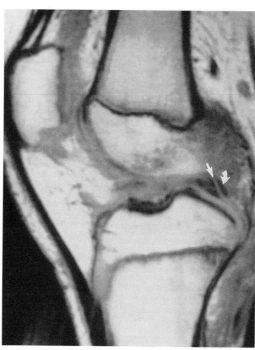

FIGURE 4–92. Ligament of Wrisberg (*small arrows*) and the posterior cruciate ligament (*large arrows*) are seen on a T1-weighted posterior coronal image. The ligament of Wrisberg's attachments to the posterior horn of the lateral meniscus (M) and posteromedial femoral condyle (FC) are evident.

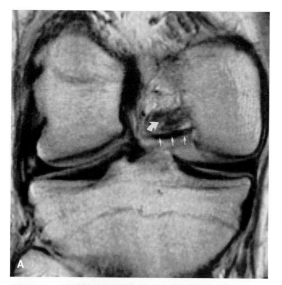

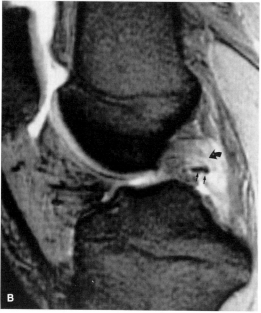

FIGURE 4–94. A pseudotear (*straight arrow*) is seen as a linear band of increased signal intensity on a T1-weighted sagittal image. This band is located between the superior articular surface of the posterior horn of the lateral meniscus and the meniscofemoral ligament (*curved arrow*).

FIGURE 4–93. (**A**) Intermediate-weighted coronal and (**B**) T2*-weighted sagittal images show the anatomy of the ligament of Humphrey (*straight arrows*). A complete tear of the posterior cruciate ligament is also present (*curved arrow*).

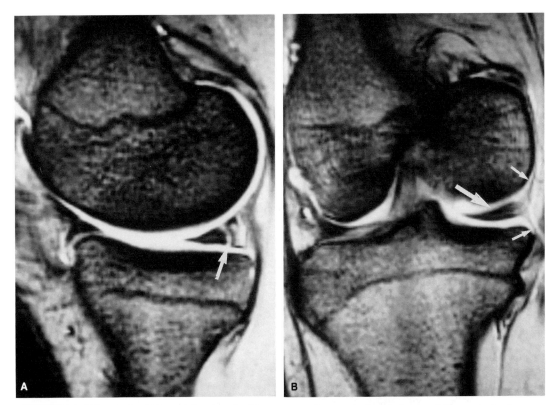

FIGURE 4–95. (**A**) A T2*-weighted sagittal image reveals a vertical pseudotear of the posterior horn of the medial meniscus. (**B**) The corresponding radial gradient-echo image shows normal meniscofemoral and meniscotibial attachments (*small arrows*) of the medial meniscus (*large arrow*).

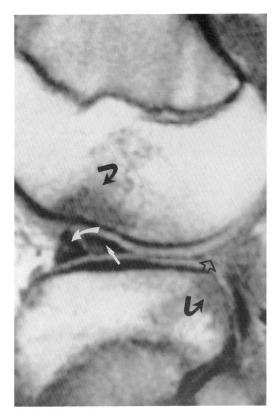

FIGURE 4–96. The posterior horn of the lateral meniscus (*open arrow*) is displaced toward (*straight arrow*) the anterior horn of lateral meniscus (*curved arrow*). Trabecular bone contusions are of low signal intensity relative to the adjacent bright fat marrow epiphysis on a T1-weighted sagittal image.

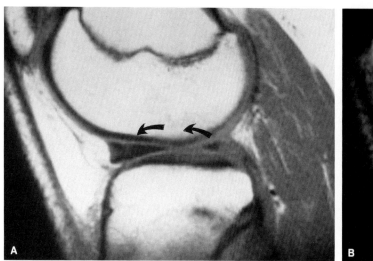
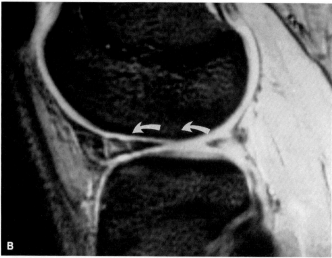

FIGURE 4–97. (**A**) Sagittal T1-weighted and (**B**) T2*-weighted images show a lateral bucket-handle meniscal tear with an anteriorly displaced posterior horn (*curved arrows*) lying in tandem with the anterior horn fibrocartilage. Note the posterior horn remnant.

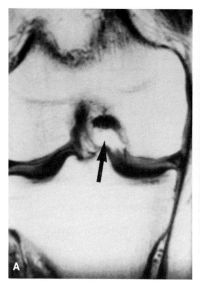
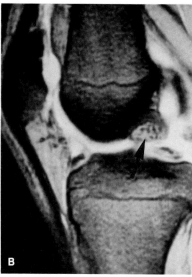

FIGURE 4–98. (**A**) A T1-weighted image shows high signal intensity intercondylar notch fat (*arrow*) beneath the posterior cruciate ligament, which mimics (**B**) intermediate signal intensity fat simulating a loose body on a T2*-weighted sagittal image.

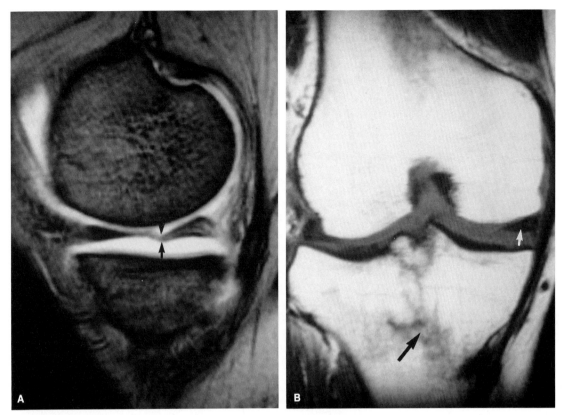

FIGURE 4–99. (**A**) A T2*-weighted sagittal image demonstrates that a wavy or folded contour may be a normal variant of the untorn medial meniscus (*arrows*). (**B**) The corresponding T1-weighted coronal image reveals low signal intensity trabecular microfractures (*black arrow*) and a normal medial meniscus (*white arrow*).

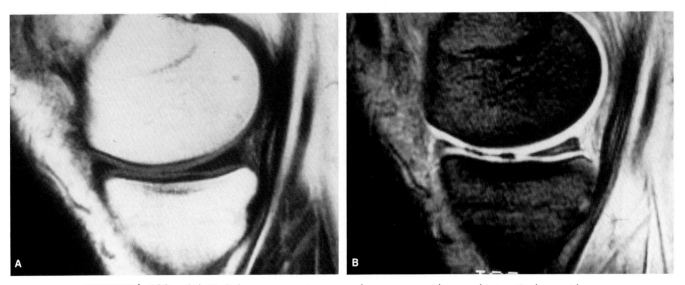

FIGURE 4–100. (**A**) Medial compartment vacuum phenomenon with normal intraarticular gas identified as a thin linear area of signal void between the femoral and tibial articular cartilage is apparent on a T1-weighted sagittal image. (**B**) A T2*-weighted sagittal image demonstrates blooming of signal void secondary to magnetic susceptibility effects of the intraarticular gas.

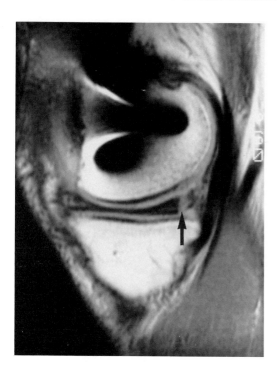

FIGURE 4–101. A T1-weighted sagittal image shows that peripheral grade 3 signal intensity (*arrow*) in a postmeniscal transplant represents suture attachment with healing—not a vertical tear.

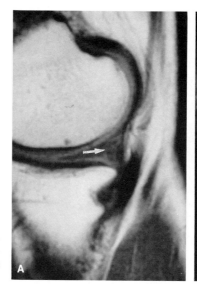 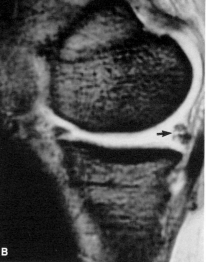

FIGURE 4–102. (**A**) Sagittal T1-weighted and (**B**) T2*-weighted images show normal residual grade 3 signal intensity (*arrow*) in a partial remnant from a posterior horn medial meniscectomy. This intensity does not represent a retear in this stable meniscal rim.

FIGURE 4–104. (**A**) A complex tear (*arrows*) that involves the posterior horn of the medial meniscus is shown on a T2*-weighted sagittal image. Superior and inferior surface extension are present. (**B**) A small, contoured posterior horn remnant (*arrow*) remains after partial meniscectomy, as demonstrated on a T2*-weighted sagittal image.

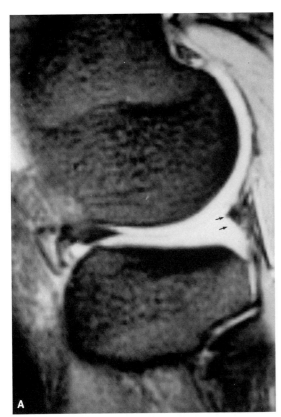

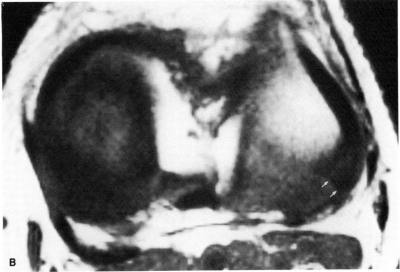

FIGURE 4–103. (**A**) A partial lateral meniscectomy with a posterior horn remnant (*arrows*) is seen on a T2*-weighted sagittal image (**B**) An abrupt lateral meniscus surgical defect (*arrow*) is revealed on a T1-weighted axial image.

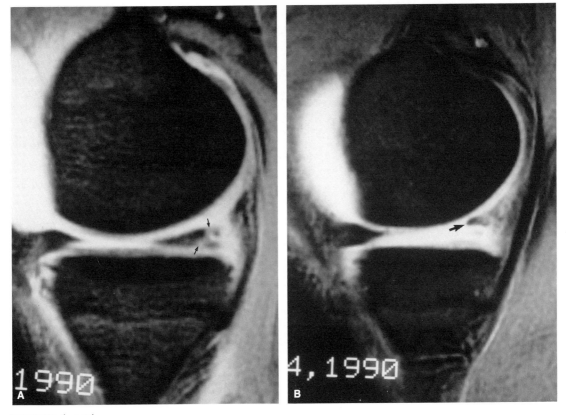

FIGURE 4–104.

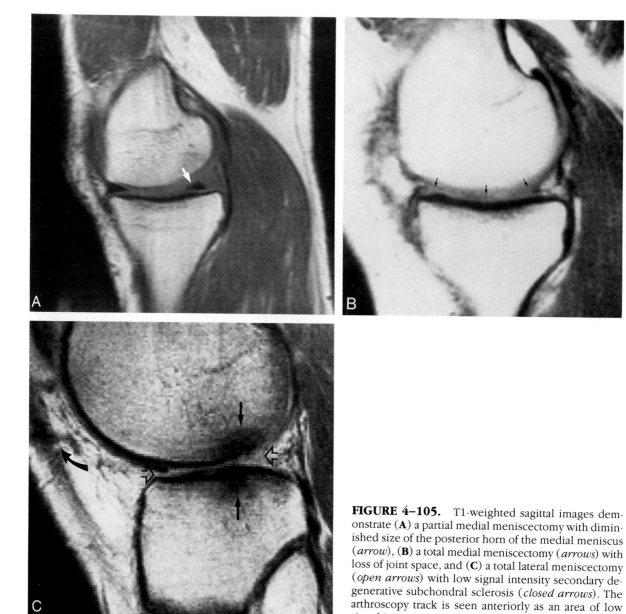

FIGURE 4–105. T1-weighted sagittal images demonstrate (**A**) a partial medial meniscectomy with diminished size of the posterior horn of the medial meniscus (*arrow*), (**B**) a total medial meniscectomy (*arrows*) with loss of joint space, and (**C**) a total lateral meniscectomy (*open arrows*) with low signal intensity secondary degenerative subchondral sclerosis (*closed arrows*). The arthroscopy track is seen anteriorly as an area of low signal intensity in part **A** (*curved arrow*).

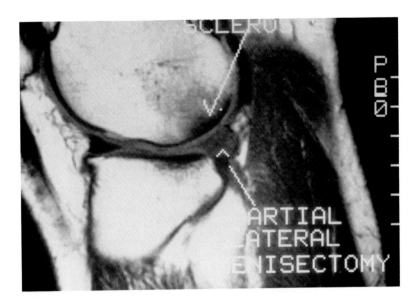

FIGURE 4-106. On a T1-weighted sagittal image, low signal intensity subchondral sclerosis is seen in the posterior lateral femoral condyle after a partial lateral meniscectomy.

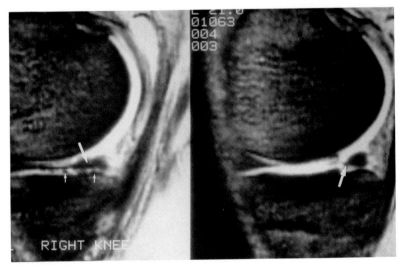

FIGURE 4-107. T2*-weighted sagittal images show focal areas of articular cartilage degeneration (*small arrows*) that occurred after partial medial meniscectomy. The posterior horn remnant demonstrates irregular contouring of its articular surfaces and apex (*large arrows*).

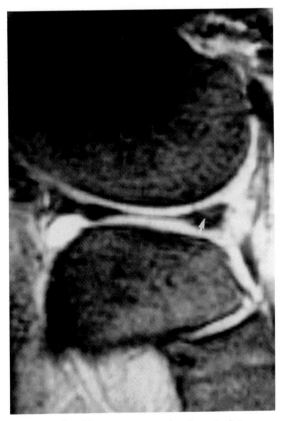

FIGURE 4-108. A T2*-weighted sagittal image made after primary repair of the lateral meniscus shows an absence of signal intensity in the posterior horn.

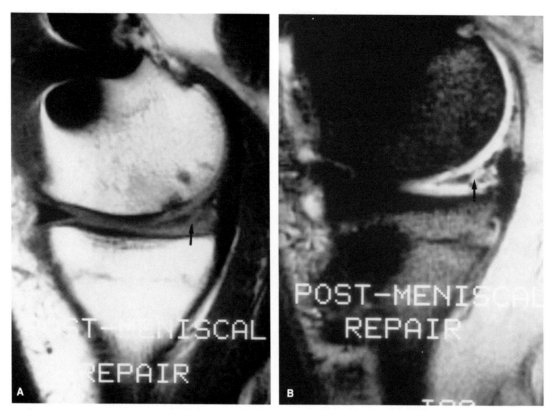

FIGURE 4–109. (**A**) Sagittal T1-weighted and (**B**) T2*-weighted images show residual grade 3 signal intensity (*arrow*) after primary repair of the meniscus. No retear was found at second-look arthroscopy.

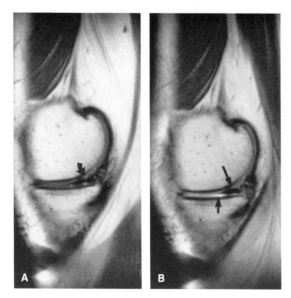

FIGURE 4–110. (**A**) Pre- and (**B**) postintraarticular gadolinium-enhanced T1-weighted sagittal images show an intact posterior horn after primary meniscal repair of a bucket-handle tear. High signal intensity gadolinium coats the articular cartilage (*small straight arrow*) adjacent to the intact posterior horn (*large straight arrow*). A suture artifact is shown on the unenhanced image (*curved arrow*).

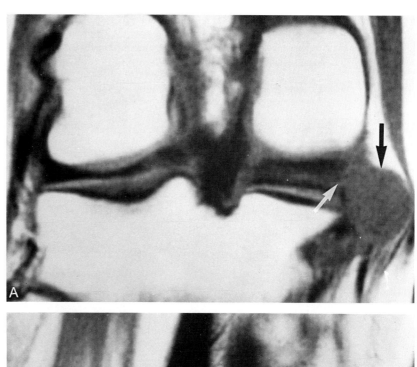

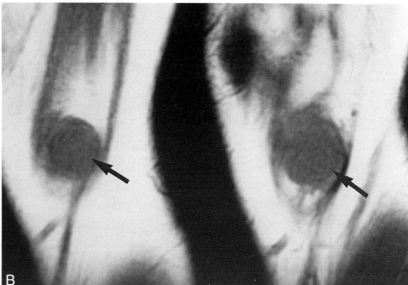

FIGURE 4–111. A medial meniscal cyst projects medial to the joint line (*black arrows*) on (**A**) coronal and (**B**) peripheral T1-weighted images. Communication between the cyst and a meniscal tear (*white arrow*) is revealed on the coronal image.

FIGURE 4-114.   (**A**) A T2*-weighted sagittal image shows a complex tear (*arrow*) of the posterior horn of the medial meniscus. The tear has both horizontal and vertical components. An associated hyperintense meniscal cyst (*curved arrow*) projects anteriorly with peripheral extension following the convex contour of the posterior horn and body of the meniscus. On 3D MR image rendering, (**B**) the superior and (**C**) the inferior surface views show a corresponding meniscal cyst (blue) in communication with a posterior horn medial meniscus tear (*arrow*).

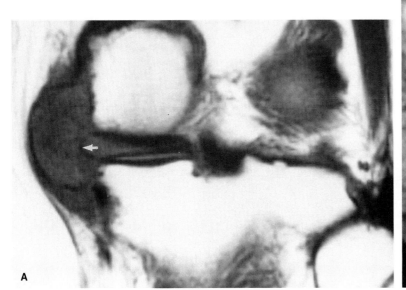

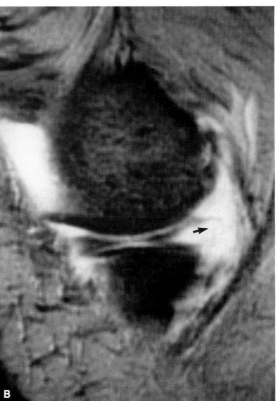

FIGURE 4-112.   A horizontal tear of the medial meniscus communicates with a posteromedial meniscal cyst. (**A**) The cyst is of low signal intensity on the T1-weighted coronal image and (**B**) is hyperintense on the T2*-weighted sagittal image.

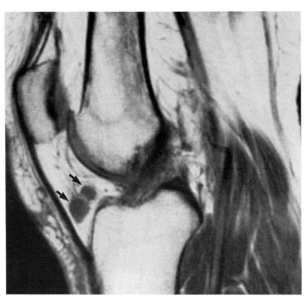

FIGURE 4-113.   A bilobed meniscal cyst (*arrows*) is seen dissecting through Hoffa's infrapatellar fat pad. The synovial fluid contents are of low signal intensity on this T1-weighted sagittal image.

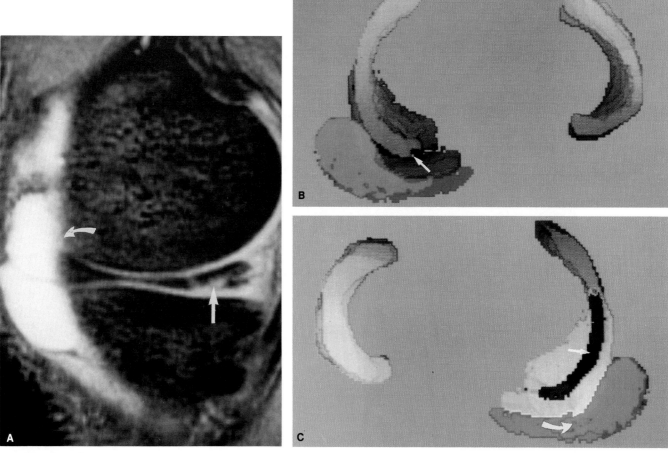

FIGURE 4–114.

FIGURE 4–115. Chondrocalcinosis. (**A**) A T1-weighted sagittal image shows grade 3 signal intensity of the posterior horn of the medial meniscus (*arrows*). (**B**) On the corresponding T2*-weighted sagittal image, chondrocalcinosis dampens the meniscal signal intensity (*arrow*) secondary to localized magnetic susceptibilities. (**C**) A T2*-weighted sagittal image through the lateral compartment displays multiple foci of calcium pyrophosphate disease deposition within the articular cartilage (*large arrows*) and the meniscus (*small arrows*). (**D**) On the corresponding lateral radiograph, chondrocalcinosis is evident in a region of meniscal fibrocartilage (*large arrows*) and articular cartilage (*small arrow*). (**E**) On a gross meniscal specimen, deposition of chondrocalcinosis is seen in the lateral meniscus (*arrow*).

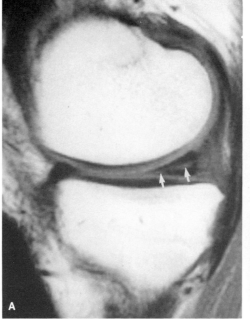

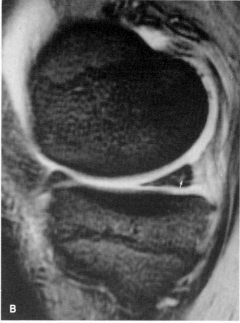

(continued)

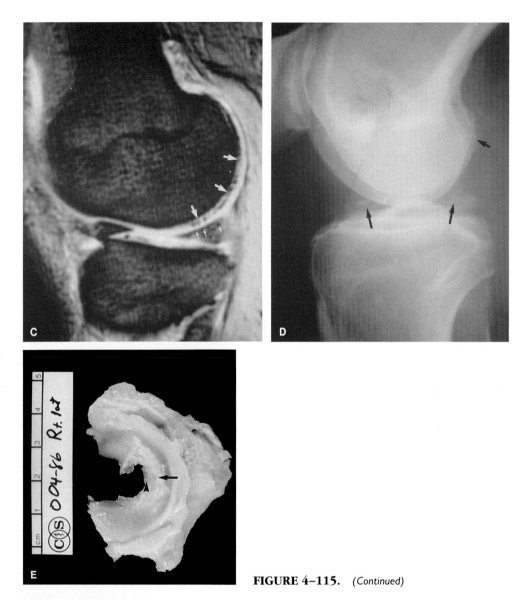

FIGURE 4–115. *(Continued)*

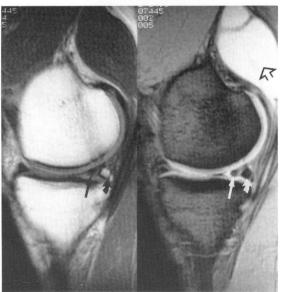

FIGURE 4–116. The meniscal ossicle (*curved arrow*) is of bright marrow fat signal intensity on a T1-weighted sagittal image (*left*) and low signal intensity on a T2*-weighted sagittal image (*right*). The blunted apex of the posterior horn is indicated (*straight arrow*). A popliteal cyst is seen at increased signal intensity on the T2*-weighted sagittal image (*open arrow*).

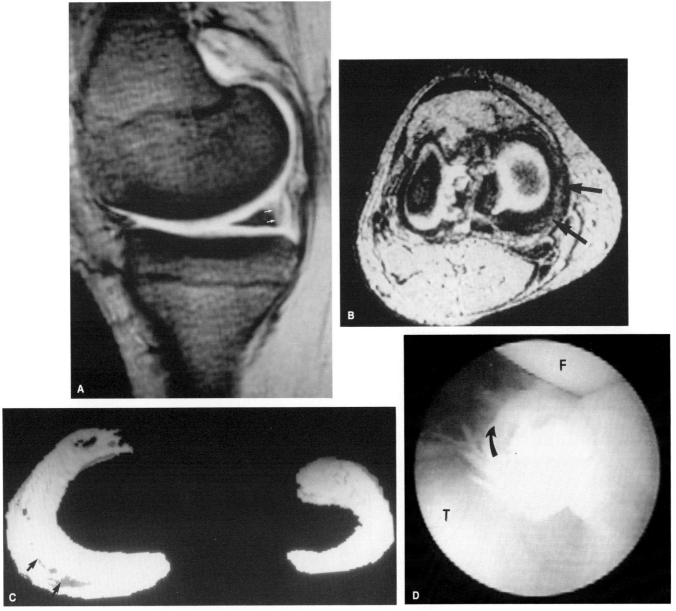

FIGURE 4–117. Meniscocapsular tear. (**A**) A T2-weighted sagittal image shows a thin linear vertical signal in the posterior horn of the medial meniscus (*arrows*). (**B**) A 0.7-mm 3D Fourier transform T2*-weighted axial image shows peripheral meniscocapsular increased signal intensity. (**C**) The corresponding 3D MR rendering reveals a meniscocapsular tear (*arrows*). (**D**) On arthroscopy, separation of the meniscus from the capsule (*curved arrow*) is seen. (F, femur; T, tibia.)

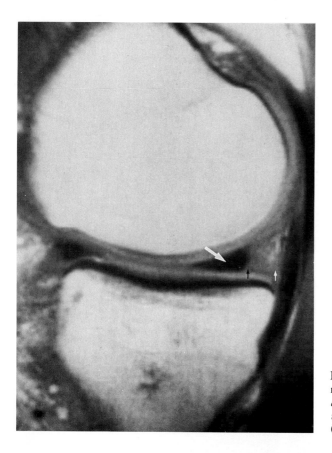

FIGURE 4–118. A T1-weighted image shows meniscocapsular separation with exposed tibial cartilage. The periphery of the meniscus (*black arrow*) should cover the periphery of the hyaline cartilage surface (*small white arrow*). The posterior horn of the medial meniscus is identified (*large white arrow*). This finding may be nonspecific.

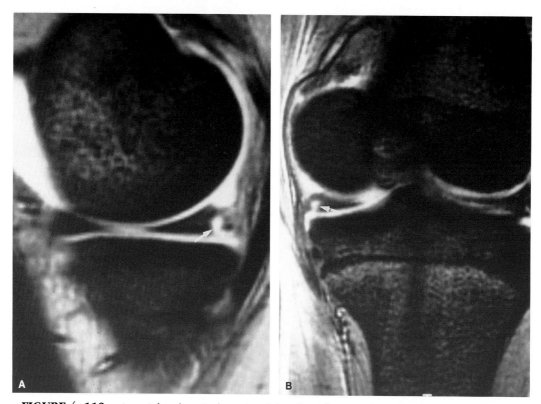

FIGURE 4–119. A peripheral vertical tear involving the inferior surface of the posterior horn of the medial meniscus as seen on T2*-weighted (**A**) sagittal and (**B**) radial images. This degree of vertical signal intensity is abnormal and does not represent a meniscal recess.

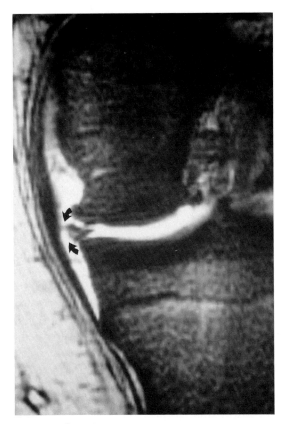

FIGURE 4–120.

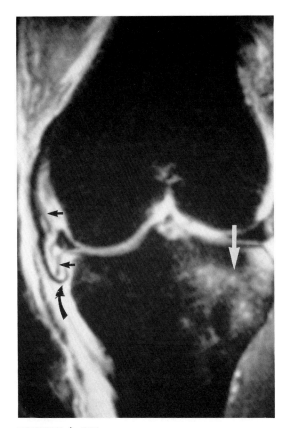

FIGURE 4–121.

FIGURE 4–120. Meniscocapsular separation may occur without peripheral capsular attachment to the medial meniscus. Fluid signal intensity extends freely between the medial collateral ligament and the meniscus (*arrows*) on all T2*-weighted radial images.

FIGURE 4–121. A complete tear (*curved arrow*) of the superficial layer of the distal medial collateral ligament is shown on a short TI inversion recovery coronal image. The deep medial capsular layer is represented by the meniscofemoral and meniscotibial attachments (*small straight black arrows*). A lateral tibial plateau contusion is also shown (*white arrow*).

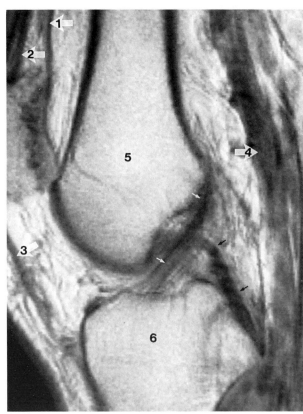

FIGURE 4–122. The sagittal intercondylar notch. (*white arrows,* anterior cruciate ligament; *black arrows,* posterior cruciate ligament; 1, suprapatellar bursa with fluid; 2, quadriceps tendon; 3, patellar tendon; 4, popliteal artery; 5, femur; 6, tibia.)

Magnetic Resonance Appearance of the Anterior Cruciate Ligament

For MR examination of the ACL, the knee should be placed in 10° to 15° of external rotation to orient the ligament with the sagittal imaging plane (Fig. 4-122). Excessive external rotation of the knee results in elongation of the anterior-to-posterior dimensions of the femoral condyles and limits accurate imaging of the meniscal cartilages. We routinely use all three planes (*i.e.*, axial, sagittal, coronal) to evaluate the ACL, although sagittal images best demonstrate the femoral and tibial attachments (Figs. 4-123 through 4-125). Although partial voluming may be minimized with thin sections, we have not found 3-mm images to be significantly more sensitive than routine 5-mm contiguous images in identifying ligamentous disruptions (Fig. 4-126). When the image is suboptimal, direct oblique imaging of the ACL is recommended, with an axial plane localizer to display the tibial and femoral attachments of the ACL (Figs. 4-127 through 4-129).[85-87] More accurate identification of ACL fibers can be achieved by using 1-mm 3DFT volume techniques on multiple sagittal images (Figs. 4-130 and 4-131).T2- or T2*-weighted images may be necessary to differentiate edema from hemorrhage in partial or complete ligamentous tears (Fig. 4-132). In the presence of joint effusion, T2 or T2* weighting is frequently necessary to visualize low signal intensity fibers that appear blurred on T1-weighted images. Kinematic imaging of the ACL in the sagittal plane has been attempted in partial ligamentous tears and reconstructions.[84]

On coronal and sagittal images, the normal ACL is seen as a band of low signal intensity with separate fiber striations visible near attachment points. Inhomogeneity of the ACL may be secondary to interposition of fat in the distal fibers. Anterior to the ACL, the ligament mucosa arises from the superior condylar notch. It may sometimes be seen as a distinct structure on MR images. Independent of partial voluming, the ACL may demonstrate a greater signal than that observed in the homogeneously dark PCL on T1-, T2- and T2*-weighted images. An intact ACL on coronal images with no increased signal intensity on corresponding T2- or T2*-weighted sagittal images differentiates between partial voluming of the ligament with the lateral femoral condyle and a proximal tear.

In complete tears of the ACL, discontinuity is present in a low signal intensity band with or without loss of the normally taut parallel margins (Fig. 4-133). Partial or complete ligamentous disruptions may be associated with blurring of the cruciate fascicles from edema or hemorrhage (Fig. 4-134). In acute tears or sprains, fluid or edema is shown with high signal intensity on T2- and T2*-weighted images. There is discontinuity of the ligament with a concave anterior margin or wavy contour, which indicates abnormal laxity (Fig. 4-135). Fluid and fiber defects, seen as masses of intermediate or increased signal intensity, may be seen in complete tears. Hemarthrosis associated with ACL tears is characterized by synovitis with an irregular free concave edge of Hoffa's infrapatellar fat pad (Fig. 4-136).

Accurate assessment of partial ligamentous tears is more difficult than the detection of complete disruptions. Posterior bowing of the ACL or buckling of the PCL may be associated with increased laxity from a partial or chronic tear of the ACL (Fig. 4-137). Absence of the ACL on both sagittal and coronal images is diagnostic for ACL disruption. Anterior displacement of the tibia on lateral sagittal images is a secondary sign of anterolateral instability (Fig. 4-138). This anterior drawer sign, however, is dependent on the degree of knee flexion, positioning, and design of the extremity coil, and its usefulness is limited by lack of comparison with the contralateral knee. On sagittal images, if the ACL is intact, a vertical line drawn at a tangent to the posterolateral femoral condyle should intersect the posterior lateral tibial plateau (Fig. 4-139). The low signal intensity ACL may be seen with horizontal orientation in subacute or chronic injuries (Figs. 4-140 and 4-141). Chronic tears are not usually associated with synovitis; thus, there is no irregular fat-pad sign. Focal angulation of the ACL or adhesion to the PCL have also been observed in chronic tears.[88]

ACL deficiency also leads to intrasubstance meniscal degeneration and tears, possibly because the menisci have to stabilize anterior tibial translation on the femur in an ACL-deficient knee (Fig. 4-142).[24] A bony ligamentous avulsion of the meniscotibial portion of the middle one-third of the lateral capsular ligament (*i.e.*, Segond fracture) is associated with rupture of the ACL.[12,89] A lateral femoral condylar notch or a low signal intensity cortical depression separate from the normal sulcus terminale may also be seen with ACL rupture (Fig. 4-143). Murphy and colleagues have found posterolateral tibial plateau (94%) and lateral femoral condyle (91%) subchondral bone impactions to be relatively specific signs of an acute complete ACL tear.[89a] This association with trabecular bone contusions is attributed to lateral femoral condyle impaction into the posterior tibia during either the initial rotary subluxation or the recoil of the lateral femoral condyle. In the author's experience, trabecular contusions in the middle-to-anterior lateral femoral condyle are more likely to be associated with ACL disruption than a posterolateral femoral condyle impaction in the presence of a posterolateral tibial plateau injury. Posterolateral capsular disruptions with fluid extravasation posterior to the popliteus tendon have been observed in acute ACL tears (Fig. 4-144).

In a review of 242 arthroscopies indicated by 3000 MR examinations, the accuracy of MR imaging in ACL diagnosis was 95%. Accuracy, sensitivity, and specificity increased when T2-weighted sequences were added.[90] In another study of arthroscopically documented ACL tears, Lee and associates reported a MR sensitivity of 94%, compared with 78% for the anterior drawer test and 89% for Lachman's test.[91] Magnetic resonance was shown to have a specificity of 100% for clinical tests of ACL instability. The use of orthogonal imaging, as compared with nonorthogonal (*i.e.*, oblique sagittal) imaging, increased accuracy from 61% to 66% and sensitivity from 70% to 100%; specificity remained at 100% for detection of ACL injuries.[87]

Treatment of Anterior Cruciate Ligament Injury

The specific treatment selected for ACL injury often depends on whether an associated meniscal injury or a second ligament injury is present. Associated meniscal tears, collateral ligament injuries, or patellofemoral instabilities are indications for anterior cruciate reconstructions.[92] Primary repair is most successful when avulsion occurs at either the femoral or tibial ACL attachment (Fig. 4–145). Avulsion or cortical low signal intensity bone with an associated subchondral marrow-containing component may be more difficult to see on T1-weighted contrast (Fig. 4–146). Patients with midsubstance interstitial tears are not good candidates for ACL repair.

Anterior Cruciate Ligament Reconstruction. The goal of ACL reconstruction is to establish sufficient isometric tension to keep the distance between the tibial and femoral attachment points from changing more than 1 to 2 mm through 0° to 90° of flexion. Surgical reconstructions are classified as extraarticular, intraarticular, or combined intra- and extraarticular.[12,93] Extraarticular procedures (*e.g.*, the MacIntosh procedure, the Ellison procedure, and the Andrews procedure) include a transfer for the pes anserinus and various lateral techniques that use the iliotibial tract to provide restraint to anterior subluxation of the lateral tibial plateau. These procedures have been used with variable success and may be associated with rotatory instability (*i.e.*, pes transfer). The results with intraarticular reconstruction, which involves the use of patellar tendon, bone, and vascular transfer, are better than those achieved with extraarticular techniques (Fig. 4–147). In these procedures, the iliotibial band may be transferred intraarticularly in a lateral over-the-top reconstruction (Fig. 4–148). Other techniques use the semitendinosus tendon and iliotibial band and either the semitendinosus tendon or the semitendinosus and gracilis tendons (Fig. 4–149).[93]

Autogenous, allographic, xenographic, and synthetic tissues have been used for ligament reconstruction in acute and chronic ACL injuries.[12,94–96] Allograft tissues in-clude the patellar and Achilles tendons (Fig. 4–150); synthetic allograft materials include carbon fiber, knitted dacron, and braided polypropylene. The use of expanded polytetrafluoroethylene or Gortex has been complicated by attenuation, rupture, and stretching of the grafts (Fig. 4–151).

To limit impingement of a graft on the anterolateral aspect of the condylar notch, especially in knee extension, an adequate notchplasty is necessary.[92] A congenitally narrow intercondylar notch may result in impingement of the ACL (Fig. 4–152). Parallel osseous tunnels through the lateral femur and the anterior tibia are created after isometric points are selected (Fig. 4–153).

Magnetic resonance imaging can be used to evaluate ACL reconstructions. Procedures using tunneling in the intercondylar notch and anterior tibia, as well as points of ligamentous fixation provided there is minimal metallic artifact, can be evaluated with MR imaging. On T2- or T2*-weighted images, torn, prosthetic, or grafted ligaments may be seen with increased signal intensity and splaying of fibers in areas of fluid accumulation around separated fascicles. Increased signal intensity without change in ligament morphology cannot be used as a primary criterion for diagnosing an ACL tear. Coronal or sagittal oblique images parallel with the reconstructed ligament may improve imaging of the entire course of the ACL (Figs. 4–154 through 4–156). We have used the MR anterior drawer sign (*i.e.*, anterior translation of the tibia relative to the femur in the lateral compartment of the knee) as well as buckling of the PCL to indicate abnormal ligament laxity in ACL reconstructions. Rak and colleagues have reported excellent correlations between MR findings and clinical examination (92%) and MR findings and second-look arthroscopy (100%) in ACL reconstructions using patellar bone–tendon–tibial bone autografts.[97] Buckling of the PCL was associated with ACL laxity in these cases. Less satisfactory results were reported by Moeser and colleagues in observing ACL reconstructions performed with fasciae latae from the iliotibial band in a MacIntosh lateral substitution over-the-top repair.[98] In 84% of cases studied by Fezoulidis and associates, carbon fiber ligament augmentation of the ACL was accurately imaged on MR scans of intra- and extraarticular grafts.[99]

In the evaluation of impinged ACL grafts, an increase in signal intensity was observed in the distal two-thirds of the grafts; this increase persists 1 to 3 years after implantation.[100] An association exists between the location of the tibial tunnel anterior to the slope of the intercondylar roof and the development of hyperintensity in suspected graft impingement. Tibial tunnels placed posterior to and parallel with the slope of the intercondylar roof were associated with unimpinged grafts.

(*text continues on page 274*)

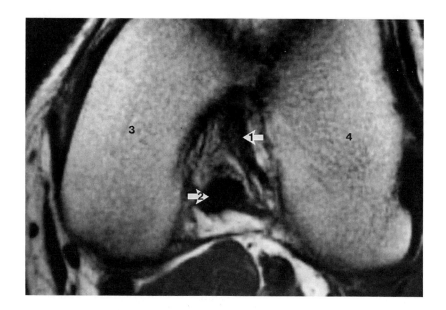

FIGURE 4–123. Axial intercondylar anatomy of the anterior and posterior cruciate ligaments. (1, anterior cruciate ligament; 2, posterior cruciate ligament; 3, medial femoral condyle; 4, lateral femoral condyle.)

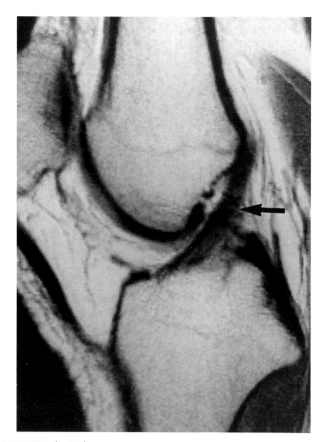

FIGURE 4–124. An intact low signal intensity anterior cruciate ligament (*arrow*) is shown on a T1-weighted sagittal image.

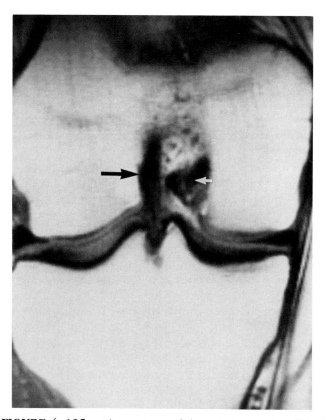

FIGURE 4–125. The anatomy of the anterior cruciate (*black arrow*) and posterior cruciate (*white arrow*) ligaments as seen on a T1-weighted coronal image. The anterior cruciate ligament is seen as a band, whereas the posterior cruciate ligament is circular in cross section.

FIGURE 4–127. Anterior cruciate oblique imaging. (**A**) The axial plane through the intercondylar notch is used as a localizer for prescribing (**B**) direct oblique sagittal 3-mm images through the anterior cruciate ligament (*arrows*).

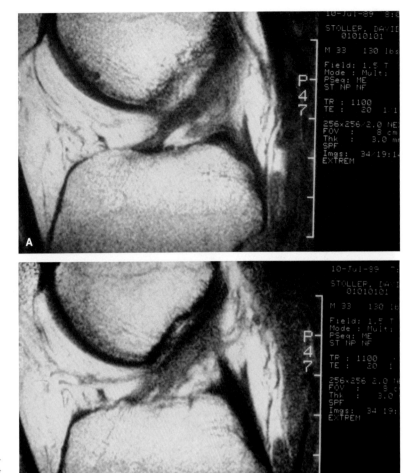

FIGURE 4–126. Small field of view T1-weighted 3-mm sagittal images of normal anterior cruciate ligament and posterior cruciate ligament anatomy from (**A**) lateral to (**B**) medial.

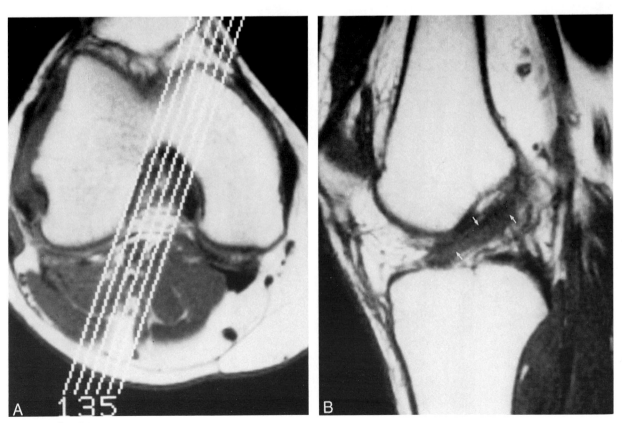

FIGURE 4–127.

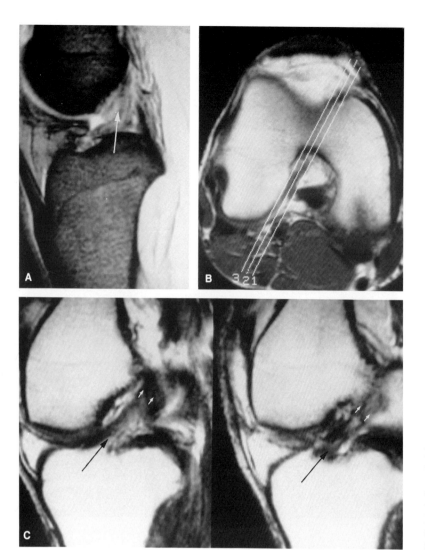

FIGURE 4–128. (**A**) A T2*-weighted sagittal image of a poorly depicted anterior cruciate ligament (*arrow*). (**B**) A T1-weighted axial image is used to prescribe sagittal oblique images. (**C**) On these T1-weighted sagittal oblique images, the intact proximal lateral femoral condylar attachments (*white arrows*) and anterior tibial attachments (*black arrows*) are splayed or fanned out.

FIGURE 4–129. (**A**) A proximal tear of the anterior cruciate ligament shows hyperintense hemorrhage of fibers in its lateral femoral condylar attachment on a T2*-weighted sagittal image (*arrow*). (**B**) The corresponding 3-mm oblique sagittal image confirms the loss of proximal anterior cruciate ligament morphology (*arrow*). (**C**) A T1-weighted sagittal oblique image of normal anatomy with intact tibial (*single arrow*) and femoral attachments (*double arrows*) is shown for comparison.

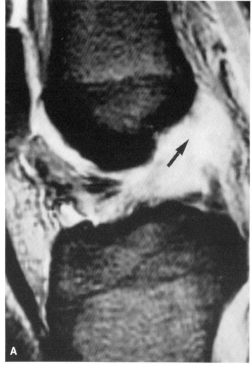

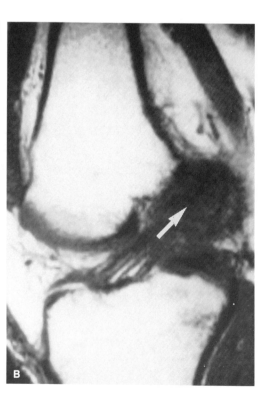

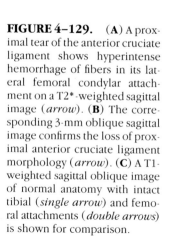

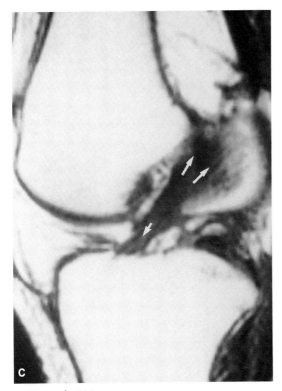

FIGURE 4–129. *(Continued)*

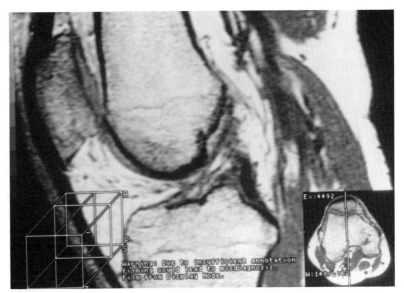

FIGURE 4–130. Precise control of image prescription is possible by reformatting in the plane of the torn anterior cruciate ligament as designated by 3D Fourier transform volume axial images.

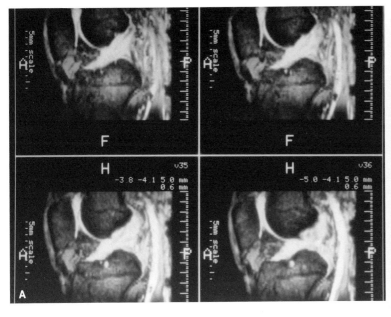

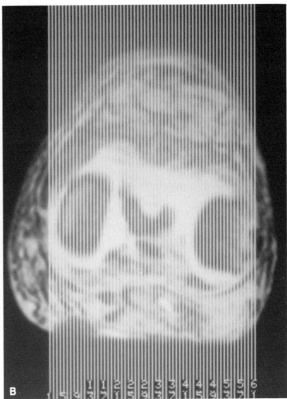

FIGURE 4–131. (**A**) These 0.6-mm sagittal reformatted images through a torn anterior cruciate ligament were generated from (**B**) a 32-slice 3D Fourier transform volume axial image.

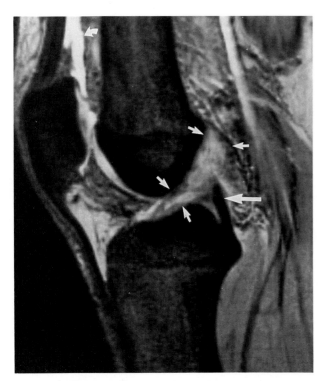

FIGURE 4–132. High signal intensity edema can be seen in a torn anterior cruciate ligament (*small straight arrows*) on a T2*-weighted image. A normal low signal intensity posterior cruciate ligament is shown in contrast (*large straight arrow*). Bright signal intensity suprapatellar effusion is also demonstrated (*curved arrow*).

FIGURE 4–133. A midsubstance tear of the anterior cruciate ligament (*arrow*) shows loss of continuity of its normally parallel margins.

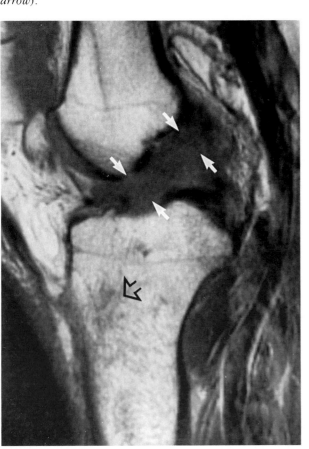

FIGURE 4–134. A T1-weighted sagittal image of a torn and edematous anterior cruciate ligament (*solid arrows*) shows blurring of the ligamentous fibers. The low signal intensity marrow edema indicates a bone contusion (*open arrow*).

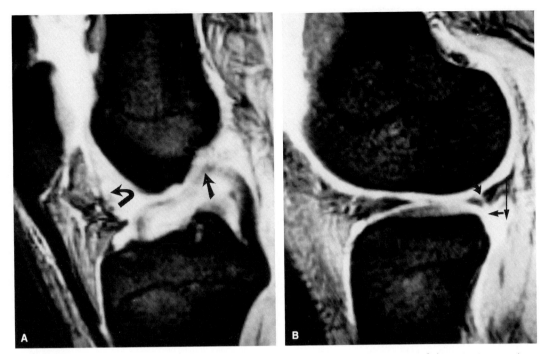

FIGURE 4–135. (**A**) A complete tear of the proximal femoral attachment of the anterior cruciate ligament (*arrow*) is seen on a T2*-weighted sagittal image. The lax anterior cruciate ligament is characterized by a wavy contour and lack of taut parallel margins. Associated synovitis is associated with an irregular contour of Hoffa's infrapatellar fat pad (*curved arrow*). (**B**) An associated vertical tear (*curved arrow*) of the posterior horn of the lateral meniscus is shown on a T2*-weighted sagittal image. Note the anterior displacement of the tibia relative to the femur (*all straight arrows*).

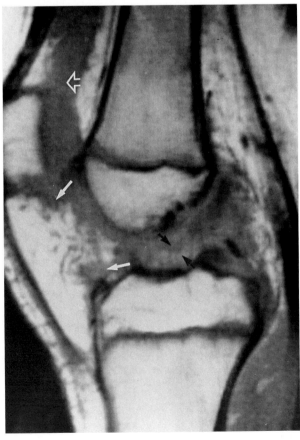

FIGURE 4–136. The presence of a disrupted anterior cruciate ligament (*solid black arrows*) associated with hemorrhagic effusion (*open white arrow*) and synovitis is implied by the irregular Hoffa's infrapatellar fat pad (*solid white arrows*).

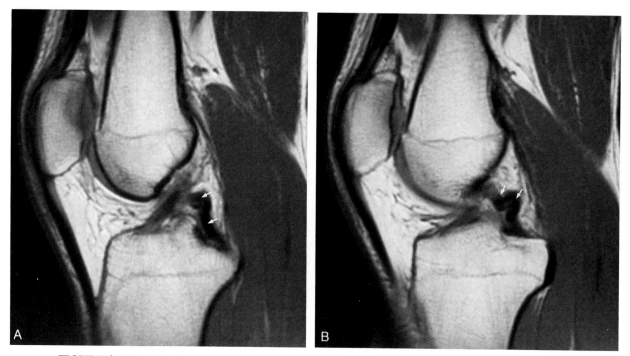

FIGURE 4–137. (**A, B**) T1-weighted images show a buckled posterior cruciate ligament. Increased laxity of the anterior cruciate ligament associated with buckling of posterior cruciate ligament (*arrows*) is secondary to forward translation of the tibia relative to the femur.

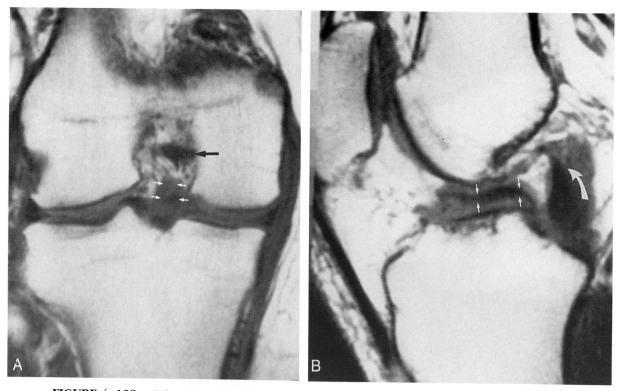

FIGURE 4–138. (**A**) A T1-weighted coronal image shows a complete tear of the anterior cruciate ligament with a tibial remnant (*white arrows*). The posterior cruciate ligament (*black arrow*) is intact. (**B**) A T1-weighted sagittal image displays a disrupted anterior cruciate ligament (*straight white arrows*) associated with buckling of the posterior cruciate ligament (*curved white arrow*). (**C**) A T1-weighted sagittal image demonstrates auto-anterior drawer sign with forward displacement of the tibia on the femur (*arrows*).

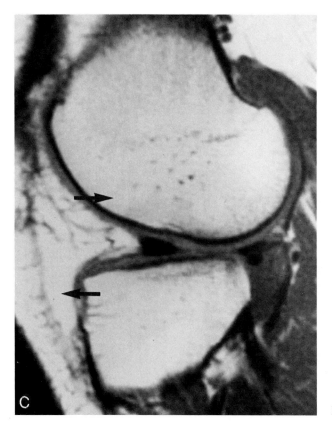

FIGURE 4–138. *(Continued)*

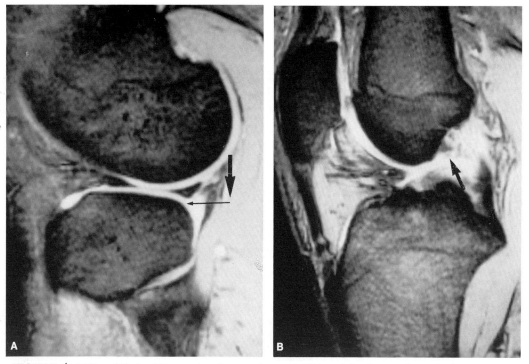

FIGURE 4–139. (**A**) An MR anterior drawer sign on a T2*-weighted sagittal image shows anterior displacement of the lateral tibial plateau (*thin arrow*) relative to a plum line dropped from the lateral femoral condyle (*thick arrow*). (**B**) Complete disruption of the anterior cruciate ligament (*arrow*) as shown on a T2*-weighted sagittal image.

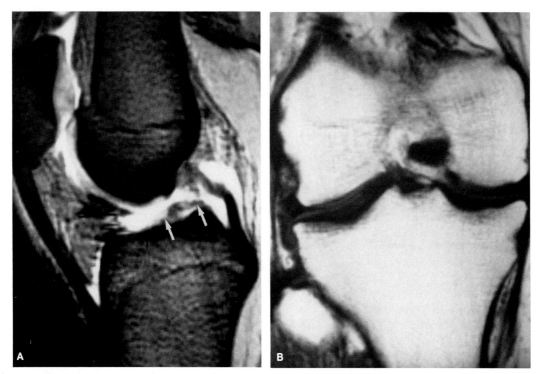

FIGURE 4–140. (**A**) A chronic anterior cruciate ligament tear with a horizontally oriented ligament (*arrows*) is seen on a T2*-weighted sagittal image. No synovitis (*i.e.,* irregular infrapatellar fat pad) or blurring of the ligament fibers is seen in this chronic injury. (**B**) The anterior cruciate ligament is absent on this T1-weighted coronal image.

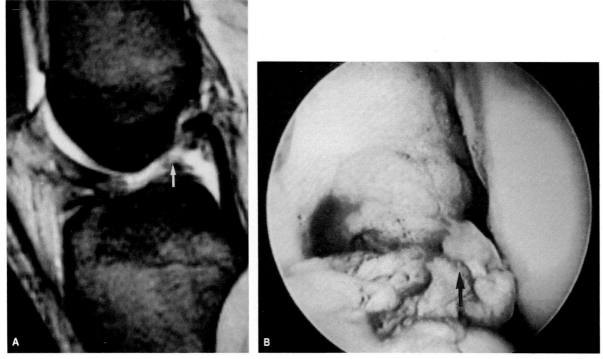

FIGURE 4–141. (**A**) A T2*-weighted sagittal image and (**B**) an intercondylar arthroscopic image of a completely disrupted anterior cruciate ligament (*arrows*).

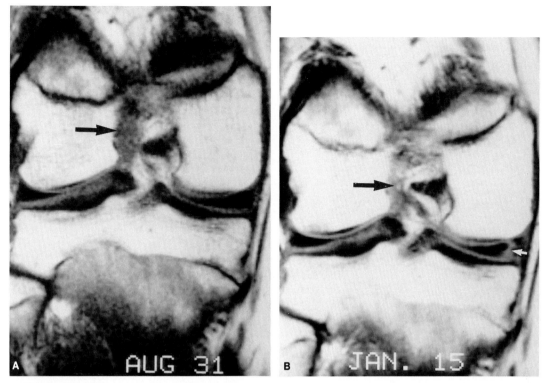

FIGURE 4–142. (**A**) An anterior cruciate ligament tear (*arrow*) is seen on a T1-weighted coronal image. (**B**) A repeat scan 4.5 months later shows an associated vertical grade 3 signal intensity medial meniscus tear (*white arrow*). The anterior cruciate ligament is absent (*black arrow*).

FIGURE 4–143. (**A**) Sagittal T1-weighted and (**B**) T2*-weighted images show an osteochondral impaction oriented directly above the anterior horn of the lateral meniscus (*straight arrows*). A posterior lateral tibial plateau contusion (*curved arrows*) is shown in association with complete rupture (*i.e.,* grade III tear) of the proximal anterior cruciate ligament fibers. With the knee fixed in flexion, external rotation of the tibia with an applied valgus force commonly produces associated bony trauma.

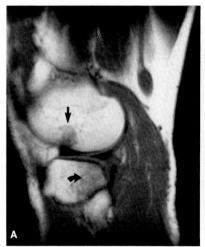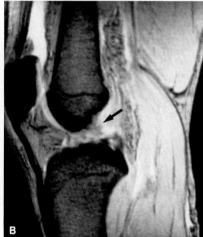

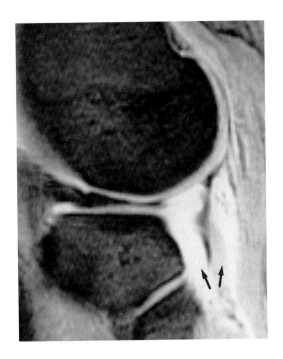

FIGURE 4–144. A posterolateral capsular tear with high signal intensity joint fluid is seen anterior and posterior to popliteus tendon (*arrows*). Anterior translation of the tibia relative to the femur was the result of an associated anterior cruciate ligament tear.

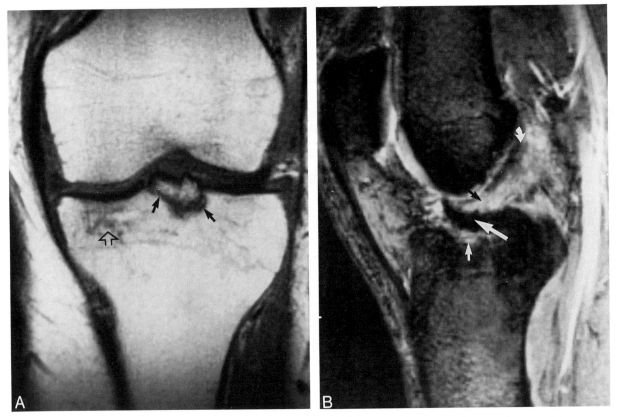

FIGURE 4–145. Anterior cruciate ligament avulsion. (**A**) A T1-weighted coronal image shows avulsion of the anterior tibial spine (*solid arrows*) caused by tension from the anterior cruciate ligament. Associated low signal intensity edema is seen in a medial tibial plateau compression fracture (*open arrow*). (**B**) The corresponding T2*-weighted image demonstrates a high signal intensity hemorrhage in the tibial portion of the anterior cruciate ligament (*black arrow*). Normal anterior cruciate ligament fibers demonstrate low signal intensity (*curved arrow*). Low signal intensity fracture avulsion (*large white arrow*) and undermining high signal intensity fluid are also shown (*small white arrow*).

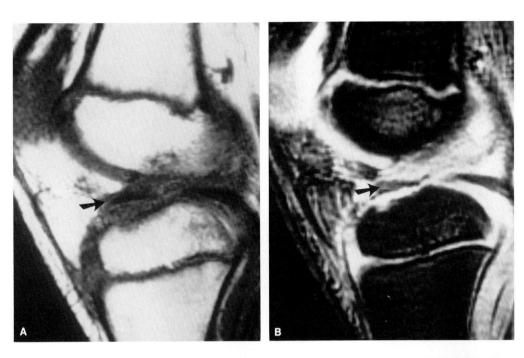

FIGURE 4–146. An avulsed anterior cruciate ligament with an attached epiphyseal fragment (*arrow*) demonstrates cortical low signal intensity on (**A**) T1-weighted and (**B**) T2*-weighted sagittal images. On T1-weighted images, the low signal intensity cortical fragment is adjacent to low signal intensity fluid and can be overlooked. Similarly, the fragment is adjacent to the low signal intensity fat pad on T2*-weighted images, and, again, can be overlooked.

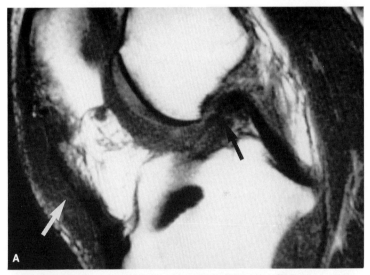

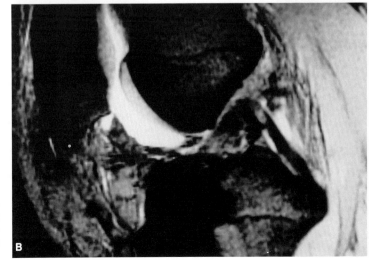

FIGURE 4–147. (**A**) A T1-weighted image of patellar tendon anterior cruciate ligament reconstruction shows the donor site (*white arrow*) and the reconstructed ligament (*black arrow*). (**B**) The corresponding T2*-weighted image is given for comparison.

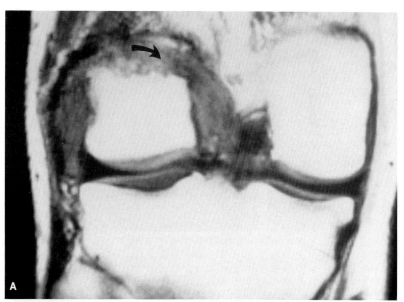

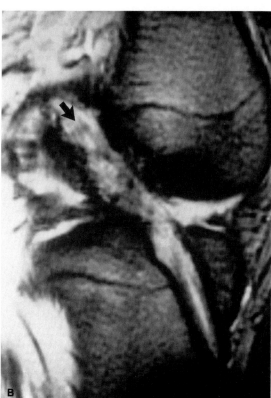

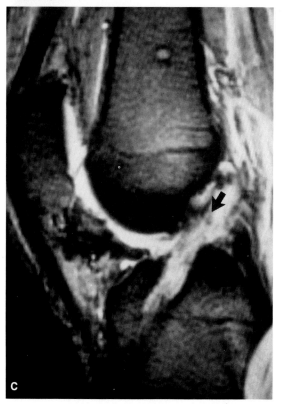

FIGURE 4–148. Lateral over-the-top repair of the anterior cruciate ligament was made using the iliotibial band. On (**A**) T1-weighted posterior coronal and (**B**) T2*-weighted radial oblique images, the reconstructed ligament (*arrow*) is seen over the lateral femoral condyle. (**C**) On a T2*-weighted sagittal image, the reconstructed ligament (*arrow*) is seen in the intercondylar notch.

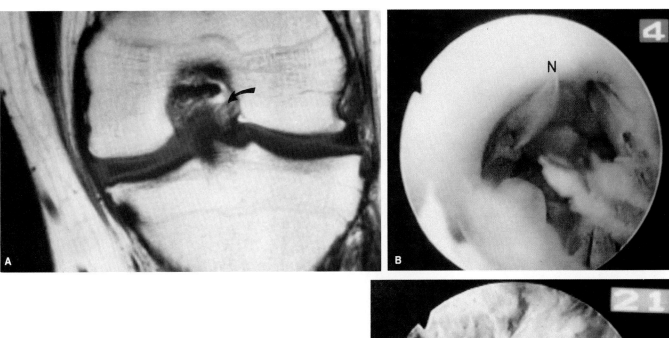

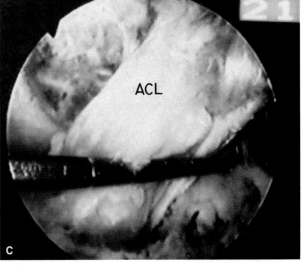

FIGURE 4–149. (**A**) The anterior cruciate ligament is absent on this T1-weighted coronal image (*curved arrow*). (**B**) An arthroscopic view shows a shredded anterior cruciate ligament in the intercondylar notch (N). (**C**) The anterior cruciate ligament (ACL) was reconstructed using the semitendinosus tendon.

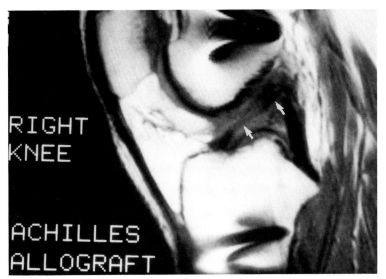

FIGURE 4–150. An Achilles tendon allograft (*arrows*) can be used for reconstruction of the anterior cruciate ligament, as seen on this T1-weighted sagittal image.

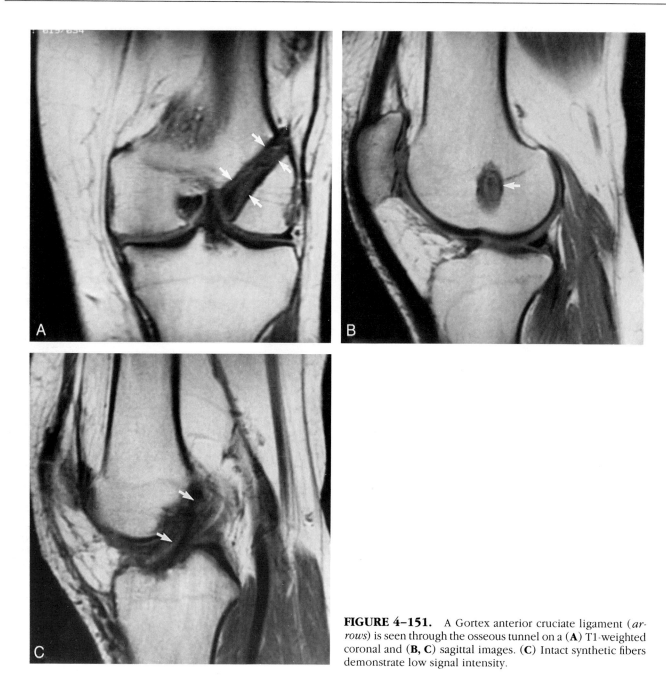

FIGURE 4–151. A Gortex anterior cruciate ligament (*arrows*) is seen through the osseous tunnel on a (**A**) T1-weighted coronal and (**B, C**) sagittal images. (**C**) Intact synthetic fibers demonstrate low signal intensity.

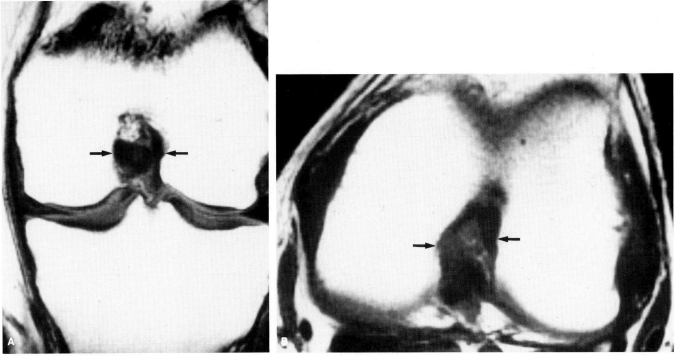

FIGURE 4–152. Congenital narrowing (*arrows*) of the intercondylar notch, as seen on (**A**) T1-weighted coronal and (**B**) axial images.

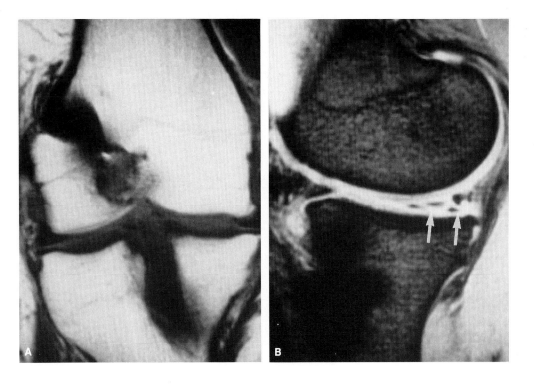

FIGURE 4–153. (**A**) Femoral and tibial osseous tunnels were created for the reconstructed anterior cruciate ligament as seen on a T1-weighted coronal image. (**B**) An associated complex tear of the posterior horn of the medial meniscus with multiple grade 3 signal intensities (*arrows*) is seen on a T2*-weighted sagittal image.

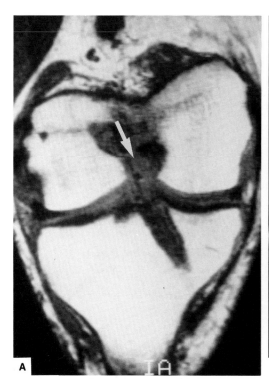

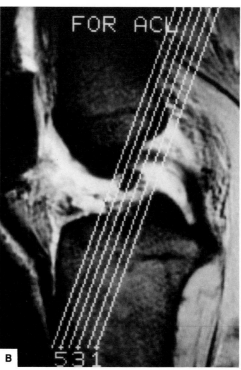

FIGURE 4–154. (**A**) A T1-weighted coronal oblique image prescribed from (**B**) a T2*-weighted sagittal localizer provides the optimal representation of the reconstructed anterior cruciate ligament (*arrow*) in the coronal plane.

FIGURE 4–155. (**A**) A coronal localizer indicates the location of (**B**) a sagittal oblique image, which shows the location of the anterior cruciate ligament reconstruction (*arrow*) on these T1-weighted images.

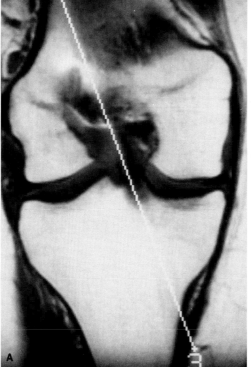

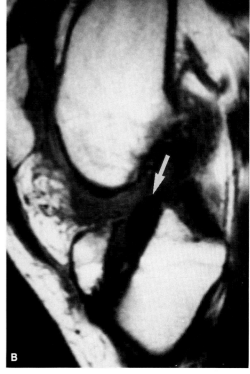

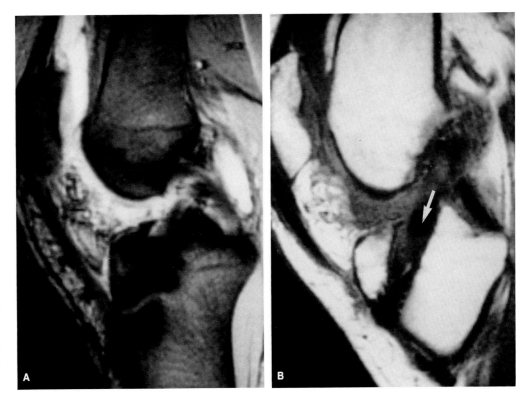

FIGURE 4–156. Intraarticular anterior cruciate ligament reconstruction (*arrow*), not evident on (**A**) a T2*-weighted sagittal image, is revealed on (**B**) a T1-weighted sagittal oblique image.

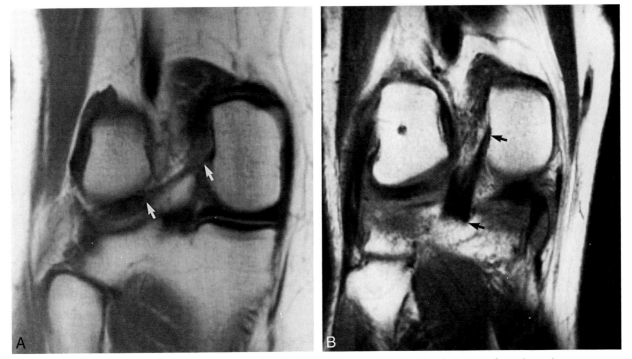

FIGURE 4–157. (**A**) A coronal image of low signal intensity shows the ligament of Wrisberg (*i.e.,* meniscofemoral ligament; *arrows*) extending from the posterior horn of the lateral meniscus to the medial femoral condyle. (**B**) The coronal anatomy of the posterior cruciate ligament (*arrows*) is seen immediately anterior to the insertion of the ligament of Wrisberg on the medial femoral condyle.

Posterior Cruciate Ligament

Functional Anatomy of the Posterior Cruciate Ligament

The PCL originates in the lateral aspect of the medial femoral condyle, crosses the ACL, and attaches to the posterior intercondyloid fossa of the tibia.[101,102] The PCL is composed of anterolateral and posteromedial bands that tighten on flexion and extension, respectively. With progressive knee flexion, the posteromedial bundle of the PCL passes anteriorly under the anterolateral bundle. The PCL is viewed as a central stabilizer of the knee, resisting posterior tibial displacement on the femur. It stabilizes the joint against excessive varus or valgus angulation and resists internal rotation of the tibia on the femur. Posterior to the PCL, the ligament of Wrisberg connects with the posterior horn of the lateral meniscus and inserts on the medial femoral condyle (Fig. 4–157). The ligament of Humphrey passes anterior to the PCL. Either the anterior or posterior meniscofemoral ligaments are found in 80% of knee-joint specimens.[103]

The ligaments of Humphrey and Wrisberg are taut in flexion and extension, respectively. With internal rotation of the tibia, both meniscofemoral ligaments tighten; therefore, the posterior drawer test should be performed in neutral or external tibial rotation.[24,104] These ligaments are considered stabilizers of the posterior horn of the lateral meniscus. The PCL is twice as strong as the ACL, with a larger cross-sectional area and higher tensile strength; these features account for a lower incidence of rupture of the PCL.[24,105,106]

Location and Mechanism of Injury of the Posterior Cruciate Ligament

Tears of the PCL are most common in the midportion (76%), followed by avulsions from the femur (36%–55%) and tibia (22%–42%).[11,107,108] Rupture can be caused by excessive rotation, hyperextension, dislocation, or by direct trauma while the knee is flexed.[109] Injuries to the PCL are usually associated with tears of either the ACL, the meniscus, or the collateral ligaments.[104,110] When there is a lateral shift in the normal center of the axis of rotation of the joint, PCL insufficiency may lead to articular cartilage degeneration in the medial compartment of the knee. A positive posterior drawer sign indicating posterior tibial displacement can be seen in up to 60% of cases.[24]

The posterolateral capsule and the popliteus complex are secondary restraints to posterior tibial displacement, with a less important contribution made by the MCL.[24]

Magnetic Resonance Appearance of the Posterior Cruciate Ligament

In the sagittal plane, the PCL is seen as a uniform dark band, usually displayed on a single sagittal image

(Fig. 4–158). The low signal intensity anterior or posterior meniscofemoral ligaments are identified in up to 60% of MR examinations. Posterior coronal or coronal oblique images demonstrate ligament attachments to the femur and tibia (Fig. 4–159). The anatomy of the PCL is not as sensitive to position as that of the ACL, and in partial knee flexion, the PCL is taut. An abnormally high arc or buckling in the PCL, however, may indicate a tear of the ACL with forward tibial displacement.

Any increase in signal, on either T1-, T2- or T2*-weighted images, within this normally low signal intensity ligament should be interpreted as abnormal (Fig. 4–160).[111] Magnetic resonance has demonstrated excellent results in allowing identification of both normal PCL morphology and tears, as confirmed by arthroscopy or arthrotomy.[111] The finding of increased signal intensity with normal PCL morphology on T1-weighted images requires additional T2- or T2*-weighted images to identify the site of ligamentous pathology (Fig. 4–161). Hemorrhage and edema, seen in acute injuries, are bright on T2- or T2*-weighted images and cause less distortion or mass effect than tears of the ACL (Fig. 4–162). Secondary extrasynovial bleeding with PCL tears may be present. Complete disruption of the PCL demonstrates a loss or gap in ligamentous continuity (Fig. 4–163). Partial tears may be more difficult to assess (Fig. 4–164). Chronic tears with fibrous scarring demonstrate intermediate signal intensity on T1- and T2-weighted images. Coronal images, with the PCL on cross-sectional display, are often helpful in identifying increased signal intensity within central fibers. The presence of a large joint effusion does not interfere with visualization of the PCL. An avulsion tear of the tibial plateau may be associated with high signal intensity ligamentous hemorrhage and a bone fragment containing marrow (Figs. 4–165 and 4–166).

Treatment of Posterior Cruciate Ligament Injury

Posterior cruciate ligament tears with tibial plateau avulsion require surgical treatment and direct repair. Midsubstance and femoral avulsions require augmentation and reconstruction with use of free or vascularized grafts from the semitendinosus and gracilis tendons, the medial head of the gastrocnemius, or patellar tendon.[24,104] PCL tears associated with ACL tears or extensive capsular disruption are also surgically treated.

COLLATERAL LIGAMENTS

Medial Collateral Ligament

Warren and Marshall have divided the medial aspect of the knee into three layers, from superficial to deep.[112] Layer 1 consists of the deep fascia surrounding the sartorius muscle and overlying the gastrocnemius. Layer 2 is the superficial MCL, and layer 3 is the medial capsular ligament (*i.e.,* the true capsule of the knee joint that forms the deep layer of the MCL in its midportion). Posteriorly, layers 2 and 3 merge to form the posterior oblique ligament.

Functional Anatomy of the Medial Collateral Ligament

The medial or tibial collateral ligament (MCL) is 8 to 10 cm long and extends from its medial epicondylar origin to attach 4 to 5 cm inferior to the tibial plateau and posterior to the pes anserinus insertion (Fig. 4–167). The insertion of the MCL on the tibia is covered by the muscle group of the pes anserinus. The MCL is considered to be composed of two layers:

1. Deep fibers corresponding to layer 3 that attach to the capsule and medial meniscus peripherally
2. More superficial fibers corresponding to layer 2.

In general, the term medial collateral ligament refers to layer 2. When the knee is extended, the fibers of the MCL are taut and limit hyperextension. When the knee is flexed, the MCL provides primary valgus stability. The MCL remains taut through flexion. The MCL is separated from the underlying capsular ligament and medial meniscus by a bursa that reduces friction during knee flexion (Fig. 4–168). MCL function is tested with applied valgus stress in partial knee flexion, with the tibia in external rotation (allowing for relaxation of the cruciates).

The medial capsular ligament (layer 3) is composed of meniscofemoral and meniscotibial attachments to the meniscus. The superficial medial collateral ligament provides the primary valgus restraint relative to the deep capsular ligament.[24] If the MCL fails at 10 to 15 mm of joint opening, the cruciate ligaments become the primary restraints to valgus stress. In the anterior-cruciate-ligament–deficient knee, the superficial MCL and medial capsule function as secondary restraints to anterior tibial translation.

Location and Mechanism of Injury of the Medial Collateral Ligament

Usually, the MCL is injured with a valgus force applied to the flexed knee. Partial ruptures or sprains frequently involve fibrous attachments to the medial femoral condyle. Complete MCL ruptures may be associated with tears of the medial and posterior capsule, the ACL, and the medial meniscus.[29] Peripheral medial meniscal tears are more common in isolated MCL injuries, whereas substance tears are seen more frequently with combined MCL and ACL injuries.[113] A contusion or fracture caused by the impact of the lateral femoral condyle on the lateral tibial plateau during valgus injury is common.

A grading system for MCL ligament injuries has been developed. Grade I lesions are minimal tears without instability. Grade II injuries are partial tears with increased instability, and grade III injuries are complete ruptures with gross instability.[24] Quantification of joint-space opening has led to an additional classification system that can be applied to partial tears or sprains. Grade I joint-space opening is 0 to 5 mm; grade II is 6 to 10 mm; grade III is 11 to 15 mm; and grade IV is 16 to 20 mm. Stress testing in an extremity coil should be performed with the knee at 25° of flexion to produce maximum medial joint-space opening (Fig. 4–169).

Magnetic Resonance Appearance of Medial Collateral Ligament Injury

Tears and Sprains. Arthrography is limited in the ability to detect MCL injuries, especially after 48 hours when extravasation of contrast media can no longer be seen. Magnetic resonance evaluation of these injuries is best accomplished with coronal images that demonstrate the low signal intensity MCL and its attachment points, where it merges with low signal intensity cortical bone. Occasionally, separation of the deep and superficial layers can be distinguished on T2-weighted images. A thin band of intermediate signal intensity, originally thought to be fat, is really an intraligamentous bursa and is often seen between the anterior portion of the MCL and the deep or medial capsular ligament complex.[114] Although this line does not represent meniscocapsular separation, increased signal intensity above or below the level of meniscus is pathologic, especially posteriorly where layers 2 and 3 fuse.

Edema and hemorrhage, which extend into subcutaneous fat, are identified parallel with the superficial MCL may occur in grade I sprains. The MCL is of normal thickness and is closely applied to underlying cortical bone. Partial tears or grade II sprains of the MCL demonstrate displacement of ligamentous fibers from adjacent cortical bone with varying degrees of edema and hemorrhage (Fig. 4–170). T2-weighted images demonstrate high signal edema, hemorrhage, or both around low signal intensity ligamentous fibers, which are superficial and deep to the medial collateral ligament. There is usually ligamentous attenuation in grade II injuries. In grade III lesions or tears, there is complete loss of continuity of the ligamentous fibers with or without extension into the capsular layer (see Fig. 4–170). Complete biomechanical failure of the MCL is associated with disruption of the medial capsular layer or ligament (Fig. 4–171).[115,116]

MCL tears may be associated with extensive joint effusion (*i.e.,* hemarthrosis) and extravasation of joint fluid, which tracks along ligament fibers (Fig. 4–172). Focal hemorrhage can be visualized at the femoral epicondylar attachment in complete ligamentous avulsions (Fig. 4–173). Subacute hemorrhage demonstrates increased signal intensity on T1- and T2-weighted images. A tear of the distal or tibial attachment may be associated with a wavy or serpiginous ligamentous contour (Fig. 4–174). Conventional T2-weighted and gradient-echo T2*-weighted images can be useful in documenting interval healing with reattachment of the torn MCL (see Fig. 4–173). Tearing of the MCL with capsular disruption may be associated with a peripheral meniscal tear and widening of the medial joint space. In response to chronic tears, the medial collateral ligament is thickened but not increased in signal intensity.

Calcification of the femoral epicondylar or proximal attachment of the MCL is thought to be the result of trauma and is referred to as Pellegrini–Stieda disease. The calcified deposit in Pellegrini–Stieda disease is low in signal intensity on T1- and T2-weighted images. Thickened ligamentous healing may be demonstrated at the same time calcification or paraarticular ossification is detected. Acute avulsions of the MCL may additionally be associated with a low signal intensity fractured cortical fragment (Fig. 4–175).

In the acute setting, nondisplaced compression fractures of the lateral tibial plateau are seen in conjunction with MCL injuries (see Fig. 4-174). These fractures or bone contusions demonstrate low signal intensity on T1-weighted images and high signal intensity on T2-weighted images and can be identified on MR scans even when radiographs are normal.[117]

Radial images of the knee have been useful in displaying attachments of the MCL and the meniscofemoral and meniscotibial ligaments. Routine orthogonal coronal images poorly display the separation of the meniscofemoral and meniscotibial components of the medial capsular ligament. Radial images, however, should not replace routine coronal images, because MCL disruptions may be misdiagnosed unless the full posterior-to-anterior extent of the ligament is identified.

Medial or Tibial Collateral Ligament Bursitis.

Medial or Tibial Collateral Ligament Bursitis. Medial or tibial collateral ligament bursitis has been demonstrated on MR studies in patients presenting with medial joint pain (Fig. 4–176). Bright signal intensity on T2- or T2*-weighted images is demonstrated between the layer 2 MCL and the layer 3 medial capsular ligament. A well-defined, elongated collection of fluid extending predominantly inferior to the joint line may be observed without associated pathology in the medial meniscus, capsular ligament, or MCL.[118]

Treatment of Medial Collateral Ligament Injury

Grades I, II, and III of isolated MCL sprains are treated with early functional rehabilitation. In isolated grade III MCL tears, operative and nonoperative treatment is equally effective. The posterior oblique ligament,

or posterior MCL, assists the MCL in resisting valgus and external rotation forces in extension and flexion; therefore, disruption of the MCL in association with the posterior oblique ligament may require surgical reconstruction. In addition, combined MCL and ACL injuries are usually treated with surgical repair.

Lateral Collateral Ligament

The lateral aspect of the knee is divided into three structural layers.[24] Layer 1 is the most superficial layer and consists of the iliotibial tract with its anterior expansion and the superficial portion of the biceps femoris with its posterior expansion. Layer 2 consists of the quadriceps retinaculum anteriorly and two patellofemoral ligaments or retinacula posteriorly. Layers 1 and 2 merge at the lateral aspect of the patella. Layer 3 is the deepest layer and consists of the lateral joint capsule, including attachments to the lateral meniscus, and the lateral capsular ligament with its meniscofemoral and meniscotibial components. The LCL is located posteriorly between the superficial and deep divisions of layer 3. The ligament itself is considered a layer 2 structure. The posterolateral complex (*i.e.,* arcuate complex) includes the LCL, the popliteus tendon, the lateral head of the gastrocnemius muscle, and the arcuate ligament.

The arcuate popliteal ligament spans the posterolateral joint and extends distally, parallel with the LCL. The arcuate ligament has attachments to the lateral meniscus and the popliteus tendon. The oblique popliteal ligament, formed by the reflected portion of the semimembranosus tendon, makes up the primary portion of the posterior capsule (Fig. 4–177).

Functional Anatomy of the Lateral Collateral Ligament

The LCL, or fibular collateral ligament, is 5 to 7 cm long. It is extracapsular and free from meniscal attachment in its course from the lateral femoral epicondyle to its conjoined insertion with the biceps femoris tendon on the fibular head.[39] The intracapsular popliteus tendon passes medial to the LCL, and the posterior fibers of the LCL blend with the deep capsule, which contributes to the arcuate popliteal ligament.

Location and Mechanism of Injury of the Lateral Collateral Ligament

The arcuate popliteal ligament and complex stabilize the posterolateral aspect of the knee against varus and external rotation. With the leg in internal rotation, an applied varus force can cause injury to the LCL and capsule. Injury or disruption of the LCL is significantly less common than injury to the MCL. Cruciate and lateral meniscal tears may be associated with lateral compartment ligamentous tears. Conventional radiographs may reveal widening of the joint space, fracture of the fibular head, and Segond fracture (*i.e.,* avulsion of the tibial insertion of the lateral capsule ligament). Segond fracture or lateral capsular sign is also associated with ACL injuries.[24]

Magnetic Resonance Appearance of the Lateral Collateral Ligament

The LCL is best seen on posterior coronal images and appears as a band of low signal intensity (Fig. 4–178). Occasionally, peripheral sagittal images demonstrate LCL anatomy at the level of the fibular head (Figs. 4–179 and 4–180). One-millimeter 3D volume protocols routinely image the LCL on at least two sagittal images. Edema and hemorrhage, although less frequent in this location, are seen as ligamentous thickening with increased signal intensity on T2-weighted images. Edema and hemorrhage may also be confirmed on peripheral sagittal images. Signal intensity is not as high in LCL injuries as in MCL disruptions, perhaps because the normal capsular separation of the LCL excludes accumulation of extravasated joint fluid. In complete disruptions, the LCL demonstrates a wavy contour and loss of ligamentous continuity (Figs. 4–181 and 4–182). Radial images have improved characterization of the LCL when 3DFT protocols are not used (Fig. 4–183). Lateral collateral ligament injuries are graded by a system similar to that described for MCL injuries.

Medial plateau compression fractures can be detected on MR scans and are associated with significant varus injuries.[117] Tears of the iliotibial band may also be associated with LCL disruptions. Inclusion of the iliotibial band on anterior coronal images is important if this structure is to be used to reconstruct the LCL. The iliotibial band, which provides lateral compartment support, is seen as a thin band of low signal intensity, parallel with the femur, with an anterolateral tibial insertion on Gerdy's tubercle. The biceps femoris muscle also plays an important role as a lateral stabilizer.

Treatment of Lateral Collateral Ligament Injury

Surgical repair of the LCL is necessary when there are associated acute ACL injuries.[24] Surgery is also used to treat grade III tears (*i.e.,* greater than 15 mm of joint-space opening) without an associated ACL tear if both the primary (*i.e.,* LCL) and secondary (*i.e.,* posterolateral or arcuate complex) restraints are injured.

PATELLOFEMORAL JOINT AND THE EXTENSOR MECHANISM

Axial images are required to characterize patellofemoral articulation. The lateral and medial patellar facets are obliquely oriented and cannot be accurately characterized on sagittal or coronal images. Patellar cartilage, the femoral groove, and retinacular attachments are defined on axial sections medial to the patellofemoral joint. The quadriceps muscles and tendon can be seen on sagittal or axial images. The patellar tendon is seen *en face* in the coronal plane, in profile in the sagittal plane, and in cross section in the axial plane.

Chondromalacia and the Extensor Mechanism

Chondromalacia patellae is characterized by patellofemoral (*i.e.,* retropatellar) joint pain, accentuated during knee flexion, and associated crepitus. Softening of the articular cartilage with associated degenerative change is responsible for the spectrum of changes seen. Chondromalacia most often affects adolescents and young adults and may either be primary and idiopathic or occur subsequent to patellar trauma.[119] In the adult form of the disease, osteoarthritic changes occur in adolescence, but no symptoms appear until middle age.

Patella alta, which consists of an increased valgus angle and femoral condylar hypoplasia, may predispose the patient to cartilage changes involving both the medial and lateral facets. Softening of the subchondral bone may be associated with articular cartilage changes including softening, edema, and fissuring. Symptoms of chondromalacia may mimic meniscal pathology. Degenerative chondromalacia secondary to osteoarthritis may affect either the medial or the lateral patellar facets, depending on the underlying cause.

The causes of acute chondromalacia include instability, direct trauma, and fracture. The causes of chronic chondromalacia include subluxation, an increased Q angle, quadriceps imbalance, post-traumatic malalignment, excessive lateral pressure syndrome, and PCL injuries. Chronic chondromalacia may also result from inflammatory arthritis, synovitis, and infection.[24]

Four arthroscopic grades of chondromalacia are classified by Outerbridge.[120,121] In grade 0 chondromalacia, the articular cartilage is normal. In grade 1, discoloration of the articular cartilage occurs and may include blistering, usually without fragmentation or fissuring. Blistering represents separation of the superficial layer of articular cartilage. Localized softening, swelling, and fibrillation is limited to an area of 0.5 cm or less in diameter. In grade 2 disease, fissuring and fibrillation within soft areas of the articular cartilage may extend to a depth of 1 to 2 mm and to an area of 1.3 cm or less in diameter. In grade 3 chondromalacia, fissuring and fibrillation may involve more than one-half the depth of the articular cartilage thickness and an area greater than 1.3 cm in diameter. The articular cartilage surface resembles crab meat, with fasciculation of multiple cartilaginous fragments attached to underlying subchondral bone. There is no involvement of subchondral bone, however. In grade 4 disease (*i.e.,* end-stage chondromalacia), complete loss or erosion of the articular cartilage surface results in exposed subchondral bone. Advanced patellofemoral arthrosis and end-stage chondromalacia have the same appearance. Medial facet cartilage surface degeneration occurs with aging and also represents a form of chondromalacia.

Magnetic Resonance Appearance of Chondromalacia

T2-, T2*, or enhanced T1-weighted axial images can be used to define the fluid–cartilage interface in the patellofemoral joint (Fig. 4–184). On axial MR images, cartilage attenuation or erosions can be seen in either the medial or lateral facets (Fig. 4–185).[122] Frequently, opposing femoral cartilage also demonstrates thinning on sagittal images. Sagittal images, which are less sensitive to cartilage erosions, may show a straightening or loss of the convex curve normally seen in patellar hyaline cartilage when viewed in profile. T2- and/or T2*-weighted sequences are useful in demonstrating inhomogeneity of the signal obtained from patellar cartilage in areas of focal edema. Subchondral low signal intensity, which represents sclerosis, may be associated with irregular surface erosions (Fig. 4–186). Low signal intensity patellar cysts sometimes may be seen in the early stags of patellar softening, before cartilage erosions occur (Fig. 4–187).

The articular cartilage surface on T1-weighted axial images is displayed with a homogeneous intermediate signal intensity (Fig. 4–188). A thin layer of fluid signal intensity, however, is often difficult to separate from the underlying articular cartilage surface. T2*-weighted images are useful in separating the fluid–cartilage interface in the thicker articular cartilage of the patellofemoral joint.[108] Joint effusions demonstrate low signal intensity on T1-weighted images and bright signal intensity on T2-weighted images, and they are commonly associated with patellofemoral chondromalacia. Cartilage erosions may be the source of loose bodies (Fig. 4–189). Associated thinning of articular cartilage on the anterolateral femoral condyle and subchondral sclerosis in the patellofemoral groove should be evaluated (Fig. 4–190).

The arthroscopic grades of chondromalacia patella have been correlated with findings on MR imaging.[123,124] On T1-weighted MR images, arthroscopic grade 1 chondromalacia, indicated by patellar softening, is characterized by focal areas of decreased signal intensity without cartilage surface or subchondral bone extension. Magnetic resonance examination may not be sensitive to certain grade 1 lesions. In grade 2 chondromalacia, indicated by blisterlike swelling, areas of decreased signal intensity extend to the articular cartilage surface. A sharp margin is preserved between the patellar and trochlear articular cartilage surfaces (Fig. 4–191). The surface irregularity

and attenuation seen in arthroscopic grade 3 disease correlates with focal areas of decreased signal intensity associated with loss of the sharp articular margin between the patellar and trochlear surfaces. T2- or T2*-weighted images may demonstrate imbibed fluid in surface articular cartilage defects as high signal intensity sites (Fig. 4–192). Ulceration and exposure of the subchondral bone seen in arthroscopic grade 4 are represented on MR images by frank articular cartilage defects, exposed subchondral bone, and undermining of fluid in subchondral bone (Figs. 4–193 through 4–195).

Correlation with pathologic specimens has also demonstrated the ability of MR imaging to characterize cartilage morphology, particularly ulcerations of the cartilage surface (*i.e.,* fibrillation).[125]

Treatment of Chondromalacia

Treatment of chondromalacia requires an initial conservative period of rehabilitation.[24] Instabilities or malalignments may require surgical intervention if conservative treatment fails. Arthroscopic shaving or removal of fibrillated and traumatized areas of articular cartilage, especially in post-traumatic chondromalacia, may improve the patient's symptoms, although results may deteriorate with time (Fig. 4–196). Treatment by shaving of the patella surface cartilage can be identified on MR studies as an artificially straight articular surface with macroscopic metallic artifacts (Fig. 4–197). Other surgical procedures include chondroplasty with subchondral drilling, spongialization realignment procedures, tibial tubercle elevation, patellectomy, and patellar resurfacing.

Patellar Subluxation and Dislocation

Patellar subluxation sometimes presents with symptoms of joint locking and may be mistaken for a torn meniscus.[126] The repetitive trauma caused by bilateral displacement of the patella accelerates articular cartilage surface degeneration (Fig. 4–198). Torn medial retinacular attachments can be identified on axial images subsequent to patellar dislocation and traumatic subluxations. Patella alta, lateral femoral condyle hypoplasia, genu valgum or recurvatum, and abnormal (*i.e.,* lateral) insertion of the patellar tendon can precipitate displacements. We have used MR imaging to identify dysplastic patellae without a medial facet or central ridges as a cause for lateral subluxation associated with a shallow or hypoplastic femoral groove. This is classified as a Wiberg type 5 (*i.e.,* Jagerhut) patella (Fig. 4–199).[127] Other patellar types are displayed on axial plane images (Fig. 4–200).

Alignment between the patella and the trochlear groove of the femur can be directly measured by the patellar congruence and tilt angles.[124] The patellar congruence angle is the angle formed by a line bisecting the femoral sulcus angle and a second line connecting the apex of the trochlea and apex of the patella. The normal congruence angle is −8° ± −6°. A positive congruence angle is associated with recurrent lateral dislocations. The patellar tilt angle is determined by a line parallel with the lateral facet and a second line parallel with the posterior femoral condylar surfaces. The normal patellar tilt angle measures more than 8°. Excessive lateral pressure syndrome may be associated with an abnormal patellar tilt angle (less than 8°).

Axial kinematic MR imaging techniques (see Chap. 10) can be used to document patellar instability in either the medial or lateral direction from 0° to 35° of knee flexion.[128-130] Medial instability, which is uncommon, has been identified as a complication of lateral retinacular release (Fig. 4–201).

Retinacular Attachments

The medial and lateral retinacula are fascicle extensions of the vastus medialis and lateralis muscle groups, respectively.[10] The retinacula reinforce and guard normal patellar tracking. On anterior coronal images, the retinacular attachments are seen as low signal intensity structures converging on the medial and lateral patellar facets. The medial and lateral retinacula, however, are best evaluated on axial images through the patellofemoral joint.

The medial retinaculum is more frequently torn than the lateral, especially after patellar dislocation (Figs. 4–202 and 4–203). Axial MR images demonstrate either a free-floating retinaculum without patellar attachment, or a masslike effect caused by compressed torn retinacular fibers or chondral fragments (Fig. 4–204). Associated edema and hemorrhage produce high signal intensity on T2- or T2*-weighted images.

A tight lateral retinaculum (*i.e.,* excessive lateral pressure syndrome) tilts the patella in a lateral direction without subluxation. A retinacular release may be performed to minimize the development of lateral facet degenerative disease. The site of retinacular division following release may be evaluated with MR studies.

Patellar Tendon Abnormalities

Tears

Patellar tendon tears, which result in loss of extension and a high-riding patella, can occur with avulsion injuries from the tibial tubercle (Fig. 4–205) or inferior pole of the patella (Fig. 4–206).[131] Bony fragments, with or with-

out the signal intensity of marrow, may be identified on sagittal MR images. T2*-weighted sagittal images are sensitive to small avulsed bone fragments that may be overlooked on T1- or conventional T2-weighted images (see Fig. 4–205). Increased tendon laxity and a wavy contour occur in acute and chronic tears (Fig. 4–207). Rupture at the inferior pole of the patella may be associated with proximal retraction of the tendon. The patellar tendon may appear thickened after arthroscopy or trauma.

Treatment of patellar tendon ruptures includes direct tendon-to-tendon repair, reconstruction with semitendinosus tendon, or cancellous reattachment.[24]

Tendinitis

Patellar tendinitis, also referred to as jumper's knee, usually affects the patellar tendon and its insertions. Malalignment of the extensor mechanism, instability associated with forces generated in jumping sports, and overuse lead to the inflammatory changes.[24] The tendinitis usually occurs in adults, and patients present with anterior knee pain.

On axial and sagittal MR images, patellar tendinitis, whether acute or chronic, demonstrates thickening of the patellar tendon (Fig. 4–208). In acute or subacute tendinitis, which may be associated with partial tendinous tearing, intratendinous areas of low signal intensity are seen on T1-weighted images and increased signal intensity is seen on T2-weighted, T2*-weighted, or STIR images. Short TI inversion recovery protocols may be more sensitive than low signal intensity T1- and conventional T2-weighted images in identifying areas of chronic edema. Focal thickening of the patellar tendon can be seen proximally in jumper's knee, as opposed to distal thickening, which may be more common in Osgood–Schlatter disease (discussed later in the chapter). In chronic tears, synovial hyperplasia, fibrinoid necrosis, and inflammation contribute to focal areas of high signal intensity.[132] Patellar tendon thickening may also occur as a sequela to arthroscopy.

Patella Alta and Baja

The patellar tendon-to-patella ratio is considered abnormal when the lengths of the patella and patellar tendon are unequal.[131] Patella alta (*i.e.,* high position of the patella) and patella baja (*i.e.,* low position of the patella) can be determined on direct sagittal images that show the entire length of the patellar tendon and the superior-to-inferior dimensions of the patella. Patella alta has been associated with subluxation, chondromalacia, Sinding–Larsen–Johansson syndrome, cerebral palsy, and quadriceps atrophy (Fig. 4–209).[133] Patella baja is seen with polio, achondroplasia, and juvenile rheumatoid (*i.e.,* chronic) arthritis (JRA; Figs. 4–210 and 4–211).

(text continues on page 306)

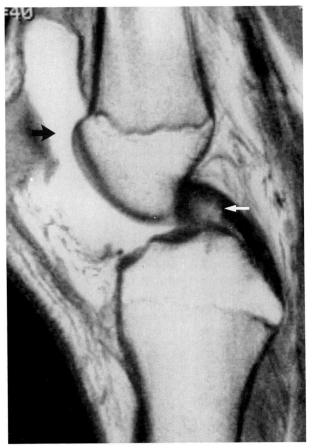

FIGURE 4–158. An intact low signal intensity posterior cruciate ligament (*white arrow*) shows adjacent high signal intensity joint effusion (*black arrow*) on a T2-weighted sagittal image.

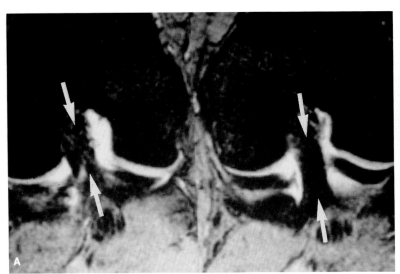

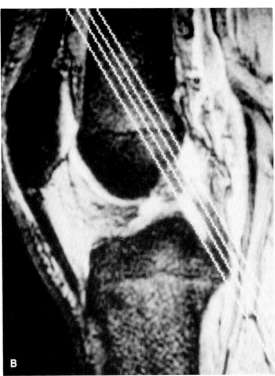

FIGURE 4–159. (**A**) Posterior cruciate ligament attachments (*arrows*) appear elongated on the T2*-weighted posterior coronal oblique image. (**B**) The corresponding T2*-weighted sagittal localizer with coronal oblique prescriptions is shown.

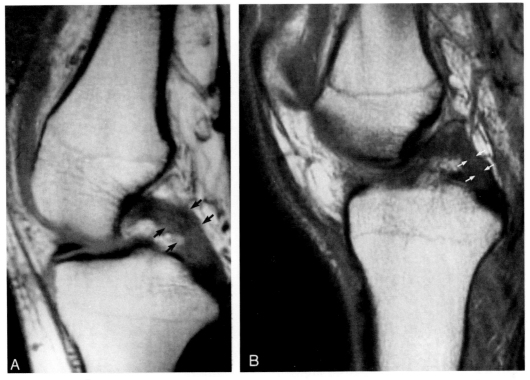

FIGURE 4–160. Low signal intensity edema and hemorrhage in a torn posterior cruciate ligament (*arrows*) are demonstrated on T1-weighted sagittal images in two separate patients.

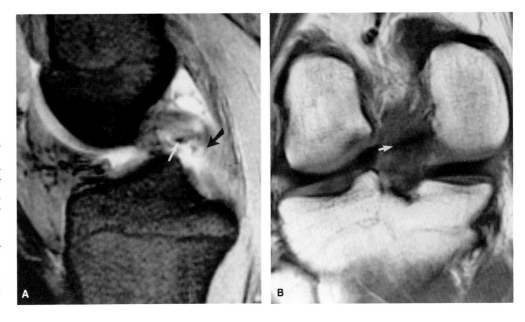

FIGURE 4–161. (**A**) A T2*-weighted sagittal image shows a hyperintense complete posterior cruciate ligament tear (*black arrow*). The ligament of Humphrey (*white arrow*) is seen anterior to the posterior cruciate ligament. (**B**) The corresponding T1-weighted coronal image shows the ligament of Humphrey (*arrow*) located anterior to the expected location of the absent posterior cruciate ligament.

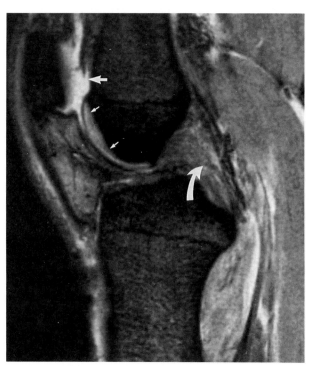

FIGURE 4–162. A posterior cruciate ligament tear with edema and hemorrhage demonstrates high signal intensity (*curved arrow*) on a T2*-weighted image. The interface between cartilage (*small white arrows*) and fluid (*large white arrows*) is shown.

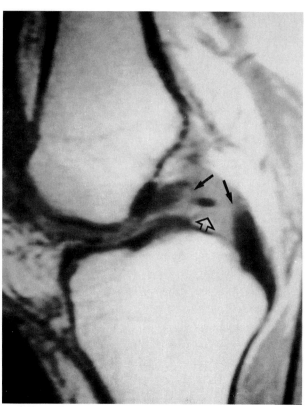

FIGURE 4–163. A T1-weighted sagittal image shows complete transection of the posterior cruciate ligament with hemorrhage (*open arrow*) and loss of ligamentous continuity (*solid arrows*).

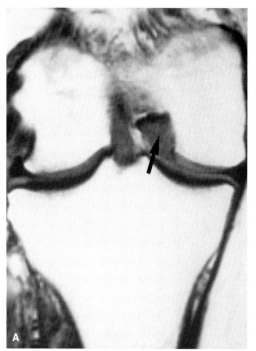

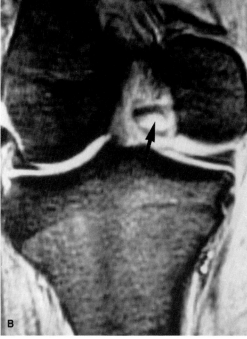

FIGURE 4–164. A grade II interstitial posterior cruciate ligament tear with widened, but not discontinuous, ligament (*arrows*) demonstrates (**A**) intermediate signal intensity on a T1-weighted image and (**B**) increased signal intensity on a T2*-weighted coronal image.

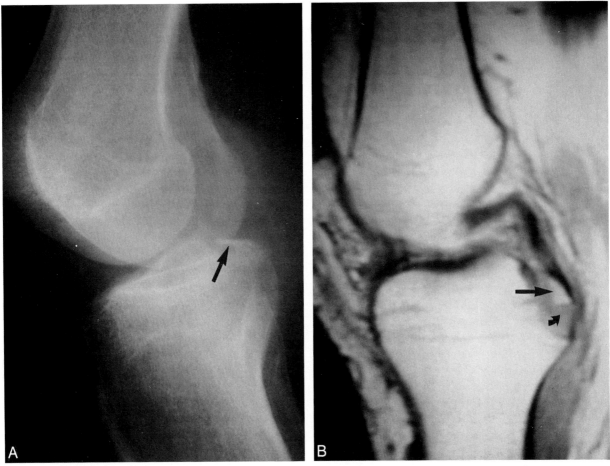

FIGURE 4–165. Posterior cruciate avulsion. (**A**) A lateral radiograph shows an avulsed bony fragment from the posterior tibial plateau (*arrow*). (**B**) The corresponding T1-weighted sagittal image shows avulsed bone containing high signal intensity yellow marrow from the attachment site of the posterior cruciate ligament (*straight arrow*). Intermediate signal intensity is generated by associated edema and hemorrhage (*curved arrow*).

FIGURE 4–166. (**A**) A posterior cruciate ligament tear is associated with an avulsed tibial bony fragment (*all arrows*) on this T1-weighted image. (**B**) A large fractured osteochondral fragment (*white arrow*) is seen anterior to the posterior cruciate ligament attachment (*black arrow*). (**C**) A posterior tibial intercondylar fracture is revealed on a T1-weighted axial image (*arrow*). *(continued)*

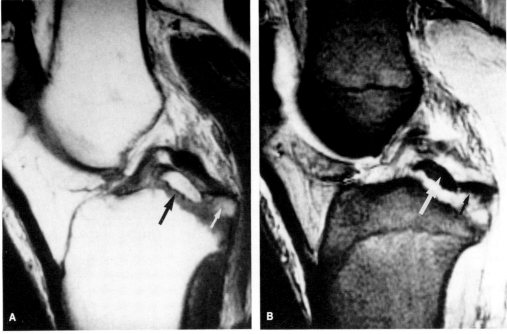

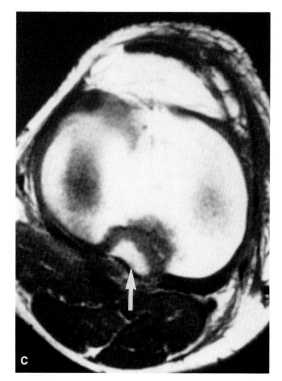

FIGURE 4–166. *(Continued)*

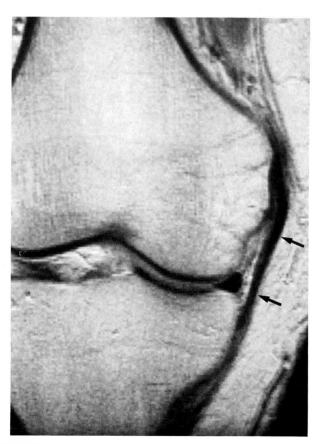

FIGURE 4–167. An intact low signal intensity superficial band represents the tibial medial collateral ligament (*arrows*) on an anterior T1-weighted coronal image. A more posterior coronal section would show attachment with the deep band of the medial collateral ligament and the periphery of the medial meniscus at the meniscocapsular insertion.

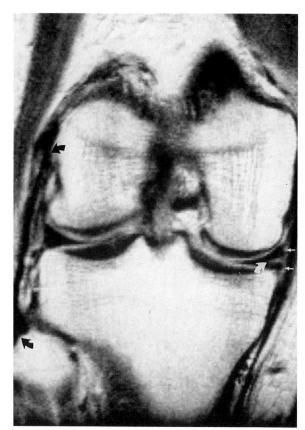

FIGURE 4–168. A normal intermediate signal intensity connection exists between the medial collateral ligament and the periphery of the medial meniscus (*straight white arrows*) on an intermediate-weighted image. Linear grade II degeneration is also demonstrated (*curved white arrow*). The intact fibular lateral collateral ligament is seen in the same coronal section (*curved black arrows*).

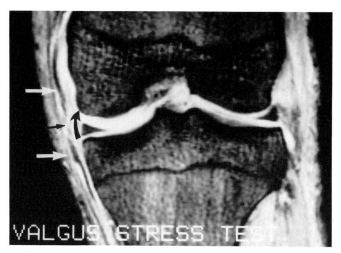

FIGURE 4–169. Applied valgus stress (*curved arrow*) produces medial compartment opening in the presence of medial collateral ligament disruption (*straight white arrows*) at the level of the joint line (*straight black arrow*) on a T2*-weighted coronal image.

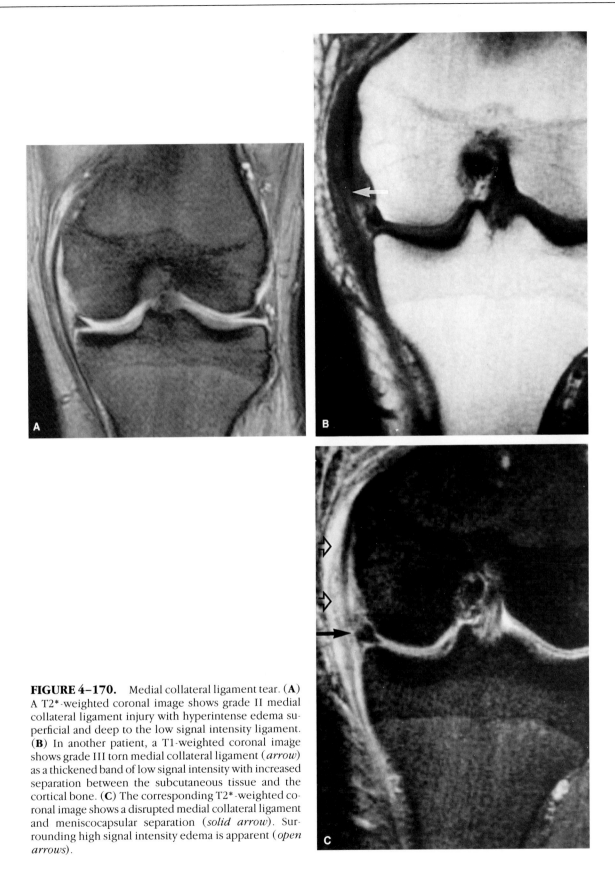

FIGURE 4–170. Medial collateral ligament tear. (**A**) A T2*-weighted coronal image shows grade II medial collateral ligament injury with hyperintense edema superficial and deep to the low signal intensity ligament. (**B**) In another patient, a T1-weighted coronal image shows grade III torn medial collateral ligament (*arrow*) as a thickened band of low signal intensity with increased separation between the subcutaneous tissue and the cortical bone. (**C**) The corresponding T2*-weighted coronal image shows a disrupted medial collateral ligament and meniscocapsular separation (*solid arrow*). Surrounding high signal intensity edema is apparent (*open arrows*).

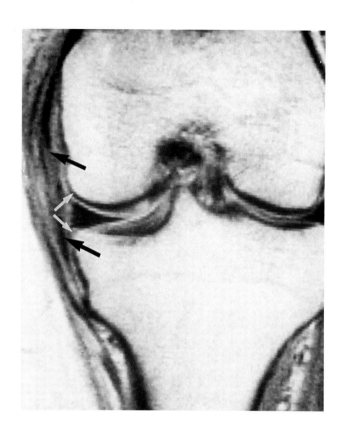

FIGURE 4–171. An intermediate-weighted coronal image of a medial collateral ligament tear (*black arrows*) shows meniscocapsular separation and valgus instability. Widening of the medial joint compartment (*white arrows*) is apparent.

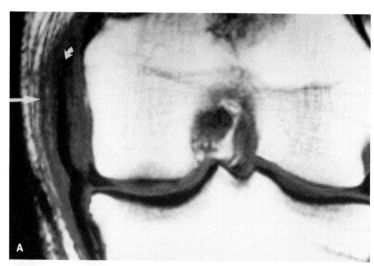

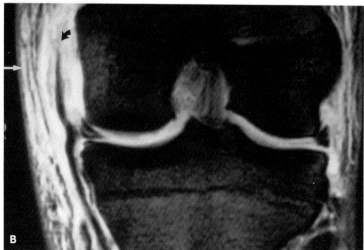

FIGURE 4–172. (**A**) Coronal T1-weighted and (**B**) T2*-weighted images show extensive extracapsular soft-tissue edema (*straight arrows*) and hemorrhage in a grade III medial collateral ligament tear (*curved arrows*). Note the increased separation between subcutaneous tissue and medullary marrow signal intensity.

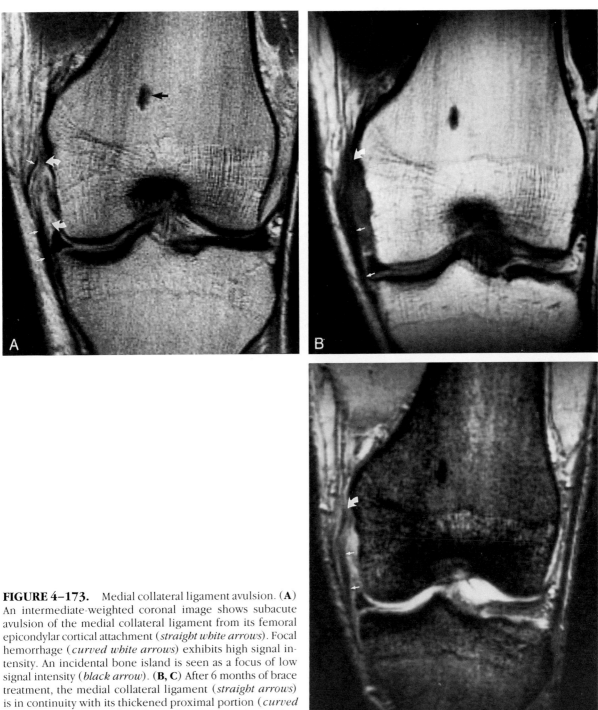

FIGURE 4–173. Medial collateral ligament avulsion. (**A**) An intermediate-weighted coronal image shows subacute avulsion of the medial collateral ligament from its femoral epicondylar cortical attachment (*straight white arrows*). Focal hemorrhage (*curved white arrows*) exhibits high signal intensity. An incidental bone island is seen as a focus of low signal intensity (*black arrow*). (**B, C**) After 6 months of brace treatment, the medial collateral ligament (*straight arrows*) is in continuity with its thickened proximal portion (*curved arrows*). Delineation of the femoral cortical attachment improves as weighting progresses from (**B**) a T1-weighted to (**C**) a T2*-weighted sequence.

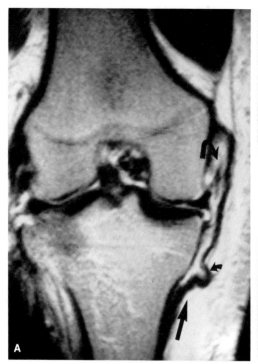 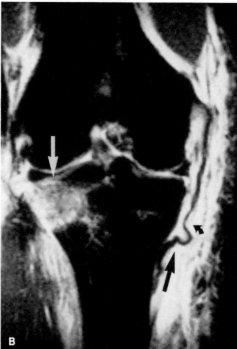

FIGURE 4–174. (**A**) Coronal T2-weighted and (**B**) short TI inversion recovery (STIR) images show avulsion of the distal tibial attachment of the medial collateral ligament with proximal ligament retraction (*straight black arrow*) and increased ligamentous laxity (*small curved arrow*). Lateral tibial plateau impaction is best demonstrated by STIR contrast with hyperintense marrow hemorrhage (*straight white arrow*). Associated disruption of the meniscofemoral attachment of the deep capsular ligament (*large curved arrow*) is present. Note the extracapsular soft-tissue edema and hemorrhage evident on the STIR image.

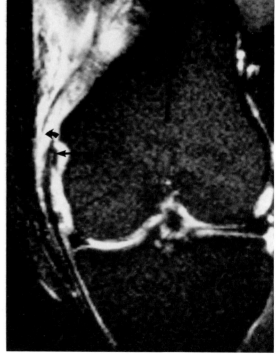

FIGURE 4–175. Grade III medial collateral ligament tear with an avulsed bone fragment (*straight arrow*) is seen on a short TI inversion recovery coronal image. The associated extracapsular hemorrhage (*curved arrow*) is hyperintense. There was no associated meniscal tear.

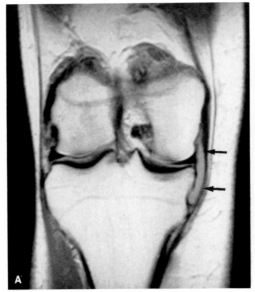
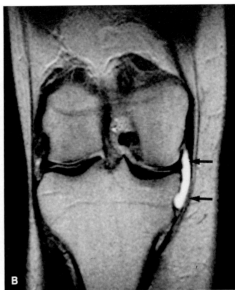

FIGURE 4-176. Coronal (**A**) intermediate-weighted and (**B**) T2-weighted images of tibial collateral ligament bursitis (*arrows*) show no associated medial meniscus or collateral ligament pathology. Fluid is hyperintense on the T2-weighted image.

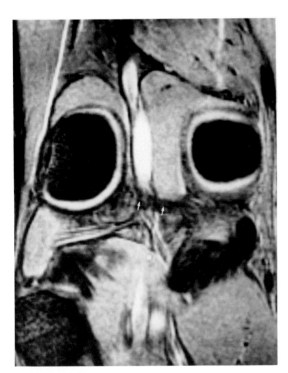

FIGURE 4-177. The oblique popliteal ligament (*arrows*) is visible on a 1-mm 3D Fourier transform volume posterior coronal T2*-weighted image. This structure would be routinely missed in 3- to 5-mm sections.

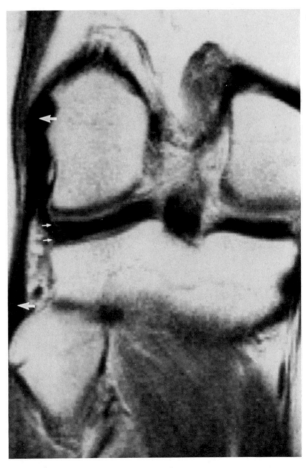

FIGURE 4-178. A intact lateral collateral ligament has low signal intensity on a T1-weighted posterior coronal image (*large arrows*). The ligament is separate from the lateral meniscus (*small arrows*).

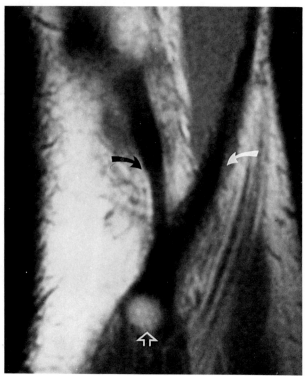

FIGURE 4–179. A T1-weighted peripheral sagittal image displays the conjoined insertion on the fibular head (*open arrow*) of the separate lateral collateral ligament (*curved black arrow*) and biceps femoris tendon (*curved white arrow*).

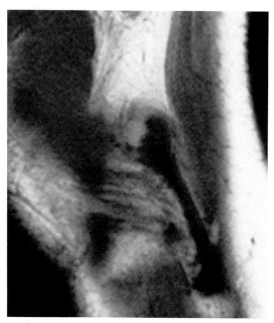

FIGURE 4–180. Low signal intensity indicates the lateral collateral ligament on a peripheral sagittal T1-weighted image.

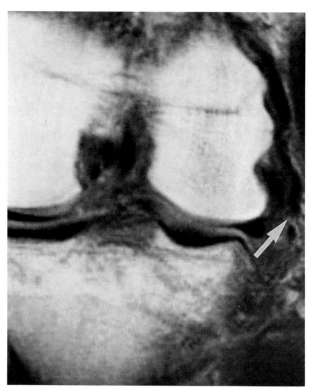

FIGURE 4–181. A complete tear of the lateral collateral ligament near its distal fibular attachment (*arrow*) can be seen on a T1-weighted coronal image. The disrupted ligament has a wavy contour.

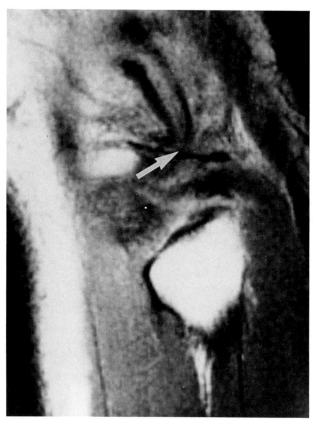

FIGURE 4–182. Complete disruption of the fibular lateral collateral ligament at the level of the joint line (*arrow*) is revealed on a T1-weighted sagittal image.

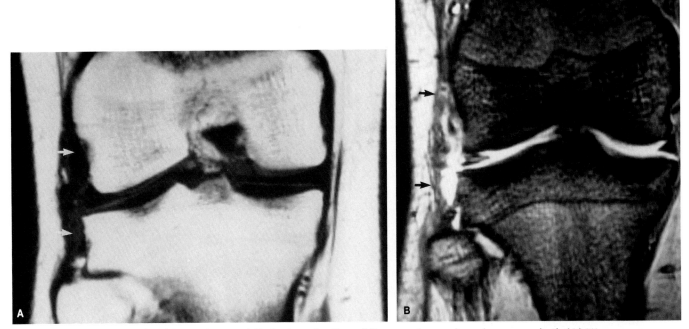

FIGURE 4–183. A disrupted fibular lateral collateral ligament (*arrows*) can be seen on both (**A**) T1-weighted coronal and (**B**) T2*-weighted radial images. Reliable imaging of the lateral collateral ligament requires thin section (*i.e.*, <5-mm) coronal radial images.

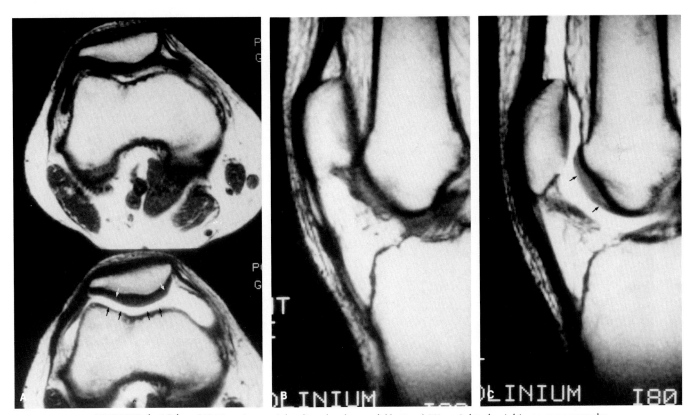

FIGURE 4–184. (**A**) Unenhanced (*top*) and enhanced (*bottom*) T1-weighted axial images accurately depict the patellofemoral articular cartilage (*white arrows*) with intraarticular gadolinium enhancement (*black arrows*). (**B**) Unenhanced and (**C**) enhanced T1-weighted sagittal images show the anterolateral femoral articular cartilage (*arrows*) with distention of suprapatellar bursa.

FIGURE 4–186. Lateral facet chondromalacia. (**A**) Lateral patellar facet cartilage degeneration (*solid arrows*) with subchondral irregularity and low signal intensity sclerosis (*open arrow*) occurred in a professional ballet dancer. (**B**) The asymptomatic knee is shown for comparison; note the thicker articular cartilage surface (*arrows*).

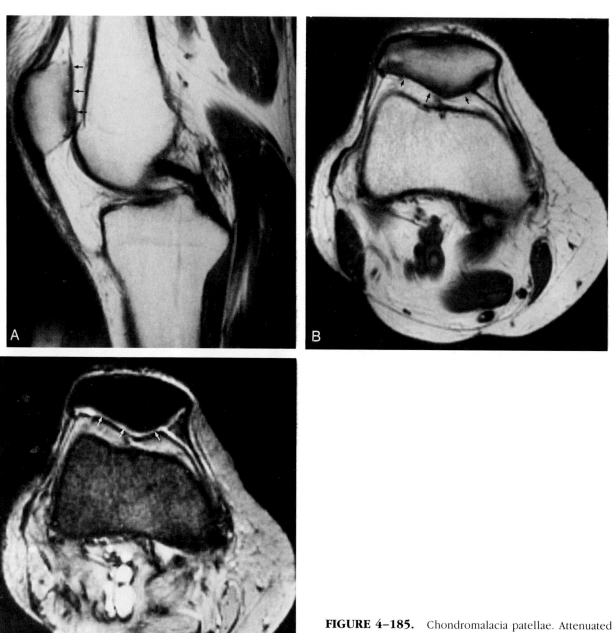

FIGURE 4–185. Chondromalacia patellae. Attenuated hyaline cartilage (*arrows*) of the patellar facets appears different on (**A**) T1-weighted sagittal and (**B**) axial images and on (**C**) T2*-weighted axial images. Thinning articular cartilage is shown with high signal intensity on the T2*-weighted sequence.

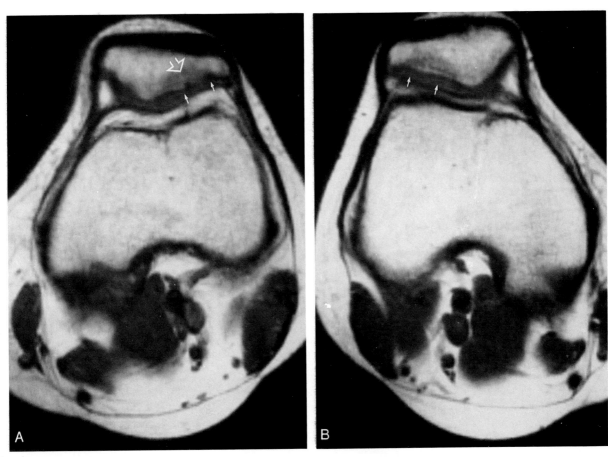

FIGURE 4–186.

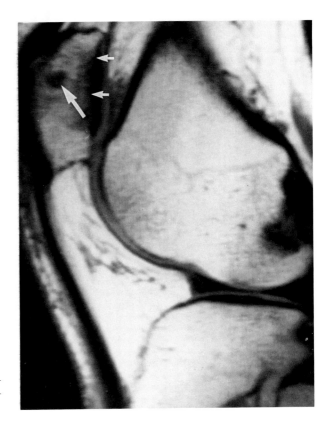

FIGURE 4–187. A T1-weighted sagittal image in a patient with chondromalacia patellae demonstrates low signal intensity subchondral sclerosis (*small arrows*) and a degenerative patellar cyst (*large arrow*).

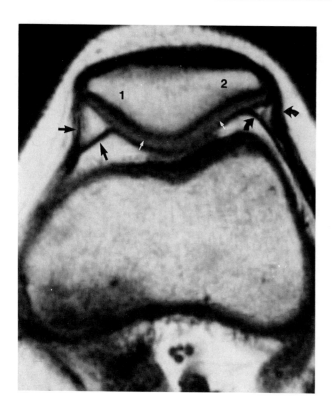

FIGURE 4–188. Axial anatomy at the level of the patellofemoral joint. Suprapatellar bursal retentions should not be confused with plica or retinacula (*inner straight and curved black arrows*). (*Outer straight black arrow,* medial retinacular attachments; *outer curved black arrow,* lateral retinacular attachments; *white arrows,* articular cartilage of medial and lateral patellar facets; 1, medial patellar facet; 2, lateral patellar facet.)

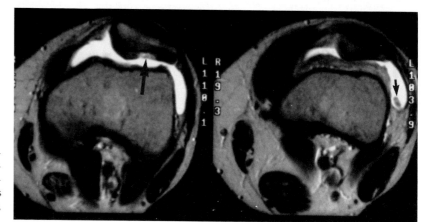

FIGURE 4–189. A T2-weighted axial image reveals a high signal intensity lateral patellar facet articular cartilage defect (*long arrow, left*) with an associated intermediate signal intensity cartilaginous loose body in the suprapatellar bursa (*short arrow, right*).

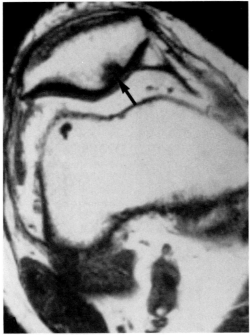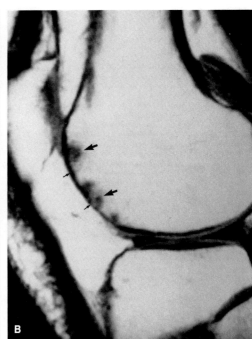

FIGURE 4–190. Patello-femoral arthrosis. (**A**) A T1-weighted axial image shows low signal intensity subchondral sclerosis (*arrow*) and the attenuated articular cartilage surface of the medial facet. (**B**) A T1-weighted sagittal image shows denuded anterolateral femoral articular cartilage surface (*small arrows*) with low signal intensity subchondral sclerotic foci (*large arrows*).

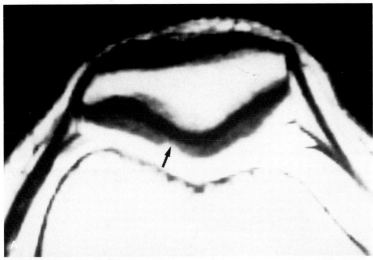

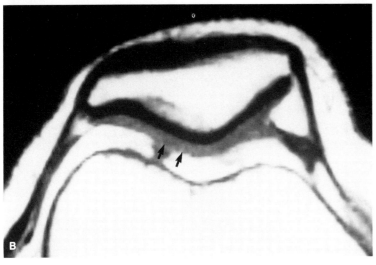

FIGURE 4–191. (**A**) Grade II chondromalacia of the lateral facet is detected as a focal area of imbibed gadolinium contrast (*arrow*) that extends to the cartilage surface on an intraarticular, enhanced T1-weighted axial image. (**B**) An unenhanced T1-weighted axial image shows normal cartilage thickness (*arrow*). Localized softening, swelling, or blistering of the articular cartilage may be associated with decreased signal intensity intracartilaginous foci on T1-weighted images.

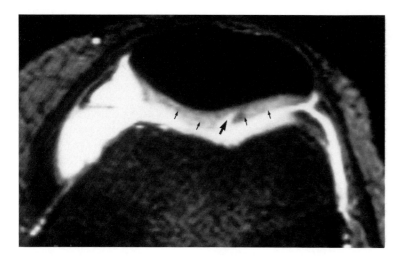

FIGURE 4–192. A T2*-weighted image demonstrates grade 3 chondromalacia with articular cartilage fissuring to the deep articular cartilage layer (*large arrow*). Degenerative attenuated lateral facet cartilage and normal thickness medial facet cartilage show high signal intensity inhomogeneity secondary to increased free water associated with fibrillation of the cartilage surface (*small arrows*).

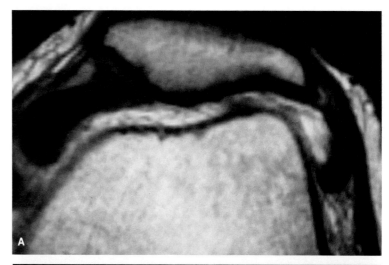

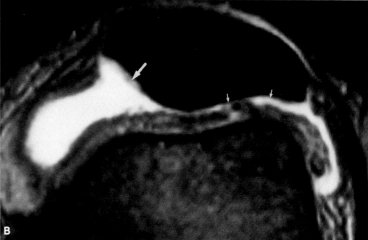

FIGURE 4–193. Denuded articular cartilage, present from the subchondral bone to the cartilage surface and involving the medial (*large arrow*) and lateral (*small arrows*) patellar facets, occurs in grade 4 chondromalacia and is seen on (**A**) T1-weighted and (**B**) T2*-weighted axial images.

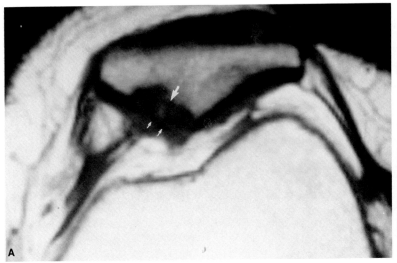

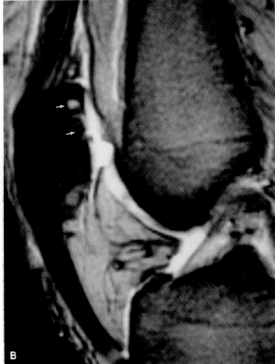

FIGURE 4–194. (**A**) A T1-weighted sagittal image shows grade 4 chondromalacia with medial facet subchondral sclerosis (*large arrow*) and denuded cartilage that extends to the subchondral bone (*small arrows*). (**B**) A T2*-weighted sagittal image reveals hyperintense subchondral imbibed fluid signal intensity (*arrows*).

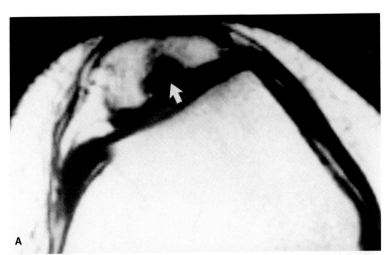

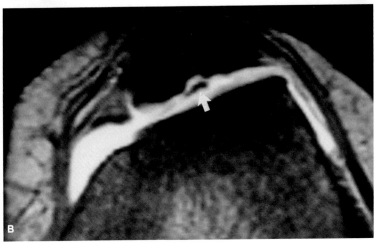

FIGURE 4–195. In grade 4 chondromalacia (*arrow*), (**A**) lateral facet subchondral sclerosis is revealed on a T1-weighted axial image, and (**B**) ulceration with fragmentation is revealed on a T2*-weighted image. More advanced grades of chondromalacia (*i.e.,* grades 3 and 4) are usually associated with low signal intensity marrow changes on T1-weighted images. Grade 4 chondromalacia is frequently associated with imbibed subchondral fluid signal intensity.

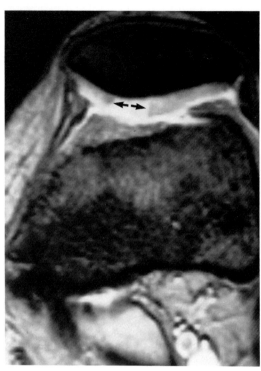

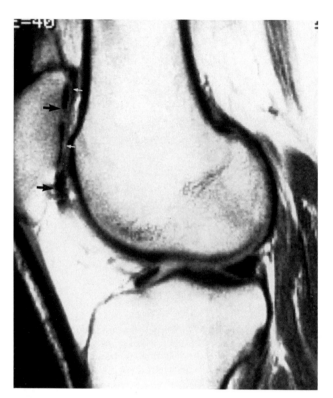

FIGURE 4-196. After surgery for grade 4 chondromalacia, the full-thickness articular cartilage defect (*arrows*) is replaced by hyperintense fluid signal intensity on a T2*-weighted axial image. Also note the surgically-produced geometric edges of the articular cartilage defect.

FIGURE 4-197. On an intermediate-weighted sagittal image, the patellar cortex (*black arrow*) demonstrates low signal intensity and a thin rim of shaved hyaline articular cartilage (*white arrows*) demonstrates intermediate signal intensity.

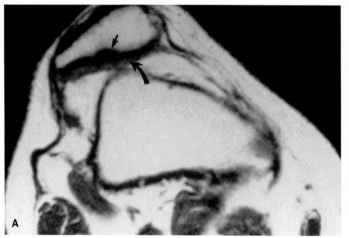

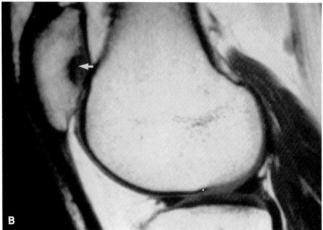

FIGURE 4-198. (**A**) A T1-weighted axial image shows lateral patellar subluxation (*curved arrow*). Subchondral sclerosis is identified (*straight arrow*). (**B**) A T1-weighted sagittal image reveals subchondral sclerotic erosion (*arrow*).

FIGURE 4-201. Medial subluxation of the patella occurred after lateral retinacular release. (**A**) An extremity coil T1-weighted axial image obtained in full extension shows the normal position of the patella. (**B**) A body coil localizer used to prescribe a kinematic series (**C** through **G**) produced from 0° to 40° of flexion when imaged at 10° increments. (*All arrows*, position of patella.)

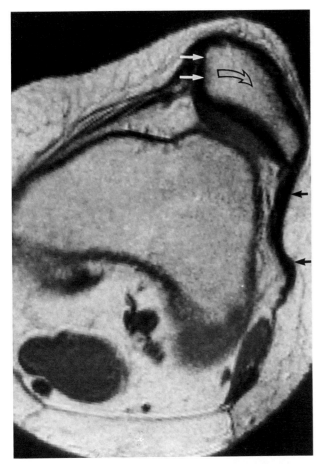

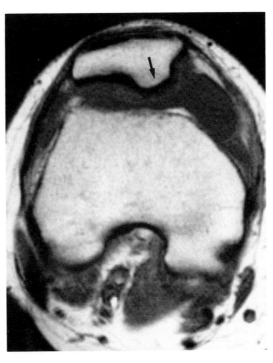

FIGURE 4–199. A T1-weighted axial image shows lateral subluxation (*curved open arrow*) of a dysplastic patella with a missing medial facet (*white straight arrows*). This defect is referred to as a Jagerhut patella. A lax lateral retinaculum is also seen (*black straight arrows*).

FIGURE 4–200. A Wiberg type 2 patella is indicated by concave surfaces, a smaller medial facet, and a prominent central ridge (*arrow*), as seen on a T1-weighted axial image.

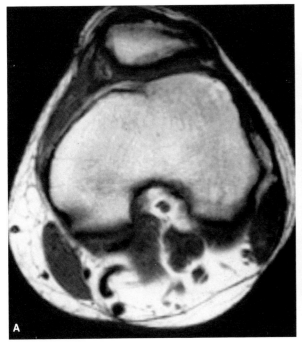

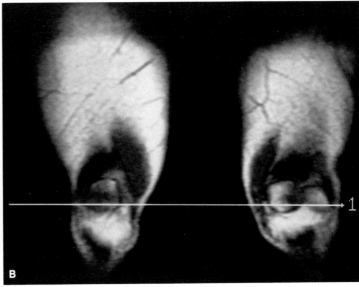

FIGURE 4–201. *(Continued)*

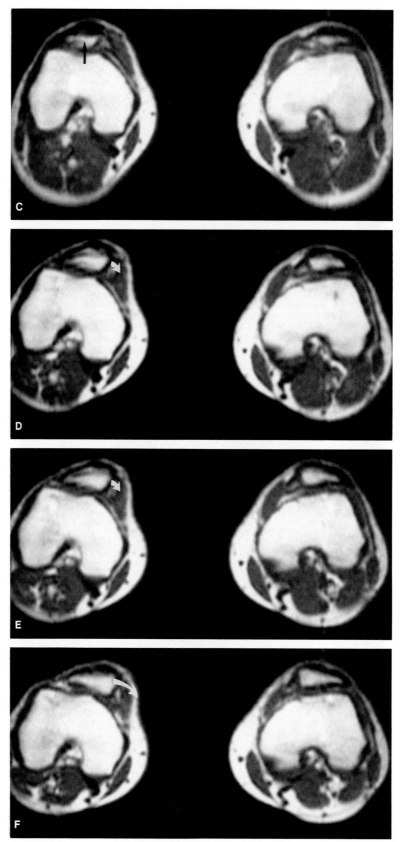

FIGURE 4–201. *(Continued)*

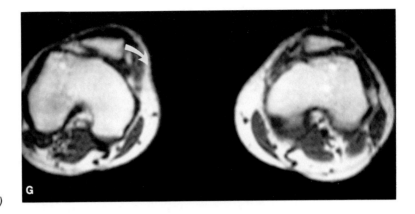

FIGURE 4–201. *(Continued)*

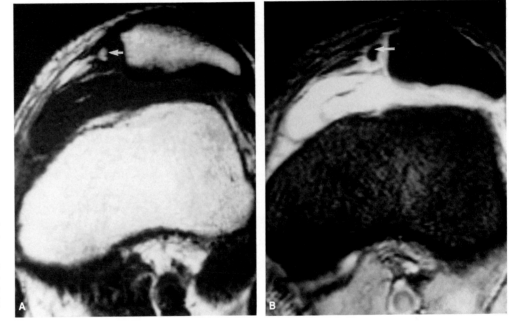

FIGURE 4–202. A medial retinacular tear with an avulsed patellar bone fragment (*arrows*) demonstrates (**A**) high signal intensity marrow fat on a T1-weighted axial image and (**B**) low signal intensity on a T2*-weighted axial image.

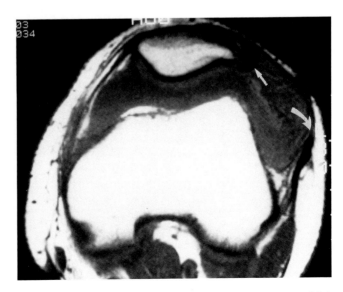

FIGURE 4–203. Traumatic disruption of the lateral patellar retinaculum is seen on a T1-weighted axial image. Torn low signal intensity fibers are revealed at the lateral aspect of the patella (*straight arrow*). A retracted vastus lateralis tendon is shown (*curved arrow*).

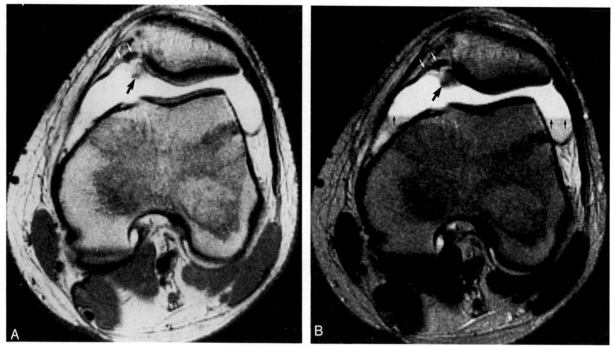

FIGURE 4–204. A medial retinacular tear (*white arrows*) with a chondral fragment (*large black arrow*) is shown on (**A**) intermediate-weighted and (**B**) T2-weighted axial images. Hemorrhagic serum-sediment fluid level can be seen on the T2-weighted image (*small black arrows*).

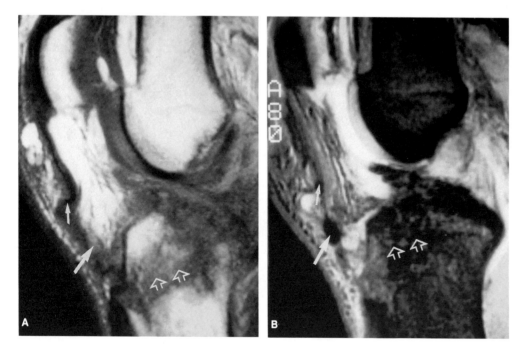

FIGURE 4–205. Sagittal (**A**) T1-weighted and (**B**) T2*-weighted images show acute rupture of the tibial insertion of the patellar tendon with proximal tendon retraction (*small straight arrow*). An avulsed bone fragment (*large straight arrows*) is best depicted as a low signal intensity focus on a T2*-weighted sagittal image. A trabecular bone contusion is indicated (*open arrows*).

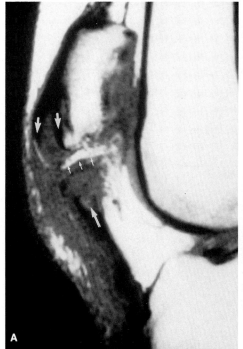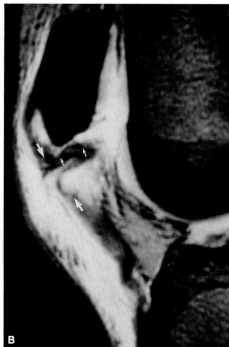

FIGURE 4–206. Sagittal (**A**) T1-weighted and (**B**) T2*-weighted images show a proximal inferior pole patellar tendon rupture with proximal retraction of the patella. Patellar tendon rupture may be associated with trauma and steroid injections. The tendon ends (*large arrows*) and tear site (*small arrows*) are shown.

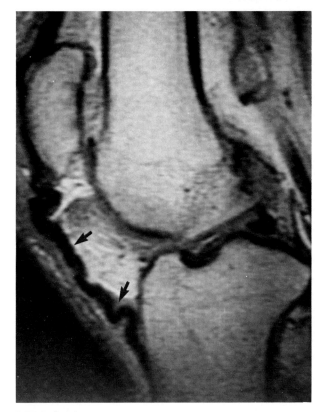

FIGURE 4–207. A T1-weighted sagittal image shows a tear of the patellar tendon that results in increased laxity and redundant contour (*arrows*).

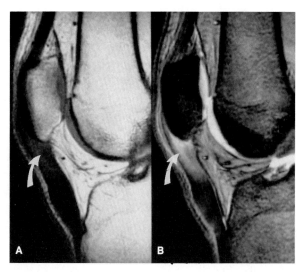

FIGURE 4–208. Patellar tendinitis (*i.e.,* jumper's knee) results in proximal patellar tendon edema (*curved arrows*). This edema exhibits (**A**) intermediate signal intensity on a T1-weighted sagittal image and (**B**) increased signal intensity on a T2*-weighted sagittal image. There is diffuse thickening of the entire patellar tendon.

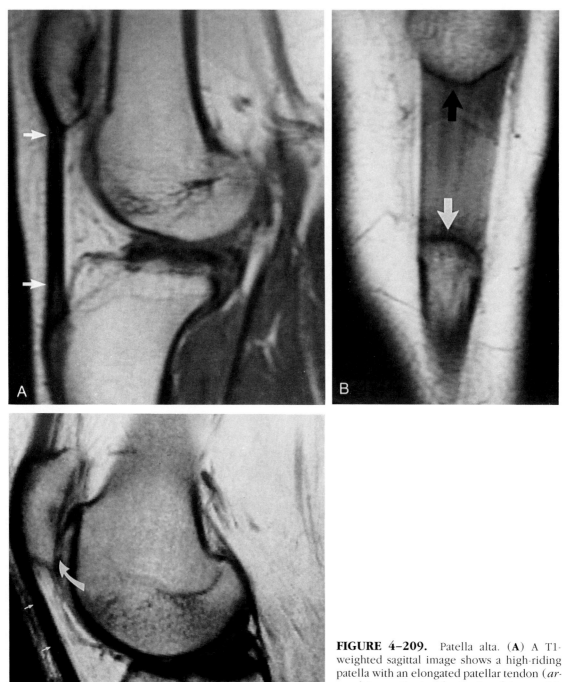

FIGURE 4–209. Patella alta. (**A**) A T1-weighted sagittal image shows a high-riding patella with an elongated patellar tendon (*arrows*) in a patient with atrophy of the quadriceps muscle. (**B**) The corresponding coronal image demonstrates a stretched patellar tendon *en face*. Patellar attachments (*black arrow*) and tibial tubercle attachments (*white arrow*) are identified. (**C**) Patella alta in a separate patient shows a lengthened patellar tendon (*straight arrows*) and patellar subluxation (*curved arrow*).

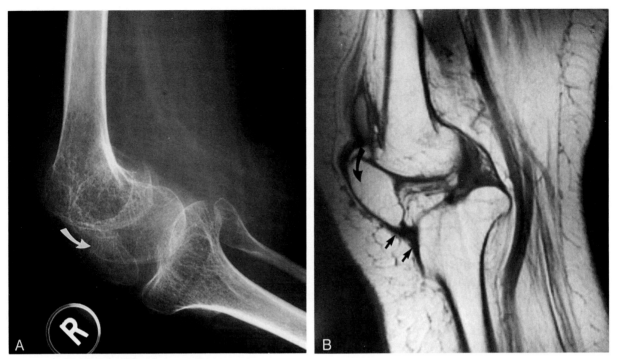

FIGURE 4–210.   Patella baja. The patella (*curved arrows*) is in a low position, and there is a shortened patellar tendon (*straight arrows*) on (**A**) a lateral radiograph and (**B**) on a T1-weighted sagittal image of this polio patient.

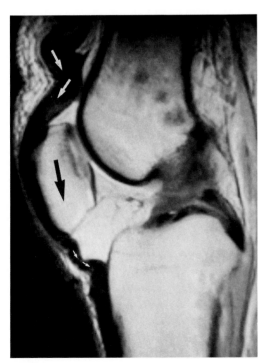

FIGURE 4–211.   A proximal quadriceps tendon rupture results in patella baja (*black arrow*), lax quadriceps tendon (*white arrows*), and foreshortened patellar tendon.

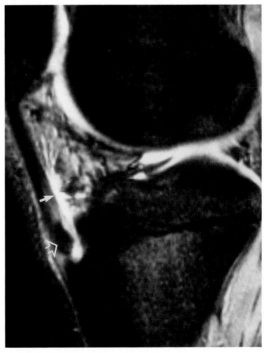

FIGURE 4–212.   Osgood–Schlatter disease causes fragmentation of the tibial tubercle (*open arrow*) and development of a hyperintense fluid directly posterior to the patellar tendon (*solid arrow*). Signal intensity is mildly increased in the adjacent fibers of the patellar tendon.

Osgood–Schlatter Disease

In Osgood–Schlatter disease, osteochondrosis of the developing tibial tuberosity (*i.e.,* apophysis) is thought to be secondary to traumatic avulsion during adolescent growth. Radiographic changes include soft-tissue edema anterior to the tibial tuberosity and avulsion and fragmentation of the tibial tubercle ossification center. Magnetic resonance findings include irregularity of the distal patellar tendon and Hoffa's infrapatellar fat pad. With Osgood–Schlatter disease, multiple small ossicles or a single fragment anterior to the tibial tuberosity display the high signal intensity of marrow fat on T1-weighted images and low signal intensity on T2*-weighted images (Figs. 4–212 and 4–213). Patellar tendon thickening and low signal intensity sclerosis in underlying subchondral bone may be other MR findings. In Sinding–Larsen–Johansson syndrome, osteochondrosis involves the distal patellar pole at the insertion of the patellar tendon (Fig. 4–214). Patellar contusion or fracture with associated diffuse marrow hemorrhage should not be mistaken for Sinding–Larsen–Johannson disease (Fig. 4–215).

Patellar Bursae

There are two anterior subcutaneous bursae—one over the patella and the other anterior to the patellar tendon. Inflammation (*i.e.,* bursitis) demonstrates low signal intensity on T1-weighted images and high signal intensity on T2-weighted images. Prepatellar bursitis and superficial infrapatellar bursitis each are seen as a single localized soft-tissue mass, anterior to the patella and proximal patellar tendon, respectively (Figs. 4–216 and 4–217). Deep infrapatellar bursitis is identified posterior to the patellar tendon and inferior to Hoffa's infrapatellar fat pad.[10]

Selected Patellofemoral Surgical Procedures

Patellectomy may be required to treat nonmanageable chondromalacia with severe pain and comminuted fractures of the patella.[24] This procedure is usually reserved for patients who are not candidates for a patellofemoral replacement or for the Maquet procedure.[134] Sagittal MR images display the absent patella and the continuity of quadriceps and patellar tendons.

The Maquet procedure, or anterior tibial tubercle elevation, is performed to decrease loading forces across the patellofemoral joint by raising the insertion of the patellar tendon.[134] It is not used as a primary treatment for patellar malalignment.

The Elmslie–Trillat procedure, or tibial tuberosity transfer, is performed as an adjunct in cases of abnormal patellar tendon obliquity to minimize lateralizing forces.[134]

Extensor Mechanism Injuries

The quadriceps muscle group is composed of the rectus femoris and vastus intermedius muscles, which insert on the base of the patella, and the vastus lateralis and medius muscles, which insert on the lateral and medial patella, respectively. Quadriceps tears or ruptures occur in the young athlete with either forced muscle contraction or direct trauma. Myositis ossificans can be a sequela to injury, especially when the vastus medialis is involved. Acute quadriceps tendon rupture is treated with direct surgical repair, with or without reinforcement of the tendon fibers.

For MR evaluation of extensor muscle tears, an initial set of coronal or sagittal images is used to display the longitudinal extent of muscle involvement (Fig. 4–218). Axial images are used to identify both the precise muscle group involved and its adjacent anatomic relations. Axial images are also useful in differentiating between complete muscle tears with diastasis and partial tears with associated atrophy. Magnetic resonance imaging is sensitive to both the acute and chronic hemorrhage in extensor muscle tears. Edema and areas of fraying in the affected muscle demonstrate intermediate signal intensity on T1-weighted images. Edema and hemorrhage demonstrate increased signal intensity on T2-weighted images. Muscle atrophy and fatty infiltration are seen as regions of increased signal intensity on T1-weighted images. A retracted proximal or distal muscle bundle can be identified as a soft-tissue mass with higher signal intensity than native muscle. Any increase in signal intensity within the quadriceps tendon is abnormal. Increases range from intrasubstance signal in degeneration or tendinitis to high signal intensity hemorrhage or edema in complete avulsions or ruptures of the tendon.

GENERAL PATHOLOGIC CONDITIONS AFFECTING THE KNEE

Arthritis

Assessment of the extent, progression, and therapeutic response in adult arthritic disorders and in JRA is enhanced by MR imaging of articular cartilage.[135] Even in patients with negative conventional radiographs, joint effusions, synovial reactions, popliteal cysts, and osteonecrosis can be demonstrated and evaluated with MR studies.

Cartilage Evaluation

Cartilage of the patellar, femoral, and tibial articular surfaces is routinely observed on T1-weighted images.[135] Due to its hydropic composition, normal hyaline cartilage demonstrates intermediate signal intensity on T1-weighted images, compared with the low signal intensity of cortex and fibrocartilaginous menisci (Fig. 4–219). On conventional T2-weighted images, hyaline cartilage maintains an intermediate signal intensity. However, with gradient-echo, chemical-shift, and fast, low-angle shot techniques, hyaline cartilage demonstrates high signal intensity, making it possible to detect early stages of hyaline cartilage degeneration (Fig. 4–220). A decrease in the signal intensity of cartilage has been attributed to a loss of water-binding proteoglycans molecules. With T2*-weighted images, articular cartilage defects less than 3 mm long have been identified in patients who suffered from trauma, arthritis, osteochondritis, or osteonecrosis (Fig. 4–221).[104] Although these defects may not be detected with conventional T1- or T2-weighted spin-echo images, conventional T2-weighted contrast does provide superior delineation of thinner cartilage surfaces (*e.g.*, the medial and lateral compartments), especially in the presence of joint fluid (Fig. 4–222).

The thicker articular cartilage of the patellofemoral joint is adequately characterized by either T2- or T2*-weighted protocols (Fig. 4–223). A chemical-shift artifact in the frequency-encoded direction may cause underestimation of the apparent thickness of the curvilinear hyaline cartilage on the femoral condylar surface. The thinner articular surface of the tibia is a less predictable indicator of disorders affecting articular congruity. With T1-weighted sequences, joint effusions reduce the definition of articular cartilage surfaces. With T2*-weighted echo techniques, better delineation of the fluid–cartilage interface is possible because effusions generate higher signal intensity than adjacent cartilage surfaces. A dual-echo gradient-echo sequence may optimize visualization of the fluid–cartilage interface. Inversion recovery sequences set at the null point of water where water appears black have also shown potential for more accurate assessment of cartilage thickness in effusions associated with arthritis and trauma. With 3D FASTER techniques, there is a high signal intensity fluid interface with intermediate signal intensity cartilage on T1-weighted contrast. T1-weighted hybrid fat-suppression images have been recommended by Chandnani and colleagues to more accurately characterize hyaline articular cartilage structures.[136]

The thicker articular cartilage in children allows an increased sensitivity in detecting focal erosions and cartilage thinning. In infants, the articular cartilage is seen prior to the appearance of the distal femoral and proximal tibial ossific nuclei, and it demonstrates higher signal intensity than the adjacent marrow (Fig. 4–224). Before any radiographic evidence of joint-space narrowing is found, focal erosions and uniform attenuation of articular cartilage can be observed in MR studies in patients with JRA, hemophilia, and degenerative joint disease. Loss of subchondral signal intensity has also been observed in patients with sclerosis in association with initial cartilage loss. Interosseous cysts and hemorrhage, which demonstrate increased signal intensity on T2-weighted images, may develop at sites of denuded hyaline cartilage.

Synovium Evaluation and the Irregular Hoffa's Infrapatellar Fat-Pad Sign

Synovial reaction and proliferation are characterized on MR images by changes in the contour of synovial reflections. Irregularity with loss of the smooth posterior concave free border of Hoffa's infrapatellar fat pad can be observed in a variety of synovial reactions and is referred to as the irregular infrapatellar fat-pad sign (Fig. 4–225).[135] Although the synovium cannot be imaged directly in early synovitis, a corrugated surface along Hoffa's infrapatellar fat pad is evident in the initial stages of synovial irritation. This irregular fat-pad sign has been seen in patients with hemophilia, rheumatoid arthritis, pigmented villonodular synovitis (PVNS), Lyme arthritis, inflammatory osteoarthritis, and hemorrhagic effusions—caused by arthritis or trauma—with reactive synovium. In addition to these synovial reactions, swelling of the retropatellar fat pad has been seen in chronic patellofemoral chondromalacia and instability.[24] Gd-DTPA-contrast–enhanced T1-weighted images are useful in the accurate identification of pannus tissue, which is demonstrated as areas of increased signal adjacent to the low signal intensity joint fluid (Fig. 4–226).[137] On T1-, T2-, and T2*-weighted protocols, synovial hypertrophy and pannus demonstrate low-to-intermediate signal intensity and are more difficult to identify (Fig. 4–227). Fluid associated with synovial masses generates increased signal intensity on T2- or T2*-weighted images.

Juvenile Rheumatoid Arthritis

In the initial stages of clinical presentation of JRA, MR studies demonstrate synovitis with irregularity of Hoffa's infrapatellar fat pad (Fig. 4–228).[138] Articular cartilage erosions and synovial hypertrophy can be identified before joint-space narrowing is evident on plain film radiography. Posterior popliteal cysts of the gastrocnemius and semimembranosus bursae, associated with JRA, demonstrate low signal intensity on T1-weighted images and uniformly high signal intensity on T2-weighted images (Fig. 4–229). Thickening of the synovium of the suprapatellar bursa can be seen with low signal intensity on T1- and T2-weighted images (Fig. 4–230). With MR studies in more advanced disease, subarticular cysts, sub-

(text continues on page 318)

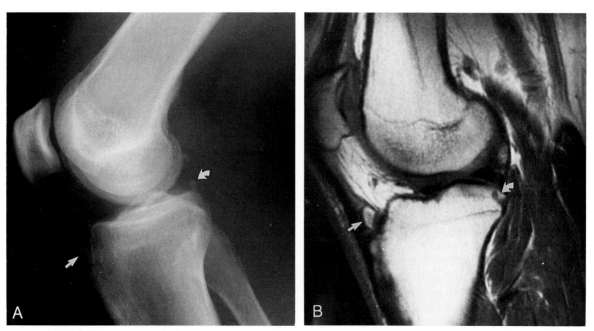

FIGURE 4–213. Unresolved or chronic Osgood–Schlatter disease is associated with avulsion and irregularity of the tibial tuberosity ossicle (*straight arrows*) (**A**) on a lateral radiograph and (**B**) on a T1-weighted sagittal image. An unrelated posterior osteochondral fragment is also identified (*curved arrows*).

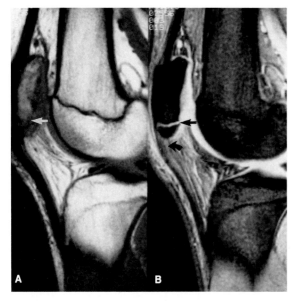

FIGURE 4–214. Sagittal (**A**) T1-weighted and (**B**) T2*-weighted images of the patella of a patient with Sinding–Larsen–Johansson disease. Note the separation of the lower pole of the patella (*straight arrows*) and mild thickening and hyperintensity of the proximal patellar tendon (*curved arrow*).

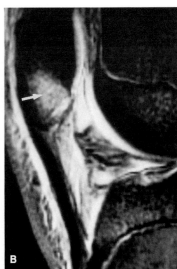

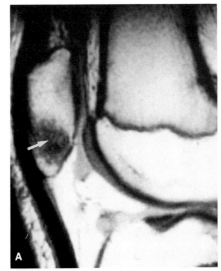

FIGURE 4–215. Marrow hemorrhage (*arrows*) in an inferior patellar pole nondisplaced trabecular fracture demonstrates (**A**) low signal intensity on a T1-weighted image and (**B**) high signal intensity on a T2*-weighted image. The diffuse morphology of marrow hemorrhage is in contrast to the sharp demarcation seen in Sinding–Larsen–Johansson disease; the two should not be confused (see Fig. 2–214).

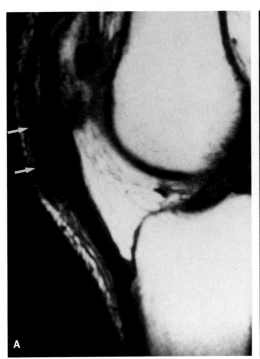

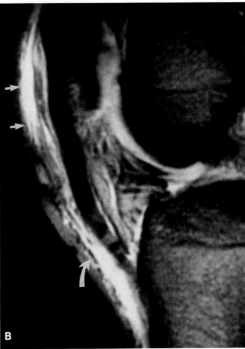

FIGURE 4–216. Prepatellar bursitis (*straight arrows*) and superficial infrapatellar bursitis (*curved arrow*) as represented on (**A**) sagittal T1-weighted and (**B**) T2*-weighted images. The prepatellar bursa is located between the skin and the anterior surface of the patella, and extends distally anterior to the proximal one-half of the patellar tendon. Prepatellar bursitis that occurs secondary to kneeling is known as housemaid's knee.

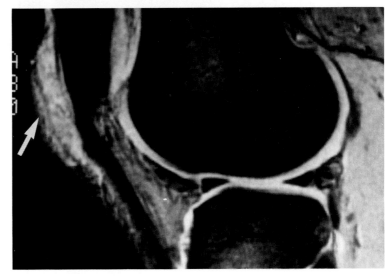

FIGURE 4–217. Chronic prepatellar bursitis with diffuse thickening and hyperintensity of tissue anterior to the patella (*arrow*) is seen on a T2*-weighted sagittal oblique image.

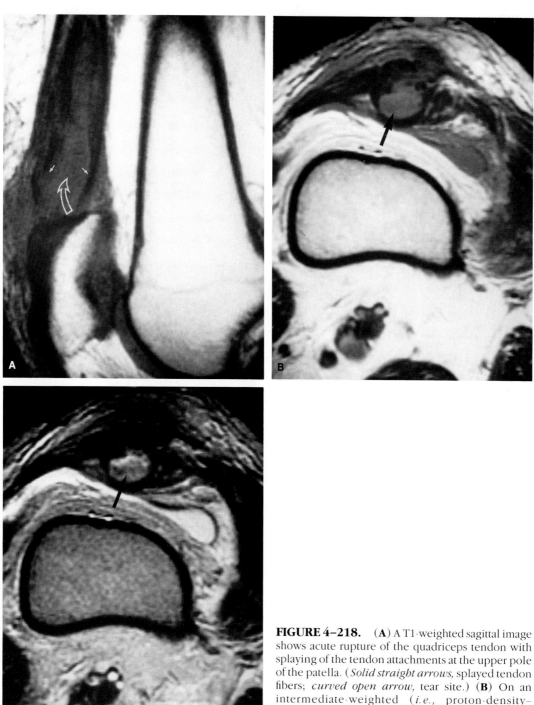

FIGURE 4–218. (**A**) A T1-weighted sagittal image shows acute rupture of the quadriceps tendon with splaying of the tendon attachments at the upper pole of the patella. (*Solid straight arrows,* splayed tendon fibers; *curved open arrow,* tear site.) (**B**) On an intermediate-weighted (*i.e.,* proton-density–weighted) axial image, the tear site exhibits low signal intensity (*arrow*). (**C**) On a T2-weighted axial image, the tear site demonstrates high signal intensity (*arrow*).

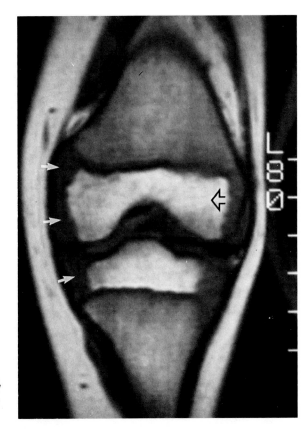

FIGURE 4–219. On a T1-weighted coronal image of the knee of a child, hyaline articular cartilage exhibits thick intermediate signal intensity (*solid white arrows*). Epiphyseal yellow marrow demonstrates bright signal intensity (*open black arrow*).

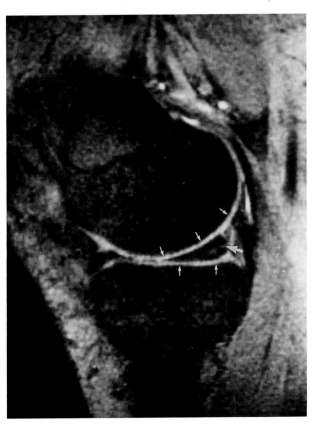

FIGURE 4–220. Articular cartilage exhibits bright signal intensity with T2* gradient-echo contrast in a sagittal location (*small arrows*). Grade 2 degeneration in the posterior horn of the medial meniscus is shown (*large arrow*).

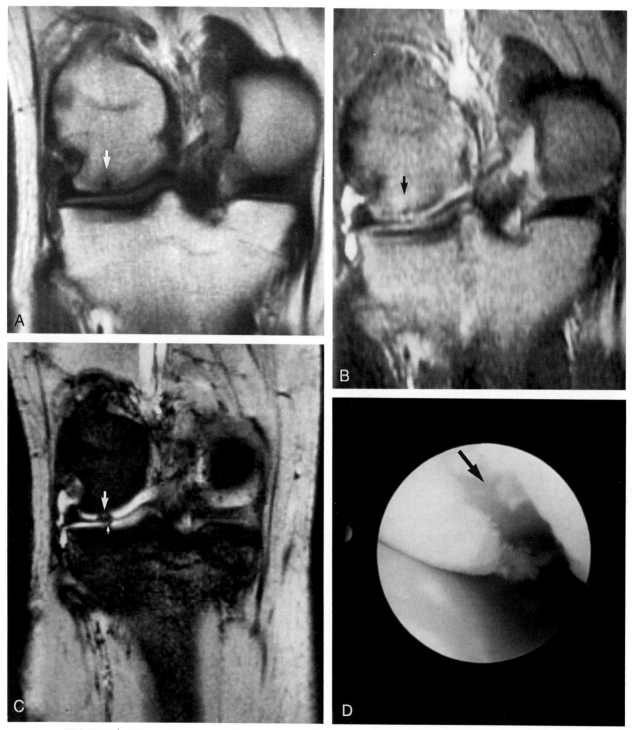

FIGURE 4–221.   Osteochondral injury in a javelin thrower. (**A**) A T1-weighted coronal image demonstrates a low signal intensity traumatic osteochondral defect that involves the posterior lateral femoral condyle (*arrow*). (**B**) The corresponding conventional T2-weighted image displays increased signal intensity within the osteochondral defect (*arrow*). (**C**) A T2*-weighted image in the same patient shows hyaline articular cartilage defects in the femoral condyle (*large arrow*) and opposing tibial plateau (*small arrow*) that were not revealed on the previous T1- or T2-weighted images. (**D**) Subsequent arthroscopy allowed identification of an articular cartilage defect in the lateral femoral condyle (*arrow*).

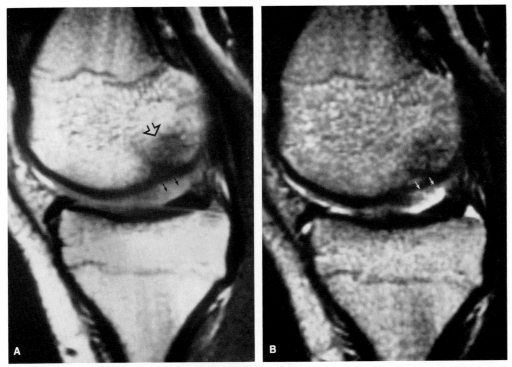

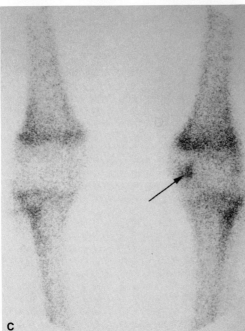

FIGURE 4–222. (**A**) T1-weighted and (**B**) T2-weighted sagittal images show articular cartilage trauma with fissuring of the articular cartilage (*small arrows*) A traumatic bone contusion is present (*open arrow*). (**C**) The corresponding bone scan shows uptake in the medial femoral condyle (*arrow*).

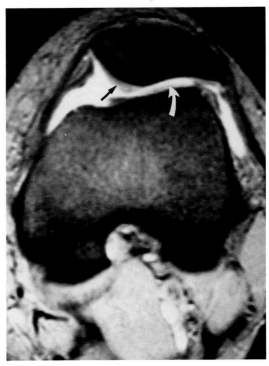

FIGURE 4–223. A T2*-weighted axial image will define the fluid–cartilage interface (*straight arrow*) that occurs in chondromalacia. Note the fluid surfaces in areas of denuded articular cartilage (*curved arrow*).

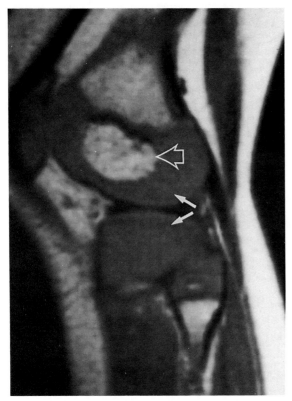

FIGURE 4–224. Normal thick hyaline articular cartilage demonstrates intermediate signal intensity (*solid arrows*) on a T1-weighted sagittal image. The femoral ossific nucleus is seen with high signal intensity marrow fat (*open arrow*). The tibial ossific nucleus has not yet developed.

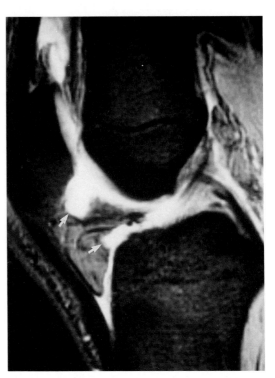

FIGURE 4–225. Confirmed hemorrhagic joint effusion results in synovial irritation with an irregular Hoffa's infrapatellar fat pad concave free edge (*arrows*) seen on a T2*-weighted sagittal image. In the absence of arthritis or infection, a non-hemorrhagic effusion will not result in a positive Hoffa's infrapatellar fat-pad sign.

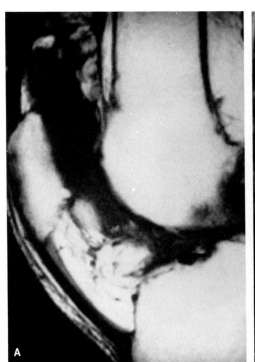
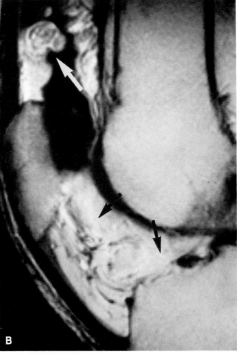

FIGURE 4–226. Lateral compartment pannus is shown (**A**) before and (**B**) after intravenous gadolinium administration. A comparison of these T1-weighted sagittal images demonstrates selective high signal intensity enhancement of pannus tissue. The suprapatellar synovium (*white arrow*) and hypertrophied synovium posterior to Hoffa's infrapatellar fat pad (*black arrows*) are shown.

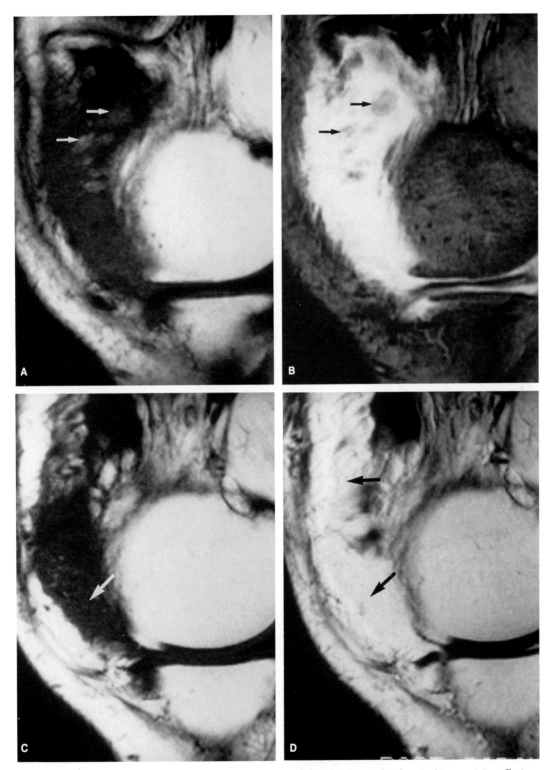

FIGURE 4–227. Medial compartment pannus tissue. (**A**) On a T1-weighted sagittal image, joint effusion with irregular focal areas of suprapatellar fat (*arrows*) demonstrates high signal intensity. (**B**) The corresponding T2*-weighted sagittal image shows hyperintense joint effusion and lower signal intensity fat (*arrows*). (**C**) A T1-weighted sagittal image displays low signal intensity joint effusion (*arrow*) prior to intravenous gadolinium injection. (**D**) The corresponding contrast-enhanced T1-weighted sagittal image shows pannus tissue at a high signal intensity (*arrows*).

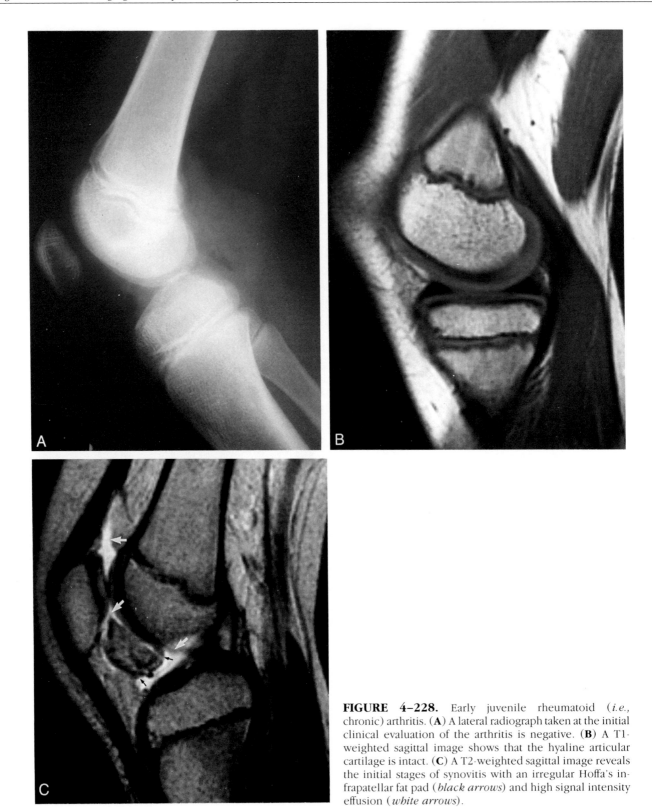

FIGURE 4–228. Early juvenile rheumatoid (*i.e.,* chronic) arthritis. (**A**) A lateral radiograph taken at the initial clinical evaluation of the arthritis is negative. (**B**) A T1-weighted sagittal image shows that the hyaline articular cartilage is intact. (**C**) A T2-weighted sagittal image reveals the initial stages of synovitis with an irregular Hoffa's infrapatellar fat pad (*black arrows*) and high signal intensity effusion (*white arrows*).

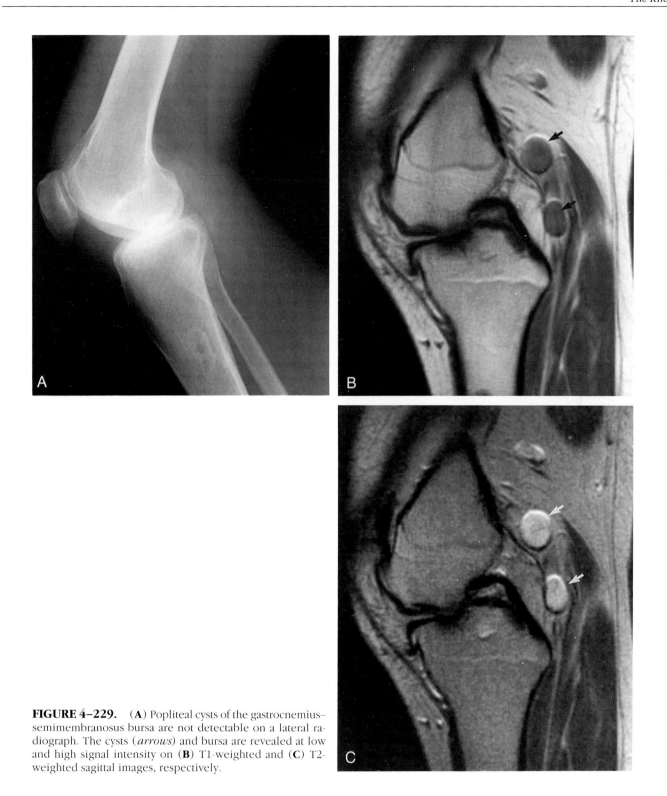

FIGURE 4–229. (**A**) Popliteal cysts of the gastrocnemius–semimembranosus bursa are not detectable on a lateral radiograph. The cysts (*arrows*) and bursa are revealed at low and high signal intensity on (**B**) T1-weighted and (**C**) T2-weighted sagittal images, respectively.

chondral sclerosis, and osteonecrosis can be detected on both femoral and tibial surfaces (Figs. 4–231 and 4–232). These changes are frequently not evident on conventional radiographs. Hypoplastic menisci with smaller anterior and posterior horns and body have also been observed on MR studies in JRA patients. This finding might be related to an alteration in the fluid composition of synovial fluid that impairs normal fibrocartilage development.

Rheumatoid Arthritis

In adult patients with rheumatoid arthritis, bicompartmental and tricompartmental disease is displayed on MR images through the medial and lateral femorotibial compartments and patellofemoral joint (Fig. 4–233).[135] Marginal and subchondral erosions with diffuse loss of hyaline articular cartilage are evident on both medial and lateral femoral articular surfaces. Large joint effusions with popliteal cysts are commonly seen and demonstrate uniform high signal intensity on T2- and T2*-weighted images. Less frequently, signs of degenerative arthritis with osteophytosis and subchondral sclerosis demonstrate low signal intensity on MR scans. An irregular fat pad may be seen in the more active stages of the disease. Hypertrophied synovial masses remain low in signal intensity on T1- and T2-weighted contrast images.

Gd-DTPA-contrast–enhanced images can be used to identify pannus tissue in rheumatoid arthritis.[139,140] Contrast-enhanced images are more effective than nonenhanced T1-, T2-, or T2*-weighted images for separating joint fluid from adjacent pannus tissue. The ability to map out pannus is useful in evaluating patients with severe inflammatory arthritis for synovectomy prior to total joint arthroplasty.

Osteonecrosis and infarcts in rheumatoid patients can be seen by MR evaluation before corresponding radiographic changes are evident.

Pigmented Villonodular Synovitis

Pigmented villonodular synovitis is a monarticular synovial proliferative disorder. It usually presents as a nonpainful soft-tissue mass, and the knee is a common site of involvement, especially in the diffuse form of the disease. Hemosiderin-laden macrophages are frequently deposited in hyperplastic synovial masses, and sclerotic bone lesions may be associated.

Several reports have correlated MR findings in PVNS with surgically confirmed pathologic changes.[141–143] The hemosiderin-infiltrated synovial masses demonstrate low signal intensity on T1-, T2-, and T2*-weighted images because of the paramagnetic effect of iron (Figs. 4–234 and 4–235). Adjacent synovial fluid, however, may be seen with increased signal intensity on T2-weighted images. Hemosiderin deposits may be observed in thick-

ened synovial reflections superior to Hoffa's infrapatellar fat pad. Condylar erosions may be associated with a synovial mass and fibrous tissue (Fig. 4–236). A more localized nodular form of PVNS, seen as a well-described mass, may be within Hoffa's infrapatellar fat pad.

Hemophilia

In MR studies in patients with hemophilic arthropathy, hemosiderin and fibrous tissue—formed from repeated episodes of joint hemorrhage—demonstrate low signal intensity on T1- and T2-weighted images (Fig. 4–237).[144,145] Irregular fat pads and markedly thickened, hemosiderin-laden synovial reflections of low signal intensity are common findings (Fig. 4–238). Although conventional radiographs are normal, articular cartilage irregularities and erosions can be detected on MR scans.

Subchondral and intraosseous cysts or hemorrhage can be identified on coronal and sagittal MR images (Fig. 4–239). Fluid-filled cysts generate high signal intensity on T2- or T2*-weighted images. Areas of fibrous tissue remain low in signal intensity on T1-, T2-, and T2*-weighted images, and low signal intensity synovial effusions can be differentiated from adjacent hemosiderin and fibrous depositions on T2-weighted sequences. Articular and subchondral abnormalities of the femoral condylar and tibial surfaces were common findings, seen in 75% to 85% of cases (Fig. 4–240).

Lyme Arthritis

Lyme disease and resultant arthritis are transmitted by the *Ixodes* sp. tick and are characterized by the delayed appearance of an oligo- or polyarticular inflammatory arthritis.[146] The knee is most commonly affected, with development of inflammatory synovial effusions, synovial hypertrophy, infrapatellar fat-pad edema, and, in severe chronic cases, cartilage erosions. In one patient, studied 3 months after a documented tick bite, MR scans revealed an extensive joint effusion and an irregular, corrugated Hoffa's infrapatellar fat pad (Fig. 4–241).[135] After the MR studies, contrast material was injected into the joint to confirm scalloping of the synovium, characteristic of synovitis, which was first identified on MR imaging. No cartilage erosions were identified. In another patient with Lyme arthritis, an irregular fat pad was seen in association with popliteal cysts present for several years. There was no associated intraarticular pathology.

Osteoarthritis

The MR findings in degenerative arthrosis vary from osteophytic spurring, which demonstrates the bright signal intensity of marrow, to compartment collapse, denuded articular cartilage, torn and degenerative meniscal fibrocartilage, and diminished marrow signal intensity in areas of subchondral sclerosis (Fig. 4–242).[147] The ability to accurately assess hyaline cartilage surfaces gives MR imaging an advantage over plain film radiography in preoperative planning for joint replacement procedures, especially in unicondylar arthroplasties for osteoarthritis.[148] Chondral fragments, of intermediate signal intensity, and loose bodies, with the high signal intensity of marrow fat, may be associated with more advanced degenerative disease (Figs. 4–243 and 4–244). Marrow-fat contrast of osteochondral fragments is decreased on T2*-weighted images (Fig. 4–245). In addition to the patellofemoral, medial, and lateral compartments of the knee, the tibiofibular joint may be affected by degenerative arthrosis, ganglia, or trauma (Figs. 4–246 and 4–247).

In synovial chondromatosis, multiple synovium-based chondral fragments demonstrate low-to-intermediate signal intensity (Fig. 4–248). In primary chondromatosis, the metaplastic fragments are usually similar to one another in size, while in secondary chondromatosis, they occur in a variety of sizes. Synovitis in inflammatory osteoarthritis may simulate multiple loose bodies in visualizing the irregular, corrugated fat-pad surfaces (Fig. 4–249).

Osteonecrosis and Related Disorders

Spontaneous osteonecrosis of the knee typically affects older, predominantly female patients who present with acute medial joint pain.[42,149,150] spontaneous osteonecrosis most often involves the weight-bearing surface of the medial femoral condyle (Fig. 4–250); however, cases have been described in which the medial and lateral tibial plateaus and the lateral femoral condyle were involved (Fig. 4–251).[151] In tibial involvement, the weight-bearing surface may or may not be affected. Meniscal tears are often associated with this condition.

Conventional radiographs are not sensitive in evaluating the osteonecrotic focus prior to the development of sclerosis and osseous collapse. Even in patients with negative radiographs, however, a low signal intensity focus can be detected on T1- and T2-weighted MR images.[152,153] Normal high signal intensity marrow fat replaces the low signal intensity necrotic focus after lateral osteotomy (Fig. 4–252). Subchondral sclerosis may be masked on T2*-weighted images. We have also observed a more diffuse pattern of low signal intensity in the early stages of the disease and better demarcation of the lesion with time. The overlying articular cartilage and status of the meniscus can be evaluated on T1-weighted images or on T2*-weighted images. We have documented osteonecrosis in both the medial and lateral tibial plateaus with MR imaging. In one patient with JRA, osteonecrosis

of the tibial plateau was observed on MR images and confirmed at biopsy.

Osteochondritis dissecans differs from spontaneous osteonecrosis of the knee in that it primarily affects male patients and involves the non-weight-bearing surface of the medial femoral condyle (Fig. 4–253).[154–156] A history of knee trauma is found in up to 50% of patients. In older patients, the morphology and location of osteochondritis dissecans may overlap with the spectrum of MR findings seen in spontaneous osteonecrosis.

A staging system for osteochondritis has been developed based on arthroscopic findings. In stage 1, the lesion is 1 to 3 cm and the articular cartilage is intact. Stage 2 is characterized by an articular cartilage defect without a loose body. In stage 3, a partially detached osteochondral fragment, with or without fibrous tissue interposition, is found. Stage 4 demonstrates a loose body with a crater filled with fibrous tissue.[24,155]

On MR images, the focus of osteochondritis demonstrates low signal intensity on T1- and T2-weighted images before it can be detected on conventional radiographs (Fig. 4–254). Overlying defects in the articular cartilage are generally appreciated on T2*-weighted images, where cartilage contrast is high; however, STIR contrast is more sensitive to subchondral bone changes (Figs. 4–255 and 4–256). Magnetic resonance imaging is particularly valuable in demonstrating associated free and loose osseous and chondral fragments. Imbibed high signal intensity subchondral fluid implies fissuring of the overlying articular cartilage and has a high correlation with lesion instability (Fig. 4–257).[157] Focal cystic regions deep to the lesion are also associated with instability of the fragment. Healed lesions do not demonstrate a bright signal intensity interface between the fragment and femur and show the return of marrow-fat signal intensity (Fig. 4–258). When the skeleton is mature, nonseparated lesions are treated by drilling (Fig. 4–259). Loose osteochondrotic fragments are removed, and partially detached fragments are treated with debridement prior to reduction and stabilization.[24]

Bone infarcts are usually metaphyseal in location, but have been identified in more epiphyseal or diaphyseal locations (Figs. 4–260 and 4–261). The MR appearance of a bone infarct is characteristic, with a serpiginous low signal border of reactive bone and a central component of high signal intensity equivalent to yellow marrow. On T2-weighted images, a chemical-shift artifact may be seen as a linear segment of high signal intensity paralleling the outline of the infarct. Bone infarcts can be differentiated from enchondromas on MR images. The latter lack a serpiginous border and on T1-weighted images have a central region of low signal intensity that increases with progressive T2 weighting. Calcified bone infarcts, how-

(text continues on page 338)

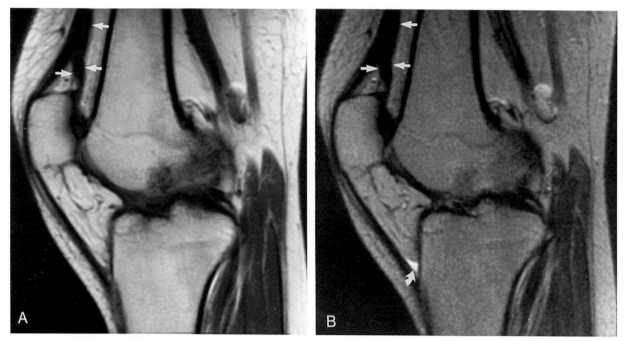

FIGURE 4–230. Juvenile rheumatoid (*i.e.,* chronic) arthritis causes suprapatellar synovial hypertrophy (*white arrows*), seen at low signal intensity on (**A**) T1-weighted and (**B**) T2-weighted sagittal images. In contrast, a focus of fluid demonstrates bright signal intensity (*curved arrow*) on the T2-weighted image.

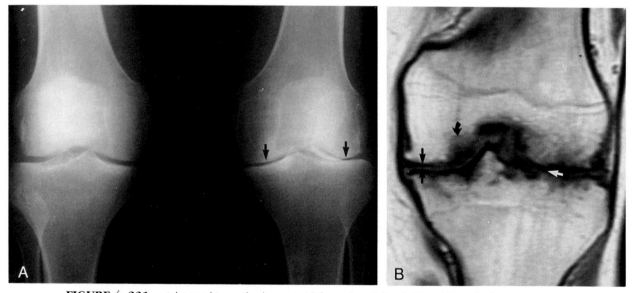

FIGURE 4–231. Advanced juvenile rheumatoid (*i.e.,* chronic) arthritis with marked joint-space narrowing (*black arrows*) is seen on (**A**) an anteroposterior radiograph and (**B**) a T1-weighted coronal image. Articular cartilage erosion (*white arrow*) and subchondral sclerosis (*curved arrow*) are best imaged by MR scan.

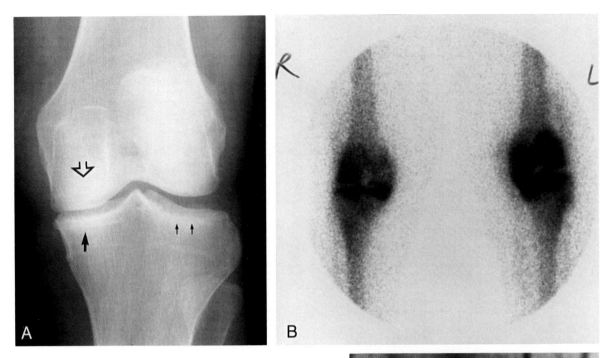

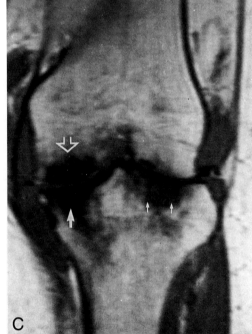

FIGURE 4–232. Juvenile rheumatoid (*i.e., chronic*) arthritis with steroid-induced osteonecrosis. (**A**) An anteroposterior radiograph shows subchondral sclerosis in the medial femoral (*open arrow*) and tibial (*large solid arrow*) condyles and in the lateral tibial plateau (*small solid arrows*). (**B**) The corresponding ^{99m}TC-MDP bone scan shows increased uptake of bone tracer in the left femur and tibia. (**C**) A T1-weighted coronal image demonstrates three separate foci of low signal intensity necrotic bone in the medial femoral condyle (*open arrow*) and medial (*large solid arrow*) and lateral (*small solid arrows*) tibial plateaus. All three sites of osteonecrosis were confirmed at biopsy.

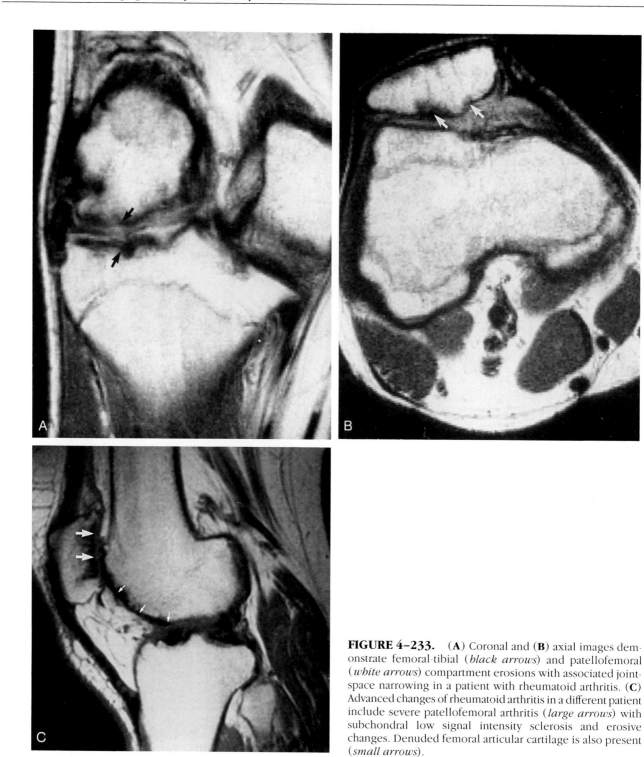

FIGURE 4–233. (**A**) Coronal and (**B**) axial images demonstrate femoral-tibial (*black arrows*) and patellofemoral (*white arrows*) compartment erosions with associated joint-space narrowing in a patient with rheumatoid arthritis. (**C**) Advanced changes of rheumatoid arthritis in a different patient include severe patellofemoral arthritis (*large arrows*) with subchondral low signal intensity sclerosis and erosive changes. Denuded femoral articular cartilage is also present (*small arrows*).

FIGURE 4–234. (**A**) Anteroposterior and (**B**) lateral radiographs of the distal femur and proximal tibia are unremarkable in a patient with pigmented villonodular synovitis. (**C**) On an intermediate-weighted coronal image, a low signal intensity hyperplastic synovium is revealed on the lateral aspect of the knee (*arrows*). (**D**) On a T2-weighted sagittal image, a synovial mass of fibrous tissue and hemosiderin (*white arrows*) remains low in signal intensity whereas an adjacent effusion demonstrates bright signal intensity (*black arrow*). (**E**) On another T2-weighted sagittal image, low signal intensity hemosiderin has been deposited in a thickened synovial reflection along the concave surface of Hoffa's infrapatellar fat pad (*arrows*). (**F**) Intermediate-weighted and (**G**) T2-weighted axial images of the posterior hemosiderin-laden synovial mass demonstrate no change in signal intensity (*open arrows*). A suprapatellar effusion (*solid arrows*) increases in signal intensity on a T2-weighted image.

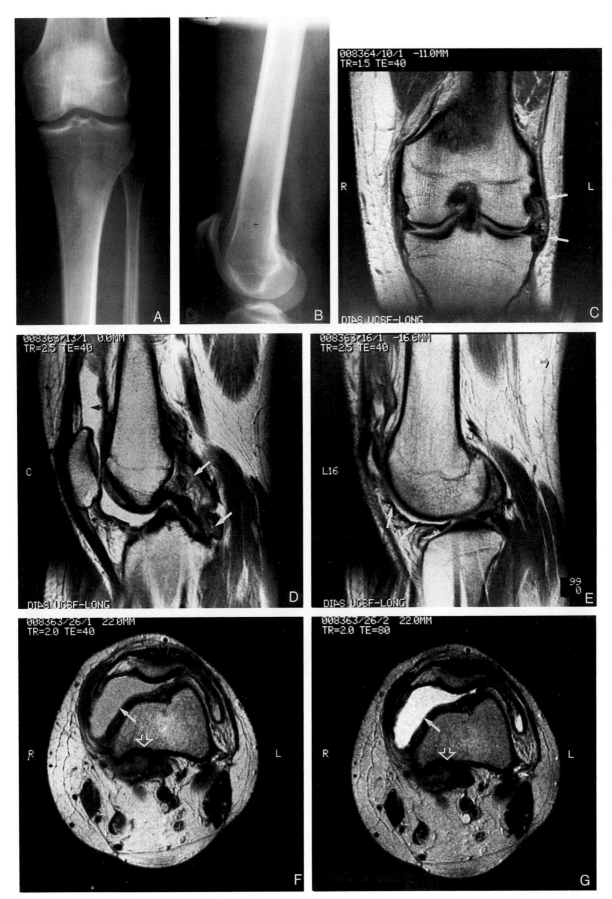

FIGURE 4–234.

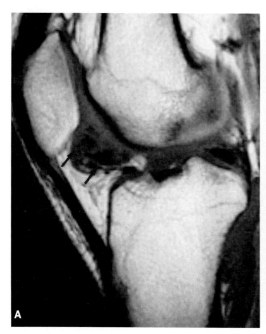

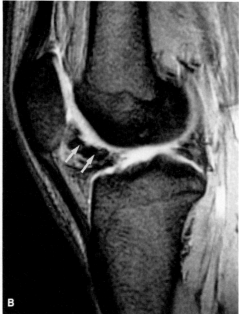

FIGURE 4-235. (**A**) On sagittal T1-weighted and (**B**) T2*-weighted images, pigmented villonodular synovitis is characterized by low signal intensity hemosiderin deposits in thickened synovium along the free edge of Hoffa's infrapatellar fat pad (*arrows*). The paramagnetic effect of hemosiderin results in a decreased T2 relaxation time.

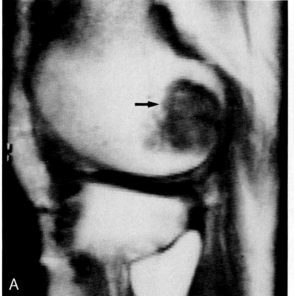

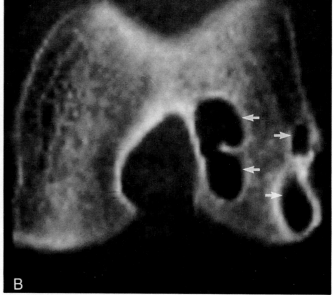

FIGURE 4-236. (**A**) On a T1-weighted sagittal image, a pigmented villonodular synovitis mass (*black arrow*) is seen in the posterolateral femoral condyle. (**B**) On an axial CT scan, femoral erosion (*white arrows*) is demonstrated.

FIGURE 4-238. The knee of a hemophiliac patient shows early cartilage erosions (*small arrows*) and a thickened hemosiderin-laden synovium that demonstrates low signal intensity (*large arrows*) on (**A**) T1-weighted and (**B**) T2-weighted images. Irregularity of Hoffa's infrapatellar fat pad indicates synovial irritation.

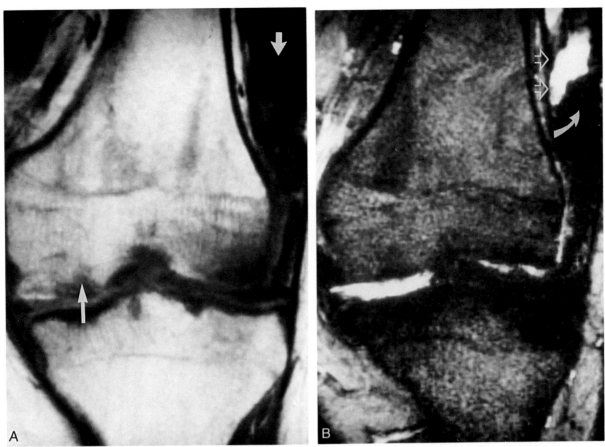

FIGURE 4–237. (A) A T1-weighted coronal image demonstrates erosive changes (*long arrow*) and surrounding low signal intensity areas along the lateral femur (*short arrow*) in a hemophiliac. (B) A T2*-weighted image distinguishes high signal intensity fluid or hemorrhage (*open arrows*) from chronic hemosiderin deposition (*curved arrow*).

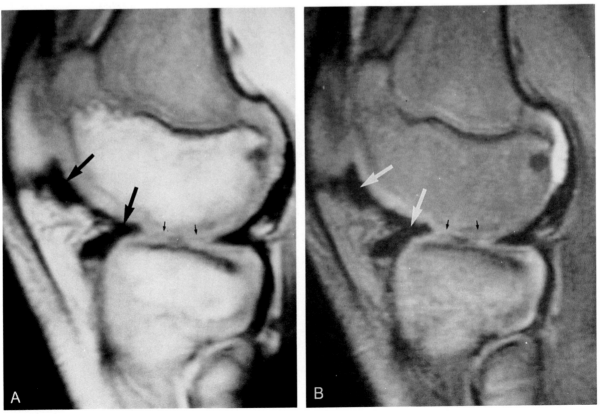

FIGURE 4–238.

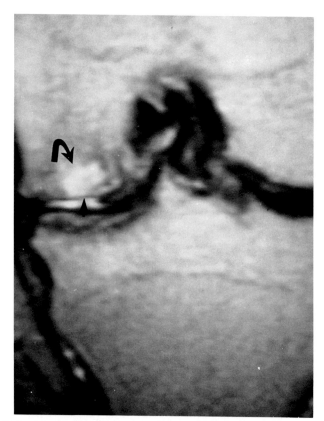

FIGURE 4–239. An intraosseous cyst (*curved arrow*) has formed through a defect in the femoral articular cartilage (*straight arrow*) in this hemophiliac patient. The cyst demonstrates high signal intensity on a T2-weighted coronal image.

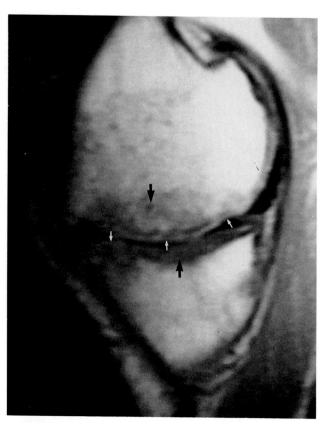

FIGURE 4–240. The knee of an adult hemophiliac shows low signal intensity subchondral sclerosis (*black arrows*) and denuded articular cartilage (*white arrows*) on a T1-weighted sagittal image.

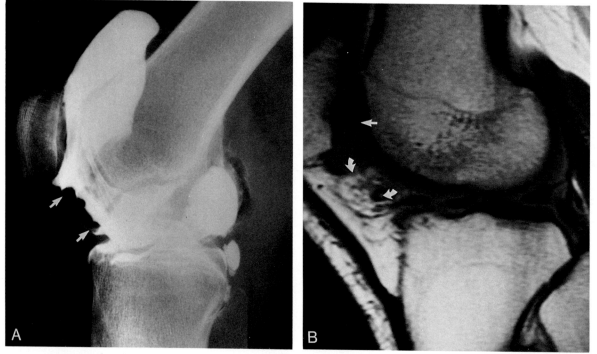

FIGURE 4–241. Lyme arthritis. (**A**) A lateral view arthrogram demonstrates a scalloped appearance of contrast (*arrows*) that indicates synovitis. (**B**) T1-weighted and (**C**) T2-weighted sagittal images show an irregular Hoffa's infrapatellar fat pad (*curved arrows*) with interdigitation of synovial effusion (*straight arrow*). Joint effusion is bright on the T2-weighted image. (**D**) On an intermediate-weighted sagittal image, the asymptomatic knee in the same patient displays the normal concave contour of the free edge of Hoffa's infrapatellar fat pad (*arrows*).

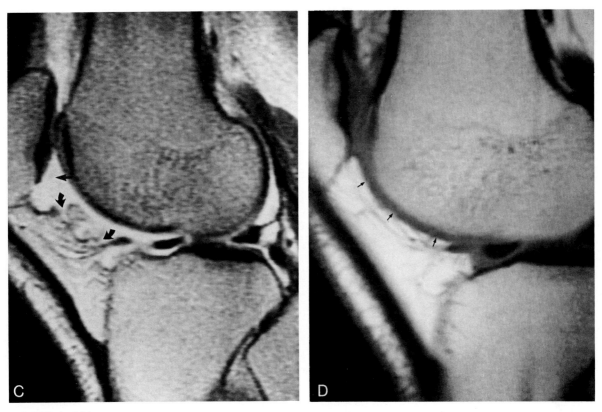

FIGURE 4–241. *(Continued)*

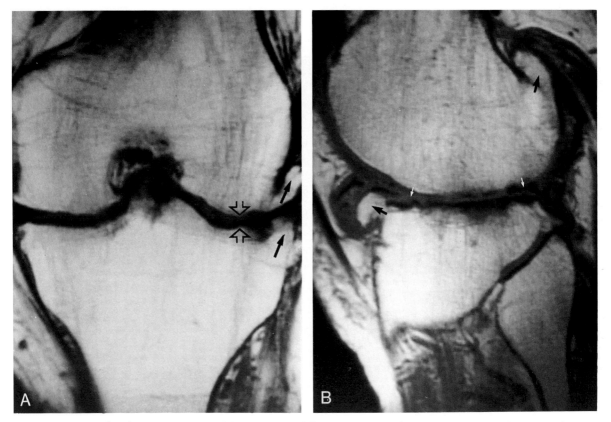

FIGURE 4–242. T1-weighted (**A**) coronal and (**B**) sagittal images of degenerative osteoarthritis reveal fat-marrow–containing osteophytes (*solid black arrows*), joint-space narrowing (*open black arrows*), eroded hyaline articular cartilage (*solid white arrows*) and macerated menisci.

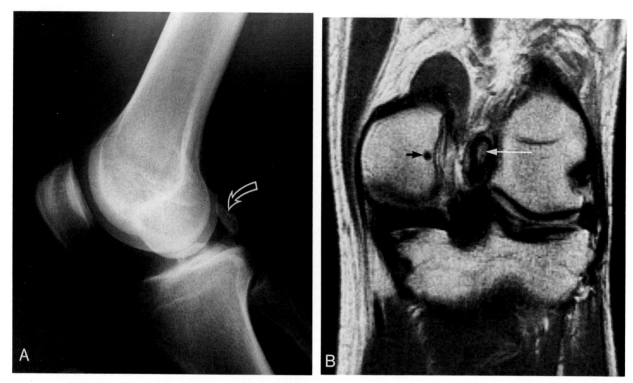

FIGURE 4–243. (**A**) On a plain film lateral radiograph, an intraarticular loose body is identified posteriorly (*curved open arrow*). (**B**) On a T1-weighted coronal image, the loose body is seen in the intercondylar notch (*white arrow*). The free fragment demonstrates high central marrow signal intensity and low peripheral cortical signal intensity. An incidental bone island is seen as a focus of low signal intensity in compact bone (*black arrow*).

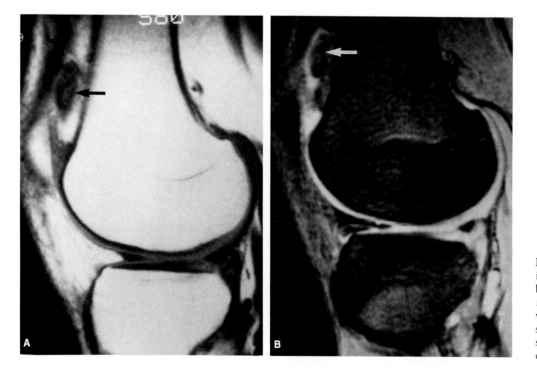

FIGURE 4–244. A low signal intensity cartilaginous loose body in suprapatellar bursa (*arrows*) is revealed on (**A**) T1-weighted and (**B**) T2*-weighted sagittal images. No fat marrow signal intensity occurs in pure cartilaginous lesions.

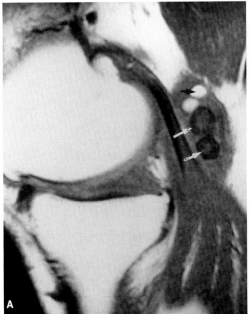
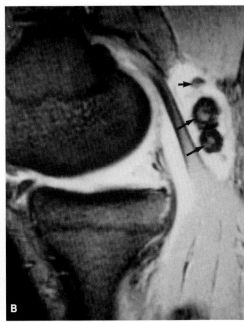

FIGURE 4–245. Sagittal (**A**) T1-weighted and (**B**) T2*-weighted images show multiple fat marrow (*small arrows*) and sclerotic (*large arrows*) loose bodies in a popliteal cyst located adjacent to the medial head of gastrocnemius muscle. The conspicuity of fat marrow signal intensity is lost on the T2*-weighted image.

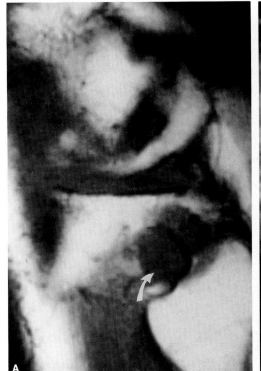
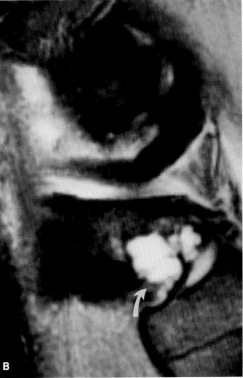

FIGURE 4–246. A degenerative synovial fluid-filled cyst (*curved arrows*) of the superior tibiofibular joint demonstrates (**A**) low signal intensity on a T1-weighted image and (**B**) high signal intensity on a T2*-weighted image. The lateral meniscus is completely absent, and there is associated joint-space narrowing.

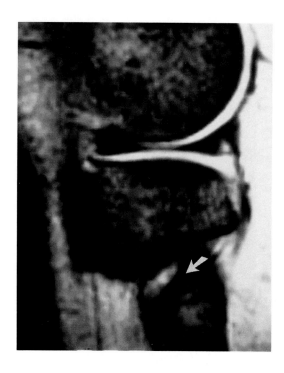

FIGURE 4–247. Anterior subluxation of the fibula (*arrow*) at the superior tibiofibular joint is demonstrated on a T2*-weighted sagittal image.

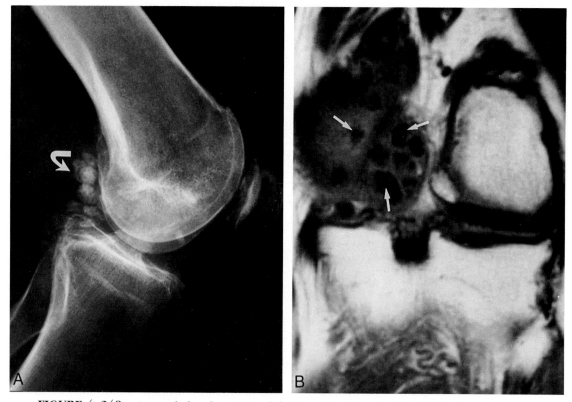

FIGURE 4–248. Synovial chondromatosis. (**A**) A lateral radiograph shows multiple calcified loose bodies (*curved arrow*). (**B**) On a T1-weighted coronal image, osteochondral loose bodies (*arrows*) are seen collecting in the posteromedial joint capsule. (**C**) On T1-weighted and (**D**) T2*-weighted sagittal images, synovium-based osteochondral fragments (*arrows*) are revealed. The surrounding joint effusion demonstrates bright signal intensity with T2*-weighted contrast.

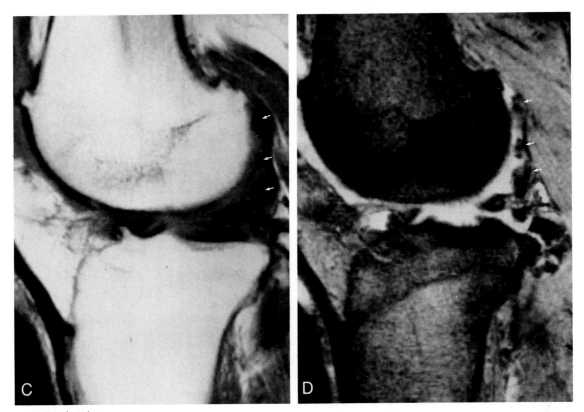

FIGURE 4–248. *(Continued)*

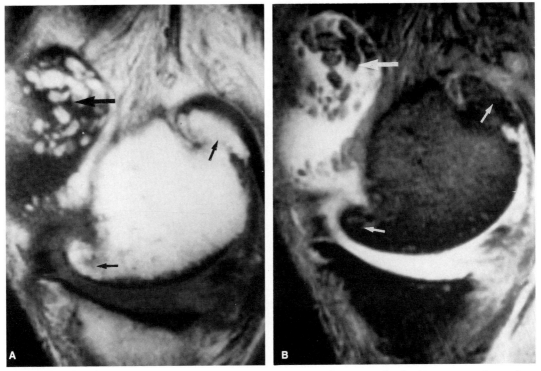

FIGURE 4–249. Synovitis with a fragmented appearance of suprapatellar fat (*large arrows*) may be mistaken for loose osteochondral fragments on (**A**) T1-weighted and (**B**) T2*-weighted sagittal images. Medial femoral condylar osteophytes (*small arrows*) are present.

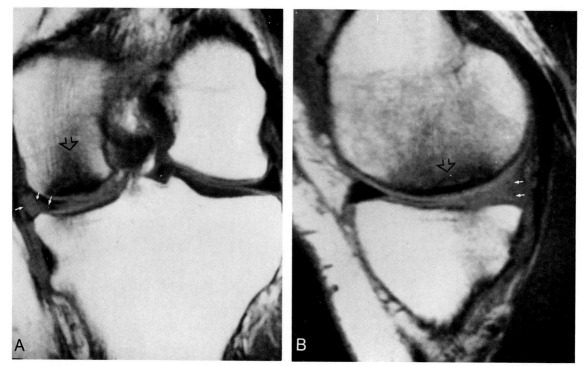

FIGURE 4–250. Spontaneous osteonecrosis of the medial femoral condyle demonstrates low signal intensity (*open arrow*) on (**A**) T1-weighted coronal and (**B**) sagittal images. The posterior horn of the medial meniscus is macerated and torn (*white arrows*).

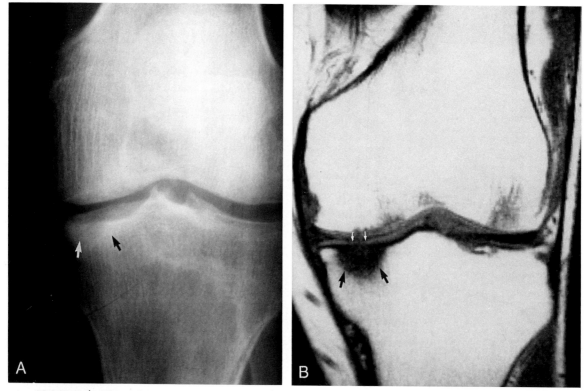

FIGURE 4–251. (**A**) On an anteroposterior radiograph, a sclerotic focus in the medial tibial plateau (*arrows*) indicates osteonecrosis. (**B**) On a T1-weighted coronal image, a well-defined region of sub-chondral low signal intensity is seen in the medial tibial plateau (*black arrows*). Thinning of overlying hyaline articular cartilage is also observed (*white arrows*).

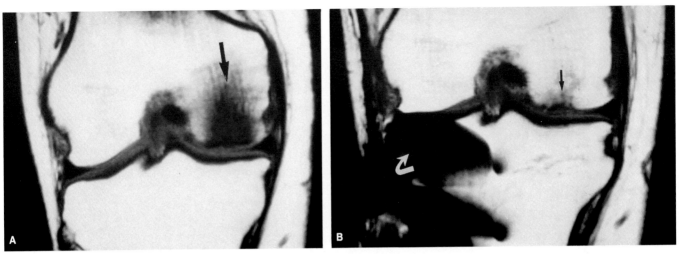

FIGURE 4–252. Medial femoral condyle osteonecrosis (*straight arrows*) (**A**) prior to and (**B**) after lateral tibial osteotomy (*curved arrow*). Resolution of the low signal necrotic marrow after osteotomy is significant.

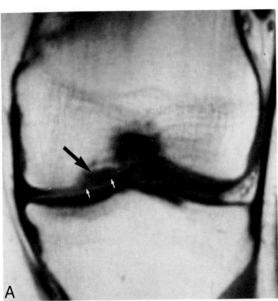

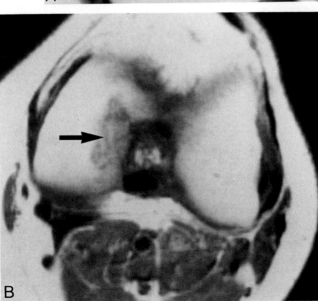

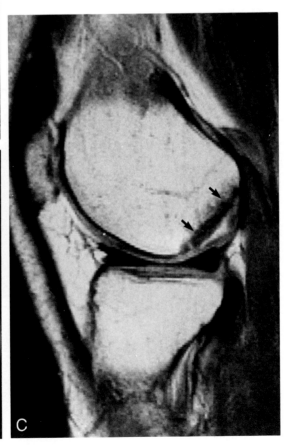

FIGURE 4–253. Osteochondritis dissecans (*black arrows*) involves the lateral aspect of the medial femoral condyle on (**A**) T1-weighted coronal and (**B**) axial images of this patient. The overlying hyaline articular cartilage is bowed (*white arrows*). (**C**) On a T1-weighted sagittal image of another patient with osteochondritis dissecans, the low signal intensity focus of devitalized bone is in the non-weight-bearing portion of the medial femoral condyle (*arrows*).

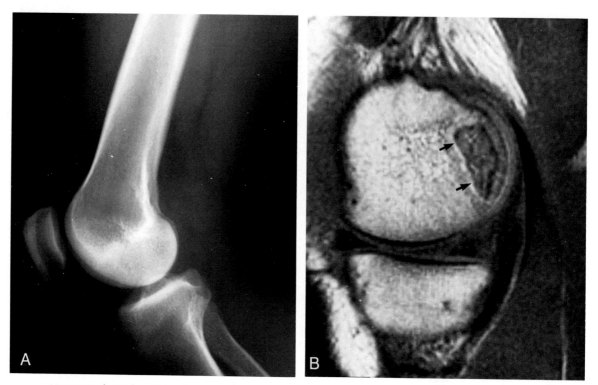

FIGURE 4–254. (**A**) A lateral radiograph is negative for osteochondritis dissecans. (**B**) On a T1-weighted sagittal image, however, a low signal intensity focus of osteochondritis dissecans is revealed in the posterior medial femoral condyle (*arrows*).

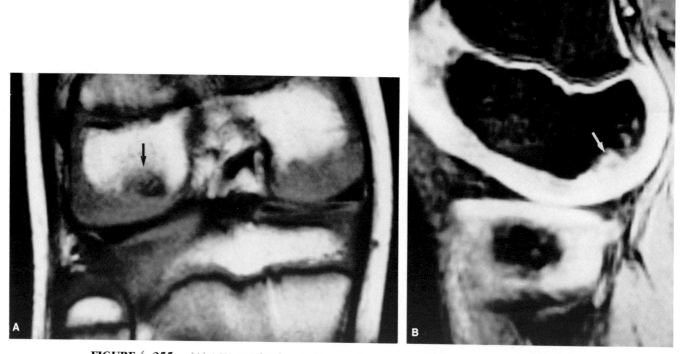

FIGURE 4–255. (**A**) A T1-weighted sagittal image displays osteochondritis dissecans with low signal intensity focus (*black arrow*) in the posterior lateral femoral condyle. (**B**) On a T2*-weighted sagittal image, subchondral hyperintensity is seen in an area of cartilage fissuring (*white arrow*).

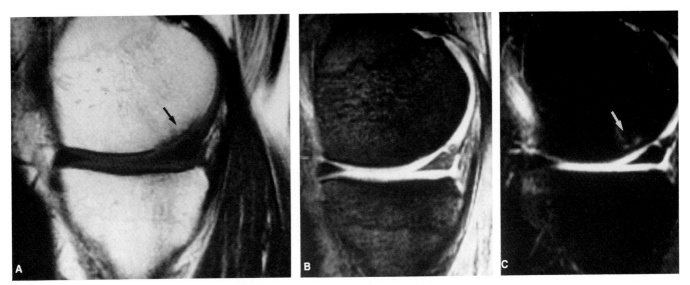

FIGURE 4–256. (**A**) On a T1-weighted image, medial femoral condyle osteochondritis dissecans is indicated by a low signal intensity subchondral focus (*arrow*). (**B**) Short TI inversion recovery contrast reveals a small subchondral region of hyperintensity (*arrow*). (**C**) The corresponding T2*-weighted image is normal.

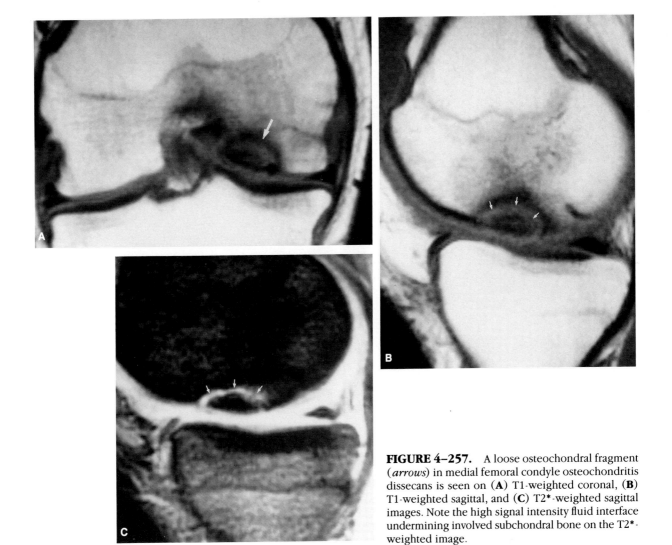

FIGURE 4–257. A loose osteochondral fragment (*arrows*) in medial femoral condyle osteochondritis dissecans is seen on (**A**) T1-weighted coronal, (**B**) T1-weighted sagittal, and (**C**) T2*-weighted sagittal images. Note the high signal intensity fluid interface undermining involved subchondral bone on the T2*-weighted image.

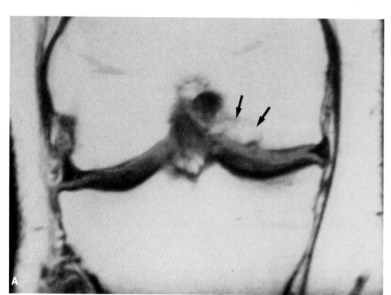
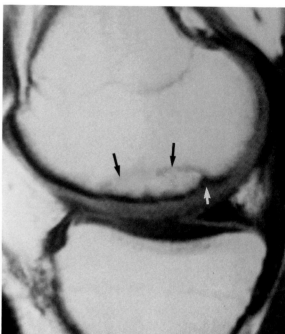

FIGURE 4–258. Healed focus of osteochondritis dissecans (*black arrows*) is seen on (**A**) T1-weighted coronal and (**B**) sagittal images. There is normal marrow fat signal intensity in the involved ovoid segment. No undermining fluid interface is seen. Residual irregularity of the low signal intensity cortical surface (*white arrow*) is present.

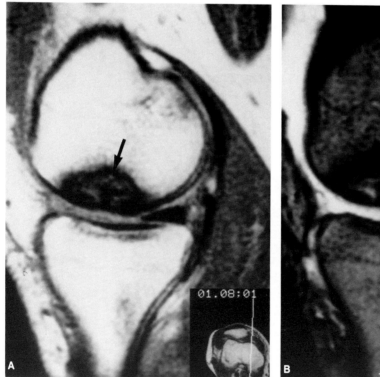
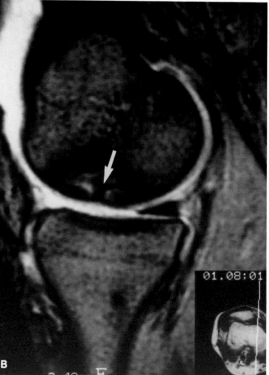

FIGURE 4–259. Medial femoral condylar osteochondritis dissecans (*arrows*) demonstrates a (**A**) low signal intensity focus on a T1-weighted sagittal image and (**B**) increased signal intensity in areas of subchondral bone on a T2*-weighted sagittal image. (**C**) This finding, in association with attenuated overlying articular cartilage, is confirmed on the corresponding arthroscopic photograph before (frame 9) and after (frames 10, 11, and 12) arthroscopic drilling.

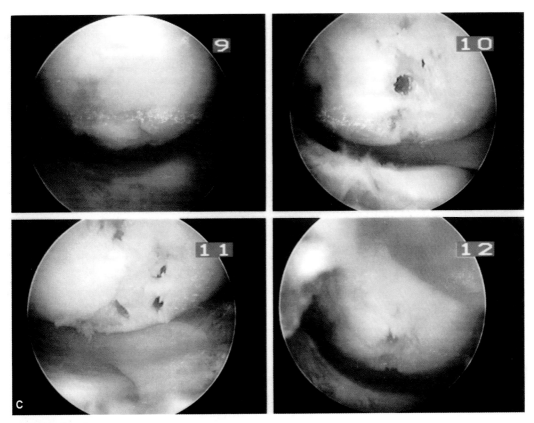

FIGURE 4–259. *(Continued)*

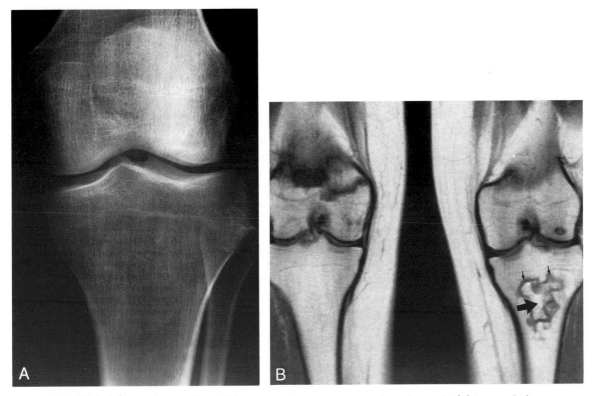

FIGURE 4–260. A bone infarct, (**A**) not seen in an anteroposterior radiograph, (**B**) is revealed on a T1-weighted coronal image with characteristic serpiginous low signal intensity peripheral sclerosis (*small arrows*) and a high signal intensity central portion (*large arrow*).

ever, demonstrate low signal intensity on T1- and T2-weighted images (Fig. 4–262). Bone infarcts may be seen in association with steroid therapy, as in part of a chemotherapy protocol (Fig. 4–263).

Joint Effusions

Joint effusions are characterized by low signal intensity on T1-weighted images and bright signal intensity on corresponding T2-weighted images (Fig. 4–264). With the knee in 10° of external rotation, the effusion may be more prominent in the lateral compartment of the knee, simulating an artificial *ballottement*. With the patient in the supine position, the posterior capsule is preferentially distended and collects fluid before suprapatellar bursal distention occurs. Layers of postaspiration fat–fluid, fluid–fluid, and air–fluid levels can be demonstrated in suprapatellar fluid collections. When MR imaging is performed after arthrography, contrast material can be seen coating the articular cartilage and extending into the suprapatellar recess. On T2-weighted images, fluid, initially trapped between meniscal surfaces, is seen with a bright signal intensity interface that does not interfere with evaluation of the meniscal fibrocartilage.

Inflammatory and noninflammatory effusions are indistinguishable in MR appearance. Our experience is that T1-weighted sequences are adequate for detecting small effusions, and there is no need for longer T2 protocols. Coronal images are complementary, with the distribution of fluid in the medial and lateral gutters extending into the suprapatellar bursa taking on a saddle-bag appearance (Fig. 4–265).

Popliteal Cysts

Classically, popliteal cysts (*i.e.,* Baker's cysts) of the gastrocnemiosemimembranosus bursae arise between the medial and lateral heads of the gastrocnemius muscle and the more lateral semimembranosus muscle (Fig. 4–266).[158,159] These cysts demonstrate low signal intensity on T1-weighted images and uniformly increased signal intensity on T2-weighted images. Septations that divide the cysts into compartments may also be seen, usually in atypical cyst locations. A narrow neck connecting the cyst to the joint is usually identified on axial images. Popliteal cysts are frequently seen in association with tears of the posterior horn of the medial meniscus (Fig. 4–267). Intraarticular communication and associated pathology are seen on contiguous sagittal images. Hemorrhagic joint effusions may be observed with a fluid–fluid level in the cyst. Loose bodies may collect in a posterior popliteal cyst (Fig. 4–268). The dissecting or ruptured popliteal cyst with subacute hemorrhage demonstrates increased

signal intensity on T1- and T2-weighted images due to the presence of blood (Fig. 4–269). Susceptibility artifact is shown as areas of low signal intensity in subacute and chronic hemorrhage on gradient-echo images.

Atypical locations for popliteal cysts include the tibiofibular joint and the bursa between the lateral head of the gastrocnemius and biceps femoris. These cysts may also present as soft-tissue masses proximal and distal to the popliteal fossa (Fig. 4–270). In very young children, popliteal cysts may occur as a primary disorder in the absence of concurrent intraarticular pathology (Fig. 4–271).[160] The cysts are frequently seen in patients with JRA or adult rheumatoid arthritis. With MR evaluation, a cyst can be differentiated from a popliteal artery aneurysm (Fig. 4–272) or venous malformation (Fig. 4–273), which may present with a similar clinical picture. Magnetic resonance offers the advantage of evaluating both popliteal and intraarticular pathology, areas of limited diagnostic accuracy, with ultrasound or conventional radiography. We have used intravenous Gd-DTPA to show lack of enhancement in a popliteal cyst with poorly defined margins (Fig. 4–274). Rarely, intraarticular Gd-DTPA or conventional arthrography is required to document communication with the joint. Treatment of underlying joint pathology in conjunction with excision of the cyst prevents recurrence.

Plicae

Synovial plicae are embryologic remnants of the septal division of the knee into three compartments.[161,162] They may be found as a normal variant in 20% to 60% of adult knees. The common plicae are suprapatellar, medial patellar, and infrapatellar (Figs. 4–275 and 4–276). Medial patellar and infrapatellar plicae are best seen on axial images, whereas the suprapatellar plica is seen on sagittal images traversing the suprapatellar bursa (Fig. 4–277). Plica tissue is seen with low signal intensity on T1-, T2-, and T2*-weighted images. The infrapatellar plica is the most common and can be confused with the ACL on arthrography. In patients presenting with a suprapatellar soft-tissue mass, MR studies may reveal the presence of a persistent plica dividing the suprapatellar bursa into two separate compartments containing hemorrhagic synovial fluid and debris (Fig. 4–278).

An inflamed medial patellar plica thickens and may interfere with normal quadriceps function. Erosion or abrasion of femoral condylar or patellar articular cartilage can occur as the plica loses its flexibility and gliding motion. On axial MR images, an abnormal medial patellar plica may be seen as a thickened band of low signal intensity with underlying irregularity of the medial patellar facet cartilage surface. Sagittal images through the medial compartment of the knee show the longitudinal orientation of the medial plica extending toward Hoffa's infrapatellar fat pad, anterior to the anterior horn of the medial meniscus. Although plical thickness is not measured, fibrotic hypertrophy secondary to chronic irritation can be identified and is considered symptomatic when impingement on the medial femoral condyle in knee flexion is present.

Fractures

Fractures about the knee can involve the femoral condyle, the tibial plateau surface, or the patella.[117] Tibial plateau fractures are the most common and predominantly occur with lateral plateau involvement (Fig. 4–279).[163] The most common mechanism of injury is impaction of the anterior portion of the lateral femoral condyle in a valgus mechanism of injury. Axial loading, or pure compressive force, produces an impaction or compression fracture of the plateau, whereas a pure valgus force results in a split condylar fracture. A valgus compressive force is responsible for the frequent occurrence of lateral tibial condylar plateau fractures with tears of the medial meniscus, ACL, and MCL. Fractures of the knee can be identified on MR scans in patients with acute or chronic knee pain and negative conventional radiographs (Fig. 4–280). Subsequent plain film radiography often shows areas of sclerosis or periosteal reaction at the fracture site that was initially identified on MR images. The most common MR pattern of fracture is sharp, well-defined, linear segments of decreased signal intensity in the distal femur or proximal tibia.

In an acute fracture, associated fluid or hemorrhage demonstrates increased signal intensity on T2- or T2*-weighted images. Fractures with diffuse areas of associated low signal intensity on T1-weighted images demonstrate increased signal intensity with long TR and TE settings. This reflects the prolonged T2 values in edematous or hemorrhagic marrow. Short TI inversion recovery images are more sensitive than gradient-echo T2*-weighted images in identifying subacute fractures with associated edema (Fig. 4–281). T2*-weighted contrast may, however, be useful in displaying acute fracture morphology when excessive marrow hemorrhage obscures detail on T1-weighted or STIR images (Fig. 4–282). Chronic fractures remain low in signal intensity with variable TR and TE parameters.

In animal models, post-traumatic growth-plate abnormalities, including changes in cartilage, transphyseal vascularity, and bony bridge formation, can be detected with MR imaging.[164] The metaphyseal–epiphyseal junction in the physis should not be mistaken for a transverse linear fracture (Fig. 4–283). Discontinuity of the physis may occur with trauma or epiphysiodesis (Fig. 4–284).

In the adult, the physeal line or scar does not demonstrate increased signal intensity on T2-weighted images. In a child, a chemical-shift artifact may display bright signal intensity parallel with the physis.

Magnetic resonance imaging is also used to differentiate stress fractures, common in the proximal tibia, from neoplastic processes (Fig. 4–285). The linear segment of the stress fracture in the knee is usually accompanied by marrow edema. The lack of a soft-tissue mass, cortical destruction, and characteristic marrow extension effectively excludes a tumor from the differential diagnosis. Rarely, a stress fracture is obscured on MR scans by reactive edema, and high-resolution and thin section CT is required to identify it.

A diffuse or localized pattern of low signal intensity on T1-weighted images without a defined fracture is seen with bone bruises or contusions at sites of microtrauma or impaction of trabecular bone (Fig. 4–286).[165] Recognition of occult subcortical fractures is important because osteochondral sequelae with significant cartilage damage may develop.[166] In an acute or subacute setting, increased signal intensity is seen on T2-, T2*-weighted, or STIR images prior to the appearance of sclerosis on plain film radiographs (Figs. 4–287 and 4–288). Normal metaphyseal–diaphyseal low signal intensity red marrow inhomogeneity should not be mistaken for a contusion. This marrow pattern is frequently seen in female patients and should not cross the physeal scar into subchondral bone. Short TI inversion recovery images or heavily T2-weighted images (TR > 3000 msec) may demonstrate varying degrees of increased signal intensity. The morphology of bone contusions has been characterized into three types based on T1- or intermediate-weighted images.[167] In type I lesions, findings included a diffuse decrease in signal intensity in metaphyseal and epiphyseal areas (Fig. 4–289). In type II, injury interruption of the low signal intensity cortical line is found (Fig. 4–290). In type III, a localized decrease in signal intensity in subchondral bone is seen (Fig. 4–291). Type I and II lesions are difficult to detect on radiography and arthroscopy and are frequently associated with tears of the ACL and contralateral collateral ligament. A pathologic fracture may be complicated by internal hemorrhage that obscures the underlying lesion (Fig. 4–292).

Hohl has classified tibial plateau fractures as minimally displaced (i.e., less than 4 mm of depression or displacement) or displaced.[168] Displaced fractures are further subdivided into local compression (Fig. 4–293), split compression (Fig. 4–294), total condylar depression, split, rim, and bicondylar fractures. Magnetic resonance allows multiplanar fracture and articular cartilage characterization, which is not possible with CT (Fig. 4–295).

Patellar fractures should be differentiated from bi-

(text continues on page 360)

FIGURE 4–264. Suprapatellar effusion. Joint effusion, (**A**) demonstrating low signal intensity on a T1-weighted sagittal image and (**B**) high signal intensity on a T2-weighted sagittal image, distends the suprapatellar bursa (*large arrows*) and the anterior capsule (*small arrows*) without obscuring the lateral meniscus.

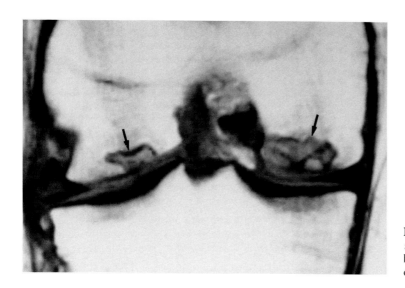

FIGURE 4–261. Bilateral femoral condylar infarcts (*arrows*) have characteristic low signal intensity serpiginous borders. Bone infarcts and osteonecrosis may have similar clinical presentations.

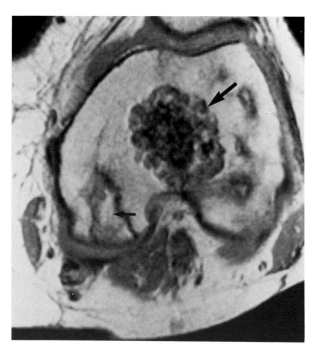

FIGURE 4–262. A calcified bone infarct is seen with multiple central punctate areas of low signal intensity (*large arrow*) on a T1-weighted axial image. The central portion of an adjacent non-calcified bone infarct is isointense with yellow marrow (*small arrow*).

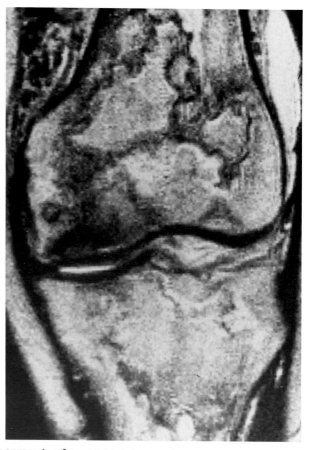

FIGURE 4–263. Multiple bone infarcts may occur in a leukemic patient taking steroids.

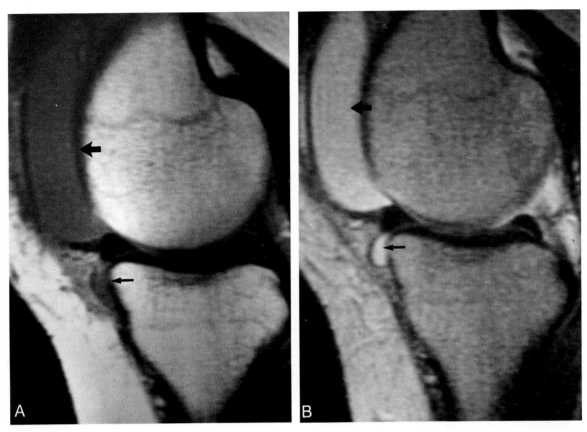

FIGURE 4–264.

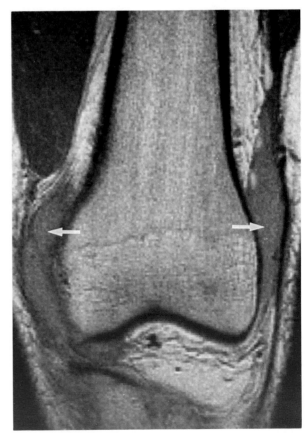

FIGURE 4–265. The saddle-bag distribution of joint effusion in the medial and lateral buttes of the suprapatellar bursae (*arrows*) is seen on an intermediate-weighted coronal image.

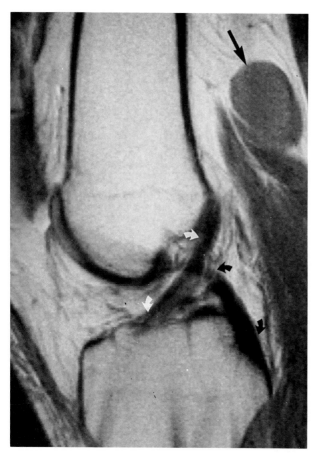

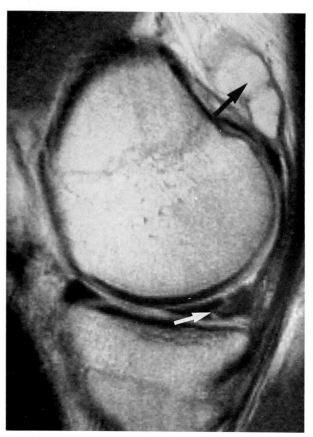

FIGURE 4–266. The popliteal cyst is characteristically located medial to the medial head of the gastrocnemius muscle (*straight black arrow*). Cyst contents demonstrate intermediate signal intensity on an intermediate-weighted sagittal image. Normal anterior (*curved white arrows*) and posterior (*curved black arrows*) cruciate ligament anatomy is also shown.

FIGURE 4–267. A T2-weighted sagittal image reveals increased signal intensity synovial fluid in a popliteal cyst (*black arrow*) and a vertical tear in the posterior horn of the medial meniscus (*white arrow*).

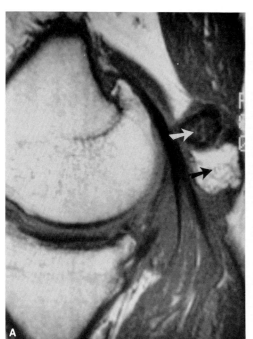

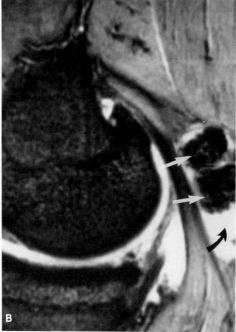

FIGURE 4–268. Popliteal cysts. (**A**) A T1-weighted sagittal image reveals a low signal intensity sclerotic loose body (*white arrow*) and a high signal intensity loose body (*black arrow*) that contains marrow fat. (**B**) Fat contrast is lost on a T2*-weighted sagittal image (*straight white arrows*, loose bodies; *curved black arrow*, popliteal cyst.)

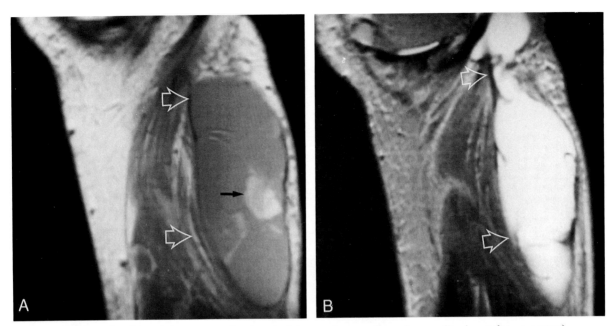

FIGURE 4–269. (**A**) A T1-weighted sagittal image shows a dissecting popliteal cyst (*open arrows*) with area of high signal intensity subacute hemorrhage (*solid arrow*). (**B**) On a T2-weighted sagittal image, the high signal intensity cyst (*open arrows*) is traceable to the joint line.

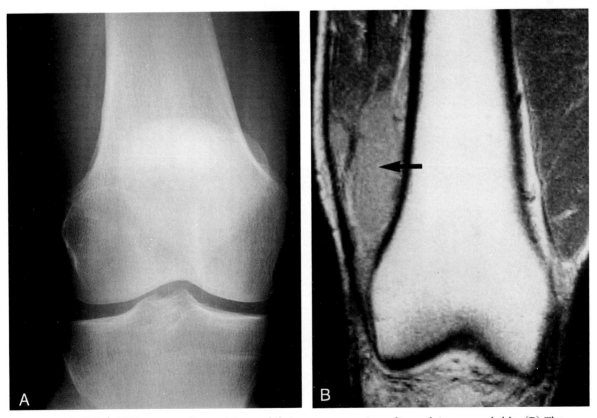

FIGURE 4–270. Atypical synovial cyst. (**A**) An anteroposterior radiograph is unremarkable. (**B**) The corresponding intermediate-weighted coronal image reveals a synovial cyst located along the distal lateral femur (*arrow*). The septate (*small arrow*) atypical popliteal cyst (*large arrow*) demonstrates (**C**) intermediate signal intensity on a balanced weighted axial image and (**D**) high signal intensity on a T2-weighted axial image. (**E**) In comparison, a T2-weighted axial image shows a more typical location for the popliteal cyst (*straight arrow*), medial to the medial head of the gastrocnemius muscle (*curved arrow*).

(continued)

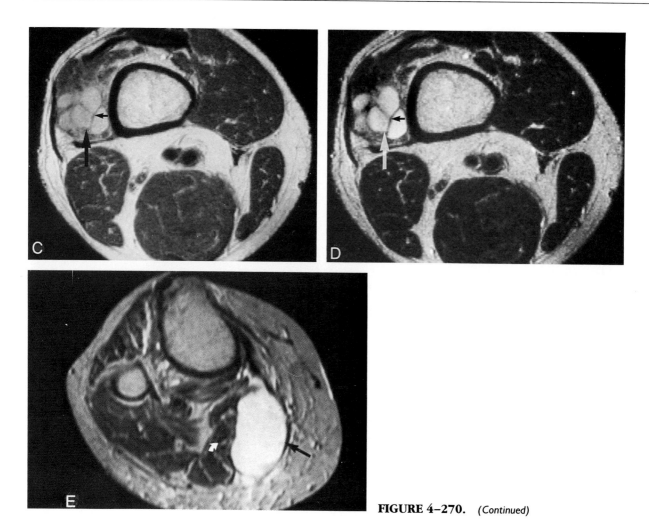

FIGURE 4–270. *(Continued)*

FIGURE 4–271. A popliteal cyst (*arrow*) occurred without intraarticular communication in this child. No associated joint pathology was present when examined on a T2*-weighted sagittal image.

FIGURE 4–273. Venous malformation. (**A**) A venous angiogram shows a serpiginous tangle of vessels (*arrow*). (**B**) T1-weighted and (**C**) T2-weighted coronal images demonstrate inhomogeneity, with generalized increased signal intensity seen on the T2-weighted image. Low signal intensity foci represent vessels with faster flowing blood (*curved arrows*).

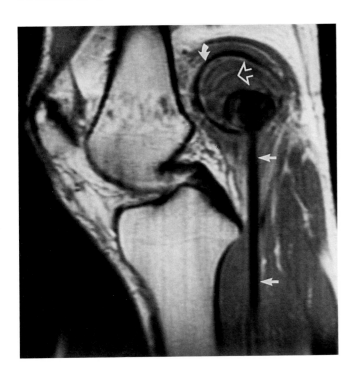

FIGURE 4–272. A T1-weighted sagittal image demonstrates an enlarged aneurysm of the popliteal artery. The normal low signal intensity popliteal artery (*solid arrows*), intermediate signal intensity thrombus (*open arrow*), and low signal intensity peripheral rim of calcification (*curved arrow*) are identified.

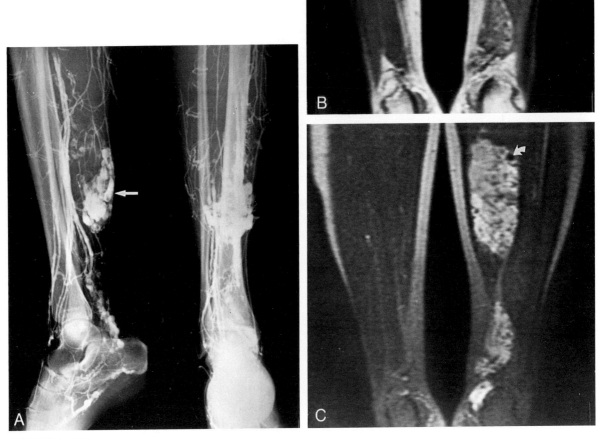

FIGURE 4–273.

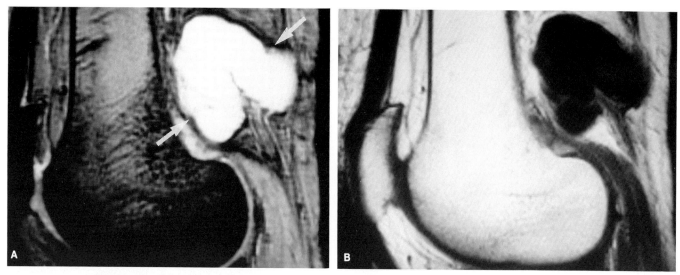

FIGURE 4–274. (**A**) An atypical lateral popliteal cyst (*arrow*) is hyperintense on a T2*-weighted sagittal image. (**B**) Lack of enhancement on an intravenous gadolinium T1-weighted sagittal image is characteristic of cystic fluid collections, not primary soft-tissue masses.

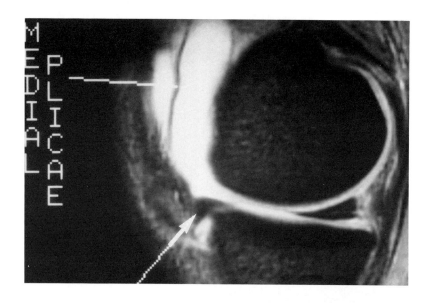

FIGURE 4–275. A thick low signal intensity medial patellar plica on a T2*-weighted sagittal image. The protruding anterior horn of the medial meniscus (*arrow*) should not be mistaken for a tear in this peripheral sagittal image.

FIGURE 4–276. Medial patellar plica (*arrows*) in (**A**) a T2*-weighted sagittal image and (**B**) the corresponding T1-weighted axial image.

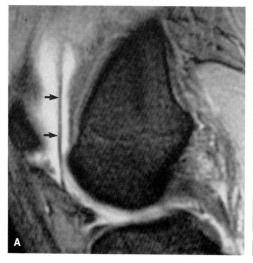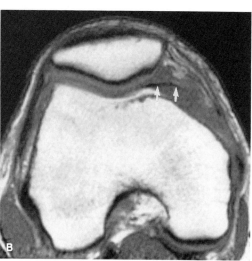

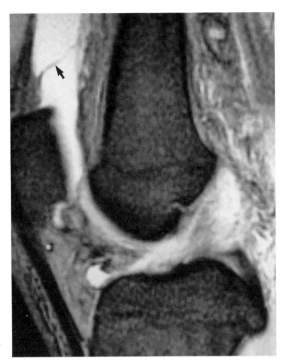

FIGURE 4–277. A low signal intensity suprapatellar plica (*arrow*) is seen on a T2*-weighted sagittal image. Effusion demonstrates bright signal intensity.

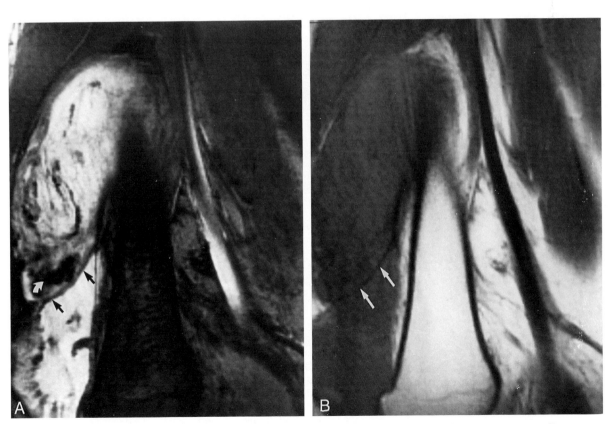

FIGURE 4–278. Division of the suprapatellar bursa into two compartments with an intact suprapatellar plica is seen as a low signal intensity band (*solid arrows*) on (**A**) T2*-weighted and (**B**) T1-weighted sagittal images. On the T2*-weighted image, low signal intensity hemosiderin deposits (*curved arrow*) contrast with the surrounding bright signal intensity hemorrhagic fluid.

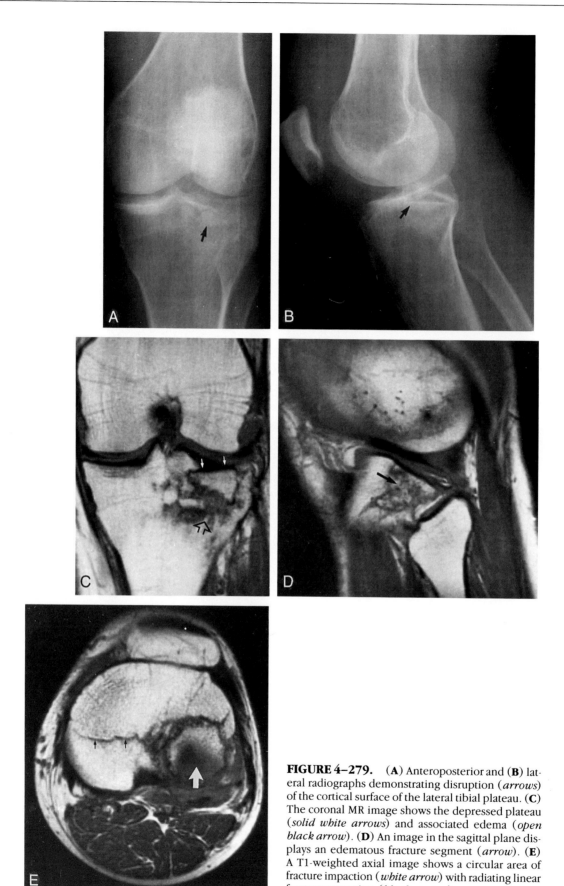

FIGURE 4–279. (**A**) Anteroposterior and (**B**) lateral radiographs demonstrating disruption (*arrows*) of the cortical surface of the lateral tibial plateau. (**C**) The coronal MR image shows the depressed plateau (*solid white arrows*) and associated edema (*open black arrow*). (**D**) An image in the sagittal plane displays an edematous fracture segment (*arrow*). (**E**) A T1-weighted axial image shows a circular area of fracture impaction (*white arrow*) with radiating linear fracture extension (*black arrows*).

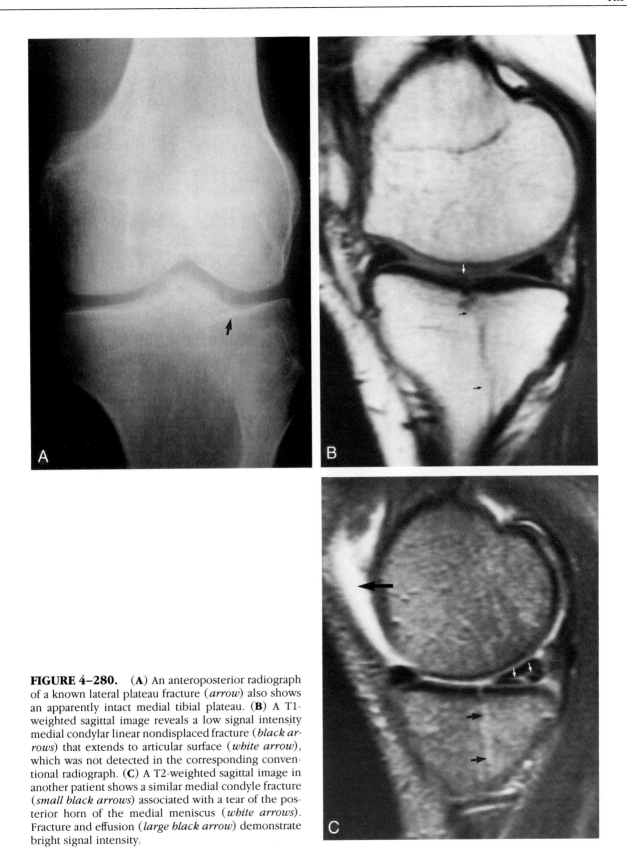

FIGURE 4–280. (**A**) An anteroposterior radiograph of a known lateral plateau fracture (*arrow*) also shows an apparently intact medial tibial plateau. (**B**) A T1-weighted sagittal image reveals a low signal intensity medial condylar linear nondisplaced fracture (*black arrows*) that extends to articular surface (*white arrow*), which was not detected in the corresponding conventional radiograph. (**C**) A T2-weighted sagittal image in another patient shows a similar medial condyle fracture (*small black arrows*) associated with a tear of the posterior horn of the medial meniscus (*white arrows*). Fracture and effusion (*large black arrow*) demonstrate bright signal intensity.

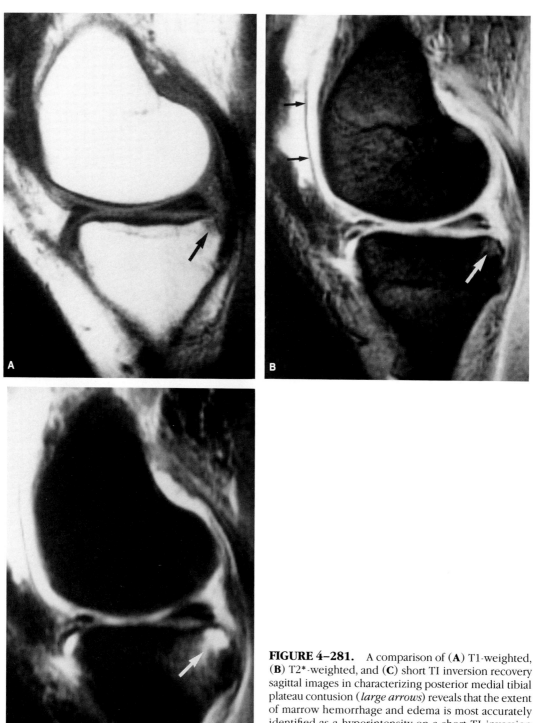

FIGURE 4–281. A comparison of (**A**) T1-weighted, (**B**) T2*-weighted, and (**C**) short TI inversion recovery sagittal images in characterizing posterior medial tibial plateau contusion (*large arrows*) reveals that the extent of marrow hemorrhage and edema is most accurately identified as a hyperintensity on a short TI inversion recovery contrast image. Medial plica (*small arrows*) is seen on the T2*-weighted sagittal image.

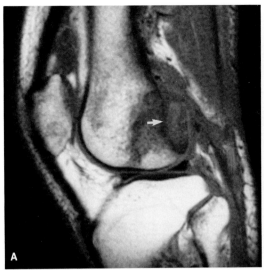

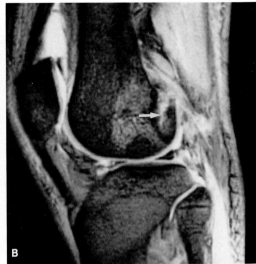

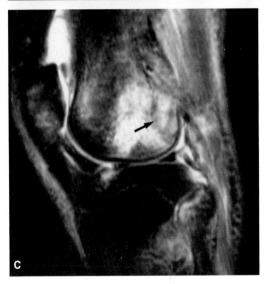

FIGURE 4–282. A condylar fracture of the distal femur (*arrows*) is seen on (**A**) T1-weighted, (**B**) T2*-weighted, and (**C**) short TI inversion recovery (STIR) images. Marrow hemorrhage demonstrates low signal intensity on the T1-weighted image and is hyperintense on the T2*-weighted and STIR images. Detail of the fracture morphology is best seen on T2* contrast, where marrow hyperemia is minimized and low signal intensity sclerotic bone at the fracture site is highlighted.

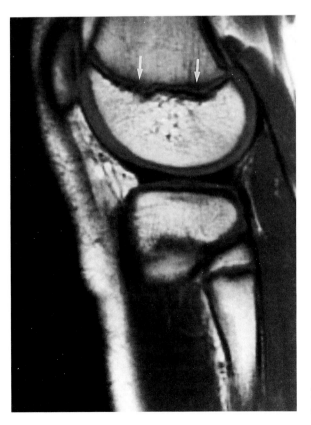

FIGURE 4–283. A normal low signal intensity physeal line is seen at the metaphyseal–epiphyseal junction (*arrows*).

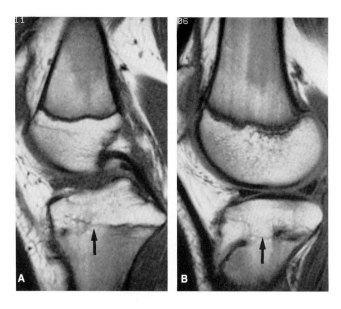

FIGURE 4–284. Epiphysiodesis is used to treat leg length inequality. Interruption (*arrows*) of the normal low signal intensity physeal plates in the (**A**) medial and (**B**) lateral aspect of the proximal tibia is seen on T1-weighted sagittal images.

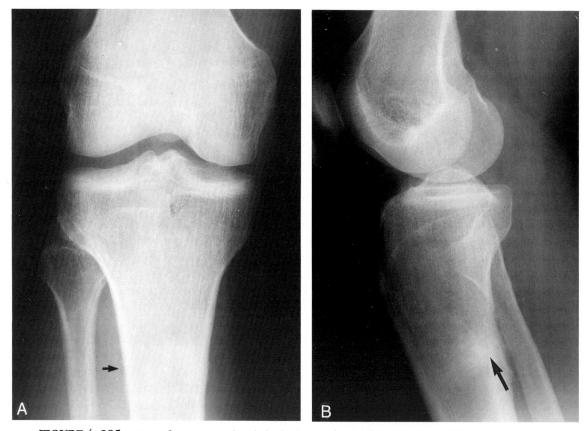

FIGURE 4–285. Stress fracture. Localized tibial sclerosis (*arrows*) is apparent on (**A**) anteroposterior and (**B**) lateral radiographs. (**C**) On a T1-weighted coronal image, the low signal intensity transverse fracture (*arrow*) is located in the proximal tibia.

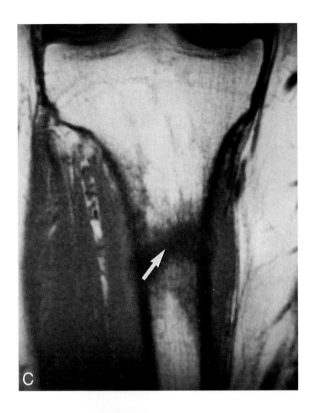

FIGURE 4–285. *(Continued)*

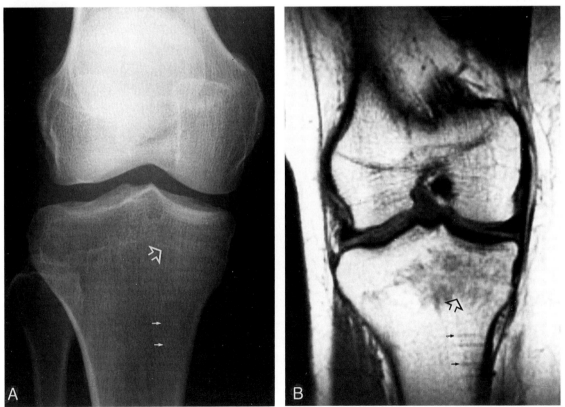

FIGURE 4–286. Bone contusion. (**A**) An anteroposterior radiograph shows minimal sclerosis in the medial tibial condyle (*open arrow*). Normal transverse growth lines of trabecular condensation are present in the proximal tibia (*solid arrows*). (**B**) On a T1-weighted coronal image, a diffuse region of low-signal intensity marrow edema is identified in area of bone contusion without discrete fracture (*open arrow*). Adjacent stress or growth lines can be identified by their parallel arrangement and transverse orientation (*small solid arrows*).

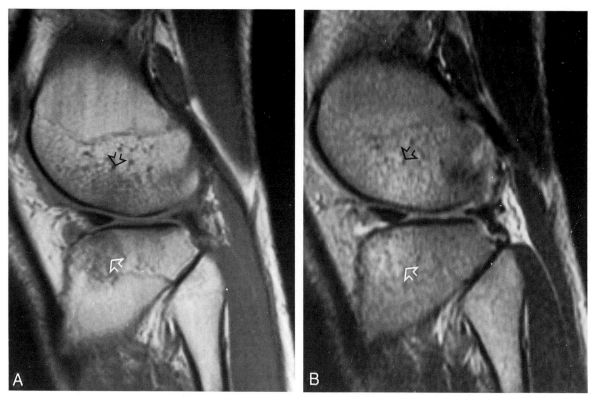

FIGURE 4–287. (**A**) T1-weighted and (**B**) T2-weighted sagittal images demonstrate low and high signal intensity, respectively, in marrow edema and hemorrhage in the subchondral bone of the proximal tibia (*white open arrows*) and distal femur (*black open arrows*). In the absence of any radiographic abnormality, this appearance was consistent with the patient's history of trauma and corresponding pain and tenderness.

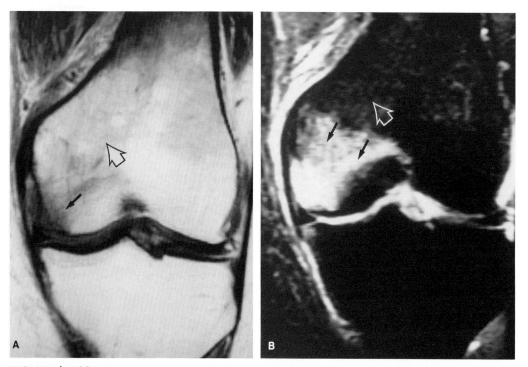

FIGURE 4–288. Marrow hemorrhage (*solid arrows*) must be differentiated from normal metaphyseal red marrow (*open arrows*). (**A**) A T1-weighted coronal image shows low signal intensity trabecular contusion and metaphyseal marrow. (**B**) A short TI inversion recovery coronal image is used to identify hyperintense marrow hemorrhage. On T1-weighted images, low signal intensity red marrow inhomogeneity is a normal finding in females, as long as it does not extend across the physeal scar. (**C**) A T1-weighted coronal image in another patient demonstrates metaphyseal and diaphyseal red marrow inhomogeneity (*arrow*).

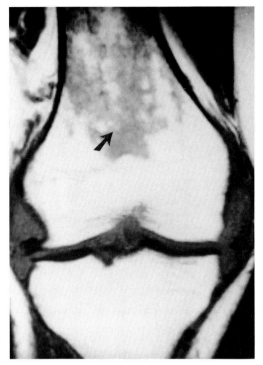

FIGURE 4–288. *(Continued)*

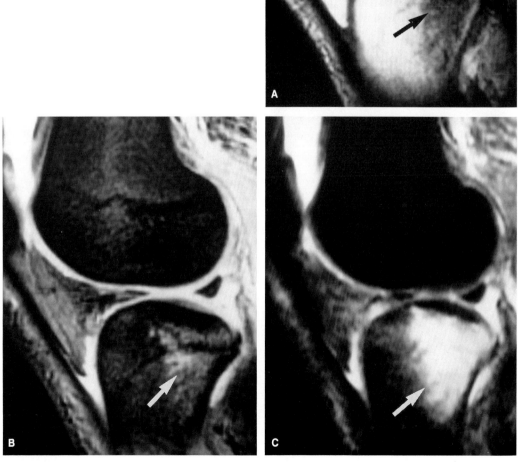

FIGURE 4–289. (**A**) A lateral plateau contusion marrow hemorrhage (*i.e.,* type I lesion; *arrows*) is seen as a diffuse region of hyperemia demonstrating   low signal intensity on a T1-weighted sagittal image and (**C**) severe hyperintensity on a short TI inversion recovery image. Type I bone injuries appear as diffuse or reticulated low signal intensity areas in metaphyseal and epiphyseal regions of trabecular bone without cortical fracture.

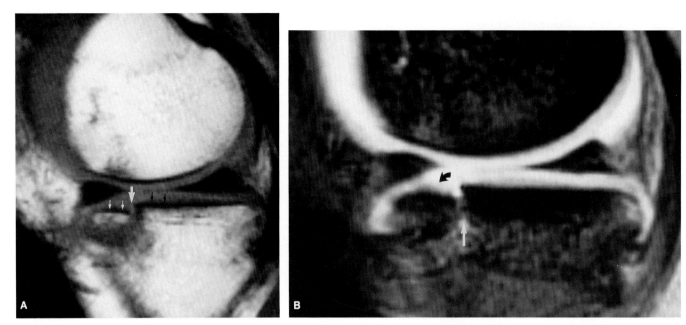

FIGURE 4–290.   A type II bone injury is revealed on (**A**) T1-weighted and (**B**) T2*-weighted sagittal images of a medial tibial plateau fracture (*large arrow*) with a depression of tibial cortex smaller than 3 mm (**A,** *small arrows;* **B,** *curved arrow*). Note the associated low signal intensity marrow hemorrhage on the T1-weighted image. No abnormality was detected on conventional radiographs.

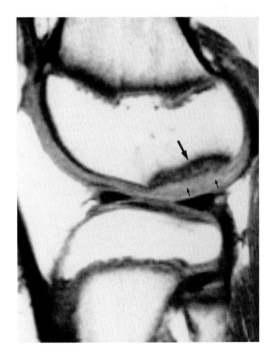

FIGURE 4–291.   A T1-weighted sagittal image shows a type III bone lesion with flattening of the intermediate signal intensity articular cartilage (*small arrows*) overlying a low signal intensity focus of osteochondritis dissecans (*large arrow*). Osteonecrosis, osteochondritis dissecans, and degenerative sclerosis are all considered type III lesions not related to acute trauma.

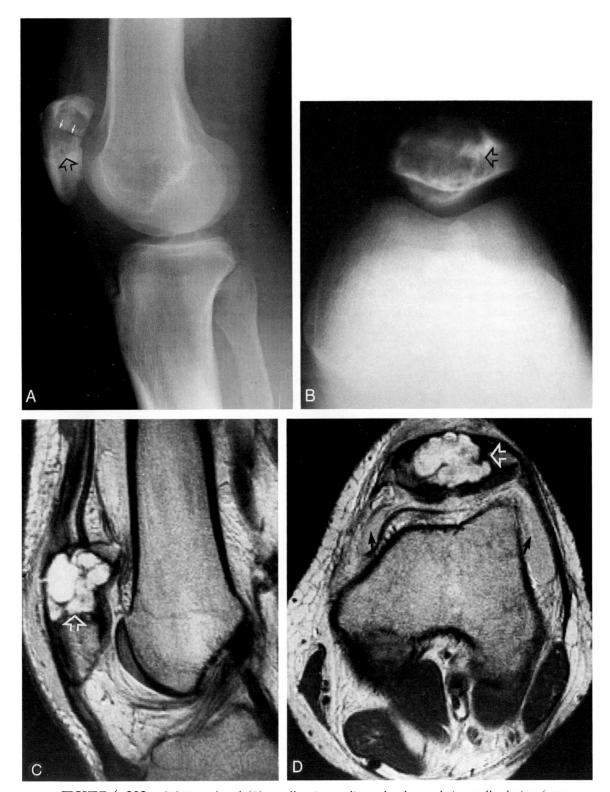

FIGURE 4–292. (**A**) Lateral and (**B**) patellar-view radiographs show a lytic patellar lesion (*open arrows*) and pathologic fracture of the patella (*closed arrows*). (**C**) Intermediate-weighted sagittal and (**D**) axial images show a high signal intensity lesion (*open arrows*) with areas of internal septation. This lesion represents organizing subacute hemorrhage and eosinophilic granuloma tissue after patellectomy. Associated joint effusion is indicated (*solid arrows*). In the presence of extensive hemorrhage, MR failed to delineate the fracture segment.

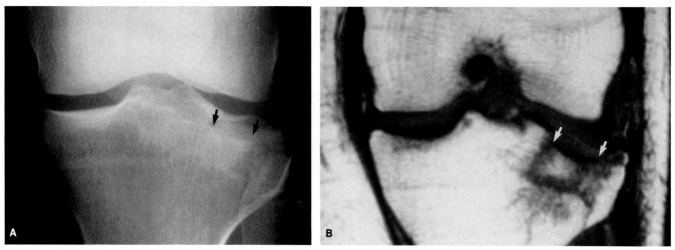

FIGURE 4–293. A local, central-depression–type lateral tibial plateau fracture (*arrows*) is seen on (**A**) an anteroposterior radiograph and (**B**) a T1-weighted coronal image. Fracture morphology and subchondral marrow hemorrhage are best demonstrated on an MR image.

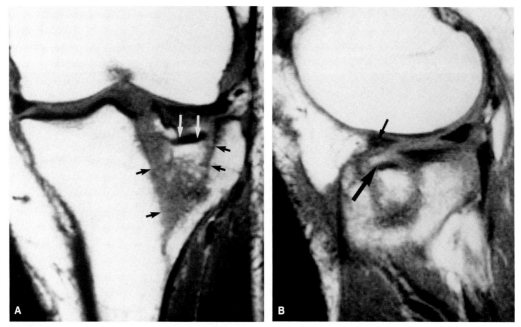

FIGURE 4–294. (**A**) A T1-weighted coronal image shows a vertical wedge (*black arrows*) tibial plateau fracture with a central depression component (*white arrows*) involving the lateral tibial condyle. (**B**) T1-weighted and (**C**) T2*-weighted sagittal images demonstrate cortical depression (*large arrow*) and associated meniscal tear of the anterior horn of the lateral meniscus (*small arrow*). (**D**) A T1-weighted axial image shows the anterior-to-posterior extent of the plateau fracture and the central depression (*arrows*). (**E**) A 3D CT image displays a vertical fracture segment (*small thick arrows*) with intra-articular involvement (*long thin arrow*).

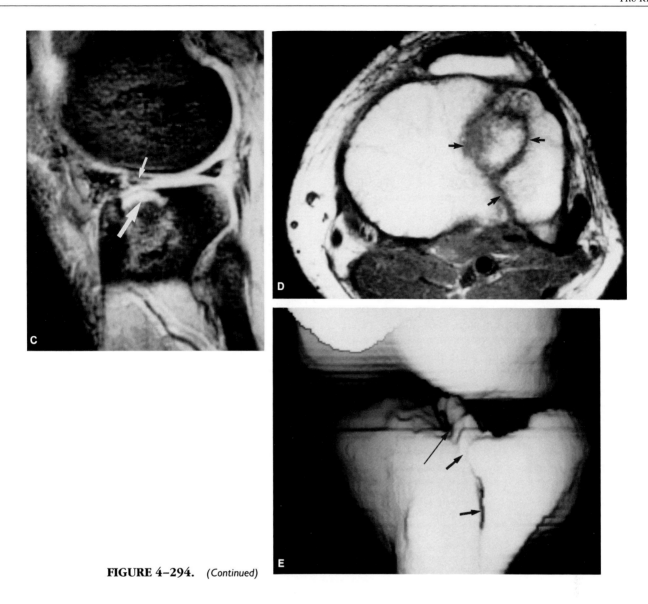

FIGURE 4–294. *(Continued)*

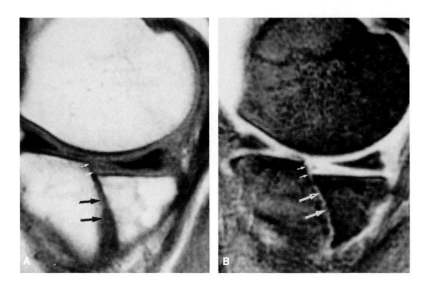

FIGURE 4–295. A displaced medial tibial plateau fracture (*large arrows*) with depressed and offset articular cartilage surfaces (*small arrows*) can be seen on (**A**) T1-weighted and (**B**) T2*-weighted sagittal images.

partite patellar morphology (Fig. 4–296). Patellar fractures are vertical, transverse, or comminuted. The bipartite patella is a developmental variant that involves accessory ossification of the superolateral margin, and not a fracture (Fig. 4–297).

A lipohemarthrosis may be identified in fractures involving the patella, femur, or tibia. T1- and T2-weighted images are useful in identifying fluid–fluid layers (Fig. 4–298).

Compartment syndrome, a known complication of trauma, including fracture, has been identified with edema, which is limited to a specified muscle group (Fig. 4–299).[169] Edema may be replaced with fatty atrophy after denervation (Fig. 4–300). Sudeck's atrophy or reflex sympathetic dystrophy can also occur as a complication of fracture (Fig. 4–301). Diffuse juxtaarticular low signal intensity on T1-weighted images is seen as patients develop aggressive osteoporosis with or without the presence of an associated fracture.[170] On STIR images, reflex sympathetic dystrophy demonstrates increased signal intensity secondary to hyperemic bone marrow edema.[171] Short TI inversion recovery imaging sequences are more sensitive and may define increased signal intensity in hyperemic bone in patients with negative T2- or T2*-weighted images (Fig. 4–302).

Infection

Capsular distention and joint effusions can be seen on MR scans of infected joints, but are nonspecific findings.[172]

A septic joint may be further characterized by intraarticular debris and synovitis from hematogenous seeding. In osteomyelitis in the immature skeleton, a mottled pattern of yellow marrow stores may be identified in the epiphyseal center of the femur or tibia. This appearance should not be confused with the coarsened trabecular pattern seen in Paget's disease.[173] In one case of osteomyelitis involving the distal femur, MR studies revealed collections of infected fluid confined by elevated periosteum (Fig. 4–303). Plain film radiography and nuclear bone scans were negative in this case, which was surgically debrided on the basis of the MR findings.

An infectious tract with fluid may simulate pathologic fracture or stress fracture and, when associated with extensive surrounding edema, can be confused with tumor (Fig. 4–304). In a patient with multifocal osteomyelitis, seeding of the distal femur and proximal humerus was identified on MR scans as a central nidus of high intensity marrow and calcified sequestra of low signal intensity (Fig. 4–305). Marrow infiltration and soft-tissue extension of osteomyelitis can also be demonstrated using STIR sequences (Fig. 4–306). Cellulitis is best identified on STIR protocols (Fig. 4–307). The STIR sequence, however, may be sensitive to reactive marrow changes in the absence of active infection and in the presence of normal marrow signal intensity on T2-weighted images.[174] A low signal intensity "rim sign" has been described in chronic infection resulting from trauma.[174] This rim of fibrous tissue or reactive bone is of low signal intensity on T1-, T2-, and STIR-weighted images and surrounds the area of active bone disease.

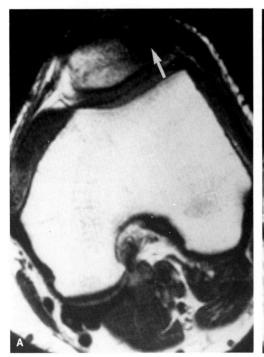
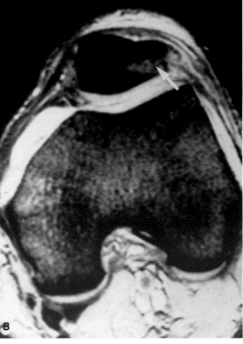

FIGURE 4–296. A lateral patellar contusion (*arrows*) demonstrates (**A**) low signal intensity on a T1-weighted axial image and (**B**) linear increased signal intensity on a T2*-weighted axial image.

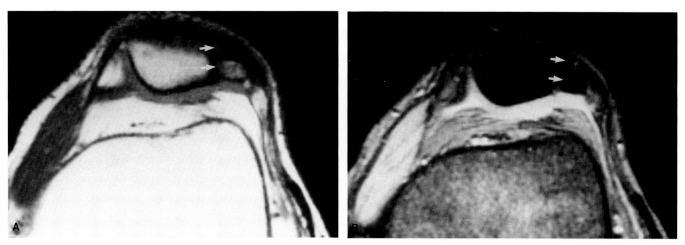

FIGURE 4–297. (**A**) T1-weighted and (**B**) T2*-weighted axial images show bipartite patella involving the superolateral margin of the patella. The anterior-to-posterior dividing line represents a developmental anomaly of the accessory ossification center (*arrows*).

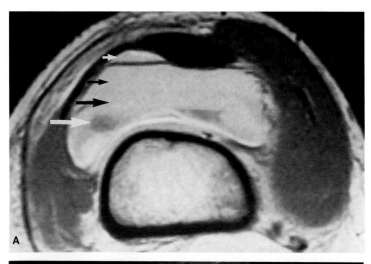

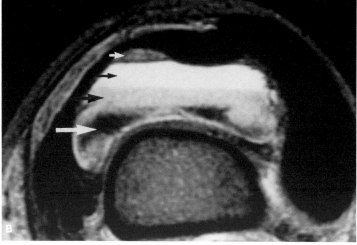

FIGURE 4–298. Lipohemarthrosis with fat–serum–cellular layering is identified in hemorrhagic effusion. (*Large black arrow,* cellular layer; *small black arrow,* serum layer; *small white arrow,* fat layer.) Deep layering of hemosiderin elements (*large white arrow*) is shown on (**A**) intermediate-weighted and (**B**) T2-weighted axial images. Hemarthrosis is commonly seen in anterior cruciate ligament tears and osteochondral fractures. The supernatant layer of hemorrhage is bright in long TR/TE protocols, whereas the cellular layer is dark on short and long TR/TE protocols.

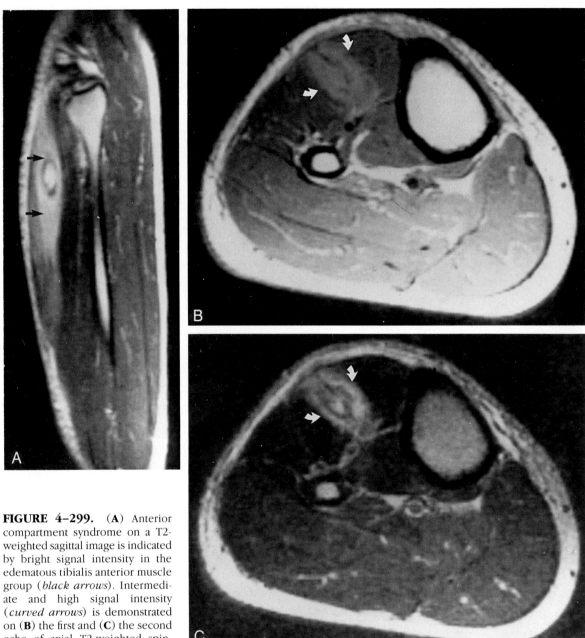

FIGURE 4–299. (**A**) Anterior compartment syndrome on a T2-weighted sagittal image is indicated by bright signal intensity in the edematous tibialis anterior muscle group (*black arrows*). Intermediate and high signal intensity (*curved arrows*) is demonstrated on (**B**) the first and (**C**) the second echo of axial T2-weighted spin-echo sequences.

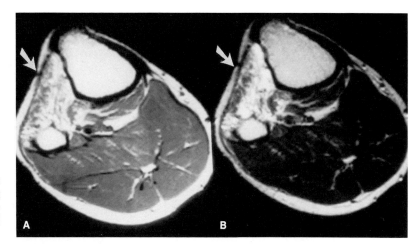

FIGURE 4–300. Fatty atrophy (*arrows*) of the muscles of the anterior fascial compartment of the leg secondary to peroneal nerve injury is seen on (**A**) intermediate-weighted and (**B**) T2-weighted axial images.

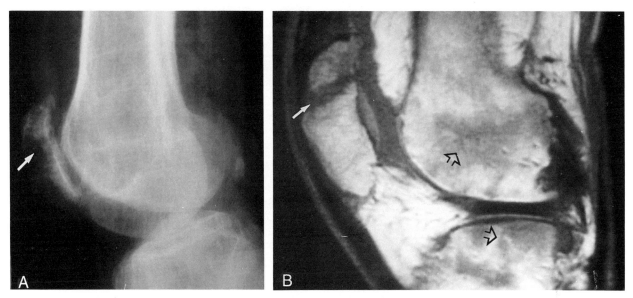

FIGURE 4–301. (**A**) A lateral radiograph shows patellar fracture (*arrow*) and diffuse osteoporosis. (**B**) A T1-weighted sagittal image shows the transverse patellar fracture (*solid white arrow*) and patchy juxtaarticular low signal intensity (*open black arrows*) that corresponds to aggressive osteoporosis in reflex sympathetic dystrophy.

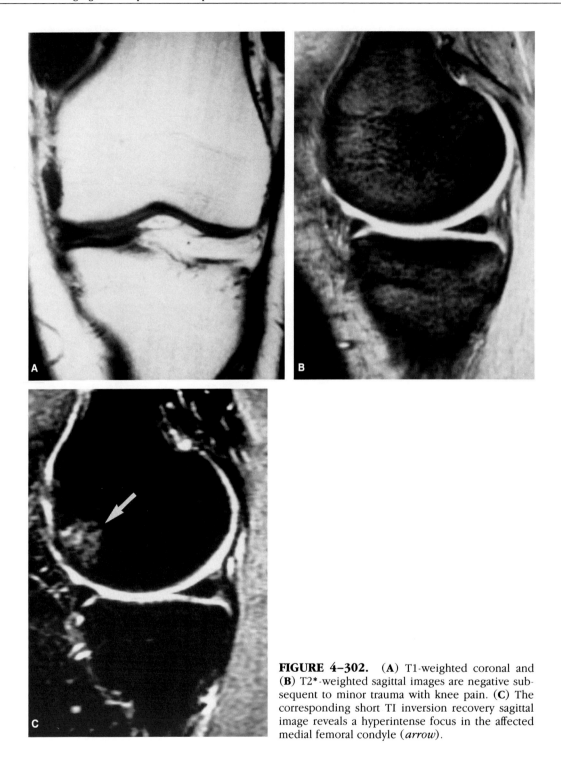

FIGURE 4–302. (**A**) T1-weighted coronal and (**B**) T2*-weighted sagittal images are negative subsequent to minor trauma with knee pain. (**C**) The corresponding short TI inversion recovery sagittal image reveals a hyperintense focus in the affected medial femoral condyle (*arrow*).

FIGURE 4–303. Staphylococcal osteomyelitis was not identified on (**A**) conventional radiographs and (**B**) bone scintigraphy. (**C**) Sagittal T2-weighted and (**D**) axial intermediate-weighted and (**E**) T2-weighted images demonstrate purulent fluid (*white arrows*), necrotic tissue (*small black arrows*), and elevated low signal intensity periosteum (*large black arrows*). Purulent debris (*i.e.,* fluid) demonstrates increased signal intensity on T2-weighted images (*small white arrows*).

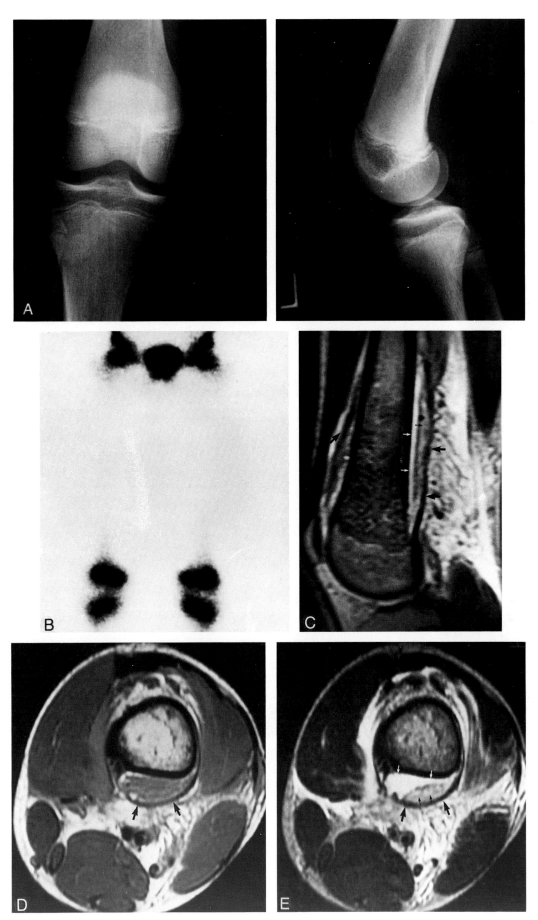

FIGURE 4–303.

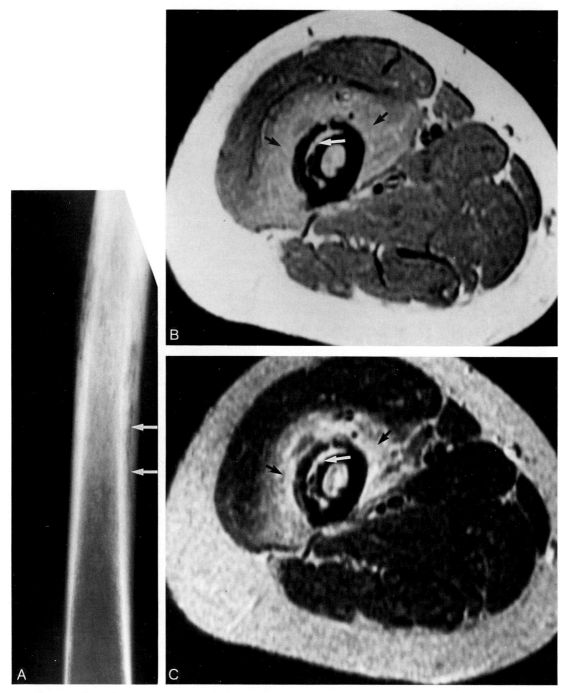

FIGURE 4–304. Osteomyelitis can simulate Ewing's sarcoma. (**A**) An anteroposterior radiograph of the midfemur demonstrates periosteal reaction and longitudinal cortical lucency (*arrows*). (**B**) Intermediate-weighted and (**C**) T2-weighted axial images reveal a corresponding high signal intensity infectious track (*white arrows*) with surrounding perilesional edema (*black arrows*). Edema demonstrates increased signal intensity in a T2-weighted image.

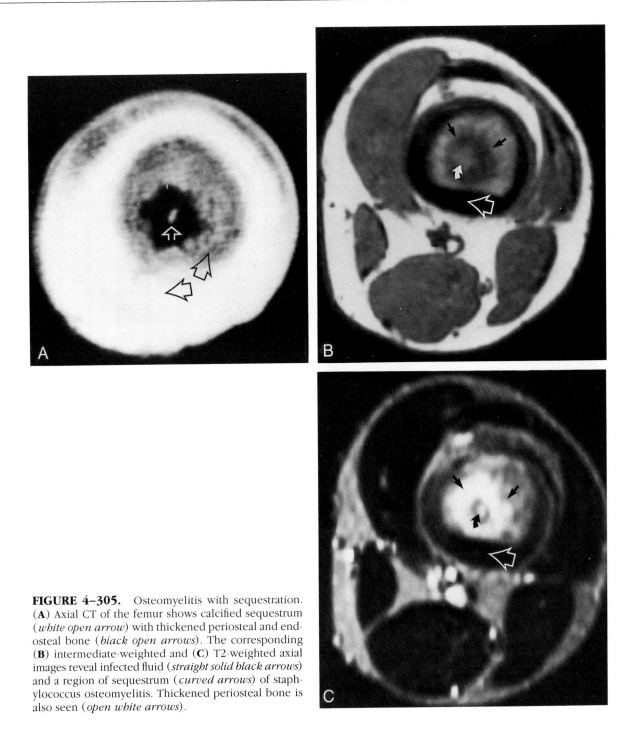

FIGURE 4–305. Osteomyelitis with sequestration. (**A**) Axial CT of the femur shows calcified sequestrum (*white open arrow*) with thickened periosteal and endosteal bone (*black open arrows*). The corresponding (**B**) intermediate-weighted and (**C**) T2-weighted axial images reveal infected fluid (*straight solid black arrows*) and a region of sequestrum (*curved arrows*) of staphylococcus osteomyelitis. Thickened periosteal bone is also seen (*open white arrows*).

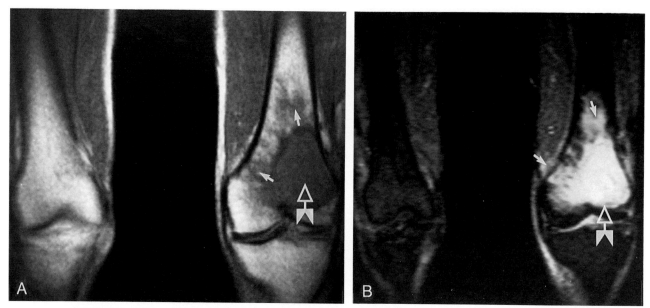

FIGURE 4–306. (**A**) T1-weighted and (**B**) short TI inversion recovery (STIR) coronal images display the focus of staphylococcal osteomyelitis in the femoral metaphysis (*flagged arrows*). Marrow infiltration and extension (*solid arrows*) demonstrate low signal intensity on the T1-weighted image and high signal intensity on the STIR image.

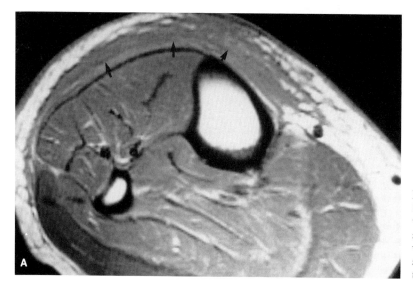

FIGURE 4–307. Soft-tissue cellulitis (*arrows*) is (**A**) intermediate in signal intensity on a proton-density–weighted image, (**B**) is mildly bright on a T2-weighted axial image, and (**C**) is hyperintense on a short TI inversion recovery (STIR) image. STIR contrast is more sensitive to inflammatory soft-tissue disorders than other types of imaging.

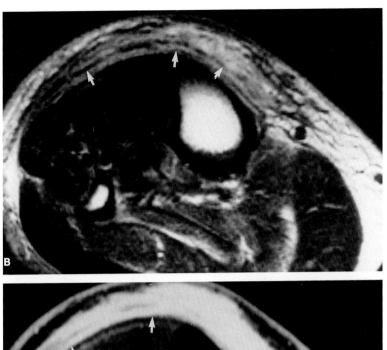

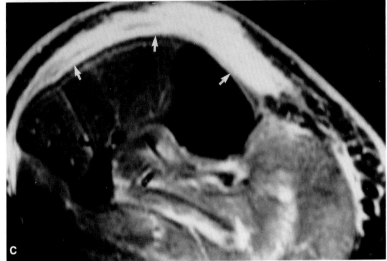

FIGURE 4–307. *(Continued)*

REFERENCES

1. Stoller DW, Genant HK. Magnetic resonance imaging of the knee and hip. Arthritis Rheum 1990;33(3):441.
2. Kursunoglu-Brahme S, Resnick D. Magnetic resonance imaging of the knee. Orthop Clin North Am 1990;21(3):561.
3. Mink JH, Deutsch AL. Magnetic resonance imaging of the knee. Clin Orthop 1989;244:29.
4. Burk DL Jr, Mitchell DG, Rifkin MD, Vinitski S. Recent advances in magnetic resonance imaging of the knee. Radiol Clin North Am 1990;28(2):379.
5. Reicher MA, et al. High resolution magnetic resonance imaging of the knee joint: normal anatomy. AJR 1985;145:895.
6. Reicher MA, et al. MR imaging of the knee. Part 1: traumatic disorders. Radiology 1987;162:547.
7. Hartzman MD, et al. MR imaging of the knee. Part II. Chronic disorders. Radiology 1987;162:553.
8. Buckwalter KA, Pennas DR. Anterior cruciate ligament: oblique sagittal MR imaging. Radiology 1990;175(1):276.
9. Adam G, Bohndorf K, Drobnitzky M, Guenther RW. MR imaging of the knee: three-dimensional volume imaging combined with fast processing. J Comput Assist Tomogr 1989;13(6):984.
10. Crues JV and Shellock FG. Technical considerations. In: Mink JH, Reicher MA, Crues JY, eds. Magnetic resonance imaging of the knee. New York: Raven Press, 1987:3.
11. Li DKB, et al. Magnetic resonance imaging of the ligaments and menisci of the knee. Radiol Clin North Am 1986;24:209.
12. Bessette GC, Hunter RE. The anterior cruciate ligament. Orthopaedics 1990;13(5):551.
13. Grigis FG, et al. The cruciate ligaments of the knee joint. Clin Orthop 1975;106:216.
14. Watanabe AT, et al. Normal variations in MR imaging of the knee: appearance and frequency. AJR 1987;153:341.
15. Stoller DW, et al. Meniscal tears: pathological correlation with MR imaging. Radiology 1987;163:452.
16. Stoller DW, et al. Gradient echo MR imaging of the knee. Radiology 1987;165(P).
17. Mandelbaum BR, et al. Magnetic resonance imaging as a tool for evaluation of traumatic knee injuries: anatomical and pathoanatomical correlations. Am J Sports Med 1986;14:361.

18. Harms SE, Flamig DP, Fisher CF, Fulmer JM. New method for fast MR imaging of the knee. Radiology 1989;173:743.

19. Spritzer CE, et al. MR imaging of the knee: preliminary results with a 3DFT GRASS pulse sequence. AJR 1988;150(3):597.

20. Arnoczky SP, et al. Microvasculature of the human meniscus. AM J Sports Med 1982;10:90.

21. Arnoczky SP, et al. The microvasculature of the meniscus and its response to injury. Am J Sports Med 1983;11:31.

22. Kaplan EB. The embryology of the menisci of the knee joint. Bull Hosp Joint Dis 1955;16:111.

23. Voto S. A nomenclature system for meniscal lesions of the knee. Surgical Rounds for Orthopaedics. 1989;October:34.

24. Chernye S. Disorders of the knee. In: Dee R, et al, eds. Principles of orthopaedic practice. vol 2. New York: McGraw-Hill, 1989: 1283.

25. Wilson R, et al. Arthroscopic anatomy. In: Scott W, et al, eds. Arthroscopy of the knee. Philadelphia: WB Saunders, 1990:49.

26. Yocum LA, et al. Isolated lateral meniscectomy: a study of 26 patients with isolated tears. J Bone Joint Surg [Am] 1979;61(3): 338.

27. Hallen L, et al. The "screw-home" movement in the knee joint. Acta Orthop Scand 1966;37:97.

28. Shaw JA, et al. The longitudinal axis of the knee and the role of the cruciate ligaments in controlling transverse rotation. J Bone Joint Surg [Am] 1974;56:1603.

29. Turek SL. Orthopaedics: principles and their applications, 4th ed. Philadelphia: JB Lippincott, 1984:1269.

30. Krause WR, et al. Mechanical changes in the knee after meniscectomy. J Bone Joint Surg [Am] 1976;58(5):599.

31. Warren RF, et al. Meniscal lesions associated with anterior cruciate ligament injury. Clin Orthop 1983;172:32.

32. Crues JV III, et al. Meniscal tears of the knee: accuracy of MR imaging. Radiology 1987;164:445.

33. Jackson DW, Jennings LD, Maywood RM, Berger PE. Magnetic resonance imaging of the knee. Am J Sports Med 1988;16(1):29.

34. Polly DW Jr, Callaghan JJ, Sikes RA, et al. The accuracy of selective magnetic resonance imaging compared with the findings of arthroscopy of the knee. J Bone Joint Surg [Am] 1988;70(2):192.

35. Glashow JL, Katz R, Schneider M, Scott W. Double-blind assessment of the value of magnetic resonance imaging in the diagnosis of anterior cruciate and meniscal lesions. J Bone Joint Surg [Am] 1989;71(1):113.

36. Crues JV, Ryu R, Morgan FW. Meniscal pathology. The expanding role of magnetic resonance imaging. Clin Orthop 1990;252:90.

37. Mink JH, et al. MR imaging of the knee: technical factors, diagnostic accuracy, and further pitfalls. Radiology 1987;165(P):175.

38. Tyrrell R, et al. Fast three-dimensional MR imaging of the knee: a comparison with arthroscopy. Radiology 1987;166:865.

39. Fischer SP, et al. Accuracy of diagnosis from magnetic resonance imaging of the knee. J Bone Joint Surg [Am] 1991;73(1):2.

40. Beltran J, et al. Meniscal tears: MR demonstration of experimentally produced injuries. Radiology 1986;158:691.

41. Koenig SH, et al. The importance of motion of water for magnetic resonance imaging. Invest Radiol 1985;20:297.

42. Tobler TH. Makroskopische und histologische Befund am kniegelnk Meniscus in verschiedenen Lebensaitern. Schweiz Med Wochenschr 1926;56:1359.

43. Roca FA, Vilalta A. Lesions of the meniscus. I: macroscopic and histologic findings. Clin Orthop 1980;146:289.

44. Roca FA, Vilalta A. Lesions of the meniscus. II: horizontal cleavages and lateral cysts. Clin Orthop 1980;146:301.

45. Kornick JK, et al. Meniscal abnormalities in the asymptomatic population at MR imaging. Radiology 1990;177:463.

46. Kursunoglu-Brahme S, et al. Jogging causes acute changes in the knee joint: an MR study in normal volunteers. AJR 1990;154(6): 1233.

47. Reinig JW, McDevitt ER, Ove PN. Progress of meniscal degenerative changes in collage football players: evaluation with MR imaging. Radiology 1991;181:255.

48. Smillie LS. Diseases of the knee joint. 2nd ed. London: Churchill-Livingstone, 1980:340.

49. Mink JH. The knee. In: Mink JH, Deutsch A, eds. MRI of the musculoskeletal system. A teaching file. 1990:251.

50. Ricklin P, et al. Meniscus lesions: diagnosis, differential diagnosis and therapy. 2nd ed. New York: Stratton, 1983.

51. Levinsohn ME, Baker BE. Prearthrotomy diagnostic evaluation of the knee: review of 100 cases diagnosed by arthrography and arthroscopy. AJR 1980;134:107.

52. Watts I, et al. Pitfalls in double contrast knee arthrography. Br J Radiol 1980;53:754.

53. Stoller DW, et al. Three dimensional rendering and classification of meniscal tears disarticulated from 3-D FT images. In: Abstracts of 9th Annual Scientific Meeting and Exhibition of the Society of Magnetic Resonance in Medicine. vol 1. New York: 1990:346.

54. Singson RD, et al. MR imaging of displaced bucket-handle tear of the medial meniscus. AJR 1991;156:121.

55. Weiss KL. Sagittal MR images of the knee: a low signal. AJR 1991;156:117.

56. Rosenberg TD. Arthroscopic diagnosis and treatment of meniscal disorders. In: Scott W, et al, eds. Arthroscopy of the knee. Philadelphia: WB Saunders, 1990:67.

57. Rosenberg TD, et al. Arthroscopic surgery of the knee. In: Chapman W, et al, eds. Operative orthopaedics. Philadelphia: JB Lippincott, 1988:1585.

58. Kaplan EB. Discoid lateral meniscus of the knee joint. J Bone Joint Surg [Am] 1957;39:77.

59. Dickason JM, et al. A series of ten discoid medial menisci. Clin Orthop 1982;168:75.

60. Weiner B, Rosenberg N. Discoid medial meniscus: associations with bone changes in the tibia. J Bone Joint Surg [Am] 1974;56: 171.

61. Barnes CL, McCarthy RE, VanderSchilden JL, McConnell JR. Discoid lateral meniscus in a young child: case report and review of the literature. J Pediatr Orthop 1988;8(6):707.

62. Howe MA, Buckwalter KA, Braunstein EM, Wojtys EM. Case report 483: discoid lateral meniscus (DLM), medially displaced with complex tear. Skeletal Radiol 1988;17(4):293.

63. Silverman JM, Mink JH, Deutsch AL. Discoid menisci of the knee: MR imaging appearance. Radiology 1989;173(2):351.

64. Mink JR, et al. MR imaging of the knee: pitfalls in interpretation. Radiology 1987;165(P):239.

65. Kaplan PA, et al. MR of the knee: the significance of high signal in the meniscus that does not clearly extend to the surface. AJR 1991;156:333.

66. Herman LJ, et al. Pitfalls in MR imaging of the knee. Radiology 1988;167(3):775.

67. Vahey TN, et al. MR imaging of the knee: pseudotear of the lateral meniscus caused by the meniscofemoral ligament. AJR 1990;154(6):1237.

68. Turner DA, Rapoport MI, Erwin WD, et al. Truncation artifact: a potential pitfall in MR imaging of the menisci of the knee. Radiology 1991;179:629.

69. Garrett JC, et al. Meniscal transplantation in the human knee: a preliminary report. Arthroscopy 1991;7(1):57.

70. Smith DK, et al. The knee after partial meniscectomy: MR imaging features. Radiology 1990;176(1):141.

71. Deutsch AL, et al. Peripheral meniscal tears: MR findings after conservative treatment of arthroscopic repair. Radiology 1990;176(2):485.

72. Gallimore GW, Harms SE. Knee injuries: high resolution MR imaging. Radiology 1986;160:457.

73. Burk DL, et al. Meniscal and ganglion cysts of the knee: MR evaluation. AJR 1988;150:331.

74. Coral A, et al. Imaging of the meniscal cyst of the knee in three cases. Skeletal Radiol 1989;18(6):451.

75. Strobel M. Anatomy, proprioception and biomechanics in diagnostic evaluation of the knee. Berlin: Springer-Verlag, 1990:2.

76. Kennedy JC, et al. The anatomy and function of the anterior cruciate ligament. J Bone Joint Surg [Am] 1974;56:223.

77. Feagin JA, Curl WW: Isolated tear of the anterior cruciate ligament: 5-year follow-up study. Am J Sports Med 1976;4:95.

78. Fetto JF, et al. The natural history and diagnosis of anterior cruciate ligament insufficiency. Clin Orthop 1980;147:29.

79. Kennedy JC, et al. The anatomy and function of the anterior cruciate ligament as determined by clinical and morphological studies. J Bone Joint Surg [Am] 1974;56:223.

80. Cerabona F, et al. Patterns of meniscal injury with acute anterior cruciate ligament tears. Am J Sports Med 1988;16(6):603.

81. Indelicato PA, et al. A perspective of lesions associated with ACL insufficiency of the knee. A review of 100 cases. Clin Orthop 1985;198:77.

82. Warren RF. Meniscectomy and repair in the anterior cruciate ligament-deficient patient. Clin Orthop 1990;242:55.

83. McDaniel WJ. Untreated ruptures of the anterior cruciate ligament. J Bone Joint Surg [Am] 1980;62:696.

84. Niitsu M, et al. Tears of the cruciate ligaments and menisci: evaluation with cine MR imaging. Radiology 1991;178:859.

85. Buckwalter KA, et al. Anterior cruciate ligament: oblique sagittal MR imaging. Radiology 1990;175:276.

86. Mesgarzadah M, et al. Magnetic resonance imaging of the knee and correlation with normal anatomy. Radiographics 1988;8(4):707.

87. Vellet AD, et al. Accuracy of nonorthogonal magnetic resonance imaging in acute disruption of the anterior cruciate ligament. Arthroscopy 1989;5(4):287.

88. Vahey TN, Broome DR, et al. Acute and chronic tears of the anterior cruciate ligament: differential features at MR imaging. Radiology 1991;181:251.

89. Weber WN, Neumann CH, Barakos JA, et al. Lateral tibial rim (Segond) fractures: MR imaging characteristics. Radiology 1991;180:731.

89a. Murphy BJ, Smith RL, et al. Bone signal abnormalities in the posterolateral tibia and lateral femoral condyle in complete tears of the anterior cruciate ligament: a specific sign? Radiology 1992;182:221.

90. Mink JH, et al. Tears of the anterior cruciate ligament and menisci of the knee: MR imaging evaluation. Radiology 1988;167:769.

91. Lee JK, et al. Anterior cruciate ligament tears: MR imaging compared with arthroscopy and clinical tests. Radiology 1988;166:861.

92. Karzel RP, et al. Arthroscopic diagnosis and treatment of cruciate and collateral ligament injuries. In: Scott W, et al, eds. Arthroscopy of the knee. Philadelphia: WB Saunders, 1990:131.

93. Boden BP, et al. Arthroscopically-assisted anterior cruciate ligament reconstruction: a follow-up study. Contemp Orthop 1990;20(2):187.

94. Arnoczky SP, et al. Replacement of the anterior cruciate ligament using patellar tendon allograft. J Bone Joint Surg [Am] 1986;68:376.

95. Fox JM, et al. Techniques and preliminary results in arthroscopic anterior cruciate prosthesis. Presented at the 53rd annual meeting of the American Academy of Orthopaedic Surgeons, New Orleans, February 20, 1986.

96. Zarins B, et al. Combined anterior cruciate ligament reconstruction using semitendinosus tendon and iliotibial tract. J Bone Joint Surg [Am] 1968;68:160.

97. Rak KM, et al. Anterior cruciate ligament reconstruction: evaluation with MR imaging. Radiology 1991;178:553.

98. Moeser P, et al. MR imaging of anterior cruciate ligament repair. J Comput Assist Tomogr 1989;13(1):105.

99. Fezoulidis I, et al. MRI of the status following augmentation plasty of the anterior cruciate ligament using carbon fibers. Radiology 1989;29(1):550.

100. Howell SM, Berns GS, Farley TE. Unimpinged and impinged anterior cruciate ligament grafts: MR signal intensity measurements. Radiology 1991;179:639.

101. Hughston JC, et al. Classification of knee ligament instabilities, part I: the medial compartment and cruciate ligaments. J Bone Joint Surg [Am] 1976;58:159.

102. Kennedy JC. The posterior cruciate ligament. J Trauma 1967;7:367.

103. Williams PL, et al. Gray's anatomy. 37th ed. Edinburgh: Churchill-Livingstone, 1989:527.

104. Clancy WG, et al. Treatment of knee joint instability secondary to rupture of the posterior cruciate ligament: report of a new procedure. J Bone Joint Surg [Am] 1983;65(3):310.

105. Kennedy JC, Grainger RW: The posterior cruciate ligament. J Trauma 1966;7(3):367.

106. Kennedy JC, et al. Tension studies of human knee ligament. J Bone Joint Surg [Am] 1976;58:350.

107. Turner, et al. Acute injury of the ligaments of the knee: magnetic resonance evaluation. Radiology 1985;154:717.

108. Loos WC, et al. Acute posterior cruciate ligament injuries. Am J Sports Med 1981;9(2):86.

109. Seebacher JR, et al. The structures of the postero-lateral aspect of the knee. J Bone Joint Surg [Am] 1982;64:536.

110. Hughston JC, et al. Acute tears of the posterior cruciate ligament: results of operative treatment. J Bone Joint Surg [Am] 1980;62(3):438.

111. Grover JS, et al. Posterior cruciate ligament: MR imaging. Radiology 1990;174:527.

112. Cherney S. The knee. In: Dee R, et al, eds. Principles of orthopaedic practice. New York: McGraw-Hill, 1989:1054.

113. Fetto JF, et al. Medial collateral ligament injuries of the knee: a rationale for treatment. Clin Orthop 1978;132:206.

114. Anderson JE eds. Grant's atlas of anatomy. Baltimore: Williams & Wilkins, 1983.

115. Indelicato PA, et al. Nonoperative management of complete tears of the medial collateral ligament. Orthop Rev. 1989;18(8):947.

116. Kennedy JC, et al. Medial and anterior instability of the knee. An anatomical and clinical study using stress machines. J Bone Joint Surg [Am] 1971;53:1257.

117. Stoller DW, Mink J. MRI detection of knee fractures. American Roentgen Ray Society (abstracts). Miami, Florida, April 15–May 1, 1987.

118. Lee JK, et al. Tibial collateral ligament bursa: MR imaging. Radiology 1991;178:855.

119. Resnick D, Niwayama G. Diagnosis of bone and joint disorders. 2nd ed. vol 3. Philadelphia: WB Saunders, 1988:1455.

120. Outerbridge RE. The etiology of chondromalacia patellae. J Bone Joint Surg [Br] 1961;43:752.

121. Lombardo SJ, Bradley JP. Arthroscopic diagnosis and treatment of patellofemoral disorders. In: Scott W, et al, eds. Arthroscopy of the knee. Philadelphia: WB Saunders, 1990:155.

122. Stoller DW. MRI of the patella and patellofemoral joint. Presented to the American Roentgen Ray Society, San Francisco, California, May 8, 1988.

123. Yulish BS, et al. Chondromalacia patellae: assessment with MR imaging. Radiology 1987;164:763.

124. Conway WF, Hayes CW, et al. Cross-sectional imaging of the patellofemoral joint and surrounding structures. RadioGraphics 1991;11:195.

125. Hayes CW, et al. Patellar cartilage lesions: in vitro detection and staging with MR imaging and pathologic correlation. Radiology 1990;176:479.

126. Resnick D, Niwayama GL. Diagnosis of bone and joint disorders. 2nd ed. vol 5. Philadelphia: WB Saunders, 1988:2896.

127. Resnick D, Niwayama GL. Diagnosis of bone and joint disorders. 2nd ed. vol 5. Philadelphia: WB Saunders, 1988:722.

128. Shellock FG, et al. Technical developments and instrumentation. Radiology 1988;168:551.

129. Shellock FG, et al. Patellar tracking abnormalities: clinical experience with kinematic MR imaging in 130 patients. Radiology 1989;172:799.

130. Nitsu M, et al. Moving knee joint: technique for kinematic MR imaging. Radiology 1990;174:569.

131. Rockwood CA, Green CP, eds. Fractures. Philadelphia: JB Lippincott, 1975.

132. Bodne D, et al. Magnetic resonance imaging of chronic patellar tendinis. Skeletal Radiol 1988;17:24.

133. Weissman BNW, Sledge CB. Orthopaedic radiology. Philadelphia: WB Saunders, 1986;497.

134. Grelsamer RP, Cartier P. Comprehensive approach to patellar pathology. Orthopaedics 1990;20(5):493.

135. Stoller DW, Genant HK. MR Imaging of knee arthritides. Radiology 1987;165(P):233.

136. Chandnani VP, Ho C, et al. Knee hyaline cartilage evaluated with MR imaging: a cadaveric study involving multiple imaging sequences and intraarticular injection of gadolinium and saline solution. Radiology 1991;178:557.

137. Björkengren AG, Geborek P, Rydholm U, et al. MR imaging of the knee in acute rheumatoid arthritis: synovial uptake of gadolinium-DOTA. AJR 1990;155:329.

138. Stoller DW. MRI in juvenile rheumatoid (chronic) arthritis. Presented to the Association of University Radiologists, Charleston, South Carolina, March 22, 1987.

139. Konig H, et al. Rheumatoid arthritis: evaluation of hypervascular and fibrous pannus with dynamic MR imaging enhanced with Gd-DTPA. Radiology 1990;176:473.

140. Adam G, et al. Rheumatoid arthritis of the knee: value of gadopentetate dimeglumine-enhanced MR imaging. AJR 1991;156:125.

141. Stoller DW, Genant HK. MRI of pigmented villonodular synovitis. American Roentgen Ray Society (abstracts). San Francisco, California, May 8, 1988.

142. Kottal RA, et al. Pigmented villonodular synovitis: report of MR imaging in two cases. Radiology 1987;163:551.

143. Poletti SC, et al. The use of magnetic resonance imaging in the diagnosis of pigmented villonodular synovitis. Orthopaedics 1990;13(2):185.

144. Kulkarni MV, et al. MR imaging of hemophiliac arthropathy. J Comput Assist Tomogr 1986;10:445.

145. Yulish BS, et al. Hemophilic arthropathy: assessment with MR imaging. Radiology 1987;164:759.

146. Johnston YE, et al. Lyme arthritis: spirochetes found in synovial microangiopathic lesions. Am J Pathol 1985;118:26.

147. Kindynis P, et al. Osteophytosis of the knee: anatomic, radiologic and pathologic investigation. Radiology 1990;174:841.

148. Elia EA, Lotke PA, Ecker ML. Unicondylar arthroplasty for osteoarthritis of the knee. Surgical Rounds for Orthopaedics. January 17, 1990.

149. Burk DL, et al. 1.5T surface-coil MRI of the knee. AJR 1986;147:293.

150. Williams JL, et al. Spontaneous osteonecrosis of the knee. Radiology 1973;107:15.

151. Lotke PA, Ecker ML. Osteonecrosis-like syndrome of the medial tibial plateau. Clin Orthop 1983;176:148.

152. Bjorkengren AG, et al. Spontaneous osteonecrosis of the knee: value of MR imaging in determining prognosis. AJR 1990;154:331.

153. Kursunoglu-Brahme S, et al. Osteonecrosis of the knee after arthroscopic surgery: diagnosis with MR imaging. Radiology 1991;178:851.

154. Linden B. The incidence of osteochondritis dissecans in the condyles of the femur. Acta Orthop Scand 1976;47:664.

155. Mesgarzadah M, et al. Osteochondritis dissecans: analysis of mechanical stability with radiography, scintigraphy and MR imaging. Radiology 1987;165:775.

156. Resnick D, Niwayama G. Diagnosis of bone and joint disorders. 2nd ed. vol 5. Philadelphia: WB Saunders, 1988:3313.

157. De Smet AA, et al. Osteochondritis dissecans of the knee: value of MR imaging in determining lesion stability and presence of articular cartilage defects. AJR 1990;155:549.

158. Guerra J, et al. Gastrocnemius-semimembranosus bursal region of the knee. AJR 1981;136:593.

159. Lindgree PG, Willen R. Gastrocnemius-semimembranosus bursa and its relation to the knee joint. Anatomy and histology. Acta Radiol (Diagn) 1977;18:497.

160. Edmonson AS, Crenshaw AH, eds. Campbell's operative orthopaedics. vol 2. St. Louis: CV Mosby, 1980:1408.

161. Apple JS, et al. Synovial plicae of the knee. Skeletal Radiol 1982;7:251.

162. Calvo RD, et al. Managing plica syndrome of the knee. Phys Sports Med 1990;18(7):64.

163. Berquist TH. Imaging of orthopaedic trauma and surgery. Philadelphia: WB Saunders, 1986:293.

164. Jaramillo D, et al. Posttraumatic growth-plate abnormalities: MR imaging of bony-bridge formation in rabbits. Radiology 1990;175:767.

165. Mink JH, et al. Occult cartilage and bone injuries of the knee: detection, classification and assessment with MR imaging. Radiology 1989;170:823.

166. Vellet AD, et al. Occult posttraumatic osteochondral lesions of the knee: prevalence, classification and short-term sequelae evaluated with MR imaging. Radiology 1991;178:271.

167. Lynch TCP, et al. Bone abnormalities of the knee: prevalence and significance of MR imaging. Radiology 1989;171:761.

168. Hohl M. Managing the challenge of tibial plateau fractures. J Musc Med 1991;October:70.

169. Berquist TH, et al. Magnetic resonance imaging of the musculoskeletal system. New York: Raven Press, 1987;127.

170. Kressel HY, ed. Magnetic resonance imaging annual. New York: Raven Press, 1986;1.

171. Resnick D, Niwayama G. Diagnosis of bone and joint disorders. 2nd ed. vol 1. Philadelphia: WB Saunders, 1988:228.

172. Resnick D, Niwayama G. Diagnosis of bone and joint disorders. 2nd ed. vol 1. Philadelphia: WB Saunders, 1988:2037.

173. Roberts MC, et al. Paget disease: MR imaging findings. Radiology 1989;173:341.

174. Erdman WA, Tamburro F, Jayson HT, et al. Osteomyelitis: characteristics and pitfalls of diagnosis with MR imaging. Radiology 1991;180:533.

C H A P T E R 5

David W. Stoller

The Ankle and Foot

Standard radiographic evaluation of the ankle joint requires anteroposterior (AP), lateral, and mortise radiographs. In patients with foot trauma, an additional oblique view may be obtained. Less frequently, arthrography and tonography may be used, primarily in the evaluation of ligamentous tears and articular cartilage defects. In tarsal coalitions and sustentacular trauma, computed tomography (CT) scans have been used to delineate talocalcaneal, transverse tarsal, and tibiotalar joint anatomy.[1]

Computed tomography is limited, however, to the specific plane of section (*i.e.,* axial or angled coronal) and is dependent on reformatted images for visualization in the other orthogonal planes. Magnetic resonance (MR) imaging of the ankle and foot provides high tissue contrast and excellent spatial resolution, affording superior depiction of complex soft-tissue anatomy (*e.g.,* muscles, ligaments, tendons).[2-8] In addition, marrow and cortical bone definition permit increased sensitivity in the detection of fractures, cysts, infections, and trauma.[9] The unique ability of MR to directly display hyaline articular cartilage has made it valuable in assessing arthritis and transchondral fractures and in identifying intraarticular loose bodies.

IMAGING PROTOCOLS FOR THE ANKLE AND FOOT

High resolution anatomic images of the ankle and foot are obtained with a dedicated extremity surface coil using a 12- to 16-cm field of view (FOV) and a 256 × 256 (192) acquisition matrix (Fig. 5–1). Routine T1-weighted axial, sagittal, and coronal images are obtained with a repetition time (TR) of 500 to 600 msec and an echo time (TE) of 15 to 20 msec. Thin (*i.e.,* 3- to 4-mm) sections, either contiguous interleaved or with a 1-mm interslice gap, are preferred. T2-weighted axial protocols are obtained with a TR of 2000 msec and a TE of 20 and 80 msec. With the use of an extremity or head coil to optimize the signal-to-noise ratio, T1- and T2-weighted sequences can be performed at 1 excitation.

Effective T2*-weighted contrast can be generated from a T2-weighted image with gradient-echo techniques using a partial flip angle of less than 90° (20° to 30°). Two-dimensional Fourier transform (2DFT) multiplanar gradient-echo protocols use a TR of 400 to 600 msec, a TE of 15 to 20 msec, and a flip angle of 20° to 30°. Coronal or sagittal plane images are preferred with a T2*-weighted protocol. Axial three-dimensional Fourier transform (3DFT) T2*-volume images with a 1- to 2-mm slice thickness have been used to evaluate medial or lateral ligamentous structures. Short TI inversion recovery (STIR) images provide superior contrast in evaluating transchondral fractures, bone contusions, and tendinitis.

To image the forefoot, the patient is placed in a prone position to orient the long axis of the foot with the orthogonal axial imaging plane or with the oblique image prescriptions parallel with the long axes of the metatarsals and cuneiform bones.

By placing both legs within the circular extremity coil, comparison with the contralateral ankle and foot can be achieved. Alternatively, when smaller FOVs are needed, the extremities may be imaged one at a time by repositioning the surface coil. The foot is usually placed in a neutral position, although partial plantar flexion may be useful when comparing MR images to a CT ankle examination that was performed with 45° of tibiotalar angulation. A wrist coil provides adequate anatomic coverage for imaging the toes and distal metatarsal. Thin (*i.e.,* 3-mm) axial T1- and T2*-weighted or STIR images are most useful. Kinematic techniques are used in inversion and eversion in the coronal plane, plantar and dorsiflexion in the sagittal plane, and internal or external rotation in the coronal or axial planes (Fig. 5–2). Re-

stricted range of motion, ligamentous instabilities, and tendon subluxations may necessitate the use of kinematic protocols (Figs. 5–3 and 5–4).

ANATOMY OF THE ANKLE AND FOOT

Gross Anatomy

Compartments of the Leg

Anterior and posterior intermuscular septa and the interosseous membrane define the three major compartments of the lower leg (Fig. 5–5). The anterior compartment of the leg consists of the tibialis anterior, the extensor hallucis longus, the extensor digitorum longus, and the peroneus tertius muscles. The neurovascular bundle contains the deep peroneal nerve and the anterior tibial artery. The posterior compartment is divided into superficial and deep sections by deep transverse fascia. The superficial posterior compartment consists of the gastrocnemius, plantaris, and soleus muscles. The deep posterior compartment contains the popliteus, flexor digitorum longus, flexor hallucis longus, and tibialis posterior muscles. The neurovascular supply is provided by the tibial nerve and posterior tibial artery. The anterolateral compartment contains the peroneus longus and peroneus brevis muscles. The neurovascular supply is from the superficial peroneal nerve and branches of the peroneal artery.

Distal Tibiofibular Joint

The distal or inferior tibiofibular joint is a fibrous joint strongly connected by the interosseous ligament, which is continuous with the crural interosseous membrane (Fig. 5–6). The stronger anterior and posterior tibiofibular ligaments reinforce the joint anterior and posterior to the interosseous ligament. The inferior transverse ligament represents the distal deep fibers of the posterior tibiofibular ligament.

Ankle Joint

The ankle or tibiotalar joint is a synovial articulation formed by the distal tibia and fibula. It is often described as a hinge joint between the talus and the mortise (Fig. 5–7); however, the apex of rotation of the ankle joint is not fixed, as in a simple hinge joint. In fact, the apex of rotation changes during extremes of plantar flexion and dorsiflexion. The articular surfaces of the tibiotalar joint are covered with hyaline cartilage (Fig. 5–8). The fibrous capsule attaches to the articular margins of the tibia, fibula, and talus, with an anterior extension onto the talar neck. The capsule, which is thin anteriorly and posteri-

(text continues on page 381)

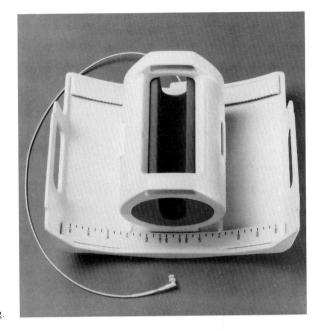

FIGURE 5–1. An extremity coil is used for ankle and foot imaging.

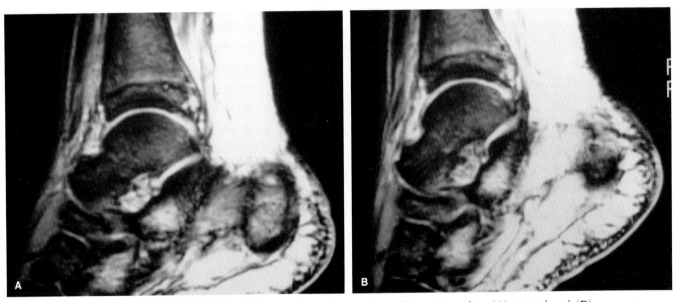

FIGURE 5–2. Kinematic imaging is performed with the ankle positioned in (**A**) neutral and (**B**) extreme plantar flexion. T2*-weighted sagittal images provide the best contrast.

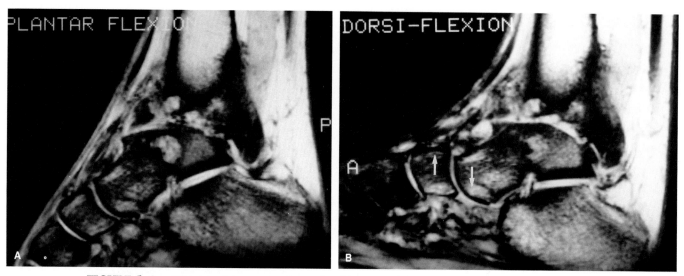

FIGURE 5–3. Tibiotalar joint motion is restricted between (**A**) plantar flexion and (**B**) dorsiflexion. Note the relative motion (*arrows*) at the talonavicular joint in dorsiflexion as seen on T2*-weighted images.

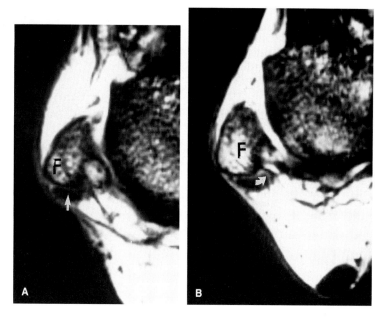

FIGURE 5–4. T2*-weighted axial images show normal movement of the peroneal tendons from (**A**) eversion to (**B**) inversion. A shallow peroneal groove or notch may result in tendon subluxation. (F, fibula.)

FIGURE 5–5. A transverse section through the midcalf shows the anterior and lateral compartments and their contents.

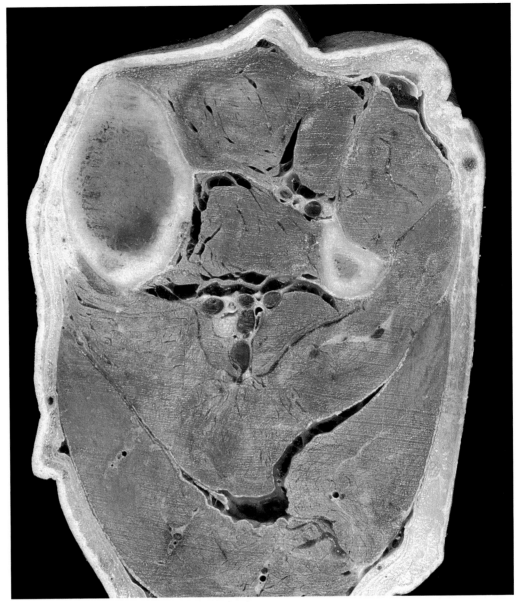

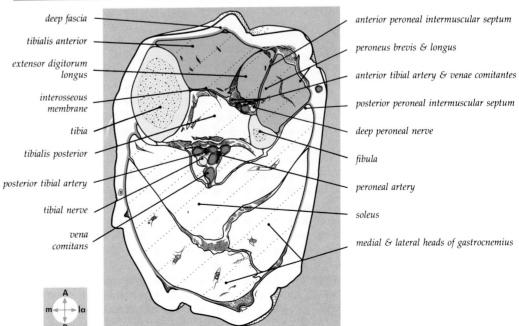

deep fascia

tibialis anterior

extensor digitorum
longus

interosseous
membrane

tibia

tibialis posterior

posterior tibial artery

tibial nerve

vena
comitans

anterior peroneal intermuscular septum

peroneus brevis & longus

anterior tibial artery & venae comitantes

posterior peroneal intermuscular septum

deep peroneal nerve

fibula

peroneal artery

soleus

medial & lateral heads of gastrocnemius

A
m ⟷ la
P

FIGURE 5–5.

377

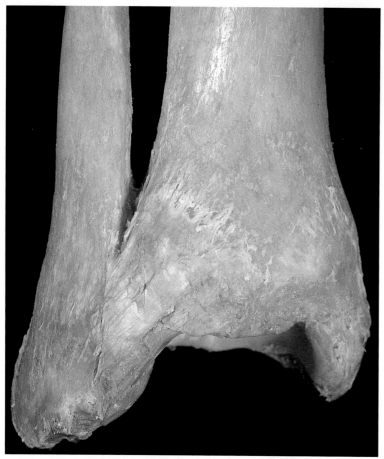

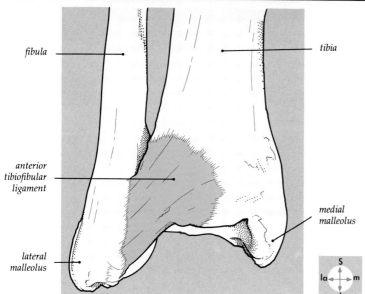

FIGURE 5-6. The inferior tibiofibular joint is a fibrous joint.

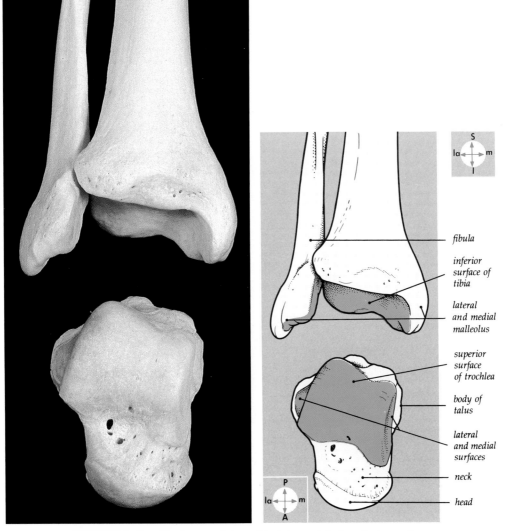

FIGURE 5–7. The bones of the ankle joint and their articular surfaces.

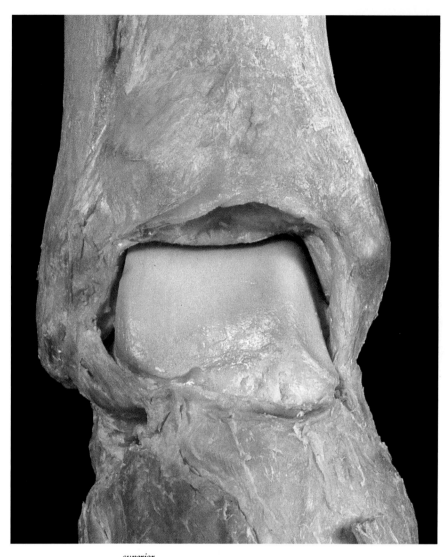

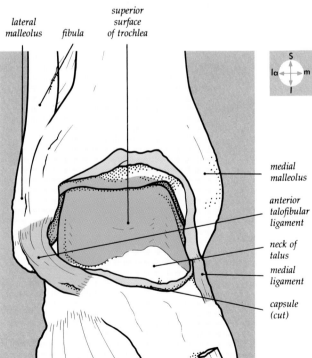

lateral malleolus   *fibula*   *superior surface of trochlea*

medial malleolus

anterior talofibular ligament

neck of talus

medial ligament

capsule (cut)

FIGURE 5–8. An anterior view of the ankle joint and its articular surfaces is revealed by removal of the capsule.

orly, is reinforced by strong collateral ligaments. The socket, framed by the distal tibia and medial and lateral malleoli, is wider anteriorly than posteriorly and is completed posteriorly by the transverse tibiofibular ligament (Fig. 5–9). The synovial membrane is attached to all articular margins and covers the intracapsular part of the talar neck.

Ligaments

Deltoid Ligament. The medial or deltoid ligament is a strong band attached by its apex to the border of the medial malleolus (Fig. 5–10). The triangular, superficial part of the deltoid is formed by the tibionavicular fibers anteriorly, the tibiocalcaneal fibers medially, and the posterior tibiotalar fibers posteriorly. Behind the navicular tuberosity, tibionavicular fibers blend with the medial margin of the plantar calcaneonavicular or spring ligament. The deep part of the deltoid, which is rectangular, consists of the anterior tibiotalar fibers (Fig. 5–11).

Lateral Ligament. Three distinct bands make up the weaker lateral ligament of the ankle (Fig. 5–12). These ligamentous bands are the anterior talofibular ligament, the calcaneofibular ligament, and the posterior talofibular ligament. The posterior tibiofibular ligament lies superior to the horizontally oriented posterior talofibular ligament. The inferior part of the posterior tibiofibular ligament is also referred to as the inferior transverse ligament (Figs. 5–13 and 5–14). In dorsiflexion, the posterior talofibular and tibiofibular ligaments diverge like the blades of a scissors, and in plantar flexion, they lie edge to edge.

Tarsal Joints

Subtalar Joint. The subtalar or talocalcaneal joint is the posterior articulation between the talus and the calcaneus. Functionally, the subtalar joint includes the talocalcaneal part of the talocalcaneonavicular joint (Fig. 5–15). The strong talocalcaneal or interosseous ligament attaches to the sulcus tali and sulcus calcanei. The capsule is strengthened by the medial and lateral talocalcaneal ligaments.

Talocalcaneonavicular Joint. The talocalcaneonavicular joint is a multiaxial articulation between the triple-faceted anterior–inferior talar surface with the talar head, the posterior concavity of the navicular bone, the middle and anterior talar facets of the calcaneus, and the fibrocartilaginous superior surface of the plantar calcaneonavicular (*i.e.,* spring) ligament (see Fig. 5–15). The talonavicular, plantar calcaneonavicular, and calcaneonavicular parts of the bifurcated ligament support the osseous components of this joint.

Calcaneocuboid Joint. The calcaneocuboid joint is a separate joint with its own capsule between the anterior calcaneus and the posterior surface of the cuboid. The calcaneocuboid and talonavicular part of the talocalcaneonavicular joint forms the midtarsal joint (Fig. 5–16). Support is provided by the fibrous capsule, the calcaneocuboid part of the bifurcated ligament, and the long plantar and plantar calcaneocuboid (*i.e.,* short plantar) ligaments. The bifurcated ligament is a strong, Y-shaped ligament on the dorsal surface of the joint, with attachments to the anterior dorsal calcaneal surface proximally, and to the dorsomedial aspect of the cuboid and dorsolateral aspect of the navicular bone distally. The long plantar ligament is a strong ligament located along the plantar surface. It is attached to the undersurface of the calcaneus, the cuboid, and the bases of the 3rd, 4th, and 5th metatarsal bones. A tunnel for the peroneus longus is created as it bridges the tendon's groove on the cuboid's plantar surface. The plantar calcaneocuboid, or short plantar ligament, is a wide, short band attached to the anterior tubercle on the plantar aspect of the calcaneus and the adjacent surface of the cuboid.

Other Tarsal Joints. The cuneonavicular synovial joint is formed by the navicular bone and the three cuneiform bones (see Fig. 5–16). The cuboideonavicular joint is a fibrous joint. The intercuneiform and cuneocuboid joints are synovial joints continuous with the cuneonavicular joint cavity.

Regional Anatomy of the Ankle

Retinacula

The extensor (Fig. 5–17) and flexor retinacula (Fig. 5–18) are formed by thickened deep fascia and maintain the position of long tendons crossing the ankle. The superior extensor retinaculum attaches to the distal anterior fibula and tibia and invests the tibialis anterior tendon medially. The Y-shaped inferior extensor retinaculum attaches to the anterolateral part of the calcaneus (*i.e.,* stem) and extends to the medial malleolus (*i.e.,* upper limb) and medial plantar fascia (*i.e.,* lower limb; see Fig. 5–17). The tibialis anterior, the extensor hallucis longus, the extensor digitorum longus, and the peroneus tertius tendons divide the upper limb of the retinaculum into superficial and deep layers. The flexor retinaculum extends inferiorly and posteriorly from the medial malleolus to the medial calcaneal surface (see Fig. 5–18). The tendons of the deep calf muscles (*e.g.,* flexor digitorum longus, flexor hallucis longus, and tibialis posterior) and the neurovascular structures in the posterior compartment pass underneath the flexor retinaculum before entering the foot.

The superior peroneal retinaculum extends inferiorly and posteriorly from the lateral malleolus to the lateral calcaneal surface, binding the peroneus longus and brevis tendons (see Fig. 5–17). The inferior peroneal retinaculum is attached to the peroneal trochlea and calcaneus above and below the peroneal tendons.

Anterior Structures. The saphenous nerve, the great saphenous vein, and the medial and lateral branches of the superficial peroneal nerve pass anterior to the extensor retinaculum in a medial-to-lateral direction. The tibialis anterior tendon, the extensor hallucis longus tendon, the anterior tibial artery with venae comitantes, the deep peroneal nerve, the extensor digitorum longus tendon, and the peroneus tertius pass deep to or through the extensor retinaculum in a medial-to-lateral direction (Figs. 5–19 and 5–20).

Posterior Structures. The tibialis posterior tendon, the flexor digitorum longus, the posterior tibial artery with venae comitantes, the tibial nerve, and the flexor hallucis longus flow in a medial-to-lateral direction and are located posterior to the medial malleolus and deep to the flexor retinaculum (see Fig. 5–20). The sural nerve and the small saphenous vein pass posterior to the lateral malleolus, superficial to the superior peroneal retinaculum. The peroneus longus and brevis tendons course posterior to the lateral malleolus deep to the superior peroneal retinaculum (see Fig. 5–20). The pre-Achilles fat pad and the Achilles tendon are located posterior to the ankle.

Foot

Muscles of the Sole of the Foot

Deep to the plantar aponeurosis (Fig. 5–21), the muscles of the sole of the foot are divided into four layers from superficial to deep. The first layer consists of the abductor hallucis, the flexor digitorum brevis, and the abductor digiti minimi (Fig. 5–22). The second layer consists of the quadratus plantae, the lumbricals, the flexor digitorum longus tendons, and the flexor hallucis longus tendons (Fig. 5–23). The third layer includes the flexor hallucis brevis, the adductor hallucis, and the flexor digiti minimi brevis (Fig. 5–24). The fourth layer is made up of the interossei plantares (Fig. 5–25), the peroneus longus tendon, and the tibialis posterior tendon (Fig. 5–26).

Arches of the Foot

The arches of the foot provide support for bipedal motion and forward propulsion. The medial and lateral longitudinal arches are formed by the tarsal and meta-

tarsal bones (Fig. 5–27). The higher, medial arch, which forms the instep of the foot, is formed by the calcaneus, the talus, the navicular, the three cuneiform bones, and the medial three metatarsals (see Fig. 5–27; Fig. 5–28). The plantar calcaneonavicular (*i.e.,* spring) ligament helps support the head of the talus, which articulates with the navicular anteriorly and the sustentaculum tali posteriorly (Fig. 5–29). The lateral arch consists of the calcaneus, the cuboid, and the lateral two metatarsals. Body weight is transmitted through the anterior and posterior pillars of the arches. The posterior pillar of the medial and lateral arches are the tubercles on the inferior calcaneal surface. The anterior pillars of the medial and lateral arches are formed by their respective metatarsal heads. The transverse arch of the foot consists of the five metatarsal bones and the adjacent cuboid bones and cuneiform bones.

Metatarsophalangeal and Interphalangeal Joints of the Foot

The metatarsophalangeal joints are ball-and-socket articulations between the metatarsal head and the base of the proximal phalanx and the fibrocartilaginous plantar plate (Figs. 5–30 through 5–32). The interphalangeal joints are hinge joints that permit flexion and extension (see Fig. 5–30; Fig. 5–33).

Normal Magnetic Resonance Appearance of the Ankle and Foot

Axial Images

In the axial plane, the low signal intensity bands of the anterior and posterior tibiofibular ligaments are demonstrated at the level of the tibial plafond (Fig. 5–34). The inferior extensor retinaculum is identified anterior to and at its attachment to the medial malleolus, and represents the upper limb of this Y-shaped band of deep fascia. On axial images through the tibiotalar joint, the tendons of the tibialis anterior, extensor hallucis longus, extensor digitorum longus, and peroneus tertius muscles occupy the anterior compartments in a medial-to-lateral direction. The peroneus brevis muscle and tendon and the more lateral peroneus longus tendon are located posterior to the lateral malleolus. The tendons of the tibialis posterior, flexor digitorum longus, and flexor hallucis longus can be identified posteriorly, running from a medial position posterior to the medial malleolus to a lateral position posterior to the tibial plafond and talar dome. Posterior and medial to the greater saphenous vein, the anterior tibionavicular fibers of the deltoid ligament blend with the low signal cortex of the anterior surface of the medial malleolus.

The Achilles tendon is identified in cross section as a

(text continues on page 417)

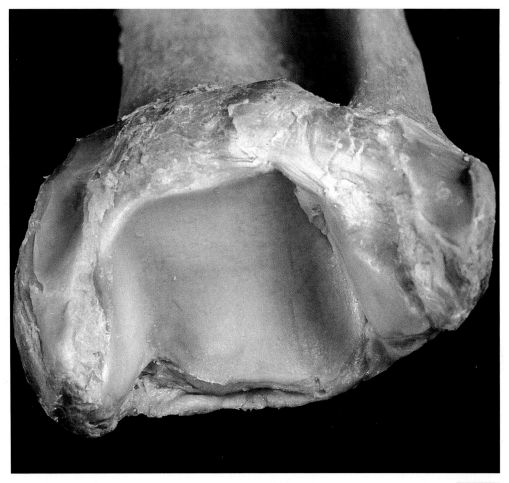

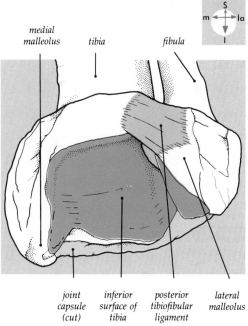

FIGURE 5–9. An oblique view of the wedge-shaped articular socket of the ankle joint.

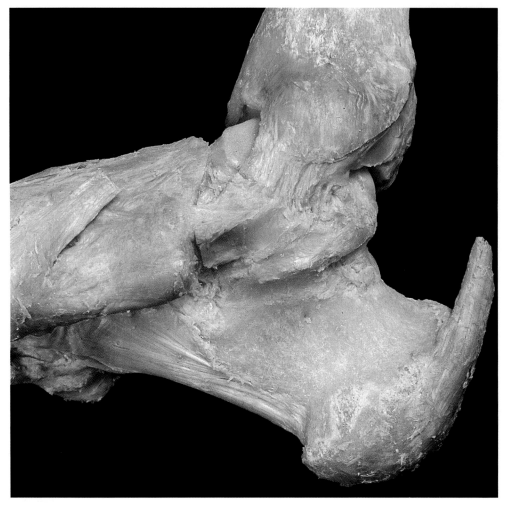

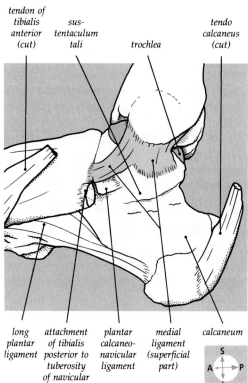

tendon of tibialis anterior (cut)   sus-tentaculum tali   trochlea   tendo calcaneus (cut)

long plantar ligament   attachment of tibialis posterior to tuberosity of navicular   plantar calcaneo-navicular ligament   medial ligament (superficial part)   calcaneum

FIGURE 5–10. The medial collateral ligament of the ankle joint can be seen after removal of the capsule.

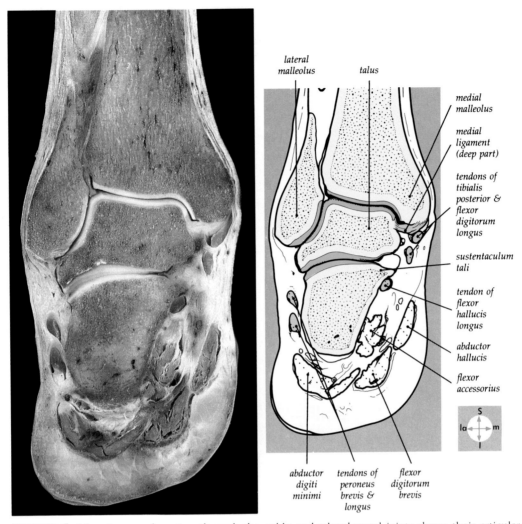

FIGURE 5–11. A coronal section through the ankle and talocalcaneal joints shows their articular surfaces.

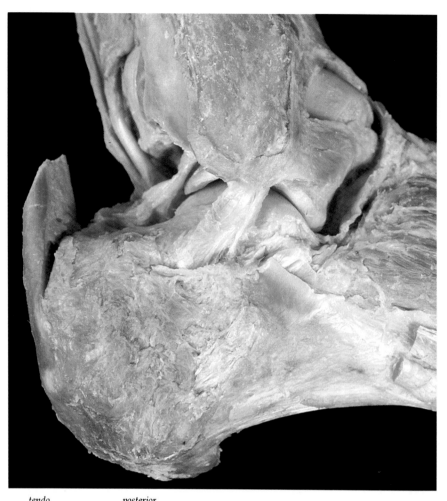

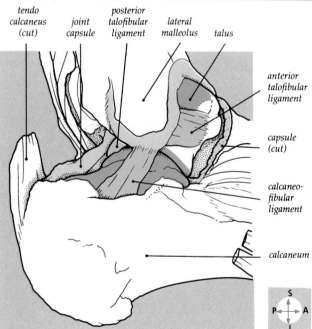

tendo calcaneus (cut)

joint capsule

posterior talofibular ligament

lateral malleolus

talus

anterior talofibular ligament

capsule (cut)

calcaneo-fibular ligament

calcaneum

FIGURE 5–12. The lateral collateral ligament of the ankle joint can be seen after removal of the capsule.

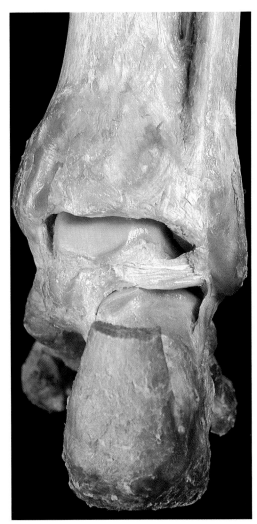

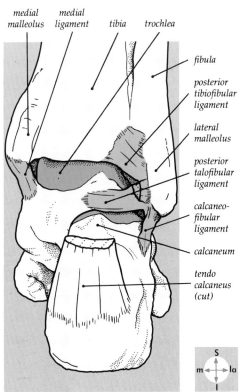

medial
malleolus | medial
ligament | tibia | trochlea

fibula

posterior
tibiofibular
ligament

lateral
malleolus

posterior
talofibular
ligament

calcaneo-
fibular
ligament

calcaneum

tendo
calcaneus
(cut)

FIGURE 5–13. The posterior view of the ankle joint shows the articular surface of the talus after removal of the capsule.

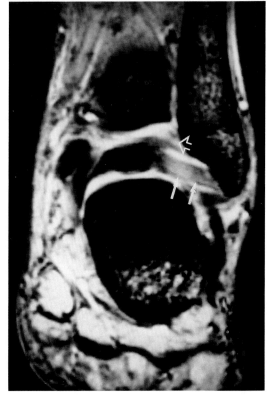

FIGURE 5–14. Transverse tibiofibular (*open arrow*) and posterior talofibular (*solid arrows*) ligaments are seen on a T2*-weighted coronal image.

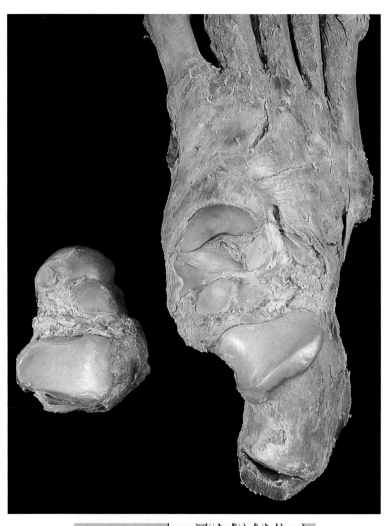

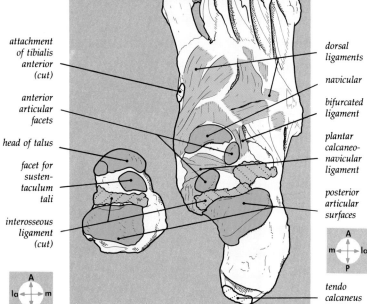

attachment
of tibialis
anterior
(cut)

anterior
articular
facets

head of talus

facet for
susten-
taculum
tali

interosseous
ligament
(cut)

dorsal
ligaments

navicular

bifurcated
ligament

plantar
calcaneo-
navicular
ligament

posterior
articular
surfaces

tendo
calcaneus
(cut)

FIGURE 5–15. In this gross photograph of the talocal-caneal and talonavicular joints, the talus has been disarticulated and turned over.

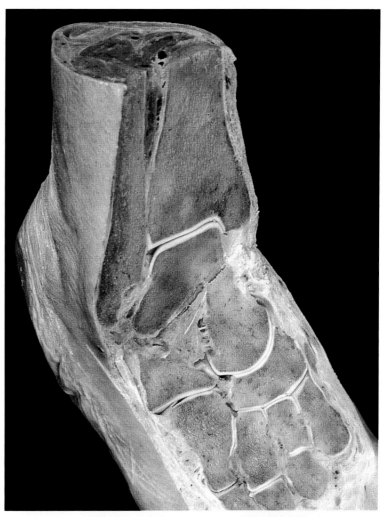

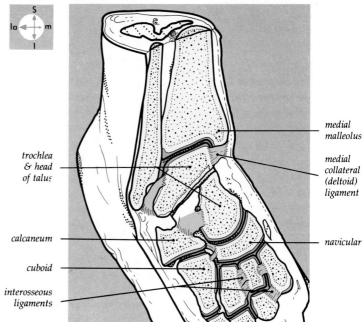

FIGURE 5–16. Vertical and horizontal sectioning of the foot and ankle reveals the interrelationships of the tarsal joints.

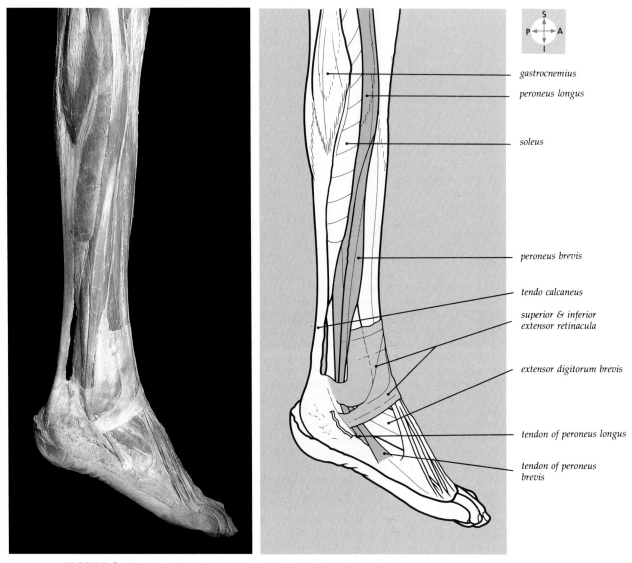

FIGURE 5–17. The lateral aspect of the ankle and foot shows the peroneal tendons and the retinacula.

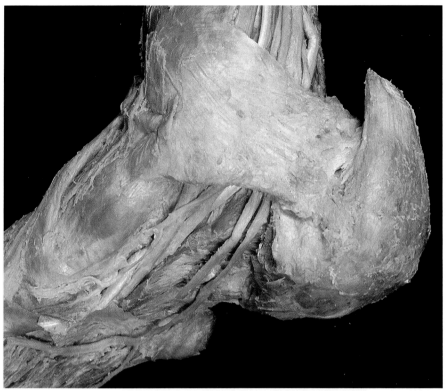

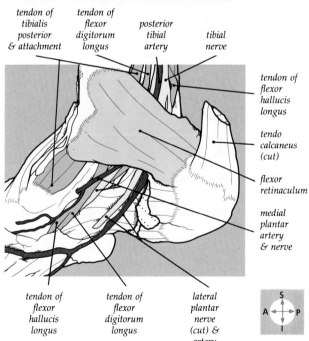

tendon of tibialis posterior & attachment

tendon of flexor digitorum longus

posterior tibial artery

tibial nerve

tendon of flexor hallucis longus

tendo calcaneus (cut)

flexor retinaculum

medial plantar artery & nerve

tendon of flexor hallucis longus

tendon of flexor digitorum longus

lateral plantar nerve (cut) & artery

FIGURE 5–18. The long tendons and the principal vessels and nerves from the posterior compartment of the leg pass deep to the flexor retinaculum to enter the sole of the foot.

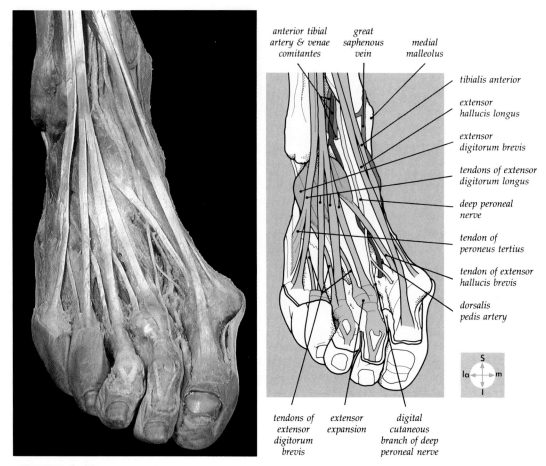

anterior tibial
artery & venae
comitantes

great
saphenous
vein

medial
malleolus

tibialis anterior

extensor
hallucis longus

extensor
digitorum brevis

tendons of extensor
digitorum longus

deep peroneal
nerve

tendon of
peroneus tertius

tendon of extensor
hallucis brevis

dorsalis
pedis artery

tendons of
extensor
digitorum
brevis

extensor
expansion

digital
cutaneous
branch of deep
peroneal nerve

FIGURE 5–19. Principal structures in the dorsum of the ankle and foot can be seen after removal of the extensor retinaculum.

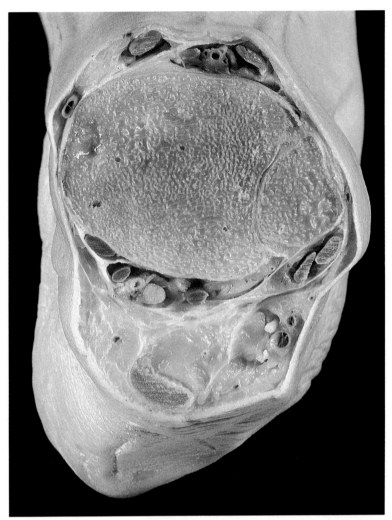

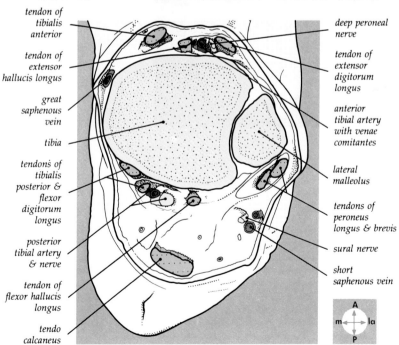

tendon of
tibialis
anterior

tendon of
extensor
hallucis longus

great
saphenous
vein

tibia

tendons of
tibialis
posterior &
flexor
digitorum
longus

posterior
tibial artery
& nerve

tendon of
flexor hallucis
longus

tendo
calcaneus

deep peroneal
nerve

tendon of
extensor
digitorum
longus

anterior
tibial artery
with venae
comitantes

lateral
malleolus

tendons of
peroneus
longus & brevis

sural nerve

short
saphenous vein

FIGURE 5–20. A transverse section through the ankle immediately above the joint cavity shows its anterior and posterior relations.

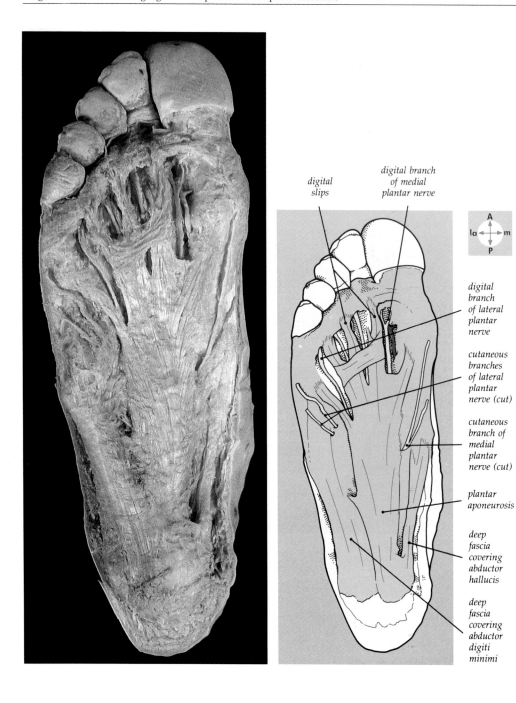

FIGURE 5-21. Plantar aponeurosis, deep fascia, and a cutaneous nerve are revealed by removing the skin of the sole of the foot.

Labels on figure:
digital slips
digital branch of medial plantar nerve
digital branch of lateral plantar nerve
cutaneous branches of lateral plantar nerve (cut)
cutaneous branch of medial plantar nerve (cut)
plantar aponeurosis
deep fascia covering abductor hallucis
deep fascia covering abductor digiti minimi

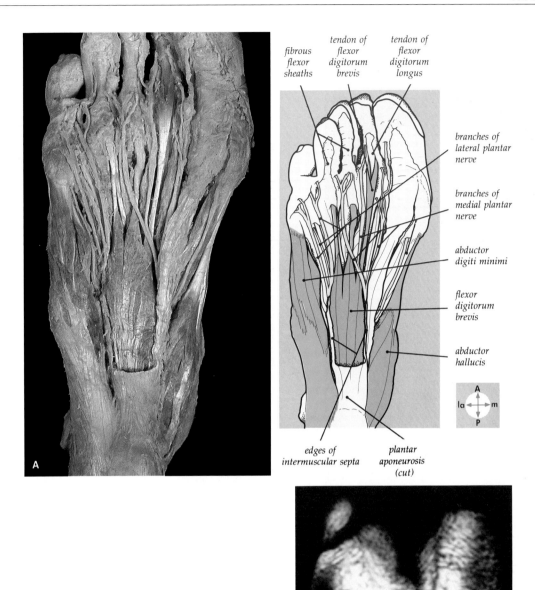

fibrous flexor sheaths

tendon of flexor digitorum brevis

tendon of flexor digitorum longus

branches of lateral plantar nerve

branches of medial plantar nerve

abductor digiti minimi

flexor digitorum brevis

abductor hallucis

edges of intermuscular septa

plantar aponeurosis (cut)

FDB

FIGURE 5–22. (**A**) Superficial intrinsic muscles and plantar nerves are shown after removal of the deep fascia, part of the plantar aponeurosis, and the second fibrous tendon sheath. In this specimen, the flexor digitorum brevis has only three tendons. (**B**) The flexor digitorum brevis (FDB) muscle and the tendons of the first layer of plantar muscles are shown on a T1-weighted axial image.

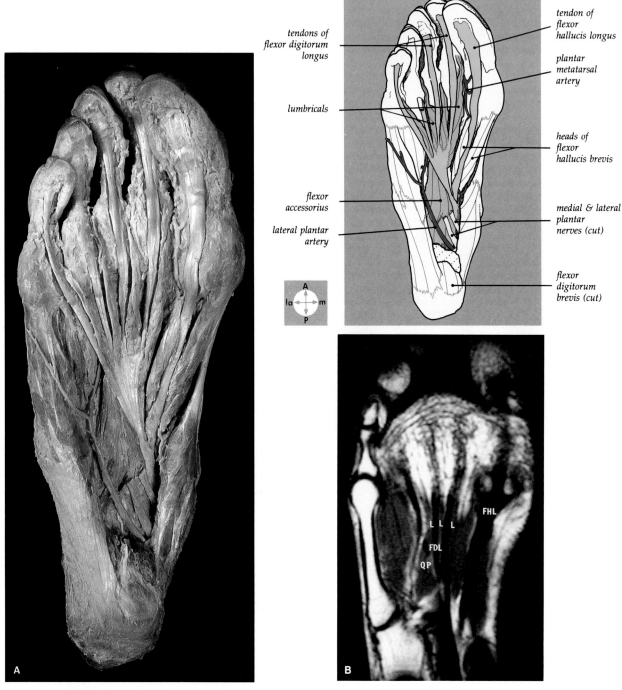

FIGURE 5–23. (**A**) The tendons of the flexor digitorum longus, flexor hallucis longus, flexor accessorius, and the lumbricals can be seen after removal of the medial and lateral plantar nerves and the tendons of the flexor digitorum brevis. (**B**) The quadratus plantae muscle (QP), lumbrical muscles (L), tendons of the flexor digitorum longus (FDL), and tendon of the flexor hallucis longus (FHL), all of the second layer of plantar muscles, are shown on a T1-weighted axial image.

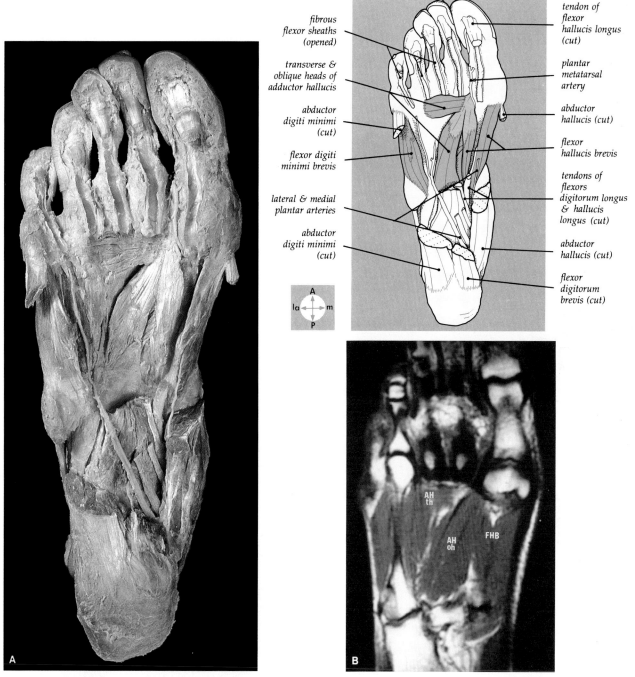

FIGURE 5–24. (**A**) The deep intrinsic muscles are revealed by removal of the long flexor tendon and abductors of the great and little toes. (**B**) The transverse head (th) and oblique head (oh) of the adductor hallucis muscle (AH) and the flexor hallucis brevis muscle (FHB) of the third layer of plantar muscles are shown on a T1-weighted axial image.

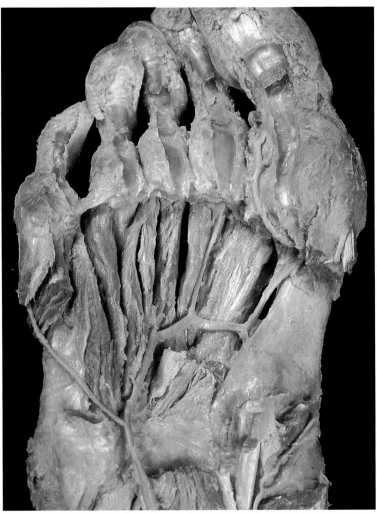

FIGURE 5–25. (**A**) The interosseous muscles and the plantar arterial arch are exposed by removal of the adductor hallucis. (**B**) The dorsal interosseous muscles (I) of the fourth layer of plantar muscles are shown on a T1-weighted axial image.

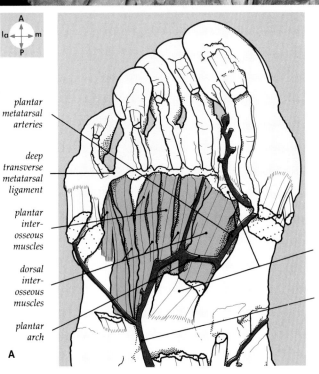

plantar metatarsal arteries

deep transverse metatarsal ligament

plantar interosseous muscles

dorsal interosseous muscles

plantar arch

adductor hallucis (cut)

lateral & medial plantar arteries

A

B

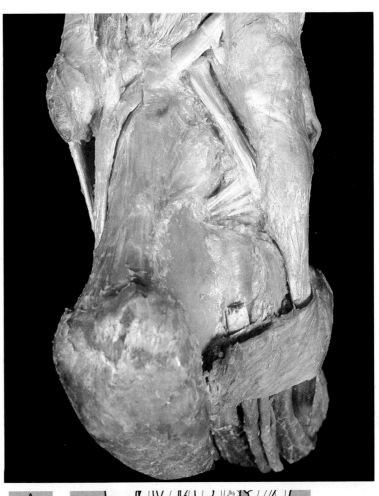

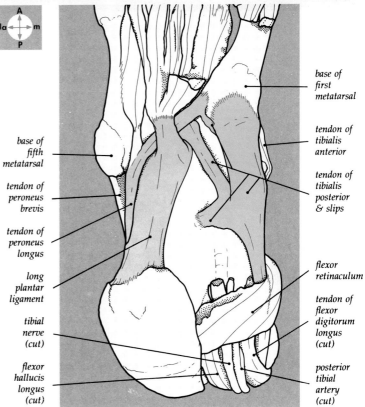

base of
first
metatarsal

tendon of
tibialis
anterior

tendon of
tibialis
posterior
& slips

flexor
retinaculum

tendon of
flexor
digitorum
longus
(cut)

posterior
tibial
artery
(cut)

base of
fifth
metatarsal

tendon of
peroneus
brevis

tendon of
peroneus
longus

long
plantar
ligament

tibial
nerve
(cut)

flexor
hallucis
longus
(cut)

FIGURE 5–26. The tendons of the peroneus longus and the tibialis posterior lie deep in the sole of the foot. The long plantar ligament has been preserved.

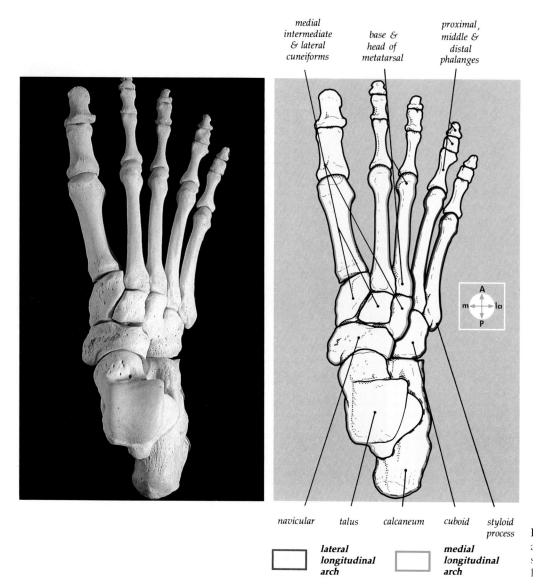

FIGURE 5–27. The dorsal aspect of the bones of the foot shows the medial and lateral longitudinal arches.

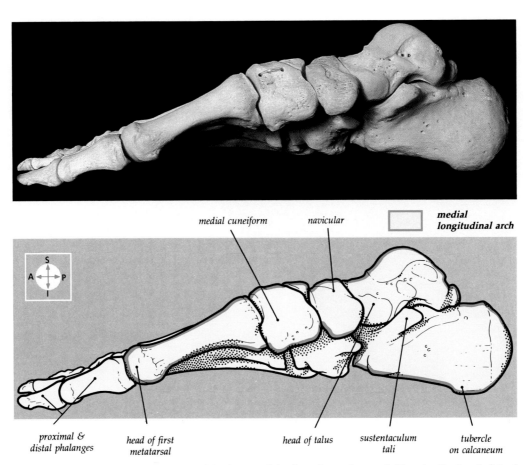

FIGURE 5–28. The medial aspect of the bones of the foot shows the medial longitudinal arch (blue).

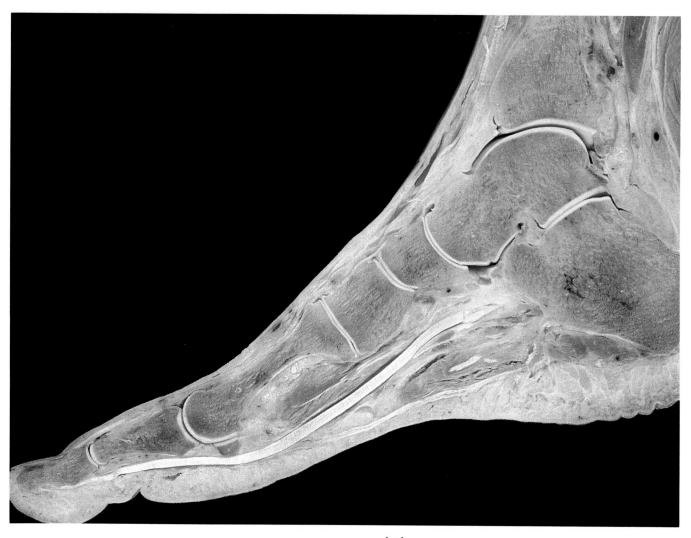

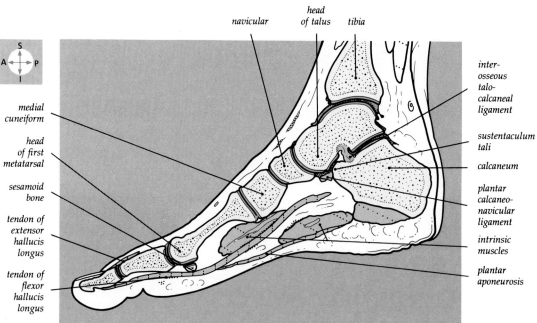

FIGURE 5–29. A sagittal section of the foot shows the medial longitudinal arch.

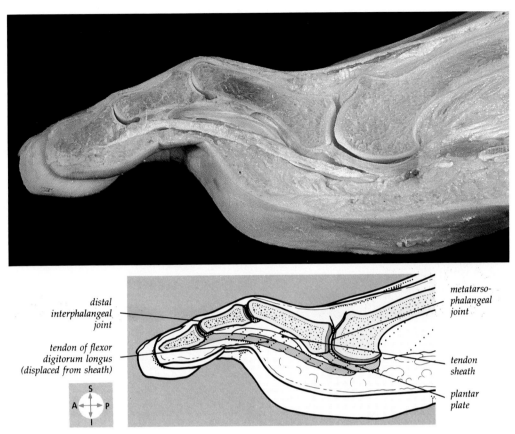

FIGURE 5–30. A sagittal section through the 3rd toe shows the metatarsophalangeal and interphalangeal joints.

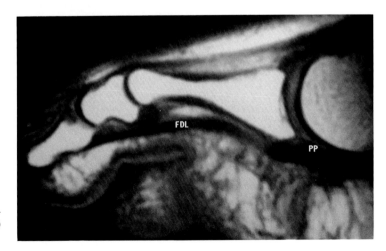

FIGURE 5–31. A T1-weighted sagittal image demonstrates the tendon of the flexor digitorum longus (FDL) and the plantar plate (PP).

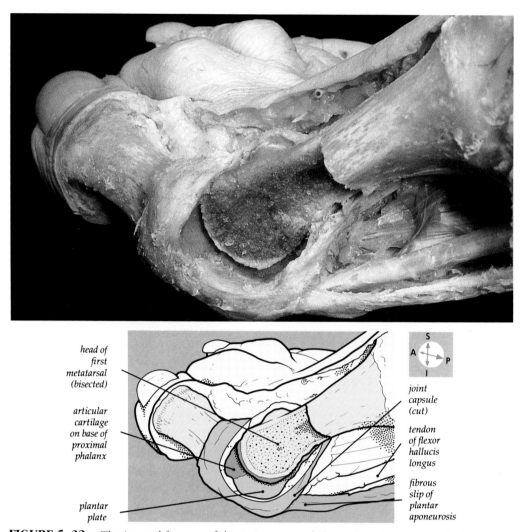

head of
first
metatarsal
(bisected)

articular
cartilage
on base of
proximal
phalanx

plantar
plate

joint
capsule
(cut)

tendon
of flexor
hallucis
longus

fibrous
slip of
plantar
aponeurosis

FIGURE 5–32. The internal features of the 1st metatarsophalangeal joint are revealed when part of the capsule and the distal part of the metatarsal bone are removed.

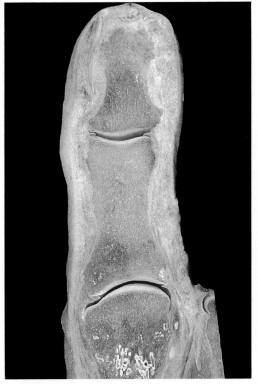

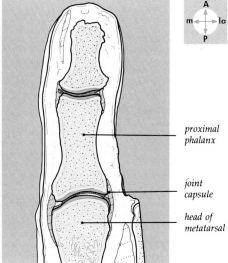

proximal phalanx

joint capsule

head of metatarsal

FIGURE 5–33. A longitudinal section through the great toe shows its joints.

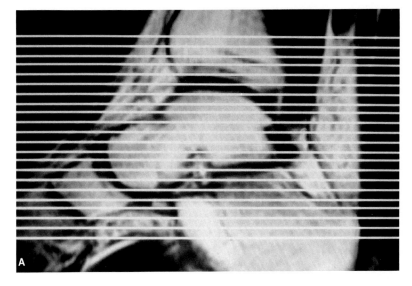

FIGURE 5–34. Normal axial MR anatomy. **(A)** This T1-weighted sagittal localizer was used to prescribe axial image locations from **(B)** superior to **(W)** inferior.

(continued)

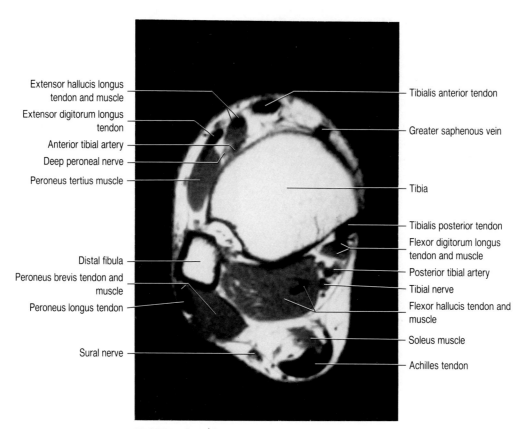

Extensor hallucis longus tendon and muscle

Extensor digitorum longus tendon

Anterior tibial artery

Deep peroneal nerve

Peroneus tertius muscle

Distal fibula

Peroneus brevis tendon and muscle

Peroneus longus tendon

Sural nerve

Tibialis anterior tendon

Greater saphenous vein

Tibia

Tibialis posterior tendon

Flexor digitorum longus tendon and muscle

Posterior tibial artery

Tibial nerve

Flexor hallucis tendon and muscle

Soleus muscle

Achilles tendon

FIGURE 5–34B.

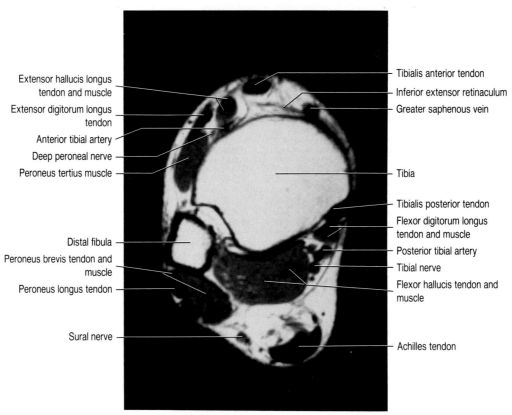

Extensor hallucis longus tendon and muscle

Extensor digitorum longus tendon

Anterior tibial artery

Deep peroneal nerve

Peroneus tertius muscle

Distal fibula

Peroneus brevis tendon and muscle

Peroneus longus tendon

Sural nerve

Tibialis anterior tendon

Inferior extensor retinaculum

Greater saphenous vein

Tibia

Tibialis posterior tendon

Flexor digitorum longus tendon and muscle

Posterior tibial artery

Tibial nerve

Flexor hallucis tendon and muscle

Achilles tendon

FIGURE 5–34C.

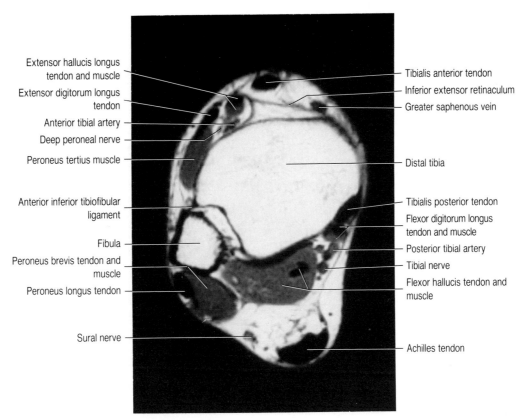

Extensor hallucis longus tendon and muscle
Extensor digitorum longus tendon
Anterior tibial artery
Deep peroneal nerve
Peroneus tertius muscle
Anterior inferior tibiofibular ligament
Fibula
Peroneus brevis tendon and muscle
Peroneus longus tendon
Sural nerve

Tibialis anterior tendon
Inferior extensor retinaculum
Greater saphenous vein
Distal tibia
Tibialis posterior tendon
Flexor digitorum longus tendon and muscle
Posterior tibial artery
Tibial nerve
Flexor hallucis tendon and muscle
Achilles tendon

FIGURE 5–34D.

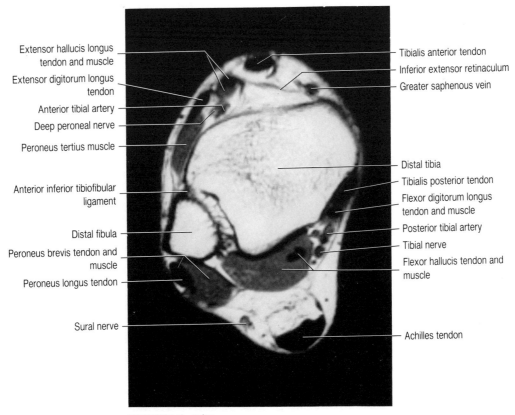

Extensor hallucis longus tendon and muscle
Extensor digitorum longus tendon
Anterior tibial artery
Deep peroneal nerve
Peroneus tertius muscle
Anterior inferior tibiofibular ligament
Distal fibula
Peroneus brevis tendon and muscle
Peroneus longus tendon
Sural nerve

Tibialis anterior tendon
Inferior extensor retinaculum
Greater saphenous vein
Distal tibia
Tibialis posterior tendon
Flexor digitorum longus tendon and muscle
Posterior tibial artery
Tibial nerve
Flexor hallucis tendon and muscle
Achilles tendon

FIGURE 5–34E.

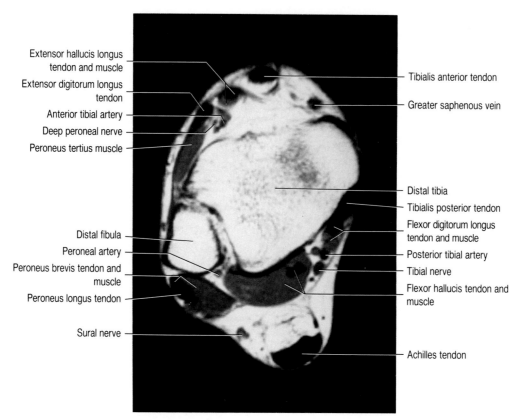

Extensor hallucis longus tendon and muscle
Extensor digitorum longus tendon
Anterior tibial artery
Deep peroneal nerve
Peroneus tertius muscle

Distal fibula
Peroneal artery
Peroneus brevis tendon and muscle
Peroneus longus tendon

Sural nerve

Tibialis anterior tendon
Greater saphenous vein

Distal tibia
Tibialis posterior tendon
Flexor digitorum longus tendon and muscle
Posterior tibial artery
Tibial nerve
Flexor hallucis tendon and muscle

Achilles tendon

FIGURE 5–34F.

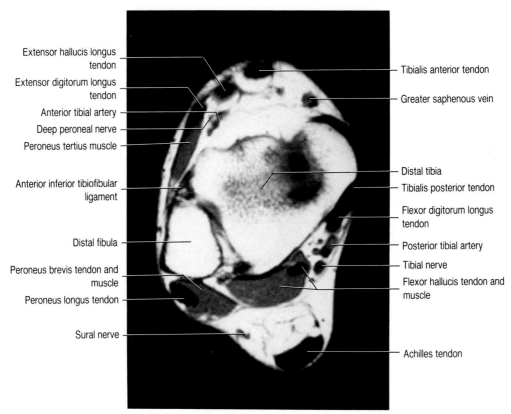

Extensor hallucis longus tendon
Extensor digitorum longus tendon
Anterior tibial artery
Deep peroneal nerve
Peroneus tertius muscle

Anterior inferior tibiofibular ligament

Distal fibula

Peroneus brevis tendon and muscle
Peroneus longus tendon

Sural nerve

Tibialis anterior tendon
Greater saphenous vein

Distal tibia
Tibialis posterior tendon
Flexor digitorum longus tendon
Posterior tibial artery
Tibial nerve
Flexor hallucis tendon and muscle

Achilles tendon

FIGURE 5–34G.

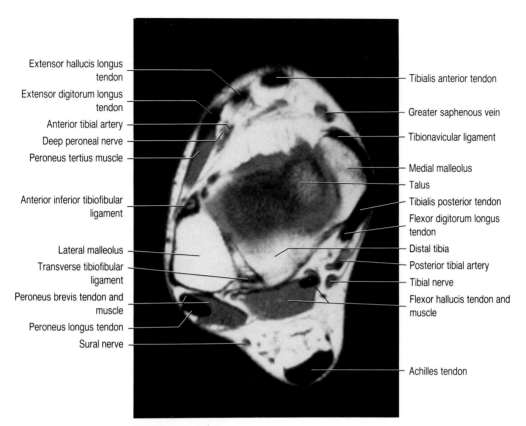

Extensor hallucis longus tendon
Extensor digitorum longus tendon
Anterior tibial artery
Deep peroneal nerve
Peroneus tertius muscle
Anterior inferior tibiofibular ligament
Lateral malleolus
Transverse tibiofibular ligament
Peroneus brevis tendon and muscle
Peroneus longus tendon
Sural nerve

Tibialis anterior tendon
Greater saphenous vein
Tibionavicular ligament
Medial malleolus
Talus
Tibialis posterior tendon
Flexor digitorum longus tendon
Distal tibia
Posterior tibial artery
Tibial nerve
Flexor hallucis tendon and muscle
Achilles tendon

FIGURE 5–34H.

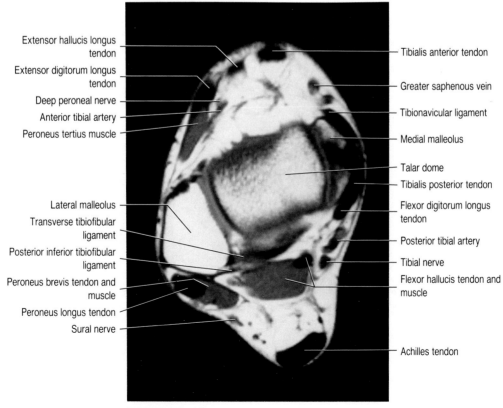

Extensor hallucis longus tendon
Extensor digitorum longus tendon
Deep peroneal nerve
Anterior tibial artery
Peroneus tertius muscle
Lateral malleolus
Transverse tibiofibular ligament
Posterior inferior tibiofibular ligament
Peroneus brevis tendon and muscle
Peroneus longus tendon
Sural nerve

Tibialis anterior tendon
Greater saphenous vein
Tibionavicular ligament
Medial malleolus
Talar dome
Tibialis posterior tendon
Flexor digitorum longus tendon
Posterior tibial artery
Tibial nerve
Flexor hallucis tendon and muscle
Achilles tendon

FIGURE 5–34I.

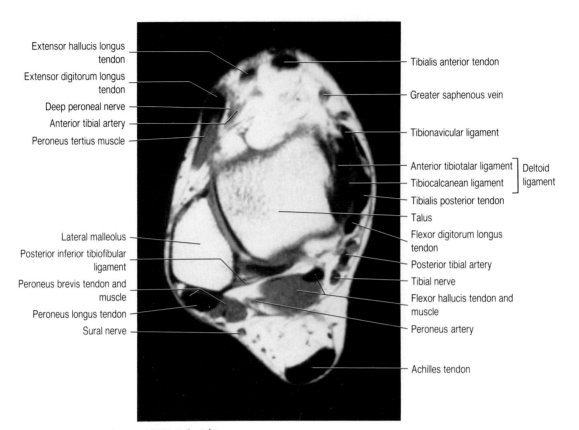

Extensor hallucis longus tendon

Extensor digitorum longus tendon

Deep peroneal nerve

Anterior tibial artery

Peroneus tertius muscle

Lateral malleolus

Posterior inferior tibiofibular ligament

Peroneus brevis tendon and muscle

Peroneus longus tendon

Sural nerve

Tibialis anterior tendon

Greater saphenous vein

Tibionavicular ligament

Anterior tibiotalar ligament ⎤ Deltoid
Tibiocalcanean ligament ⎦ ligament

Tibialis posterior tendon

Talus

Flexor digitorum longus tendon

Posterior tibial artery

Tibial nerve

Flexor hallucis tendon and muscle

Peroneus artery

Achilles tendon

FIGURE 5–34J.

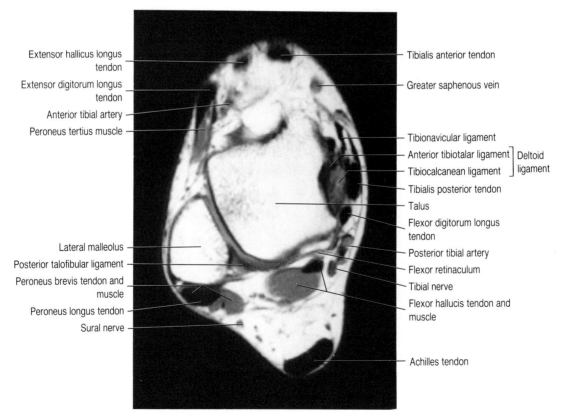

Extensor hallicus longus tendon

Extensor digitorum longus tendon

Anterior tibial artery

Peroneus tertius muscle

Lateral malleolus

Posterior talofibular ligament

Peroneus brevis tendon and muscle

Peroneus longus tendon

Sural nerve

Tibialis anterior tendon

Greater saphenous vein

Tibionavicular ligament

Anterior tibiotalar ligament ⎤ Deltoid
Tibiocalcanean ligament ⎦ ligament

Tibialis posterior tendon

Talus

Flexor digitorum longus tendon

Posterior tibial artery

Flexor retinaculum

Tibial nerve

Flexor hallucis tendon and muscle

Achilles tendon

FIGURE 5–34K.

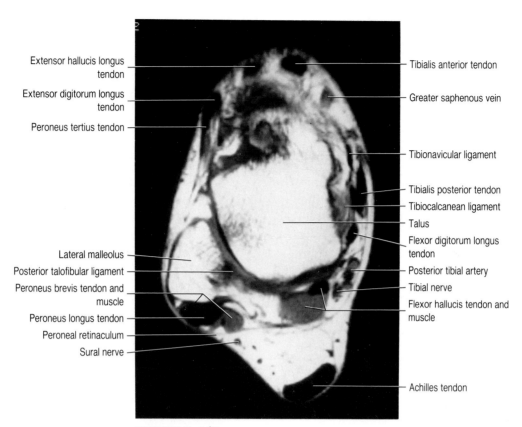

Extensor hallucis longus tendon

Extensor digitorum longus tendon

Peroneus tertius tendon

Lateral malleolus

Posterior talofibular ligament

Peroneus brevis tendon and muscle

Peroneus longus tendon

Peroneal retinaculum

Sural nerve

Tibialis anterior tendon

Greater saphenous vein

Tibionavicular ligament

Tibialis posterior tendon

Tibiocalcanean ligament

Talus

Flexor digitorum longus tendon

Posterior tibial artery

Tibial nerve

Flexor hallucis tendon and muscle

Achilles tendon

FIGURE 5–34L.

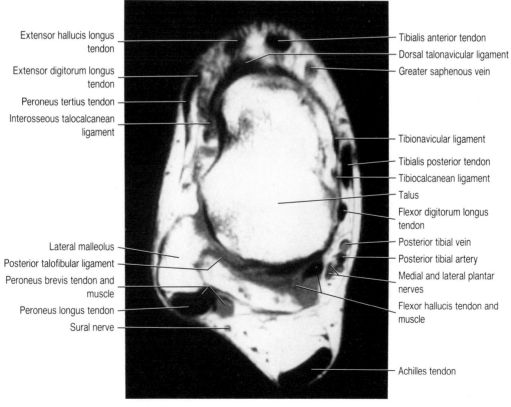

Extensor hallucis longus tendon

Extensor digitorum longus tendon

Peroneus tertius tendon

Interosseous talocalcanean ligament

Lateral malleolus

Posterior talofibular ligament

Peroneus brevis tendon and muscle

Peroneus longus tendon

Sural nerve

Tibialis anterior tendon

Dorsal talonavicular ligament

Greater saphenous vein

Tibionavicular ligament

Tibialis posterior tendon

Tibiocalcanean ligament

Talus

Flexor digitorum longus tendon

Posterior tibial vein

Posterior tibial artery

Medial and lateral plantar nerves

Flexor hallucis tendon and muscle

Achilles tendon

FIGURE 5–34M.

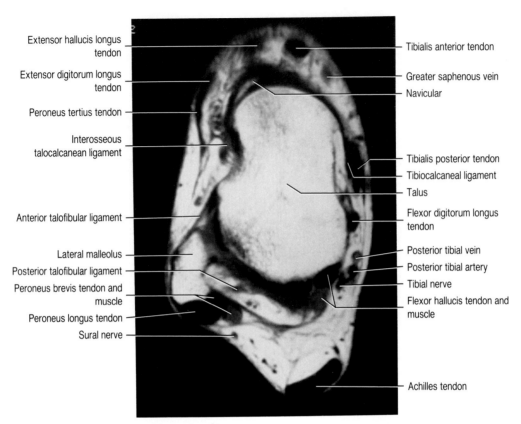

Extensor hallucis longus tendon

Extensor digitorum longus tendon

Peroneus tertius tendon

Interosseous talocalcanean ligament

Anterior talofibular ligament

Lateral malleolus

Posterior talofibular ligament

Peroneus brevis tendon and muscle

Peroneus longus tendon

Sural nerve

Tibialis anterior tendon

Greater saphenous vein

Navicular

Tibialis posterior tendon

Tibiocalcaneal ligament

Talus

Flexor digitorum longus tendon

Posterior tibial vein

Posterior tibial artery

Tibial nerve

Flexor hallucis tendon and muscle

Achilles tendon

FIGURE 5–34N.

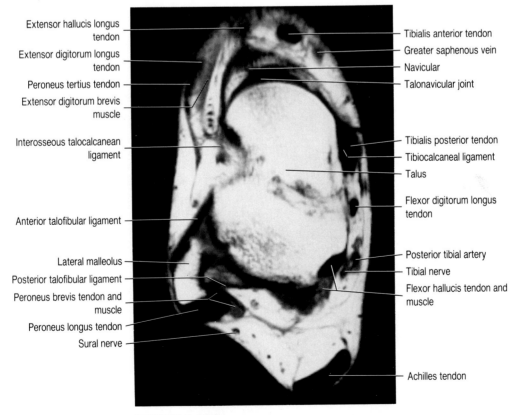

Extensor hallucis longus tendon

Extensor digitorum longus tendon

Peroneus tertius tendon

Extensor digitorum brevis muscle

Interosseous talocalcanean ligament

Anterior talofibular ligament

Lateral malleolus

Posterior talofibular ligament

Peroneus brevis tendon and muscle

Peroneus longus tendon

Sural nerve

Tibialis anterior tendon

Greater saphenous vein

Navicular

Talonavicular joint

Tibialis posterior tendon

Tibiocalcaneal ligament

Talus

Flexor digitorum longus tendon

Posterior tibial artery

Tibial nerve

Flexor hallucis tendon and muscle

Achilles tendon

FIGURE 5–34O.

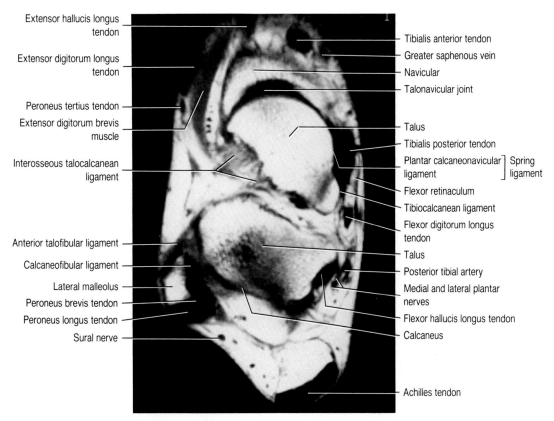

Extensor hallucis longus tendon
Extensor digitorum longus tendon
Peroneus tertius tendon
Extensor digitorum brevis muscle
Interosseous talocalcanean ligament
Anterior talofibular ligament
Calcaneofibular ligament
Lateral malleolus
Peroneus brevis tendon
Peroneus longus tendon
Sural nerve

Tibialis anterior tendon
Greater saphenous vein
Navicular
Talonavicular joint
Talus
Tibialis posterior tendon
Plantar calcaneonavicular ligament ⎦ Spring ligament
Flexor retinaculum
Tibiocalcanean ligament
Flexor digitorum longus tendon
Talus
Posterior tibial artery
Medial and lateral plantar nerves
Flexor hallucis longus tendon
Calcaneus
Achilles tendon

FIGURE 5–34P.

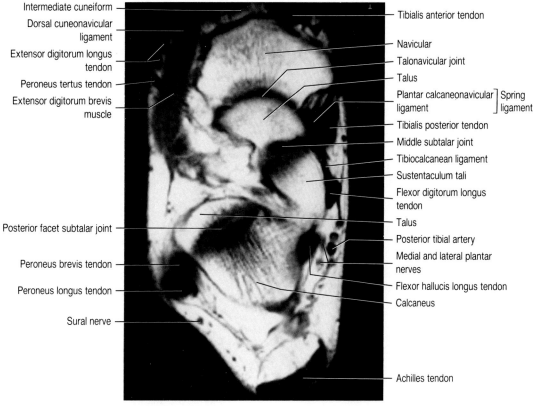

Intermediate cuneiform
Dorsal cuneonavicular ligament
Extensor digitorum longus tendon
Peroneus tertus tendon
Extensor digitorum brevis muscle
Posterior facet subtalar joint
Peroneus brevis tendon
Peroneus longus tendon
Sural nerve

Tibialis anterior tendon
Navicular
Talonavicular joint
Talus
Plantar calcaneonavicular ligament ⎦ Spring ligament
Tibialis posterior tendon
Middle subtalar joint
Tibiocalcanean ligament
Sustentaculum tali
Flexor digitorum longus tendon
Talus
Posterior tibial artery
Medial and lateral plantar nerves
Flexor hallucis longus tendon
Calcaneus
Achilles tendon

FIGURE 5–34Q.

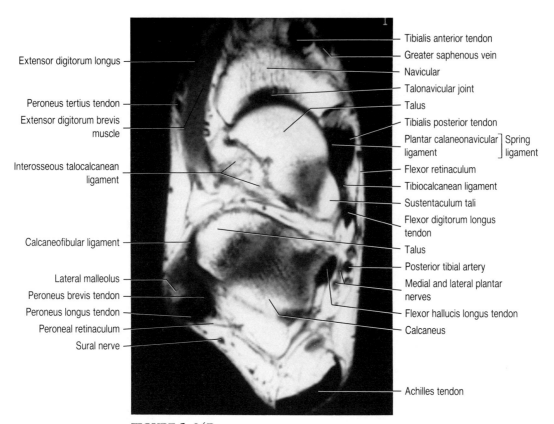

Extensor digitorum longus

Peroneus tertius tendon

Extensor digitorum brevis muscle

Interosseous talocalcanean ligament

Calcaneofibular ligament

Lateral malleolus
Peroneus brevis tendon
Peroneus longus tendon
Peroneal retinaculum
Sural nerve

Tibialis anterior tendon
Greater saphenous vein
Navicular
Talonavicular joint
Talus
Tibialis posterior tendon
Plantar calaneonavicular ligament ⎤ Spring
⎦ ligament
Flexor retinaculum
Tibiocalcanean ligament
Sustentaculum tali
Flexor digitorum longus tendon
Talus
Posterior tibial artery
Medial and lateral plantar nerves
Flexor hallucis longus tendon
Calcaneus

Achilles tendon

FIGURE 5–34R.

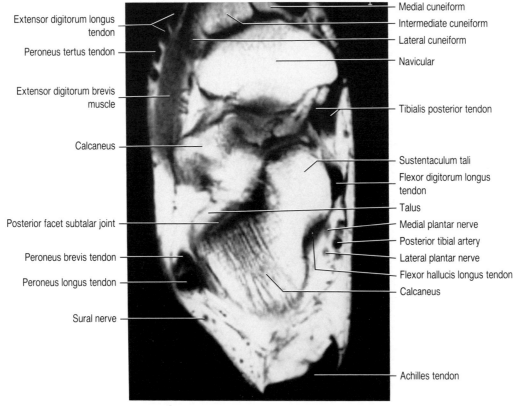

Extensor digitorum longus tendon

Peroneus tertus tendon

Extensor digitorum brevis muscle

Calcaneus

Posterior facet subtalar joint

Peroneus brevis tendon

Peroneus longus tendon

Sural nerve

Medial cuneiform
Intermediate cuneiform
Lateral cuneiform
Navicular

Tibialis posterior tendon

Sustentaculum tali
Flexor digitorum longus tendon
Talus
Medial plantar nerve
Posterior tibial artery
Lateral plantar nerve
Flexor hallucis longus tendon
Calcaneus

Achilles tendon

FIGURE 5–34S.

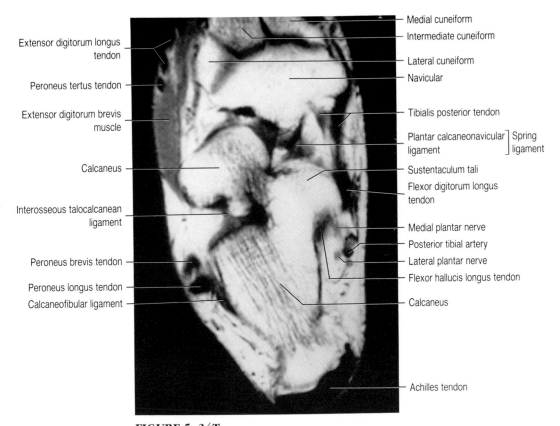

Extensor digitorum longus tendon

Peroneus tertus tendon

Extensor digitorum brevis muscle

Calcaneus

Interosseous talocalcanean ligament

Peroneus brevis tendon

Peroneus longus tendon

Calcaneofibular ligament

Medial cuneiform

Intermediate cuneiform

Lateral cuneiform

Navicular

Tibialis posterior tendon

Plantar calcaneonavicular ligament] Spring ligament

Sustentaculum tali

Flexor digitorum longus tendon

Medial plantar nerve

Posterior tibial artery

Lateral plantar nerve

Flexor hallucis longus tendon

Calcaneus

Achilles tendon

FIGURE 5–34T.

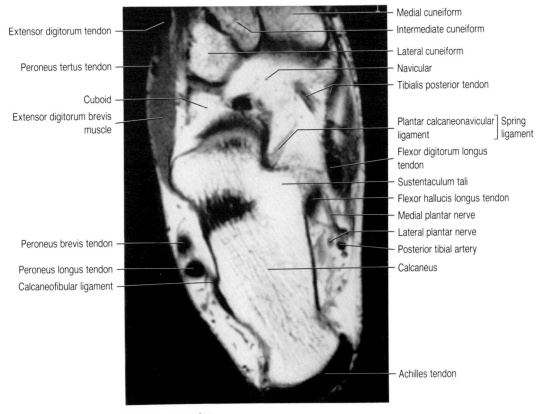

Extensor digitorum tendon

Peroneus tertus tendon

Cuboid

Extensor digitorum brevis muscle

Peroneus brevis tendon

Peroneus longus tendon

Calcaneofibular ligament

Medial cuneiform

Intermediate cuneiform

Lateral cuneiform

Navicular

Tibialis posterior tendon

Plantar calcaneonavicular ligament] Spring ligament

Flexor digitorum longus tendon

Sustentaculum tali

Flexor hallucis longus tendon

Medial plantar nerve

Lateral plantar nerve

Posterior tibial artery

Calcaneus

Achilles tendon

FIGURE 5–34U.

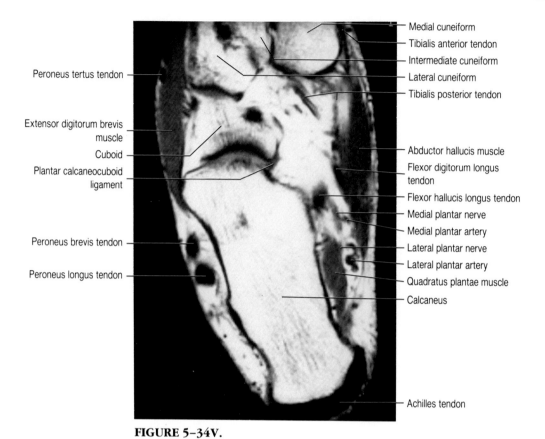

Peroneus tertus tendon

Extensor digitorum brevis muscle

Cuboid

Plantar calcaneocuboid ligament

Peroneus brevis tendon

Peroneus longus tendon

Medial cuneiform

Tibialis anterior tendon

Intermediate cuneiform

Lateral cuneiform

Tibialis posterior tendon

Abductor hallucis muscle

Flexor digitorum longus tendon

Flexor hallucis longus tendon

Medial plantar nerve

Medial plantar artery

Lateral plantar nerve

Lateral plantar artery

Quadratus plantae muscle

Calcaneus

Achilles tendon

FIGURE 5–34V.

Peroneus tertus tendon

Extensor digitorum brevis muscle

Cuboid

Peroneus brevis tendon

Peroneus longus tendon

Medial cuneiform

Intermediate cuneiform

Lateral cuneiform

Tibialis posterior tendon

Abductor hallucis muscle

Flexor digitorum longus tendon

Flexor hallucis longus tendon

Medial plantar nerve

Medial plantar artery

Lateral plantar nerve

Lateral plantar artery

Quadratus plantae muscle

Calcaneus

Achilles tendon

FIGURE 5–34W.

thick structure of low signal intensity with a convex posterior surface and a flattened anterior surface. The posterior Achilles tendon represents the convergence of the gastrocnemius, plantaris, and soleus muscles. The soleus muscle group that is present at the level of the distal tibia is not seen at the tibiotalar joint level. Sections through the level of the distal lateral malleolus demonstrate the anterior and posterior talofibular ligaments. Medially, the tibionavicular and tibiocalcaneal parts of the deltoid ligament are also shown at this level. The peroneal retinaculum can be seen coursing medial and posterior to the lateral malleolus. The interosseous talocalcaneal ligament is posterolateral to either the anterior talus or the talar head. The plantar calcaneonavicular ligament, or spring ligament, is located inferior to the lateral malleolus between the lateral talus and tibialis posterior tendon.

The calcaneofibular ligament is optimally seen with the foot in 40° of plantar flexion, and on neutral axial images it can be seen lateral to the posterior inferior talus and anterior and medial to the peroneus brevis tendon. The sural nerve, intermediate in signal intensity, is located posteromedial to the peroneus brevis muscle. The tibial nerve is medial to the flexor hallucis longus tendon and continues distally as the medial and lateral plantar nerves. The flexor retinaculum is superficial to the tendons of the deep muscles on the medial side of the ankle. In the foot, the tendons of the flexor hallucis brevis and longus muscles are seen posterior to the 1st metatarsal and cuneiform. The longitudinally oriented quadratus plantae and abductor hallucis muscles are medial to the calcaneus and cuboid. The peroneus longus tendon—a fourth-layer muscle of the sole of the foot—enters the foot by passing posterior to the lateral malleolus and can be seen obliquely crossing the foot to its insertion onto the base of the 1st metatarsal and medial cuneiform.

The anterior neurovascular bundle, composed of the anterior tibial artery and vein and deep peroneal nerve, is located posterior to the extensor tendons, whereas the posterior neurovascular bundle, composed of the posterior tibial artery, vein, and tibial nerve, is located posterior to the flexor digitorum and flexor hallucis longus tendons.

Sagittal Images

On sagittal planar images, the long axis of tendons crossing the ankle joint can be seen (Fig. 5–35).

Medial Sagittal Images. In the plane of the medial malleolus, the tibialis posterior and flexor digitorum longus tendons are directly posterior to the medial malleolus. The tibialis posterior tendon enters the foot by passing deep to the flexor retinaculum and superior to the sustentaculum tali to its insertion on the tuberosity of the navicular bone. The flexor digitorum longus tendon

also enters the foot after passing posterior to the medial malleolus and deep to the flexor retinaculum. This tendon is divided into four segments after crossing the flexor hallucis longus tendon, which contributes slips to the medial two divisions. These segments insert onto the bases of the distal phalanges. The quadratus plantae muscle inserts at the division of the flexor hallucis into four tendons. Distally, each tendon is an origin for the lumbrical muscles.

The deltoid ligament, composed of the tibiocalcaneal, tibionavicular, and anterior and posterior tibiotalar ligaments, appears as a wide band of low signal intensity radiating from the distal tibia (*i.e.,* medial malleolus) to the tuberosity of the navicular bone and the sustentaculum tali. The flexor hallucis longus tendon is located posterior to the tibialis posterior tendon and the flexor digitorum longus. It passes posterior to the medial malleolus, deep to the flexor retinaculum. The low signal intensity tendon grooves the posterior talar process and inferior surface of the sustentaculum tali proximal to its insertion onto the base of the distal phalanx of the great toe.

The plantar flexor digitorum brevis—a first-layer muscle of the sole of the foot—and the quadratus plantae—a second-layer muscle of the sole of the foot—are displayed on medial sagittal images. The adductor hallucis—a first-layer muscle—inserts onto the medial proximal phalanx of the first toe and is seen between the 1st and 2nd metatarsals on medial sagittal images. The tibialis anterior tendon crosses the dorsal surface of the talus before it inserts on the medial cuneiform bone and the bone of the 1st metatarsal.

Midplane Sagittal Images. The middle subtalar joint, the tarsal sinus, and the posterior subtalar joint are demonstrated on sagittal images medial to the midsagittal plane. The anterior subtalar joint is shown in the plane of the cuboid and calcaneocuboid joint. The peroneus longus, which extends anteriorly along the lateral inferior surface of the calcaneus and is inferior to the peroneal tubercle, enters the foot at the lateral inferior margin of the cuboid. The extensor hallucis longus tendon is identified along the dorsum of the foot and extends to insert onto the distal phalanx of the first toe. The interosseous talocalcaneal ligament, with its associated high signal intensity fat, is bordered anteriorly by the anterior process of the calcaneus and posteriorly by the lateral process of the talus. On T1-weighted sequences, the pre-Achilles fat pad of high signal intensity is located directly anterior to the low spin density Achilles tendon.

Lateral Sagittal Images. In the plane of the fibula, the peroneus brevis and longus tendons pass posterior to the lateral malleolus. The peroneus brevis lies anterior to the peroneus longus tendon and is in direct contact with the lateral malleolus. The peroneus brevis can be followed to its insertion on the base of the 5th metatarsal bone. The peroneus longus tendon disappears inferior and medial to the peroneus brevis tendon and enters the cuboid sulcus; therefore, it appears shorter than the peroneus brevis tendon on lateral sagittal images.

Coronal Images

Figure 5–36 provides examples of various coronal images in the foot and ankle.

Posterior Coronal Images. The thick, low signal intensity Achilles tendon is clearly displayed on posterior coronal images, and its attachment to the calcaneal tuberosity can be observed. The soleus muscle, with its inverted-V–shaped origin from the soleal line of the tibia and posterior fibula, contributes to the calcaneal tendon (or Achilles tendon), along with the gastrocnemius and plantaris. The peroneus brevis and flexor hallucis longus muscles are identified lateral to the soleus muscle, and the peroneal tendons are located inferior to the lateral malleolus. The flexor digitorum longus muscle and tendon cross superficially, in a medial-to-lateral direction, to the tibialis posterior in the distal calf. The tibialis posterior tendon is located medial to the posterior malleolus. The posterior talofibular and inferior tibiofibular ligaments are shown on coronal images at the level of the posterior malleolus and posterior process of the talus. The plantar aponeurosis is superficial to the flexor digitorum brevis muscle, whereas the quadratus plantae muscle lies deep to this muscle.

Midplane Coronal Images. The calcaneofibular ligament is best imaged at the level of the posterior subtalar joint and lateral malleolus. The lateral process of the talus can be seen in the same sections as the anterior lateral malleolus. The middle subtalar joint is formed by the sustentaculum tali and the inferior medial talar surface. This is the best plane for evaluating talocalcaneal coalitions. The peroneus brevis and longus tendons course laterally, superior and inferior, respectively, to the peroneal groove of the calcaneus.

Anterior Coronal Images. The tibiotalar and tibiocalcaneal fibers of the deltoid ligament extend obliquely to the talus and vertically to the sustentaculum tali, respectively. The tibialis posterior tendon is medial to the deltoid ligament and superior to the sustentaculum tali, and can be used as a landmark. The flexor digitorum longus tendon enters the foot, having crossed superficially in a medial-to-lateral direction to both the tibialis posterior and the flexor hallucis longus tendons, which are parallel. The flexor digitorum longus tendon is located medial to the sustentaculum tali. The anterior compartment tendons of the tibialis anterior, the extensor hallucis longus, and the extensor digitorum longus tendons, are displayed on the anterior surface of the distal tibia, medially and laterally. The anterior tibiotalar fibers of the deltoid ligament are also seen in the plane of the anterior tibia.

Anatomic Variants

A number of normal anatomic variants of the ankle as seen on MR images may be misleading. These have been characterized in studies of asymptomatic patients.[10] In the posterior tibiotalar joint, a low signal intensity cortical irregularity may mimic the appearance of osteonecrosis (Figs. 5–37 and 5–38). The posterior tibiofibular ligament may be mistaken for a loose body in the posterior capsule on midsagittal images (see Fig. 5–38). Occasionally, the intact posterior talofibular ligament may appear as an attenuated structure with signal inhomogeneity. Less frequently, fluid in the peroneal tendon sheath may be confused with a longitudinal tendon tear. In one patient, axial planar images revealed marked asymmetry and hypertrophy of the peroneus brevis muscle and tendon as a normal anatomic variant (Fig. 5–39). An accessory soleus muscle is an anatomic variant that may present as a mass in the distal calf or medial ankle.[11]

PATHOLOGY OF THE ANKLE AND FOOT

Transchondral Fractures

Transchondral fracture is the accepted term for several osteochondral lesions including osteochondral fracture, osteochondritis dissecans, and talar dome fracture. Transchondral fractures of the medial and lateral talar dome involve the articular cartilage and subchondral bone, and have a high association with antecedent trauma (*i.e.,* torsional impaction).

Diagnosis and Staging

Conventional radiographs are not sensitive to early lesions, and as a result, immobilization and surgery may be delayed. This situation is associated with a 50% rate of arthritis. Magnetic resonance imaging of the talar dome is more accurate than CT scanning, and complements diagnostic arthroscopic examination of the tibiotalar joint in early diagnosis (Fig. 5–40).

Forced inversion and dorsiflexion produces a lateral lesion (*i.e.,* impingement between the lateral margin of the talar dome and the fibular styloid; Figs. 5–41 and 5–42). Forced inversion and plantar flexion with external

(text continues on page 447)

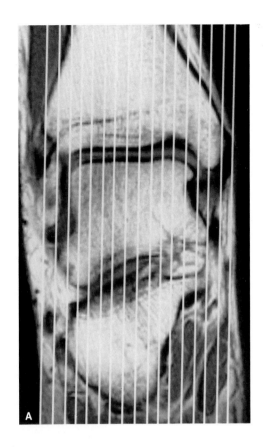

FIGURE 5–35. Normal sagittal MR anatomy. (**A**) This T1-weighted coronal localizer was used to prescribe sagittal images from (**B**) medial to (**R**) lateral.

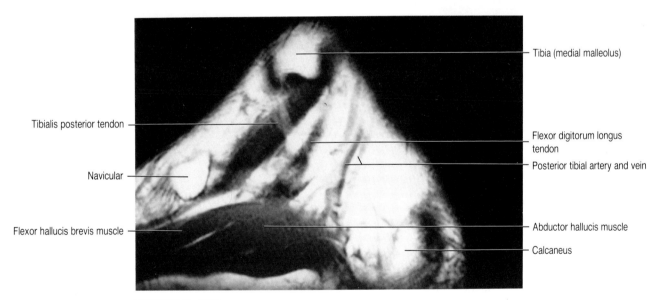

Tibialis posterior tendon

Navicular

Flexor hallucis brevis muscle

Tibia (medial malleolus)

Flexor digitorum longus tendon

Posterior tibial artery and vein

Abductor hallucis muscle

Calcaneus

FIGURE 5–35B.

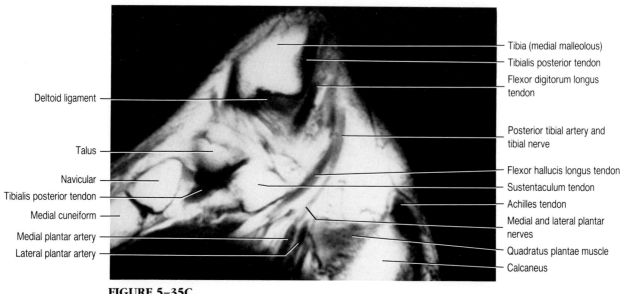

Tibia (medial malleolous)

Tibialis posterior tendon

Flexor digitorum longus tendon

Posterior tibial artery and tibial nerve

Flexor hallucis longus tendon

Sustentaculum tendon

Achilles tendon

Medial and lateral plantar nerves

Quadratus plantae muscle

Calcaneus

Deltoid ligament

Talus

Navicular

Tibialis posterior tendon

Medial cuneiform

Medial plantar artery

Lateral plantar artery

FIGURE 5–35C.

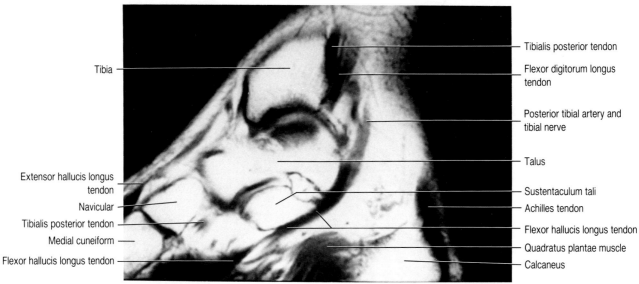

Tibialis posterior tendon

Flexor digitorum longus tendon

Posterior tibial artery and tibial nerve

Talus

Sustentaculum tali

Achilles tendon

Flexor hallucis longus tendon

Quadratus plantae muscle

Calcaneus

Tibia

Extensor hallucis longus tendon

Navicular

Tibialis posterior tendon

Medial cuneiform

Flexor hallucis longus tendon

FIGURE 5–35D.

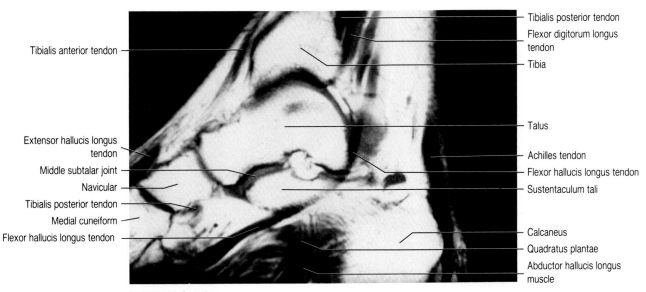

Tibialis anterior tendon —

Extensor hallucis longus tendon —

Middle subtalar joint —

Navicular —

Tibialis posterior tendon —

Medial cuneiform —

Flexor hallucis longus tendon —

— Tibialis posterior tendon

— Flexor digitorum longus tendon

— Tibia

— Talus

— Achilles tendon

— Flexor hallucis longus tendon

— Sustentaculum tali

— Calcaneus

— Quadratus plantae

— Abductor hallucis longus muscle

FIGURE 5–35E.

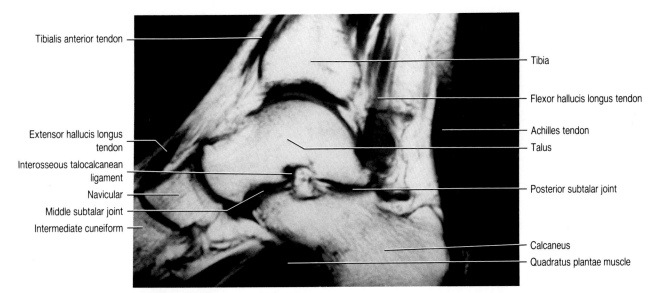

Tibialis anterior tendon —

Extensor hallucis longus tendon —

Interosseous talocalcanean ligament —

Navicular —

Middle subtalar joint —

Intermediate cuneiform —

— Tibia

— Flexor hallucis longus tendon

— Achilles tendon

— Talus

— Posterior subtalar joint

— Calcaneus

— Quadratus plantae muscle

FIGURE 5–35F.

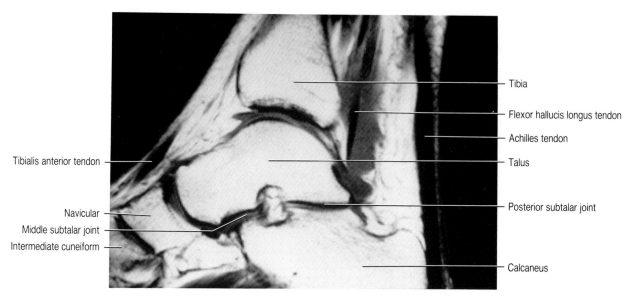

Tibia

Flexor hallucis longus tendon

Achilles tendon

Talus

Posterior subtalar joint

Calcaneus

Tibialis anterior tendon

Navicular

Middle subtalar joint

Intermediate cuneiform

FIGURE 5–35G.

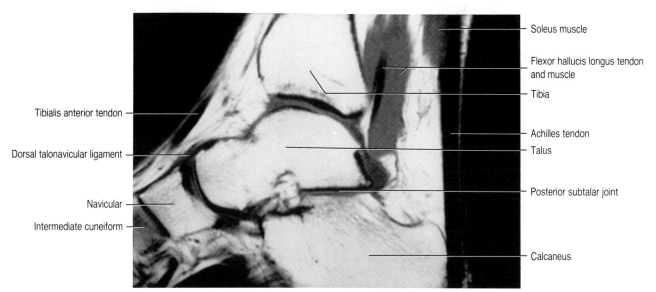

Soleus muscle

Flexor hallucis longus tendon and muscle

Tibia

Achilles tendon

Talus

Posterior subtalar joint

Calcaneus

Tibialis anterior tendon

Dorsal talonavicular ligament

Navicular

Intermediate cuneiform

FIGURE 5–35H.

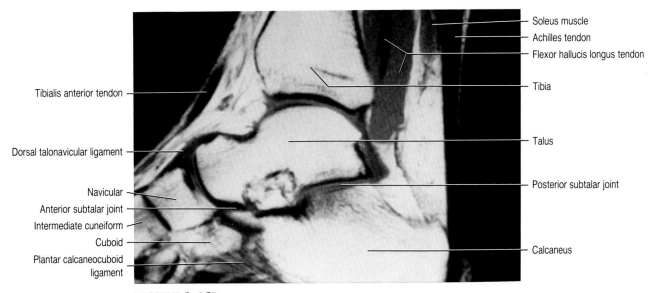

Soleus muscle

Achilles tendon

Flexor hallucis longus tendon

Tibia

Talus

Posterior subtalar joint

Calcaneus

Tibialis anterior tendon

Dorsal talonavicular ligament

Navicular

Anterior subtalar joint

Intermediate cuneiform

Cuboid

Plantar calcaneocuboid ligament

FIGURE 5–35I.

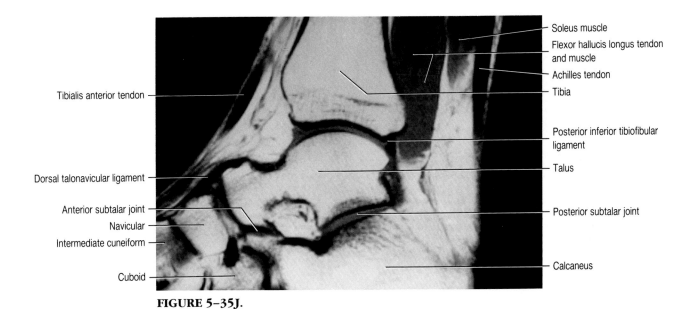

Soleus muscle

Flexor hallucis longus tendon and muscle

Achilles tendon

Tibia

Posterior inferior tibiofibular ligament

Talus

Posterior subtalar joint

Calcaneus

Tibialis anterior tendon

Dorsal talonavicular ligament

Anterior subtalar joint

Navicular

Intermediate cuneiform

Cuboid

FIGURE 5–35J.

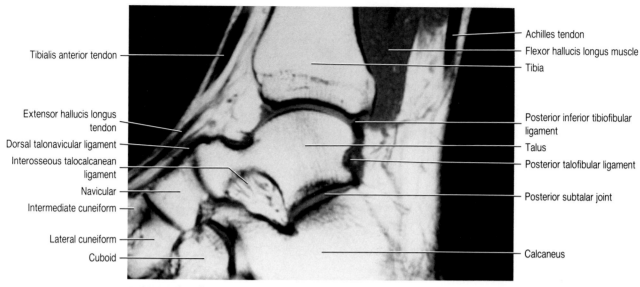

Tibialis anterior tendon

Extensor hallucis longus tendon

Dorsal talonavicular ligament

Interosseous talocalcanean ligament

Navicular

Intermediate cuneiform

Lateral cuneiform

Cuboid

Achilles tendon

Flexor hallucis longus muscle

Tibia

Posterior inferior tibiofibular ligament

Talus

Posterior talofibular ligament

Posterior subtalar joint

Calcaneus

FIGURE 5–35K.

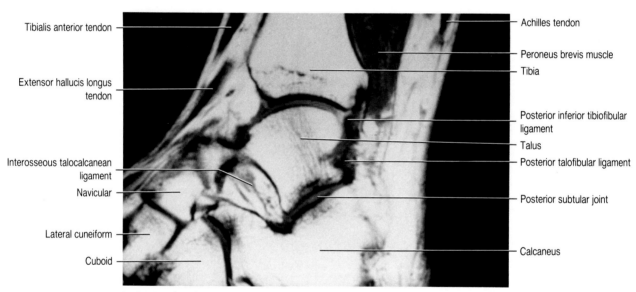

Tibialis anterior tendon

Extensor hallucis longus tendon

Interosseous talocalcanean ligament

Navicular

Lateral cuneiform

Cuboid

Achilles tendon

Peroneus brevis muscle

Tibia

Posterior inferior tibiofibular ligament

Talus

Posterior talofibular ligament

Posterior subtular joint

Calcaneus

FIGURE 5–35L.

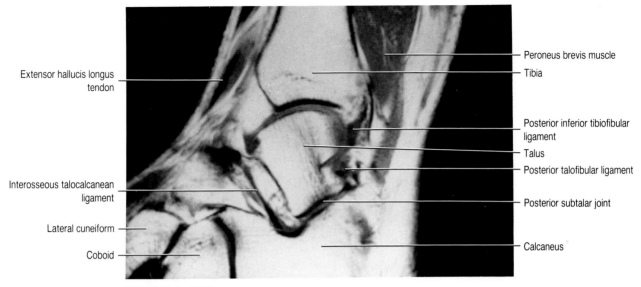

Extensor hallucis longus tendon

Peroneus brevis muscle

Tibia

Posterior inferior tibiofibular ligament

Talus

Posterior talofibular ligament

Posterior subtalar joint

Interosseous talocalcanean ligament

Lateral cuneiform

Coboid

Calcaneus

FIGURE 5–35M.

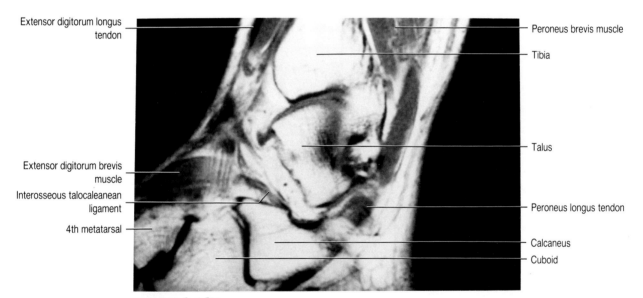

Extensor digitorum longus tendon

Peroneus brevis muscle

Tibia

Talus

Extensor digitorum brevis muscle

Interosseous talocaleanean ligament

4th metatarsal

Peroneus longus tendon

Calcaneus

Cuboid

FIGURE 5–35N.

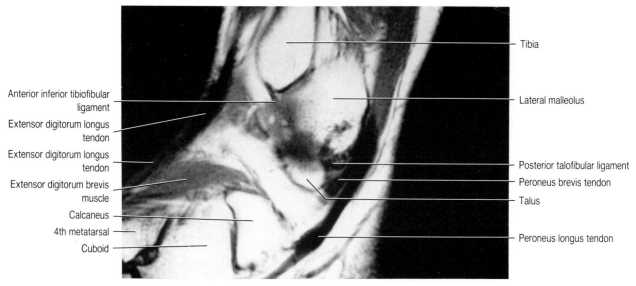

Tibia

Anterior inferior tibiofibular ligament

Lateral malleolus

Extensor digitorum longus tendon

Extensor digitorum longus tendon

Posterior talofibular ligament

Extensor digitorum brevis muscle

Peroneus brevis tendon

Calcaneus

Talus

4th metatarsal

Cuboid

Peroneus longus tendon

FIGURE 5–35O.

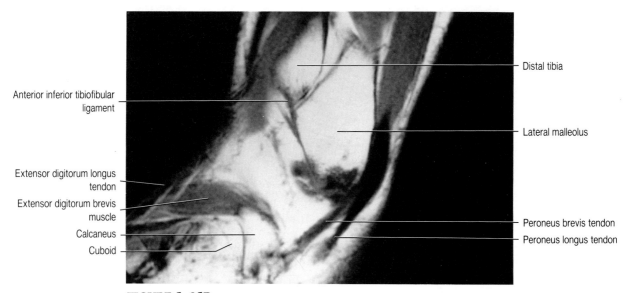

Anterior inferior tibiofibular ligament

Distal tibia

Lateral malleolus

Extensor digitorum longus tendon

Extensor digitorum brevis muscle

Calcaneus

Peroneus brevis tendon

Cuboid

Peroneus longus tendon

FIGURE 5–35P.

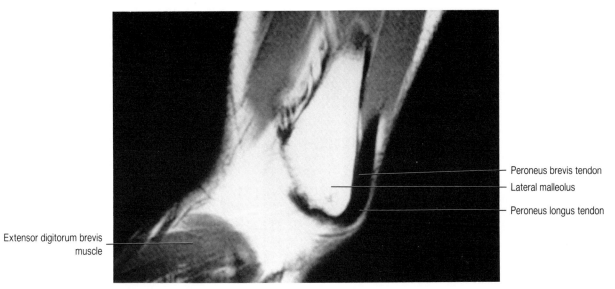

Peroneus brevis tendon

Lateral malleolus

Peroneus longus tendon

Extensor digitorum brevis
muscle

FIGURE 5–35Q.

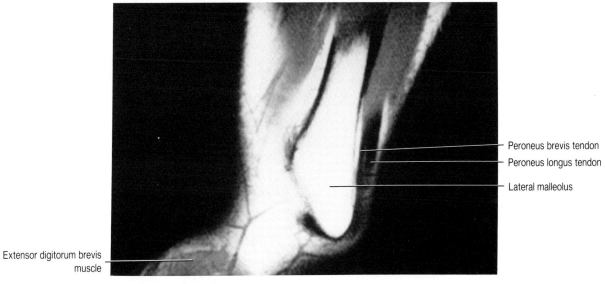

Peroneus brevis tendon

Peroneus longus tendon

Lateral malleolus

Extensor digitorum brevis
muscle

FIGURE 5–35R.

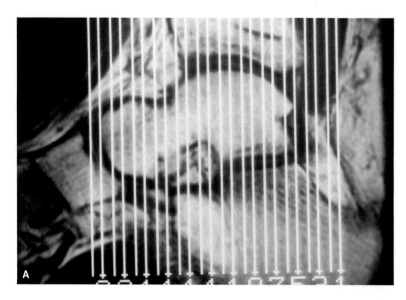

FIGURE 5–36. Normal coronal MR anatomy. (**A**) This T1-weighted sagittal localizer was used to prescribe coronal images from (**B**) posterior to (**U**) anterior.

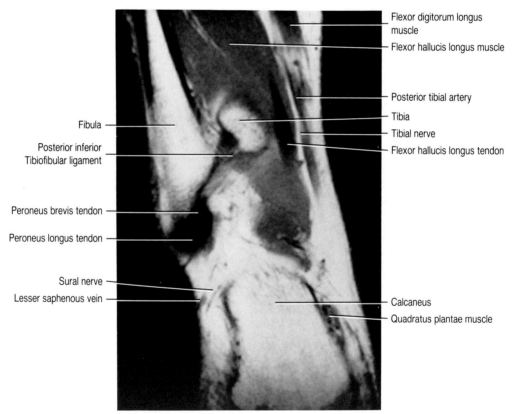

Flexor digitorum longus muscle

Flexor hallucis longus muscle

Posterior tibial artery

Tibia

Tibial nerve

Flexor hallucis longus tendon

Fibula

Posterior inferior Tibiofibular ligament

Peroneus brevis tendon

Peroneus longus tendon

Sural nerve

Lesser saphenous vein

Calcaneus

Quadratus plantae muscle

FIGURE 5–36B.

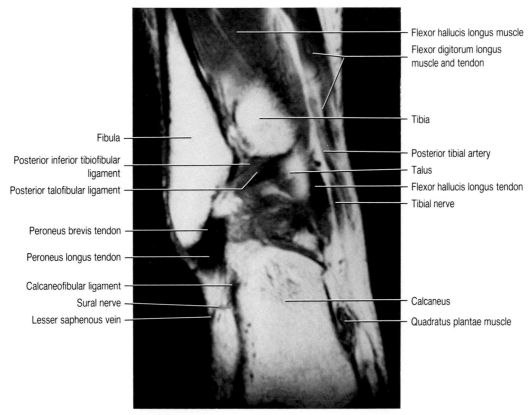

Flexor hallucis longus muscle

Flexor digitorum longus muscle and tendon

Tibia

Fibula

Posterior inferior tibiofibular ligament

Posterior talofibular ligament

Posterior tibial artery

Talus

Flexor hallucis longus tendon

Tibial nerve

Peroneus brevis tendon

Peroneus longus tendon

Calcaneofibular ligament

Sural nerve

Lesser saphenous vein

Calcaneus

Quadratus plantae muscle

FIGURE 5–36C.

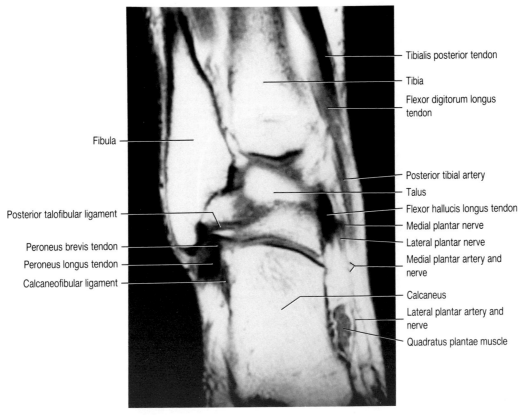

Tibialis posterior tendon

Tibia

Flexor digitorum longus tendon

Fibula

Posterior talofibular ligament

Peroneus brevis tendon

Peroneus longus tendon

Calcaneofibular ligament

Posterior tibial artery

Talus

Flexor hallucis longus tendon

Medial plantar nerve

Lateral plantar nerve

Medial plantar artery and nerve

Calcaneus

Lateral plantar artery and nerve

Quadratus plantae muscle

FIGURE 5–36D.

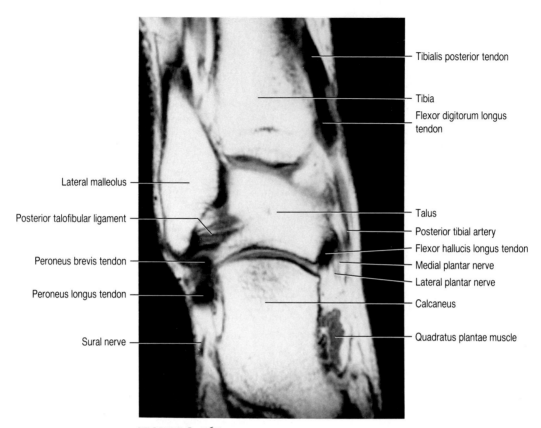

Tibialis posterior tendon

Tibia

Flexor digitorum longus tendon

Lateral malleolus

Posterior talofibular ligament

Talus

Posterior tibial artery

Peroneus brevis tendon

Flexor hallucis longus tendon

Medial plantar nerve

Peroneus longus tendon

Lateral plantar nerve

Calcaneus

Sural nerve

Quadratus plantae muscle

FIGURE 5–36E.

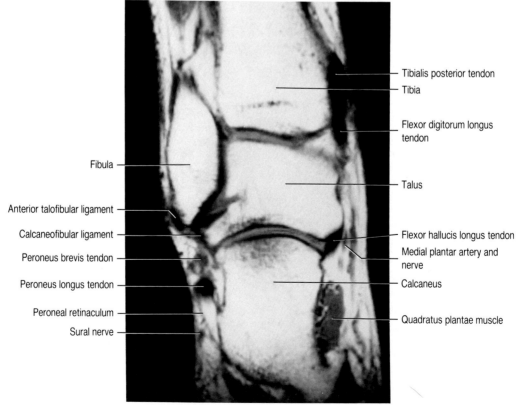

Tibialis posterior tendon

Tibia

Flexor digitorum longus tendon

Fibula

Anterior talofibular ligament

Talus

Calcaneofibular ligament

Peroneus brevis tendon

Flexor hallucis longus tendon

Medial plantar artery and nerve

Peroneus longus tendon

Peroneal retinaculum

Calcaneus

Sural nerve

Quadratus plantae muscle

FIGURE 5–36F.

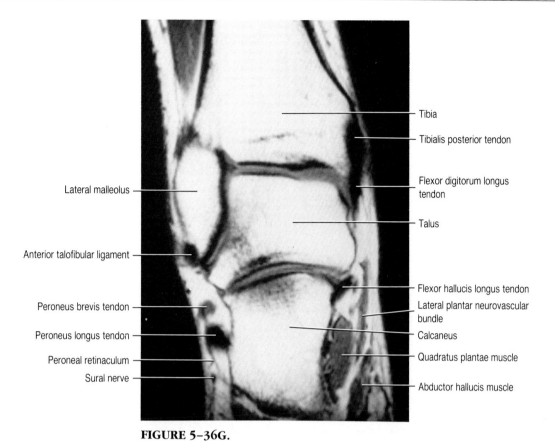

Tibia

Tibialis posterior tendon

Flexor digitorum longus tendon

Talus

Flexor hallucis longus tendon

Lateral plantar neurovascular bundle

Calcaneus

Quadratus plantae muscle

Abductor hallucis muscle

Lateral malleolus

Anterior talofibular ligament

Peroneus brevis tendon

Peroneus longus tendon

Peroneal retinaculum

Sural nerve

FIGURE 5–36G.

Tibia

Tibialis posterior tendon

Deltoid ligament (posterior tibiotalar ligament)

Flexor digitorum longus tendon

Talus

Medial plantar neurovascular structures

Flexor hallucis longus tendon

Calcaneus

Lateral plantar neurovascular bundle

Quadratus plantae muscle

Abductor hallucis muscle

Lateral malleolus

Anterior talofibular ligament

Peroneus brevis tendon

Peroneus longus tendon

Sural nerve

FIGURE 5–36H.

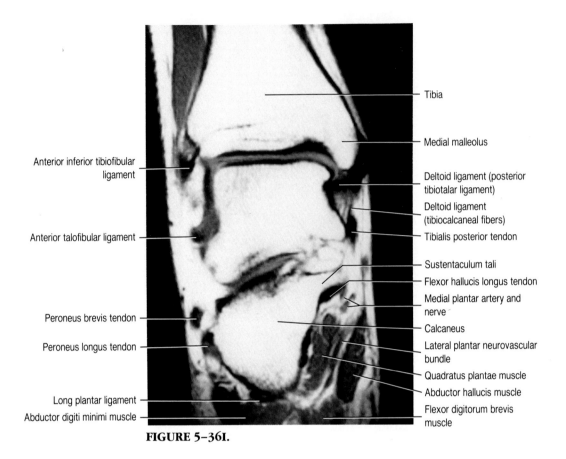

Anterior inferior tibiofibular ligament

Anterior talofibular ligament

Peroneus brevis tendon

Peroneus longus tendon

Long plantar ligament

Abductor digiti minimi muscle

Tibia

Medial malleolus

Deltoid ligament (posterior tibiotalar ligament)

Deltoid ligament (tibiocalcaneal fibers)

Tibialis posterior tendon

Sustentaculum tali

Flexor hallucis longus tendon

Medial plantar artery and nerve

Calcaneus

Lateral plantar neurovascular bundle

Quadratus plantae muscle

Abductor hallucis muscle

Flexor digitorum brevis muscle

FIGURE 5–36I.

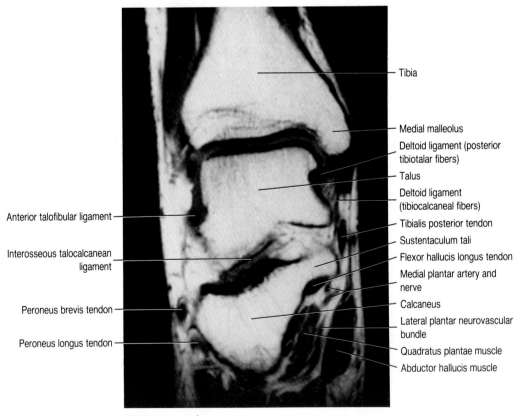

Anterior talofibular ligament

Interosseous talocalcanean ligament

Peroneus brevis tendon

Peroneus longus tendon

Tibia

Medial malleolus

Deltoid ligament (posterior tibiotalar fibers)

Talus

Deltoid ligament (tibiocalcaneal fibers)

Tibialis posterior tendon

Sustentaculum tali

Flexor hallucis longus tendon

Medial plantar artery and nerve

Calcaneus

Lateral plantar neurovascular bundle

Quadratus plantae muscle

Abductor hallucis muscle

FIGURE 5–36J.

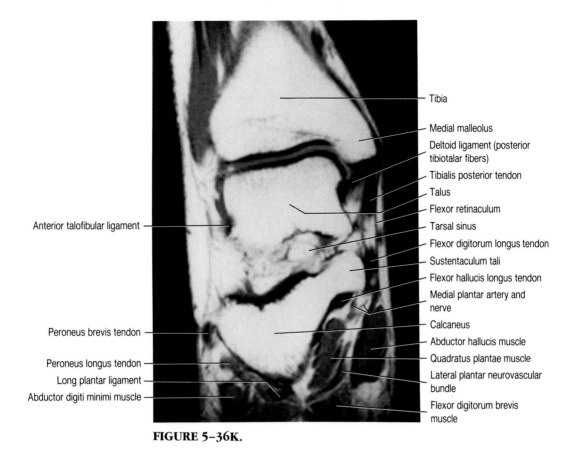

Anterior talofibular ligament

Peroneus brevis tendon

Peroneus longus tendon

Long plantar ligament

Abductor digiti minimi muscle

Tibia

Medial malleolus

Deltoid ligament (posterior tibiotalar fibers)

Tibialis posterior tendon

Talus

Flexor retinaculum

Tarsal sinus

Flexor digitorum longus tendon

Sustentaculum tali

Flexor hallucis longus tendon

Medial plantar artery and nerve

Calcaneus

Abductor hallucis muscle

Quadratus plantae muscle

Lateral plantar neurovascular bundle

Flexor digitorum brevis muscle

FIGURE 5–36K.

Anterior talofibular ligament

Calcaneus

Peroneus brevis tendon

Peroneus longus tendon

Long plantar ligament

Abductor digiti minimi muscle

Tibia

Medial malleolus

Deltoid ligament (tibiotalar fibers)

Deltoid ligament (tibiocalcaneal fibers)

Tibialis posterior tendon

Talus

Sustentaculum tali

Flexor digitorum longus tendon

Flexor hallucis longus tendon

Medial plantar artery and nerve

Quadratus plantae muscle

Abductor hallucis muscle

Lateral plantar neurovascular bundle

Flexor digitorum brevis muscle

FIGURE 5–36L.

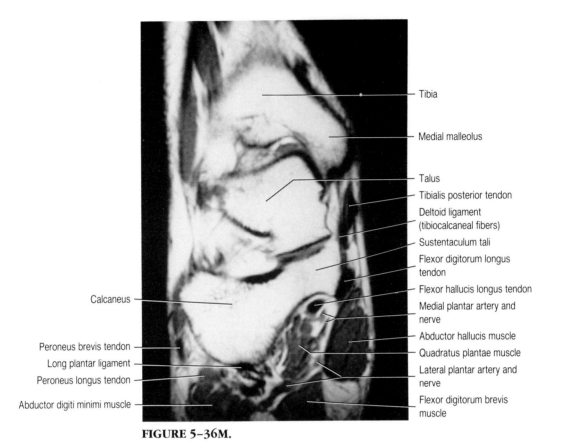

Tibia

Medial malleolus

Talus

Tibialis posterior tendon

Deltoid ligament (tibiocalcaneal fibers)

Sustentaculum tali

Flexor digitorum longus tendon

Flexor hallucis longus tendon

Medial plantar artery and nerve

Abductor hallucis muscle

Quadratus plantae muscle

Lateral plantar artery and nerve

Flexor digitorum brevis muscle

Calcaneus

Peroneus brevis tendon

Long plantar ligament

Peroneus longus tendon

Abductor digiti minimi muscle

FIGURE 5–36M.

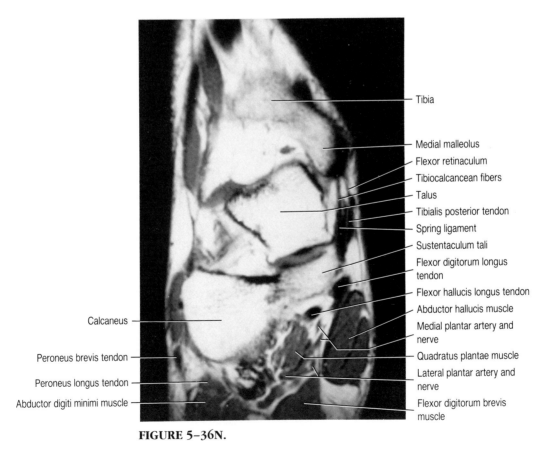

Tibia

Medial malleolus

Flexor retinaculum

Tibiocalcancean fibers

Talus

Tibialis posterior tendon

Spring ligament

Sustentaculum tali

Flexor digitorum longus tendon

Flexor hallucis longus tendon

Abductor hallucis muscle

Medial plantar artery and nerve

Quadratus plantae muscle

Lateral plantar artery and nerve

Flexor digitorum brevis muscle

Calcaneus

Peroneus brevis tendon

Peroneus longus tendon

Abductor digiti minimi muscle

FIGURE 5–36N.

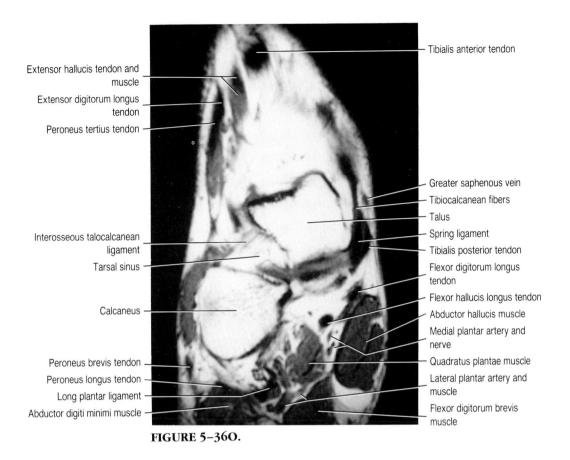

Extensor hallucis tendon and muscle

Extensor digitorum longus tendon

Peroneus tertius tendon

Interosseous talocalcanean ligament

Tarsal sinus

Calcaneus

Peroneus brevis tendon

Peroneus longus tendon

Long plantar ligament

Abductor digiti minimi muscle

Tibialis anterior tendon

Greater saphenous vein

Tibiocalcanean fibers

Talus

Spring ligament

Tibialis posterior tendon

Flexor digitorum longus tendon

Flexor hallucis longus tendon

Abductor hallucis muscle

Medial plantar artery and nerve

Quadratus plantae muscle

Lateral plantar artery and muscle

Flexor digitorum brevis muscle

FIGURE 5–36O.

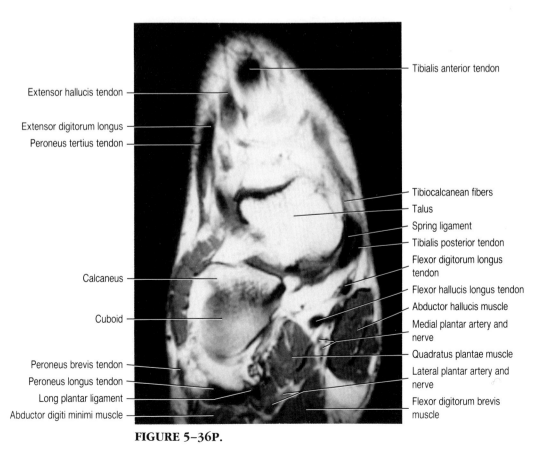

Extensor hallucis tendon

Extensor digitorum longus

Peroneus tertius tendon

Calcaneus

Cuboid

Peroneus brevis tendon

Peroneus longus tendon

Long plantar ligament

Abductor digiti minimi muscle

Tibialis anterior tendon

Tibiocalcanean fibers

Talus

Spring ligament

Tibialis posterior tendon

Flexor digitorum longus tendon

Flexor hallucis longus tendon

Abductor hallucis muscle

Medial plantar artery and nerve

Quadratus plantae muscle

Lateral plantar artery and nerve

Flexor digitorum brevis muscle

FIGURE 5–36P.

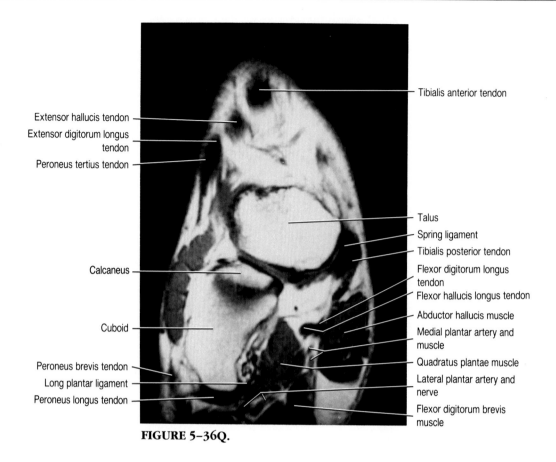

Extensor hallucis tendon

Extensor digitorum longus tendon

Peroneus tertius tendon

Calcaneus

Cuboid

Peroneus brevis tendon

Long plantar ligament

Peroneus longus tendon

Tibialis anterior tendon

Talus

Spring ligament

Tibialis posterior tendon

Flexor digitorum longus tendon

Flexor hallucis longus tendon

Abductor hallucis muscle

Medial plantar artery and muscle

Quadratus plantae muscle

Lateral plantar artery and nerve

Flexor digitorum brevis muscle

FIGURE 5–36Q.

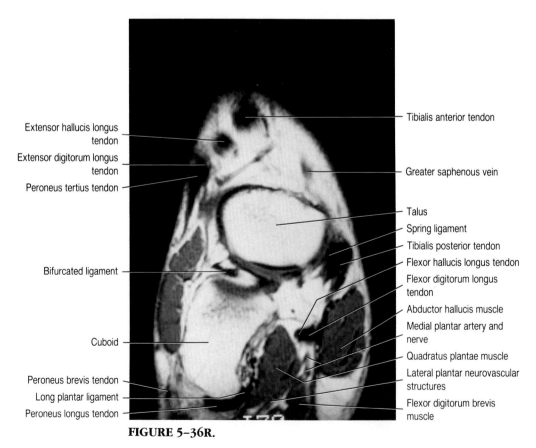

Extensor hallucis longus tendon

Extensor digitorum longus tendon

Peroneus tertius tendon

Bifurcated ligament

Cuboid

Peroneus brevis tendon

Long plantar ligament

Peroneus longus tendon

Tibialis anterior tendon

Greater saphenous vein

Talus

Spring ligament

Tibialis posterior tendon

Flexor hallucis longus tendon

Flexor digitorum longus tendon

Abductor hallucis muscle

Medial plantar artery and nerve

Quadratus plantae muscle

Lateral plantar neurovascular structures

Flexor digitorum brevis muscle

FIGURE 5–36R.

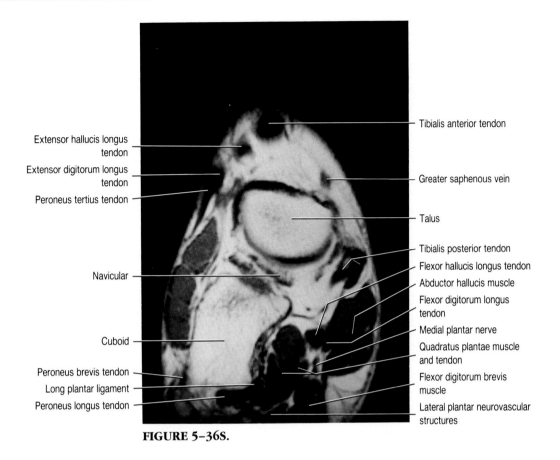

Extensor hallucis longus tendon

Extensor digitorum longus tendon

Peroneus tertius tendon

Navicular

Cuboid

Peroneus brevis tendon

Long plantar ligament

Peroneus longus tendon

Tibialis anterior tendon

Greater saphenous vein

Talus

Tibialis posterior tendon

Flexor hallucis longus tendon

Abductor hallucis muscle

Flexor digitorum longus tendon

Medial plantar nerve

Quadratus plantae muscle and tendon

Flexor digitorum brevis muscle

Lateral plantar neurovascular structures

FIGURE 5–36S.

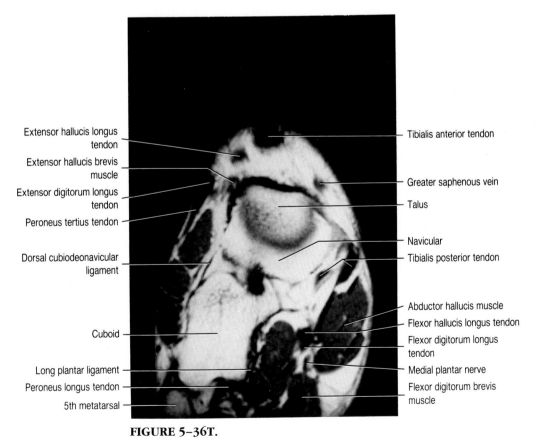

Extensor hallucis longus tendon

Extensor hallucis brevis muscle

Extensor digitorum longus tendon

Peroneus tertius tendon

Dorsal cubiodeonavicular ligament

Cuboid

Long plantar ligament

Peroneus longus tendon

5th metatarsal

Tibialis anterior tendon

Greater saphenous vein

Talus

Navicular

Tibialis posterior tendon

Abductor hallucis muscle

Flexor hallucis longus tendon

Flexor digitorum longus tendon

Medial plantar nerve

Flexor digitorum brevis muscle

FIGURE 5–36T.

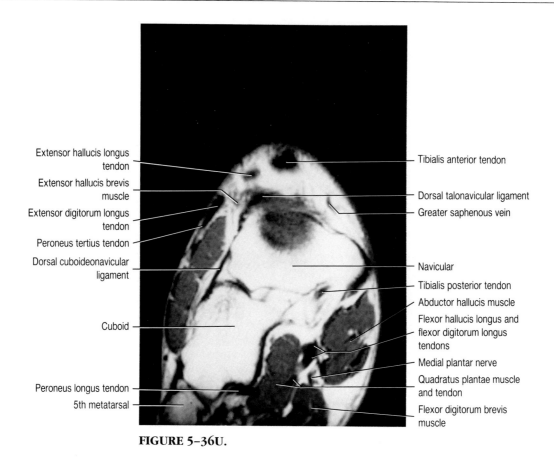

Extensor hallucis longus tendon

Extensor hallucis brevis muscle

Extensor digitorum longus tendon

Peroneus tertius tendon

Dorsal cuboideonavicular ligament

Cuboid

Peroneus longus tendon

5th metatarsal

Tibialis anterior tendon

Dorsal talonavicular ligament

Greater saphenous vein

Navicular

Tibialis posterior tendon

Abductor hallucis muscle

Flexor hallucis longus and flexor digitorum longus tendons

Medial plantar nerve

Quadratus plantae muscle and tendon

Flexor digitorum brevis muscle

FIGURE 5–36U.

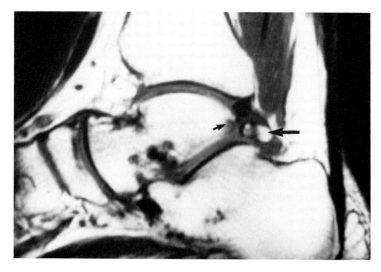

FIGURE 5–37. Low signal intensity irregular posterior talar cortex (*small black arrow*) as a normal variant. Normal fat signal intensity is present in os trigonum (*large black arrow*). T1-weighted sagittal image.

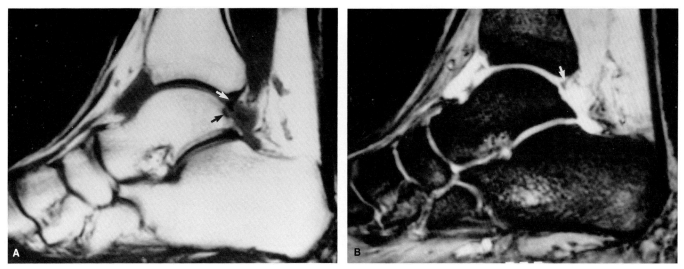

FIGURE 5–38. (**A**) A T1-weighted sagittal image demonstrates focal low signal intensity irregularity mimicking a transchondral fracture of the posterior talar cortex (*black arrow*). The low signal intensity posterior tibiofibular ligament is located posterior to the tibiotalar joint and is not a loose body (*white arrow*). (**B**) A T2*-weighted sagittal image shows the posterior tibiofibular ligament (*white arrow*) in contrast to high signal intensity joint effusion.

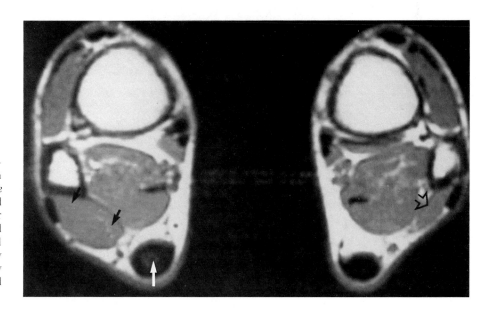

FIGURE 5–39. Asymmetric hypertrophy of the peroneus brevis muscle can occur as a normal anatomic variant (*black arrows*). The contralateral, normal-sized peroneus brevis muscle is shown for comparison (*open arrow*). Associated Achilles tendinitis demonstrates a central area of intermediate signal intensity within an enlarged, low-signal intensity tendon (*white arrow*) on a T1-weighted axial image.

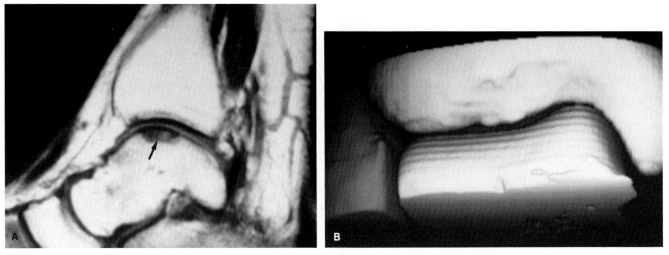

FIGURE 5–40. **(A)** A T1-weighted sagittal image shows a stage I transchondral fracture with a low signal intensity compression fracture (*arrow*) of the talus. **(B)** Preservation of tibiotalar joint surfaces can be seen on a 3D CT image.

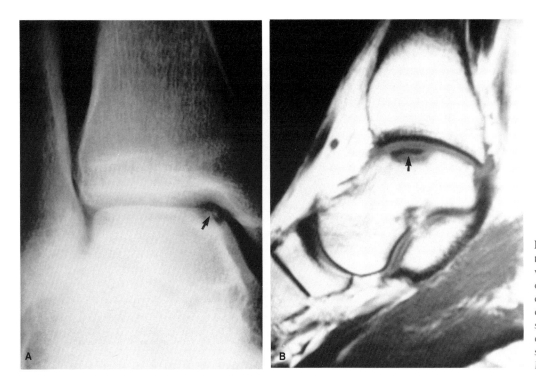

FIGURE 5–41. Stage III transchondral fracture (*arrow*) with a complete nondisplaced osteochondral fragment is seen on **(A)** an anteroposterior radiograph and **(B)** a T1-weighted sagittal image. The osteochondral fragment demonstrates low signal intensity sclerosis on the MR image.

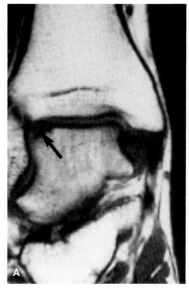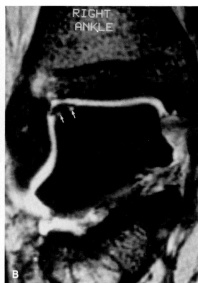

FIGURE 5–42. A stage III transchondral fracture of the lateral talar dome is seen on (**A**) T1-weighted (*black arrow*) and (**B**) T2*-weighted (*white arrows*) coronal images. High signal intensity joint fluid undermines the osteochondral fracture on the T2*-weighted image.

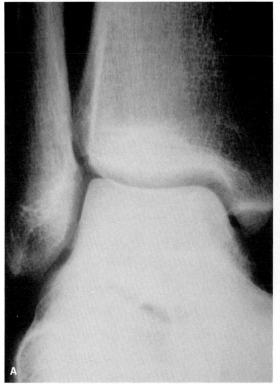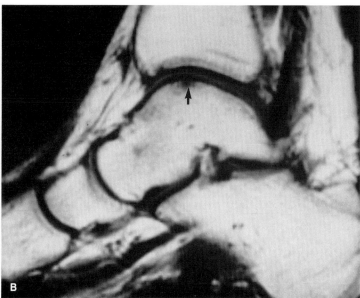

FIGURE 5–43. (**A**) An anteroposterior radiograph taken in internal rotation is negative for fracture. (**B**) A T1-weighted image reveals a stage I transchondral compression fracture (*arrow*) with a low signal intensity subchondral focus. The overlying low signal intensity cortex and intermediate signal intensity articular cartilage are intact.

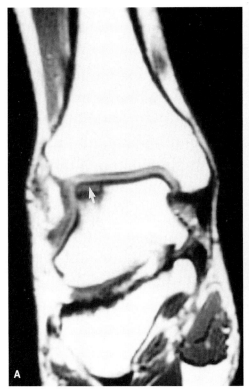

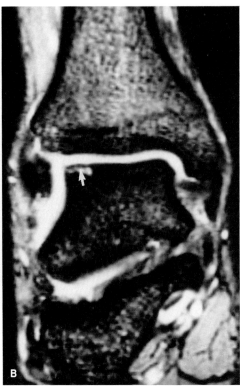

FIGURE 5–44. A stage II lesion with a partial osteochondral fracture (*arrow*) involving the lateral talar dome can be seen on (**A**) T1-weighted and (**B**) T2*-weighted coronal images. The hyperintense fluid undermines the lateral aspect of the osteochondral lesion in the T2*-weighted image.

FIGURE 5–45. (**A**) A T1-weighted coronal image shows a stage III transchondral fracture with a low signal intensity, complete, nondisplaced osteochondral fracture (*straight arrow*). Note the associated diffuse low signal intensity subchondral talar marrow hyperemia (*curved arrow*). (**B**) High signal intensity talar hyperemia (*curved arrow*) is displayed on a short TI inversion recovery sagittal image. Tibiotalar joint effusion distends the anterior and posterior capsules.

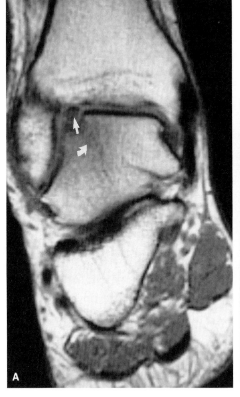

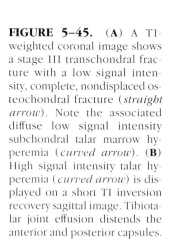

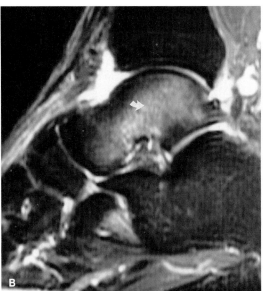

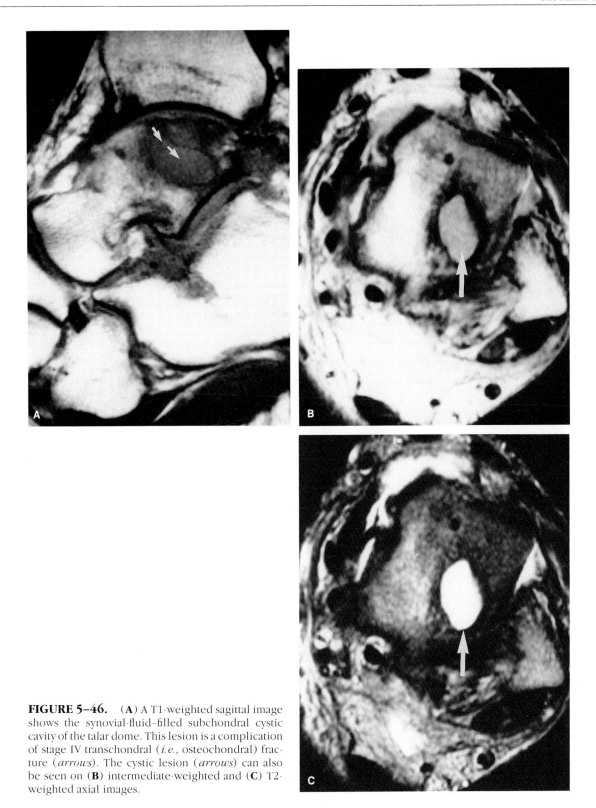

FIGURE 5–46. (**A**) A T1-weighted sagittal image shows the synovial-fluid–filled subchondral cystic cavity of the talar dome. This lesion is a complication of stage IV transchondral (*i.e.,* osteochondral) fracture (*arrows*). The cystic lesion (*arrows*) can also be seen on (**B**) intermediate-weighted and (**C**) T2-weighted axial images.

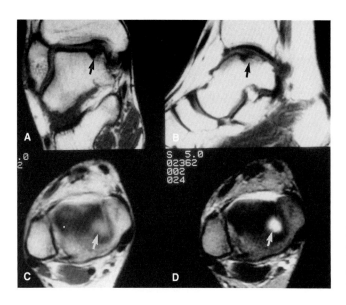

FIGURE 5–47. A transchondral fracture (*arrow*) demonstrates subchondral and cortical irregularity on (**A**) coronal and (**B**) sagittal T1-weighted images. Fluid imbibed through the traumatized articular cartilage surface is shown on (**C**) intermediate-weighted and (**D**) T2-weighted axial images.

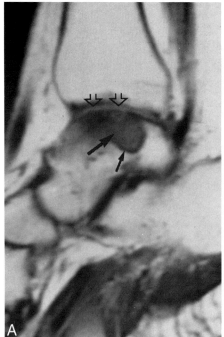

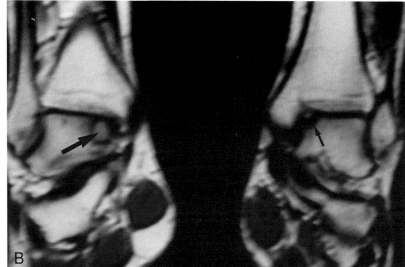

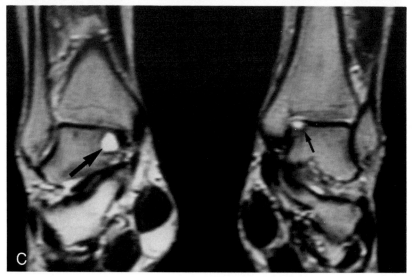

FIGURE 5–48. (**A**) In a transchondral fracture, a T1-weighted sagittal image shows a medial talar osteochondral defect with a low signal intensity periphery of reactive bone (*small solid arrow*) and intermediate signal intensity viscous synovial fluid contents (*large solid arrow*). The overlying hyaline articular cartilage is intact (*open arrows*). On corresponding T2-weighted coronal spin-echo sequence images, the talar cavity (*large arrows*) demonstrates (**B**) intermediate signal intensity on a balanced weighted image and (**C**) uniform high-signal intensity fluid in second echo. A contralateral smaller talar defect is shown (*small arrows*).

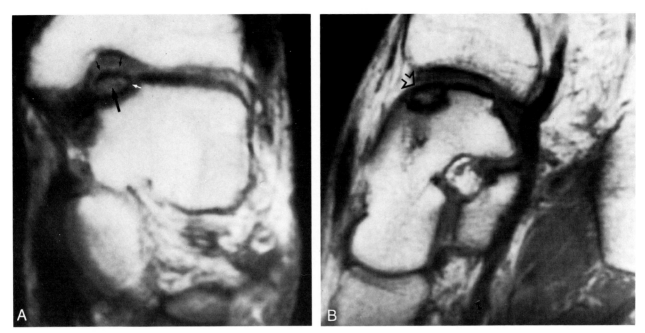

FIGURE 5–49. (**A**) In a transchondral fracture, a T1-weighted coronal image shows an osteochondral talar lesion (*large black arrow*) with upward bowing of the medial talar hyaline articular cartilage surface (*small black arrows*). Intermediate signal intensity fluid is seen undermining transchondral defect (*white arrow*). (**B**) A T1-weighted sagittal image demonstrates attenuated articular cartilage overlying the transchondral fracture (*open arrow*).

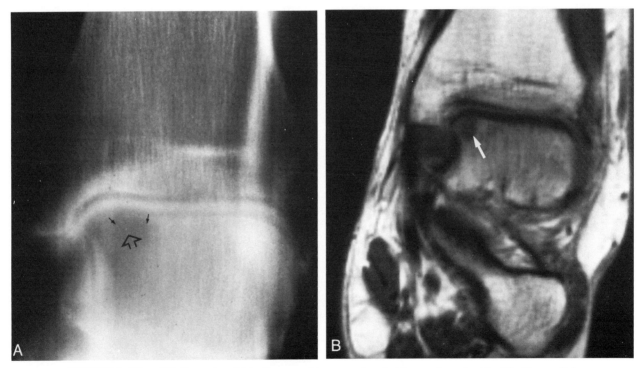

FIGURE 5–50. (**A**) Osteochondritis dissecans (*i.e.,* transchondral fracture) can be identified by medial talar lucency (*open arrow*) on an anteroposterior tomogram. The superior outline is defined (*small arrows*). (**B**) A T1-weighted coronal image shows a low signal intensity osteochondral defect (*arrow*). (**C**) A T2*-weighted image demonstrates a fluid-filled osteochondral cavity (*open arrow*) and overlying cartilage disruption (*solid arrow*). *(continued)*

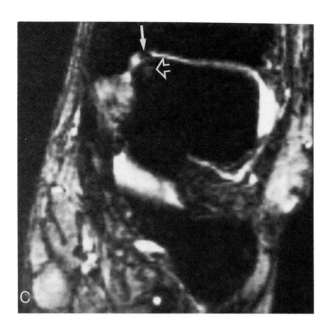

FIGURE 5–50. *(Continued)*

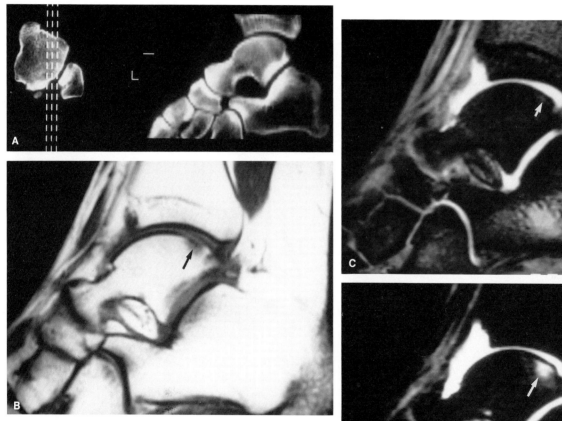

FIGURE 5–51. (**A**) Axial CT (*left*) and 2D reformatted CT (*right*) images are negative for transchondral fracture. (**B**) The low signal intensity posterolateral transchondral fracture is revealed on a T1-weighted sagittal image (*arrow*). (**C**) Minimal signal abnormality is seen on a T2*-weighted sagittal image (*arrow*). (**D**) The hyperintense osteochondral lesion is more accurately displayed on a short TI inversion recovery image (*arrow*). Note that the area of increased signal intensity is greater than that seen on T1- and T2*-weighted sagittal images.

rotation of the tibia causes a medial lesion (*i.e.,* impact between the posteromedial tibia and medial talar margin). The medial and lateral surfaces of the talus are involved in 56% and 44% of transchondral fractures, respectively. The medial lesion, is usually cup-shaped and deeper than the lateral lesion. The medial lesion is not as strongly associated with a history of antecedent trauma as the lateral lesion, which tends to be wafer-shaped and thin.

If the fibular collateral ligament fails to rupture because articular surfaces are contacted, the presentation of pain may be minimal. More severe injuries are accompanied by ligamentous tearing. Berndt and Harty have developed a four-part staging system for characterizing transchondral fractures based on plain radiographs.[12] In stage I, there is a subchondral compression fracture of the talus with no ligamentous sprain (Fig. 5–43). Radiographs are negative, and lesions in this stage may be painless. Stage II lesions involve a partially detached osteochondral fragment with a hinge or flap of articular cartilage (Fig. 5–44). A T2- or T2*-weighted image may be necessary to identify the osteochondral fragment. In stage III lesions, a complete nondisplaced fracture remains within the bony crater (Fig. 5–45). Stage IV lesions are characterized by detachment with a loose osteochondral fragment (Fig. 5–46). Although stage II to IV lesions are themselves painless, they may be associated with a painful sprain or rupture of the collateral ankle ligaments.

Magnetic Resonance Findings

As mentioned, early x-rays of transchondral fracture may be negative until a necrotic focus is observed.[13] Necrosis is characterized by increased bone density of the necrotic focus and surrounding demineralization secondary to increased vascularization. In addition, it is not possible to assess the integrity of hyaline articular cartilage surfaces in osteocartilaginous defects with conventional radiographs or CT scans. With MR imaging, however, tibiotalar anatomy can be displayed in the coronal, axial, or sagittal plane to identify the talar defect and presence of an avulsed body fragment.[14] Subchondral marrow and articular cartilage surfaces are uniquely demonstrated on MR images.

The hyaline articular cartilage surface of the talar dome demonstrates intermediate signal intensity on T1- or T2-weighted images and high signal intensity on T2*-weighted images. A detached cortical fragment, on the other hand, remains low in signal intensity. Adherent hyaline articular cartilage, reparative fibrocartilage, or associated fibrous tissue demonstrates intermediate signal intensity. On T1-weighted images, the bony defect of the talus demonstrates low or intermediate signal intensity, depending on the composition of synovial fluid and fibrous tissue, respectively. On T2-weighted images, synovial fluid contents generate increased signal intensity. Peripheral areas of low signal intensity within the subchondral bone on T1- and T2-weighted images have been correlated with reactive bone sclerosis on plain radiographs.

Abnormalities of the articular surface include regions of cartilage thinning, bowing, nodularity, or disruption.[15] The accumulation of high intensity joint fluid at or undermining the cartilage surface indicates small fissures or breaks in articular cartilage (Figs. 5–47 and 5–48).

On sagittal or coronal images, a focal, upward bowing of the hyaline cartilage overlying the bony defect may be demonstrated (Fig. 5–49). The cartilage may be deformed or bowed without disruption, and it frequently shows softening at surgery. A postsurgical fibrocartilaginous scar may appear as an intermediate intensity focal area of thickening, bridging a cartilaginous defect. T2*-weighted images are useful for identification of small areas of cartilage disruption (Fig. 5–50).[16] Fluid, edema, and hyperemia in subchondral bone can be identified on STIR images with greater sensitivity than with corresponding T2- or T2*-weighted images (Fig. 5–51). De Smet and colleagues have correlated the stability of the osteochondral fragment with signal intensity using T2-weighted images.[17] They found that an irregular high signal intensity zone at the fragment–talar interface was observed in partially attached fragments, whereas a complete ring of fluid signal intensity surrounding the lesion occurred in unattached fragments.

Treatment

Treatment protocols for transchondral fracture vary, depending on the stage of the lesion. Immobilization with conservative treatment may be used except in lateral stage II and stage IV fractures, which often require free fragment excision, curettage, and drilling. Stage II and III lesions should be treated with curetting or drilling and Kirschner wire pinning (Fig. 5–52). A drilled or abraded base permits fibrocartilaginous ingrowth in lesions with a nonreplaceable fragment. Complications, including locking of the joint, which occurs with larger bone fragments; degenerative arthritis, which is more likely to occur with lateral, often symptomatic, lesions; and nonunion of the fracture, often lead to traumatic osteoarthritis. Arthroscopic techniques have relatively low morbidity and complication rates in the treatment of talar dome fractures.[18]

Value of Magnetic Resonance Imaging

Although conventional radiographic techniques should remain the choice for the initial evaluation of patients with suspected osteochondral defects, MR offers the ability to assess both the talar defect and the integrity of overlying cartilage surfaces. The presence of an intact articular surface could obviate the need for surgical excision and curettage, in favor of more conservative treatments such as drilling.

Injuries to the Tendons

A variety of studies have confirmed the usefulness of MR imaging in the evaluation of tendinous and ligamentous structures about the ankle. Intact tendons and ligaments demonstrate low signal intensity on all pulsing sequences. The thicker tendons of the ankle can be studied in multiple planes, and smaller ligamentous bands may be seen in only one orthogonal plane.

Achilles Tendon Rupture

The Achilles tendon is the largest tendon in the body and is formed by the confluence of the gastrocnemius and soleus muscle complexes. Injuries to this tendon secondary to athletic activity are frequent in middle-aged males.[19,20] There may be a predisposition to disruption of the Achilles tendon in the already weakened connective tissue and collagen fibers of patients with disorders such as rheumatoid arthritis, systemic lupus erythematosus, diabetes mellitus, and gout. The Achilles tendon is most susceptible to rupture 2 to 6 cm superior to the os calcis. Acute rupture is associated with forced dorsiflexion of the foot against a contracting force generated by the triceps surae group. Rupture of the contracted musculotendinous unit may occur secondary to direct trauma.

Diagnosis. With clinical examination alone, rupture of the Achilles tendon is missed in up to 25% of cases, perhaps because the other tendons of the posterior calf maintain plantar flexion and allow a tendinous gap to be missed on clinical examination. Clinical assessment by the Thompsen test is performed in the prone position. In Achilles tendon rupture, squeezing the calf does not produce the normal response of plantar flexion.

Lateral radiography and xerography have not been effective in identifying abnormalities in the Achilles tendon. Although tendon thickening in inflammation and discontinuities in tears have been observed with some success using real time ultrasonography, this technique is limited in soft-tissue contrast discrimination, FOV, and inability to accurately evaluate both adjacent soft-tissue and bony structures.

Magnetic Resonance Imaging Technique. The Achilles tendon can be demonstrated on sagittal, axial, and thin section coronal MR images.[21] A routine examination of the tendon uses a 14- to 16-cm FOV and sections 3 to 4 mm thick. A T1-weighted sequence is performed in the sagittal plane through the Achilles tendon. T2*-weighted or STIR images show associated hemorrhage or edema in the tendinous or peritendinous soft-tissue structures. T2- or T2*-weighted axial sequences reveal fluid, hemorrhage, or inflammatory tendon changes, and to evaluate the integrity of other tendons and ligaments supporting the ankle. Thin section (3-mm) coronal images display the width of the Achilles tendon and the condition of disrupted tendon fibers.

Magnetic Resonance Findings. The normal Achilles tendon demonstrates uniform low signal intensity. Axial images show the tendon in cross section with a mildly flattened anterior surface and a convex posterior surface. In ruptures of the Achilles tendon, the relationship of the proximal and distal portions of the torn tendon can be seen in MR studies either before or after application of a plaster cast (Fig. 5–53). High signal intensity fat may be interposed at the tear site in complete tendinous disruptions (Fig. 5–54). Fraying or corkscrewing of the tendon edges is frequently associated with proximal tendon retraction (Fig. 5–55). In the absence of overlapping tendon edges, no tendon fibers can be seen at the tear site on axial images (Figs. 5–56 and 5–57). In one study of preoperative MR imaging findings that included tendon morphology, orientation of torn fibers, and measurement of tendon diastasis, all correlated with surgical findings during tendon repair.[22] Associated hemorrhage within peritendinous soft tissues is revealed on axial or sagittal sections. Subacute hemorrhage generates high signal intensity on T1-weighted images. Areas of edema or inflammation demonstrate increased signal intensity on T2- or T2*-weighted images.

Treatment. As more patients with tendon tears are conservatively managed with serial casting, MR has become invaluable in documenting the degree of apposition in the disrupted proximal and distal tendon fragments. Retracted tendon sections are less likely to heal with conservative management, and MR evaluation allows early identification of these patients, who are candidates for surgical intervention (Fig. 5–58). Fibrous bridging also appears to be more tenuous with increased tendon separation. A bulbous contour may be demonstrated in the proliferating ends of a torn Achilles tendon, and it increases with greater tendon diastasis. Fibrous healing, with approximation of torn fibers, can be evaluated with MR imaging performed at monthly intervals.

The Achilles tendon and overlying skin are relatively avascular and may become infected after surgery with implanted material or autogenous tendon. The incidence of complications with surgical repair is reported to be 20%. Rerupture of the Achilles tendon is frequently seen in athletic patients within months of surgical repair. Nonsurgical treatment associated with a shorter morbidity

(text continues on page 461)

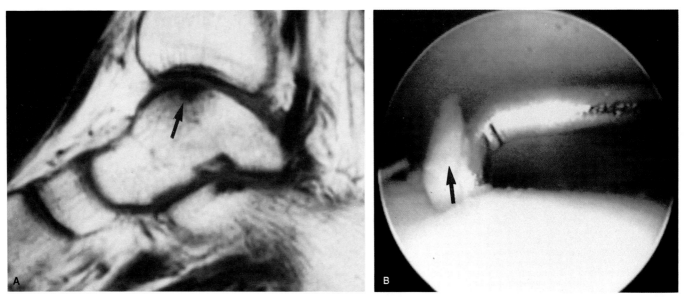

FIGURE 5–52. (**A**) A low signal intensity transchondral fracture extends to the talar cortex (*arrow*) as seen on a T1-weighted sagittal image. (**B**) The partially detached cartilaginous flap (*arrow*) is mobilized during arthroscopy of the tibiotalar joint.

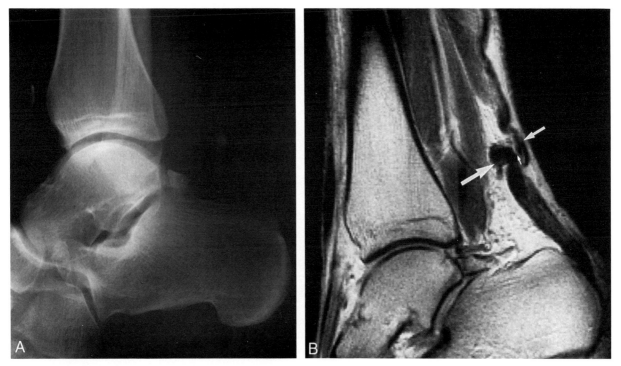

FIGURE 5–53. (**A**) On an anteroposterior radiograph performed after acute injury to the Achilles tendon, minimal posterior soft-tissue swelling is present. (**B**) A T1-weighted sagittal image reveals complete rupture of the Achilles tendon with proximal (*medium arrow*) and distal (*large arrow*) tendon fibers identified in close approximation (*small arrow*). (**C**) On a T1-weighted sagittal image taken after 4 months of cast treatment, complete fibrous healing with apposition of the torn tendon can be seen (*arrows*). *(continued)*

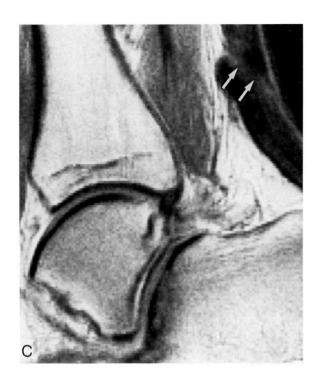

FIGURE 5–53. *(Continued)*

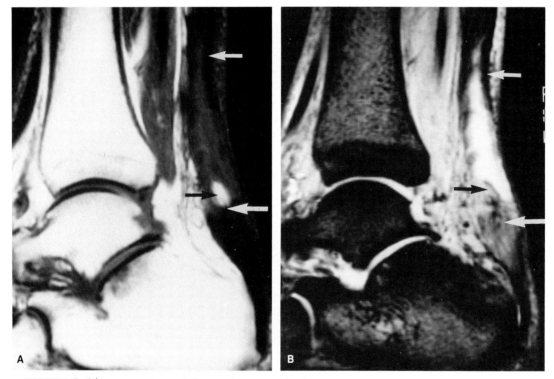

FIGURE 5–54. A complete Achilles tendon tear with a large tendinous gap (*white arrows*). Interposed fat demonstrates (**A**) bright signal intensity on a T1-weighted image and (**B**) intermediate signal intensity on a T2*-weighted image. (**C**) On a 3-mm T1-weighted posterior coronal image, the proximal (*single arrow*) and distal (*double arrow*) tendon edges are indicated with interposed high signal intensity fat (F). (**D**) On intermediate-weighted (*left*) and T2-weighted (*right*) axial images, a high signal intensity hemorrhagic tear site (*straight arrows*) with unattached low signal intensity anterior tendon fibers (*curved arrows*) is revealed at the level of the distal tibia.

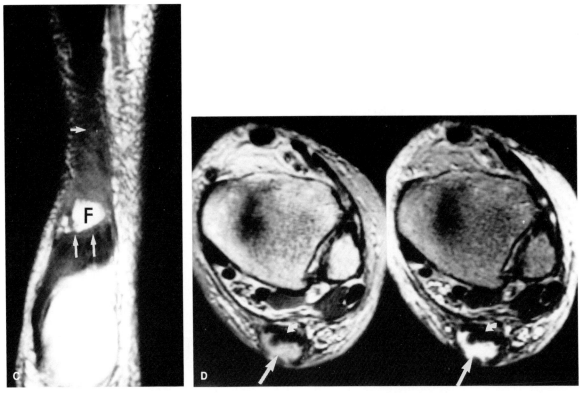

FIGURE 5–54. *(Continued)*

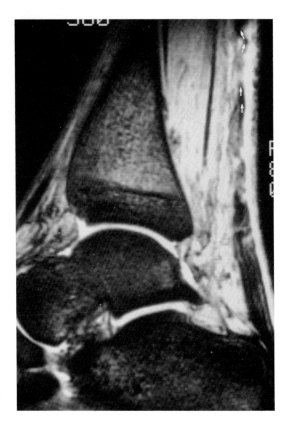

FIGURE 5–55. Fraying of the torn, retracted, proximal Achilles tendon can be seen on a T2*-weighted sagittal image (*arrows*). Repositioning of the surface coil is frequently required to locate retracted proximal fibers.

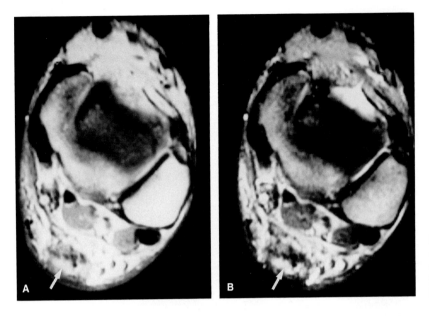

FIGURE 5–56. No tendon fibers are present (*arrow*) at the level of the tibiotalar joint in a patient with a complete Achilles rupture as seen on (**A**) intermediate-weighted and (**B**) T2-weighted axial images.

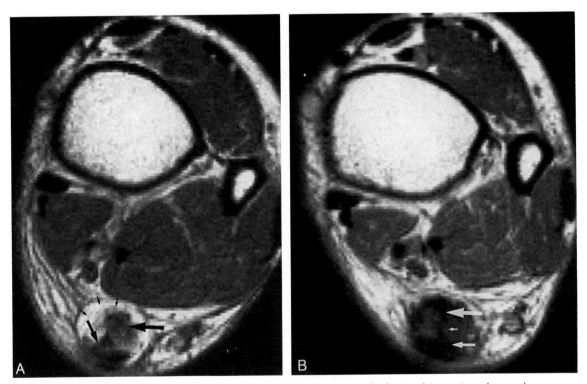

FIGURE 5–57. (**A**) A T1-weighted axial image demonstrates a high signal intensity subacute hemorrhage (*small arrows*) in a patient with rupture of the Achilles tendon. The proximal tendon (*large arrow*) is anterior to the distal tendon (*medium arrow*). (**B**) An intermediate signal intensity fibrous union (*small arrow*) between the proximal (*large arrow*) and distal (*medium arrow*) tendon ends is indicated on a T1-weighted axial image.

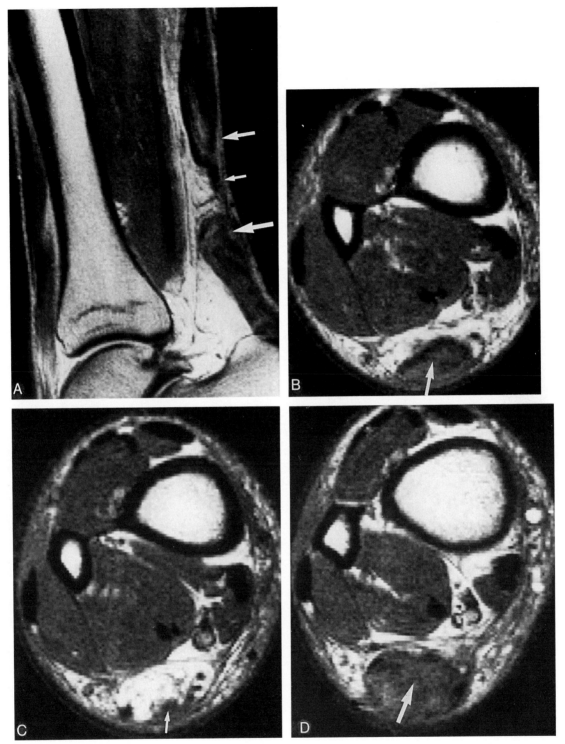

FIGURE 5–58. (**A**) T1-weighted sagittal and corresponding (**B**) superior, (**C**) mid-, and (**D**) inferior axial images demonstrate a healing Achilles tendon with an enlarged proximal end (*medium arrow*), tenuous union (*small arrow*), and bulbous distal tendon (*large arrow*). These signs indicate suboptimal Achilles tendon union.

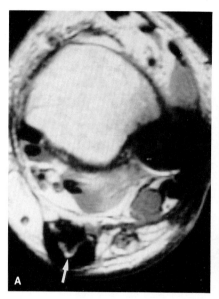
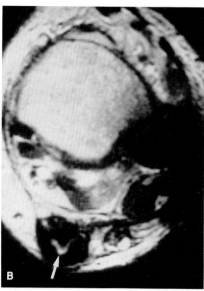

FIGURE 5–59. A postoperative high signal intensity suture artifact (*arrows*) is seen on (**A**) intermediate-weighted and (**B**) T2-weighted axial images of a thickened Achilles tendon.

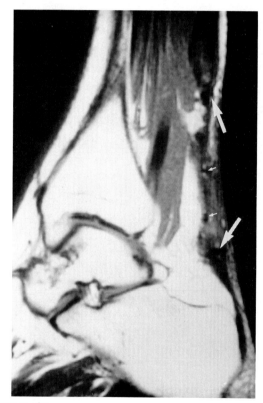

FIGURE 5–60. A T1-weighted sagittal image shows retear of an Achilles tendon repair with postoperative suture artifact (*small arrows*) and tendon discontinuity (*large arrows*).

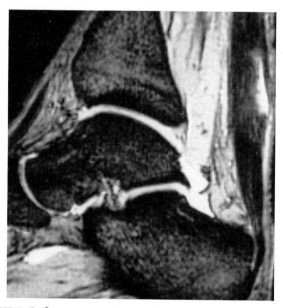

FIGURE 5–61. A partial tear of the posterior aspect of the Achilles tendon is seen on a T2*-weighted sagittal image. High signal intensity fluid is demonstrated in the longitudinally oriented tear. Associated diffuse thickening of the tendon is present.

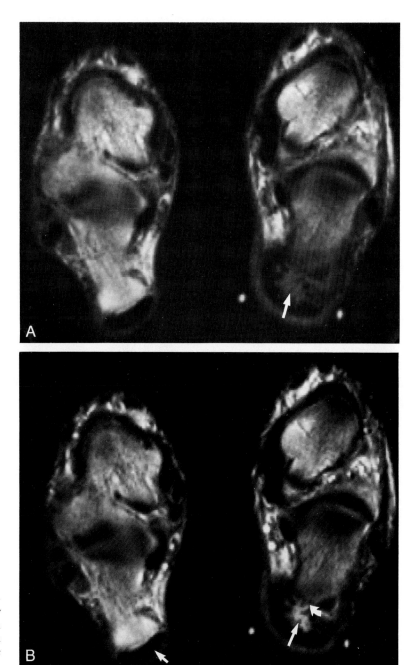

FIGURE 5–62. A partial tear of the left Achilles tendon (*long arrows*) demonstrates (**A**) low signal intensity on T1-weighted images and (**B**) high signal intensity on T2-weighted images. An intact right Achilles tendon (*short arrow*) is shown for comparison. Erosion of the posterior calcaneal surface has occurred (*curved arrow*).

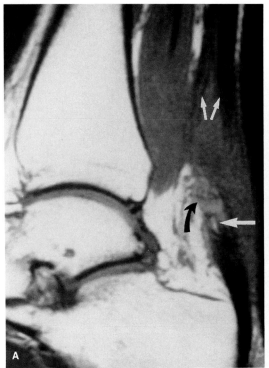

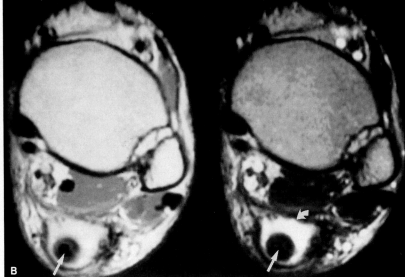

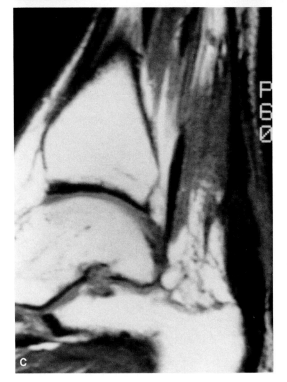

FIGURE 5–63. (**A**) A T1-weighted sagittal image shows what appears to be a complete Achilles tendon tear. Proximal (*double white arrows*) and distal (*single white arrow*) splayed tendon fibers are indicated. Intermediate signal intensity fat (*curved black arrow*) is interposed at tear site. (**B**) At the level of the distal tibia, however, a persistent band of tendon fibers with circular morphology (*straight arrows*) can be seen. High signal intensity hemorrhage is present anterior to the torn tendon (*curved arrow*) as seen on intermediate-weighted (*left*) and T2-weighted (*right*) axial images. (**C**) The corresponding T1-weighted parasagittal image documents the remaining intact tendon fibers.

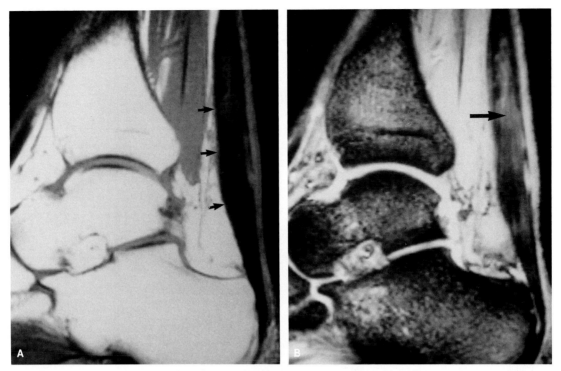

FIGURE 5–64. Achilles tendinitis is demonstrated in (**A**) T1-weighted and (**B**) T2*-weighted sagittal images. Note the diffuse Achilles tendon thickening (*small arrows*) and longitudinally directed hyper-intensity (*large arrow*).

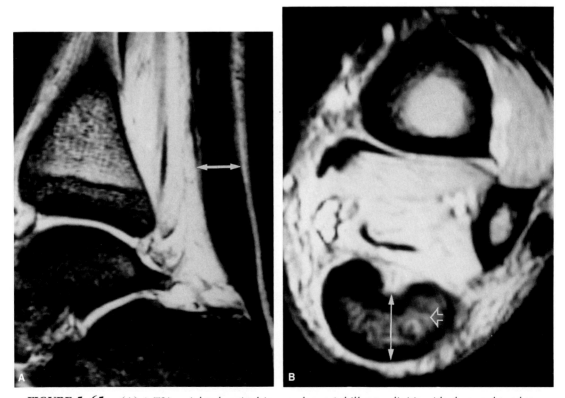

FIGURE 5–65. (**A**) A T2*-weighted sagittal image shows Achilles tendinitis with abnormal tendon thickening (*double-headed arrow*) and convexity to the anterior tendon margin. (**B**) A T2*-weighted axial image demonstrates high signal intensity tendinitis (*open arrow*) and diffuse thickening (*double-headed arrows*) without tendon discontinuity. Without a true synovial sheath, the Achilles tendon responds to inflammation with tendon thickening and intrasubstance signal change. The paratenon, or loose con-nective tissue anterior to the Achilles tendon, may show associated edematous changes.

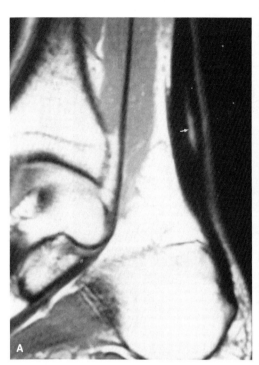

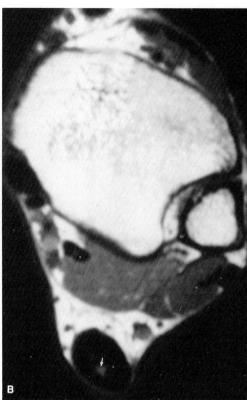

FIGURE 5–66. A linear area of high signal intensity mucinous degeneration and inflammation (*arrows*) occurs in a thickened Achilles tendon, as seen on T1-weighted (**A**) sagittal and (**B**) axial images.

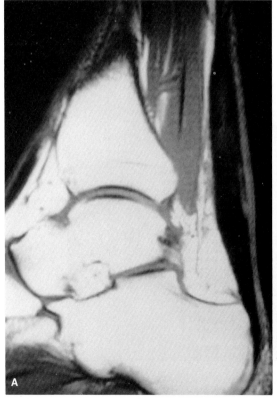

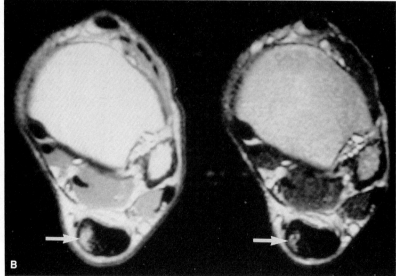

FIGURE 5–67. (**A**) A T1-weighted image shows a thickened Achilles tendon. (**B**) Achilles tendon degeneration or tendinitis (*arrow*) is revealed on an intermediate-weighted image (*left*), but appears without significant increased signal intensity on a T2-weighted image (*right*).

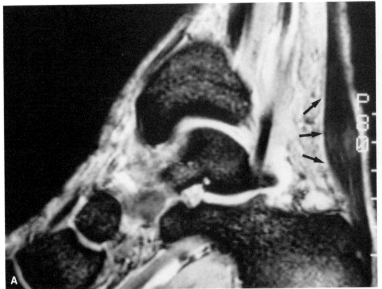

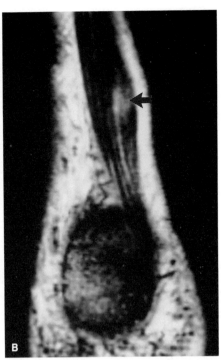

FIGURE 5–68. (**A**) A T2*-weighted sagittal image shows focal Achilles tendinitis with localized thickening and anterior convexity (*arrows*). (**B**) A T2*-weighted coronal image demonstrates tendon hyperintensity (*arrow*).

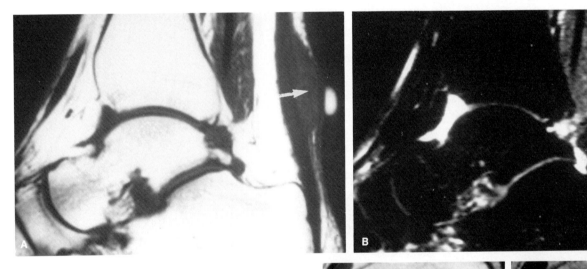

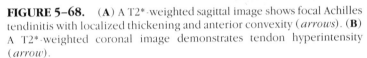

FIGURE 5–69. A soft-tissue sodium urate deposit (*i.e.,* tophus) located posterior to the Achilles tendon (*arrows*) demonstrates (**A**) low signal intensity on a T1-weighted sagittal image and (**B**) high signal intensity on a short TI inversion recovery sagittal image. The corresponding (**C**) intermediate-weighted and (**D**) T2-weighted axial images show no significant increase in signal intensity in the gouty deposit.

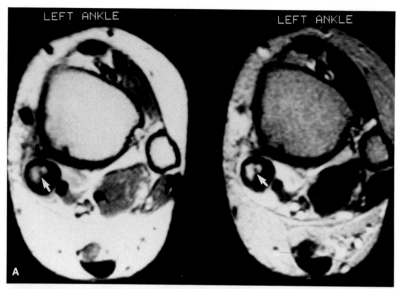

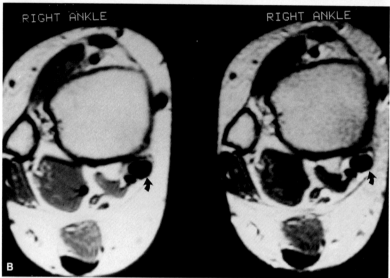

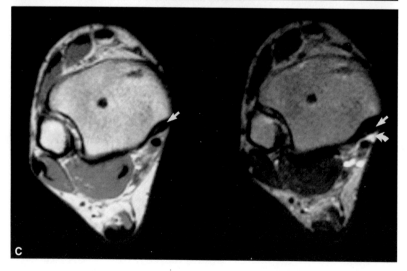

FIGURE 5–70. (**A**) A type 1 (*i.e.,* incomplete) tear of the tibialis posterior tendon is characterized by tendon thickening and central high signal intensity (*arrow*) on intermediate-weighted (*left*) and T2-weighted (*right*) axial images of the left ankle. (**B**) Normal morphology, size, and low signal intensity of the tendon (*curved arrow*) of the uninjured right ankle is shown for comparison on intermediate-weighted (*left*) and T2-weighted (*right*) axial images. (**C**) A type 2 lesion (partial tear, *curved arrow*) demonstrates associated tendon attenuation (*straight arrows*) and an adjacent hyperintense fluid signal intensity.

may be complicated by rerupture, venous thrombosis, and prolonged immobilization in cast therapy. Surgery is the preferred treatment for rerupture in the athlete who requires the strongest possible healing. Chronic thickening of the Achilles tendon or residual inflammatory changes are demonstrated on axial and sagittal MR images. Tendons repaired with strands of a polymer of lactic acid (PLA) show a thickened fusiform tendon with moderate signal intensity streaks on T1-weighted images (Fig. 5–59).[23] Changes in signal intensity were attributed to the PLA implant and surrounding collagenogenic response.

Magnetic resonance may be valuable in the selection of patients best suited for conservative therapy, thereby improving the present statistics for rerupture with conservative treatment (10%) compared with surgical treatment (4%).[24,25] Retear of a primary repaired tendon shows residual suture artifact (Fig. 5–60).

Partial Tendon Tears. Partial tendon tears are also defined on MR images in the sagittal and axial planes. Linear or focal regions of increased signal and thickening of fibers without a tendinous gap are characteristic of partial tears of the Achilles tendon (Figs. 5–61 and 5–62). Without inflammatory reaction, tendinitis—a common affliction among joggers—can be recognized by a thickening of the tendon complex. Incomplete tears may also be present with partial continuity of a portion of tendon fibers on at least one sagittal image (Fig. 5–63).

Achilles Tendinitis

Overuse of the calf muscles may lead to tenosynovitis of the Achilles tendon. Swelling of the tendon sheath may be present with effusion and crepitus. In stenosing tenosynovitis, chronic inflammation of the peritenon is found. Partial tearing, intrasubstance cysts from chronic partial tears, or nodules may also be identified. New collagen formation and associated fibrillation, nodularity, degeneration, and discoloration contribute to constriction of the peritenon.

Magnetic resonance findings include focal or fusiform thickening of the Achilles tendon and diffuse or linear increased signal intensity on T2-weighted, T2*-weighted, or STIR images (Figs. 5–64 and 5–65).[32] Inflammatory changes may coexist with mucinous or myxoid degeneration, which may or may not demonstrate similar increases in signal intensity on T2-weighted images (Figs. 5–66 and 5–67). Anterior convexity of the enlarged tendon may be revealed on sagittal images, and proximal extension of fluid in the retrocalcaneal bursa may also be seen (Fig. 5–68). It may be difficult to distinguish areas of tendinitis from intrasubstance tendon tears without documenting discontinuity in tendon tears. A healed Achilles tendon tear displays thickening without associated increased signal intensity.

If treatment by immobilization is not successful, stripping and excision of the thickened peritenon and granulation tissue are performed. The use of steroids may weaken the tendon and produce rupture. In gout, deposition of tophaceous material may also lead to spontaneous rupture of the Achilles tendon (Fig. 5–69). Tophi appear similar to nodular myxoidlike degeneration and demonstrate intermediate and increased signal inhomogeneity on T2-weighted, T2*-weighted, or STIR images.

Tibialis Posterior Injuries

Diagnosis. Rupture of the tibialis posterior tendon can occur spontaneously and is associated with prior synovitis, steroid injection, or trauma. Chronic tibialis tendon rupture usually occurs in middle-aged females in their fifth or sixth decades. Clinically, a unilateral flatfoot deformity develops, often with no history of trauma.[26] Intrinsic degeneration of the tendon occurs, and the typical site of rupture is either at or within 6 cm proximal to its navicular insertion. Collapse of the medial longitudinal arch creates the characteristic flatfoot deformity with associated heel valgus, talar plantar flexion, and forefoot abduction. Failure of calcaneal inversion in standing on tiptoe with a valgus heel is observed on clinical examination. In some cases, as many as 43 months have elapsed between clinical presentation and diagnosis.

Edema or soft-tissue thickening may be demonstrated inferior to the medial malleolus, although conventional radiographs do not demonstrate tendon pathology. Loss of a convex arch may be observed on weight-bearing views through the talonavicular or naviculocuneiform joint.

Magnetic Resonance Findings. Magnetic resonance demonstrates complete disruption of the tibialis posterior tendon with or without abnormal morphology of the ends of the tendon. A partial or chronic tear or a retracted tendon may present with enlargement of the affected tendon. T2-weighted axial images that extend inferior to the medial malleolus should demonstrate the normal tibialis posterior tendon anterolateral *medial* to the flexor digitorum longus tendon.

Partial tears of the posterior tibial tendon are classified either as hypertrophied (*i.e.,* type 1) regions with heterogeneous signal intensity in vertical splits (Fig. 5–70) or partial rupture with attenuated sections of tendon (*i.e.,* type 2).[27] Complete tears (*i.e.,* type 3) are delineated by a tendinous gap (Fig. 5–71). When MR findings were correlated with CT scans and surgical exploration, MR was shown to be superior to CT in detecting the spectrum of early partial tendon ruptures, longitudinal tearing, and the presence of synovial fluid.[28] Subtle areas of associated periostitis were more readily delineated with CT.

Intrinsic degenerations usually demonstrate varying degrees of increased internal signal intensity with fusiform enlargement. Fluid in the tendon sheath, demonstrating increased signal intensity on T2- or T2*-weighted images, may be observed in patients with tenosynovitis.

Treatment. Conservative treatment, which frequently fails, involves support of the medial longitudinal arch with orthoses. Surgical treatment consists of either osseous stabilization (*i.e.,* double or triple arthrodesis) with hindfoot arthrodesis, repair, or replacement of the ruptured tendon. A side-to-side anastomosis to the flexor digitorum longus or transfer of the flexor digitorum longus with suturing of its distal stump to the flexor hallucis longus have been attempted.

Other Tendon Injuries

The peroneal tendons may rupture secondary to trauma or laceration of the lateral aspect of the ankle. Magnetic resonance defines the position of the peroneal tendons and the fibular and retinacular anatomy.[29] Absence of the low signal intensity tendon within the peroneal tendon sheath may be observed on sagittal or axial images (Fig. 5–72).[30] The peroneal tendons are also involved in partial or complete dislocations. An absent or convex peroneal canal in the distal fibula may be a contributing factor. Dislocation of the tendons may be associated with stripping of the loosely attached superior peroneal retinaculum.

Rupture of the tibialis anterior tendon can occur between the extensor retinaculum and the insertion onto the medial first cuneiform and adjacent base of the 1st metatarsal. Weakness of dorsiflexion, localized tenderness, and dropfoot gait are observed on clinical evaluation.

Tearing of the flexor hallucis longus has been demonstrated on axial MR images at the level of the musculotendinous junction (Fig. 5–73).[31] The flexor hallucis longus is a plantar flexor of the first toe and participates in plantar flexion and inversion of the foot. Rupture of this tendon may be difficult to identify on clinical examination without the assistance of MR localization. Tearing of muscle fibers of the flexor digitorum brevis or quadratus plantae at the level of the flexor digitorum longus tendons may present clinically as tenderness over the plantar aponeurosis (Fig. 5–74).

Tenosynovitis

Tenosynovitis, either inflammatory or infectious, affects the tendons and synovial sheaths. The flexor hallucis longus tendon is susceptible to tendinitis and rupture where it passes through the tarsal tunnel. This injury is common in ballet dancers and presents with swelling and tenderness posterior to the medial malleolus. Flexor hallucis tendon pathology may be misdiagnosed as tendinitis of the tibialis posterior or flexor digitorum longus tendons. T2-weighted axial images show areas of increased fluid signal intensity in the tendon sheath. However, a normal communication with the ankle joint occurs in 10% to 15% of normal studies (Fig. 5–75). A low signal intensity tendon on scans with a long TR and TE excludes partial tear.

Tenosynovitis also involves the tibialis posterior and peroneal tendons (Figs. 5–76 and 5–77). Tibialis posterior tenosynovitis is associated with rheumatoid arthritis and planovalgus foot and usually occurs in an older age group. Peroneal tenosynovitis is associated with spastic flatfoot and is usually found in a younger population, often with a history of trauma. In acute tenosynovitis, findings usually include a synovial effusion without a thickened tendon or sheath. In chronic tenosynovitis, an effusion is accompanied by a thickened tendon and synovial sheath. On T2-weighted images, synovial sheath thickening demonstrates intermediate signal intensity (Fig. 5–78).

Ligamentous Injuries

Pathogenesis. Injuries to the ligaments about the ankle usually result from inversion and internal rotation of the foot combined with ankle plantar flexion.[33] When the foot is positioned in neutral or plantar flexion, the orientation of the anterior talofibular ligament is 45° to the horizontal, and it functions as a restraint to internal rotation (Fig. 5–79).[33] The vertically oriented calcaneofibular ligament primarily protects against varus force, and offers little resistance to internal rotation. The anterior talofibular ligament is the weakest and usually the first ligament to rupture with forced inversion and plantar flexion.[34] Even when inversion and plantar flexion forces cause rupture of the calcaneofibular ligament, the posterior talofibular ligament may remain uninjured, except in severe ankle trauma with dislocation.[34]

If all three ligaments are ruptured, the ankle is unstable. With complete disruption of the anterior talofibular ligament, forward displacement of the talus in the ankle mortise is present. With sequential rupture of the anterior talofibular and calcaneofibular ligaments, medial tilting of the talus is found with progressive widening of the lateral joint space. The strong deltoid ligament, or medial collateral ligament, consists of the tibionavicular, anterior tibiotalar, tibiocalcaneal, and posterior tibiotalar ligaments and rarely ruptures. Avulsion fracture of the medial malleolus and disruption of the anterior tibiofibular ligament are associated with abduction and laterally directed forces.[34]

Diagnosis. Ankle sprains are classified into three clinical grades.[33] In a grade I sprain, there is stretching or partial tearing of anterior talofibular ligament fibers. Grade II represents a moderate sprain associated with significant edema in which there is partial tearing of the anterior talofibular ligament with stretching of the cal-

(text continues on page 473)

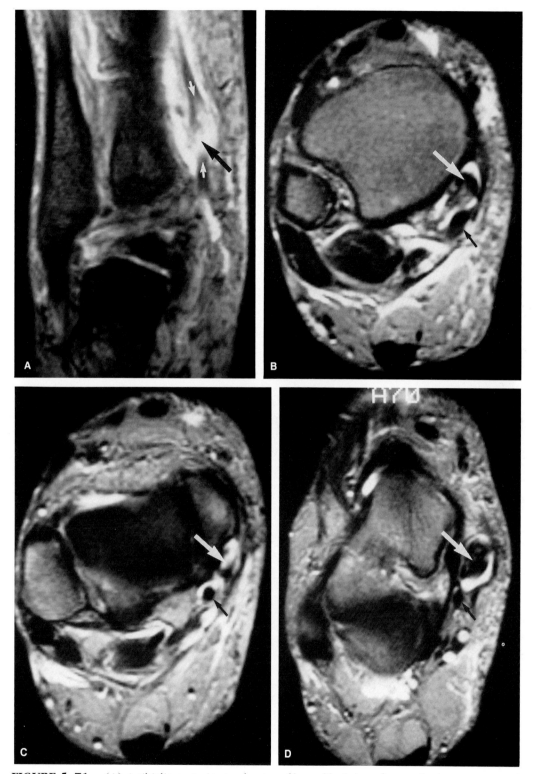

FIGURE 5–71. (**A**) A tibialis posterior tendon tear (*large black arrow*), type 3, shows a retracted proximal tendon (*white arrow*) and distal tendon segment (*white arrow*) on a T2*-weighted posterior coronal image. Three separate T2-weighted axial images demonstrate tendon morphology (*large white arrows*) (**B**) proximal to the tear site, (**C**) at the tear site, and (**D**) distal to the tear site. Note the absence of the tibialis posterior tendon at the tear site and the low signal intensity thickened tendon proximal and distal to the area of disruption. The normal flexor digitorum longus tendon is indicated (*small black arrows*).

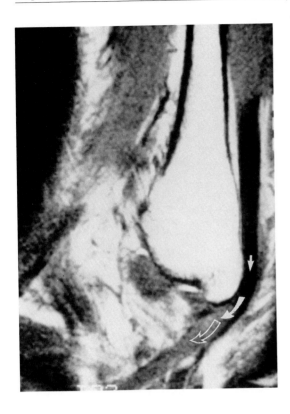

FIGURE 5–72. In a peroneus longus tendon tear, the peroneus longus tendon is absent distal and inferior to the lateral malleolus (*curved arrows*). The peroneus longus tendon is posterior to the lateral malleolus (*small arrow*), as seen on a T1-weighted sagittal image.

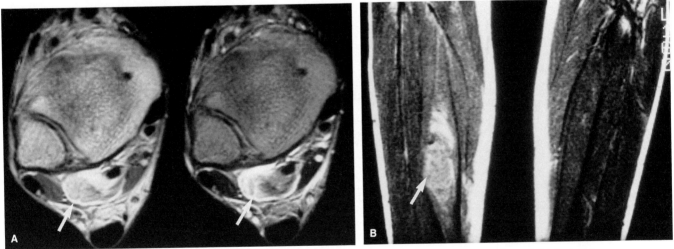

FIGURE 5–73. (**A**) A grade 2 (*i.e.,* partial) tear of the flexor hallucis longus muscle with high signal intensity hemorrhage (*arrow*) is seen on intermediate-weighted (*left*) and T2-weighted (*right*) axial images. (**B**) The subacute hemorrhage (*arrow*) is bright on a T1-weighted coronal image.

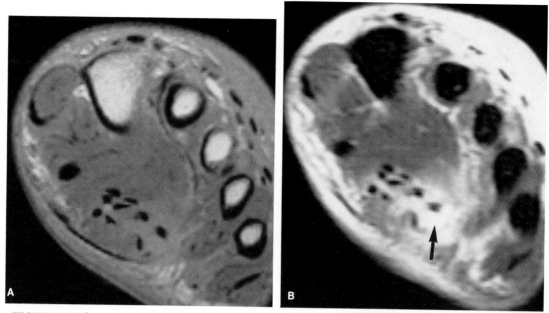

FIGURE 5-74. A grade 1 to 2 muscle tear with localized hemorrhage and edema involving the flexor digitorum brevis (*straight arrow*) and quadratus plantar muscle groups occurred due to a windsurfing accident. Edema and hemorrhage are (**A**) isointense compared with muscle on an intermediate-weighted coronal image and (**B**) hyperintense on a short TI inversion recovery coronal image.

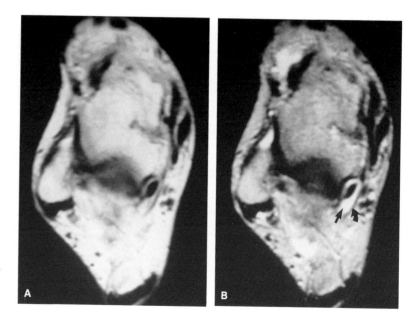

FIGURE 5-75. Flexor hallucis longus tenosynovitis with high signal intensity effusion (*straight arrow*) and without associated tendon sheath thickening (*curved arrow*) is demonstrated on (**A**) intermediate-weighted and (**B**) T2-weighted axial images.

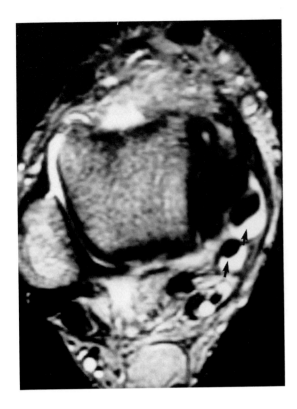

FIGURE 5–76. High signal intensity tenosynovitis involving the tibialis posterior and flexor digitorum longus tendons (*arrows*) is seen on a T2-weighted axial image.

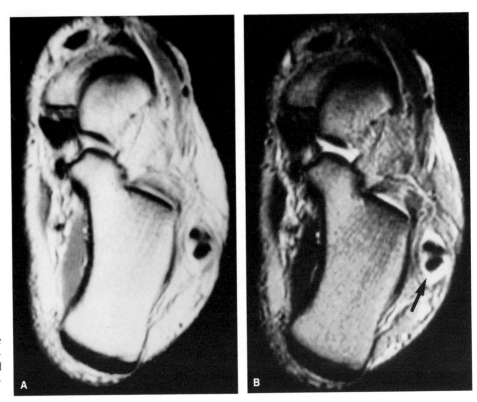

FIGURE 5–77. Tenosynovitis of the peroneal tendons is seen on (**A**) intermediate-weighted and (**B**) T2-weighted axial images (*arrow*). Fluid is hyperintense on the T2-weighted image.

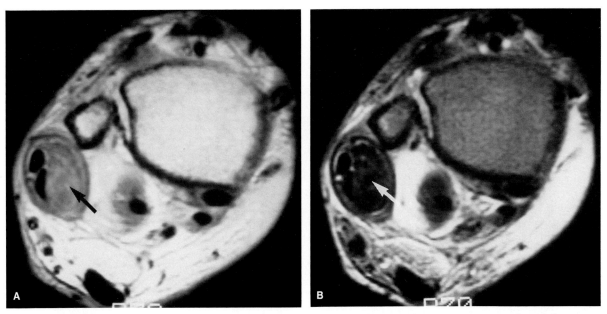

FIGURE 5–78. In chronic peroneal tenosynovitis, thickened low signal intensity synovium (*arrows*) encases the peroneus brevis and longus tendons. There is no increased signal intensity within synovial tissue on (**A**) intermediate-weighted or (**B**) T2-weighted axial images.

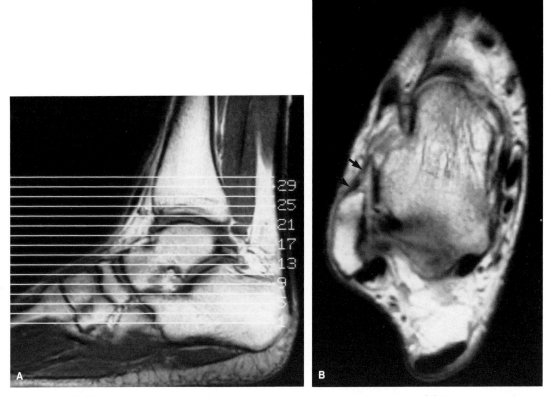

FIGURE 5–79. (**A**) A sagittal localizer with orthogonal axial prescriptions and (**B**) the corresponding T1-weighted axial image allow identification of the anterior talofibular ligament (*arrows*). (**C**) A sagittal localizer with axial oblique prescriptions oriented along the short axis of the navicular and (**D**) the corresponding T1-weighted axial oblique image allow identification of the anterior talofibular ligament (*solid arrow*) and the navicular attachment of the tibialis posterior tendon (*open arrow*). *(continued)*

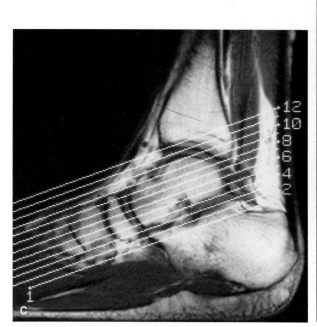

FIGURE 5–79. *(Continued)*

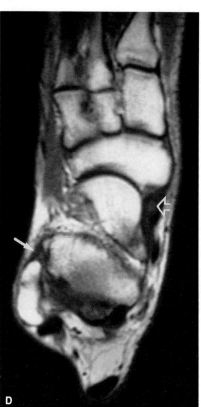

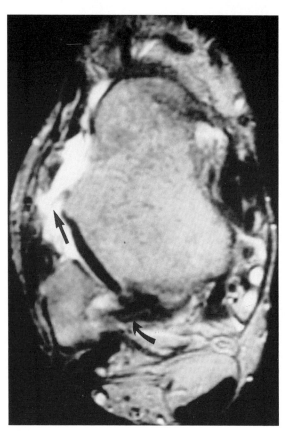

FIGURE 5–80. Disruption of the anterior talofibular ligament results in its replacement by high signal intensity fluid (*straight arrow*). The low signal intensity posterior talofibular ligament is intact (*curved arrow*), as seen on a T2-weighted axial image.

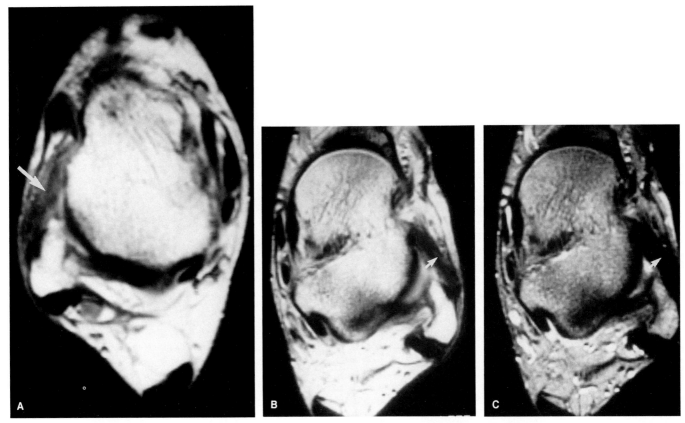

FIGURE 5–81. (**A**) A T1-weighted axial image shows a chronically thickened intermediate signal intensity anterior talofibular ligament (*arrow*). The normal thickness is 2 to 3 mm. Thickening is secondary to a previous inversion injury. A different patient shows a healed anterior talofibular ligament tear (*arrows*), which is seen as a low signal intensity thickened ligament on axial (**B**) intermediate-weighted and (**C**) T2-weighted images.

FIGURE 5–82. An association exists between chronic anterior talofibular ligament tear and subtalar joint degeneration arthrosis. (**A**) The chronic anterior talofibular ligament tear (*curved arrows*) is seen on intermediate-weighted (*right*) and T2-weighted (*left*) axial images. (**B**) Low signal intensity posterior subtalar sclerosis (*arrows*) is best depicted on the T1-weighted image; whereas (**C**) a synovium-filled subchondral cyst (*arrow*) is seen on the T2*-weighted sagittal image.

(continued)

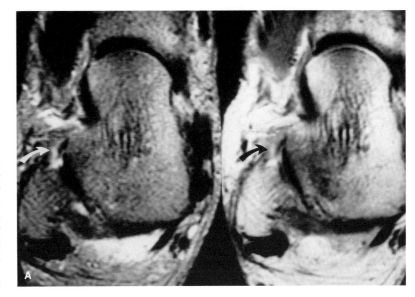

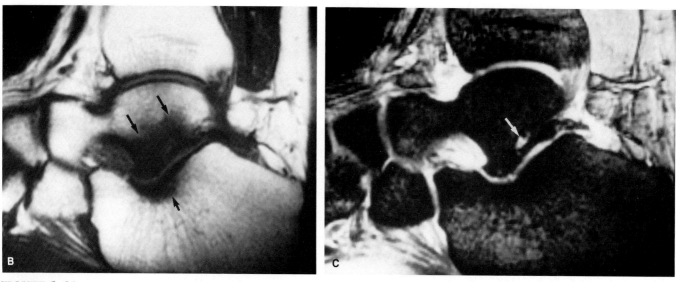

FIGURE 5–82. *(Continued)*

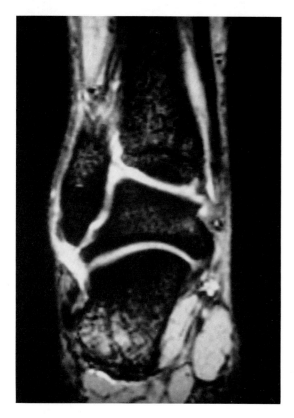

FIGURE 5–83. There is an absence of ligamentous fibers on this T2*-weighted coronal image of calcaneofibular ligament disruption.

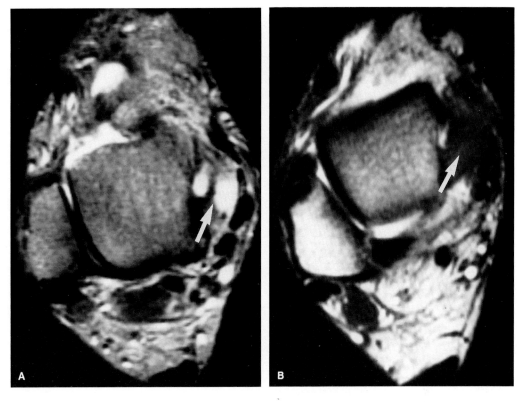

FIGURE 5–84. (**A**) A T2-weighted axial image shows a partial deltoid ligament tear (*arrow*) with high signal intensity hemorrhage in the tibiotalar and tibiocalcaneal fibers. (**B**) Another T2-weighted axial image of a normal low signal intensity deltoid ligament (*arrow*) is shown for comparison.

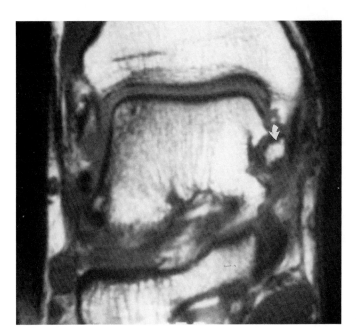

FIGURE 5–85. An old medial malleolar avulsion fracture (*arrow*) with disruption of tibiotalar ligament fibers is seen on a T1-weighted coronal image.

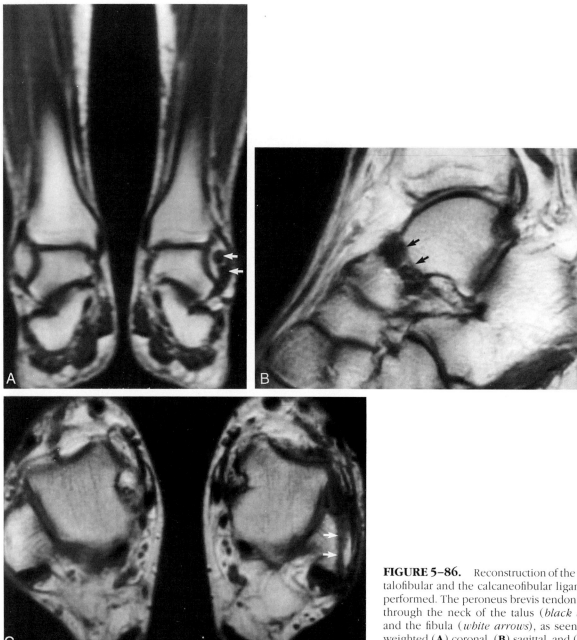

FIGURE 5–86. Reconstruction of the anterior talofibular and the calcaneofibular ligaments is performed. The peroneus brevis tendon tunnels through the neck of the talus (*black arrows*) and the fibula (*white arrows*), as seen on T1-weighted (**A**) coronal, (**B**) sagittal, and (**C**) axial images.

caneofibular ligament. In a grade III injury, ankle instability is present with tearing of the anterior talofibular and calcaneofibular ligaments.

Magnetic Resonance Findings. The normal ligamentous anatomy of the ankle is clearly demonstrated on MR images, although indications for the use of MR as a primary modality for evaluation of patients with ligament sprains or ruptures has not been established. Magnetic resonance imaging provides direct visualization of ankle ligaments not possible with conventional radiographs, arthrography, or CT. Clinical assessment of ligament injury is frequently difficult in the presence of soft-tissue swelling and a joint effusion. Results of stress positioning with conventional radiographs may be variable, and the patient frequently requires anesthesia to limit pain and guarding. Comparison views with the opposite ankle are also necessary. Magnetic resonance is particularly useful in assessing the tibial plafond and talar dome. Subchondral and articular damage to the superior talar dome may occur with subluxation of the ankle (*i.e.,* talar displacement in plantar flexion) secondary to anterior talofibular ligament interruption.

The anatomy of the anterior talofibular ligament is best displayed on axial or axial oblique planar images with T2- or T2*-weighted contrast. At the level of the distal lateral malleolus, the anterior talofibular ligament is seen as a prominent, low signal intensity, 2- to 3-mm band, oriented anteromedially and extending to its talar attachment. Axial oblique images perpendicular to the talonavicular joint may be used to demonstrate anterotalofibular ligament fibers more parallel with the plane of section. Acute tears are associated with either partial ligamentous disruption or complete absence of the ligament (Fig. 5–80). T2- or T2*-weighted images identify localized high signal intensity fluid or hemorrhage. Chronically torn talofibular ligament fibers often form a meniscoid lesion with tissue interposed between the talus and the fibula. This finding should be helpful in evaluating patients with lateral ankle pain and a history of ligament disruption. Chronic or healed ligamentous disruptions show generalized thickening of the ligament (Fig. 5–81).

We have observed an association between anterior talofibular ligament tears and isolated subtalar joint arthrosis (Fig. 5–82). In five of seven patients, low signal intensity subchondral sclerosis and attenuation of articular cartilage was demonstrated in the posterior subtalar joint in the presence of a subacute or chronic anterior talofibular ligament injury. Although traditionally, chronic subtalar instability was thought to be associated with lateral ankle sprains, conventional radiographs alone are inadequate for displaying this anatomy.[33,35]

Calcaneofibular ligament tears, when seen in association with anterior talofibular ligament injuries, are best seen on coronal plane images through the lateral malleolus (Fig. 5–83).[34] Posterior oblique (*i.e.,* anterior superior to posterior inferior) axial images or axial images performed with the foot in plantar flexion also display calcaneofibular ligament fibers.[36] Tearing of the calcaneofibular ligament may result in a communication between the ankle joint and the peroneal tendon sheaths.[33]

On axial plane images, deltoid ligament injuries usually demonstrate inflammatory or edematous changes without complete ligament disruptions (Fig. 5–84). On coronal plane images, however, it is often possible to identify associated avulsions of the medial malleolus and to separate tibiotalar from tibiocalcaneal fibers (Fig. 5–85). Focal areas of increased signal intensity on T2- or T2*-weighted images are more commonly seen than complete absence of the ligament. Kinematic and stress positioning of the ankle may be effective in showing rupture, thinning, and lengthening of the ligament. In a patient with a Watson–Jones reconstruction of the lateral ligaments (*e.g.,* anterior talofibular), the mobilized peroneus brevis tendon, rerouted through the fibula, was intact (Fig. 5–86). Disruption of the anterior talofibular ligament is confirmed in other lateral ligament reconstructions (Fig. 5–87). The clinical diagnosis of anteroinferior tibiofibular ligament injuries, which may occur in football and downhill skiing, may be difficult because acute swelling is uncommon in the setting of distal anterior tibiofibular syndesmosis pain. Therefore, identification of an intact or disrupted ligament on MR scans may be particularly useful in diagnosing and treating an ankle injury.

Fractures

Ankle Fractures

The classification of ankle fractures by the Lauge–Hansen system is based on the position of the foot and the direction of the injuring force. Four categories of fracture are recognized:

1. Supination–external rotation injuries
2. Supination–adduction injuries
3. Pronation–external rotation injuries
4. Pronation–abduction injuries.[37]

Magnetic resonance complements conventional radiographic and CT evaluation, allowing more specific demonstration of soft-tissue ligamentous injuries. For example, in the supination–external rotation mechanism, injury progresses through four stages:

1. Stage 1: anterior tibiofibular ligament rupture
2. Stage 2: oblique spiral fracture of the lateral malleolus
3. Stage 3: a posterior lip or margin fracture of the tibia (Fig. 5–88)
4. Stage 4: avulsion fracture of the medial malleolus or deltoid ligament rupture.

The pronation–external rotation injury starts with fracture of the medial malleolus and progresses clockwise through injuries similar to those outlined for supination–external rotation fractures. In supination–external rotation injuries, fracture of the fibula usually occurs within 2.5 cm of the ankle mortise. In pronation–external rotation injuries, the fracture is usually 8 to 9 cm proximal to the tip of the lateral malleolus (more than 2.5 cm from the ankle joint). Adduction forces usually result in horizontal transverse fractures of the lateral malleolus and vertical oblique fracture of the medial malleolus, whereas abduction forces produce a horizontal fracture of the medial malleolus and an oblique distal fibular fracture.[33,37] Additionally, MR may have a role in identifying early periosteal trauma and hemorrhage prior to the development of stress fractures (Fig. 5–89).

Fractures of the Foot

Calcaneus. Calcaneal fractures are divided into intraarticular and extraarticular types according to the involvement of the subtalar joint.[37,38] Extraarticular fractures that do not involve the subtalar joint include fractures of the tuberosity, the anterior process, the sustentaculum tali, or the body.[37] Intraarticular fractures, which are more common, are classified by Essex–Lopresti into two categories—a tongue-type injury and a depression-type injury—based on the secondary fracture pattern seen in association with the primary or oblique fracture segment.[37] The tongue-type fracture is transverse and extends to the posterior tuberosity (Fig. 5–90). The depression-type fracture has a secondary fracture line that runs from the body of the calcaneus directly posterior to the subtalar joint (Fig. 5–91). Both MR and CT are useful in demonstrating joint alignment, fragment displacement, and involvement of the subtalar joint. Prognosis is better for extraarticular fractures that do not involve the subtalar joint.[38]

Talus. Since the ankle mortise protects the talus from direct injury, talar fractures usually result from transmuted forces.[37] Fractures of the talus can involve the neck (Fig. 5–92), the body (Figs. 5–93 and 5–94), the head, and the posterior and lateral processes. Avascular necrosis is a known complication of talar neck fractures, and with MR it is possible to assess adjacent bone marrow for signs of this process and to demonstrate nondisplaced fracture morphology.[39] The articular cartilage surfaces can also be directly evaluated on MR studies.

Navicular. Navicular fractures are characterized by ligamentous capsular avulsions and fractures of the tuberosity and body.[37] Sagittal plane MR images are particularly useful for identification of stress fractures involving one or both cortices (Fig. 5–95). Axial images, however, may be required to display fracture lines parallel with the sagittal plane (Fig. 5–96). Although avascular necrosis is not common, MR is also helpful in demonstrating subchondral sclerosis prior to the appearance of increased radiographic density. Cuneiform fractures are less common and are associated with direct trauma (Fig. 5–97).

Tarsometatarsal or Lisfranc Fractures. The homolateral and divergent types of Lisfranc fractures are best evaluated by standard radiographs or coronal reformatted 1.5-mm CT scans (Fig. 5–98). The medial border of the middle or intermediate cuneiform and the lateral border of the medial cuneiform should be in line with or directly congruent with their respective metatarsals. The role of MR may be limited to evaluating soft-tissue and capsular structures when radiographic or CT examinations are negative.

Metatarsal Stress Fractures. Magnetic resonance and CT have been used for early diagnosis of metatarsal stress fractures prior to positive findings with conventional radiography (Fig. 5–99). Ballet dancers are particularly prone to developing stress injuries involving the base of the 2nd and 3rd metatarsals. ^{99m}TC-MDP scintigraphy may not be specific for fracture as opposed to degenerative arthrosis in these cases. STIR protocols have characterized marrow hyperemia in recurrent injuries in the presence of negative or unchanged radiographs or CT evaluations (Fig. 5–100). Cast immobilization or nonweight-bearing is necessary in dancers who have significant pain.

Tarsal Coalition

Tarsal coalition represents either a congenital or acquired fibrous, cartilaginous, or bony fusion of the tarsal bones.[40] Calcaneonavicular coalition is the most common type, reported in 53% of cases; talocalcaneal coalitions represent 37%.[41] Talonavicular and calcaneocuboid types are infrequent. Although coalitions are present at birth, radiographic detection is difficult because ossification of the fibrous or cartilaginous connection does not occur until the second decade.[40] Tarsal coalition is also associated with a painful pes planus or flatfoot in a child or adolescent.[41] Forefoot abduction and hindfoot valgus can result in tension in the peroneal muscles and tendons (*i.e.,* peroneal spastic flatfoot).

Computed tomography scanning with 1.5-mm sections has been used to complement specialized radiographic studies (AP, lateral, 45° lateral oblique, and 45° views) to better distinguish the facets and coalitions (Fig. 5–101). Computed tomography demonstrates fibrous coalitions indirectly by displaying irregular or roughened cortical surfaces. However, CT is limited in that direct multiplanar scanning is not possible and reformatted sagittal and coronal scans must be performed. The close

(text continues on page 487)

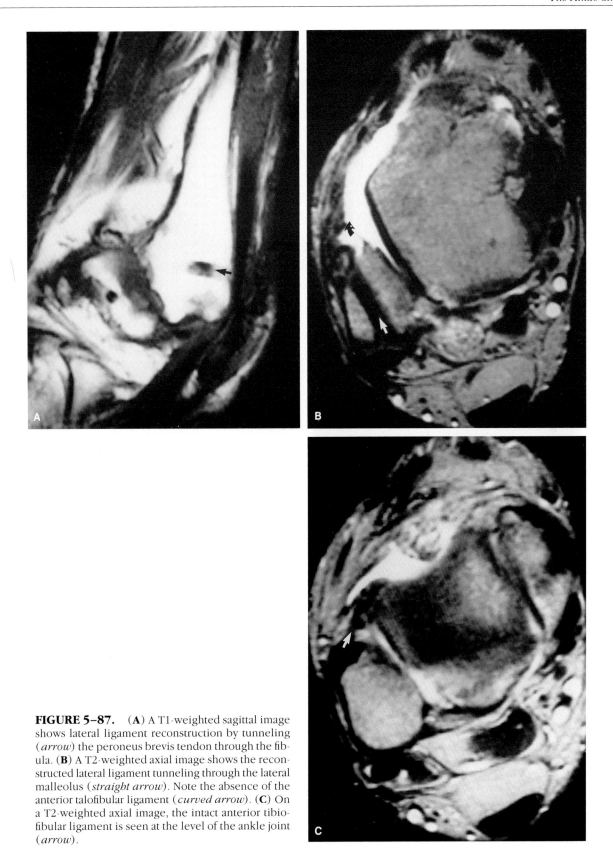

FIGURE 5–87. (**A**) A T1-weighted sagittal image shows lateral ligament reconstruction by tunneling (*arrow*) the peroneus brevis tendon through the fibula. (**B**) A T2-weighted axial image shows the reconstructed lateral ligament tunneling through the lateral malleolus (*straight arrow*). Note the absence of the anterior talofibular ligament (*curved arrow*). (**C**) On a T2-weighted axial image, the intact anterior tibiofibular ligament is seen at the level of the ankle joint (*arrow*).

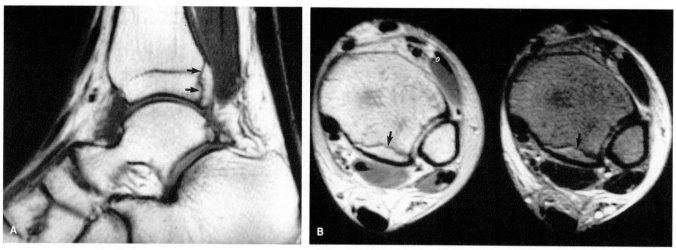

FIGURE 5–88. An old posterior malleolar fracture (*arrows*) with a sclerotic low signal intensity segment is identified in (**A**) T1-weighted sagittal and (**B**) T2-weighted axial images. Continuity of the tibial plafond and the posterior tibial cortex indicate a united fracture.

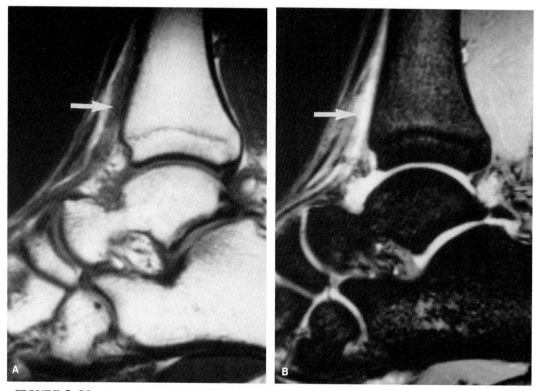

FIGURE 5–89. Reactive edema parallel with the distal anterior tibial periosteum has occurred in a runner with symptomatic shin splints (*arrows*). No stress fracture was identified. Soft-tissue edema demonstrates (**A**) low signal intensity on a T1-weighted sagittal image and bright signal intensity on both (**B**) T2*-weighted sagittal and (**C**) T2-weighted axial images.

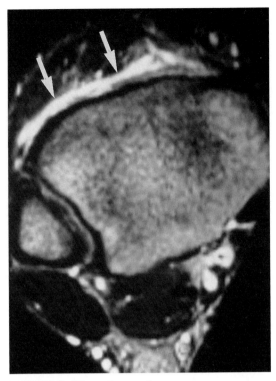

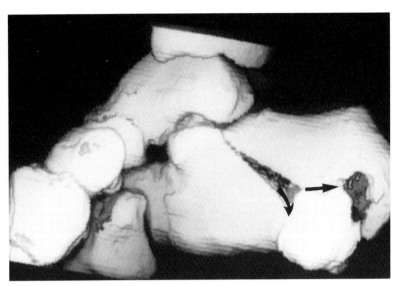

FIGURE 5–90. A 3D CT image shows a primary fracture (*curved arrow*) and a posterior secondary fracture line (*straight arrow*) with a resulting tongue fragment.

FIGURE 5–89. *(Continued)*

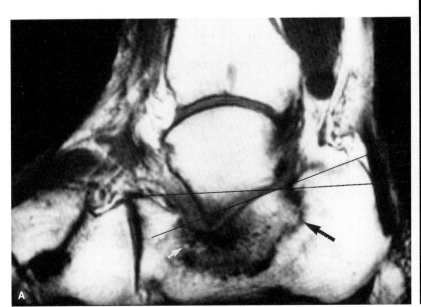

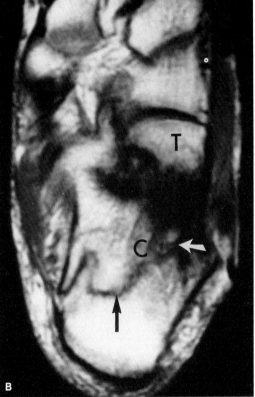

FIGURE 5–91. (**A**) A T1-weighted sagittal image shows a joint-depression type intraarticular calcaneal fracture with a secondary fracture line (*black arrow*) exiting the body posterior to the subtalar joint. The primary fracture component is more anterior (*white arrow*) relative to the secondary fracture line. Depression of the fracture fragment causes a decrease in Bohler's angle (*crossed lines*), which is normally between 20° and 40°. (**B**) A T1-weighted axial image shows subtalar joint extension (*white arrow*) of a calcaneal fracture (*black arrow*). (C, calcaneus; T, talus.)

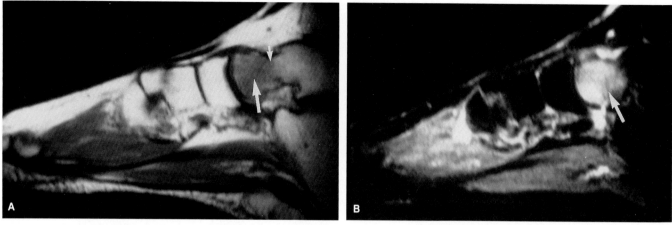

FIGURE 5–92. A nondisplaced fracture of the talar neck (*small arrow*) with hemorrhage and marrow hyperemia (*large arrows*) is seen on (**A**) T1-weighted and (**B**) short TI inversion recovery sagittal images. Hyperemia of the distal talus (*i.e.,* talar head and neck) may be related to interruption of the blood vessels that enter dorsally and laterally on the surface of the talar neck.

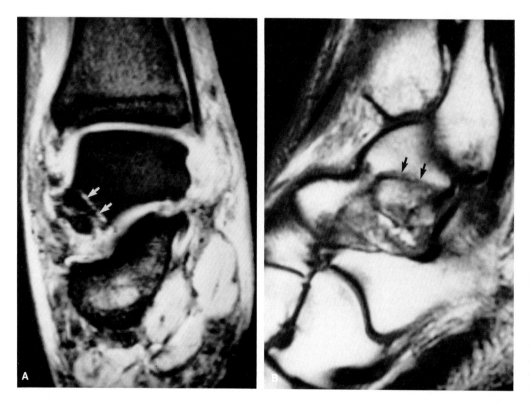

FIGURE 5–93. A fracture of the talar body involving the lateral tubercle (*arrows*) is seen on (**A**) T2*-weighted coronal and (**B**) T1-weighted sagittal images. Talar body fractures are less common than talar neck fractures and are associated with a fall from a height.

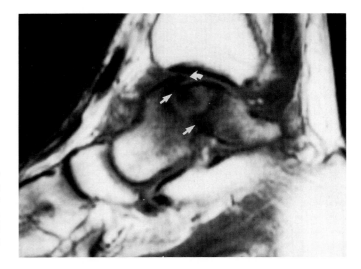

FIGURE 5–94. A coronal shearing fracture of the talar body (*straight arrows*) is associated with discontinuity of the talar dome cortex (*curved arrow*). Low signal intensity subchondral marrow hyperemia and hemorrhage is displayed on a T1-weighted sagittal image. Displaced fractures of the talar body may be complicated by avascular necrosis, although this complication is more common in talar neck fractures.

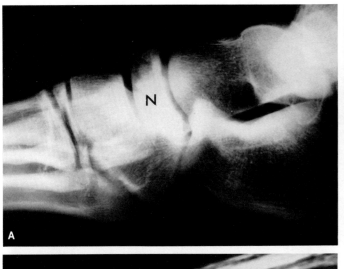

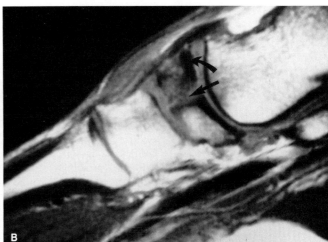

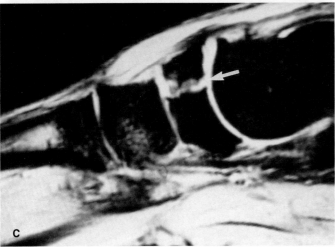

FIGURE 5–95. A navicular stress fracture with involvement of proximal and distal cortices occurred in a world class sprinter. (**A**) A lateral radiograph of the foot does not show the fracture of the navicular (N). (**B**) A T1-weighted sagittal image reveals low signal intensity sclerosis of the dorsal fragment (*curved arrow*). (*Straight arrow*, fracture segment). (**C**) High signal intensity fluid extension across the fracture site is revealed on a T2*-weighted sagittal image (*arrow*).

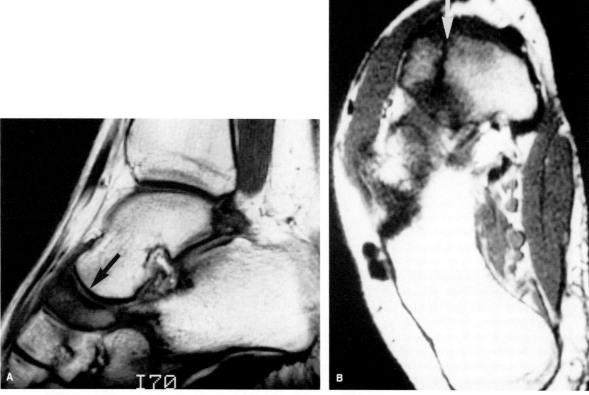

FIGURE 5–96. A navicular fracture (*arrow*) that was not recognized by conventional radiography is shown with associated marrow hemorrhage and hyperemia demonstrating (**A**) diffuse low signal intensity on a T1-weighted sagittal image and (**B**) as a linear fracture line (*arrow*) on a T1-weighted axial image. Fracture morphology is best seen in the axial plane when the plane of injury is sagittally oriented.

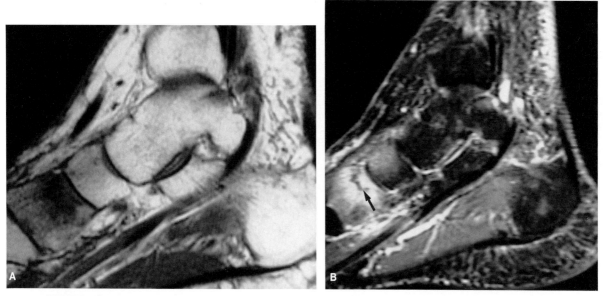

FIGURE 5–97. A nondisplaced medial cuneiform fracture with associated marrow hyperemia demonstrates (**A**) low signal intensity in a T1-weighted sagittal image and (**B**) high signal intensity (*arrow*) in a short TI inversion recovery image. Isolated injuries of the cuneiforms are usually the result of direct trauma.

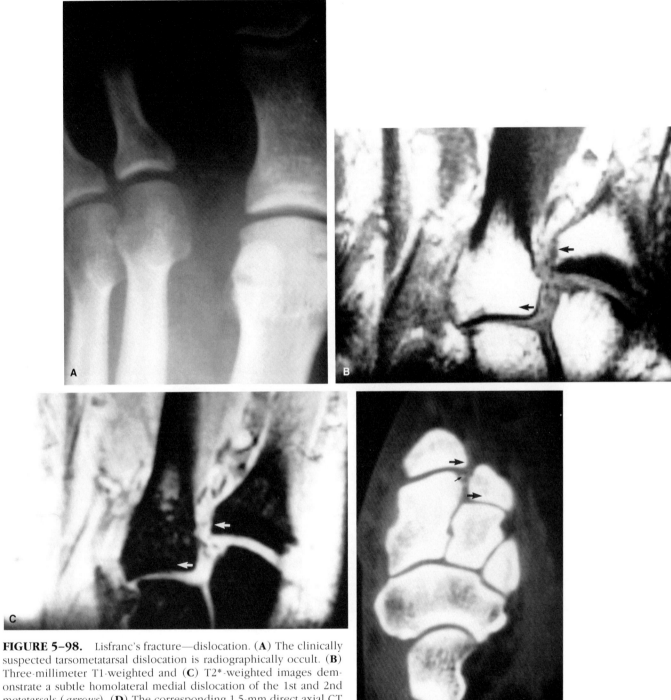

FIGURE 5–98. Lisfranc's fracture—dislocation. (**A**) The clinically suspected tarsometatarsal dislocation is radiographically occult. (**B**) Three-millimeter T1-weighted and (**C**) T2*-weighted images demonstrate a subtle homolateral medial dislocation of the 1st and 2nd metatarsals (*arrows*). (**D**) The corresponding 1.5-mm direct axial CT image reveals medial displacement of the metatarsals relative to the cuneiforms (*large arrows*) and small avulsed cortical fragments (*small arrow*).

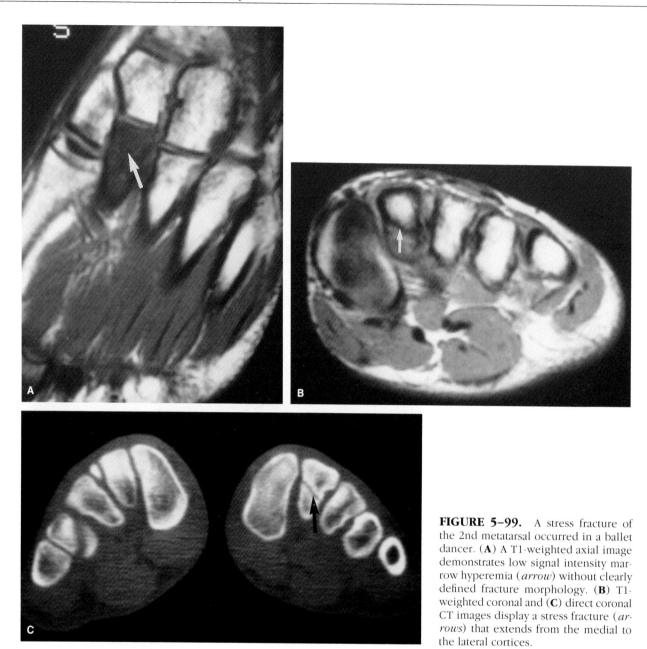

FIGURE 5–99. A stress fracture of the 2nd metatarsal occurred in a ballet dancer. (**A**) A T1-weighted axial image demonstrates low signal intensity marrow hyperemia (*arrow*) without clearly defined fracture morphology. (**B**) T1-weighted coronal and (**C**) direct coronal CT images display a stress fracture (*arrows*) that extends from the medial to the lateral cortices.

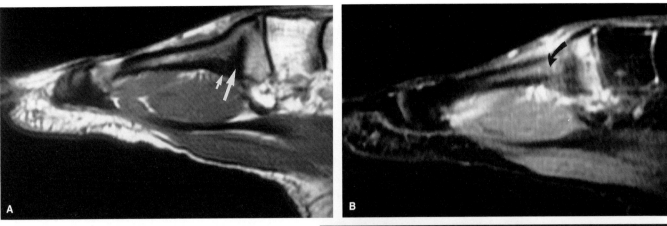

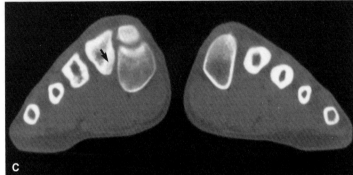

FIGURE 5–100. (**A**) A T1-weighted sagittal image shows reinjury of a 2nd metatarsal stress fracture with a sclerotic, healed fracture line (*large arrow*) and thickened, solid periosteum (*small arrow*). (**B**) A short TI inversion recovery sagittal image highlights hyperintense marrow hyperemia in a painful metatarsal base (*curved arrow*). (**C**) The corresponding coronal CT image indicates an area of healed sclerotic cortex (*arrow*) without providing information regarding the marrow cavity.

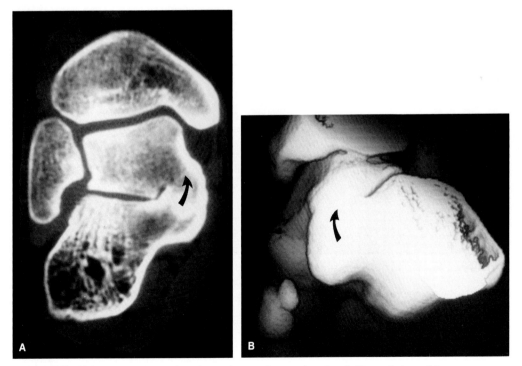

FIGURE 5–101. Talocalcaneal coalition (*curved arrows*) with solid bony fusion of the sustentaculum tali and talus is shown on (**A**) direct coronal CT and (**B**) 3D CT image. (**C, D**) The corresponding T1-weighted coronal images demonstrate continuity of the talar (T) and calcaneal (C) marrow across the sustentaculum tali (*curved arrows*).

(continued)

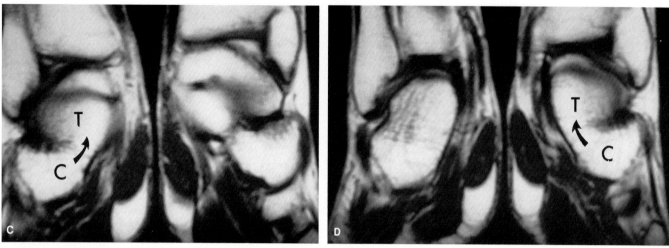

FIGURE 5–101. *(Continued)*

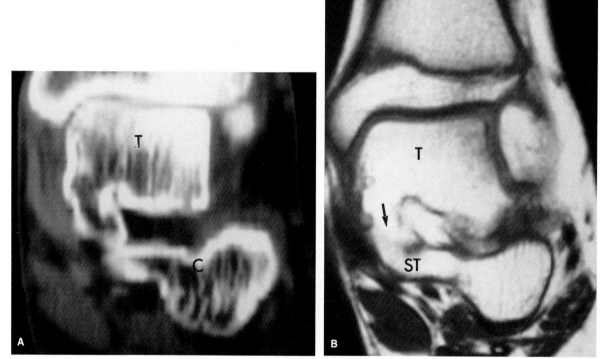

FIGURE 5–102. Talocalcaneal coalition. (**A**) A 2D reformatted CT image is not diagnostic for bony fusion between the talus (t) and calcaneus (c). (**B**) The corresponding 3-mm T1-weighted coronal image demonstrates continuity (*arrow*) of marrow fat from the tali (T) through the sustentaculum tali (ST). (**C, D**) T1-weighted sagittal images show secondary signs of talocalcaneal coalition with talar beaking (*arrow;* **C**) and degenerative changes at the calcaneal cuboid joint (*arrow;* **D**). (N, navicular; T, talus.)

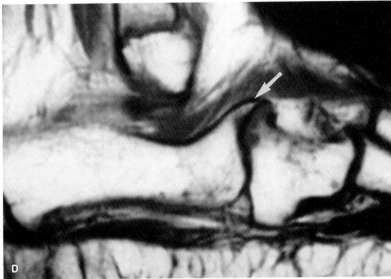

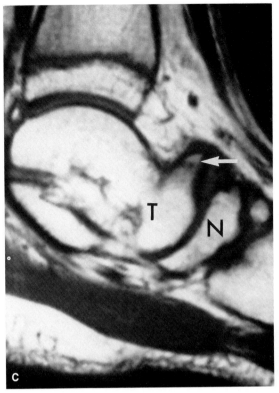

FIGURE 5-102. (Continued)

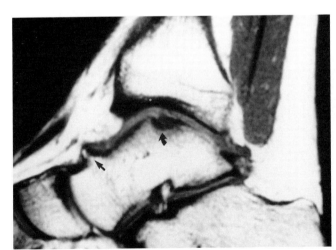

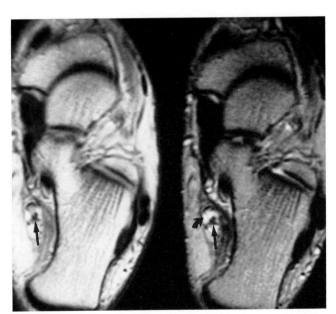

FIGURE 5-103. A normal talar ridge (*straight arrow*) in the dorsal aspect of the distal talar neck is located proximal to the distal articular surface of the talus. This is the attachment site of the joint capsule, which may become enlarged with traction. The talar ridge should not be mistaken for the talar beak of the talocalcaneal coalitions, which is located more anterior at the talonavicular joint margin. A transchondral fracture crater is shown (*curved arrow*).

FIGURE 5-104. Tarsal tunnel syndrome with venous enlargement (*curved arrow*) at the level of the lateral plantar nerve and posterior tibial artery (*straight arrow*) is seen on intermediate-weighted (*left*) and T2-weighted (*right*) axial images of a long-distance runner.

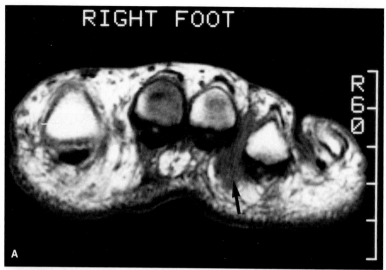

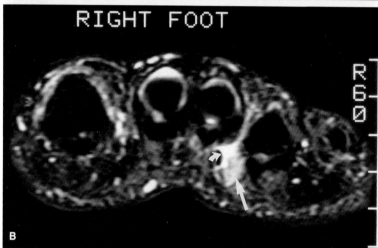

FIGURE 5–105. Morton's neuroma (*straight arrow*), located between the 3rd and 4th metatarsal heads, is (**A**) isointense with adjacent inflammation on a T1-weighted coronal image and is (**B**) mildly hyperintense on a short TI inversion recovery (STIR) coronal image. Inflammatory soft-tissue edema demonstrates greater hyperintensity (*curved arrow*) than reactive connective-tissue proliferation and associated nerve degeneration. The STIR protocols are more sensitive for Morton's neuroma than either T1- or T2-weighted images.

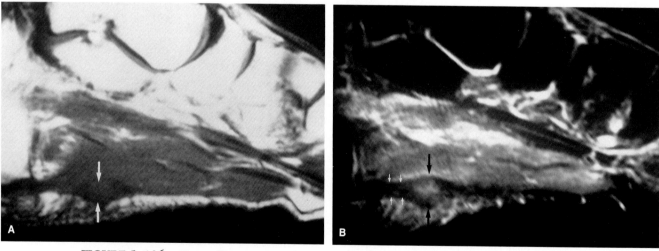

FIGURE 5–106. Plantar fibromatosis with nodular thickening (*large arrows*) in plantar aponeurosis demonstrates (**A**) low signal intensity on a T1-weighted sagittal image and (**B**) central increased signal intensity in an area of proliferating fibroblasts on a short TI inversion recovery sagittal image. The normal thickness of an adjacent plantar aponeurosis is shown (*small arrows*).

proximity of the sustentaculum tali and talus may produce a pseudocoalition on coronal reformations in talocalcaneal coalitions (Fig. 5–102).

We have used coronal, sagittal, and axial 3-mm T1-weighted MR images to successfully identify the continuity of marrow signal intensity in bony coalitions. Fibrous tissue maintains low signal intensity on T1-, T2-, and T2*-weighed images. Three-dimensional volume acquisitions allow greater operator control in designating optimal planes for reformatting suspected coalitions. Secondary signs of calcaneonavicular coalition include hypoplasia of the head of the talus and abnormal close approximation of the navicular bone and the calcaneus, with irregularity of opposing cortical surfaces. Secondary signs of a talocalcaneal coalition are talar beaking adjacent to the talonavicular articulation, a broadening lateral talar process, and a ball-and-socket ankle joint (see Fig. 5–102).[40] The normal talar ridge should not be confused with talar beaking (Fig. 5–103). Talocalcaneal coalitions usually occur through the sustentaculum tali in the middle facet.

Tarsal Tunnel Syndrome

Tarsal tunnel syndrome is an entrapment or compression neuropathy of the posterior tibial nerve as it passes through the fibro-osseous tunnel deep to the flexor retinaculum and posterior and inferior to the medial malleolus.[34] The neurovascular bundle is located between the compartments containing the flexor digitorum longus and the flexor hallucis longus tendons. Within 1 cm of the medial malleolus, the posterior tibial nerve trifurcates into the medial and lateral plantar nerves and sensory calcaneal branches.[41]

Symptoms of tarsal tunnel syndrome are pain, sensory deficits of the sole of the foot and toes, and intrinsic muscle weakness. Etiologies of compression neuropathy in this region include lipomas, varicose veins, ganglia, neurilemmomas, scarring, and tenosynovitis (Fig. 5–104).[41] Common surgical findings are entrapment of the flexor retinaculum or fibrous origin of the abductor hallucis muscle, tenosynovitis, and post-traumatic (*i.e.,* postfracture) fibrosis.[42,43] In initial MR studies of tarsal tunnel syndrome, findings of a ganglion cyst originating from the flexor hallucis longus tendon sheath, post-traumatic fibrosis, and neuroma have been documented with surgical correlation.[44] The anatomy of the tarsal tunnel is effectively displayed with MR, including the posterior tibial nerve and its branches.[45]

Comparison with the opposite ankle may be useful when a space-occupying lesion is not identified. If conservative treatment is not successful, surgical decompression is performed, with division of the retinaculum and mobilization of the medial and lateral plantar nerves and the fibrous origin of the abductor hallucis.[42]

Morton's Neuroma

Morton's neuroma is a metatarsalgia that involves localized enlargements of the interdigital nerve and begins between the 4th and 5th metatarsal heads. The lateral branch of the medial plantar nerve to the third cleft and the second and third interspaces are also commonly involved.[46] This condition occurs more frequently in women 40 to 60 years of age. Plantar foot pain and tenderness in the involved interspace is characteristic.

Histologic findings include deposition of eosinophilic material and degeneration of nerve fibers, attributed to entrapment neuropathy.[46] Frequently, no palpable mass is clinically apparent; MR axial or sagittal T1- and T2-weighted images have been used to identify these lesions.[47] T1- and T2-weighted images usually demonstrate a low to intermediate signal intensity mass arising between the plantar aspects of the involved metatarsal heads. Fibrosis of the epineurium and perineurium may contribute to the intermediate signal intensity on T2-weighted images. However, we have observed greater increases in signal intensity on T2*-weighted and STIR images (Fig. 5–105). This is in contrast to a conventional neuroma or neurofibroma, which displays bright signal intensity on T2- and T2*-weighted images. Surgical treatment involves excision of the neuroma or swelling proximal to the site of digital nerve bifurcation.[46]

Plantar Fibromatosis

Plantar fibromatosis is characterized by the development of fibrous nodules in the plantar aponeurosis similar to Dupuytren's contracture of the palmar aponeurosis.[34] Single or multiple nodules in thickened plantar fascia are found in non-weight-bearing surfaces of the foot, with lesions frequently identified in the longitudinal arch.[46] Histologic findings include proliferating fibroblasts and an acellular collagenous stroma.[34]

The nodules demonstrate low signal intensity on T1- and T2-weighted images. Central areas of intermediate signal intensity may be seen on T2*-weighted or STIR images (Fig. 5–106). Adjacent inflammatory edema is not present in plantar fibromatosis. The differential diagnosis, including a ganglion neurofibroma or fibrosarcoma, can be made by the presence of increased signal intensity on T2-weighted images.

Freiberg's Infraction

In Freiberg's infraction, osteochondrosis of the 2nd metatarsal head prior to closure of the epiphyseal plate occurs during the second decade of life. Aseptic necrosis of the metatarsal epiphysis is attributed to repeated trauma with microfracture at the metaphyseal physeal junction.[34] Deformity of the metatarsal head, shaft hypertrophy, and secondary osteoarthritis of the metatarsophalangeal joint result from repeated weight-bearing trauma.

In a patient with normal or widened joint space, MR imaging allows early identification of Freiberg's infraction through low signal intensity changes of subchondral sclerosis that occur prior to radiographic signs of increased density and fragmentation of the epiphysis (Fig. 5–107). An undiagnosed stress fracture can also be excluded using T1-weighted and STIR images. The increased signal intensity of the articular cartilage surface is best shown on T2*-weighted images. Irregularity and flattening of the epiphysis with spurring are more advanced changes, as are loss of joint space and low signal intensity metatarsal shaft hypertrophy. Treatment is directed at unloading weight-bearing forces before consideration is given to surgical management.

Clubfoot

Talipes equinovarus or congenital clubfoot deformity involves forefoot plantar flexion with inversion of the heel and forefoot. The plantar aspect of the foot faces medially, and the calcaneus is turned in a plantar direction. For characterization of complex spatial deformities, I prefer 3D CT rendering to MR, because orthogonal or oblique images are difficult to interpret because key structures pass in and out of the plane of section (Fig. 5–108). In addition, 3D display reveals the following abnormalities:

- medially and inferiorly displaced navicular bone with associated wedge deformity of the cuneiforms and cuboid
- medially displaced anterior calcaneus
- cavus deformity
- medially curved metatarsals
- flattening of the talar dome
- hypertrophy of the talar head
- internal tibial torsion.[48]

Magnetic resonance studies are being used to study Achilles tendon lengthening techniques in spastic equinus foot.[49]

Neuropathic Foot

A Charcot or neuropathic joint develops secondary to underlying neuropathic processes, commonly diabetes associated with repetitive microtrauma. The end result is articular cartilage and bone fragmentation, disintegration and dislocation of the involved joint, and new bone formation (Fig. 5–109).[50] The ankle and midfoot, including the metatarsophalangeal and midtarsal joints, are frequently involved in diabetic neuropathy. Clinically, the differential diagnosis includes superimposed or associated infection. When there is extensive involvement of all midtarsal joints and pathologic fractures, the cause is likely to be neuropathic involvement.[46]

Magnetic resonance is sensitive to the underlying marrow hyperemia in the ankle, subtalar, midtarsal, and metatarsophalangeal joints (Fig. 5–110). Areas that demonstrate diffuse or patchy low signal intensity show increased signal intensity on T2-weighted, T2*-weighted, and especially STIR images. Early destructive changes, such as periarticular fractures and associated soft-tissue reactions, are frequently detected with MR.[51] A more localized region or focus of increased subchondral or medullary signal intensity may be associated with osteomyelitis. A more periarticular marrow signal alteration is seen in reflex sympathetic dystrophy (Fig. 5–111). STIR contrast is required to demonstrate any significant marrow hyperintensity.

Yeh and colleagues have reported a higher sensitivity and specificity with MR than with ^{99m}TC-MDP bone scans for detecting osteomyelitis in diabetic patients.[52] Wang and associates used T1-weighted and STIR images to study diabetic osteomyelitis and reported a sensitivity rate of 99%, a specificity rate of 81%, and an accuracy rate of 94% with histologic correlation of MR findings.[53] Chemical-shift imaging has been used to assess the water content of the sural nerve; this technique may help to identify patients with acute neuropathic changes.[54]

Plantar Fasciitis

Inflammation of the plantar aponeurosis may be associated with a calcaneal spur. Inflammatory changes or thickening of the plantar aponeurosis adjacent to the calcaneus are frequently identified on sagittal T2-weighted, T2*-weighted, and STIR images (Fig. 5–112). T1-weighted sagittal images display the low signal intensity fascia in contrast to high signal intensity superficial fat.

Infection

Early detection and treatment of osteomyelitis and joint sepsis are critical in preserving joint function before cartilage breakdown and local or hematogenous spread occurs.[55] Changes on conventional radiographs are frequently nonspecific, with effusion (*i.e.*, capsular distention) or disruption of soft-tissue planes as the only findings. Often, no evidence of cortical destruction is found until marrow involvement is extensive, possibly up to 10 to 14 days after initial infection.

Magnetic resonance imaging is useful in the early detection of musculoskeletal infections. Although appli-

(text continues on page 507)

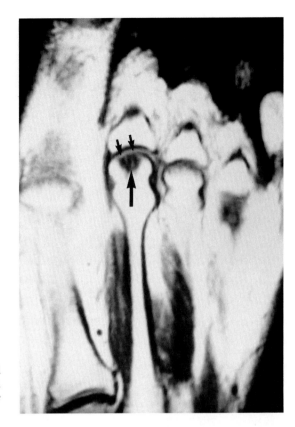

FIGURE 5–107. Freiberg's infraction with early flattening (*small arrow*) and low signal intensity osteochondrosis is detected in the 2nd metatarsal head on a T1-weighted axial image (*large arrow*). No sclerosis was revealed on the corresponding radiographs at this stage of the disease.

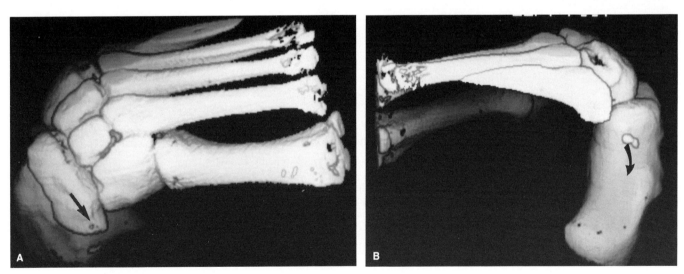

FIGURE 5–108. (**A, B**) Three-dimensional CT images show the talipes equinovarus with inferomedial displacement of the navicular (*straight arrow*), high arch or cavus deformity (*curved arrow*), inversion and adduction of the forefoot, and medial curving of the metatarsals.

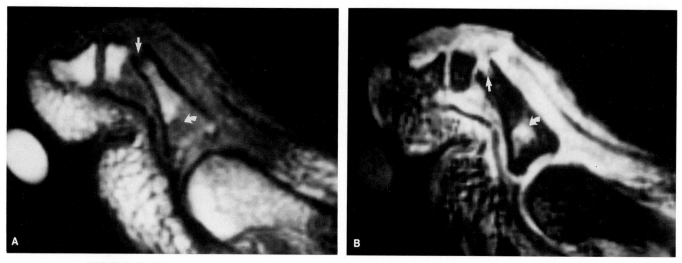

FIGURE 5–109. A neuropathic fracture of the distal aspect of the proximal phalanx (*straight arrows*) is seen on (**A**) T1-weighted and (**B**) T2*-weighted sagittal images. Note the irregular cortical edge and the subluxation at the proximal metaphalangeal joint. Abnormal marrow hyperemia is seen in the proximal aspect of phalanx (*curved arrows*).

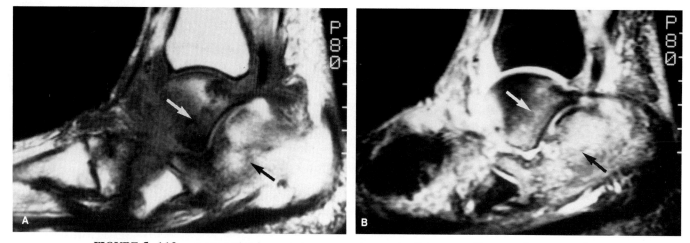

FIGURE 5–110. Neuropathic hyperemic marrow changes in diabetes mellitus are characterized by (**A**) low signal intensity areas within the talus (*white arrow*) and calcaneus (*black arrow*) on a T1-weighted sagittal image and (**B**) relative hyperintensity (*arrows*) on a short TI inversion recovery (STIR) sagittal image. The differentiation between neuroarthropathy and osteomyelitis may be more difficult when using STIR contrast. Neuropathic marrow changes, however, usually do not produce similar increases in signal intensity on T2- or T2*-weighted images when compared with STIR protocols. In osteomyelitis, affected marrow spaces produce increased signal intensity on T2-, T2*-, and STIR-weighted images.

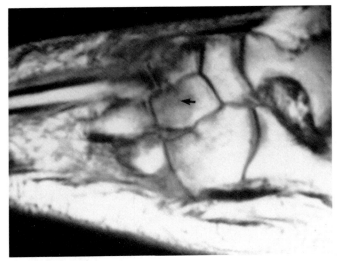

FIGURE 5–111. Low signal intensity subchondral marrow changes (*arrow*) in reflex sympathetic dystrophy can be detected on a T1-weighted sagittal image.

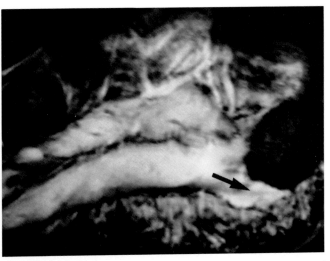

FIGURE 5–112. Plantar fasciitis with hyperintensity and loss of definition of calcaneal attachment of plantar aponeurosis (*arrow*) is seen on a T2*-weighted sagittal image.

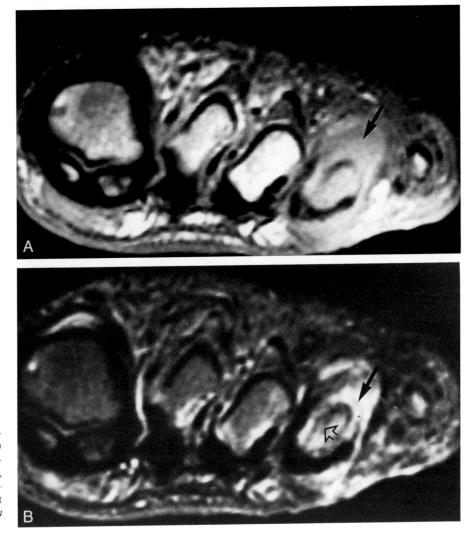

FIGURE 5–113. Staphylococcal osteomyelitis of the 4th metatarsal (*solid arrow*) demonstrates (**A**) intermediate signal intensity on a balanced, weighted axial image, and with (**B**) high signal intensity on a T2-weighted axial image. Marrow involvement is seen on the T2-weighted image (*open arrow*).

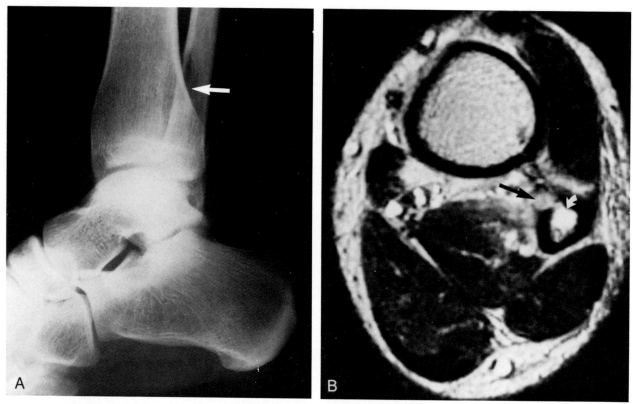

FIGURE 5–114. Osteomyelitis of the fibula. (**A**) A lateral radiograph shows localized osteopenia in the distal fibula (*arrow*). (**B**) A T2-weighted axial image demonstrates a high signal intensity infectious tract (*straight arrow*) and marrow (*curved arrow*).

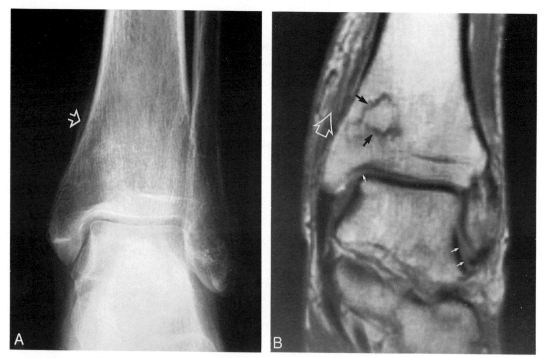

FIGURE 5–115. (**A**) An anteroposterior radiograph of osteomyelitis of the ankle demonstrates a nonspecific, uninterrupted periosteal reaction (*arrow*). The corresponding coronal images delineate the focus of osteomyelitis as intraosseous tracts (*black arrows*) with adjacent soft-tissue edema (*open arrow*). The associated joint effusion (*small arrows*) demonstrates (**B**) low signal intensity on a T1-weighted image and (**C**) high signal intensity on a T2-weighted image.

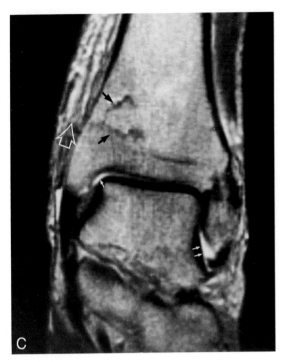

FIGURE 5–115. *(Continued)*

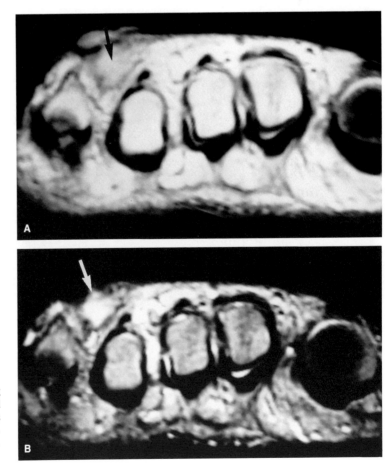

FIGURE 5–116. Soft-tissue abscess (*arrow*) involving the dorsum of the foot is seen on (**A**) intermediate-weighted and (**B**) T2-weighted coronal images. The abscess displays hyperintensity on the T2-weighted coronal image. No alterations in metatarsal marrow signal intensity and no interruptions in cortical contours occur.

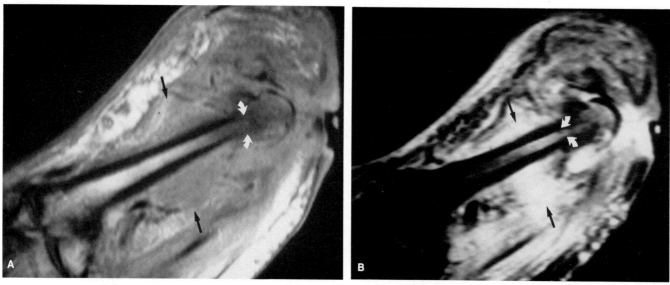

FIGURE 5–117. Osteomyelitis of the distal metatarsal occurred in a diabetic patient. (**A**) A T1-weighted sagittal image shows a low signal intensity soft-tissue mass (*straight black arrows*) and hyperemia (*curved white arrows*) with associated loss of normal medullary fat signal intensity. (**B**) With short TI inversion recovery contrast, the hyperintense soft-tissue infection (*straight black arrows*) and marrow involvement (*curved white arrows*) are evident. Attenuation of distal cortices is best seen on the T1-weighted image.

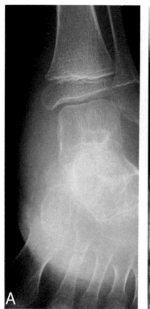
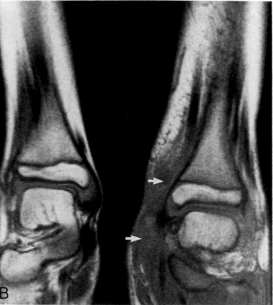

FIGURE 5–118. (**A**) An anteroposterior radiograph of the ankle shows diffuse soft-tissue swelling in a child with a chronic granulomatous infection. (**B**) The corresponding T1-weighted coronal image identifies low signal intensity fluid (*arrows*) distending the supporting capsule. Pockets of fluid (*large solid arrows*) adjacent to the thickened tendon sheaths of the tibialis posterior and flexor digitorum longus muscles (*small solid arrows*) demonstrate (**C**) low signal intensity on T1-weighted images and (**D**) high signal intensity on T2-weighted images. Septations (*small black arrow*) and necrotic-granulomatous tissue (*open arrow*) can be seen on the T2-weighted image.

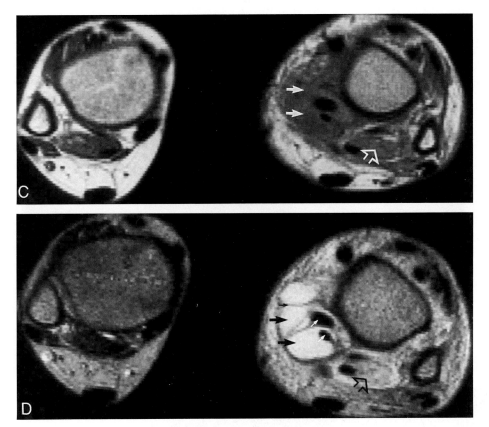

FIGURE 5–118. *(Continued)*

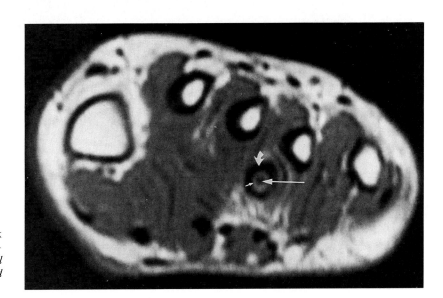

FIGURE 5–119. A low signal intensity toothpick (*long straight arrow*) incites a foreign-body reaction with an intermediate signal intensity rim (*small straight arrow*) and a fibrous periphery (*curved arrow*) as seen on a T1-weighted coronal image.

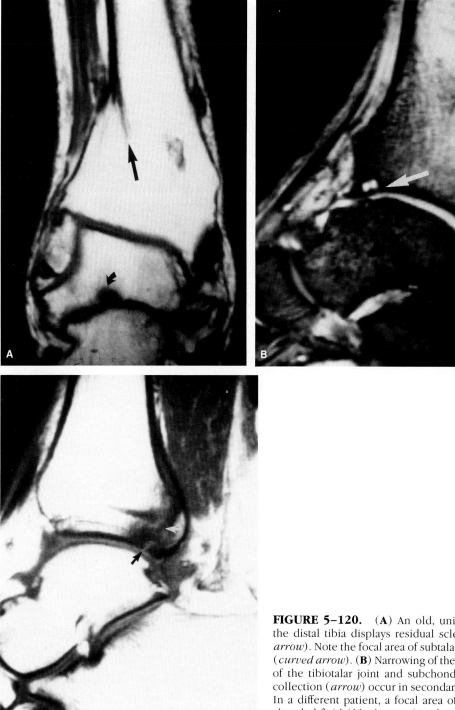

FIGURE 5–120. (**A**) An old, united fracture of the distal tibia displays residual sclerosis (*straight arrow*). Note the focal area of subtalar joint sclerosis (*curved arrow*). (**B**) Narrowing of the anterior aspect of the tibiotalar joint and subchondral cystic fluid collection (*arrow*) occur in secondary arthrosis. (**C**) In a different patient, a focal area of imbibed subchondral fluid (*black arrow*) with extension to the tibial plafond articular cartilage is seen in an old posterior malleolar fracture (*white arrow*).

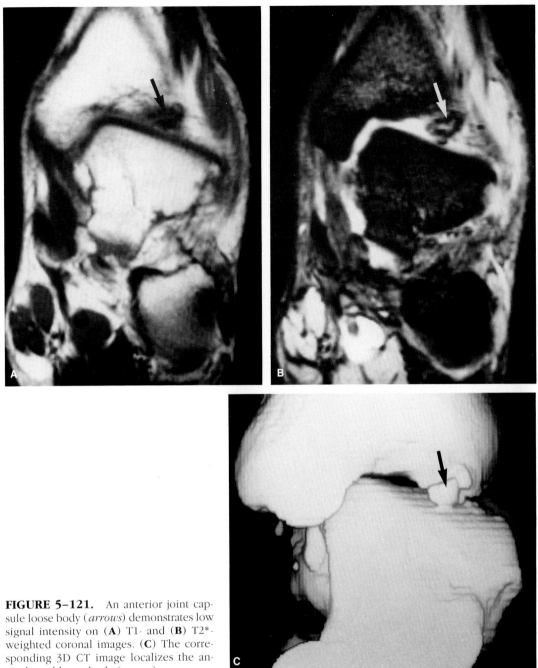

FIGURE 5–121. An anterior joint capsule loose body (*arrows*) demonstrates low signal intensity on (**A**) T1- and (**B**) T2*-weighted coronal images. (**C**) The corresponding 3D CT image localizes the anterolateral loose body (*arrow*).

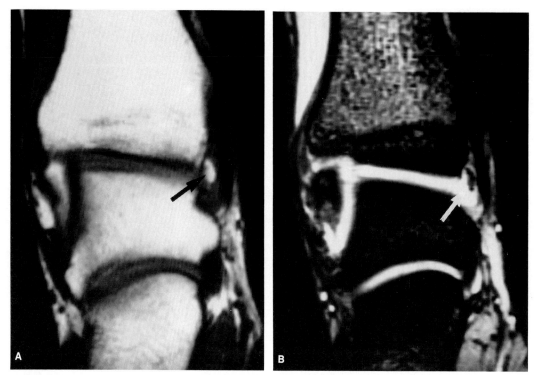

FIGURE 5–122. A marrow-containing loose body (*arrows*) demonstrates (**A**) fat signal intensity on a T1-weighted coronal image and (**B**) low signal intensity on a T2*-weighted coronal image. Localized fluid surrounds the osteochondral fragment.

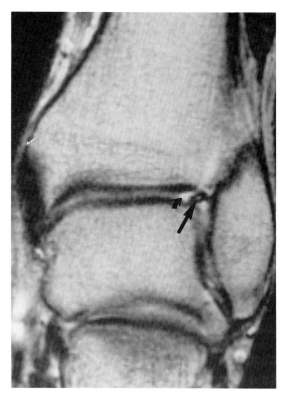

FIGURE 5–123. A low signal intensity corticated loose body (*straight arrow*) and adjacent high signal intensity fluid (*curved arrow*) are seen in the lateral aspect of the tibiotalar joint on a conventional T2-weighted coronal image.

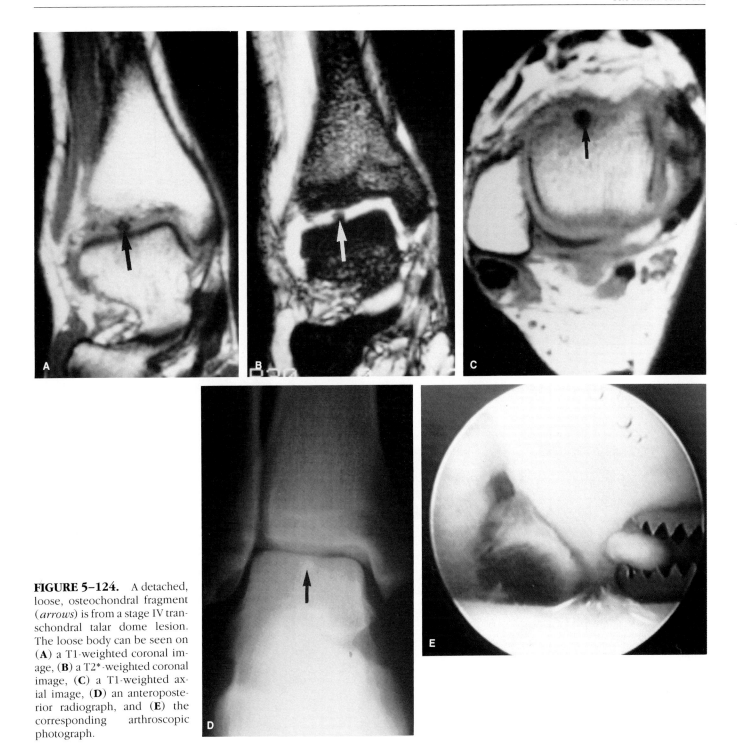

FIGURE 5–124. A detached, loose, osteochondral fragment (*arrows*) is from a stage IV transchondral talar dome lesion. The loose body can be seen on (**A**) a T1-weighted coronal image, (**B**) a T2*-weighted coronal image, (**C**) a T1-weighted axial image, (**D**) an anteroposterior radiograph, and (**E**) the corresponding arthroscopic photograph.

FIGURE 5–125. (**A**) Degenerative erosions and narrowing of the talonavicular space (*arrows*) are seen on a T1-weighted sagittal image in a patient with talonavicular arthrosis. Osteophytic overgrowth (*arrow*) is revealed on (**B**) 2D and (**C**) 3D CT images. (N, navicular; T, talar.)

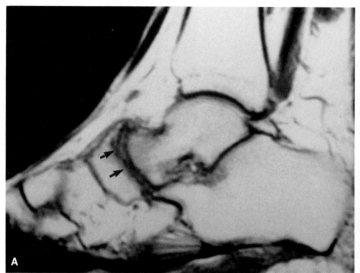

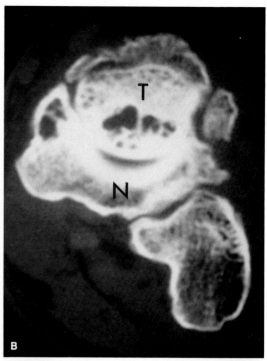

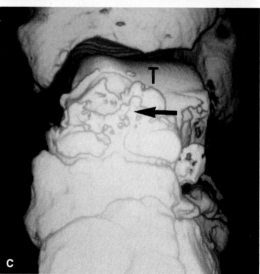

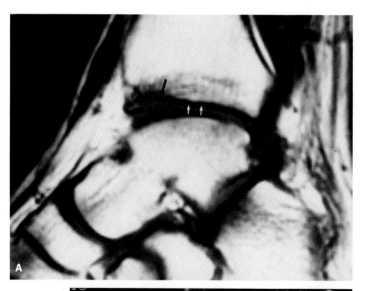

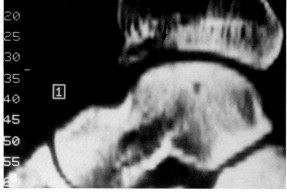

FIGURE 5–126. (**A**) A T1-weighted sagittal image shows discontinuity of the low signal intensity tibial plafond cortex (*white arrows*) in an area of subchondral erosion (*black arrow*). (**B**) The corresponding reformatted CT image demonstrates loss of the cortical margin (*arrow*).

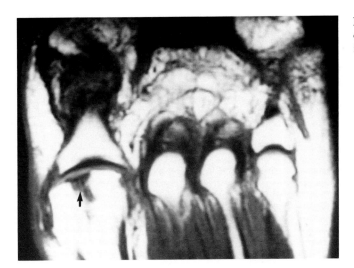

FIGURE 5–127. On a T1-weighted axial image of a springboard diver, a low signal intensity subchondral sclerosis (*arrow*) is seen in the distal aspect of the 1st metatarsal.

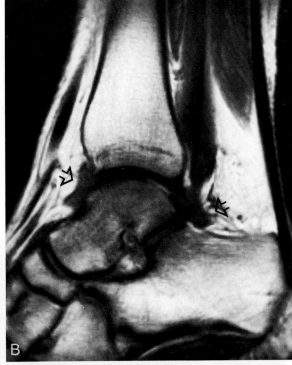

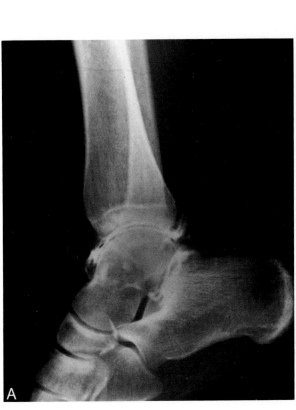

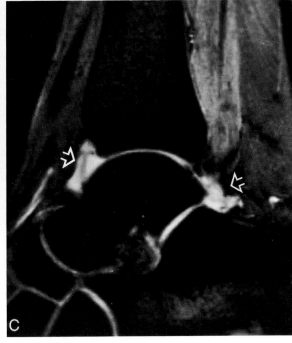

FIGURE 5–128. Ankle effusion. (**A**) A lateral radiograph shows the distribution of arthrographic contrast within the tibiotalar joint. On corresponding sagittal images, the effusion (*open arrows*) demonstrates (**B**) low signal intensity on T1-weighted images and (**C**) high signal intensity on T2*-weighted images. Anterior and posterior capsule distention is evident on the MR images.

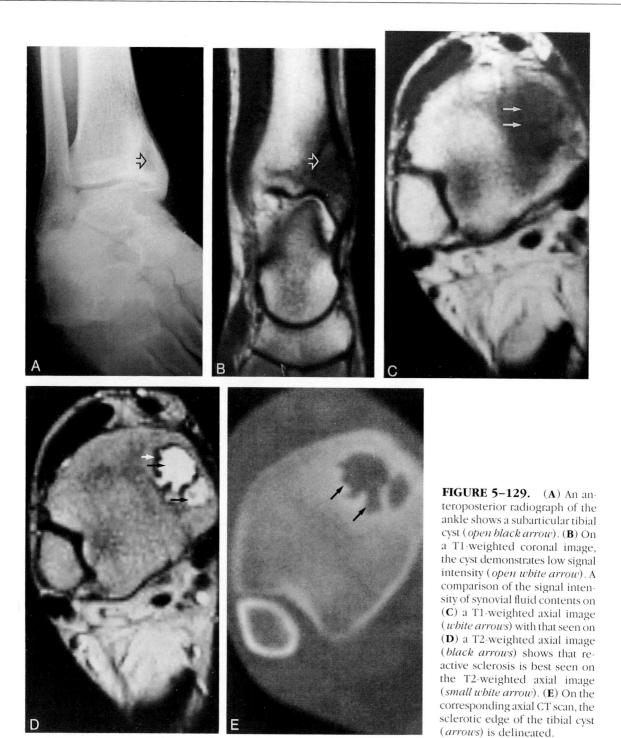

FIGURE 5–129. (**A**) An anteroposterior radiograph of the ankle shows a subarticular tibial cyst (*open black arrow*). (**B**) On a T1-weighted coronal image, the cyst demonstrates low signal intensity (*open white arrow*). A comparison of the signal intensity of synovial fluid contents on (**C**) a T1-weighted axial image (*white arrows*) with that seen on (**D**) a T2-weighted axial image (*black arrows*) shows that reactive sclerosis is best seen on the T2-weighted axial image (*small white arrow*). (**E**) On the corresponding axial CT scan, the sclerotic edge of the tibial cyst (*arrows*) is delineated.

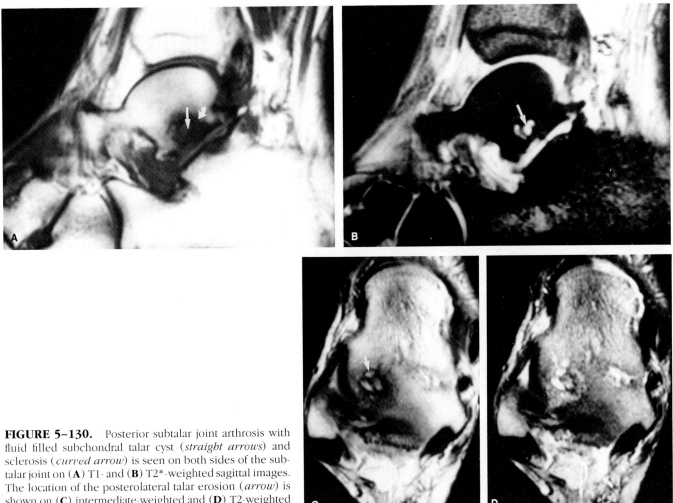

FIGURE 5–130. Posterior subtalar joint arthrosis with fluid filled subchondral talar cyst (*straight arrows*) and sclerosis (*curved arrow*) is seen on both sides of the subtalar joint on (**A**) T1- and (**B**) T2*-weighted sagittal images. The location of the posterolateral talar erosion (*arrow*) is shown on (**C**) intermediate-weighted and (**D**) T2-weighted axial images.

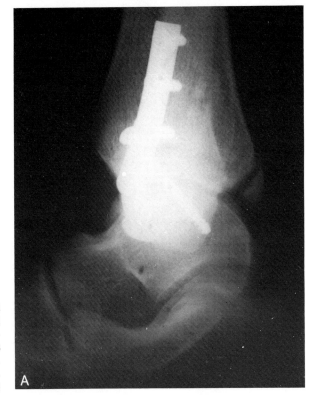

FIGURE 5–131. (**A**) A fibular screw plate fixation device is seen on a lateral radiograph. (**B**) A T1-weighted parasagittal image through the lateral ankle shows the localized metallic artifact (*arrows*). (**C**) A midsagittal section in the same patient demonstrates subarticular degenerative changes (*large black arrow*) and metaphyseal bone infarcts (*small black arrows*). Anterior capsule distention with ankle effusion is also seen (*open arrow*).

(continued)

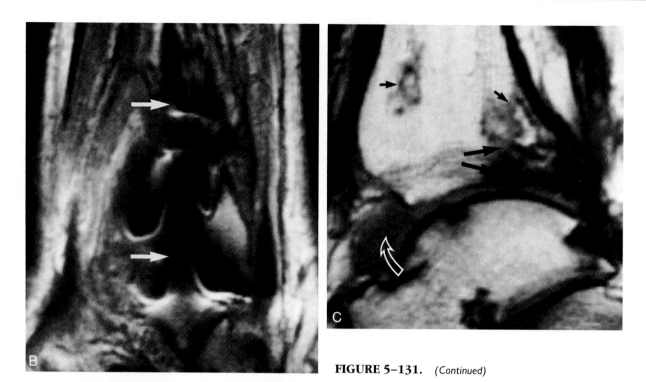

FIGURE 5–131. *(Continued)*

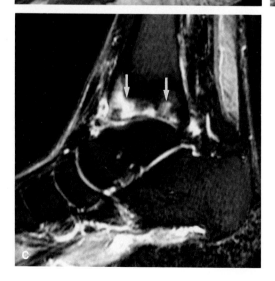

FIGURE 5–132. Loss of tibiotalar joint space. Subchondral marrow reactive hyperemia (*arrows*) demonstrates low signal intensity on (**A**) T1-weighted and (**B**) T2*-weighted sagittal images and (**C**) high signal intensity on short TI inversion recovery sagittal image.

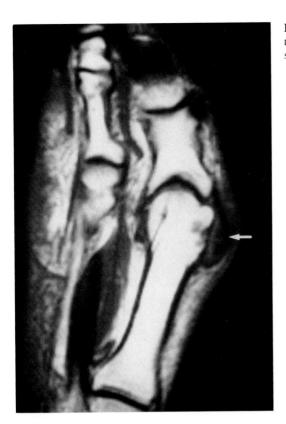

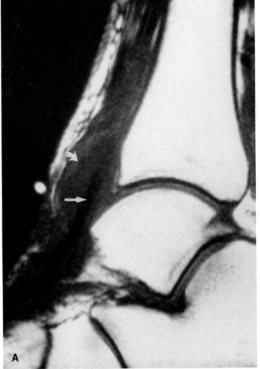

FIGURE 5–133. A hallux valgus deformity with bony low signal intensity soft-tissue prominence (*arrow*) over the medial aspect of the 1st metatarsal head is seen on a T1-weighted axial image.

FIGURE 5–134. A recurrent ganglion (*curved arrows*) of the extensor digitorum longus tendon (*straight arrows*) is seen on (**A**) a T1-weighted sagittal image and (**B**) T1-weighted and (**C**) T2*-weighted axial images. The cystic synovial fluid collection demonstrates homogeneity, well-defined margins, and hyperintensity on the T2*-weighted image.

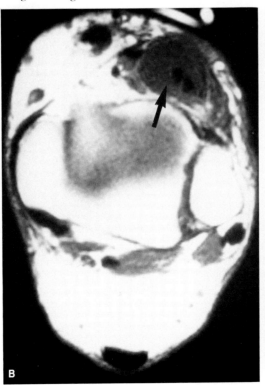

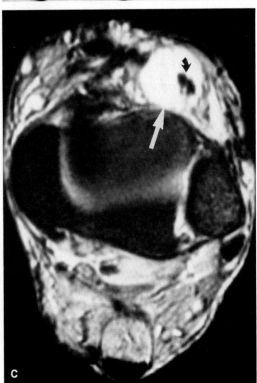

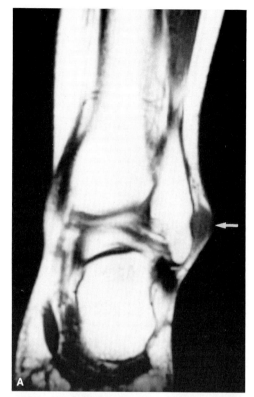

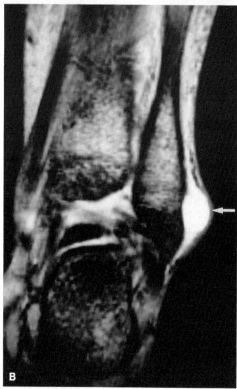

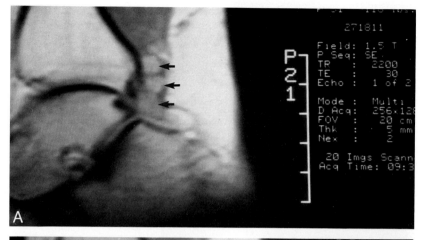

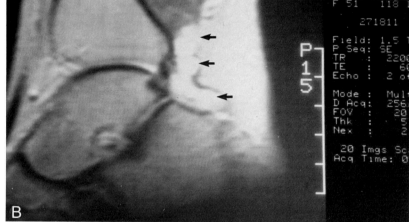

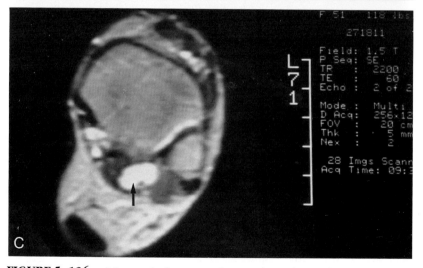

FIGURE 5–136. A juxtaarticular septated synovial cyst (*arrows*) is present posterior to the tibiotalar joint. The lesion demonstrates (**A**) low signal intensity on an intermediate-weighted sagittal image and high signal intensity on T2-weighted (**B**) sagittal and (**C**) axial images.

FIGURE 5–135. A cystic ganglion (*arrows*) projects laterally to the lateral malleolus and demonstrates (**A**) uniform low signal intensity on a T1-weighted coronal image and (**B**) high signal intensity on a T2*-weighted coronal image.

cations in the ankle and foot are preliminary, new clinical indications are being developed. The capability to detect skip lesions; to obtain high soft-tissue contrast in a multiplanar format; and to evaluate marrow, cartilage, and cortex separately shows great potential for the further use of MR for detection and monitoring of infection targeting the foot and ankle.

Infection causes an alteration in the ratio of free water to bound water that prolongs T1 and T2 tissue relaxation times; therefore, infected regions demonstrate low signal intensity on T1-weighted images and high signal intensity on T2-weighted images. Although this provides the basis for diagnostic sensitivity, neoplastic tissue undergoes similar T1 and T2 relaxation changes. Therefore, secondary characteristics such as location, distribution, extent, and morphology of signal intensity assume an important role in improving diagnostic specificity.

Osteomyelitis

Early osteomyelitis demonstrates low signal intensity on T1-weighted images and high signal intensity on T2-weighted images (Fig. 5–113). Acute and chronic osteomyelitis have been studied in the calcaneus, the cuboid, the metatarsals, and the distal tibia and fibula.[56] On T2-weighted sequences in the acute or subacute phase, a diffuse or patchy increase of signal intensity in the medullary bone indicates marrow involvement (Fig. 5–114). A peripheral rim of low signal intensity, representing reactive bone, may demarcate the focus over time. Alterations in signal intensity may also be seen at sites of cortical transgression, periosteal reaction, soft-tissue masses, and sequestrae.

In a patient with staphylococcal osteomyelitis involving the distal tibial metaphysis, a stellate pattern of signal change that mimics the MR appearance of a stress fracture was observed. Infected material in serpiginous tracts was seen on T2-weighted images as linear segments of high signal intensity (Fig. 5–115). Infectious soft-tissue (Fig. 5–116) and osseous (Fig. 5–117) involvement are successfully identified using a combination of T1-, T2-, T2*-weighted, and STIR protocols.[57]

Other Infections

Magnetic resonance evaluation of a 5-month-old child detected chronic granulomatous involvement of the ankle joint and surrounding tendons (Fig. 5–118). Synovial sheath distention and pockets of fluid demonstrated increased signal intensity on T2-weighted images, and necrotic granulomatous areas of involvement demonstrated intermediate signal intensity. Subsequent surgical exploration failed to confirm a septic etiology, although nonspecific giant cells were found on histologic examination.

In selected cases, MR may be indicated to identify the location and composition of foreign bodies. In one case, a foreign body (*i.e.*, toothpick) with a surrounding inflammatory capsule was identified by MR (Fig. 5–119). This lesion was missed both on radiography and surgical exploration.

Arthritis

To date, most experience with MR imaging of ankle arthritis has been restricted to cases of osteoarthritis and post-traumatic arthritis and to infectious and hemophiliac arthropathies (Fig. 5–120).[58]

In osteoarthritis, including cases of post-traumatic etiology, thinning of the tibiotalar and subtalar hyaline cartilage surfaces can be appreciated on coronal and sagittal T1-weighted images. As discussed earlier (see Transchondral Fractures), identification of loose bodies, possible on T1-weighted images, may require T2 weighting to create contrast with the surrounding synovial fluid, which demonstrates high signal intensity on T2-weighted sequences (Figs. 5–121 through 5–124). Osteophytic spurs with marrow contents are seen as areas of bright signal intensity isointense with fat, with a cortical rim of low signal intensity (*i.e.*, anterior tibial border) (Fig. 5–125). Cortical and subchondral irregularities can be seen in association with denuded articular cartilage (Fig. 5–126). In one case of primary osteoarthritis of the first metatarsophalangeal joint, secondary to excessive biomechanical loading in a springboard diver, MR demonstrated subchondral low signal intensity on coronal images through the foot in the absence of radiographic findings (Fig. 5–127).

The presence of an acute or chronic joint effusion— of low signal intensity on T1-weighted images—can also be determined with MR scans (Fig. 5–128). Subchondral or juxtaarticular cysts, which possess gelatinous synovial fluid, demonstrate uniformly increased signal intensity with progressive T2 weighting (Fig. 5–129). Magnetic resonance is particularly useful in assessing subtalar joint arthrosis displaying the anterior, middle, and posterior facets separately (Fig. 5–130). Subchondral and metaphyseal infarcts may coexist with joint-space narrowing and arthrosis (Fig. 5–131). STIR images are more sensitive than T2*-weighted images in documenting subchondral fluid through fissured articular cartilage (Fig. 5–132). We have not routinely used MR to document uncomplicated osteoarthritis or hallux valgus (Fig. 5–133).

On MR images, hemophilic arthropathy is indicated by low signal intensity synovial hypertrophy with paramagnetic hemosiderin deposits. On gradient-echo images, hyaline cartilage demonstrates high signal intensity, permitting identification of subtle cartilage irregularities.[58]

Ganglions arising from tendon sheaths, tibiotalar joints, or subtalar joints, with or without septations, are of uniform low signal intensity on T1-weighted images and high signal intensity on T2- and T2*-weighted images (Figs. 5–134 and 5–135). Posterior subtalar joint ganglions may be mistaken for effusion with capsular distention (Fig. 5–136). Further evidence with inflammatory and noninflammatory arthritides is required before routine use of MR imaging is indicated in the evaluation of ankle and foot articulations.

REFERENCES

1. Yousem DM, Scott WW Jr. The foot and ankle. In: Scott WW, et al, eds. Computed tomography of the musculoskeletal system. New York: Churchill-Livingston, 1987:113.

2. Crim JR, et al. Magnetic resonance imaging of the hindfoot. Foot Ankle 1989;10(1):1.

3. Rosenberg ZS, et al. Computed tomography scan and magnetic resonance imaging of the ankle tendons: an overview. Foot Ankle 1988;8(6):297.

4. Kneeland JB, et al. MR imaging of the normal ankle: correlation with anatomic sections. AJR 1988;151(1):117.

5. Solomon MA, et al. Magnetic resonance imaging in the foot and ankle. Clin Podiatr Med Surg 1988;5(4):945.

6. Sartoris DJ, Resnick D. Cross-sectional imaging of the foot: test of anatomical knowledge. J Foot Surg 1988;27(4):374.

7. Kingston S. Magnetic resonance imaging of the ankle and foot. Clin Sports Med 1988;7(1):15.

8. Noto AM, et al. MR imaging of the ankle: normal variants. Radiology 1989;170:121.

9. Kerr R, et al. Magnetic resonance imaging of foot and ankle trauma. Orthop Clin North Am 1990;21(3):591.

10. Noto AM. MR imaging of the ankle. Normal variants. Radiology 1987;165:148.

11. Ekstrom JE, et al. MR imaging of accessory soleus muscle. J Comput Assist Tomogr 1990;14(2):239.

12. Berndt A, Harty M. Transchondral fractures (osteochondritis dissecans) of the talus. J Bone Joint Surg [Am] 1959;41:988.

13. Anderson IF, et al. Osteochondral fractures of the dome of the talus. J Bone Joint Surg [Am] 1989;71(8):1143.

14. Nelson DW, et al. Osteochondritis dissecans of the talus and knee: prospective comparison of MR and arthroscopic classifications. J Comput Assist Tomogr 1990;14(5):804.

15. Yulish BS, et al. MR imaging of osteochondral lesions of the talus. J Comput Assist Tomogr 1987;11:296.

16. Stoller DW, et al. Fast MR improves imaging of musculoskeletal system. Diagn Imaging 1988:98.

17. De Smet AA, et al. Value of MR imaging in staging osteochondral lesions of the talus (osteochondritis dissecans): results in patients. AJR 1990;154(3):555.

18. Alexander AH, et al. Arthroscopic technique in talar dome fracture. Surg Rounds Orthop 1990:27.

19. Hattrup SJ, Johnson KA. A review of ruptures of the Achilles tendon. Foot Ankle 1985;6:34.

20. Willis CA, et al. Achilles tendon rupture: a review of the literature comparing surgical versus nonsurgical treatment. Clin Orthop 1986;207:156.

21. Quinn SF, et al. Achilles tendon: MR imaging at 1.5T. Radiology 1987;164:767.

22. Keene JS, et al. Magnetic resonance imaging of Achilles tendon ruptures. Am J Sports Med 1989;17(3):333.

23. Liem MD, et al. Repair of Achilles tendon ruptures with polylactic acid implant: assessment with MR imaging. AJR 1991;156:769.

24. Alanen A. Magnetic resonance imaging of hematomas in a 0.02T magnetic field. Acta Radiol (Diagn) 1986;27:589.

25. Kellam JF, et al. Review of the operative treatment of Achilles tendon rupture. Clin Orthop 1985;201:80.

26. Downey DJ, et al. Tibialis posterior tendon rupture: a cause of rheumatoid flat foot. Arthritis Rheum 1988;31(3):441.

27. Rosenberg ZS. Chronic tears of the posterior tibial tendon: a correlative study of CT, MR imaging, and surgical exploration. Radiology 1987;165(P):149.

28. Rosenberg ZS, et al. Rupture of posterior tibial tendon: CT and MR imaging with surgical correlation. Radiology 1988;169(1):229.

29. Zeiss J, et al. MR imaging of the peroneal tunnel. J Comput Assist Tomogr 1989;13(5):840.

30. Kerr R, Henry D. Radiologic case study: posterior tibial tendon rupture. Orthopedics 1989;12(10):1394.

31. Berquist TH, et al. Musculoskeletal trauma. In: Berquist TH, et al, eds. Magnetic resonance of the musculoskeletal system. New York: Raven, 1987:127.

32. Panageas E, et al. Magnetic resonance imaging of pathologic conditions of the Achilles tendon. Orthopedics 1990;19(11):975.

33. Berquist TH. Imaging of orthopaedic trauma and surgery. Philadelphia: WB Saunders, 1986:408,

34. Turek SL. The foot and ankle. In: Turek SL, ed. Orthopaedics: principles and their application. 4th ed. Philadelphia: JB Lippincott, 1984:1407.

35. Brantigan JW, et al. Instability of the subtalar joint. J Bone Joint Surg [Am] 1977;59:321.

36. Erickson SJ, et al. MR imaging of the lateral collateral ligament of the ankle. AJR 1991;156:131.

37. Levin PE. Traumatic injury to the lower limb in adults. In: Dee R, ed. Principles of orthopaedic practice. New York: McGraw-Hill, 1989;1209.

38. Johnson EE. Intraarticular fractures of the calcaneus: diagnosis and surgical management. Orthopedics 1990;13(10):1091.

39. Canale ST. Fractures of the neck of the talus. Orthopedics 1990;13(10):1105.

40. Kricun ME. Congenital foot deformities. In: Kricun ME, ed. Imaging of the foot and ankle, Rockville: Aspen Publications, 1988:47.

41. Gruber MA, et al. Congenital and developmental abnormalities of the foot in children. In: Dee R, ed. Principles of orthopaedic practice. New York: McGraw-Hill, 1989;1138.

42. Misoul C. Nerve injuries and entrapment syndromes of the lower extremity. In: Dee R, ed. Principles of orthopaedic practice. New York: McGraw-Hill, 1989;1420.

43. Takakura Y, et al. Tarsal tunnel syndrome. J Bone Joint Surg [Am] 1991;73(1):125.

44. Erickson SJ, et al. MR imaging of the tarsal tunnel and related spaces: normal and abnormal findings with anatomic correlation. AJR 1990;155(2):323.

45. Zeiss J, et al. Normal magnetic resonance anatomy of the tarsal tunnel. Foot Ankle 1990;10(4):214.

46. Dee R: Miscellaneous disorders of the foot. In: Dee R, ed. Principles of orthopaedic practice. New York: McGraw-Hill, 1989:1431.

47. Sartoris DJ, et al. Magnetic resonance images. Interdigital or Morton's neuroma. J Foot Surg 1989;28(1):78.

48. Turek SL: Congenital deformities. In: Turek SL, ed. Orthopaedics: principles and their application. 4th ed. Philadelphia: JB Lippincott, 1984:283.

49. Villani C, et al. Nuclear magnetic resonance as a contribution to the choice of technique in lengthening the Achilles tendon in a spastic equinus foot. Ital J Orthop Traumatol 1989;15(1):103.

50. Forrester DM. Arthritis. In: Kricun ME, ed. Imaging of the foot and ankle. Rockville: Aspen Publications, 1988:129.

51. Sartoris DJ, et al. Magnetic resonance imaging of tendons in the foot and ankle. J Foot Surg 1989;28(4):370.

52. Yeh WT, et al. Osteomyelitis of the foot in diabetic patients: evaluation with plain film, ^{99m}Tc-MDP bone scintigraphy, and MR imaging. AJR 1989;152(4):795.

53. Wang A, et al. MRI and diabetic foot infections. MRI 1990;8:805.

54. Griffey RH, et al. Correlation of magnetic resonance imaging and nerve conduction for the early detection of diabetic neuropathy in humans. In: Abstracts of the Meeting of the Society of Magnetic Resonance in Medicine, New York City, August 17, 1987 p 125.

55. Tang JSH, et al. Musculoskeletal infection of the extremities. Evaluation with MR imaging. Radiology 1988;166:205.

56. Berquist TH. Musculoskeletal infection. In: Berquist TH, et al, eds. Magnetic resonance of the musculoskeletal system. New York: Raven, 1987:109.

57. Harms SE, Greenway G. Musculoskeletal system. In: Stark DD, Bradley WG, eds. Magnetic resonance imaging. St. Louis: CV Mosby, 1988:1323.

58. Beltran J, et al. Ankle: surface coil MR imaging at 1.5T. Radiology 1986;161:203.

CHAPTER 6

David W. Stoller
Eugene M. Wolf

The Shoulder

Standard radiographic techniques demonstrate the osseous structure of the shoulder girdle but provide only limited evaluation of soft-tissue anatomy including the rotator cuff, the ligamentous attachments of the glenoid labrum capsule, and the subacromial space. Conventional radiographs do not allow direct visualization of the rotator cuff tendons, their defects and abnormalities, and their relationship to the undersurface of the acromion and the acromioclavicular (AC) joint. As a result, impingement disorders are difficult to characterize on plain film radiographic studies.

With single contrast and double contrast arthrography, the extension of contrast into the subacromial–subdeltoid bursa, superior and lateral to the greater tu-

berosity, depicts complete tears of the rotator cuff.[1] Arthrography is limited in assessing the size and morphology of cuff tears, and is even less well suited for displaying partial tears, especially those involving the superior or bursal surface of the supraspinatus tendon. Arthrography cannot assess the degree of retraction of the cuff tendons or the status of cuff musculature.

Contrast computed arthrotomography has been used to visualize the glenoid labrum and capsule through the intraarticular injection of air and contrast material (Fig. 6–1).[2–4] Limited soft-tissue contrast and spatial resolution in reformatted scans limit the usefulness of this technique for routine assessment of the rotator cuff and subacromial space in impingement disorders.

Ultrasonography has also been used to visualize areas of increased echogenicity in the rotator cuff.[5-7] This technique is operator-dependent and poorly delineates the individual tendons of the rotator cuff. Vick and colleagues report a low sensitivity rate (67%) and accuracy rate (85%) for sonographic detection of rotator cuff tears.[8]

Magnetic resonance (MR) imaging of the rotator cuff provides direct coronal oblique images parallel with the course of the supraspinatus tendon as localized on axial plane images (Fig. 6–2).[9-23] Axial plane images through the glenohumeral joint display capsular and labral anatomy. Sagittal oblique plane images demonstrate acromial anatomy and display the coracoacromial and coracohumeral ligaments. Two- and three-dimensional (2D, 3D) gradient-echo images provide axial coverage from the AC joint through the glenohumeral joint. Contrast enhancement with intraarticular gadolinium diethylenetriamine pentacetic acid (Gd-DTPA) shows potential in improving diagnostic accuracy in partial tears of the rotator cuff, in distinguishing severe tendinitis from rotator cuff tears, and in better defining the capsulolabral anatomy of the glenohumeral joint.[15,16,18] T1-weighted Gd-DTPA images also minimize the effect of magnetic susceptibility that is seen with gradient-echo images in the postoperative rotator cuff. With or without gadolinium enhancement, MR affords superior visualization of both soft-tissue and osseous pathology not possible with conventional arthrography or computed tomography (CT; Fig. 6–3).

IMAGING PROTOCOLS FOR THE SHOULDER

Improvements in surface coil design, such as coupled pair coils and custom-curved coils that conform to the shoulder apex, have resulted in more uniform signal intensity than was possible with a planar circular coil placed posterior to the shoulder (Fig. 6–4). Off-axis capability is required to eliminate the need to position the shoulder isocenter with respect to the magnet, and direct oblique axis prescriptions replace the need to bolster the affected shoulder to align the supraspinatus tendon parallel with the coronal imaging plane. Until recently, aliasing, or wrap-around artifact, was often the limiting factor in image quality when the field of view was smaller than 20 cm. Software advances have eliminated phase wrap, however, by allowing the acquisition of data in a 512 × 512 matrix format.

The shoulder is positioned in external rotation to tighten anterior capsular structures. The use of a fixed arm board facilitates positioning of the humeral head in external rotation while limiting transmitted respiratory excursions to the arm and shoulder.

Routine shoulder evaluations are performed with a T1-weighted axial localizer to identify the anatomic area from the AC joint through the glenohumeral joint. T1- and T2- or T2*-weighted coronal oblique images parallel with the tendon of the supraspinatus are acquired at 4 mm with a 192 matrix. One- to two-mm 3D Fourier transform (3DFT) or 4-mm 2D Fourier transform (2DFT) T2*-weighted axial images are used to evaluate the glenohumeral capsule and labrum. Sagittal oblique T1-weighted or T2*-weighted images provide an additional plane in which to evaluate the conjoined insertion of the supraspinatus and infraspinatus tendons. A 3DFT sagittal sequence is acquired as nonoblique volume images (Fig. 6–5).

Magnetic resonance gadolinium-enhanced evaluations are obtained with T1-weighted axial and coronal oblique images pre- and postintraarticular injection. Unenhanced T2*-weighted coronal oblique images and postinjection sagittal oblique images are also obtained. The spin-echo T1-weighted protocol uses a repetition time (TR) of 400 msec and an echo time (TE) of 20 msec. A short TR maximizes the bright signal intensity contrast of gadolinium on T1-weighted images. Alternatively, a fat-saturation protocol can be used in conjunction with intraarticular gadolinium studies to improve the contrast of high signal intensity gadolinium and to eliminate the bright signal intensity of fat-containing structures (Fig. 6–6).

In a special technique developed for evaluating glenohumeral anterior instability and multidirectional instabilities, the arm is placed in abduction to tighten the inferior glenohumeral ligament (IGL) labral complex (Fig. 6–7). This technique evaluates tears or laxity of the anterior superior band of the IGL. O'Brien and colleagues have reclassified the bands of the IGL into anterior and posterior, and the band formerly termed superior is now referred to as the anterior band.[24]

On axial images, the brachial plexus can be identified adjacent to the subclavian vessels, which are used as landmarks for off-axis coronal images (Figs. 6–8 and 6–9). Axial T2*-weighted or conventional T2-weighted images of both upper extremities are obtained to demonstrate any extrinsic effacement of the brachial plexus from either soft-tissue or osseous encroachment or secondary increased signal intensity from nerve trauma.

NORMAL ANATOMY OF THE SHOULDER

Shoulder girdle articulations include the glenohumeral joint, the AC joint, and the sternoclavicular joint (Fig. 6–10). The humeral head articulates with a relatively shallow glenoid fossa of the scapula and is dependent on muscular, ligamentous, and labral integrity for its stability (Fig. 6–11).[25]

Glenohumeral Joint and Capsular Gross Anatomy

The glenoid labrum, wedge-shaped in cross section, is a ring of fibrous tissue with transitional fibrocartilage attached to the margins of the glenoid cavity (Fig. 6–12).[26] Labral tissue deepens the depression of the glenoid fossa. The anatomic configuration of the glenohumeral joint allows a greater range of motion than any other joint in the body. Glenohumeral motion depends on the congruity of the humeral head, the glenoid, the rotator cuff mechanism, and the deltoid muscle. Glenohumeral joint version or humeral retroversion projects the axis of humeral head joint surfaces 25° to 40° from the coronal plane, whereas the glenoid surface is retroverted 4° to 12° with respect to the scapula.[25]

Glenoid Labrum

The glenoid labrum represents the fibrous attachment of the glenohumeral ligaments and capsule to the glenoid rim (Figs. 6–13 through 6–15).[27] The labrum has the ovoid anatomy of an essentially kidney-shaped glenoid rim. It is 3 mm high and 4 mm wide, but its size, shape, and configuration vary considerably.

The anterior glenoid labrum is formed primarily from the anterior band of the IGL (see Fig. 6–15).[24] The middle glenohumeral ligament (MGL) also contributes the more superior aspects of the anterior glenoid labrum.

The glenoid labrum is more mobile above the epiphyseal line (*i.e.,* the junction of the upper and middle one-thirds of the glenoid). It provides stability for the glenohumeral joint and functions with the biceps tendon as a mobile "biceps labral complex" that slides over the cartilaginous superior pole of the glenoid (Figs. 6–16 and 6–17). Tension on the biceps tendon increases the depth of the labrum and makes it more cup-shaped, thus stabilizing the humeral head.

Glenohumeral Ligaments

The glenohumeral ligaments are thickened bands of the joint capsule and consist of the superior, middle, and inferior glenohumeral ligaments.[27] The IGL represents the largest and most important of the glenohumeral ligaments, and contributes to the formation of the anterior and posterior glenoid labrum. The normally lax glenohumeral ligaments can be thought of as check reins on extremes of motion for the glenohumeral joint.[25] The subscapularis, the MGL and IGL labral complex provide anterior stability for the glenohumeral joint.

Inferior Glenohumeral Ligament. The IGL consists of anterior and posterior bands and an axillary pouch that attaches to the inferior two-thirds of the glenoid by means of the labrum (Figs. 6–18 through 6–21).[24] The

IGL is lax in the adducted position. With increasing abduction, the IGL tightens and the anterior band moves superiorly with respect to the humeral head. At 90° of abduction, the IGL is the primary restraint for anterior and posterior dislocations.[28]

Middle Glenohumeral Ligament. The MGL attaches to the anterior aspect of the anatomic neck of the humerus, medial to the lesser tuberosity (Fig. 6–22).[27] It arises from the glenoid by way of the labrum and the scapular neck. This structure can be identified between the subscapularis tendon and the anterior band of the IGL (Figs. 6–23 and 6–24). The MGL plays a role in the stability of the joint from 0° to 45° of abduction. The presence of the MGL is less consistent than the IGL and is absent in approximately 15% of specimens.[29]

Superior Glenohumeral Ligament. The superior glenohumeral ligament (SGL) is the smallest and least understood of the glenohumeral capsular structures.[27] The SGL originates from the upper pole of the glenoid cavity and base of the coracoid process, and is attached to the MGL, to the biceps tendon, and to the labrum. It inserts onto the anterior superior aspect of the anatomic neck of the humerus (Fig. 6–25). A normal foramen or opening often exists between the SGL and MGL, allowing communication with subscapularis bursa.[30] The SGL is closely related to the extraarticular coracohumeral ligament. The coracohumeral ligament originates on the lateral aspect of the coracoid process and inserts on the greater tuberosity. The SGL and coracohumeral ligament contribute to the stabilization of the glenohumeral joint and prevent posterior and inferior translocation of the humeral head.

Rotator Cuff and Long Head of the Biceps

The supraspinatus, infraspinatus, teres minor, and subscapularis muscles constitute the rotator cuff (Figs. 6–26 through 6–28). Their primary function is to centralize the humeral head, limiting its superior translation during abduction. The supraspinatus, infraspinatus, and teres minor tendons insert on the greater tuberosity, whereas the subscapularis tendon inserts on the lesser tuberosity. The superior portion of the subscapularis tendon is intraarticular.[27] The subscapularis tendon lies on the anterior aspect of the anterior capsule of the glenohumeral joint. The subscapularis bursa lies between the subscapularis tendon and the scapula. The long head of the biceps tendon attaches to the superior glenoid and exits the joint in the bicipital groove in the hiatus between the subscapularis and supraspinatus tendons.[27] Fibers of the biceps contribute to the posterior superior labrum and anterior

(text continues on page 534)

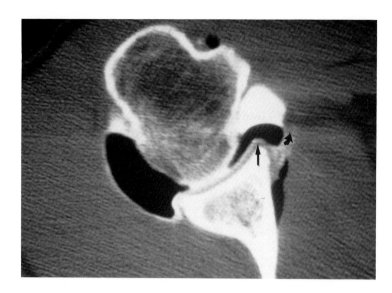

FIGURE 6–1. The anterior labrum (*straight arrow*) and middle glenohumeral ligament (*curved arrow*) can be seen on an air contrast CT study.

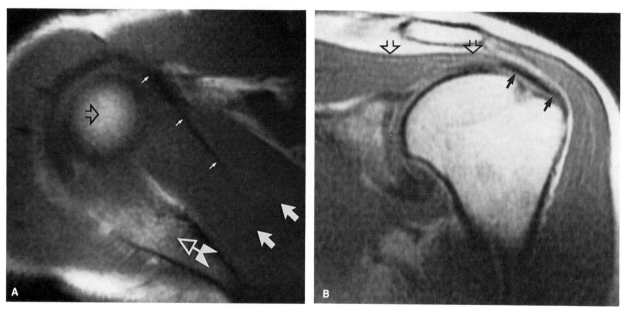

FIGURE 6–2. Localization of the supraspinatus tendon. (**A**) A T1-weighted superior axial image demonstrates an intact supraspinatus muscle (*large white arrows*) and low signal intensity tendon (*small white arrows*). The humeral head (*open black arrow*) and acromion (*flagged white arrow*) are also shown. (**B**) A T1-weighted coronal oblique image shows an intact intermediate signal intensity supraspinatus muscle (*open arrows*) and low signal intensity supraspinatus tendon (*solid arrows*).

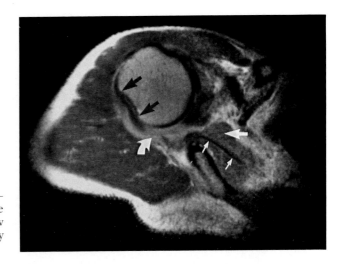

FIGURE 6–3. A rotator cuff tear (*large white arrow*) and a Hill–Sachs fracture (*black arrows*) are displayed on a superior axial image through the shoulder. The supraspinatus tendon displays disrupted low signal intensity (*small white arrows*), and intermediate signal intensity joint effusion (*curved white arrow*) is present.

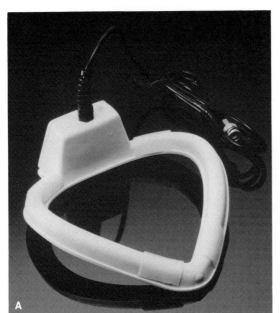

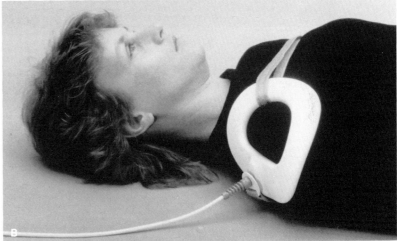

FIGURE 6–4. (**A**) General Electric (Milwaukee, WI) and (**B**) Medical Advances (Milwaukee, WI) surface coils conform to the curved shoulder girdle. Alternatively, a dual surface coil array set up in a Helmholtz configuration anterior and posterior to the shoulder can be used to image the joint.

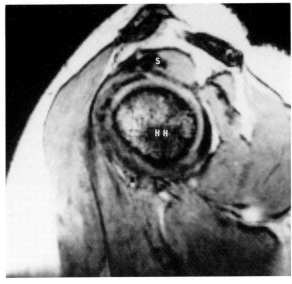

FIGURE 6–5. A 1-mm 3D Fourier transform volume image acquired on the sagittal oblique plane. (HH, humeral head; S, supraspinatus tendon.)

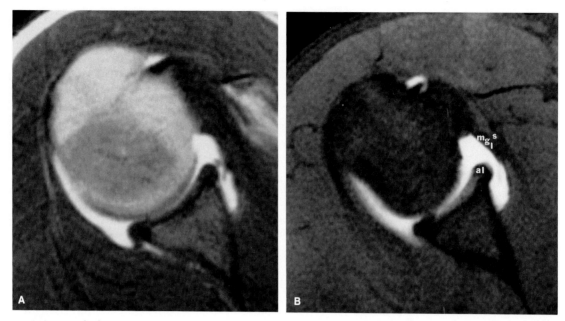

FIGURE 6–6. Intraarticular gadolinium contrast in the glenohumeral joint in (**A**) T1-weighted and (**B**) fat-suppression axial images. Note the superior contrast resolution among the labrum, capsular structures, and gadolinium on the fat-suppression image. (al, anterior labrum; mgl, middle glenohumeral ligament; s, subscapularis tendon.)

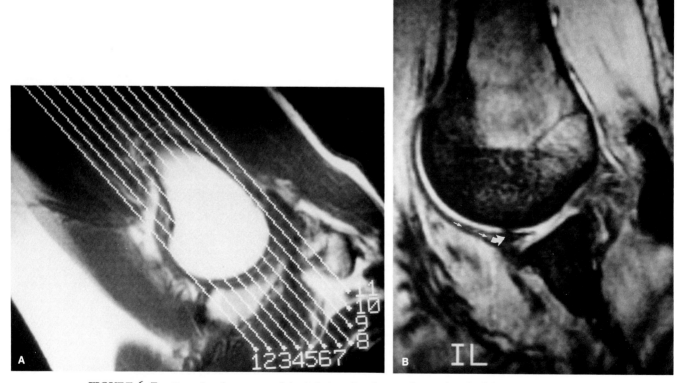

FIGURE 6–7. Functional anatomy of the inferior glenohumeral joint (IGL). (**A**) A coronal localizer is shown, with the arm placed in 90° of abduction (*i.e.,* the position of function of the IGL) and external rotation. (**B**) The corresponding axial images through the glenohumeral joint show a taut IGL (*small straight arrows*) and intact anterior IGL (*curved arrow*).

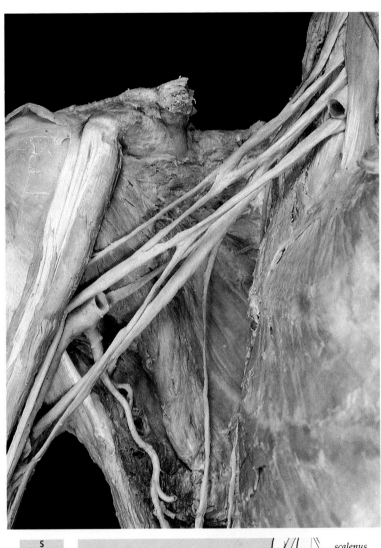

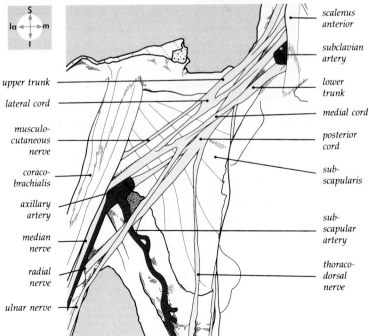

scalenus
anterior

subclavian
artery

upper trunk

lower
trunk

lateral cord

medial cord

musculo-
cutaneous
nerve

posterior
cord

coraco-
brachialis

sub-
scapularis

axillary
artery

sub-
scapular
artery

median
nerve

thoraco-
dorsal
nerve

radial
nerve

ulnar nerve

FIGURE 6–8. The components of the brachial plexus. The veins and most of the axillary artery have been removed.

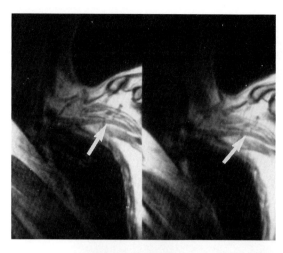

FIGURE 6–9. T1-weighted coronal oblique images through the trunks and cords of the brachial plexus (*arrows*).

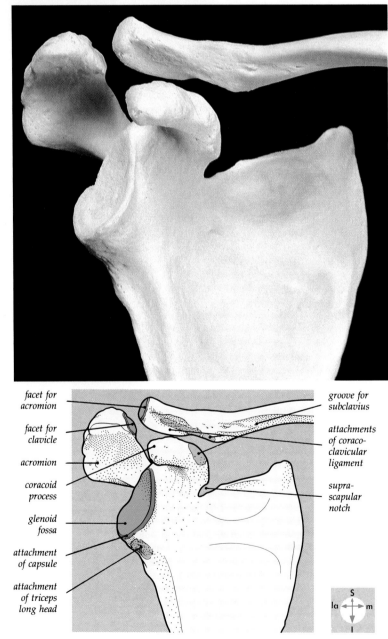

facet for
acromion

facet for
clavicle

acromion

coracoid
process

glenoid
fossa

attachment
of capsule

attachment
of triceps
long head

groove for
subclavius

attachments
of coraco-
clavicular
ligament

supra-
scapular
notch

FIGURE 6–10.

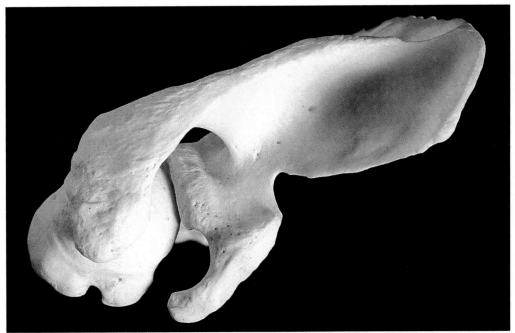

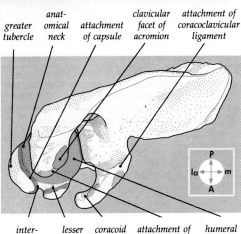

greater tubercle · anat-omical neck · attachment of capsule · clavicular facet of acromion · attachment of coracoclavicular ligament

inter-tubercular sulcus · lesser tubercle · coracoid process · attachment of coracoacromial ligament · humeral head

FIGURE 6–11. A superior view of the scapula and the upper end of the humerus. The acromion and the coracoacromial ligament prevent upward displacement of the humeral head.

FIGURE 6–10. An oblique anterior view of the scapula and lateral part of the clavicle. The bones have been separated to show the articular surfaces of the acromioclavicular joint and the sites of attachment of the coracoclavicular ligament.

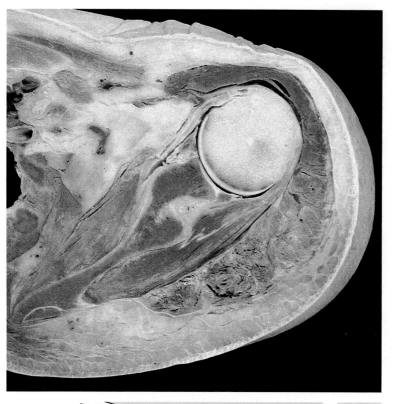

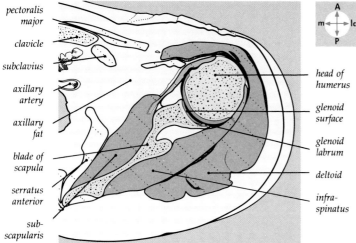

pectoralis
major

clavicle

subclavius

axillary
artery

axillary
fat

blade of
scapula

serratus
anterior

sub-
scapularis

head of
humerus

glenoid
surface

glenoid
labrum

deltoid

infra-
spinatus

FIGURE 6–12. A transverse section at the level of the humeral head shows the relations of the shoulder joint.

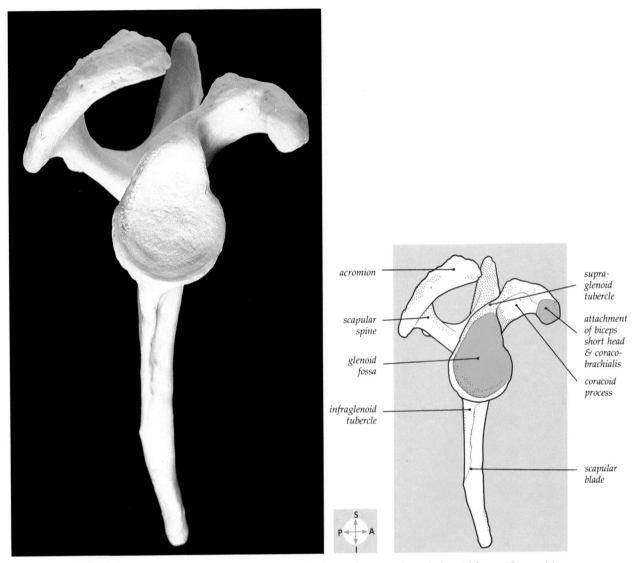

FIGURE 6–13. The lateral aspect of the scapula shows the pear-shaped glenoid fossa. The positions of the supraspinatus, infraspinatus, and subscapular fossae can be seen.

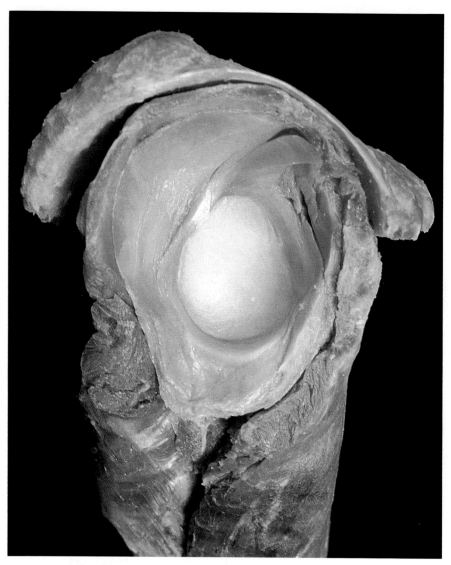

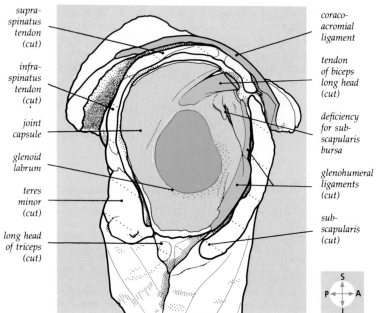

supra-
spinatus
tendon
(cut)

infra-
spinatus
tendon
(cut)

joint
capsule

glenoid
labrum

teres
minor
(cut)

long head
of triceps
(cut)

coraco-
acromial
ligament

tendon
of biceps
long head
(cut)

deficiency
for sub-
scapularis
bursa

glenohumeral
ligaments
(cut)

sub-
scapularis
(cut)

FIGURE 6–14. The scapular component of a disarticulated shoulder joint shows the relations and internal features of the joint.

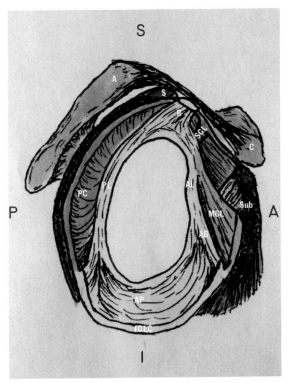

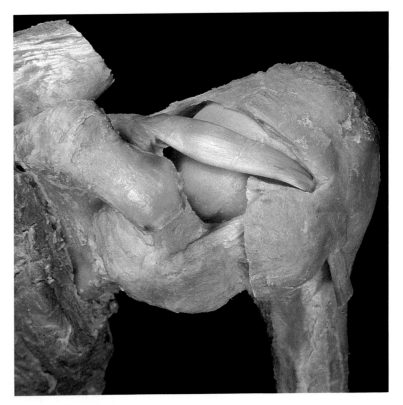

FIGURE 6–15. Glenohumeral capsular anatomy. (A, acromion; AB, anterior band of inferior glenohumeral ligament; AL, anterior labrum; AP, axillary pouch of inferior glenohumeral ligament; B, biceps tendon; C, coracoid; IGLC, inferior glenohumeral ligament complex; MGL, middle glenohumeral ligament; PC, posterior capsule; PL, posterior labrum; S, supraspinatus tendon; SGL, superior glenohumeral ligament; Sub, subscapularis tendon.)

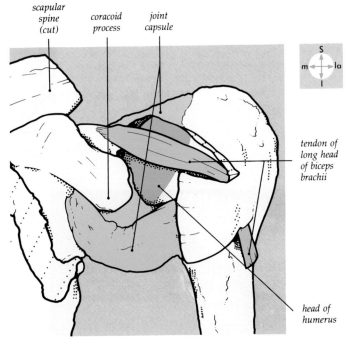

FIGURE 6–16. Removal of part of the shoulder joint capsule reveals the intracapsular but extrasynovial tendon of the long head of the biceps brachii.

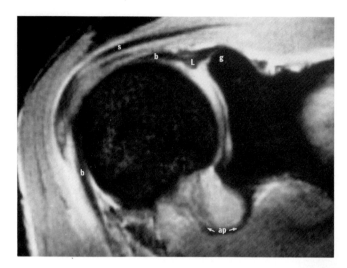

FIGURE 6–17. The biceps origin can be located on a T2*-weighted coronal oblique image. The glenoid origin of the long head of the biceps (b) can be seen, and the attachment to the anterior labrum (l) and superior glenoid (g) are shown. The biceps courses laterally and exits the joint between the supraspinatus (s) and subscapularis tendons. The axillary pouch (ap) of the inferior glenohumeral ligament is indicated. The tendon of the long head of the biceps enters the intertubercular groove under the transverse ligament.

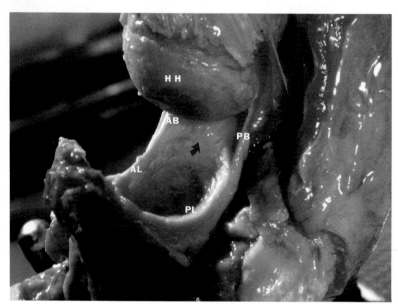

FIGURE 6–18. A gross shoulder specimen illustrates the structure of the inferior glenohumeral ligament (IGL) complex. With abduction of the humerus, the IGL structures are more prominent and taut in position. Coronal oblique MR images routinely show the axillary pouch of the IGL lax when the humerus is in the adducted position. (*Curved arrow,* axillary pouch; AB, anterior band; AL, anterior labrum; HH, humeral head; PB, posterior band; PL, posterior labrum.)

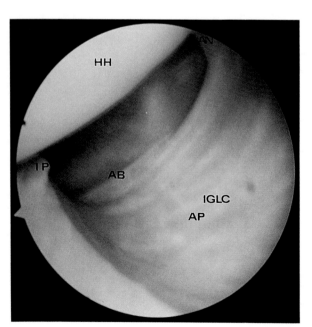

FIGURE 6–19. The inferior glenohumeral ligament complex. An arthroscopic photograph shows the anterior band (AB) and axillary pouch (AP) components of the inferior glenohumeral ligament (IGL) complex. The inferior pole of the glenoid (IP) and the anatomic neck (AN) attachments of the IGL complex are shown as viewed from the axillary pouch. (HH, humeral head.)

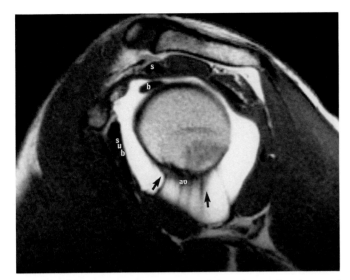

FIGURE 6–20. The axillary pouch of the inferior glenohumeral ligament is seen on an enhanced T1-weighted sagittal image. (*Arrows,* ap, axillary pouch of inferior glenohumeral ligament; b, biceps tendon; s, supraspinatus tendon; sub, subscapularis tendon.)

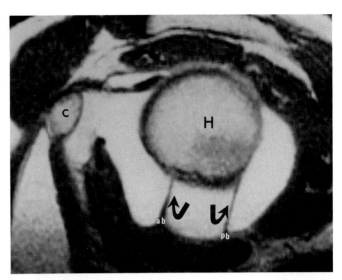

FIGURE 6–21. The anterior band (ab) and posterior band (pb) of the inferior glenohumeral ligament (*curved arrows*) extend from the glenoid origin to the humeral attachment, as seen on an enhanced T1-weighted sagittal oblique image. (C, coracoid; H, humeral head.)

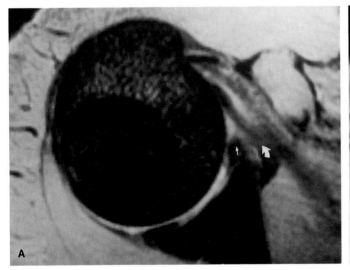

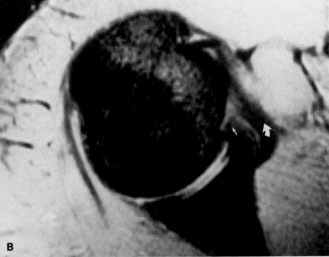

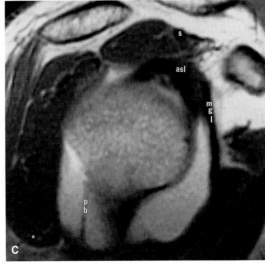

FIGURE 6–22. (**A**) T2*-weighted axial images at and below (**B**) the level of the subscapularis show the normal middle glenohumeral ligament (MGL; *curved arrows*), its medial origin from the glenoid and neck of the scapula, and its attachment to the lesser tuberosity (*small straight arrows,* anterior labrum). (**C**) An enhanced T1-weighted sagittal oblique image shows the attachment of the MGL (mgl) to the anterior superior glenoid labrum (asl). The MGL arises from the labrum below the superior glenohumeral ligament and from the neck of the scapula. The humeral attachment of the MGL is located medial to the lesser tuberosity. The MGL may arise only from the labrum or may have no attachment to it as normal anatomic variants. (pb, posterior band of IGL; s, supraspinatus tendon.)

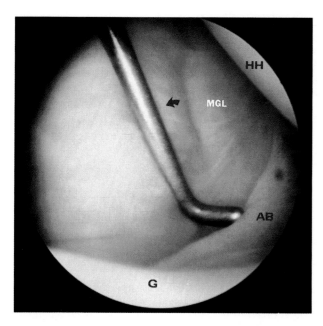

FIGURE 6–23. An arthroscopic photograph shows the anterior band (AB) of the inferior glenohumeral ligament. The subscapularis tendon (*arrow*) is located beneath the middle glenohumeral ligament (MGL) and is not directly seen. (G, glenoid; HH, humeral head.)

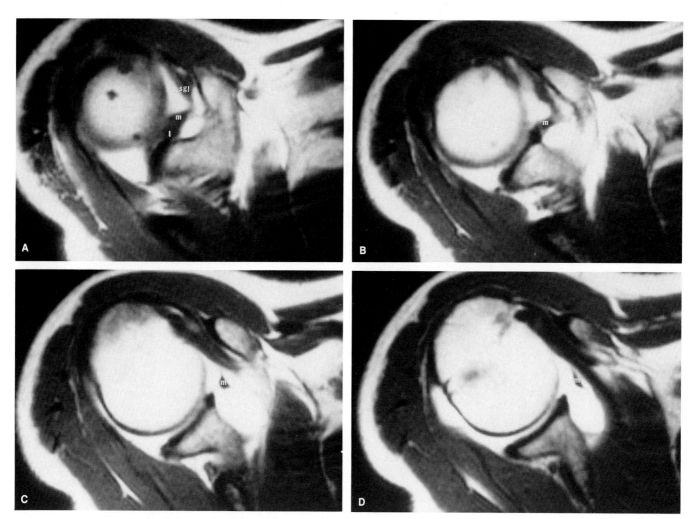

FIGURE 6–24. Gadolinium-enhanced T1-weighted axial images show the normal anatomy of the middle glenohumeral ligament (m) from (**A**) the anterior superior glenoid labrum (l) to (**F**) the level of the subscapularis. (sgl, superior glenohumeral ligament.)

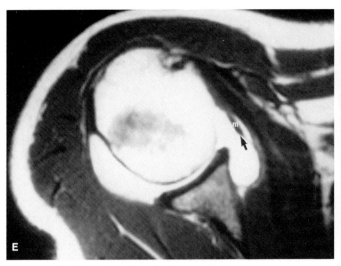

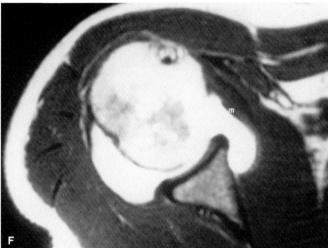

FIGURE 6–24. *(Continued)*

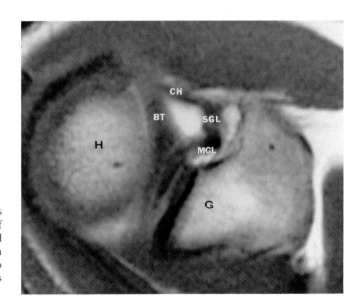

FIGURE 6–25. The superior glenohumeral ligament (SGL) is seen on an enhanced T1-weighted axial image above the level of the coracoid. The extraarticular coracohumeral ligament (CH) and intraarticular SGL are closely related structures. The middle portion of the CH crosses the SGL. The SGL is oriented perpendicular to the middle glenohumeral ligament (MGL) as shown. (BT, biceps tendon; G, glenoid; H, humeral head.)

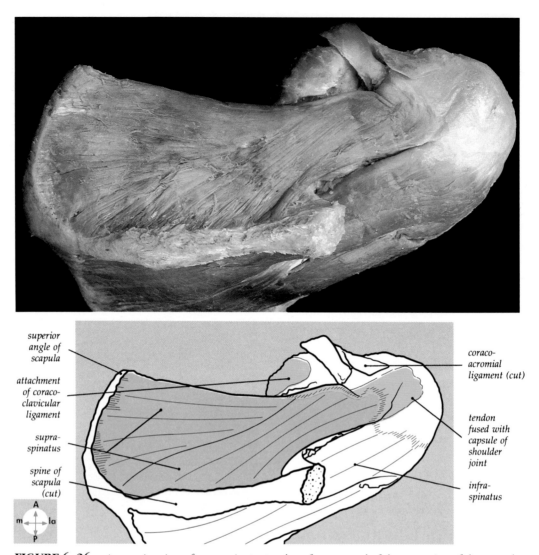

FIGURE 6–26. A superior view of supraspinatus tendon after removal of the acromion of the scapula.

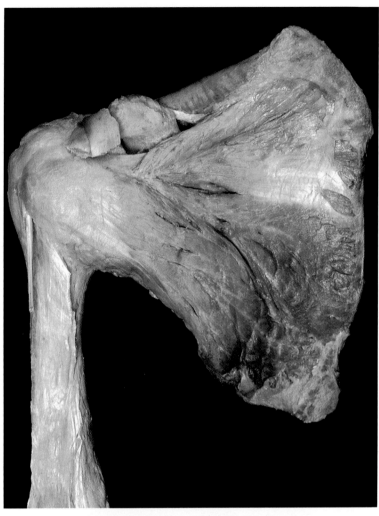

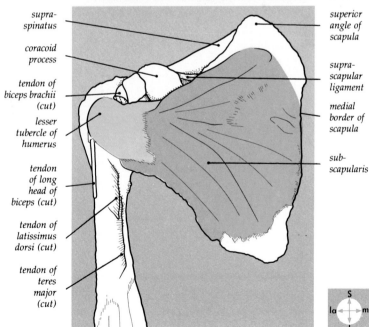

supra-
spinatus

coracoid
process

tendon of
biceps brachii
(cut)

lesser
tubercle of
humerus

tendon
of long
head of
biceps (cut)

tendon of
latissimus
dorsi (cut)

tendon of
teres
major
(cut)

superior
angle of
scapula

supra-
scapular
ligament

medial
border of
scapula

sub-
scapularis

FIGURE 6–27.   An anterior view of the subscapularis.
The attachment of the serratus anterior to the medial border
of the scapula has been excised.

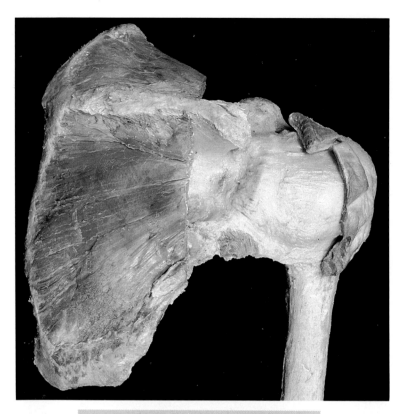

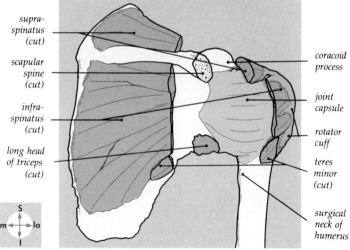

supra-
spinatus
(cut)

scapular
spine
(cut)

infra-
spinatus
(cut)

long head
of triceps
(cut)

coracoid
process

joint
capsule

rotator
cuff

teres
minor
(cut)

surgical
neck of
humerus

FIGURE 6–28. The posterior aspect of the shoulder joint. The acromion and parts of the rotator cuff muscles have been excised to reveal the joint capsule.

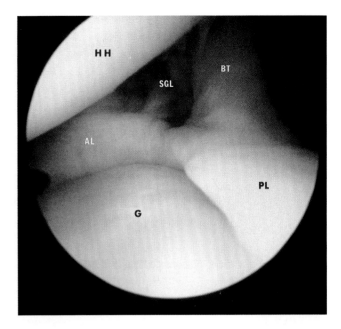

FIGURE 6–29. The biceps tendon (BT) contributes to the superior anterior labrum (AL) and the superior posterior labrum (PL) in the biceps labral complex. One component of the long head of the BT attaches to the supraglenoid tubercle. Extraarticular fibers attach to the lateral edge of the base of the coracoid process. The intraarticular portion of the long head of the BT is oriented at an approximate right angle to the surface of the glenoid (G). (HH, humeral head; SGL, superior glenohumeral ligament.)

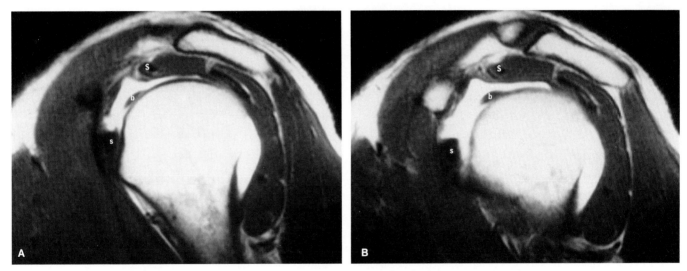

FIGURE 6–30. Intraarticular gadolinium-enhanced MR images show the normal biceps labral complex (blc) from (**A**) lateral to (**E**) medial. (*Arrows,* ap, axillary pouch of IGL; al, anterior labrum; b, biceps tendon; ch, coracohumeral ligament; mgl, middle glenohumeral ligament; S, supraspinatus tendon; s, subscapularis tendon.) (**F**) A corresponding T2*-weighted coronal image. (S, supraspinatus tendon.) (**G**) A corresponding anteroposterior arthrographic view and (**H**) enhanced T1-weighted coronal oblique image. (AP, axillary pouch; b, biceps tendon; l, labrum; S, supraspinatus tendon.) *(continued)*

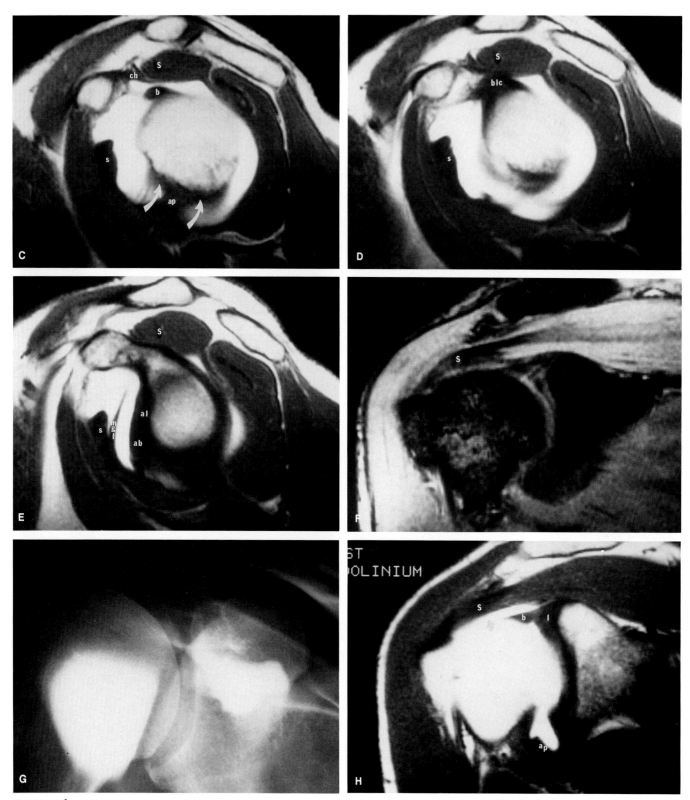

FIGURE 6–30. *(Continued)*

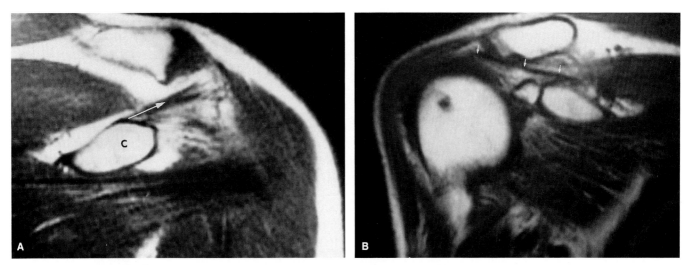

FIGURE 6–31. (**A**) A T1-weighted coronal oblique image shows an intact, low signal intensity coracoacromial ligament (*arrow*) with a broad inferior acromial attachment. (C, coracoid.) (**B**) A T1-weighted coronal oblique image shows subacromial-space narrowing with buffering of the superior ascent of the humeral head by the coracoacromial ligament (*arrows*). Development of a subacromial spur is associated with chronic impingement of the greater tuberosity on the coracoacromial ligament.

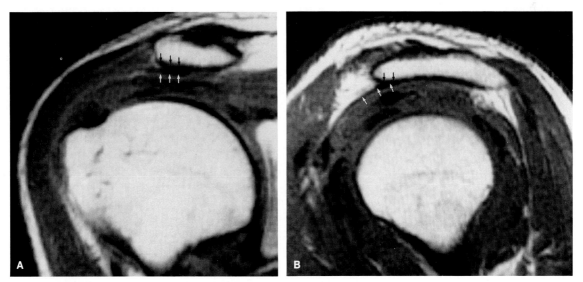

FIGURE 6–32. Pseudospur. Normal broad attachment of the coracoacromial ligament to the inferior surface of the acromion on (**A**) T1-weighted coronal oblique and (**B**) sagittal oblique images. Low signal intensity acromial cortex (*black arrows*) and adjacent coracoacromial ligament attachment (*white arrows*) give the false impression of a small subacromial spur in the coronal plane, which should not be misinterpreted as impingement. Unnecessary acromioplasties may be performed on patients with a normal coracoacromial ligament attachment and no associated acromial spurs.

superior labrum (Figs. 6–29 and 6–30). The long head of the biceps, with the biceps labral complex, functions to centralize and stabilize the joint, as does the rotator cuff.

Coracoacromial Arch

Coracoacromial Ligament

The coracoacromial ligament is the key structure of the coracoacromial arch and plays an important role in the spectrum of impingement disorders of the shoulder (Fig. 6–31). This ligament attaches to the anterior, lateral, and inferior surfaces of the acromion. Anterior acromial spurs, or traction spurs, caused by mechanical action of the humerus against this ligamentous structure, can form within the acromial portion of the coracoacromial ligament, but are relatively rare.[25] More frequently, anterior acromial spurs are identified adjacent to the acromial attachment of the coracoacromial ligament. The normal low signal intensity acromial attachment of the coracoacromial ligament is frequently mistaken for an anterior acromial spur on coronal oblique MR images. The additive thickness of the coracoacromial ligament and the inferior acromial cortex produces this "pseudospur" (Fig. 6–32). In acromioplasty performed for chronic impingement (see Shoulder Impingement Syndrome; Treatment), the coracoacromial ligament is resected.

Acromioclavicular Joint

The AC joint is a synovial joint with articular surfaces covered by fibrocartilage like the sternoclavicular joint.[31] The articular capsule is reinforced by superior and inferior AC ligaments. The articular surfaces are separated by a wedge-shaped articular disk. The coracoclavicular ligament, with its conoid and trapezoid components, provides major stability to the joint (see Fig. 6–10).

Subacromial Bursa

The subacromial bursa extends under the acromion and coracoacromial ligament. Laterally, the bursa lies over the superior surface of the supraspinatus and infraspinatus tendons and extends beyond the lateral and anterior aspects of the acromion under the deltoid. The bursa serves as a gliding surface between the rotator cuff and the teres major muscles.[32] Although communication exists between the subacromial and subcoracoid bursae, there is no communication between the subcoracoid and subscapularis bursae (Figs. 6–33 and 6–34).[33,34] Therefore, an inadvertent gadolinium injection into the subcoracoid bursa does not allow visualization of capsular structures because the subscapularis bursa is not distended. In this situation, gadolinium contrast in the subacromial bursa is not related to rotator cuff pathology.

NORMAL MAGNETIC RESONANCE APPEARANCE OF THE SHOULDER

Axial Images

On superior axial images, the normal oblique course of the supraspinatus muscle is displayed with intermediate signal intensity (Fig. 6–35). The supraspinatus tendon, from its insertion on the capsule and greater tuberosity posterior to the bicipital groove to the supraspinatus fossa of the scapula, is displayed with low signal intensity. The supraspinatus muscle appears gray on T2*-weighted images, demonstrating low signal intensity with its tendinous fibers. High signal intensity marrow fat is present in the acromion, localized laterally and parallel with the supraspinatus. At the level of the superior coracoid process, the long axis of the infraspinatus originates from the posterior inferior surface of the scapula, crosses the glenohumeral joint posterior to the supraspinatus, and inserts on the lateral aspect of the greater tuberosity. As it approaches the greater tuberosity posterolaterally, the low signal intensity infraspinatus tendon merges with the low signal intensity cortex of the humerus. The spine of the scapula separates the supraspinatus and infraspinatus muscles. The teres minor is posterolateral to the infraspinatus, originating at the axillary border of the scapula and inserting on the inferior facet of the greater tuberosity.

In cross section, the tendon of the long head of the biceps is seen as a low signal intensity structure within the bicipital groove and is sometimes associated with a small amount of high signal intensity fat. The suprascapular artery and nerve are located posterior and medial to the superior glenoid rim. The dark, low signal intensity labrum is located at the level of glenohumeral articulation, inferior to the coracoid. Normally, the anterior and posterior labrum have well-defined triangular shapes. With internal rotation, however, the anterior labrum appears to be larger than the posterior. Glenohumeral articular cartilage follows the concave shape of the glenoid cavity and demonstrates intermediate signal intensity on T1-weighted images and bright signal intensity on T2*-weighted images. Anterolateral to the glenoid, the subscapularis muscle arises from the subscapularis fossa and inserts on the lesser tuberosity. The low signal intensity subscapularis can then be identified anterior to the apex of the anterior glenoid labrum. The subscapularis tendon is present at the level of the middle and superior glenohumeral joint. Lying on this tendon, the MGL is present as a thin, low signal intensity band. The SGL is identified at the level of the coracoid and biceps tendon.

On axial images through the inferior glenohumeral joint, the IGL can be partially seen as a lax structure. The subacromial–subdeltoid bursa and the deltoid muscle can be identified between the rotator cuff and the acromion.

Coronal Images

In rotator cuff evaluations, supraspinatus tendon anatomy is best displayed on coronal oblique planar images (Fig. 6-36). On anterior and midcoronal oblique images, the supraspinatus muscle and its central tendon are seen in continuity. The low spin density supraspinatus tendon is defined at its insertion on the greater tuberosity. The subacromial bursa is interposed between the rotator cuff and the acromion. A fibrofatty layer lies between the acromion, the AC joint, and the superior bursal layer.

On anterior coronal images, the subscapularis muscle fibers and multitendinous fibers can be identified where they converge on the lesser tuberosity. Anterior coronal oblique images display the coracohumeral and coracoacromial ligaments as thin black structures. With neutral or internal rotation of the humeral head, the long head of the biceps tendon is seen in the bicipital groove on anterior coronal oblique images. The long head of the biceps enters the capsule inferior to the supraspinatus tendon and can be followed to its insertion on the superior rim of the glenoid. Coracoclavicular ligaments are also displayed on anterior coronal oblique images. The anatomy of the AC articulation is best displayed at the level of the supraspinatus tendon. The inferior glenoid labrum and axillary pouch are clearly demonstrated on these oblique images.

On midcoronal images, the muscle belly of the supraspinatus extends laterally beyond the glenoid before its central tendon reaches the musculotendinous junction of the rotator cuff.

On midcoronal to posterior coronal sections, there is a subtle transition between the supraspinatus and the conjoined insertion of the infraspinatus tendon. Posterior to the AC joint, the supraspinatus tendon forms a conjoined attachment to the greater tuberosity with the infraspinatus tendon. On the more posterior sections, the infraspinatus tendon may be mistaken for the supraspinatus tendon, which may be out of the plane of section. Humeral head articular cartilage, intermediate in signal intensity on T1-weighted images, is interposed between the low signal intensity supraspinatus tendon superiorly and the cortex inferiorly. The posterior circumflex humeral artery and the axillary nerve are identified medial to the coracobrachialis, the latissimus dorsi, and the teres major muscles and tendons. The teres minor muscles and tendons are shown on more posterior coronal oblique images at the level of the scapular spine where the teres minor attaches to the greater tuberosity.

Sagittal Images

The muscle groups of the deltoid, supraspinatus, infraspinatus, teres minor, teres major, subscapularis, and coracobrachialis are defined on sagittal plane MR images (Fig. 6-37). On midsagittal and lateral sagittal images, the supraspinatus and infraspinatus and the conjoined cuff tendons demonstrate low signal intensity between the acromion and the superior articular surfaces of the humeral head. The thickened tendon seen in the anterior one-half of the sagittal image is the supraspinatus component, whereas the fatter tendon that arches over the posterior one-half of the humeral head is the infraspinatus component. The long head of the biceps tendon is identified anterior and inferior to the supraspinatus tendon on lateral sagittal images. Toward the glenoid, the coracoacromial ligament is seen as a low signal intensity band that arches over the anterior aspect of the rotator cuff from the acromion and coracoid. Medial sagittal sections display the clavicle and AC joint in profile. The oblique transverse-oriented physis is also delineated on sagittal images. Marrow inhomogeneity, seen frequently as red-to-yellow marrow conversion, may not be complete distal to the physis in the metadiaphyseal region.

The low signal intensity glenoid labrum is also defined on sagittal images that transect the glenohumeral joint. Medial sagittal images demonstrate the coracoclavicular ligaments. The low spin density tendon of the supraspinatus is identified in the anterior portion of the supraspinatus muscle. The pectoralis minor and coracobrachialis muscles are anterior to the coracoid process. The axillary artery, vein, and brachial plexus are anterior to the subscapularis muscle and deep to the pectoralis minor. The subscapularis muscle and tendon are anterior to the capsule of the glenohumeral joint. The long head of the biceps tendon enters the joint capsule superiorly, anterior and inferior to the supraspinatus tendon. The SGL lies anterior to the humeral head and glenoid and inferior to the long head of the biceps tendon. The MGL is anterior to the medial humeral head, or lateral glenoid. The thick inferior glenoid labrum is identified as a low signal intensity structure along the inferior aspect of the glenoid.

PATHOLOGY OF THE SHOULDER

Shoulder Impingement Syndrome

Pathogenesis

Degenerative changes develop where the tendinous fibers of the rotator cuff attach to the greater tuberosity, most often in the area of the insertion of the supraspinatus tendon. This tendon, anatomically confined and compressed between bony structures at both its inferior and superior surfaces, is at risk for acute injury and chronic wear. Bursal inflammation and tendinitis produced by this compression may lead to degeneration and tearing. A type 3 hooked acromion or an anterior spur may

(text continues on page 562)

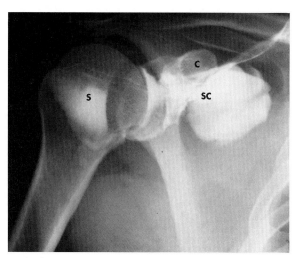

FIGURE 6–33. Separate contrast injections into the subcoracoid (SC) and subscapularis bursa (S) were performed. (C, coracoid.) The subcoracoid and subacromial bursa are seen to communicate, whereas no communication occurs between the subacromial and subscapularis bursae.

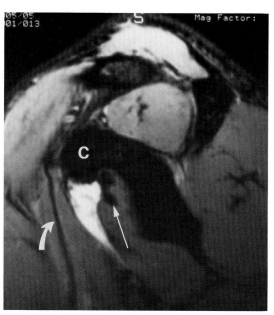

FIGURE 6–34. A gadopentetate–saline subcoracoid bursagram T2*-weighted sagittal oblique image demonstrates filling of the subcoracoid bursa anterior to the subscapularis tendon (*straight arrow*) and posterior to the conjoined tendon of the coracobrachialis and short head of the biceps (*curved arrow*). (C, coracoid.)

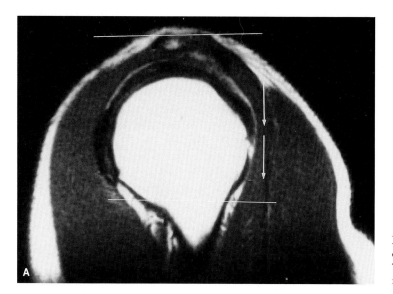

FIGURE 6–35. Normal axial MR anatomy. (**A**) This sagittal oblique localizer was used to graphically prescribe 18 axial T1-weighted image locations from (**B**) superior to (**S**) inferior.

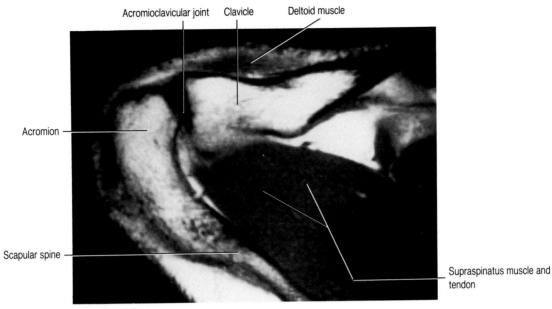

Acromioclavicular joint   Clavicle   Deltoid muscle

Acromion

Scapular spine

Supraspinatus muscle and tendon

FIGURE 6–35B.

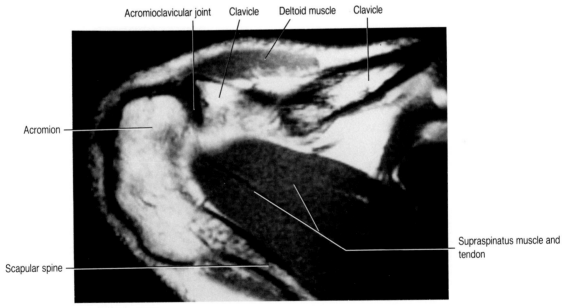

Acromioclavicular joint   Clavicle   Deltoid muscle   Clavicle

Acromion

Scapular spine

Supraspinatus muscle and tendon

FIGURE 6–35C.

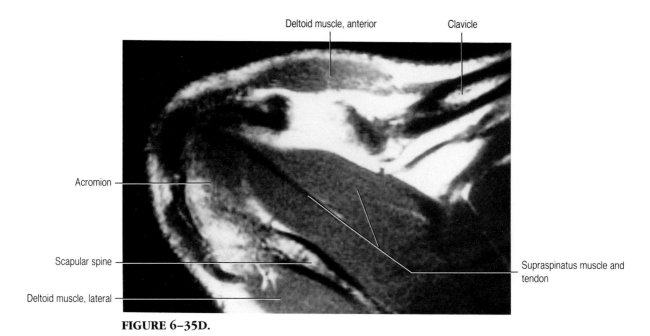

Deltoid muscle, anterior   Clavicle

Acromion

Scapular spine

Deltoid muscle, lateral

Supraspinatus muscle and tendon

FIGURE 6–35D.

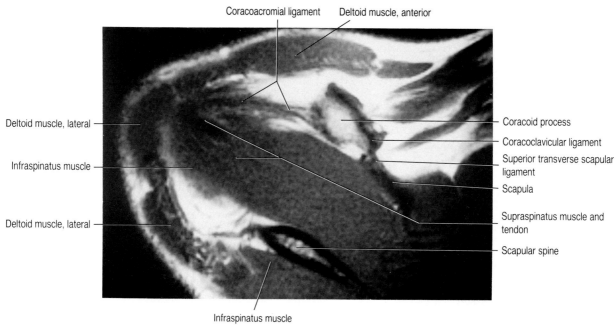

Coracoacromial ligament   Deltoid muscle, anterior

Deltoid muscle, lateral

Infraspinatus muscle

Deltoid muscle, lateral

Coracoid process

Coracoclavicular ligament

Superior transverse scapular ligament

Scapula

Supraspinatus muscle and tendon

Scapular spine

Infraspinatus muscle

FIGURE 6–35E.

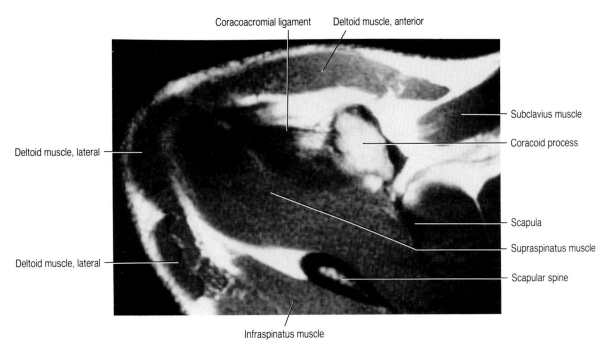

Coracoacromial ligament · Deltoid muscle, anterior

Subclavius muscle

Coracoid process

Deltoid muscle, lateral

Deltoid muscle, lateral

Scapula

Supraspinatus muscle

Scapular spine

Infraspinatus muscle

FIGURE 6–35F.

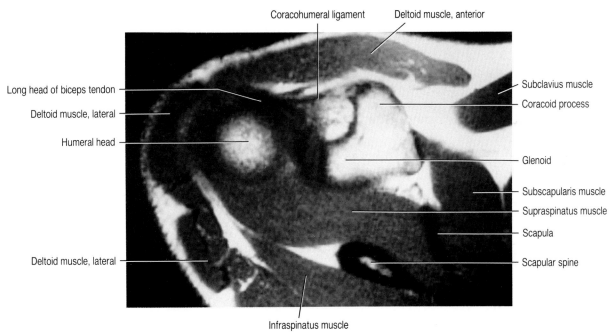

Coracohumeral ligament · Deltoid muscle, anterior

Long head of biceps tendon

Deltoid muscle, lateral

Humeral head

Subclavius muscle

Coracoid process

Glenoid

Subscapularis muscle

Supraspinatus muscle

Scapula

Deltoid muscle, lateral

Scapular spine

Infraspinatus muscle

FIGURE 6–35G.

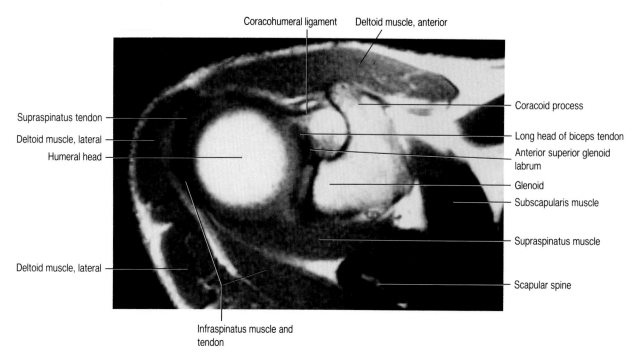

Coracohumeral ligament — Deltoid muscle, anterior

Supraspinatus tendon —

Deltoid muscle, lateral —

Humeral head —

Deltoid muscle, lateral —

— Coracoid process

— Long head of biceps tendon

— Anterior superior glenoid labrum

— Glenoid

— Subscapularis muscle

— Supraspinatus muscle

— Scapular spine

Infraspinatus muscle and tendon

FIGURE 6–35H.

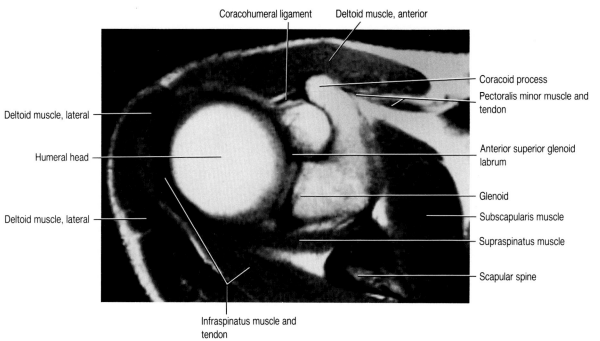

Coracohumeral ligament — Deltoid muscle, anterior

Deltoid muscle, lateral —

Humeral head —

Deltoid muscle, lateral —

— Coracoid process

— Pectoralis minor muscle and tendon

— Anterior superior glenoid labrum

— Glenoid

— Subscapularis muscle

— Supraspinatus muscle

— Scapular spine

Infraspinatus muscle and tendon

FIGURE 6–35I.

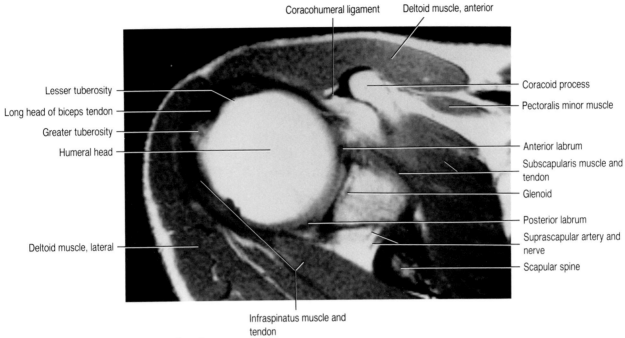

Coracohumeral ligament — Deltoid muscle, anterior

Lesser tuberosity

Long head of biceps tendon

Greater tuberosity

Humeral head

Deltoid muscle, lateral

Coracoid process

Pectoralis minor muscle

Anterior labrum

Subscapularis muscle and tendon

Glenoid

Posterior labrum

Suprascapular artery and nerve

Scapular spine

Infraspinatus muscle and tendon

FIGURE 6–35J.

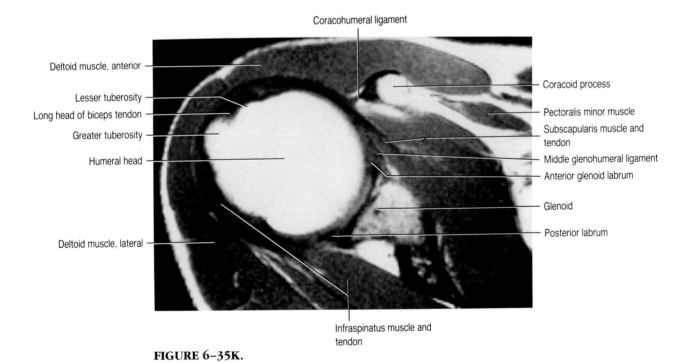

Coracohumeral ligament

Deltoid muscle, anterior

Lesser tuberosity

Long head of biceps tendon

Greater tuberosity

Humeral head

Deltoid muscle, lateral

Coracoid process

Pectoralis minor muscle

Subscapularis muscle and tendon

Middle glenohumeral ligament

Anterior glenoid labrum

Glenoid

Posterior labrum

Infraspinatus muscle and tendon

FIGURE 6–35K.

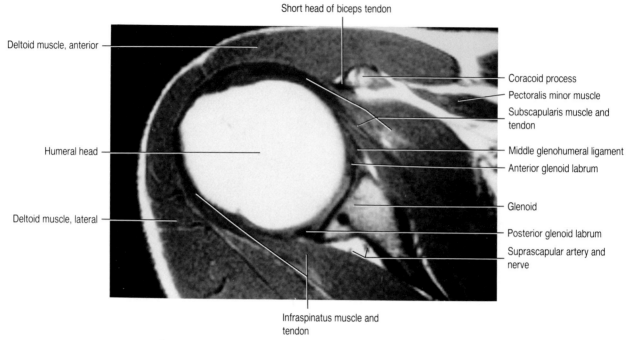

Short head of biceps tendon

Deltoid muscle, anterior

Coracoid process

Pectoralis minor muscle

Subscapularis muscle and tendon

Humeral head

Middle glenohumeral ligament

Anterior glenoid labrum

Deltoid muscle, lateral

Glenoid

Posterior glenoid labrum

Suprascapular artery and nerve

Infraspinatus muscle and tendon

FIGURE 6–35L.

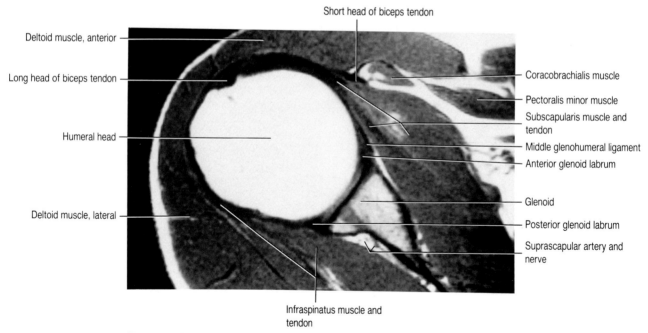

Short head of biceps tendon

Deltoid muscle, anterior

Long head of biceps tendon

Coracobrachialis muscle

Pectoralis minor muscle

Subscapularis muscle and tendon

Humeral head

Middle glenohumeral ligament

Anterior glenoid labrum

Deltoid muscle, lateral

Glenoid

Posterior glenoid labrum

Suprascapular artery and nerve

Infraspinatus muscle and tendon

FIGURE 6–35M.

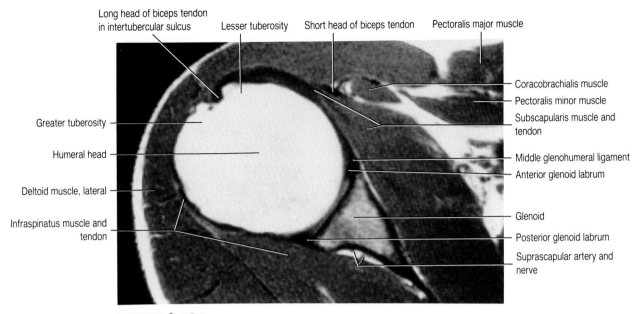

Long head of biceps tendon in intertubercular sulcus

Lesser tuberosity

Short head of biceps tendon

Pectoralis major muscle

Coracobrachialis muscle

Pectoralis minor muscle

Subscapularis muscle and tendon

Greater tuberosity

Humeral head

Middle glenohumeral ligament

Anterior glenoid labrum

Deltoid muscle, lateral

Infraspinatus muscle and tendon

Glenoid

Posterior glenoid labrum

Suprascapular artery and nerve

FIGURE 6–35N.

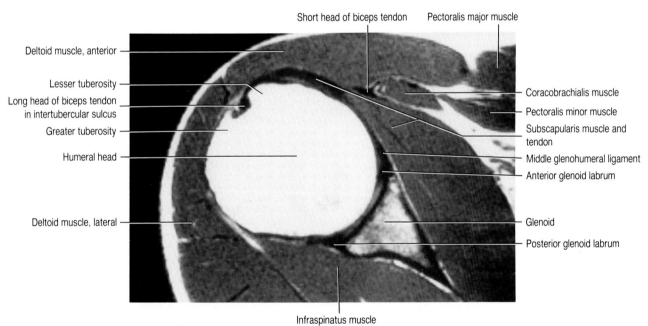

Short head of biceps tendon

Pectoralis major muscle

Deltoid muscle, anterior

Lesser tuberosity

Long head of biceps tendon in intertubercular sulcus

Greater tuberosity

Humeral head

Coracobrachialis muscle

Pectoralis minor muscle

Subscapularis muscle and tendon

Middle glenohumeral ligament

Anterior glenoid labrum

Deltoid muscle, lateral

Glenoid

Posterior glenoid labrum

Infraspinatus muscle

FIGURE 6–35O.

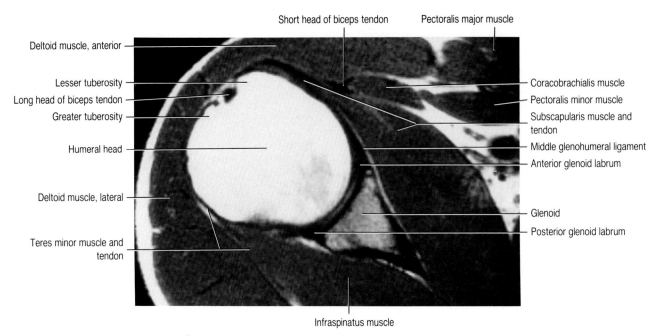

Deltoid muscle, anterior

Short head of biceps tendon

Pectoralis major muscle

Lesser tuberosity

Long head of biceps tendon

Greater tuberosity

Humeral head

Deltoid muscle, lateral

Teres minor muscle and tendon

Coracobrachialis muscle

Pectoralis minor muscle

Subscapularis muscle and tendon

Middle glenohumeral ligament

Anterior glenoid labrum

Glenoid

Posterior glenoid labrum

Infraspinatus muscle

FIGURE 6–35P.

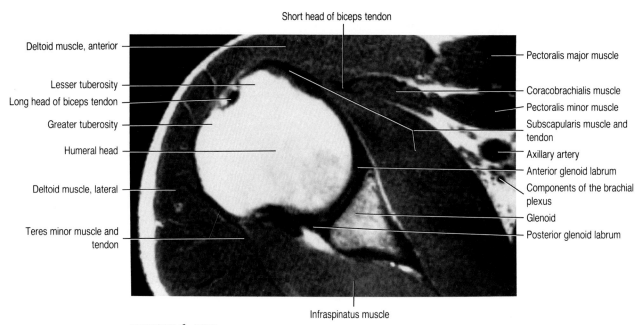

Short head of biceps tendon

Deltoid muscle, anterior

Lesser tuberosity

Long head of biceps tendon

Greater tuberosity

Humeral head

Deltoid muscle, lateral

Teres minor muscle and tendon

Pectoralis major muscle

Coracobrachialis muscle

Pectoralis minor muscle

Subscapularis muscle and tendon

Axillary artery

Anterior glenoid labrum

Components of the brachial plexus

Glenoid

Posterior glenoid labrum

Infraspinatus muscle

FIGURE 6–35Q.

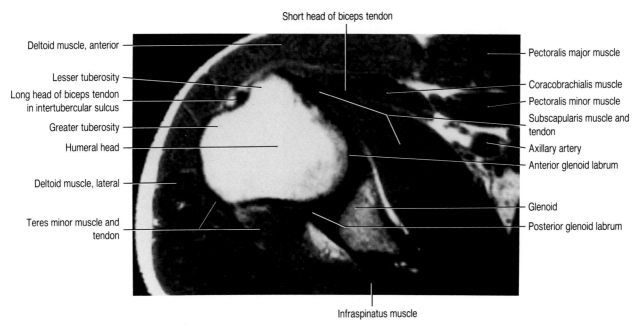

Short head of biceps tendon

Deltoid muscle, anterior —

Lesser tuberosity —

Long head of biceps tendon in intertubercular sulcus

Greater tuberosity —

Humeral head —

Deltoid muscle, lateral —

Teres minor muscle and tendon

— Pectoralis major muscle

— Coracobrachialis muscle

— Pectoralis minor muscle

— Subscapularis muscle and tendon

— Axillary artery

— Anterior glenoid labrum

— Glenoid

— Posterior glenoid labrum

Infraspinatus muscle

FIGURE 6–35R.

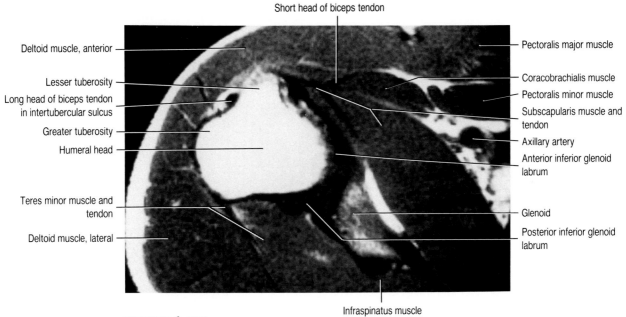

Short head of biceps tendon

Deltoid muscle, anterior —

Lesser tuberosity —

Long head of biceps tendon in intertubercular sulcus

Greater tuberosity —

Humeral head —

Teres minor muscle and tendon

Deltoid muscle, lateral —

— Pectoralis major muscle

— Coracobrachialis muscle

— Pectoralis minor muscle

— Subscapularis muscle and tendon

— Axillary artery

— Anterior inferior glenoid labrum

— Glenoid

— Posterior inferior glenoid labrum

Infraspinatus muscle

FIGURE 6–35S.

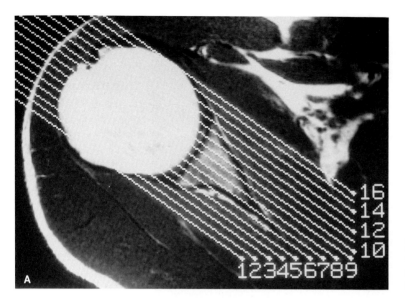

FIGURE 6–36. Normal coronal MR anatomy. (**A**) This axial localizer was used to graphically prescribe 16 coronal oblique T1-weighted image locations from (**B**) anterior to (**Q**) posterior.

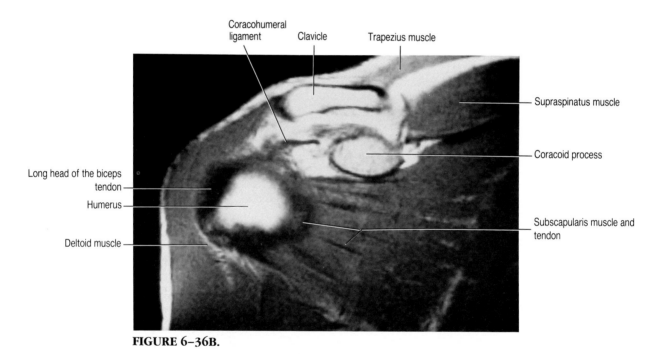

FIGURE 6–36B.

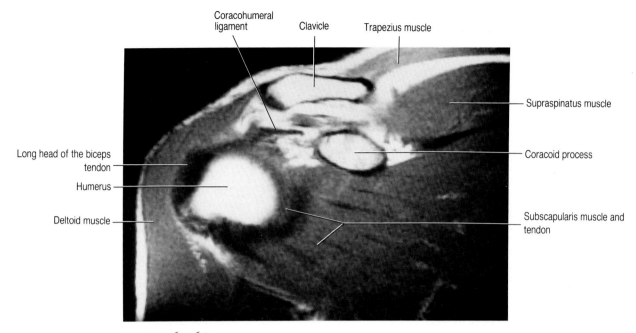

Coracohumeral ligament

Clavicle

Trapezius muscle

Supraspinatus muscle

Long head of the biceps tendon

Coracoid process

Humerus

Deltoid muscle

Subscapularis muscle and tendon

FIGURE 6–36C.

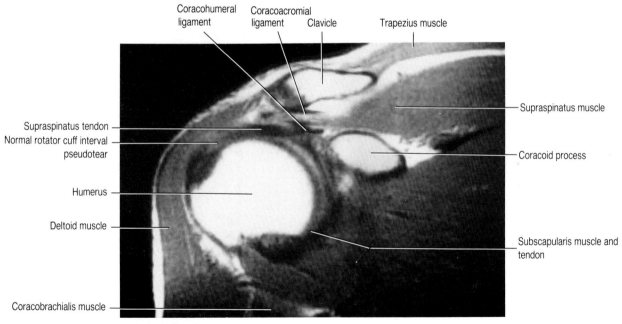

Coracohumeral ligament

Coracoacromial ligament

Clavicle

Trapezius muscle

Supraspinatus muscle

Supraspinatus tendon

Normal rotator cuff interval pseudotear

Coracoid process

Humerus

Deltoid muscle

Subscapularis muscle and tendon

Coracobrachialis muscle

FIGURE 6–36D.

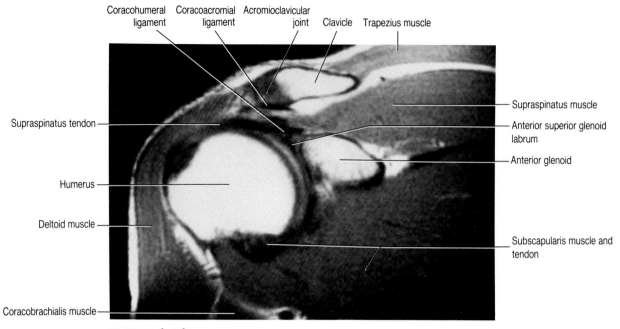

FIGURE 6–36E.

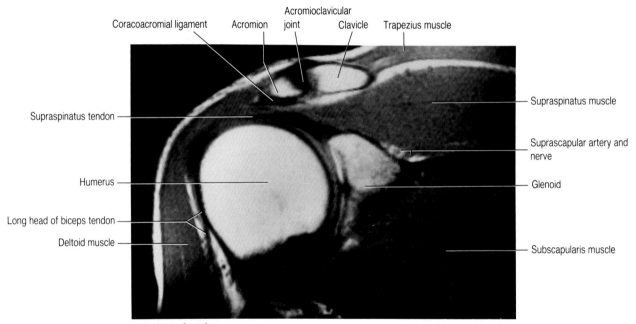

FIGURE 6–36F.

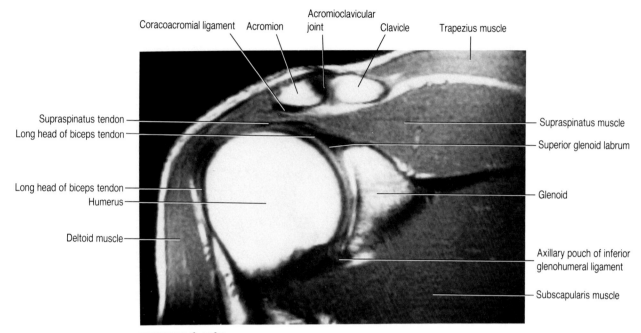

FIGURE 6–36G.

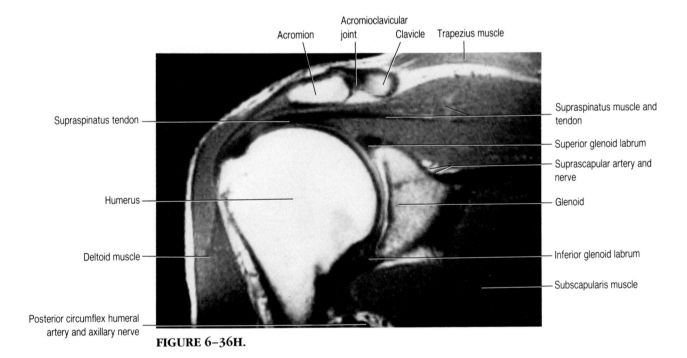

FIGURE 6–36H.

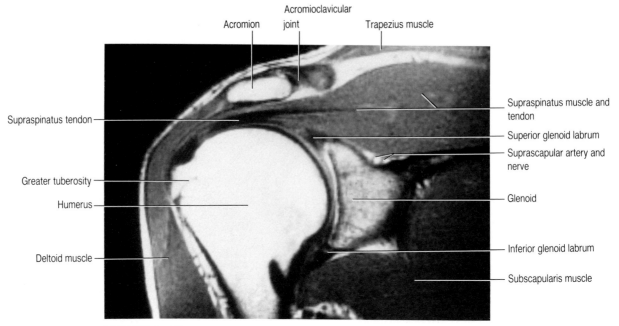

Acromion

Acromioclavicular joint

Trapezius muscle

Supraspinatus tendon

Supraspinatus muscle and tendon

Superior glenoid labrum

Suprascapular artery and nerve

Greater tuberosity

Humerus

Glenoid

Deltoid muscle

Inferior glenoid labrum

Subscapularis muscle

FIGURE 6–36I.

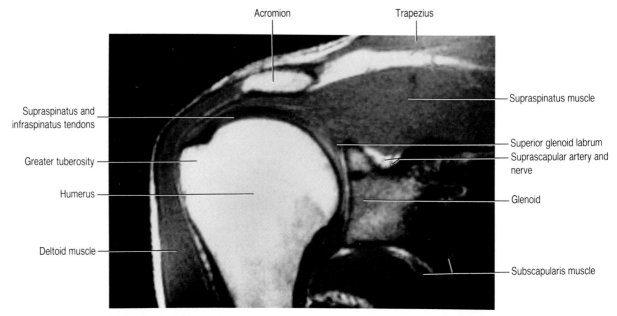

Acromion

Trapezius

Supraspinatus and infraspinatus tendons

Supraspinatus muscle

Superior glenoid labrum

Suprascapular artery and nerve

Greater tuberosity

Humerus

Glenoid

Deltoid muscle

Subscapularis muscle

FIGURE 6–36J.

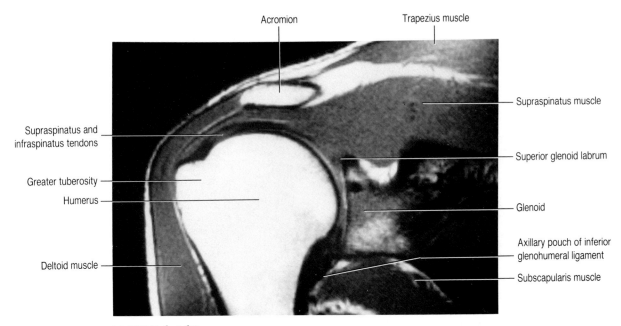

Acromion

Trapezius muscle

Supraspinatus and infraspinatus tendons

Greater tuberosity

Humerus

Deltoid muscle

Supraspinatus muscle

Superior glenoid labrum

Glenoid

Axillary pouch of inferior glenohumeral ligament

Subscapularis muscle

FIGURE 6–36K.

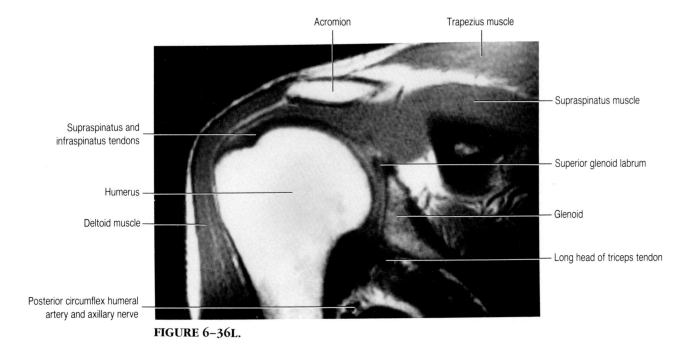

Acromion

Trapezius muscle

Supraspinatus and infraspinatus tendons

Humerus

Deltoid muscle

Posterior circumflex humeral artery and axillary nerve

Supraspinatus muscle

Superior glenoid labrum

Glenoid

Long head of triceps tendon

FIGURE 6–36L.

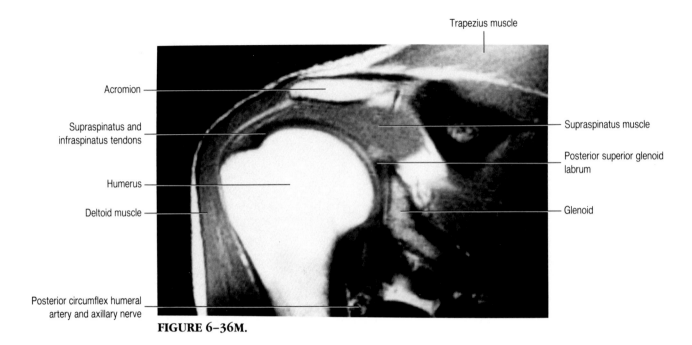

Trapezius muscle

Acromion

Supraspinatus and infraspinatus tendons

Humerus

Deltoid muscle

Posterior circumflex humeral artery and axillary nerve

Supraspinatus muscle

Posterior superior glenoid labrum

Glenoid

FIGURE 6–36M.

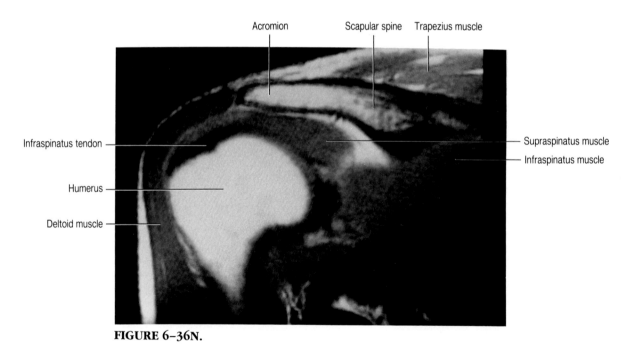

Acromion   Scapular spine   Trapezius muscle

Infraspinatus tendon

Humerus

Deltoid muscle

Supraspinatus muscle

Infraspinatus muscle

FIGURE 6–36N.

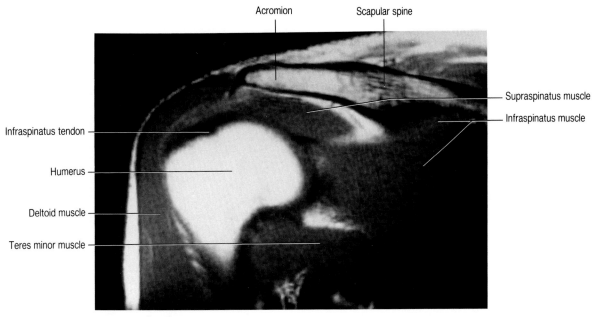

Acromion   Scapular spine

Supraspinatus muscle

Infraspinatus muscle

Infraspinatus tendon

Humerus

Deltoid muscle

Teres minor muscle

FIGURE 6–36O.

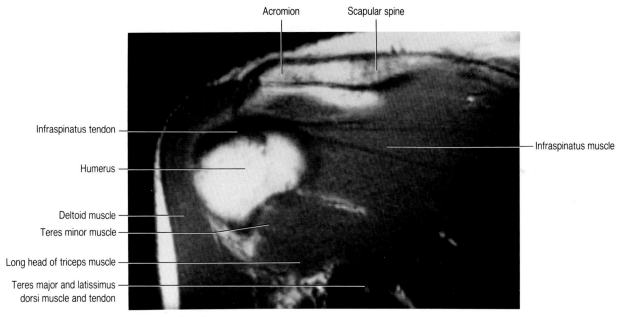

Acromion   Scapular spine

Infraspinatus muscle

Infraspinatus tendon

Humerus

Deltoid muscle

Teres minor muscle

Long head of triceps muscle

Teres major and latissimus dorsi muscle and tendon

FIGURE 6–36P.

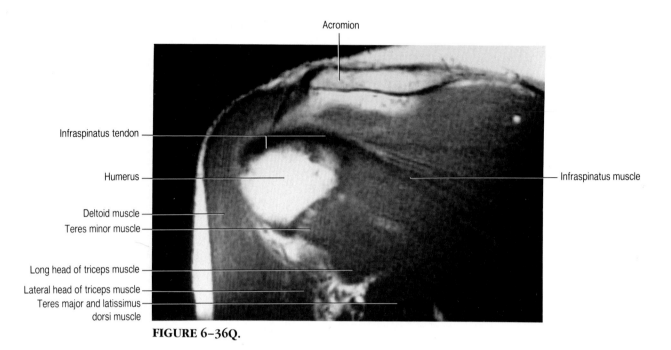

Acromion

Infraspinatus tendon

Humerus

Deltoid muscle

Teres minor muscle

Long head of triceps muscle

Lateral head of triceps muscle

Teres major and latissimus
dorsi muscle

Infraspinatus muscle

FIGURE 6–36Q.

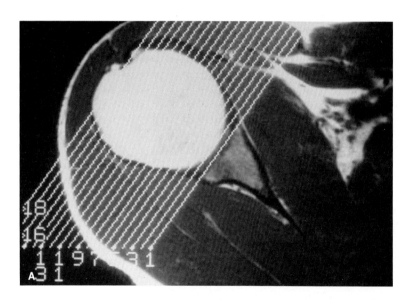

FIGURE 6–37. Normal sagittal MR anatomy. (**A**) This axial localizer was used to graphically prescribe 14 sagittal oblique T1-weighted image locations from (**B**) medial to (**O**) lateral.

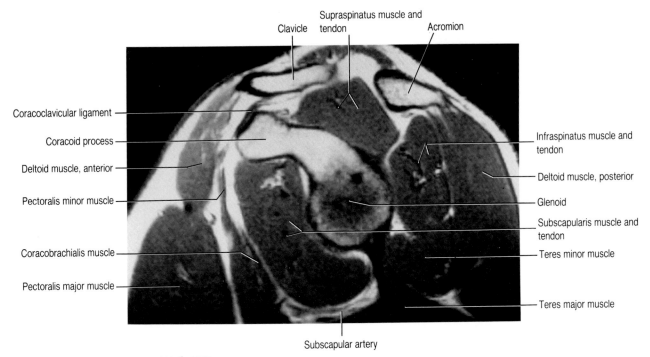

Clavicle

Supraspinatus muscle and tendon

Acromion

Coracoclavicular ligament

Coracoid process

Deltoid muscle, anterior

Pectoralis minor muscle

Coracobrachialis muscle

Pectoralis major muscle

Infraspinatus muscle and tendon

Deltoid muscle, posterior

Glenoid

Subscapularis muscle and tendon

Teres minor muscle

Teres major muscle

Subscapular artery

FIGURE 6–37B.

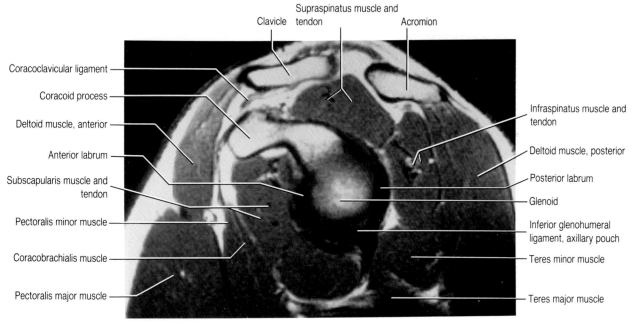

Clavicle

Supraspinatus muscle and tendon

Acromion

Coracoclavicular ligament

Coracoid process

Deltoid muscle, anterior

Anterior labrum

Subscapularis muscle and tendon

Pectoralis minor muscle

Coracobrachialis muscle

Pectoralis major muscle

Infraspinatus muscle and tendon

Deltoid muscle, posterior

Posterior labrum

Glenoid

Inferior glenohumeral ligament, axillary pouch

Teres minor muscle

Teres major muscle

FIGURE 6–37C.

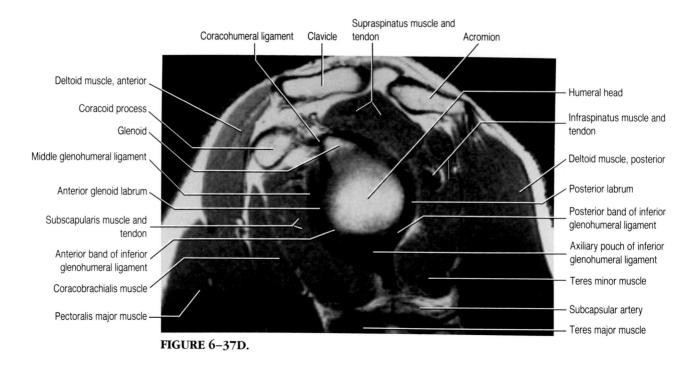

Coracohumeral ligament   Clavicle   Supraspinatus muscle and tendon   Acromion

Deltoid muscle, anterior

Coracoid process

Glenoid

Middle glenohumeral ligament

Anterior glenoid labrum

Subscapularis muscle and tendon

Anterior band of inferior glenohumeral ligament

Coracobrachialis muscle

Pectoralis major muscle

Humeral head

Infraspinatus muscle and tendon

Deltoid muscle, posterior

Posterior labrum

Posterior band of inferior glenohumeral ligament

Axiliary pouch of inferior glenohumeral ligament

Teres minor muscle

Subcapsular artery

Teres major muscle

FIGURE 6–37D.

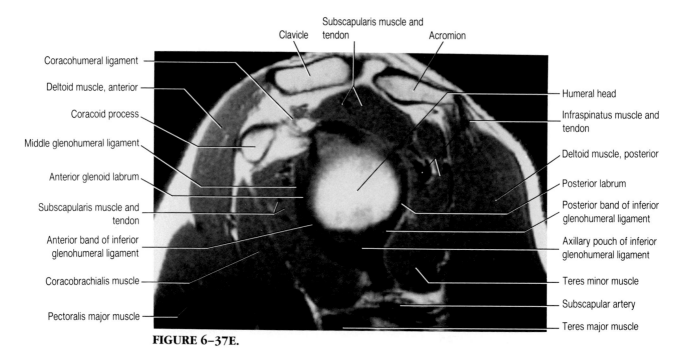

Clavicle   Subscapularis muscle and tendon   Acromion

Coracohumeral ligament

Deltoid muscle, anterior

Coracoid process

Middle glenohumeral ligament

Anterior glenoid labrum

Subscapularis muscle and tendon

Anterior band of inferior glenohumeral ligament

Coracobrachialis muscle

Pectoralis major muscle

Humeral head

Infraspinatus muscle and tendon

Deltoid muscle, posterior

Posterior labrum

Posterior band of inferior glenohumeral ligament

Axillary pouch of inferior glenohumeral ligament

Teres minor muscle

Subscapular artery

Teres major muscle

FIGURE 6–37E.

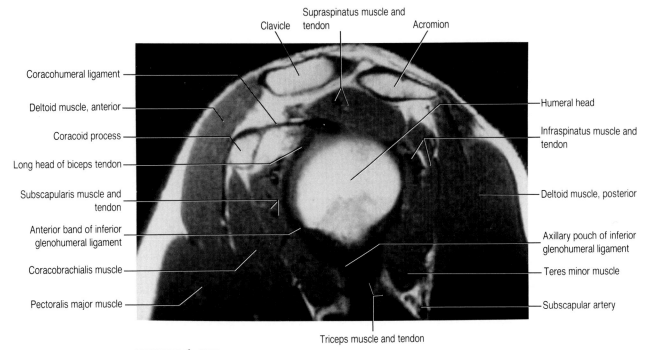

Coracohumeral ligament

Deltoid muscle, anterior

Coracoid process

Long head of biceps tendon

Subscapularis muscle and tendon

Anterior band of inferior glenohumeral ligament

Coracobrachialis muscle

Pectoralis major muscle

Clavicle

Supraspinatus muscle and tendon

Acromion

Humeral head

Infraspinatus muscle and tendon

Deltoid muscle, posterior

Axillary pouch of inferior glenohumeral ligament

Teres minor muscle

Subscapular artery

Triceps muscle and tendon

FIGURE 6–37F.

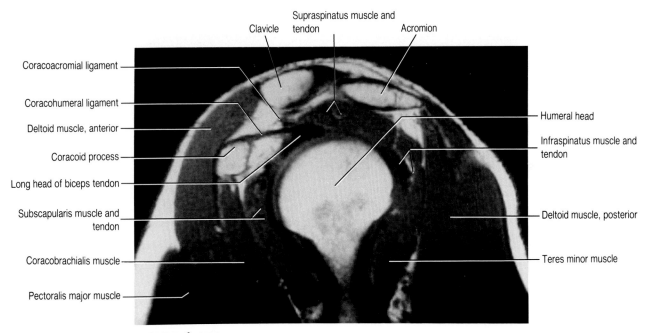

Coracoacromial ligament

Coracohumeral ligament

Deltoid muscle, anterior

Coracoid process

Long head of biceps tendon

Subscapularis muscle and tendon

Coracobrachialis muscle

Pectoralis major muscle

Clavicle

Supraspinatus muscle and tendon

Acromion

Humeral head

Infraspinatus muscle and tendon

Deltoid muscle, posterior

Teres minor muscle

FIGURE 6–37G.

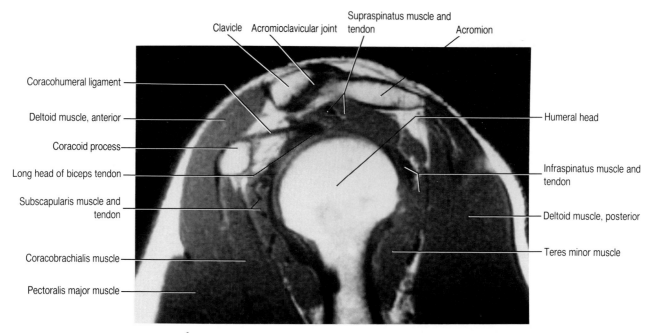

FIGURE 6–37H.

Clavicle Acromioclavicular joint Supraspinatus muscle and tendon Acromion

Coracohumeral ligament

Deltoid muscle, anterior

Coracoid process

Long head of biceps tendon

Subscapularis muscle and tendon

Coracobrachialis muscle

Pectoralis major muscle

Humeral head

Infraspinatus muscle and tendon

Deltoid muscle, posterior

Teres minor muscle

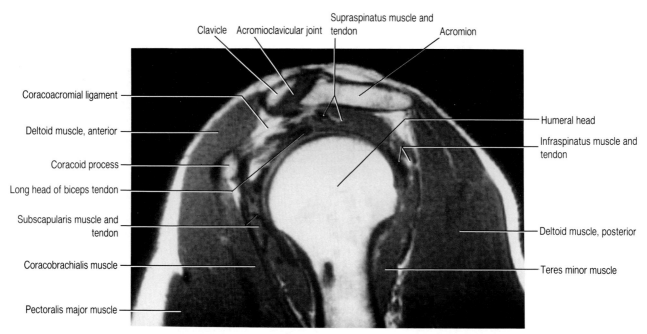

FIGURE 6–37I.

Clavicle Acromioclavicular joint Supraspinatus muscle and tendon Acromion

Coracoacromial ligament

Deltoid muscle, anterior

Coracoid process

Long head of biceps tendon

Subscapularis muscle and tendon

Coracobrachialis muscle

Pectoralis major muscle

Humeral head

Infraspinatus muscle and tendon

Deltoid muscle, posterior

Teres minor muscle

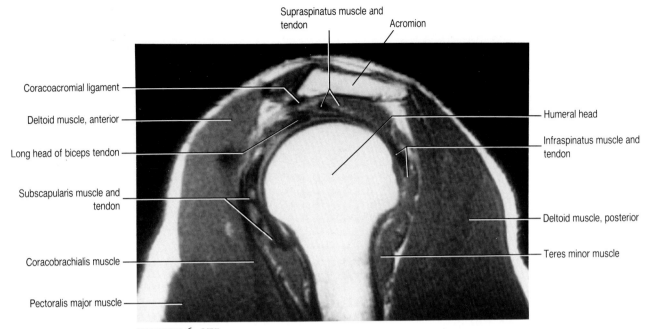

FIGURE 6–37J.

Supraspinatus muscle and tendon

Acromion

Coracoacromial ligament

Deltoid muscle, anterior

Long head of biceps tendon

Subscapularis muscle and tendon

Coracobrachialis muscle

Pectoralis major muscle

Humeral head

Infraspinatus muscle and tendon

Deltoid muscle, posterior

Teres minor muscle

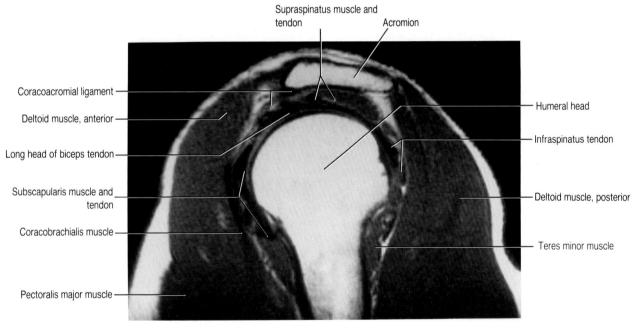

FIGURE 6–37K.

Supraspinatus muscle and tendon

Acromion

Coracoacromial ligament

Deltoid muscle, anterior

Long head of biceps tendon

Subscapularis muscle and tendon

Coracobrachialis muscle

Pectoralis major muscle

Humeral head

Infraspinatus tendon

Deltoid muscle, posterior

Teres minor muscle

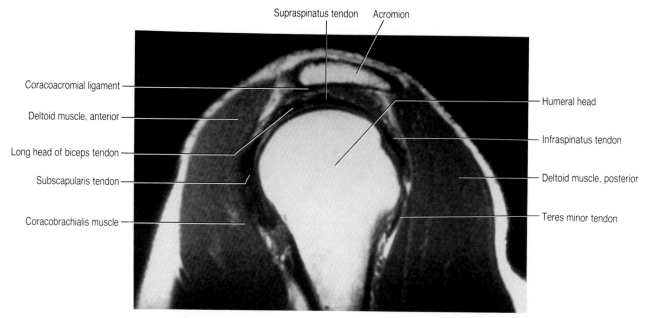

Supraspinatus tendon   Acromion

Coracoacromial ligament

Deltoid muscle, anterior

Long head of biceps tendon

Subscapularis tendon

Coracobrachialis muscle

Humeral head

Infraspinatus tendon

Deltoid muscle, posterior

Teres minor tendon

FIGURE 6–37L.

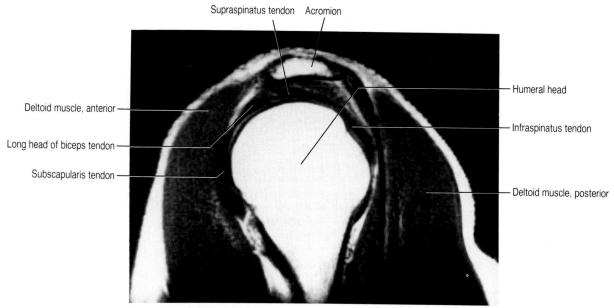

Supraspinatus tendon   Acromion

Deltoid muscle, anterior

Long head of biceps tendon

Subscapularis tendon

Humeral head

Infraspinatus tendon

Deltoid muscle, posterior

FIGURE 6–37M.

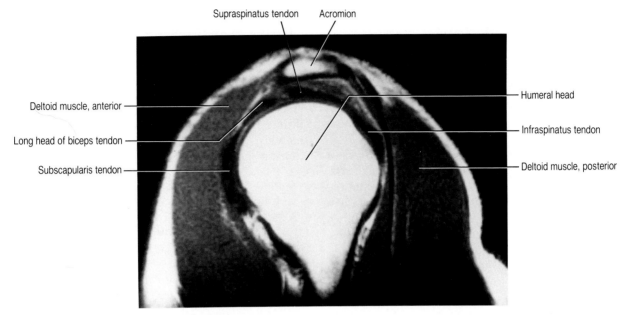

Supraspinatus tendon   Acromion

Deltoid muscle, anterior

Long head of biceps tendon

Subscapularis tendon

Humeral head

Infraspinatus tendon

Deltoid muscle, posterior

FIGURE 6–37N.

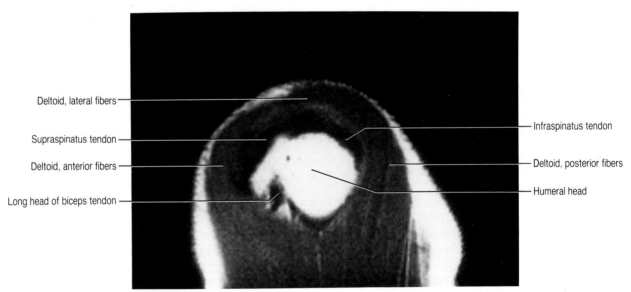

Deltoid, lateral fibers

Supraspinatus tendon

Deltoid, anterior fibers

Long head of biceps tendon

Infraspinatus tendon

Deltoid, posterior fibers

Humeral head

FIGURE 6–37O.

contribute to impingement in the subacromial space (Fig. 6–38).[31]

The pathogenesis of rotator cuff tears includes acute or chronic shoulder impingement or both.[35–39] Some semantic controversy exists as to whether chronic mechanical impingement proceeds development of complete rotator cuff lesions or whether primary degeneration of the cuff results in tears leading to chronic impingement syndrome.[36,39]

There is an important relationship among the rotator cuff, the long head of the biceps, the subacromial bursa, the AC joint, the acromion, and the humeral head in the spectrum of impingement disorders.[32,40] The most common location for impingement is between the anterior one-third of the acromion and the underlying tendons. Impingement here is called the supraspinatus outlet impingement syndrome; it is the most common etiology in rotator cuff lesions. The importance of the lateral edge of the acromion has been minimized, and the posterior portion of the acromion is no longer thought to be implicated in impingement.

Etiology

A variety of etiologies have been proposed in the painful shoulder impingement syndrome, including hypovascularity in the supraspinatus tendon, mechanical wear, sudden macrotrauma, or repetitive microtrauma from overuse—especially from throwing sports or work activities that emphasize overhand motions.[41,42]

Additional etiologies in outlet impingement include anterior acromial spurs, the shape of the acromion (*e.g.,* curved morphology, overhanging edge), the slope of the acromion, and the morphology of the AC joint (*e.g.,* hypertrophic bone, callus formation).[32,43,44] The shape of the acromion, as seen on sagittal oblique MR images or on the outlet view on plain film radiographs, has been classified into three different types by Bigliani (Fig. 6–39).[43] Type 1 acromion is flat; type 2 acromion is more curved in shape. In type 3 impingement, there is anterior hooking of the acromion, which is thought to indicate a greater predisposition to and association with rotator cuff tears (*i.e.,* tears involving the critical zone immediately proximal to the greater tuberosity insertion of the supraspinatus tendon). The slope of the acromion can also be assessed in sagittal oblique images. An association exists between impingement and rotator cuff tears, as well as a decrease or flattening of the acromial angle as measured by a tangent to the acromial surface.[45] Crues uses the terms "negatively sloped acromion" and "positively sloped acromion," to characterize open and flat acromial angles, respectively (Figs. 6–40 and 6–41).[46] An inferior lateral-sloping acromion can be evaluated separately in the coronal oblique plane and is independent of the acromial slope in the sagittal plane discussed above (Figs. 6–42 and 6–43).

Nonoutlet impingement syndrome can be caused by a prominent greater tuberosity, rotator cuff tears, biceps tendon ruptures, and tuberosity fractures. Disruption of the biomechanical function of the glenohumeral joint can be seen in patients with destructive rheumatoid arthritis or ligamentous laxity. Subacromial bursitis with calcific deposits produces a painful impingement syndrome. An unfused (*i.e.,* invisible) acromial epiphysis may also cause impingement and rotator cuff tears requiring surgical excision or epiphysiodesis.[47,48]

Classification

Neer Classification of Impingement. Neer has developed a three-stage classification system for impingement.[39] In Neer's system, subacromial impingement is presented as a mechanical process of progressive wear (*i.e.,* pretear impingement lesion) that causes 90% of rotator cuff tears.[35–37,39] The degeneration, thinning, and full-thickness tearing of the supraspinatus may extend to involve the long head of the biceps and infraspinatus tendons.

In stage 1 of Neer's classification, tendon edema and hemorrhage are present. Stage 2 is characterized by fibrosis and tendinitis. No radiographic findings nor reversible changes are found in stage 1 or stage 2 impingement. In stage 3, a partial or complete rupture or tear of the rotator cuff is found, often in association with anterior acromial spurring or greater tuberosity excrescence. When present, radiographic changes include greater tuberosity sclerosis and hypertrophic bone formation. Bursal thickening and fibrosis and partial tears in the superficial rotator cuff may be present.

Arthroscopic Classification of Impingement. With the advent of diagnostic and therapeutic arthroscopy, it is now possible to classify the different stages of the painful impingement syndrome based on arthroscopic findings in the subacromial bursa as well as on the articular surface of the rotator cuff. Arthroscopy allows identification of all the structures involved in the impingement syndrome and determination of the cause and effect of the pathology in each case. Arthroscopic classification also allows more precise communication among clinicians, which has contributed to the development of a well-defined approach to treatment (see Shoulder Impingement Syndrome; Treatment).

In type 1 impingement, signs of tendon wear or inflammation on the articular or bursal surface are seen, with associated fraying or irregularities of either articular or bursal structures. Type 1 is subdivided into type 1a (*i.e.,* articular) or type 1b (*i.e.,* bursal) findings. Type 1 also includes any signs of wear or inflammation of any of the structures in the bursa (*e.g.,* coracoacromial ligament erosion or fraying).

In type 2 impingement, tendon wear or inflammatory signs are seen, plus partial thickness tears of the articular surface in type 2a or the bursal surface in type 2b.

Type 3 impingement is characterized by a full-thickness tear of the cuff. Without retraction of the cuff, the tear is classified as type 3a; with retraction of the cuff, it is type 3b.

Magnetic Resonance Appearance

The spectrum of MR changes in shoulder impingement has also been characterized and documented.[15,35,49,50] Seeger has classified impingement into several types based on coronal plane MR images.[35] In Seeger's classification, type 1 impingement is characterized by the presence of subacromial bursitis, which is shown as a thickening of the normal high signal intensity across the subacromial–subdeltoid line. On T1-weighted images, this thickening may be of intermediate signal intensity relative to fat associated with the synovial lining. In our experience, however, the effacement of the subdeltoid–subacromial fat line is a poor indicator of impingement and has been overused. Signal intensity in the supraspinatus muscle and tendon remains unchanged. On gradient-echo images, areas of increased internal signal intensity with normal morphology of the supraspinatus tendon have been demonstrated in type 1 impingement.

In type 2 impingement, the supraspinatus tendon demonstrates high signal intensity on conventional T1-weighted images. Increased or high signal intensity of the tendon on T2-weighted images indicates a type 2b change and may represent a partial tear.

Type 3 impingement is characterized by a complete tear of the rotator cuff, with or without supraspinatus retraction. Proximal retraction of the muscle tendon junction is an indication of a significant tear, but is not specific for irreparable tears. Complete tears exist only in type 3 impingement; therefore, high signal intensity of the supraspinatus tendon on conventional T2-weighted images is considered pathognomonic for a cuff tear in this classification.

Magnetic Resonance Correlation With Arthroscopic Findings. We prefer to correlate MR changes with the three types of impingement identified by arthroscopic surgical findings (Fig. 6–44). In this classification, inflammation or degenerative tendon wear in type 1 impingement displays increased signal intensity on T1- and T2*-weighted images, with relative preservation of articular and bursal tendon surface outlines (Fig. 6–45).

Zlatkin's grading system for characterization of the rotator cuff tendons, which consists of grades 0 to 3, differentiates between tendinitis with normal morphology (grade 1) and tendinitis or tendon degeneration with abnormal morphology (grade 2).[17] Associated tendinous enlargement, which may be seen in the more acute stages

of impingement, is still considered normal morphology because normal tendon outlines are preserved. In both grade 1 and grade 2 tendons, increased signal intensity on T1-weighted and intermediate-weighted images are found. A grade 3 tendon demonstrates a tendinous defect and displays increased signal intensity on T2-weighted images. Zlatkin specifically uses the term "degeneration" to designate surface morphologic changes (*i.e.,* thinning, irregularity, or both) of the tendon, separate from histologic findings of degeneration. In this classification, a grade 2 tendon with abnormal morphology by definition may represent tendinitis with tendon degeneration or a rotator cuff tear. The association of small amounts of fluid in the subacromial bursa or loss of the subacromial–subdeltoid fat plane on T1-weighted images, however, are not reliable secondary signs for making a distinction between tendinitis or degeneration and a tear. In stage 1 impingement, increased signal intensity in the distal supraspinatus tendon may be seen on intermediate-weighted images.

No increase in signal intensity of the tendon is seen in conventional T2-weighted or long TR/TE images in type 1 impingement. The increased sensitivity of T2*-weighted images in detecting increases in tendon signal intensity may be secondary to increased proton density or prolonged T1 and T2 values. Careful evaluation of any associated change or alteration in bursal and articular surface tendon outlines should be evaluated to identify the possible development of a partial tear. The continuum between severe inflammation or degeneration and partial tear may be difficult to distinguish without identifying a focal discontinuity or defect with tracking of fluid across a tendinous surface. A histologic biopsy specimen showing inflammation and mucoid degeneration is thought to correlate with the increased signal intensity on short TR/TE images and intermediate images.[49] Rafii and colleagues have proposed that areas of increased signal intensity in the supraspinatus tendon on intermediate-weighted images may, in fact, represent degeneration (*e.g.,* eosinophilic, fibrillar, mucoid) and scarring rather than active inflammation.[51,52] This supports our observation of increased signal intensity in the supraspinatus tendon in some asymptomatic patients on short TR/TE images, intermediate-weighted images, and T2*-weighted images.

Thus, the common use of the term tendinitis, which implies active inflammation, may be imprecise in characterizing tendon signal intensity alterations without surgical confirmation. Kjellin and colleagues have suggested the designation of tendinosis or tendinopathy in such cases.[52] Additionally, in arthroscopic evaluation of impingement, we have observed that tendon wear (*i.e.,* degeneration) is a more common finding than active inflammation. Rafii has suggested that tendinous enlargement associated with an inhomogeneous signal pat-

(text continues on page 568)

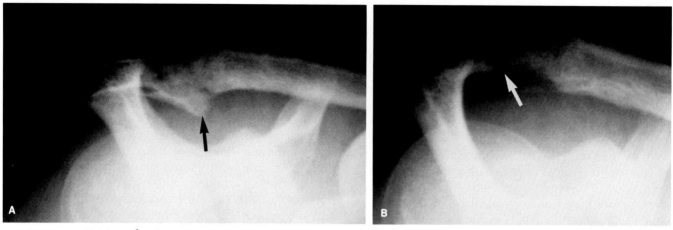

FIGURE 6-38. The outlet view (*i.e.,* lateral view of the scapula) shows the anterior acromial spur encroaching upon the supraspinatus outlet (**A**) prior to (*black arrow*) and (**B**) after (*white arrow*) acromioplasty.

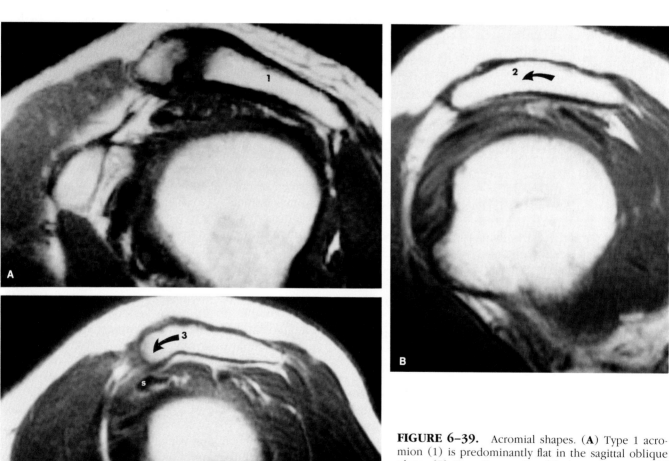

FIGURE 6-39. Acromial shapes. (**A**) Type 1 acromion (1) is predominantly flat in the sagittal oblique plane. (**B**) Type 2 acromion (2) demonstrates a mild symmetric curve or arc relative to the humeral head (*arrow*). (**C**) Type 3 acromion (3) with anterior hook morphology narrows the acromiohumeral distance (*arrow*). (s, supraspinatus tendon.) Type 3 acromion is thought to be associated with critical zone tears of the rotator cuff immediately proximal to the greater tuberosity insertion of the supraspinatus tendon.

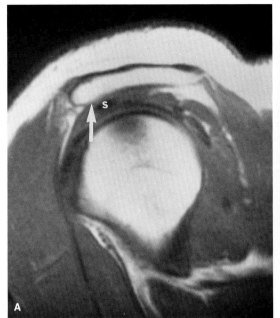

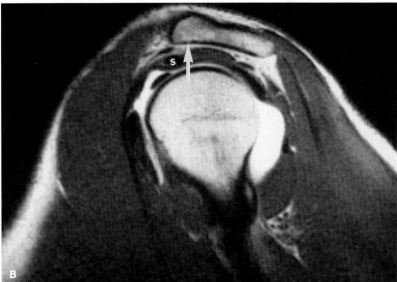

FIGURE 6–40. Acromial slope. (**A**) A T1-weighted sagittal oblique image demonstrates the positively sloped acromion (*arrow*) with the anterior inferior cortex projecting inferior to the posterior aspect of the acromion. The relative encroachment on the supraspinatus outlet may lead to impingement. The low signal intensity humeral area represents early avascular necrosis. (S, supraspinatus tendon.) (**B**) An enhanced T1-weighted sagittal oblique image shows a mildly negatively sloped acromion (*arrow*) with the anterior inferior cortex projecting superior to the posterior aspect of the acromion. (S, supraspinatus tendon.)

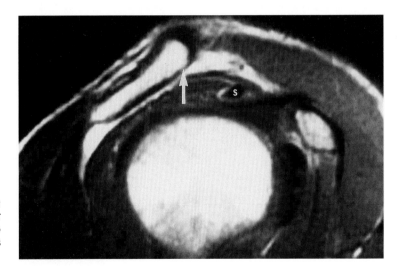

FIGURE 6–41. A T1-weighted sagittal oblique image shows a negatively sloped acromion with anterior inferior cortex (*arrow*) superiorly or cranially oriented relative to the posterior aspect of the acromion. (S, supraspinatus tendon.)

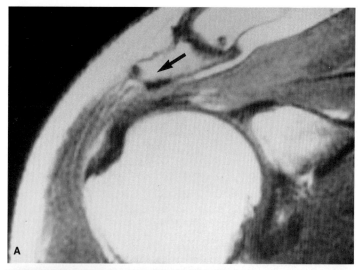

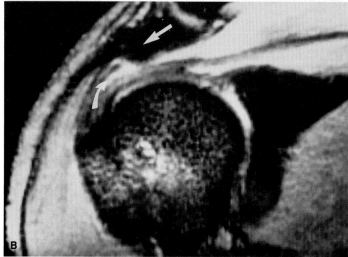

FIGURE 6–42. An inferior, lateral-sloping acromion (*straight arrow*) with bursal surface inflammation (*curved arrow*) of the supraspinatus tendon (*i.e.,* type 1 impingement) is seen on (**A**) T1-weighted and (**B**) T2*-weighted coronal oblique images.

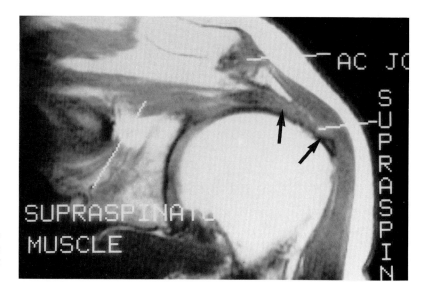

FIGURE 6–43. A T1-weighted coronal oblique image shows discontinuity of supraspinatus tendon in complete rotator cuff tear (*arrows*). Note the inferior lateral-sloping acromion.

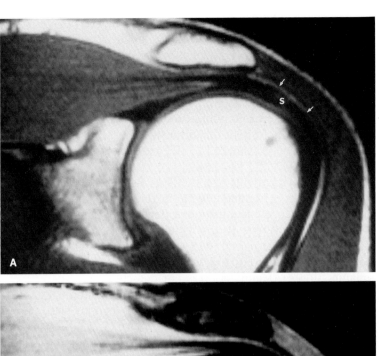

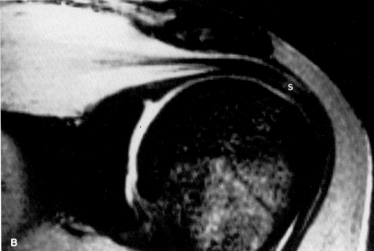

FIGURE 6-44. Normal supraspinatus tendon (S) morphology demonstrates low signal intensity contrast on (**A**) coronal oblique T1-weighted and (**B**) T2*-weighted images. The subacromial–subdeltoid fat plane is also shown (*arrow*). The subacromial space is not narrowed.

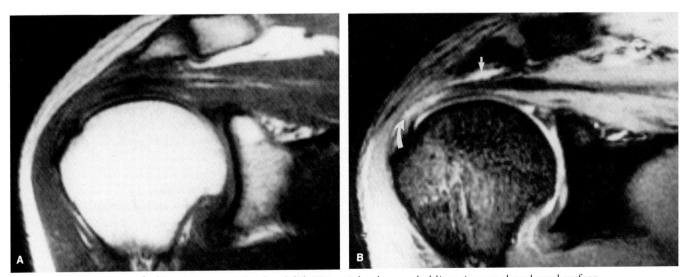

FIGURE 6-45. (**A**) T1-weighted and (**B**) T2*-weighted coronal oblique images show bursal surface inflammation (*curved arrow*) of the supraspinatus tendon without tear at arthroscopy (*i.e.,* type 1b impingement). There is a small amount of subacromial–subdeltoid bursal fluid (*straight arrow*) in the absence of a rotator cuff tear.

tern and bursitis, however, implies active tendinitis.[51] Although the subacromial peribursal fat plane is usually preserved on T1-weighted images in the early stages of impingement, it may be effaced by bursal surface inflammation in the absence of a rotator cuff tear.[53] The injection of a long-acting steroid and local anesthetic may produce an area of increased signal intensity on T2-weighted sequences with long repetition and echo times; this technique should be considered to decrease false-positive interpretations.[49]

In addition to articular (type 1a; Fig. 6–46) and bursal (type 1b; Fig. 6–47) inflammation or tendon degeneration, intrasubstance inflammation or degeneration, which we will refer to as type 1c and which may be associated with intrasubstance partial tears (Figs. 6–48 through 6–50), can be identified on MR scans. Such intrasubstance inflammation or degeneration is not detected and thus cannot be confirmed on arthroscopic surface evaluations. Conventional and gadolinium-enhanced MR imaging are negative in type 1 impingement.

Type 2 impingement lesions, with signs of inflammation or degeneration and associated partial thickness tears, are also characterized on MR as partial articular (*i.e.*, type 2a) or bursal surface (*i.e.*, type 2b) tears (Figs. 6–51 and 6–52). In the presence of a surface tear, it may be difficult and redundant to classify associated intrasubstance changes, whether secondary to inflammation, degeneration, or intrasubstance tearing. Cadaveric histopathologic studies have shown that partial tears may originate from regions of tendon degeneration without associated inflammation.[52] Coronal oblique MR images show increased signal intensity in the distal supraspinatus tendon on T1-, intermediate-, T2-, and T2*-weighted images, although the signal intensity may be variable in the intermediate-weighted image. Increased signal intensity fluid within the bursal or articular surface of the cuff is characteristic of this lesion. Small amounts of fluid may be seen in the subacromial bursa, especially in bursal surface type 2b lesions, in the absence of a full-thickness or complete tear. In addition to a partial-thickness tear, associated tendon thinning and fraying in type 2 impingement may be present. Well-defined, linear, high signal intensity on T2*-weighted images, or an area of increased signal intensity on long TR/TE images that does not extend to either the articular or the bursal surface, may represent intrasubstance partial tears. Morphologic tendon changes, such as surface irregularities or thinning, help to support this diagnosis.

In type 3 impingement, MR imaging depicts a complete tear of the rotator cuff without (*i.e.*, type 3a) or with (*i.e.*, type 3b) proximal tendon retraction (Figs. 6–53 and 6–54). Without demonstration of a defined defect, retraction of the muscle belly, or extension of fluid across the supraspinatus tendon into the subdeltoid–subacromial bursa, a complete tear cannot be unequiv-

ocally diagnosed. Increased signal intensity within the tendon on T2*-weighted images in the presence of normal tendon morphology is not diagnostic of a rotator cuff tear. Therefore, the presence of small amounts of fluid within the subacromial–subdeltoid bursa should not be used as a primary sign of a rotator cuff tear unless it is associated with a direct communication of fluid from the glenohumeral joint into the subacromial–subdeltoid bursa.

Osseous Changes

Spurs of the inferior margins of the acromion and AC joint, hypertrophy of the AC joint, and downward sloping or inferior displacement of the acromion relative to the distal clavicle all have been identified on MR images.

Acromial spurs containing marrow fat demonstrate high signal intensity on T1-weighted images. Spurs may blend with adjacent acromial cortex on T2*-weighted images, obscuring their identification. Spurs of cortical bone composition demonstrate dark signal intensity on T1-, T2-, and T2*-weighted images. Anterior traction spurs are frequently best demonstrated on T1-weighted sagittal images (Fig. 6–55). Larger acromial spurs usually contain significant amounts of fatty marrow and are bright on T1-weighted images. It is important not to misinterpret the normal inferior acromial attachment of the coracoacromial ligament as an acromial spur (see Fig. 6–32).

Degenerative cysts and sclerosis of the greater tuberosity can be visualized on coronal, axial, or sagittal images. Squaring and sclerosis of the greater tuberosity are best seen on coronal images (Fig. 6–56). Acromioclavicular hypertrophy with inferior surface osteophytes is best displayed on either anterior coronal images or sagittal images at the level of the coracohumeral and coracoacromial ligaments. Glenohumeral joint degeneration in rotator cuff tear represents the end stage in the spectrum of impingement.[41,54]

Treatment

Treatment for the different types of impingement depends on the age and activity level of the patient.[32,41] In general, most patients are treated with various conservative modalities for a period of 6 months prior to surgical intervention.

Conservative Treatment. In the acute phase, analgesics, nonsteroidal antiinflammatory drugs (NSAIDs), and steroid injection are the most effective forms of treatment. In less acute situations, conservative therapies also include physical therapy modalities and, in particular, strengthening of the rotator cuff musculature with abduction and external rotation exercises. Internal rotation exercises for the subscapularis are also recommended. Subacromial bursal injections of various steroidal antiinflammatory agents are very effective, but the effect is often ephemeral and steroids may be associated with painful postinjection flares that can be rather dramatic. These flares can last for as long as 48 hours and can produce significant distress. Repeated injections of steroids in and about the rotator cuff tendons may have a destructive effect; a general rule is that not more than two or three injections should be used in this area during a 12-month period. Oral NSAIDs may prove to be effective when combined with a reduced activity level. Regardless of the specific treatment, more than 6 months of pain or dramatically decreased activity levels are often unacceptable to the patient; therefore, if pain reduction through conservative measures is not achieved, an arthroscopic approach is warranted.

Acromioplasty. Arthroscopic subacromial decompression (ASD) is now the method of choice for the treatment of chronic outlet impingement. It is rapidly replacing open acromioplasty,[32,41] because arthroscopic acromioplasty does not violate any deltoid insertions on the acromion. Arthroscopic anterior acromioplasty, as part of ASD, is indicated for alleviation of pain secondary to the impingement of the anterior inferior surface of the acromion. In ASD, the coracoacromial ligament is detached from the anterior inferior acromial surface, and any inflamed or frayed cuff tissue is debrided. A burr is used to perform an anterior acromioplasty.

Patients with type 1 impingement, with inflammation of the tendon and evidence of articular or bursal surface irregularities, are treated by ASD only. Arthroscopic findings usually include not only fraying of the articular bursal surfaces but evidence of fraying of the coracoacromial ligament that attaches to the anterior and lateral borders of the anterior inferior surface of the acromion. Kissing lesions are irregularities of the bursal surfaces of the cuff found opposite irregularities or fraying of the coracoacromial ligament. Subacromial decompression has produced good to excellent results in 85% of patients after 2-year follow-up studies.

Patients with type 2 lesions, whether partial thickness tears of the articular surface (*i.e.,* type 2a) or the bursal surface (*i.e.,* type 2b), are also treated with subacromial decompression and debridement of the partial thickness tear. Results of treatment in type 2 lesions depend on the extent of the cuff tear: the deeper and more extensive the cleavage planes and the larger the flap of cuff produced by the tear, the greater the likelihood that a simple subacromial decompression will be insufficient and either an arthroscopic or open repair of the more significantly damaged partially torn cuff will be necessary. Nonetheless, a good number of type 2 patients respond positively to subacromial decompression alone, and because of its minimal morbidity, this procedure can be tried prior to open procedures.

Type 3 full-thickness lesions of the cuff, whether type 3a (*i.e.,* without retraction) or type 3b (*i.e.,* with

retraction), present more difficult treatment dilemmas. In general, patients with full-thickness tears of the cuff require an open procedure, although arthroscopic-assisted rotator cuff repairs are possible. In the latter, a deltoid-splitting approach, without detachment of the deltoid from the acromial edge, is used to close the tear following ASD. In patients with type 3b tears (*i.e.,* considerable retraction of the rotator cuff), standard open repairs are necessary.

The information provided by MR is helpful in preoperative planning. If the MR scan shows a small tear with minimal retraction, a less invasive, arthroscopically assisted approach can be used. If the MR scan shows significant retraction of the tendon end to the level of the superior pole of the glenoid, a more extensive approach is necessary.

In patients with severe tendon retraction and MR evidence of muscle fiber changes (*e.g.,* fibrosis, atrophy), the prognosis for cuff repair is less optimistic, and the possibility that the cuff is irreparable exists.

For patients with evidence of rotator cuff arthropathy, the likelihood of a successful repair is remote. These patients are often older, and their main complaint is pain; therefore, ASD alone produces satisfactory results (*i.e.,* pain relief) in approximately 50% of cases.

Associated Arthroscopic Procedures. During subacromial decompression, the entire glenohumeral joint is evaluated, and associated lesions, such as superior labral anterior-to-posterior (SLAP) lesions, are often noted and repair procedures undertaken. Resection of the coracoacromial ligament is performed in addition to the acromioplasty.

Patients with significant degenerative changes in the AC joint need additional preoperative diagnostic tests, particularly local injections of xylocaine, to distinguish between pain emanating from a degenerative AC joint and impingement pain produced by spurs. If joint pain is associated with impingement pain, it is necessary to perform an arthroscopic Mumford procedure (*i.e.,* resection of the distal 2 cm of the clavicle) at the same time as the ASD. If a degenerative prominence of the AC joint is producing extrinsic compression on the muscle belly of the supraspinatus, it also can be removed at the same time as the acromioplasty.

The biceps tendon, a component of the rotator cuff, must also be arthroscopically evaluated intraoperatively. The tendon is pulled into the joint so that the part of the tendon that lies within the bicipital groove can be assessed. If it is significantly frayed or attenuated, the tendon is resected from its insertion at the supraglenoid tubercle, a deltoid-splitting incision is made, and a tenodesis is performed in the bicipital groove (Fig. 6–57).

(text continues on page 576)

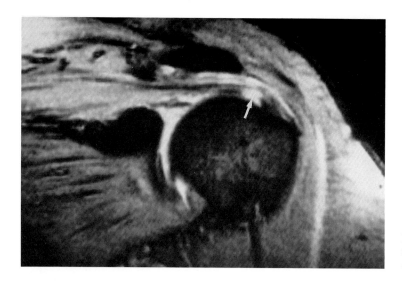

FIGURE 6–46. Articular surface hyperintensity indicative of type 1a impingement is seen on a T2*-weighted coronal oblique image (*arrow*).

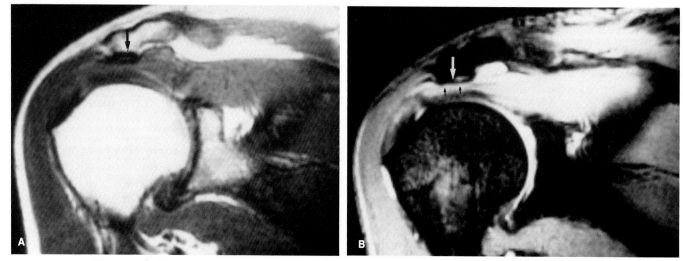

FIGURE 6–47. An anterior acromial spur (*large arrows*) in the coronal plane is seen on (**A**) T1-weighted and (**B**) T2*-weighted images. Bursal surface hyperintensity indicative of type 1b impingement is demonstrated on the T2*-weighted image (*small arrows*).

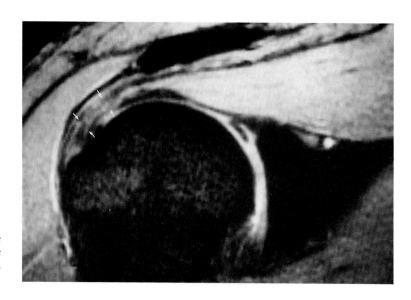

FIGURE 6–48. A T2*-weighted coronal oblique image shows intrasubstance inflammation–degeneration of the supraspinatus with normal bursal and articular tendon surface morphology (*arrows*).

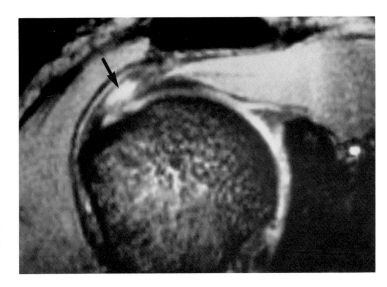

FIGURE 6–49. A high signal intensity intrasubstance tear *versus* supraspinatus tendon inflammation–degeneration is seen on a T2*-weighted coronal image. Relative preservation of the bursal and articular surface morphology is apparent.

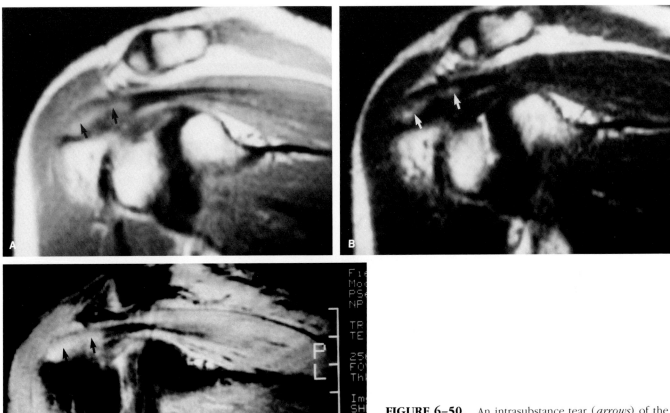

FIGURE 6–50. An intrasubstance tear (*arrows*) of the supraspinatus tendon demonstrates increased signal intensity on coronal oblique (**A**) intermediate-weighted and (**B**) T2-weighted images. There is relative preservation of the bursal and articular surface morphology, and no tendon discontinuity is present. (**C**) On the corresponding T2*-weighted coronal oblique image, the distal supraspinatus tendon (*arrow*) displays a greater degree of hyperintensity.

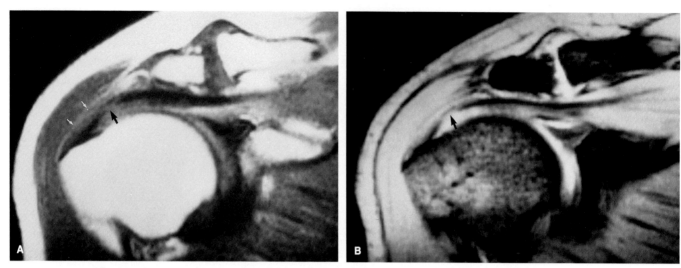

FIGURE 6–51. Type 2a impingement. Articular surface inflammation and a partial tear (*black arrows*) with high signal intensity attenuation of the inferior surface of the supraspinatus tendon are seen on (**A**) T1-weighted and (**B**) T2*-weighted images. The subacromial–subdeltoid fat line may be intact in the presence of a partial articular surface tear without bursal inflammation (*small white arrows*). Associated acromioclavicular joint arthrosis is present.

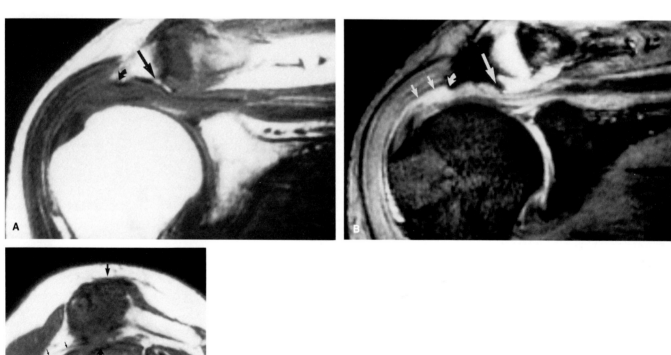

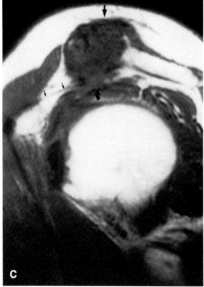

FIGURE 6–52. Type 2b impingement. (**A**) T1-weighted and (**B**) T2*-weighted coronal oblique images demonstrate an anterior inferior acromial spur (*curved arrows*) and an acromioclavicular joint osteophyte (*large straight arrows*). Subacromial-space narrowing with abnormal surface morphology in high signal intensity supraspinatus bursal surface tear (*small straight arrows*) is present. The hypertrophic acromioclavicular joint effaces the musculotendinous junction. (**C**) The corresponding T1-weighted sagittal oblique image shows a hypertrophic acromioclavicular joint (*large straight arrow*), coracoacromial ligament (*small straight arrow*), and supraspinatus tendon (*curved arrow*). The acromioclavicular joint prominence encroaches on the supraspinatus outlet.

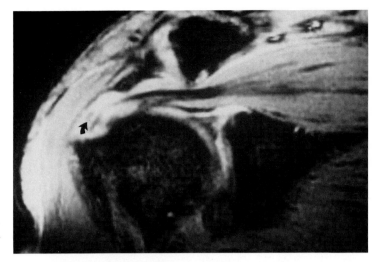

FIGURE 6-53. A rotator cuff tear (*i.e.,* type 3a impingement) with subacromial–subdeltoid bursal fluid (*arrow*) is seen on a T2*-weighted coronal oblique image.

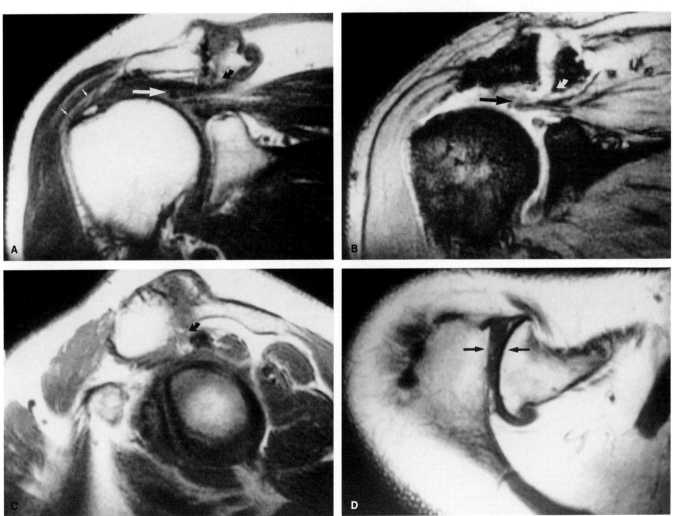

FIGURE 6-54. (**A**) T1-weighted coronal oblique, (**B**) T2*-weighted coronal oblique, and (**C**) T1-weighted sagittal oblique images demonstrate acromioclavicular joint arthrosis with hypertrophy and osteophytes (*curved arrows*) projecting from the inferior surfaces of the distal clavicle and acromion and effacing the supraspinatus musculotendinous junction. Mild cortical irregularity is present and involves the inferior surface of the anterior one-third of the acromion. Narrowing of the supraspinatus outlet is associated with a complete rotator cuff tear (*i.e.,* type 3b impingement) with proximal retraction of the supraspinatus tendon (*large straight arrows*). Note the nonspecificity of the subdeltoid fat plane (*small arrows*). (**D**) A T1-weighted superior axial image demonstrates degenerative changes at the acromioclavicular joint (*arrows*).

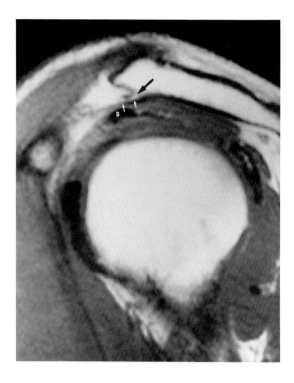

FIGURE 6–55. An anterior acromial spur (*black arrow*) effaces the proximal coracoacromial ligament (*white arrows*). Fat marrow signal intensity is shown in the acromial spur. (s, supraspinatus tendon.)

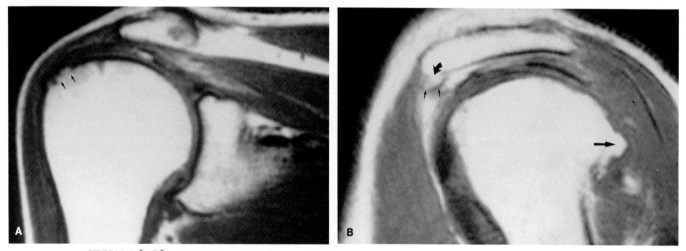

FIGURE 6–56. (**A**) A T1-weighted coronal oblique image shows early osseous evidence of impingement with osteophytic squaring of the greater tuberosity at the insertion site of the supraspinatus tendon (*arrows*). (**B**) A T1-weighted sagittal oblique image shows later changes of bony impingement with an anterior acromial spur (*curved arrow*) and humeral osteophyte (*large straight arrow*). The low signal intensity cortex of the acromial osteophyte is indicated (*small straight arrows*). The anterior acromiohumeral distance is narrowed.

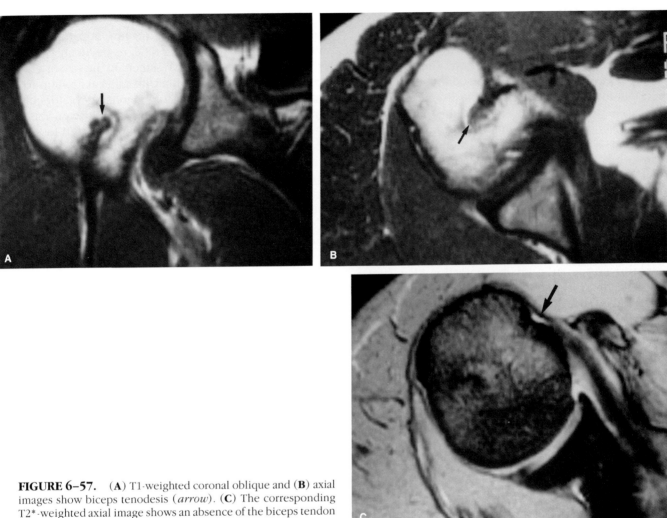

FIGURE 6–57. (**A**) T1-weighted coronal oblique and (**B**) axial images show biceps tenodesis (*arrow*). (**C**) The corresponding T2*-weighted axial image shows an absence of the biceps tendon in the bicipital groove (*arrow*).

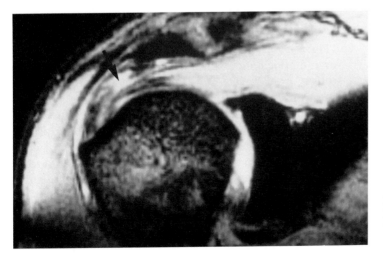

FIGURE 6–58. A partial bursal surface tear demonstrates high signal intensity on a T2*-weighted coronal oblique image. There is irregular bursal surface morphology at the tear site (*arrow*). The articular surface demonstrates continuity.

Rotator Cuff Tears

No two rotator cuff tears are alike, making their evaluation and treatment protocols complicated. The tears can be characterized as either partial or complete.[36,37] Partial tears may involve the articular or bursal surfaces in varying degrees of depth and extension into the tendon (Fig. 6–58). Intratendinous lesions may not communicate with either bursal or articular surfaces. Complete rotator cuff tears, which extend through the entire thickness of the rotator cuff, allow direct communication between the subacromial bursa and the glenohumeral joint (Fig. 6–59). A massive rotator cuff tear usually involves more than one of the rotator cuff tendons (see Fig. 6–59). Magnetic resonance images, particularly in the coronal plane, has demonstrated potential in identifying partial rotator cuff tears that escape arthrographic detection (Fig. 6–60).[55] Traumatic tears from a single episode are found in both middle-aged and older patients. In patients younger than 40 years of age, rotator cuff tears are frequently associated with acute dislocations.[32]

Magnetic Resonance Appearance

Preoperative MR studies provide important information about the size of the cuff tear, the degree of proximal or medial retraction, and the quality of the free tendon edges (Figs. 6–61 and 6–62). On T2-weighted images, most tears demonstrate increased signal intensity; partial tears usually exhibit signal characteristics similar to those described for full-thickness or complete tears (Fig. 6–63). Complete absence of the rotator cuff indicates a major tendinous disruption and is typical of rotator cuff arthropathy in which the humeral head articulates directly with the undersurface of the acromion (Fig. 6–64). Involvement of the infraspinatus or subscapularis tendons may be shown in massive rotator cuff tears (Fig. 6–65). Preoperative MR can also identify associated muscle atrophy in acute tears (Fig. 6–66). Patients with complete tears complicated by cuff arthropathy, tendon retraction, and muscle atrophy may not be candidates for primary surgical repair (Fig. 6–67).[56]

Conventional T2-weighted images with long TR/TE valves may be suboptimal in demonstrating areas of bright signal intensity in granulation tissue or hypertrophied synovium, both of which have low to intermediate signal on T1-weighted images. T2*-weighted sequences may be preferable, generating higher signal intensities in both partial and complete subacute and chronic rotator cuff tears, particularly in the absence of an associated glenohumeral joint effusion. Conventional T2-weighted images, however, frequently display superior detail of tear morphology (Fig. 6–68). Intraarticular administration of gadolinium is necessary to identify fluid superolateral to the greater tuberosity, expected in complete rotator cuff tears (Fig. 6–69).

According to reports by Zlatkin and colleagues, MR sensitivity and specificity for imaging of partial and full-thickness tears are 91% and 88%, respectively, with 89% accuracy.[17] Preoperative assessment of the size of a rotator cuff tear compared favorably with surgical findings in 95% of cases. The criteria used for diagnosing rotator cuff tear included increased tendon signal intensity with abnormal morphology or discontinuity with associated loss of the peribursal fat plane on T1-weighted images or fluid in the subacromial–subdeltoid bursa on T2-weighted images. In another study of arthroscopic or surgical correlation in complete cuff tears in 91 patients, MR had a sensitivity of 100% and a specificity of 95%.[57] Burk and colleagues reported a comparable sensitivity (92%) for both MR and arthrography in the diagnosis of rotator cuff tears.[16]

Secondary signs in rotator cuff tears, including supraspinatus muscle atrophy with bright signal intensity fatty streaks on T1-weighted images, are less conspicuous on T2*-weighted images.[50] Loss of the peribursal fat plane on T1-weighted images, fluid in the subacromial–subdeltoid bursa on T2- or T2*-weighted images, and proximal musculotendinous retraction are additional secondary signs of cuff tear, present in up to 92% of complete tears.[58] A normal supraspinatus tendon, however, may be identified in the absence of a well-defined peribursal fat plane or in the presence of small amounts of subacromial bursal fluid (Fig. 6–70). With the use of fat-suppression techniques, Mirowitz has shown that many of the established secondary criteria for diagnosis of rotator cuff tear, including obliteration of the subacromial subdeltoid fat plane and fluid in the subacromial or subdeltoid bursa, are found routinely in asymptomatic populations.[59]

In some patients, it may not be possible to differentiate severe tendinitis from a partial supraspinatus tear, whether or not T2- or T2*-weighted images are acquired (Fig. 6–71). These thickened tendons often have a macerated appearance, with a diffuse increase in signal intensity on T2*-weighted images but without a defined interruption of the tendon surface. Tendinitis, degeneration, and partial tears all are part of a spectrum of pathology in subacromial impingement—it is not surprising that they cannot always be distinguished.[50] This difficulty may discourage the use of MR in place of conventional contrast arthrography, despite its usefulness in evaluating subacromial impingement, glenohumeral labral capsular structures, and the morphology and extent of complete rotator cuff tears.

Gadolinium-Enhanced Magnetic Resonance Images.

Intraarticular administration of Gd-DTPA is useful in highlighting small partial tears involving the articular surface due to the T1-shortening effects of gadolinium. Tears are bright on T1-weighted postinjection images (Fig. 6–72).[60] Gadolinium-enhanced images accurately define tendon edges in complete rotator cuff tears (Fig. 6–73). Intraarticular gadolinium replaces the need for routine T2-weighted images, except for the evaluation of bursal surface lesions, and improves visualization of the contour or outline of the supraspinatus on postinjection T1-weighted images. Partial articular surface tears, not seen on contrast arthrograms, may be identified in gadolinium-enhanced images, especially in areas of granulation tissue in chronic tears (Fig. 6–74).[51] Partial bursal surface tears, however, may not be revealed by gadolinium-enhanced MR images (Fig. 6–75) or by conventional arthrographic examination.[60]

Gadolinium contrast enhancement is also helpful in differentiating severe tendinitis from a partial tear (Fig. 6–76). In patients with tendinitis alone, no extension of gadolinium contrast postinjection images is present, and the supraspinatus tendon can be seen to be intact. Intra-articular injection of gadolinium also distends the capsule, demonstrating labral and glenohumeral ligament anatomy.

Postoperative Rotator Cuff

Magnetic resonance imaging has also been used to evaluate postoperative rotator cuff repairs (Fig. 6–77). Gradient-echo sequences frequently show an increased magnetic susceptibility artifact; therefore, the attachment of the rotator cuff tear may not be clearly visualized. Conventional T1- or T2-weighted images minimize these artifacts while allowing visualization of increased signal intensity in cuff defects. Gadolinium-enhanced studies, with a short TR/TE T1-weighted sequence, also minimize surgical artifacts when performed postoperatively (Fig. 6–78). Sagittal images show the division of the coracoacromial ligament in acromioplasties. The rotator cuff interval between the supraspinatus and subscapularis tendons may be interrupted at surgery, allowing communication of contrast with the subacromial bursa (Figs. 6–79 and 6–80).

Surgical Management

Chronic impingement leads to complete rotator cuff tears. The repair procedure of choice is ASD, followed by a deltoid-splitting approach to gain access to the torn cuff.[36] The supraspinatus tears at its insertion on the greater tuberosity; therefore, primary repairs are fixed directly to the bone with drill holes or suture anchors. As mentioned earlier, a Mumford procedure may be performed when AC degeneration is evident.

The rotator cuff is always repaired with nonabsorbable sutures used to reattach the avulsed tendon to a denuded bed of bone. With the deltoid-splitting approach, drill holes in the acromion are not necessary, and proper subperiosteal reflection of the deltoid at the acromion permits a side-to-side closure. If extensive dissection of the deltoid from the acromion is carried out, drill holes

are necessary to repair the deltoid, which was reflected during surgery. This approach has a higher rate of morbidity, and postoperative deltoid defects are common. Most repairs can be achieved through a mini-deltoid-splitting approach.

Glenohumeral Joint Instability

The stability of the glenohumeral joint depends on the stabilizing musculotendinous structures of the rotator cuff as well as on almost all the muscles of the shoulder girdle. The importance of the glenohumeral ligament labral complex, and particularly the IGL, has been reported by Turkel.[61]

Anterior Instability

The most common of all glenohumeral joint instabilities is anterior instability, particularly that produced by lesions of the IGL labral complex (Fig. 6–81). Avulsion of the glenohumeral ligament labral complex from the glenoid rim is known as a Bankart lesion (Figs. 6–82 and 6–83). The IGL complex can also tear at its midportion or be avulsed from its humeral insertion (Fig. 6–84). The humeral avulsion of glenohumeral ligaments (*i.e.,* HAGL lesion) has been demonstrated arthroscopically and can be solely responsible for shoulder instability in some cases (Fig. 6–85). Pollock and Bigliani have shown that pathology or defects in the IGL labral complex are found at the humeral origin and within the substance of the ligament more commonly than was previously anticipated.[62] It is therefore important to evaluate the IGL labral complex from its humeral origins through its course to its labral insertions.

Measurement of IGL thickness by Bigliani and colleagues documents that the anterior band is the thickest region, followed by the anterior and posterior aspects of the axillary pouch.[62] Failure of the IGL can occur at the glenoid insertion site (40%), in the ligament substance (35%), and at the humeral insertion site (25%). Avulsions occur more frequently in the anterior band and the anterior aspect of the axillary pouch, whereas ligament substance tears are more common in the posterior aspect of the axillary pouch. Bankart avulsions represent failure of the IGL at the glenoid insertion, and IGL capsular laxity represents intrasubstance ligament failure. The tensile properties of the IGL allow for significant stretching before failure; therefore, redundancy of the IGL may be as important as avulsions of the glenoid insertion at the IGL in producing glenohumeral instabilities.

Lesions of the glenohumeral ligament labral complex can be demonstrated with contrast-enhanced CT and with MR, leading to increased identification of labral defects in patients with anterior instability.[3,58,63–67] In addition, a Hill–

(text continues on page 597)

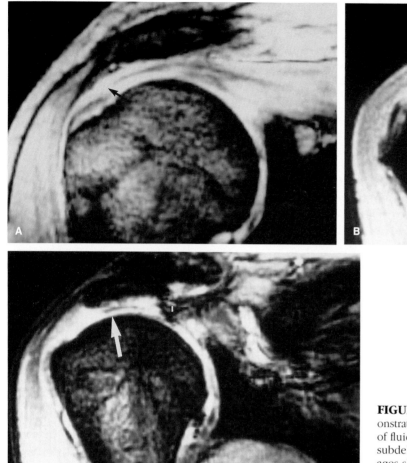

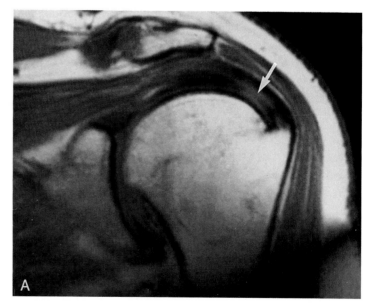

FIGURE 6–59. (**A**) A T2*-weighted coronal image demonstrates complete rotator cuff tear with direct communication of fluid between the glenohumeral joint and the subacromial subdeltoid bursa (*arrow*). T2*-weighted coronal oblique images show massive rotator cuff tear (*arrows*) with disruption of the supraspinatus (S) and infraspinatus (I) tendons both (**B**) anteriorly and (**C**) posteriorly.

FIGURE 6–60. A partial rotator cuff tear with tendinitis. Intermediate signal intensity supraspinatus edema (*arrows*) in a partial tendon tear is identified on (**A**) intermediate-weighted and (**B**) T2-weighted spin-echo sequences. (**C**) On a corresponding double contrast arthrogram (anteroposterior view), the rotator cuff lesion was missed.

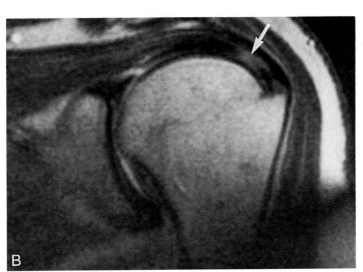

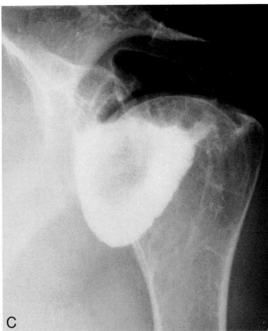

FIGURE 6–60. *(Continued)*

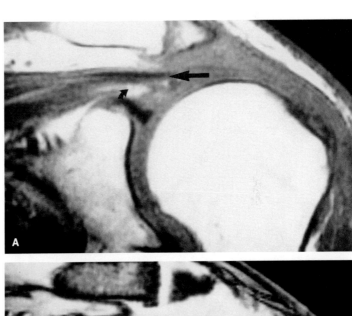

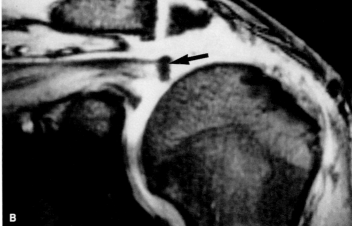

FIGURE 6–61. (**A**) T1-weighted and (**B**) T2*-weighted coronal oblique images show a complete supraspinatus tendon tear with proximal retraction of tendon edge to level of the acromioclavicular joint (*straight arrows*). Mild fatty atrophy of the supraspinatus muscle (*curved arrow*) is present.

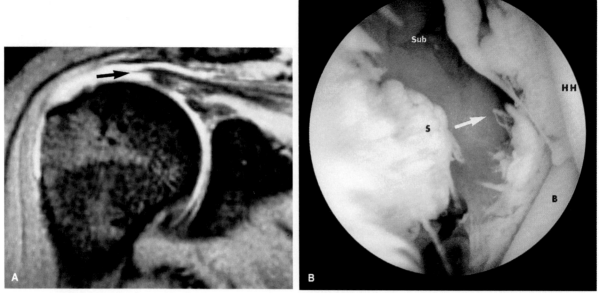

FIGURE 6–62.   Rotator cuff tear. (**A**) A T2*-weighted image shows complete tear of the supraspinatus tendon with proximal retraction (*arrow*). Glenohumeral joint fluid communicates with the subacromial–subdeltoid bursa. The retracted tendon edge is clearly depicted. (**B**) The corresponding arthroscopic view shows the articular surface of the avulsed supraspinatus tendon (*arrow;* S). (B, biceps tendon; HH, humeral head; Sub, subacromial space.)

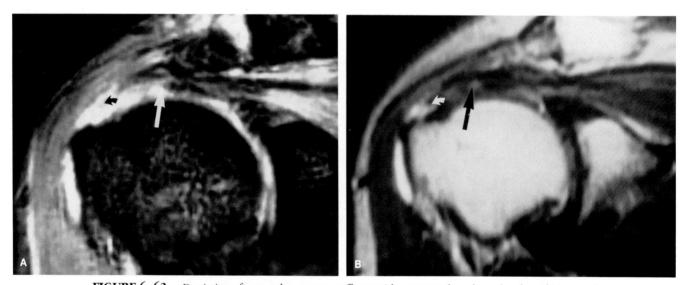

FIGURE 6–63.   Depiction of a complete rotator cuff tear with a retracted tendon edge (*straight arrows*) is better on (**A**) a T2*-weighted coronal image than on (**B**) the corresponding conventional T2-weighted coronal oblique image. The depiction of the degree of subacromial fluid extension (*curved arrows*) is also better on the T2*-weighted image.

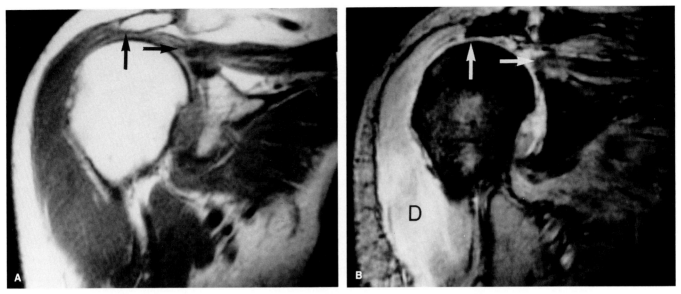

FIGURE 6–64. Rotator cuff tear. Coronal oblique (**A**) T1-weighted and (**B**) T2*-weighted images demonstrate a torn supraspinatus tendon retracted to the level of the glenoid (*horizontal arrows*). Superior ascent of the humeral head (*vertical arrows*) with decreased subacromial space is also seen. The supraspinatus muscle normally functions to prevent the ascent of the humeral head when the deltoid contracts. Deltoid muscle hemorrhage (D) is revealed on the T2*-weighted coronal oblique image.

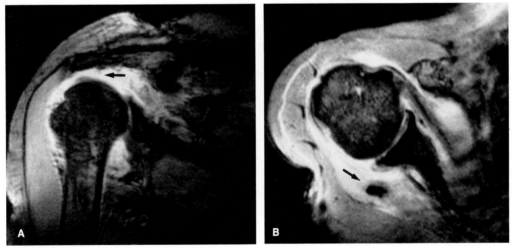

FIGURE 6–65. Infraspinatus tendon tear can occur as part of a massive rotator cuff tear. (**A**) A T2*-weighted posterior coronal oblique image shows an absence of the infraspinatus tendon (*arrow*). (**B**) A T2*-weighted image shows the retracted tendon edge of the infraspinatus (*arrow*).

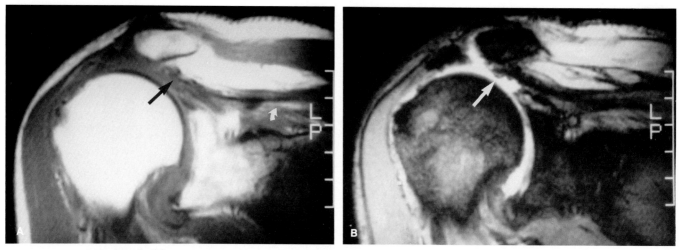

FIGURE 6–66. (**A**) T1-weighted and (**B**) T2*-weighted coronal oblique images show a rotator cuff tear. The supraspinatus tendon is completely disrupted and proximally retracted to the level of the glenoid. The tendon edges are frayed and irregular (*straight arrows*) and supraspinatus muscle atrophy is present (*curved arrow*).

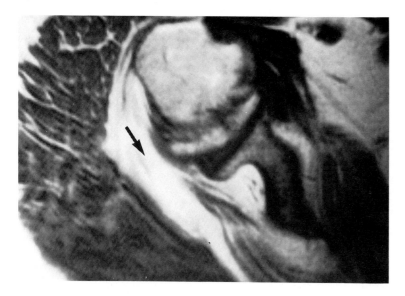

FIGURE 6–67. A chronic infraspinatus tendon tear demonstrates high signal intensity fatty atrophy (*arrow*) on a T1-weighted axial image.

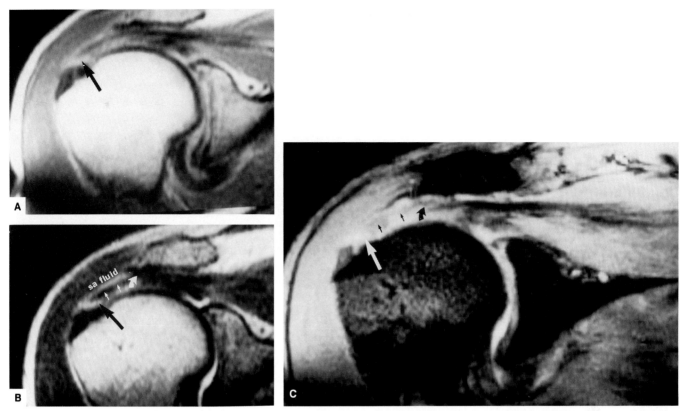

FIGURE 6-68. A rotator cuff tear on (**A**) intermediate- and (**B**) T2-weighted coronal oblique images as compared with (**C**) T2*-weighted coronal oblique image. On conventional T2-weighted images, contrast detail is greater at the tear site in the supraspinatus (*large straight arrows*), the frayed tendon edge (*small straight arrows*), and the subacromial bursal fluid (sa fluid). However, the retracted tendon edge (*curved arrows*) to the level of the acromion is equally well displayed on both the conventional and the T2*-weighted images.

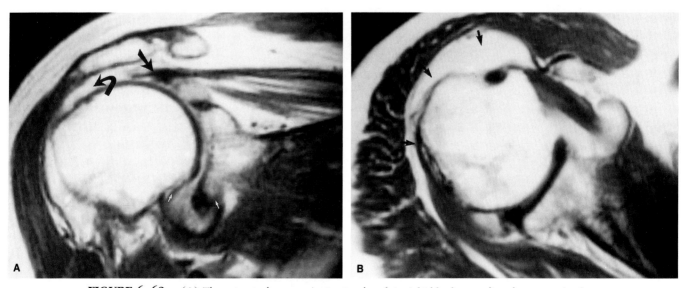

FIGURE 6-69. (**A**) The retracted supraspinatus tendon (*straight black arrow*) and communication of contrast with the subacromial bursa (*curved arrow*) are shown on a T1-weighted coronal oblique image of a large rotator cuff tear. The humeral and glenoid attachments of the inferior glenohumeral ligament are also shown (*straight white arrows*). (**B**) Lateral extension of contrast relative to the humeral head (*arrows*) represents subacromial communication, as seen on a T1-weighted axial image.

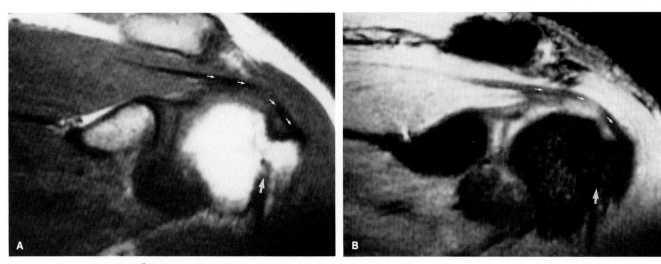

FIGURE 6–70. A normal supraspinatus tendon (*small arrows*) without an identifiable subacromial–subdeltoid fat line is seen on (**A**) T1-weighted and (**B**) T2*-weighted coronal oblique images. Note the location of the long head of the biceps tendon (*large arrow*).

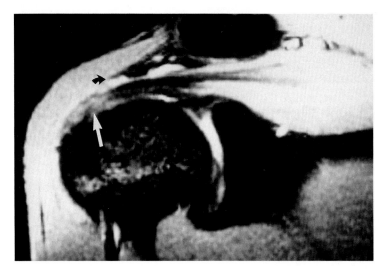

FIGURE 6–71. An attenuated, untorn supraspinatus (*straight arrow*) tendon is seen after acromioplasty. Subacromial fluid is present without an associated rotator cuff tear (*curved arrow*).

FIGURE 6–72. A partial rotator cuff tear. (**A**) On coronal oblique T1-weighted and (**B**) T2*-weighted images, a partial articular surface tear of the supraspinatus tendon is not fully visible. The focus of increased signal intensity involving the articular surface of the supraspinatus tendon (*arrow*) could also represent inflammation when seen on the T2*-weighted image. Previous acromioplasty is confirmed by the absence of the acromion in these images. (**C**) An enhanced coronal image clearly depicts high signal intensity in a partial articular surface tear (*arrow*) without extension of contrast into the subacromial–subdeltoid bursa.

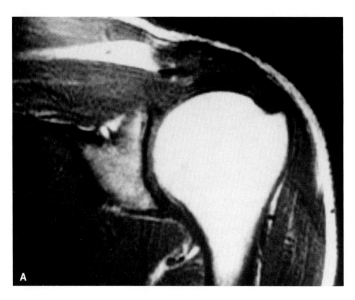

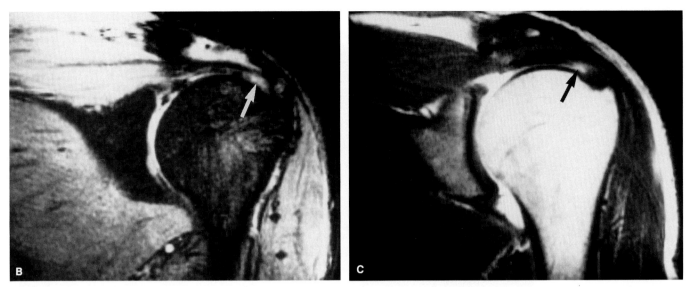

FIGURE 6–72. *(Continued)*

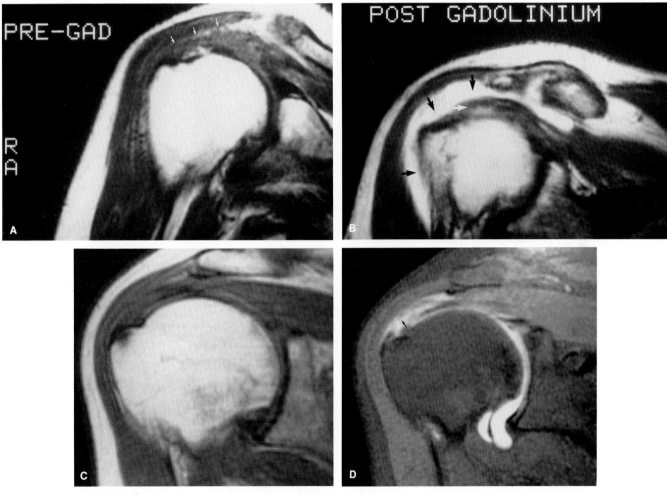

FIGURE 6–73. (**A**) On an unenhanced T1-weighted coronal image, the retracted supraspinatus tendon is not accurately depicted. The nonspecific subdeltoid fat plane is preserved in the presence of a complete rotator cuff tear (*arrows*). (**B**) An enhanced T1-weighted coronal image allows precise localization of the distal end of the torn supraspinatus tendon (*white arrow*). Gadolinium contrast fills the subacromial bursa superior and lateral to the greater tuberosity. A different patient demonstrates complete rotator cuff tear on coronal oblique (**C**) T1-weighted and (**D**) enhanced T1-weighted fat-suppression images. Tear morphology (*arrow*) and detail of the tendon edges are best displayed on the gadolinium-enhanced image. The contrast communicates with the subacromial bursa without retraction of the muscle–tendon junction.

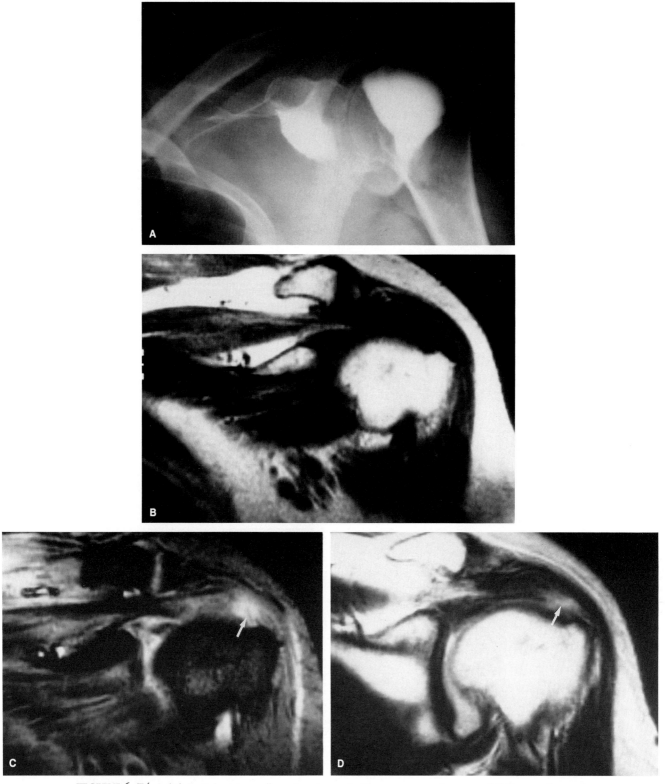

FIGURE 6–74. (**A**) Partial rotator cuff tear is not revealed by a contrast arthrogram. (**B**) A nonenhanced T1-weighted coronal oblique image of the supraspinatus tendon is also nonspecific for tear. No peribursal fat line is identified. (**C**) A T2*-weighted coronal oblique image displays a hyperintense focus in the anterior supraspinatus tendon (*arrow*) consistent with either severe inflammation or partial tear. No fluid is identified in the subacromial bursa. (**D**) An enhanced T1-weighted coronal oblique image reveals a hyperintense partial tear of the supraspinatus tendon (*arrow*).

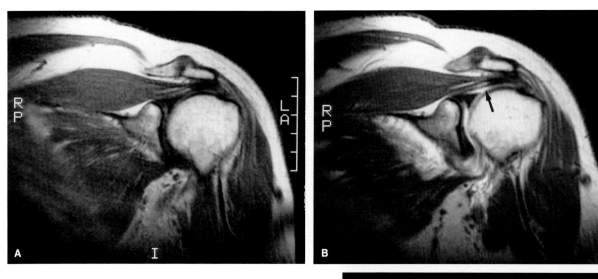

FIGURE 6–75. Partial rotator cuff tear. (**A**) Unenhanced and (**B**) enhanced T1-weighted images are false-negative studies that show no extension of contrast into the subacromial bursa (*arrow*). (**C**) The corresponding arthroscopic view reveals scar tissue in the frayed articular surface of the supraspinatus (*arrow*). A greater than 50% bursal surface tear was not detected on gadolinium-enhanced MR images. (HH, humeral head.)

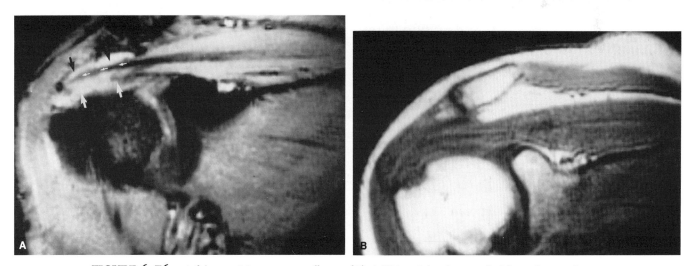

FIGURE 6–76. A false-positive rotator cuff tear. (**A**) A T2*-weighted coronal oblique image shows the supraspinatus tendon (*small white arrows*) without definition of a greater tuberosity attachment. Bursal (*black arrows*) and articular (*large white arrows*) fluid collections imply rotator cuff pathology. In a comparison of (**B**) unenhanced and (**C**) enhanced T1-weighted coronal oblique images, the enhanced coronal oblique image shows an intact supraspinatus tendon (*white arrows*) and intraarticular gadolinium contrast (*black arrow*). (**D**) The corresponding arthrogram is negative for partial or complete rotator cuff tear.

(continued)

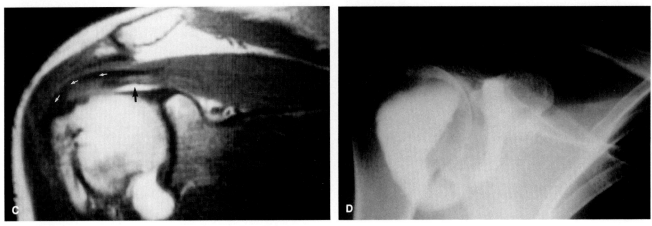

FIGURE 6–76. *(Continued)*

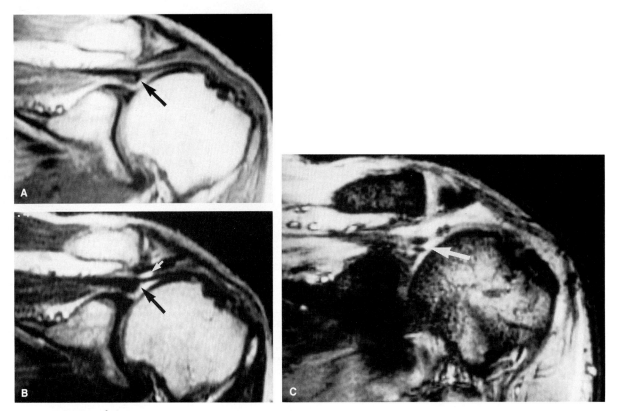

FIGURE 6–77. Chronic retear of supraspinatus tendon after rotator cuff repair is seen on (**A**) intermediate-weighted and (**B**) T2-weighted coronal images and (**C**) a T2*-weighted coronal image. The retracted tendon edge (*large arrows*) is equally well displayed on T2- and T2*-weighted images. Minimal subacromial bursal fluid (*small arrow*) is shown on the T2-weighted image. Increased magnetic susceptibility is present on the T2*-weighted image.

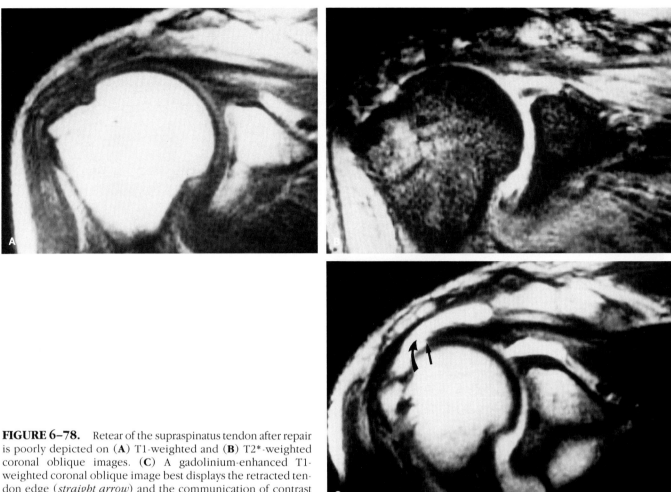

FIGURE 6–78. Retear of the supraspinatus tendon after repair is poorly depicted on (**A**) T1-weighted and (**B**) T2*-weighted coronal oblique images. (**C**) A gadolinium-enhanced T1-weighted coronal oblique image best displays the retracted tendon edge (*straight arrow*) and the communication of contrast with the subacromial bursa (*curved arrow*).

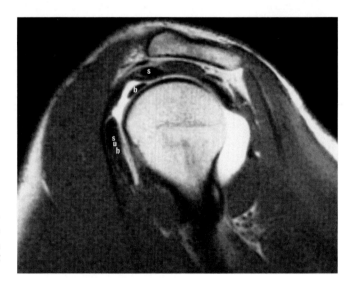

FIGURE 6–79. An intact rotator interval exists between the supraspinatus tendon (s) and subscapularis tendon (sub). The coracohumeral ligament is located on the anterior edge of the interval, whereas the long head of the biceps is located deep in the posterior aspect of the rotator interval. (b, biceps tendon.)

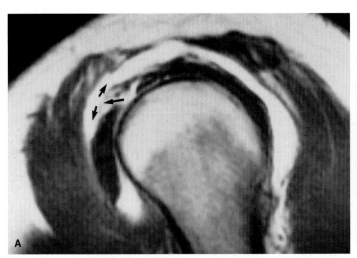 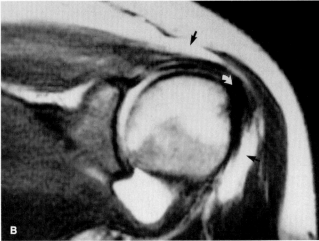

FIGURE 6–80. (**A**) A T1-weighted sagittal oblique image shows extension of intraarticular gadolinium contrast across the rotator interval (*arrows*) between the subscapularis and supraspinatus tendons, secondary to previous surgical release in entering the glenohumeral joint. (**B**) A T1-weighted coronal oblique image also demonstrates subacromial–subdeltoid gadolinium (*straight arrow*) with an intact supraspinatus tendon (*curved arrow*).

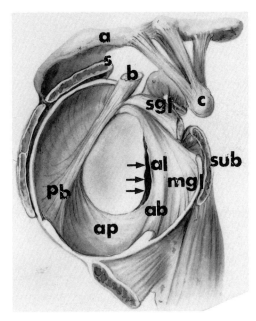

FIGURE 6–81. Anterior labral avulsion from the anterior glenoid rim (*arrows*). (a, acromion; ab, anterior band of inferior glenohumeral ligament; al, anterior labrum; ap, axillary pouch of inferior glenohumeral ligament; c, coracoid; pb, posterior band of inferior glenohumeral ligament; s, supraspinatus tendon; sgl, superior glenohumeral ligament; sub, subscapularis tendon.)

FIGURE 6–82. Avulsion of the anterior band of the inferior glenohumeral ligament (IGL). (**A**) A T2*-weighted posterior coronal image shows intact humeral (*single arrow*) and inferior glenoid pole attachments of the IGL. (p, posterior labrum.) (**B**) The more anterior T2*-weighted coronal oblique image depicts the axillary pouch of the IGL (*straight arrows*) and the avulsed anterior inferior glenoid labrum (*curved arrow*). (**C, D**) T2*-weighted axial images show the avulsed anterior labrum (*curved arrow*) and the anterior band of the IGL (*small straight arrow*). (mgl, middle glenohumeral ligament; s, subscapularis tendon.) (**E**) A T2*-weighted sagittal oblique image shows the avulsed anterior band (*arrows;* AB) of the IGL. (G, glenoid; mgl, middle glenohumeral ligament; S, subscapularis tendon.) (**F**) The corresponding arthroscopic image shows the avulsed labrum (L, *arrows*) and anterior band (AB) of the IGL. (C, articular cartilage debris; G, glenoid; MGL, middle glenohumeral ligament; S, subscapularis tendon.)

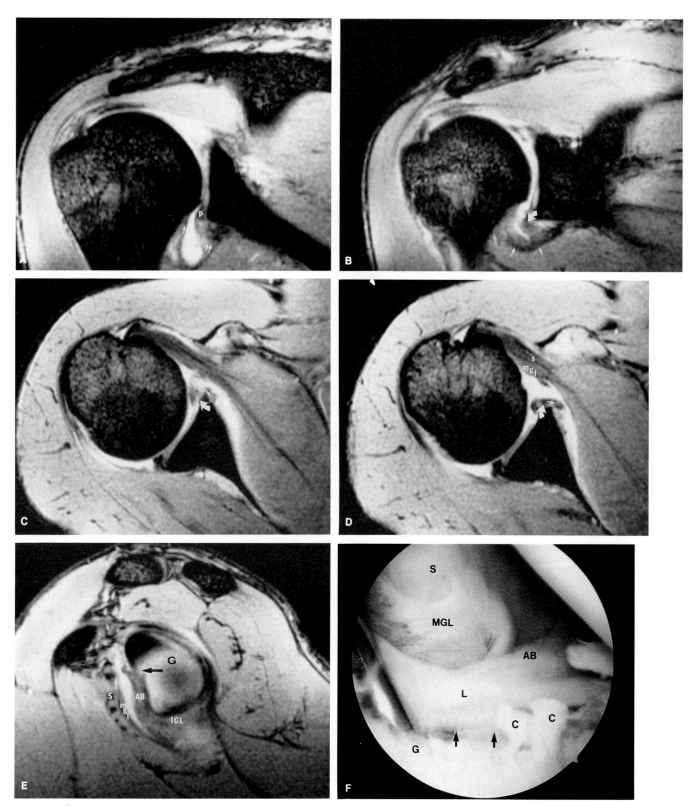

FIGURE 6–82.

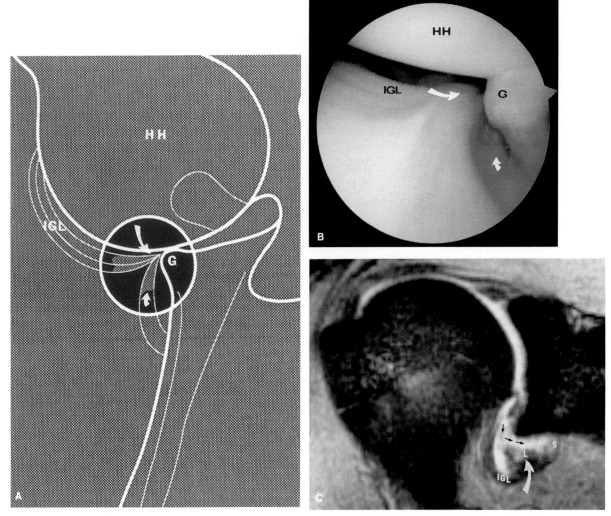

FIGURE 6–83. Bankart lesion. (**A**) A tear (*large curved arrow*) of the inferior glenoid and labral attachment of the inferior glenohumeral ligament (IGL) is present. Scarred muscle of the subscapularis is shown along the inferior glenoid neck (*small curved arrow*). The humeral head (HH) is subluxed inferiorly. (G, glenoid.) (**B**) The arthroscopic view from inferior to anterior is seen with the scope in the axillary pouch, oriented toward the anterior inferior pole of the glenoid. Note avulsed labrum from glenoid rim (G) and torn inferior pole (*large curved arrow*) attachment of IGL. (HH, humeral head.) Scarred tearing of subscapularis muscle from scapular neck is also identified (*small curved arrow*). (**C**) Avulsed anterior glenoid labrum (*curved arrow;* L) and IGL attachment are shown on a T2*-weighted coronal oblique image. Fluid extension (*straight arrows*) is identified between the inferior glenoid neck, detached labrum, and subscapularis muscle (S).

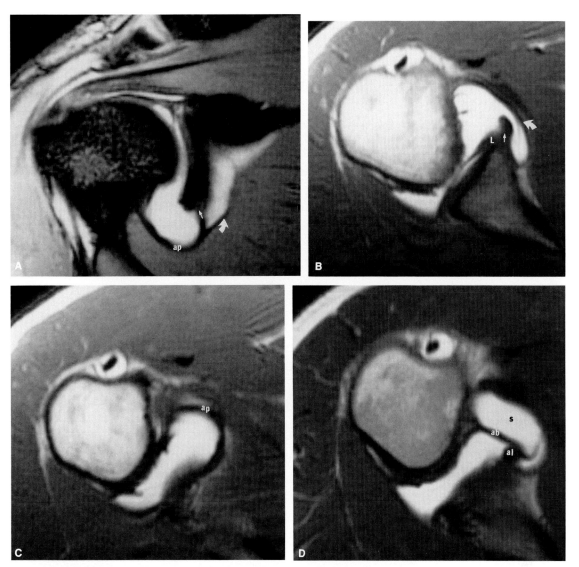

FIGURE 6–84. Inferior glenohumeral ligament labral complex. (**A**) Enhanced T2*-weighted gradient echo coronal oblique images demonstrate the normal inferior glenoid pole attachment of the axillary pouch (ap) of the inferior glenohumeral ligament (*straight arrow*). Note gadolinium contrast in normal inferior extension of subscapularis bursa (*curved arrow*). (**B**) An enhanced T1-weighted axial image identifies subscapularis bursa (*curved arrow*) and glenoid origin (*straight arrow*) of the inferior glenohumeral ligament complex (IGLC). The IGLC may originate from the glenoid, the labrum (L), or the neck of the glenoid immediately adjacent to the labrum. There is no anterior labral tear on this image. (**C**) An enhanced T1-weighted axial image below the level of the glenoid displays the normal axillary pouch (ap) of the inferior glenohumeral ligament. (**D**) An enhanced T1-weighted axial image in a different patient identifies the anterior band (ab) of the inferior glenohumeral ligament complex and its continuation as the anterior labrum (al). Gadolinium contrast is shown in the subscapularis bursa (s) anterior to the anterior band. There is no tear of the anterior inferior labrum.

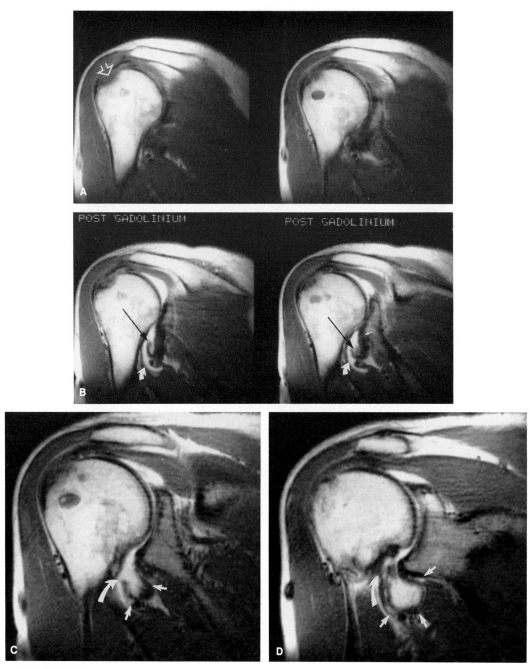

FIGURE 6–85. Humeral head avulsion of the glenohumeral ligament (HAGL lesion). T1-weighted coronal oblique images (**A**) before and (**B**) after intraarticular gadolinium administration are shown in a patient with a history of chronic anterior dislocation. A Hill–Sachs lesion is identified in the posterolateral humeral head (*open arrow*). The postgadolinium images document inferior extravasation of contrast (*curved white arrows*) through the avulsed insertion of the inferior glenohumeral ligament (IGL) to the anatomic neck of the humerus (*long black arrows*). This is diagnostic for the HAGL lesion. The IGL is also shown (*small white arrow*). (**C, D**) More anterior coronal oblique images display an abnormally capacious axillary pouch (*straight arrows*) secondary to avulsion of the IGL humeral insertion (*curved arrows*). (**E**) The corresponding arthrogram confirms extravasation of contrast (*curved arrow*) through the tear in the IGL complex (*straight arrow*). (**F**) Enhanced axial (*left*) and sagittal oblique (*right*) images demonstrate abnormal anterior and lateral displacement of the anterior band of the IGL (*curved arrow*). The sagittal oblique image shows a type 3 synovial recess with a superior subscapularis recess above the middle glenohumeral ligament (MGL, m), and an inferior subscapular recess   below the MGL. (*Large curved arrow,* axillary pouch of IGL; b, biceps tendon; S, superior subscapular recess.) (**G**) An inferior axial image shows an avulsed humeral attachment of the IGL (*large curved arrow*) and associated ligamentous and labral fraying (*small curved arrow*). (**H**) An arthroscopic image also shows the avulsed humeral attachment of the IGL (*curved arrows*). (AB, anterior band; HH, humeral head; IL, torn inferior labrum; S, subscapularis muscle).

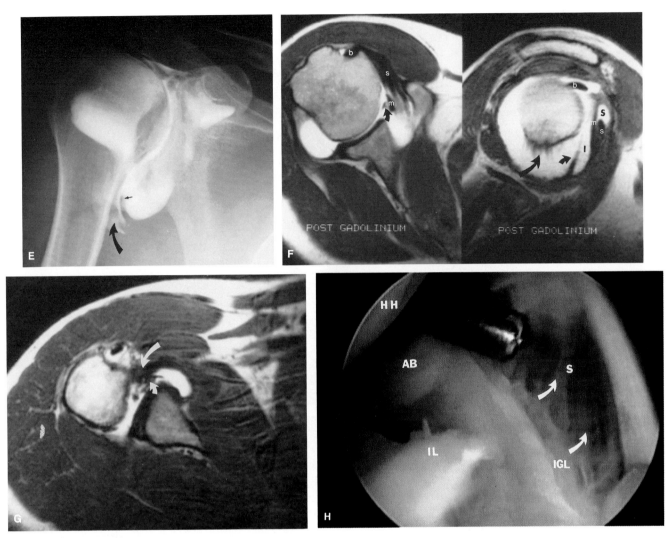

FIGURE 6–85. *(Continued)*

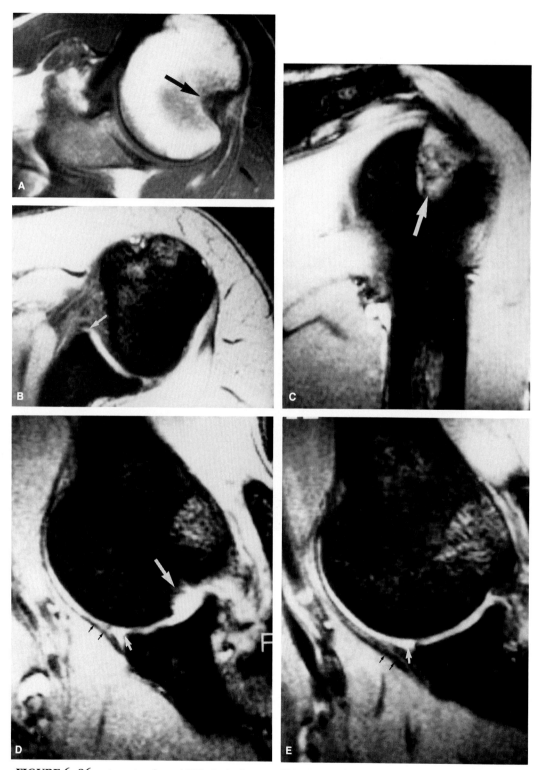

FIGURE 6–86. A posterolateral Hill–Sachs fracture (*black arrow*) and associated anterior labrum tear (*white arrow*) are seen on axial (**A**) T1-weighted and (**B**) T2*-weighted images. (**C**) A posterolateral Hill–Sachs wedge-shaped impaction (*arrow*) is seen on a T2*-weighted coronal image. Corresponding T2*-weighted axial images made on (**D**) abduction and (**E**) external rotation show a Hill–Sachs lesion (*large white arrow*), an absence of the anterior labrum (*small white arrows*), and a taut inferior gleno-humeral ligament (*small black arrows*).

Sachs posterolateral compression fracture can be seen in patients with subluxations and single or multiple episodes of dislocation (Fig. 6–86). This compression defect is identified on the posterolateral humeral head. The normal flattening of the posterior aspect of the humeral head in its inferior portion should not be mistaken for a Hill–Sachs defect. Associated Bankart lesions seen on MR images include both osseous anterior inferior glenoid rim fractures and labral tears or avulsions (Fig. 6–87).

Posterior Instability

Although posterior instability of the glenohumeral joint is relatively rare, it should be suspected in the presence of posterior labral disruption or fragmentation (Figs. 6–88 and 6–89).[68] A detailed examination with the patient under anesthesia (EUA) is critical in determining the type of instability. Examination under anesthesia must be conducted in a lateral decubitus position, with the patient's arm abducted. Axial compression and stabilization of the scapula allow the examiner to appreciate the degree of translation of the humeral head on the glenoid. Confirmation of the results of EUA and the findings on diagnostic arthroscopy determine the surgical approach.

Multidirectional Instability

In true multidirectional instability of the glenohumeral joint, force applied distally on the upper extremities with the patient's arm abducted causes inferior subluxation of the humeral head. This produces a visible sulcus (*i.e.,* the sulcus sign) between the prominence of the acromion and the inferiorly subluxed humeral head.[69] In classic multidirectional instability, the ligament laxity is bilateral and atraumatic. The index of suspicion should be high in young patients, especially young female patients with generalized joint laxities and complaints referable to the shoulders. These patients are best treated with long periods of physical therapy. Specific muscle rehabilitation, with particular attention to the shoulders, helps to provide stability to the lax joints.

No visible ligament labral lesions are seen in patients with multidirectional instability of the glenohumeral joint. The capsular ligaments are redundant, and the labrum is often hypoplastic in these patients. However, some patients with multidirectional laxity present with unidirectional pathology. These patients experience dislocation predominantly in only one direction. Arthroscopic, intra-articular findings confirm the direction of the instability.

Labral Pathology

Normal Variations

There is considerable variation in the attachment and morphology of the glenoid labrum. The most significant variation is the relative attachment, or lack thereof, to the glenoid rim in the anterior superior quadrant above the epiphyseal line (Fig. 6–90). There is frequently a sublabral foramen between the labrum and the glenoid rim, which is often cause for misinterpretation of anterior labral disruption or tears (Figs. 6–91 and 6–92). Although the glenoid labrum in the superior one-third of the glenoid above the epiphyseal line can be firmly fixed in its periphery, DePalma has shown that there is considerable variation in the anterior superior bursae and labral foramen of the complex.[29] Although the resulting different bursal configurations produce MR images that appear to demonstrate superior and anterior labral tears, these are normal anatomic variations.[24,29]

The capsule can be categorized into one of six anatomic types as described by DePalma, based on the topographic arrangements of the synovial recesses with respect to the glenohumeral ligaments (Fig. 6–93).[24,29] The six types of synovial recesses are best assessed by intra-articular-gadolinium–enhanced sagittal oblique images in which the middle and IGLs can be reliably identified (Figs. 6–94 and 6–95). In addition, a fibrous, cordlike MGL is frequently mistaken for a detached labrum above the epiphyseal line (Fig. 6–96). A filamentous extension or attachment may be identified between the cordlike MGL and the anterior labrum (Figs. 6–97 and 6–98).

In general, the labrum is more firmly attached inferior to the epiphyseal line and is continuous with the cartilaginous surface of the glenoid. DePalma demonstrated that, with increasing age and degeneration, separation of the fibrous labrum from the cartilaginous glenoid surface occurs throughout the periphery of the glenoid.[29] This is evident on arthroscopy in older patients.

Magnetic resonance also demonstrates normal variations in labral morphology, as described by Detrisac and Johnson.[27] This includes a superior wedge-shaped labrum, with the labrum firmly attached anteriorly, posteriorly, and inferiorly. Separation between the glenoid and the superior anterior labrum is a normal variation (Fig. 6–99). The posterior wedge-shaped labrum is smaller and more firmly attached to the superior glenoid (Fig. 6–100). The anterior wedge labrum is characterized by a large anterior band of the IGL, which replaces or covers a small anterior labrum (Fig. 6–101). The meniscoid labrum has a circumferentially free central margin with relatively symmetric anterior and posterior labral tissue on cross section above the epiphyseal line (Fig. 6–102).

Labral Tears

Magnetic resonance has proved to be a sensitive, specific, and accurate modality for evaluating the glenoid labrum.[65] In MR studies of labral tears with surgical or arthroscopic correlation, sensitivity was reported to be 88% and specificity 93%.[57,70] These statistics compare favorably with air contrast CT arthrography;[71,72] in addition, MR provides superior visualization of associated capsule structures and the IGL.[66] Magnetic resonance imaging protocols used to evaluate the glenoid labrum are the following:

- T1-weighted axial images
- Pregadolinium studies
- Postgadolinium studies
- T2*-weighted axial sequences using 2-mm 3DFT or 4-mm 2DFT images.

The intact fibrous labrum demonstrates low signal intensity on T1-, T2-, and T2*-weighted images. We have not found the radial MR sequence helpful in routine evaluations of the labrum.[73] The IGL labral complex has been shown on images with the arm positioned in abduction and internal rotation, however.

Tears of the IGL are usually associated with traumatic dislocation or subluxation (Figs. 6–103 and 6–104).[27,74] Labral tissue may be interposed between the humeral head and the glenoid rim, most often due to a labral tear with a relatively meniscoid and hypermobile biceps labral configuration. As the labrum becomes more meniscoid in shape, the likelihood of meniscal bucket-handle tears increases, and tissue may become interposed between the humeral head and the glenoid surface (Fig. 6–105). Snyder has described SLAP lesions, which vary from simple fraying and fragmentation of the biceps labral complex, to a bucket-handle tear, to a tricorne bucket-handle tear in which one rim of the tear actually extends up into the biceps tendon, splitting it as the rim of the tear goes up toward the bicipital groove (Fig. 6–106).[75]

Linear tears and fragmentation of the posterior labrum are less common and can be seen in patients with posterior instability with recurrent posterior subluxations (Fig. 6–107).[76,77] Associated osseous findings include an impaction fracture or defect on the anteromedial humeral head as well as fractures involving the posterior glenoid margin or lesser tuberosity.[50] Eccentric wear of the glenohumeral joint is frequently displayed as low signal intensity posterior glenoid subchondral sclerosis or as fatty marrow conversion (Fig. 6–108).

Capsular Insertions. Zlatkin and colleagues identified three types of capsular insertions: type 1, which inserts near the anterior labrum, and types 2 and 3, which insert more broadly or medially on the scapular neck and probably represent a normal variation in the scapular neck.[67] These types of insertions in fact represent normal variations in the size and morphology of the subscapular recess, which is dependent on the rotation of the shoulder and is not the result of stripping of the capsule. With internal rotation, the recess is large and the capsule appears to insert more medially on the scapular neck (Fig. 6–109). It is unlikely that the anterior pouch in the type 3 capsular insertion predisposes to anterior humeral subluxation or dislocation in a created potential space. However, in patients with histories of anterior dislocations, we have observed a capacious or enlarged subscapularis

bursa as a secondary finding. The converse may not be true.

Magnetic Resonance Appearance. Zlatkin has classified abnormal labral signal intensity into four types.[50,70]

In type 1, increased signal intensity is present within the labrum, but there is no surface extension. This corresponds to internal labral degeneration without tear.

In type 2, the blunted or frayed labrum demonstrates normal dark signal intensity (Fig. 6–110).

In type 3, T1-weighted or T2*-weighted images demonstrate increased signal intensity that extends to the surface, indicating a labral tear (Fig. 6–111).

In type 4, a labral tear is depicted by a combination of abnormal morphology with type 2 features and increased signal intensity extending to the surface of the labrum with type 3 features (Fig. 6–112).

Large tears and detachments may demonstrate a more diffuse increase in signal intensity, whereas discrete tears maintain linear morphology.[58,64-66] It is not unusual, however, for avulsed labral tissue to demonstrate low signal intensity, especially in chronic injuries (Fig. 6–113). Normal labral outlines, blunting, and avulsion of the labrum from the underlying bone are also seen. Articular cartilage, of intermediate signal intensity on T1- and T2-weighted images and increased signal intensity on T2*-weighted images, may undermine the base of anterior labral tissue and should not be mistaken for an oblique labral tear. Fluid underneath the anterior labrum at or below the level of the coracoid is a pathologic finding that represents labral tearing (Fig. 6–114). The normal sublabral foramen does not extend below the level of the coracoid process.

Gadolinium-Enhanced Magnetic Resonance Images. Intraarticular gadolinium distends the joint capsule and facilitates imaging of the glenohumeral ligaments (Fig. 6–115). Without knowledge of glenohumeral ligament anatomy, these structures may be mistaken for torn or detached labral fragments (Fig. 6–116). Gadolinium-enhanced MR imaging improves the spatial detection of avulsed labral tissue relative to the glenoid rim (Fig. 6–117). Labral tears are usually highlighted on T1-weighted axial images following intraarticular gadolinium administration. A synovial shelf may exist in the subscapularis bursa as a normal finding on enhanced studies (Fig. 6–118).[78]

Calcific Tendinitis

Calcification of the rotator cuff most commonly occurs in the supraspinatus tendon, but can occur in any of the tendons of the rotator cuff (Fig. 6–119).[79] The deposits

(text continues on page 616)

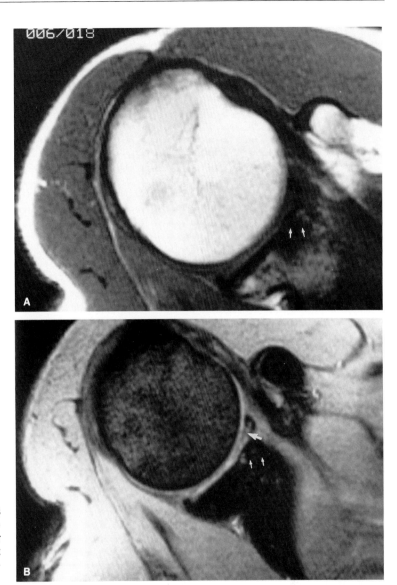

FIGURE 6–87. (**A**) A T1-weighted axial image shows an osseous Bankart lesion with fracture of the anterior inferior glenoid (*arrows*). (**B**) A linear tear of the anterior labrum (*large arrow*) is seen; however, the osseous Bankart lesion (*small arrows*) demonstrates poor contrast on a T2*-weighted axial image.

FIGURE 6–88. Posterior instability and labral tear. Multiple posterior labral tears (*black arrow*) are found on (**A**) T1-weighted and (**B**) T2*-weighted axial images. Eccentric wear of the articular cartilage (*small white arrows*) and posterior labral tears are best depicted on the T2*-weighted image, whereas posterior glenoid rim sclerosis is best depicted on the T1-weighted image (*curved arrow*). Fluid in the subcoracoid bursa was secondary to inadvertent subcoracoid injection with Gd-DTPA contrast (*open arrow*). Mild posterior subluxation of the humeral head is present.

(continued)

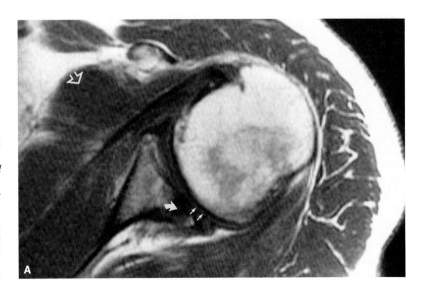

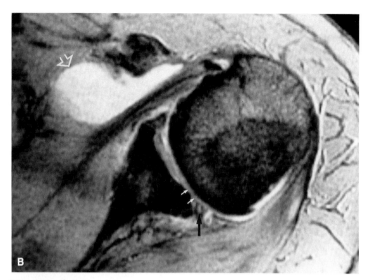

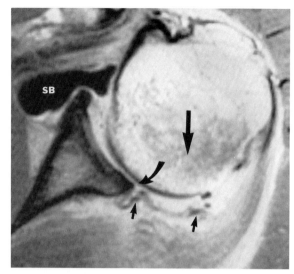

FIGURE 6–88. *(Continued)*

FIGURE 6–89.

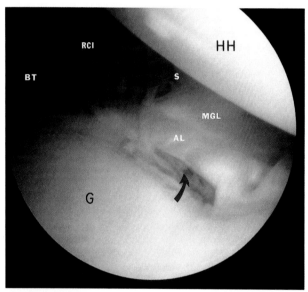

FIGURE 6–90.

FIGURE 6–91.

FIGURE 6–89. Traumatic posterior instability with complete fragmentation of the posterior labrum (*curved arrow*) and tearing of the posterior capsule (*small straight arrows*) occurred in a football player. The humeral head is posteriorly subluxed relative to the glenoid (*large straight arrow*). An intermediate-weighted axial image was performed after air contrast CT arthrography. Low signal intensity air is shown in the subscapularis bursa (SB). There was associated infraspinatus muscle–tendon disruption, demonstrated by increased signal intensity and irregularity of muscle fibers.

FIGURE 6–90. An arthroscopic photograph of a normal anatomic variant of the sublabral foramen with an absence of the anterior labrum attachment above the epiphyseal line of the glenoid (*curved arrow*). (AL, anterior labrum; BT, biceps tendon; G, glenoid; HH, humeral head; MGL, middle glenohumeral ligament; RCI, rotator cuff interval or Weitbrecht's foramen; S, subscapularis tendon.)

FIGURE 6–91. A normal anterior superior glenoid labrum (L) as seen on an enhanced T1-weighted axial image.

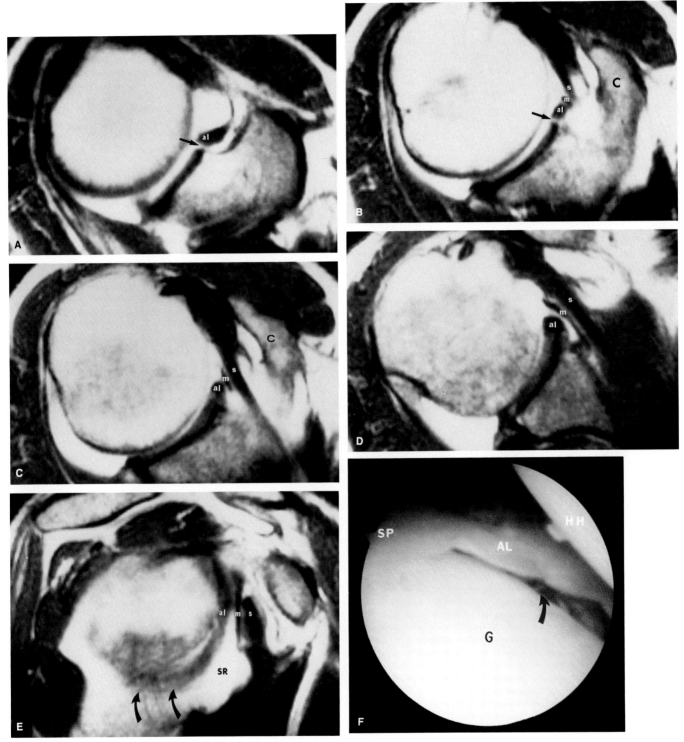

FIGURE 6–92. Sublabral foramen. (**A–D**) Enhanced T1-weighted axial images illustrate the normal anatomic relationship of subscapularis tendon (s), middle glenohumeral ligament (m), and anterior labrum (al) from anterior to posterior. Note the sublabral foramen (*arrow*) as a normal anatomic variant (**A**) above and (**B**) at the level of the superior coracoid (C). No foramen is present at the level of the (**C**) inferior coracoid or (**D**) subscapularis tendon. (**E**) The corresponding enhanced sagittal oblique image shows the subscapularis tendon (s), middle glenohumeral ligament (m), and anterior labrum (al). (*Curved arrows,* axillary pouch of inferior glenohumeral ligament; SR, subscapularis recess inferior to middle glenohumeral ligament.) (**F**) An arthroscopic image shows the sublabral foramen between the anterior superior labrum and glenoid rim (*curved arrow*). (AL, anterior labrum; G, glenoid; SP, superior pole of the glenoid.)

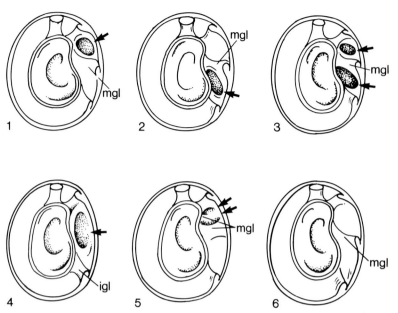

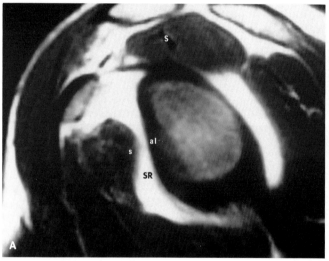

FIGURE 6–93. Six arrangements of synovial recesses (*i.e.,* joint capsule variations; *arrows*) are described by DePalma. Type 1: one synovial recess exists above the middle glenohumeral ligament. Type 2: one synovial recess exists below the middle glenohumeral ligament. Type 3: two synovial recesses exist, with a superior subscapular recess above the middle glenohumeral ligament and an inferior subscapular recess below the middle glenohumeral ligament. Type 4: no middle glenohumeral ligament is present, and one large synovial recess exists above the inferior glenohumeral ligament. Type 5: the middle glenohumeral ligament exists as two small synovial folds. Type 6: there is complete absence of the synovial recesses. (From DePalma AF. Surgery of the shoulder. Philadelphia: JB Lippincott, 1983.)

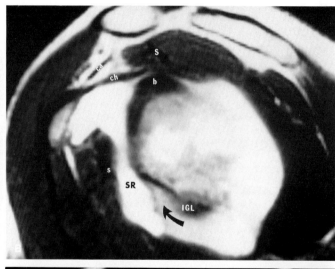

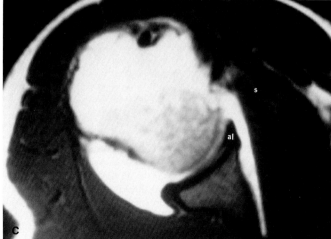

FIGURE 6–94. A single type 3 synovial recess. (**A, B**) Enhanced T1-weighted sagittal oblique images display an absence of the middle glenohumeral ligament (MGL) resulting in one large synovial recess above the inferior glenohumeral ligament (IGL). (*Curved arrow,* anterior band of IGL; al, anterior labrum; b, biceps tendon; ca, coracoacromial ligament; ch, coracohumeral ligament; S, supraspinatus tendon; SR, synovial recess; s, subscapularis tendon.) (**C**) The corresponding enhanced T1-weighted axial image shows the anterior labrum (al) and subscapularis tendon (s) without the MGL interposed between them. Contrast outlines the normal subscapularis bursa. There is no type 3 capsule.

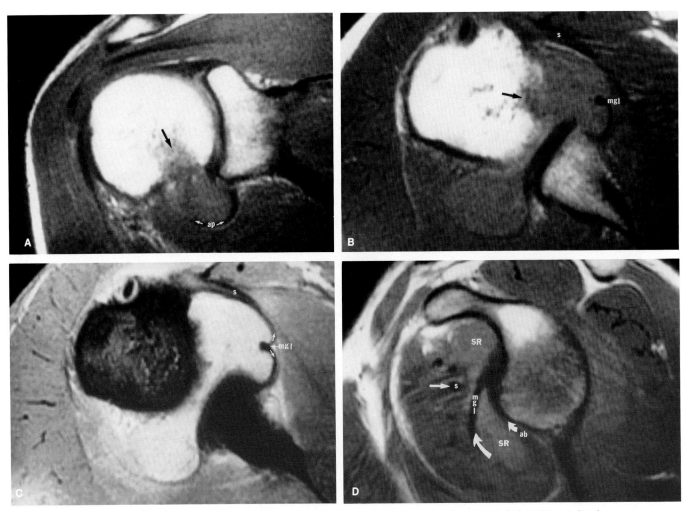

FIGURE 6-95. A type 3 synovial recess with hemorrhagic capsular distention. (**A**) A T1-weighted coronal oblique image shows the axillary pouch (ap; *white arrows*) and anteromedial humeral head contusion (*black arrow*). An impaction defect of the anteromedial humeral head is referred to as a reverse Hill–Sachs defect when associated with posterior dislocation. (**B**) T1-weighted and (**C**) T2*-weighted axial images show capsular distention with a cordlike middle glenohumeral ligament (MGL; mgl; *white arrows*) and subscapularis tendon (s). Anteromedial humeral head contusion (*black arrow*) is also shown. The anterior labrum was intact at arthroscopy. (**D**) The corresponding T1-weighted sagittal oblique image shows the subscapularis tendon (s; *straight arrow*), the MGL (mgl; *large curved arrow*), and the anterior band of the IGL (ab; *small curved arrow*). Fluid can be seen in the synovial recesses (SR) above and below the MGL.

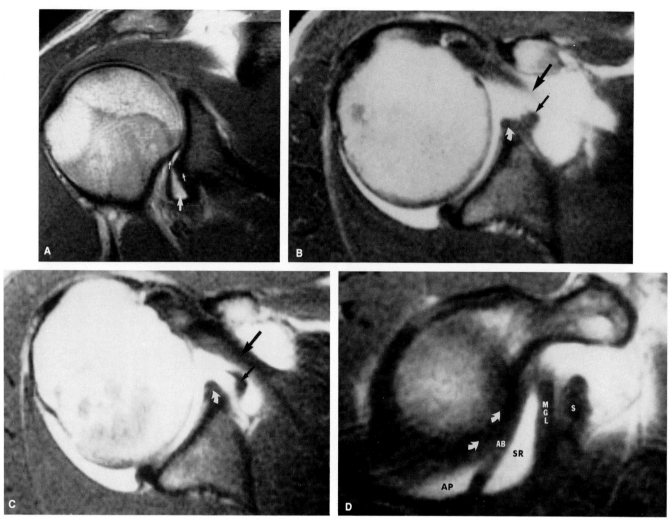

FIGURE 6–96. Cordlike middle glenohumeral ligament (MGL). (**A**) An enhanced coronal oblique T1-weighted image shows a normal axillary pouch distended with gadolinium (*large arrow*). The humeral and glenoid attachments of the inferior glenohumeral ligament (IGL; *small arrows*) are also shown. Enhanced T1-weighted axial images show a cordlike or hypertrophied MGL (*small black arrows*) that simulates an avulsion of the anterior labrum (**B**) superior to and (**C**) at the midlevel of the subscapularis tendon (*large black arrows*). The anterior labral morphology is normal (*curved white arrows*) superior to the subscapularis tendon. The MGL is closely applied to the anterior labrum. At the level of the subscapularis tendon, gadolinium contrast is seen in both the anterior and posterior surfaces of the MGL. (**D**) The corresponding enhanced T1-weighted sagittal image displays a normal anterior labrum (*curved arrows*) and anterior band of the IGL (AB). A thick, cordlike MGL and subscapularis tendon (S) can also be identified. Intraarticular gadolinium contrast is shown in the axillary pouch (AP) of the inferior glenohumeral ligament and in a synovial recess (SR) below the MGL. In the presence of a large synovial recess and cordlike MGL, the recess may be misinterpreted as a capsular rent and the ligament as a torn and displaced labrum.

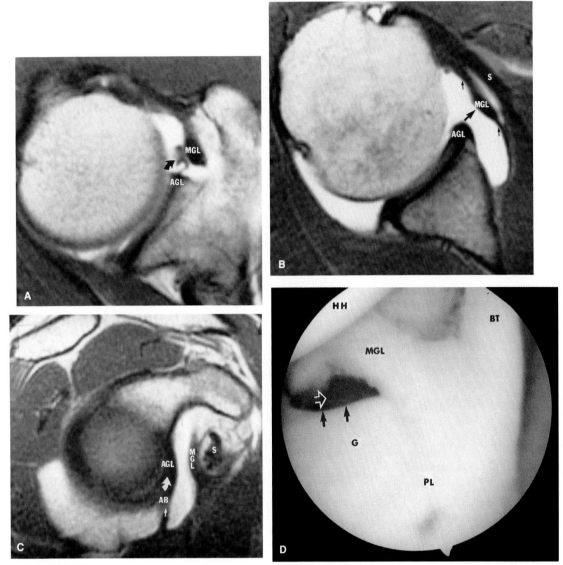

FIGURE 6–97. T1-weighted enhanced axial images (**A**) at the level of the coracoid and (**B**) inferior to the coracoid at the level of the subscapularis tendon, display a cordlike middle glenohumeral ligament (MGL). (*Curved arrow,* filamentous attachment to cordlike MGL; *large straight arrow,* cordlike portion of MGL; *small straight arrows,* thin portion of MGL; AGL, anterior glenoid labrum.) (**C**) The corresponding T1-weighted enhanced sagittal oblique image shows the relationship of the MGL to the anterior band of the IGL (AB; *straight arrow*); the anterior glenoid labrum (AGL; *curved arrow*); the middle glenohumeral ligament (MGL); and the subscapularis tendon (S). The MGL is located in the plane between the subscapularis tendon and the anterior band of the IGL or anterior glenoid labrum. (**D**) An arthroscopic view of cordlike MGL is shown. The anterior superior glenoid edge (*black arrows*) shows an absence of the labrum as a normal variant in association with prominent MGL. The MGL originates from the anteromedial femoral neck and attaches medially on the glenoid (G) and the neck of the scapula. (*Open arrow,* subscapularis recess; BT, biceps tendon; HH, humeral head; PL, posterior labrum.)

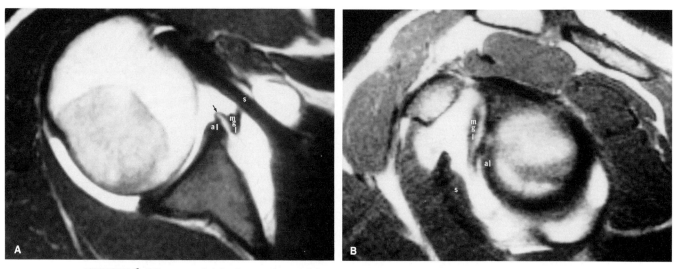

FIGURE 6–98. Pseudolabral tear. The cordlike middle glenohumeral ligament (MGL; mgl) simulates the appearance of a torn anterior labrum (al) on gadolinium-enhanced T1-weighted (**A**) axial and (**B**) sagittal oblique images. Filamentous attachment of the MGL to the anterior labrum (*black arrow*) and subscapularis tendon (s) are shown.

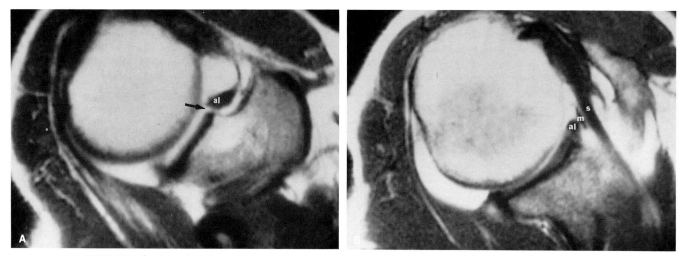

FIGURE 6–99. (**A, B**) Enhanced T1-weighted axial images show the superior wedge labrum with a firm attachment between the anterior labrum (al) and the glenoid articular surface at the level of the subscapularis tendon (s). No free central edge of the labrum is present. Normal separation of the labrum from the anterior superior glenoid rim creates a sublabral foramen (*arrow*). (m, middle glenohumeral ligament.)

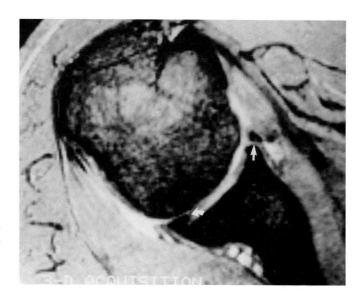

FIGURE 6–100.   Normal high signal intensity hyaline cartilage is seen where the small anterior labrum is firmly attached to the glenoid (*straight arrow*) on a 1-mm 3DFT axial T2*-weighted image. The wedge-shaped posterior labrum overlaps the articular surface and has a free central margin (*curved arrow*).

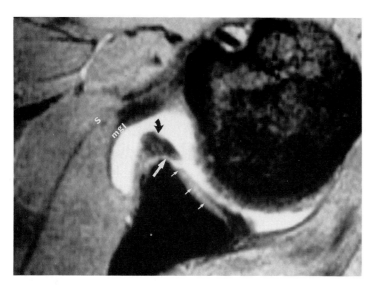

FIGURE 6–101.   Differentiating between the anterior labral tear and the anterior wedge labrum. A T2*-weighted axial image demonstrates high signal intensity fluid (*large white arrow*) undermining the detached anterior labrum (*curved black arrow*). The glenoid articular cartilage is shown tapering to the periphery at the anterior glenoid rim (*small white arrows*). Internal rotation of the humeral head results in a prominent subscapularis bursa, but no capsular stripping. An anterior wedge labrum is characterized by a large anterior band at the inferior glenohumeral ligament that replaces the anterior labrum or is associated with a hypoplastic labrum. The anterior wedge labrum could be mistaken for a labral tear, because fluid is seen beneath the free edge of the anterior band. (mgl, middle glenohumeral ligament; S, subscapularis tendon.)

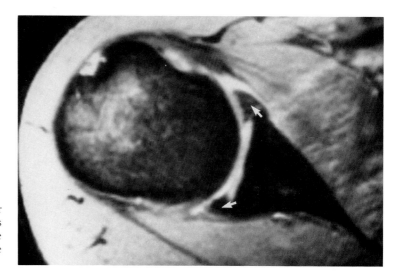

FIGURE 6–102.   Meniscal labrum. Anterior and posterior labra have symmetric meniscal morphology (*arrows*). This type of labrum has a free central margin around the entire periphery of the glenoid, usually above the epiphyseal line of the glenoid.

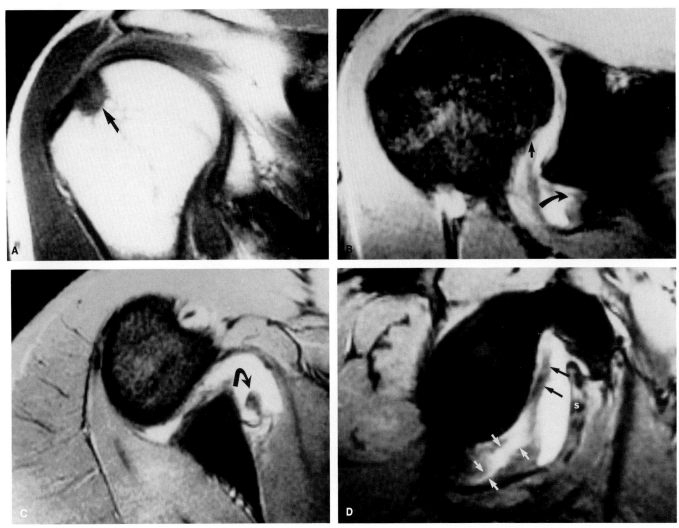

FIGURE 6–103. Traumatic anterior dislocation. (**A**) A T1-weighted coronal oblique image shows a Hill–Sachs posterolateral compression fracture (*arrow*). (**B**) A T2*-weighted coronal oblique image demonstrates avulsion of the glenoid attachment of the inferior glenohumeral ligament (IGL; *curved arrow*), which results in a deformity of the axillary pouch. The humeral attachment of the IGL (*straight arrow*) is intact. (**C**) A T2*-weighted axial image shows the medial avulsion of the anterior band and labrum (*curved arrow*). (**D**) The avulsed and medially displaced anterior labrum (*black arrows*) is seen at the level of the coracoid on a sagittal T2*-weighted image. Tear of the axillary pouch and the lower portion of the anterior band is identified by a fluid-filled gap (*white arrows*). (s, subscapularis tendon.)

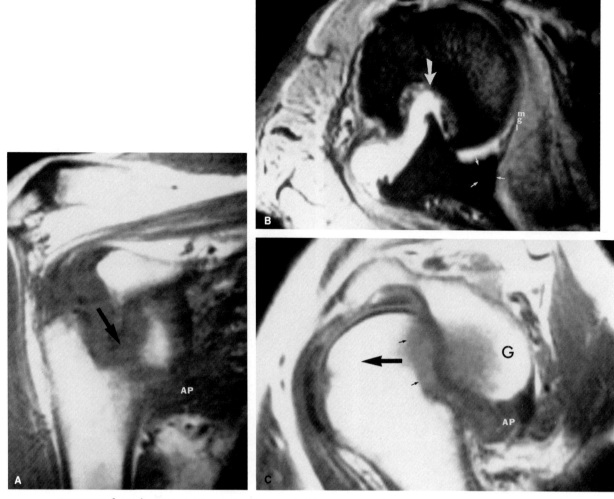

FIGURE 6–104. (**A**) A T1-weighted coronal oblique image shows anteromedial dislocation of the humeral head with a posterolateral Hill–Sachs fracture (*arrow*). Complete disruption of the axillary pouch (AP) of the inferior glenohumeral ligament has occurred. (**B**) A T2*-weighted axial image identifies the mechanism of the wedge-shaped impaction fracture (Hill–Sachs defect) as the impact of the posterolateral humeral head on the anteroinferior glenoid rim (*large arrow*). Associated osseous fragmentation is identified along the anterior surface at the scapular neck (*small arrows*). The middle glenohumeral ligament (mgl) is intact. (**C**) A T1-weighted sagittal oblique image shows anterior dislocation (*large arrow*) of the humeral head relative to the anterior glenoid (G). The Hill–Sachs fracture (*small arrows*) and torn axillary pouch (AP) are shown.

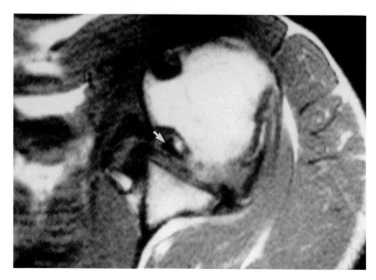

FIGURE 6–105. A fragmented anterior labrum trapped between the humeral head and glenoid (*arrow*) is revealed on a T1-weighted axial image.

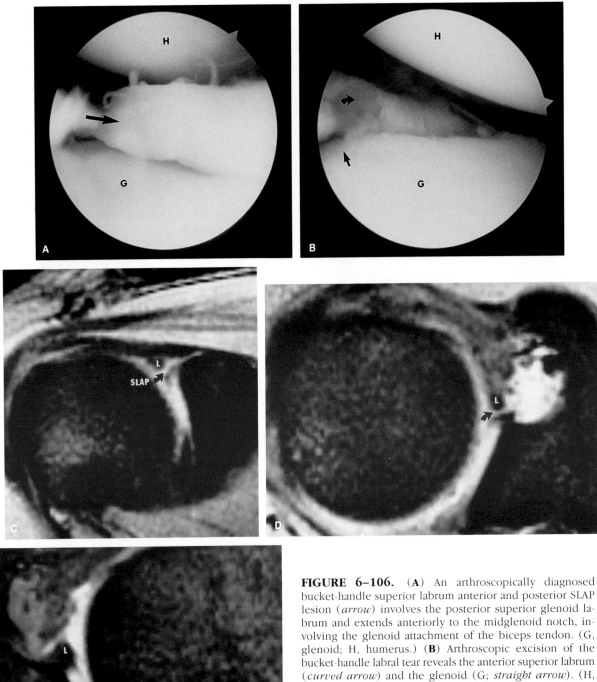

FIGURE 6–106. (**A**) An arthroscopically diagnosed bucket-handle superior labrum anterior and posterior SLAP lesion (*arrow*) involves the posterior superior glenoid labrum and extends anteriorly to the midglenoid notch, involving the glenoid attachment of the biceps tendon. (G, glenoid; H, humerus.) (**B**) Arthroscopic excision of the bucket-handle labral tear reveals the anterior superior labrum (*curved arrow*) and the glenoid (G; *straight arrow*). (H, humerus.) T2*-weighted (**C**) coronal oblique and (**D**) axial images show a SLAP lesion (*curved arrow*) that involves the anterior superior labrum (L) of the right shoulder. The avulsed labrum demonstrates linear high signal intensity, and extends completely across the base of the labrum. (**E**) A T2*-weighted axial image of the normal attachment of the anterior superior glenoid labrum (L) in the contralateral left shoulder is shown for comparison.

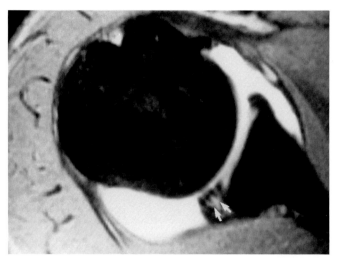

FIGURE 6–107. A T2*-weighted axial image shows multiple high signal intensity traumatic linear tears of the posterior labrum (*arrows*) in a baseball pitcher.

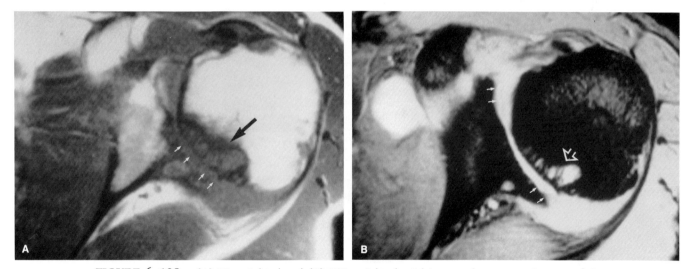

FIGURE 6–108. (**A**) T1-weighted and (**B**) T2*-weighted axial images show eccentric wear of the glenoid articular cartilage (*small arrows*). Subchondral degeneration sclerosis and cystic changes are seen in the posteriorly subluxed humeral head (*large arrow*). The posterior glenoid demonstrates decreased signal intensity in the posterior glenoid rim and is absent in the posterior labrum.

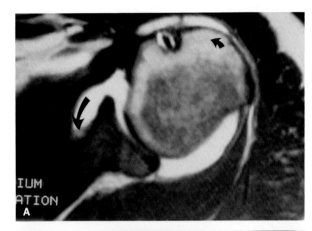

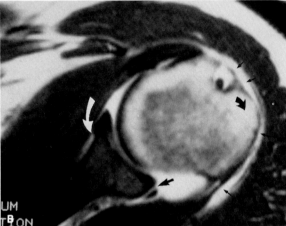

FIGURE 6–109. Normal variation in morphology of the subscapularis bursa is seen with (**A**) internal rotation and (**B**) external rotation on gadolinium-enhanced T1-weighted axial images. The subscapularis bursa has the appearance of a type 3 capsular insertion (*long black curved arrow*) in internal rotation (*short black curved arrow*) and a type 1 capsular insertion (*long curved white arrow*) in external rotation (*short black curved arrow*). Gadolinium contrast between the posterior band of the inferior glenohumeral ligament and the posterior labrum (*large straight black arrow*) and gadolinium contrast lateral to the humeral head in the subacromial bursa (*small straight black arrows*) are indicated.

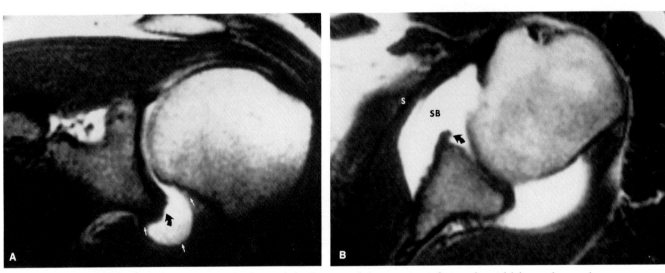

FIGURE 6–110. Anterior labral tear. (**A**) Blunting of the anterior inferior glenoid labrum (*curved arrow*) is seen on an enhanced T1-weighted coronal oblique image. Note that the anterior superior labrum is normally more wedge-shaped than the anterior inferior labrum. The axillary pouch of the inferior glenohumeral ligament (IGL) is shown (*small straight arrows*). (**B**) Partial detachment of the anterior labrum (*curved arrow*) is shown on an enhanced T1-weighted axial image. The subscapularis bursa (SB) is distended (S, subscapularis tendon). (**C**) A tear of the anterior labrum is seen (*small black arrows*) on an enhanced T1-weighted sagittal image. The axillary pouch (*curved white arrow*) and anterior band (ab) of the IGL are also shown.

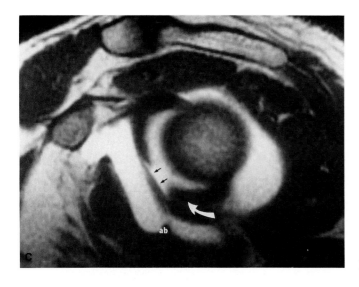

FIGURE 6–110. *(Continued)*

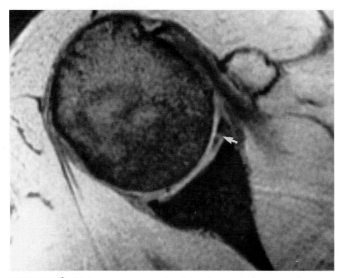

FIGURE 6–111. A T2*-weighted axial image shows surface extension of an anterior labral tear oriented perpendicular to the face of the glenoid (*arrow*).

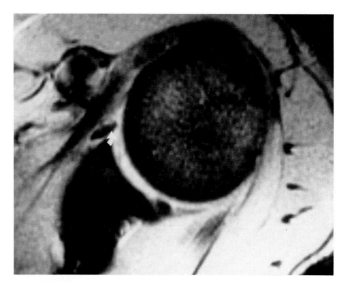

FIGURE 6–112. On a T2*-weighted axial image, a detached anterior labrum (*curved arrow*) should not be mistaken for the middle glenohumeral ligament.

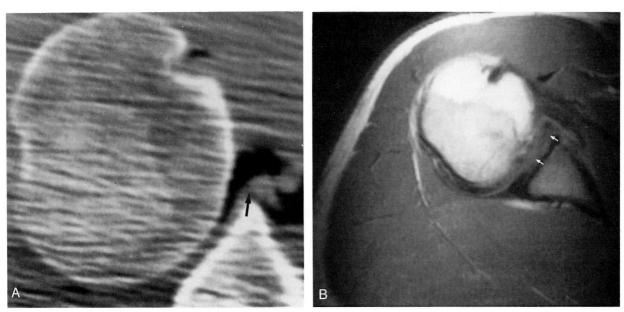

FIGURE 6–113. (**A**) Air contrast CT shows an anterior labral tear (*arrow*). (**B**) The corresponding T1-weighted axial image shows increased signal intensity in the labral tear (*arrows*).

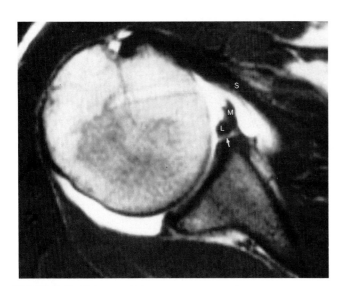

FIGURE 6–114. Gadolinium contrast undermines an anterior labral tear (*arrow*). This image was made at the level of the subscapularis tendon, inferior to the coracoid, and thus cannot represent a sublabral foramen. (L, anterior labrum; M, middle glenohumeral ligament; S, subscapularis tendon.)

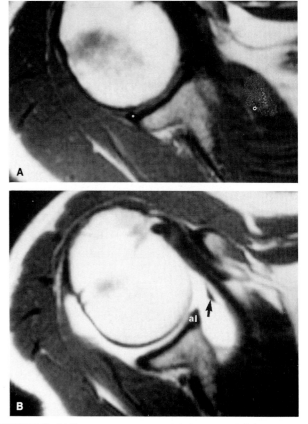

FIGURE 6–115. A comparison of (**A**) pre- and (**B**) post-gadolinium-enhanced T1-weighted axial images shows that improved identification of the anterior labrum (al) and the middle glenohumeral ligament is possible (*arrow*) on the enhanced image.

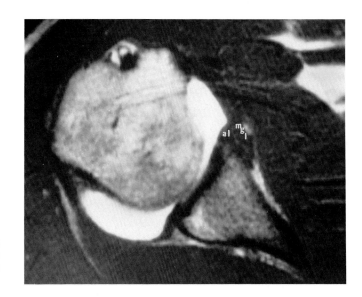

FIGURE 6–116. An enhanced T1-weighted axial image displays a middle glenohumeral ligament (mgl) that is closely applied to the anterior labrum (al), creating the appearance of an enlarged anterior labrum.

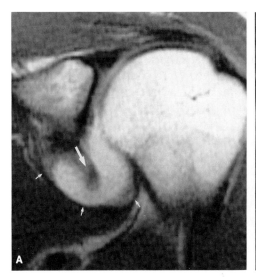 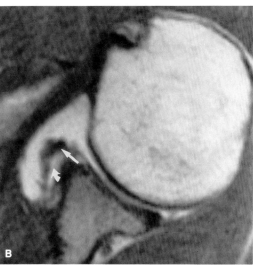

FIGURE 6–117. Labral tear. An avulsed anterior labrum (*large straight arrows*) can be seen on gadolinium-enhanced T1-weighted coronal (**A**) oblique and (**B**) axial images. Note the distended axillary pouch of the inferior glenohumeral ligament (*small straight arrows*). Contrast undermines the base of the detached labrum (*curved arrow*).

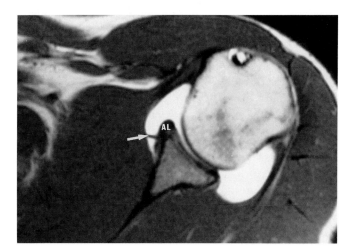

FIGURE 6–118. The synovial shelf (*arrow*) in the subscapularis bursa as it appears on a gadolinium-enhanced T1-weighted axial image. (AL, anterior labrum.)

of hydroxyapatite are seen in various views in conventional radiographs. Formation of calcific deposits in the tendinous portion of the rotator cuff is a degenerative process. The calcific build up can be extremely painful and act almost as a internal furuncle. Calcific tendinitis may exist in a subclinical or silent phase with deposits limited to the tendons of the rotator cuff (Figs. 6–120 and 6–121). In the mechanical or clinical phase, there may be elevation of the subacromial bursa as the foci of calcification increase in size.[80,81] Subbursal and intrabursal rupture may subsequently develop, with the extrusion of calcific deposits into the subacromial–subdeltoid bursa (Fig. 6–122).

Adhesive periarthritis is associated with adhesive bursitis as a complication of the tendinous calcific deposits. Nodular deposits of calcium hydroxyapatite crystals demonstrate low signal intensity on T1-, T2-, or T2*-weighted images.[82] Bursitis, or an acute inflammatory reaction with the crystal deposits in a more semiliquid state, demonstrates a more heterogeneous hyperintensity with associated scattered foci of signal void on T2- or T2*-weighted images.[83] A subacromial decompression is usually performed, along with excision and removal of the calcific deposits by dissection and debridement.

Biceps Tenosynovitis and Related Pathology

Biceps tenosynovitis, or inflammation of the biceps tendon, can be the result of trauma when it occurs in the intraarticular or extraarticular portion; however, it is most frequently a degenerative process, with inflammation occurring in the bicipital groove. Magnetic resonance frequently shows increased fluid, nonspecific for inflammation, in the biceps synovial sheath. Normally, communication exists between the joint capsule and the biceps tendon synovial sheath. Intrinsic hyperintensity may be a more specific finding for biceps tendon inflammation (Fig. 6–123) than fluid in the biceps tendon synovial sheath. Tenosynovitis demonstrates low signal intensity on T1-weighted images and high signal intensity on T2-weighted images.[84] Comparison with the opposite shoulder may be useful in assessing the significance of tendon inflammation. The Yergason test, in which forced supination produces pain in the biceps groove, is helpful in distinguishing biceps tendinitis from rotator cuff impingement. The biceps tendon lies within its groove, which makes it difficult to palpate; in fact, it is impossible to palpate the tendon in its intracapsular, intraarticular portion. The Yergason test is useful because it isolates the biceps tendon and places it under stress without placing any stress on the infraspinatus, supraspinatus, or subscapularis tendons.

Biceps tenodesis in the bicipital groove is the treatment of choice in biceps tendinitis. If tenodesis is performed prior to rupture, the tendon and muscle are fixed under proper tension and the function of the biceps muscle as well as the long head of the biceps muscle is maintained. Some controversy exists regarding whether this fixation compromises the stabilizing aspect of the glenohumeral ligament labral complex, but chronic biceps tendinitis generally occurs in older patients who are not prone to recurrent instability, therefore the use of biceps tenodesis is not usually contraindicated.

Biceps tendinitis and tenosynovitis are the earliest phases of biceps disease. Eventually, the biceps tendon may rupture and produce the classic ''Popeye'' muscle in the upper arm. Rupture of the long head of the biceps occurs in the bicipital groove. It is not approached surgically and it is best treated conservatively.

Biceps subluxations, although rare, can be seen in disease processes in which loss of the integrity of the rotator cuff has occurred or in which the biceps tendon loses the support structures that maintain it in its groove (*i.e.*, transverse ligament). The long head of the biceps tendon attaches to the supraglenoid tubercle and significantly contributes to the superior and posterior labrum. Portions of the long head fibers also support and form the anterior labrum. Internal and external rotation views in the axial plane may be useful in identifying patients with subluxation of the biceps tendon.

The dislocated biceps tendon is usually identified medial to the bicipital groove and can be seen on anterior coronal oblique, axial, and sagittal oblique images (Fig. 6–124).[85,86] Associated findings may include a shallow bicipital groove and tears of the coracohumeral ligament, subscapularis tendon, and supraspinatus tendon. The biceps tendon is located medial and anterior to the subscapularis tendon, with disruption of the transverse ligament and an intact subscapularis. The biceps tendon dislocates beneath the subscapularis tendon when associated tearing or degeneration of the subscapularis tendon insertion to the lesser tuberosity is present.

Biceps tendon ruptures occur at the top of the bicipital groove, are usually seen in patients older than 40 years of age, and are related to the spectrum of impingement (Fig. 6–125). Pure musculotendinous junction ruptures are rare and are associated with violent trauma. Neer classifies long ruptures into three types.

Type 1 is tendon rupture without retraction.
Type 2 is tendon rupture with partial recession
Type 3 is self-attaching rupture without retraction.

Clinical diagnosis of a self-attaching long head rupture without retraction is difficult prior to surgery, and these types of injuries are usually identified at the time of rotator cuff repair. Absence of the biceps tendon on axial images through the bicipital groove or on sagittal images is diagnostic (Fig. 6–126).

Fractures of the Proximal Humerus

Neer classifies upper humeral fractures into four segments:

1. Those involving the anatomic neck of the humerus
2. Those involving the greater tuberosity
3. Those involving the lesser tuberosity
4. Those involving the shaft or surgical neck of the humerus.[87]

A one-part fracture has either no displacement or angulation of any of the segments, or displacement and angulation are minimal (Fig. 6–127). A two-part fracture involves displacement of one segment. A three-part fracture involves displacement of two segments with an associated unimpacted surgical neck fracture with rotatory displacement. A four-part fracture is characterized by displacement of all four segments. Displacement is defined by fracture segment displacement of greater than 1 cm or angulation of more than 45°. Eighty percent of proximal humeral fractures have minimal or no displacement and are held together by the rotator cuff, capsule, and periosteum (Fig. 6–128). Magnetic resonance is particularly useful in identifying one-part or nondisplaced fractures not detected on conventional radiographs. Magnetic resonance also displays multiple fracture lines within any given segment (Fig. 6–129). The axial plane is important in assessing the location of the humeral head in more complex fracture–dislocations and in determining involvement of the glenohumeral joint. Short TI inversion recovery images are more sensitive than T2*-weighted protocols for the detection of areas of hemorrhage. T1-weighted images, however, adequately demonstrate the morphology of fracture segments and the congruity of articular cartilage surfaces.

Acromioclavicular Separations

There are three types of AC separations.

Type 1 is a sprain or incomplete tear of the AC joint capsule.
Type 2 represents a complete tear of the AC joint capsule with intact coracoclavicular ligaments.
Type 3 involves disruption of both the AC joint capsule and the coracoclavicular ligaments.

Widening of the AC joint space to 1.0 to 1.5 cm and a 25% to 50% increase in coracoclavicular distance is associated with tearing of the AC joint capsule and sprain of the coracoclavicular ligament (Fig. 6–130). Widening of the AC joint space to 1.5 cm or a 50% increase in the coracoclavicular distance correlates with coracoclavicular ligament disruption. Although the AC joint capsule and coracoclavicular ligaments can be directly assessed in the coronal and sagittal oblique planes, MR is usually not indicated in AC joint separations unless the status of the rotator cuff and glenoid labrum are in question.

Arthritis

Degenerative osteoarthritis of the glenohumeral joint is relatively common. It is characterized by cartilage-space narrowing, hypertrophic bone formation, subchondral cysts, and associated soft-tissue abnormalities of the rotator cuff (Figs. 6–131 through 6–133). Degenerative arthritis can be seen in younger patients, especially those who have had operative procedures for recurrent dislocation. Although the Bankart procedure and other capsular plication procedures prevent recurrent dislocation, they also significantly modify joint kinematics and may predispose the patient to degenerative joint disease. Secondary arthritis in younger patients eventually wears away the articular cartilage and produces significant joint incongruity, pain, and functional limitation. On T1-weighted images, loose bodies demonstrate the low signal intensity of sclerosis, the intermediate signal intensity of articular cartilage, or the high signal intensity of fat marrow (Fig. 6–134). Subchondral cysts with synovial fluid signal characteristics can be identified in either the distal clavicle or the acromial component of the AC joint as well as the glenohumeral joint (Fig. 6–135).

Avascular necrosis (AVN) of the humeral head can usually be differentiated from osteoarthritis by the restriction of subchondral low signal intensity ischemia (Fig. 6–136) to the humerus, without associated glenoid involvement (*i.e.,* sclerosis). Avascular necrosis of the humeral head is associated with trauma, steroid use, sickle-cell disease, and alcoholism. The Neer classification for AVN of the humerus is similar to the Ficat staging for hip osteonecrosis.[88] In stage 1, which may be asymptomatic, conventional radiographs are negative, whereas MR is positive for alterations in subchondral marrow. In stage 2 disease, which is clinically characterized by pain, the humeral head retains its spherical shape, although mild depression of the articular cartilage may be present in an area of subchondral bone. In stage 3 AVN, subchondral collapse or fracturing with overlying articular cartilage irregularity is seen. No involvement of the glenohumeral joint articular cartilage is found. Stage 4 disease leads to incongruity of the glenohumeral joint.

Rheumatoid disease of the shoulder, with its accompanying synovitis and aggressive synovial proliferation, targets the capsule of the rotator cuff and biceps tendon.[89] On T2*-weighted images, hyperplastic synovium with hemosiderin demonstrates dark signal intensity. Disruptions of the rotator cuff with loss of subacromial space are frequently demonstrated (Fig. 6–137).

(text continues on page 631)

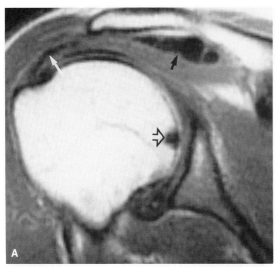

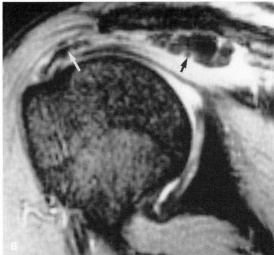

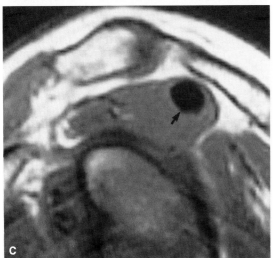

FIGURE 6–119. (**A**) T1-weighted coronal oblique, (**B**) T2*-weighted coronal oblique, and (**C**) T1-weighted sagittal oblique images show calcific tendinitis with low signal intensity calcium salt deposition in posterior supraspinatus muscle fibers (*black arrow*) and the infraspinatus tendon (*white arrow*). Infraspinatus involvement is best depicted on the T2*-weighted coronal oblique image. The etiology of calcific tendinitis may be related to local avascular changes and trauma. Calcium deposition may exist in a semiliquid form in the acute stage and as a more chalklike deposit in the chronic stages. Rotator cuff pathology and calcific tendinitis may exist independently. As calcific tendinitis progresses from the silent phase to the mechanical phase, the subacromial bursa may be elevated, followed by subbursal and then intrabursal rupture associated with pain. (*Open arrow,* subchondral sclerosis of the medial humeral head.)

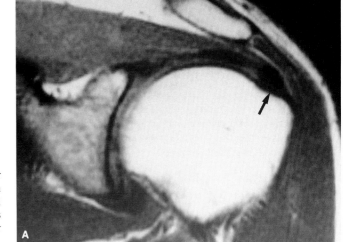

FIGURE 6–120. The subclinical or silent phase of periarticular calcium deposition (*arrows*) within the supraspinatus tendon is seen on (**A**) T1-weighted coronal oblique and (**B**) T2*-weighted axial images. (**C**) A T1-weighted coronal image in a different patient shows a calcific deposit (*large arrow*) with elevation of the bursal floor (*small arrows*) in the mechanical phase prior to subbursal rupture.

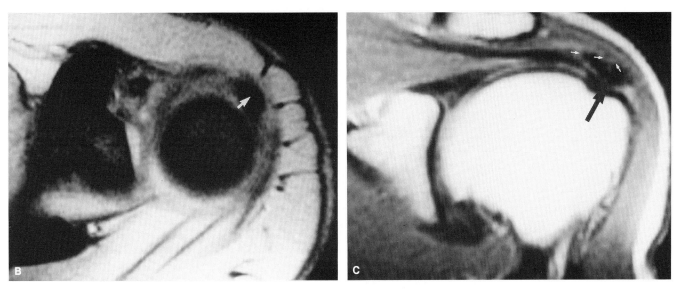

FIGURE 6–120. *(Continued)*

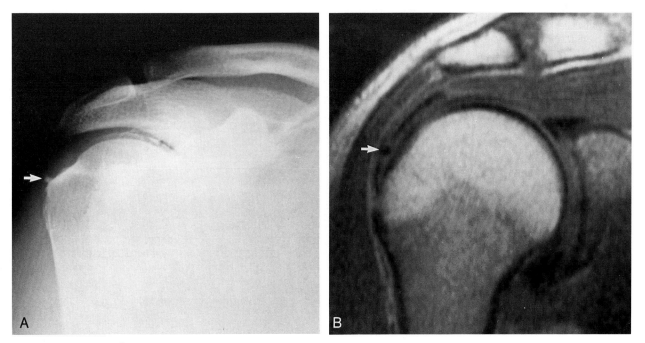

FIGURE 6–121. (**A**) On an anteroposterior radiograph, calcific density is seen in the region of the greater tuberosity (*arrow*) in a patient with calcific tendinitis. (**B**) On a T1-weighted coronal image, the calcification appears as a low signal intensity focus (*arrow*) in the supraspinatus–infraspinatus conjoined insertion.

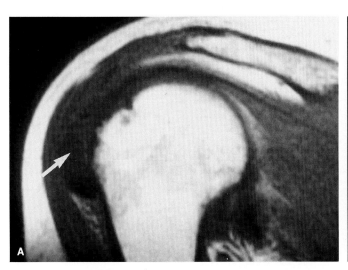

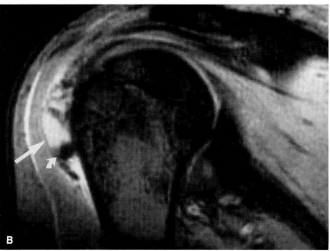

FIGURE 6–122. Low signal intensity bursal calcifications (*curved arrow*) and adjacent high signal intensity inflammatory fluid (*straight arrows*) are identified on posterior (**A**) T1-weighted and (**B**) T2*-weighted coronal oblique images in plane with the infraspinatus tendon. This finding represents the mechanical phase of calcific tendinitis with bursal extension.

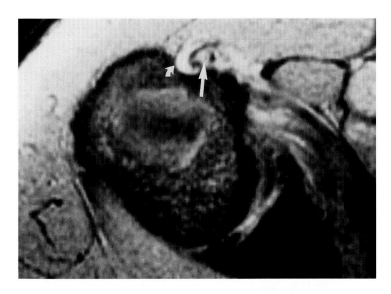

FIGURE 6–123. Bicipital tendinitis demonstrates high signal intensity in a T2*-weighted image and is centrally located within an enlarged biceps tendon (*straight arrow*). The finding of fluid in the biceps tendon sheath (*curved arrow*), however, is nonspecific, because the biceps tendon sheath normally communicates with the glenohumeral joint.

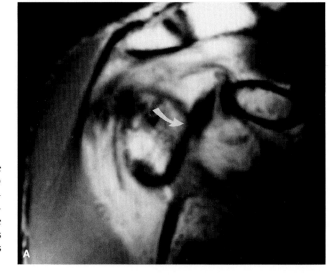

FIGURE 6–124. Dislocation of the tendon of the long head of the biceps medial to the bicipital groove (*curved arrows*) is seen on (**A**) T1-weighted coronal oblique, (**B**) T2*-weighted axial, and (**C**) T1-weighted sagittal oblique images. Degeneration and tearing of the insertion of the subscapularis tendon on the lesser tuberosity predispose the biceps to dislocate deep to the subscapularis tendon (S). There is complete rupture of the transverse ligament, which normally bridges the bicipital groove.

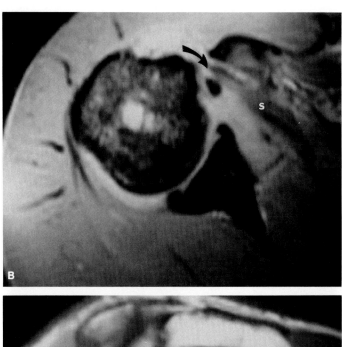

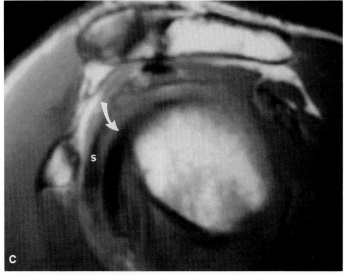

FIGURE 6–124. *(Continued)*

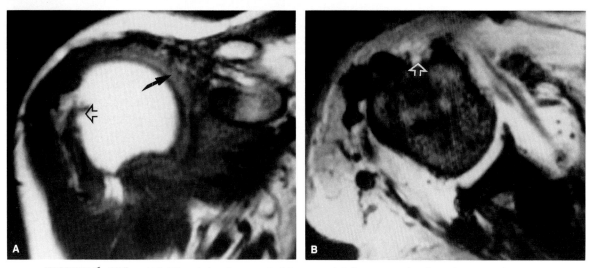

FIGURE 6–125. (**A**) T1-weighted coronal oblique and (**B**) T2*-weighted axial images show post-operative retear of the supraspinatus tendon (*solid arrow*) in association with a biceps tendon tear (*open arrows*). Retraction of the biceps occurs, and no tendon is identified in the bicipital groove at the level of the subscapularis tendon.

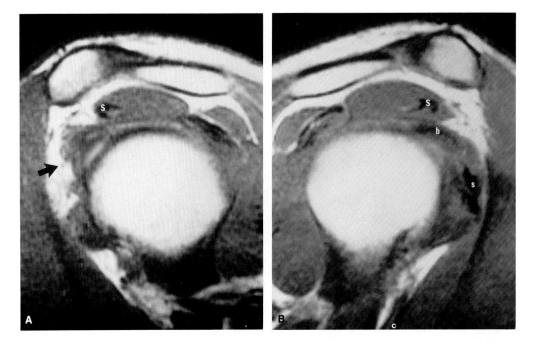

FIGURE 6–126. (**A**) A T1-weighted sagittal oblique image of the left shoulder and (**B**) a T1-weighted sagittal oblique image of the right shoulder show a tear of the left biceps (b) and subscapularis tendons (s; *arrow*). (S, supraspinatus tendon.)

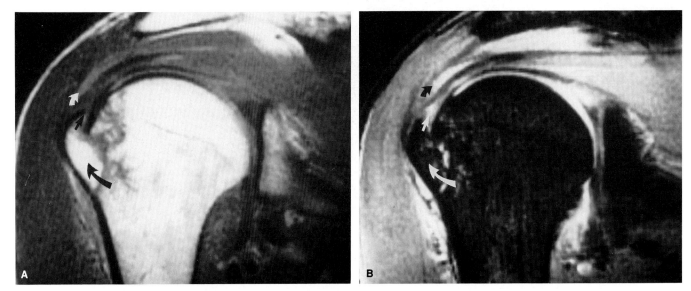

FIGURE 6–127. (**A**) T1-weighted and (**B**) T2*-weighted coronal oblique images show a greater tuberosity one-part fracture (*large curved arrows*) with an associated infraspinatus tendon tear (*straight arrows*). A small subacromial effusion is identified (*small curved arrows*). (**C**) On a T2*-weighted axial image, linear anterior labral tears (*arrows*) demonstrate high signal intensity.

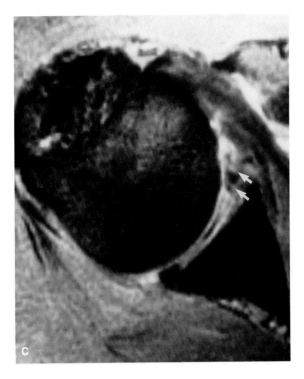

FIGURE 6–127. *(Continued)*

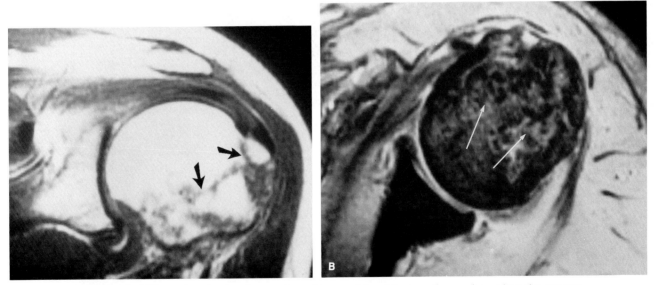

FIGURE 6–128. A nondisplaced comminuted humeral head fracture (*arrows*) involves the greater tuberosity, as seen on (**A**) T1-weighted coronal oblique and (**B**) T2*-weighted axial images.

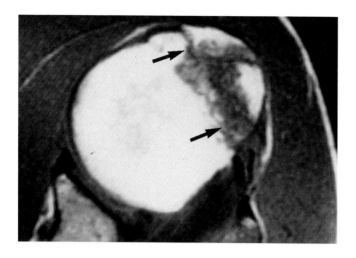

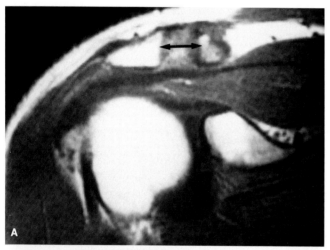

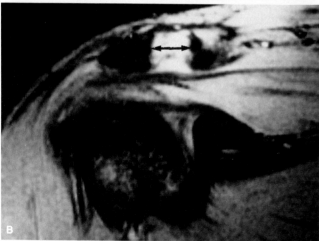

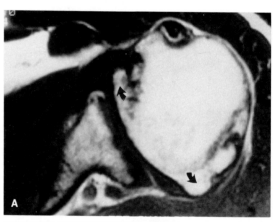

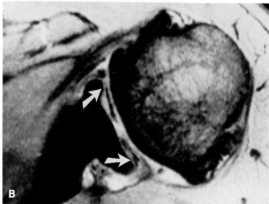

FIGURE 6–129. A T1-weighted axial image revealed a nondisplaced greater tuberosity fracture (*arrow*) in a downhill skier. The injury was not seen in conventional radiographs. A displaced fracture of the greater tuberosity may cause impingement even in the presence of a normal supraspinatus outlet.

FIGURE 6–130. (**A**) T1-weighted and (**B**) T2*-weighted coronal oblique images show a type 2 (*i.e., moderate sprain*) acromioclavicular separation (*double-headed arrows*) with widening of the acromioclavicular joint space to 10 mm. The normal acromioclavicular joint space is 3–8 mm.

FIGURE 6–131. Osteophytosis (*curved arrows*) and attenuated articular cartilage (*straight arrows*) are moderately advanced changes of osteoarthritis seen on (**A**) T1-weighted and (**B**) T2*-weighted axial images.

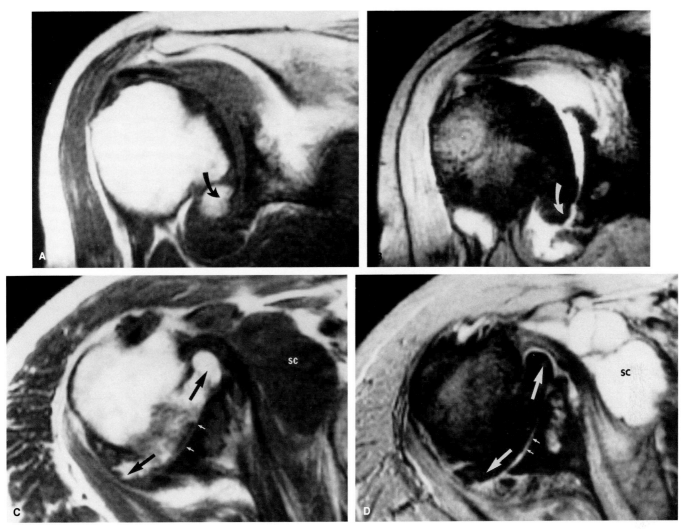

FIGURE 6–132. Advanced osteoarthritis can cause anterior and posterior osteophytosis (*large arrows and curved arrows*), denuded articular cartilage (*small arrows*), a macerated labrum, subchondral sclerosis, and cystic degeneration as seen on (**A**) a T1-weighted coronal oblique image; (**B**) a T2*-weighted coronal oblique image; (**C**) a T1-weighted axial image; and (**D**) a T2*-weighted axial image. (SC, subcoracoid fluid collection.)

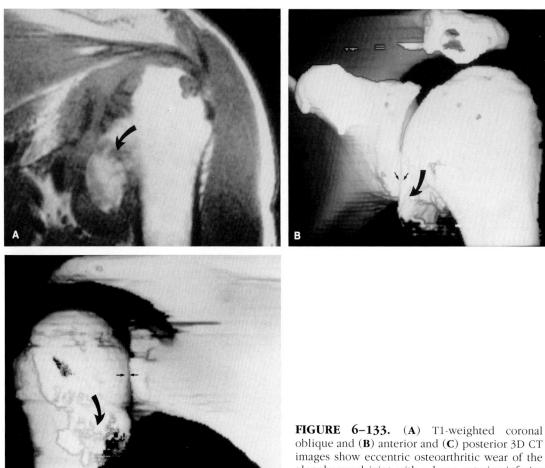

FIGURE 6–133. (**A**) T1-weighted coronal oblique and (**B**) anterior and (**C**) posterior 3D CT images show eccentric osteoarthritic wear of the glenohumeral joint with a large anterior inferior osteophyte (*curved arrows*) and preferential narrowing (*arrows*) of the anterior joint space.

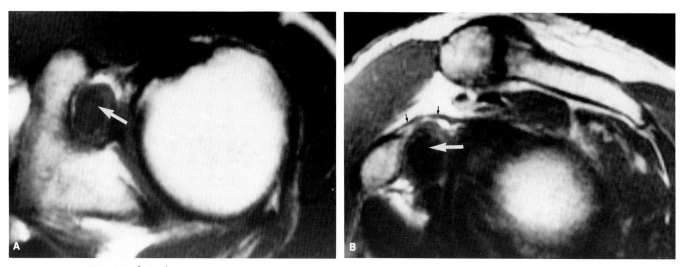

FIGURE 6–134. T1-weighted (**A**) axial and (**B**) sagittal oblique images reveal a large osseous fragment (*large arrows*) located lateral and posterior to the coracoid. Note the overlying coracohumeral ligament (*small arrows*).

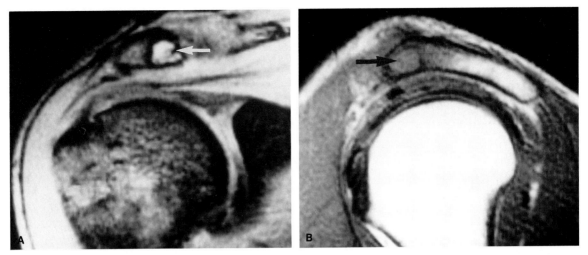

FIGURE 6–135. An acromial subchondral cyst (*arrow*) is seen in the acromioclavicular joint. (**A**) T2*-weighted coronal oblique and (**B**) T1-weighted sagittal oblique images demonstrate hooked type 3 acromion.

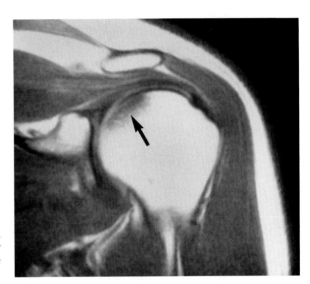

FIGURE 6–136. As shown on a T1-weighted coronal oblique image, avascular necrosis (*arrow*) of the humeral head with a focal region of low signal intensity is isolated to the humeral head and does not involve the glenoid.

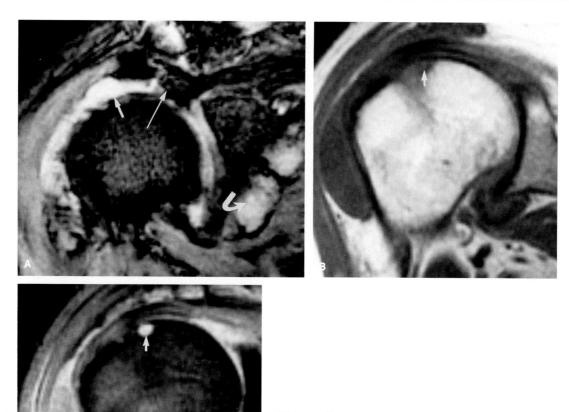

FIGURE 6–137. (**A**) Complete supraspinatus tendon tear with retraction (*long straight arrow*), subacromial fluid (*short straight arrow*), and synovitis (*curved arrow*) are seen on a T2*-weighted coronal oblique image in a patient with rheumatoid arthritis. (**B**) T1-weighted and (**C**) T2*-weighted coronal oblique images in a different patient with rheumatoid arthritis demonstrate subchondral erosion (*white arrows*) and intermediate signal intensity pannus tissue in the subacromial bursa (*black arrow*).

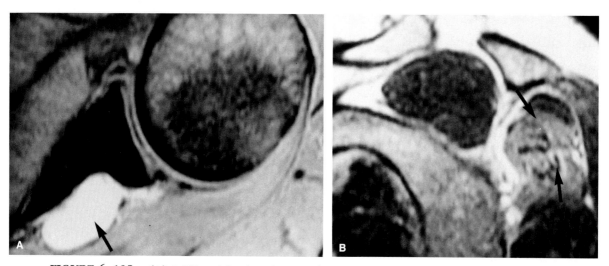

FIGURE 6–138. (**A**) A T2*-weighted axial image shows a large suprascapular ganglion (*arrow*) in the synovial fluid is compressing the suprascapular nerve. (**B**) Edema is restricted to the infraspinatus muscle, as seen on a T2-weighted sagittal image (*arrows*).

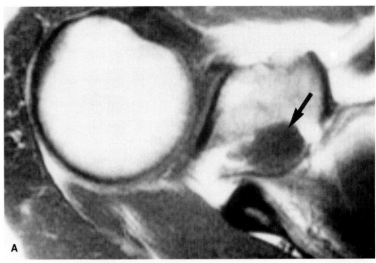

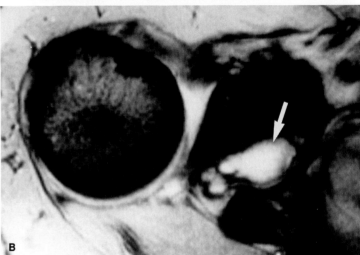

FIGURE 6–139. A suprascapular ganglion (*arrows*) demonstrates (**A**) low signal intensity on a T1-weighted axial image and (**B**) high signal intensity on a T2*-weighted axial image. There is mild fatty atrophy of the distal infraspinatus.

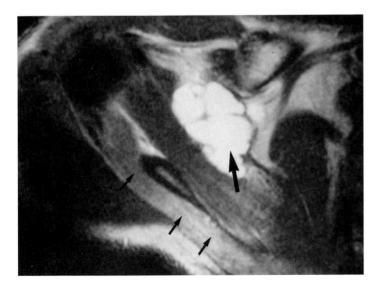

FIGURE 6–140. A T2-weighted axial image shows a suprascapular ganglion (*large arrow*) with fatty atrophy (*small arrows*) of the infraspinatus muscle.

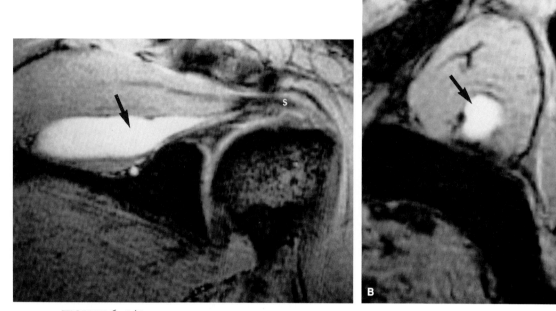

FIGURE 6–141. A supraspinatus intramuscular hemorrhage (*arrows*), which occurred secondary to weight-lifting trauma, is hyperintense on (**A**) T2*-weighted coronal oblique and (**B**) sagittal oblique images. (S, supraspinatus tendon.)

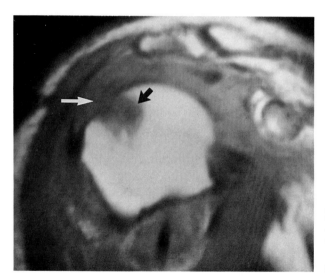

FIGURE 6–142. On a T1-weighted image, staphylococcal osteomyelitis of the right humeral head is a focus of intermediate signal intensity that transgresses cortical and trabecular bone (*black arrow*). Purulent fluid in the glenohumeral joint and subacromial–subdeltoid bursa obscures the rotator cuff insertion (*white arrow*).

Ganglions

Synovium-filled cystic ganglions involving the supra-scapular notch produce two patterns in the infraspinatus muscle secondary to suprascapular nerve compression. In the initial stage of suprascapular nerve compression, edematous changes of the infraspinatus are characterized by low to intermediate signal intensity on T1-weighted images and hyperintensity on T2- or T2*-weighted images (Fig. 6–138). Chronic compression may lead to the development of associated fatty muscle atrophy (Figs. 6–139 and 6–140). Intramuscular hemorrhage may mimic the appearance of a synovial ganglion (Fig. 6–141).

Infection

A septic joint may be associated with effusion and joint debris. Osteomyelitis may be associated with bone marrow or subchondral involvement, which demonstrate low signal intensity on T1-weighted images and high signal intensity on T2-weighted images (Fig. 6–142).

REFERENCES

1. Mink JH, Harris E, Rappaport M. Rotator cuff tears: evaluation using double contrast shoulder arthrography. Radiology 1985;157:621.
2. Rafii M, et al. Athlete shoulder injuries: CT arthrographic findings. Radiology 1987;162:559.
3. Rafii M, et al. CT arthrography of capsular structures of the shoulder. AJR 1986;146:361.
4. Resnick CS. The shoulder. In: Scott WW Jr, Majid D, Fishman EK, eds. Contemporary issues in computed tomography—CT of the musculoskeletal system. New York: Churchill-Livingstone, 1987:139.
5. Middleton WE, et al. Sonographic detection of rotator cuff tears. AJR 1985;144:349.
6. Crass DR, Craig EV, Feinberg SB. Sonography of the post-operative rotator cuff. AJR 1986;146:561.
7. Mack LA, et al. US evaluation of the rotator cuff. Radiology 1985;157:205.
8. Vick CW, et al. Rotator cuff tears: diagnosis with sonography. AJR 1990;154:121.
9. Middleton WD, et al. High resolution MR imaging of the normal rotator cuff. AJR 1987;148:559.
10. Middleton WD, et al. High resolution surface coil magnetic resonance imaging of the joints: anatomic correlation. Radiographics 1987;7:645.
11. Kieft GJ, et al. Magnetic resonance imaging of glenohumeral joint diseases. Skeletal Radiol 1987;16:285.
12. Huber DJ, et al. MR imaging of the normal shoulder. Radiology 1986;158:405.
13. Seeger LL, et al. MR imaging of the normal shoulder: anatomic correlation. AJR 1987;148:83.
14. Kieft GJ, et al. Normal shoulder: MR imaging. Radiology 1986;159:741.
15. Zlatkin MR, et al. Magnetic resonance imaging of the shoulder. Magn Reson Quart 1989;5(1):3-22.
16. Burk DL Jr, et al. Rotator cuff tears: prospective comparison of the MR imaging with arthrography, sonography, and surgery. AJR 1989;153(1):87.
17. Zlatkin MB, et al. Rotator cuff tears: diagnostic performance of MR imaging. Radiology 1989;172:223.
18. Seeger LL. Magnetic resonance imaging of the shoulder. Clin Orthop 1989;244:48.
19. Evancho AM, et al. MR imaging diagnosis of rotator cuff tears. AJR 1988;151:751.
20. Masciocchi C, et al. Magnetic resonance imaging of the shoulder: technique, anatomy, and clinical results. Radiol Med (Torino) 1989;78(5):485.
21. Tsai NC, et al. Magnetic resonance imaging of the shoulder. Radiol Clin North Am 1990;28(2):279.
22. Holt RG, et al. Magnetic resonance imaging of the shoulder: rationale and current applications. Skeletal Radiol 1990;19(1):5.
23. Meyer SJ, et al. MRI of the shoulder. Semin US CT MR 1990;11:253.
24. O'Brien SJ, et al. The anatomy and histology of the inferior glenohumeral ligament complex of the shoulder. Am J Sports Med 1990;18(5):449.
25. Neer CS. Shoulder reconstruction. Philadelphia: WB Saunders, 1990:1.
26. Moseley HF, et al. The anterior capsular mechanism in recurrent anterior dislocation of the shoulder. J Bone Joint Surg [Br] 1962;44:913,
27. Detrisac DJ, Johnson LL. Arthroscopic shoulder anatomy: pathologic and surgical implications. Thorofare, NJ: Slack, 1986.
28. Schwartz RE, et al. Capsular restraints to anterior-posterior motion of the shoulder. Trans Orthop Res Soc 1987;12:78.
29. DePalma AF. Surgery of the shoulder. Philadelphia: JB Lippincott, 1983.
30. Neer CS II, et al. Inferior capsular shift for involuntary inferior and multidirectional instability of the shoulder. A preliminary report. J Bone Joint Surg [Am] 1980;62:897.
31. McMinn RMH. Last's anatomy: regional and applied. 8th ed. Edinburgh: Churchill-Livingston, 1990:53.
32. Neer CS. Shoulder reconstruction. Philadelphia: WB Saunders, 1990:41.
33. Naimark A, Baum A. Injection of the subcoracoid bursa: a cause of technical failure in shoulder arthrography. J Canad Assoc Radiol 1989;40:170.
34. Horwitz TM, Tocantins LM. An anatomical study of the role of the long thoracic nerve and the related scapular bursae in the pathogenesis of local paralysis of the serratus anterior muscle. Anat Rec 1938;71:375.
35. Seeger LH, et al. Shoulder impingement syndrome: MR findings in 53 shoulders. AJR 1988;150:343.
36. Brems J. Rotator cuff tear: evaluation and treatment. Orthopaedics 1988;11:69,
37. Ellman H. Shoulder arthroscopy: current indications and techniques. Orthopaedics 1988;11:45.
38. Kleft GJ, et al. Rotator cuff impingement syndrome: MR imaging. Radiology 1988;166:211.
39. Neer CS. Anterior acromioplasty for the chronic impingement syndrome: a preliminary report. J Bone Joint Surg [Am] 1972;54:41.
40. Neer CS, et al. Rupture of the long head of the biceps related to subacromial impingement. Orthop Trans 1977;1:111.
41. Bigliani LU, Morrison DS. Subacromial impingement syndrome. In: Dee R, ed. Principles of orthopaedic practice. New York: McGraw-Hill, 1989:627.
42. Rathbun JB, Macnab I. The microvascular pattern of the rotator cuff. J Bone Joint Surg [Br] 1970;52:540.
43. Bigliani LU, et al. The morphology of the acromion and its relationship to rotator cuff tears. Orthop Trans 1986;10:216.
44. Ozaki J, et al. Tears of the rotator cuff of the shoulder associated

with pathologic changes in the acromion. J Bone Joint Surg [Am] 1988;70:1224.

45. Aoki M, Ishii S, Usui M. The slope of the acromion and rotator cuff impingement. Proc Am Shoulder Elbow Surg 1986.

46. Crues JV, Hyer ICC. MRI of the shoulder. Contemp Diagn Radiol 1990;13(4):1.

47. Neer CS, et al. The relationship between the unfused acromion epiphysis and subacromial impingement lesions. Orthop Trans 1983;7:138.

48. Mudge MK, et al. Rotator cuff tears associated with os acromiale. J Bone Joint Surg [Am] 1984;66:427.

49. Kieft GJ, et al. Rotator cuff impingement syndrome. MR imaging. Radiology 1988;166(1):211.

50. Zlatkin MB. MR Imaging of the shoulder: current experience and future trends. In: Kressel, HY, Modic MT, Murphy WA, eds. Syllabus special course MR. Oak Brook, IL: RSNA Publications, 1990:255.

51. Rafii M, et al. Rotator cuff lesions: signal patterns at MR imaging. Radiology 1990;177:817.

52. Kjellin I, et al. Alterations in the supraspinatus tendon at MR imaging: correlation with histopathologic findings and cadavers. Radiology 1991;181:837.

53. Mitchell MJ, et al. Peribursal fat plane of the shoulder: anatomic study and clinical experience. Radiology 1988;168:699.

54. Neer CS, Craig EU, Fukuda H. Cuff-tear arthropathy. J Bone Joint Surg [Am] 1985;65:1232.

55. Morrison DS, et al. The use of magnetic resonance imaging in the diagnosis of rotator cuff tears. Orthopedics 1990;13(6):633.

56. Buiriski G. Magnetic resonance imaging in acute and chronic rotator cuff tears. Skeletal Radiol 1990;19(2):109.

57. Iannotti JP, et al. Magnetic resonance imaging of the shoulder: sensitivity, specificity and predictive value. J Bone Joint Surg [Am] 1991;73(1):17.

58. Zlatkin MB, et al. The painful shoulder: MR imaging of the glenohumeral joint. J Comput Assist Tomogr 1988;12(6):995.

59. Mirowitz SA. Normal rotator cuff: MR imaging with conventional and fat-suppression techniques. Radiology 1991;180:735.

60. Flannigan B, et al. MR arthrography of the shoulder. AJR 1990;155:829.

61. Turkel SJ, et al. Stabilizing mechanisms preventing anterior dislocation of the glenohumeral joint. J Bone Joint Surg [Am] 1981;63:1208.

62. Pollock RG, Bigliani LU. The mechanical properties of the inferior glenohumeral ligament. Presented at the American Shoulder and Elbow Surgeons Sixth Open Meeting, New Orleans, Louisiana, February 11, 1990.

63. Singson RD, et al. CT arthrographic patterns in recurrent glenohumeral instability. AJR 1987;149:749.

64. Seeger LL, et al. Shoulder instability: evaluation with MR imaging. Radiology 1988;168(3):685.

65. Gross ML, et al. Magnetic resonance imaging of the glenoid labrum. Am J Sports Med 1990;18(3):229.

66. Kieft GJ, et al. MR imaging of recurrent anterior dislocation of the shoulder: comparison with CT arthrography. AJR 1988;150(5):1083.

67. Zlatkin MB, et al. Cross-sectional imaging of the capsular mechanism of the glenohumeral joint. AJR 1988;150:151.

68. Schwartz E, et al. Posterior shoulder instability. Orthop Clin North Am 1987;18(3):409.

69. Neer CS. Shoulder reconstruction. Philadelphia: WB Saunders, 1990:273.

70. Zlatkin MB, et al. Evaluation of rotator cuff disease and glenohumeral instability with MR imaging: correlation with arthroscopy and arthrotomy in a large population of patients. [abstr] Magn Reson Imaging 1990;8(suppl 1):78.

71. Callaghan J, et al. A prospective comparison of double contrast computed tomography (CT), arthrography and arthroscopy of the shoulder. Am J Sports Med 1988;16:13.

72. Habibian A, et al. Comparison of conventional and computed arthrotomography with MR imaging in the evaluation of the shoulder. J Comput Tomogr 1989;13:968.

73. Munk P, et al. Glenoid labrum: preliminary work with use of radial-sequence MR imaging. Radiology 1989;73(3):751.

74. Caspari RB, et al. Shoulder arthroscopy: a review of the present state of the art. Contemp Orthop 1982;4:523.

75. Snyder SJ, et al. SLAP lesions of the shoulder. Arthroscopy 1990;6(4):274.

76. Hawkins RJ, Belle RM. Posterior instability of the shoulder. Instr Course Lect 1989;38:211.

77. Norwood LA, Terry GC. Shoulder posterior subluxation. Am J Sports Med 1984;12:25.

78. Wilson AJ. Shoulder joint: arthrographic CT and long-term follow-up with surgical correlation. Radiology 1989;173:329.

79. Beltran J, et al. Tendons: high-field strength, surface coil MR imaging. Radiology 1987;162:735.

80. Hayes CW, et al. Calcium hydroxyapatite deposition disease. RadioGraphics 1990;10(6):1032.

81. Resnick D. Calcium hydroxyapatite crystal deposition disease. In: Resnick D, Niwayama G, eds. Diagnosis of bone and joint disorders. 2nd ed. Philadelphia: WB Saunders, 1988:1733.

82. Burk DL, et al. MR imaging of the shoulder: correlation with plain radiography. AJR 1990;154:549.

83. Bigliani LU. Rheumatic and degenerative disorders. In: Dee R, ed. Principles of orthopaedic practice. New York: McGraw-Hill, 1989:621.

84. Kieft GJ, et al. Magnetic resonance imaging of the shoulder in patients with rheumatoid arthritis. Ann Rheum Dis 1990;49(1):7.

85. Chan TW, et al. Biceps tendon dislocation evaluation with MR imaging. Radiology 1991;179(3):649.

86. Cervilla V, et al. Medial dislocation of the biceps brachii tendon: appearance at MR imaging. Radiology 1991;180:523.

87. Neer CS. Shoulder reconstruction. Philadelphia: WB Saunders, 1990:363.

88. Neer CS. Shoulder reconstruction. Philadelphia: WB Saunders, 1990:194.

89. Sher M, et al. Case report 578: pigmented villonodular synovitis of the shoulder. Skeletal Radiol 1990;19(2):131.

CHAPTER 7

David W. Stoller

The Elbow

Magnetic resonance (MR) applications in the evaluation of the elbow joint are limited compared with that in the other appendicular joints. Technical obstacles include the complexity of designing a surface coil to accommodate the geometry and mechanics of elbow in extension and partial flexion (*i.e.,* position of injury on locking) and the development of positioning techniques that allow imaging of the elbow joint at the patient's side without placing the shoulder joint in extension.

Although computed tomography (CT) is superior for identification of corticated or osseous loose bodies in the elbow, MR is successful in characterizing occult radial head fractures, capitellar osteochondrosis and osteochondritis dissecans, soft-tissue lesions including tears of the distal biceps tendon and ligamentous trauma, and cubital tunnel and synovial disorders.[1-6] Cartilaginous loose bodies not visible on conventional radiography or CT are frequently detected on T2- or T2*-weighted MR scans. The usefulness of CT contrast arthrography is limited by the fact that, although pooled contrast media often delineates small cartilaginous lesions and fragments, it is not possible to identify the donor site. In addition, direct imaging of the anterior and posterior fat pads, not possible with CT, may be useful in cases of trauma and arthritis. Elbow joint pathology with limited flexion and extension or pronation and supination can be studied with kinematic MR imaging techniques when applicable.

IMAGING TECHNIQUES AND PROTOCOLS FOR THE ELBOW

Extremity Coils

With the patient in the supine position, the elbow is placed by the side. A wrist coil can be used to image the elbow when limited anatomic coverage is sufficient to characterize the specific anatomic and pathologic features. The small geometry of the wrist coil, however, limits evaluation of the partially flexed or locked elbow; in this situation a knee extremity coil provides the best anatomic coverage (Fig. 7–1). By detaching the base of the knee coil, the arm can be placed off-center by the patient's side for imaging. When the elbow is splinted or locked in extreme flexion, a shoulder coil may be used with the arm placed through the coil opening (see Fig. 7–1). It is possible to optimize space for range of motion in kinematic joint imaging, because the shoulder coil is noncircumferential. A paired set of surface coils also facilitates elbow imaging with the arm placed comfortably in extension or flexion.

Pulse Parameters

T1-weighted protocols, with a short TR and TE, are used in axial, coronal, and sagittal planes of the elbow. The axial plane demonstrates the anatomy of the proximal radioulnar joint, the olecranon, and the coronoid fossa, all of which are common locations for intraarticular loose bodies. The trochlear and capitellum of the distal humerus are shown on the same image in the coronal plane. The sagittal plane displays the longitudinal course and attachment of the biceps, brachialis, and triceps tendons. The anterior and posterior fat pads are identified proximal to the trochlea on sagittal images.

T2*-weighted images are obtained in the sagittal plane to evaluate tendon rupture and in the coronal plane in cases of ligamentous injury. Either T2*-weighted or conventional T2-weighted axial images are also obtained. It is important to remember that hypertrophied synovial fat may mimic the appearance of loose bodies, especially on T2*-weighted axial images. Alternatively, three-dimensional Fourier transform (3DFT) axial images can be reformatted in other orthogonal planes. Routine protocols use 3- to 4-mm slices and a 10- to 14-cm field of view.

GROSS ANATOMY

Osseous Anatomy and Capsule

The elbow is a synovial hinge joint between the trochlea and the capitellum of the humerus, articulating with the trochlear notch of the ulna and the radial head (Fig. 7–2).[7] The joint thus forms two primary articulations (*i.e.,* the humeroulnar and humeroradial) to form a compound synovial joint.[8] The superior, or proximal, radioulnar joint represents a separate articulation in communication with the elbow joint (Fig. 7–3). The elbow does not behave as a simple uniaxial hinge throughout the range of flexion and extension. Instead, there is a changing center of rotation with sliding of joint surfaces at the extremes of joint motion.

The trochlea has a grooved surface and a prominent distal projecting medial flange. The lateral aspect of the trochlea blends with the articular surface of the capitellum. The partial sphere-shaped capitellum and the radial head are reciprocally curved. In elbow flexion, fossae superior to the capitellum and trochlea accommodate the radial head and coronal process of the ulna. In extension, the deep olecranon fossa accommodates the olecranon process. The deep concave trochlear notch of

the ulna is formed by the connection of the posterior olecranon and anterior coronoid processes. This curved ridge articulates with the grooved trochlear surface. The medial and lateral extrasynovial epicondyles and the supracondylar ridges of the humerus function as attachment points for the flexor–pronator muscles and extensor–supinator muscles, respectively.

A 40° angle is produced by the humeral shaft and the forward tilt of its condylar surfaces.[9] This relationship is important in supracondylar fractures in children and must be maintained by adequate reduction and forward angling of the trochlear ossification center. The oblique angle of the transverse axis of the epiphyses produces the carrying angle between the forearm and arm—approximately 160° in extension, adduction, and forearm supination.[9] Fracture deformity or physeal trauma may produce an accentuated carrying angle (*i.e.,* cubitus valgus) or a reverse of the carrying angle (*i.e.,* cubitus varus).

The anterior joint capsule is attached above the coronoid and radial fossae proximally, and to the coronoid process of the ulna and annular ligament encircling the radial head distally (Fig. 7–4). Posteriorly, the capsule attaches to the olecranon fossa proximally and the olecranon process of the ulna and annular ligaments distally (Fig. 7–5). The joint capsule and the annular ligament are lined by synovial membrane.

Collateral Ligaments

Medial Collateral Ligament

The triangular ulnar collateral, or medial, ligament of the elbow consists of three strong bands.[7,8] The anterior band is the strongest, and it extends from the medial epicondyle of the humerus to the medial aspect of the coronoid process in an area sometimes referred to as the sublime tubercle. The posterior band extends from the medial epicondyle of the humerus to the medial aspect or margin of the olecranon. The weaker transverse or oblique band bridges the ulnar attachments of the anterior and posterior bands.

Lateral Collateral Ligament

The triangular radial collateral, or lateral, ligament is a single band. Its apex is attached to the lateral epicondyle of the humerus and its base is attached to the upper margin of the annular ligament.[8]

Epiphysis

The epiphyseal–cartilage bone junction in the elbow is a point of structural weakness, susceptible to separation and displacement. The age of the patient and, more important, the relative sequence of identification of ossification centers is significant in recognizing epiphyseal injuries.[9] The epiphyseal maturation sequence proceeds in the following order:

1. Capitellum—1 year of age
2. Radial head—3 to 6 years of age
3. Medial epicondyle—5 to 7 years of age
4. Trochlea—9 to 10 years of age
5. Lateral epicondyle—9 to 13 years of age (Fig. 7–6).

The medial epicondyle is the last to fuse. Normally, the trochlear ossification center cannot be seen prior to the appearance of the medial epicondyle. Therefore, an avulsed and trapped medial epicondyle is diagnosed by the absence of the epicondyle coexistent with the presence of the trochlear ossification center.

Proximal Radioulnar Joint

The proximal, or superior, radioulnar joint is a synovial uniaxial pivot joint located between the circumference of the radial head and the osteofibrous ring; it consists of the annular ligament and the ulnar radial notch, otherwise known as the lesser sigmoid notch (Fig. 7–7).[8] The capsule of the radioulnar joint is continuous with the elbow joint. Pronation and supination (*i.e.,* rotatory motion) take place at the proximal and distal radioulnar joints, and each one prescribes an arc of 90°.

Annular Ligament

The annular ligament is the key structure of the proximal radioulnar joint encircling the radial head and neck without radial attachment. The radial head is thus free to rotate within the confines of the annular ligament.[7,8] The thin quadrate ligament supports the synovial membrane between the neck of the radius and ulna, distal to the radial notch. Crisscrossing fibers maintain ligament tension throughout supination and pronation. The annular ligament may become interposed between the radial head and the capitellum, causing subluxation of the radial head. This injury occurs before radial head ossification, and commonly presents at 2 years of age (Fig. 7–8).

MAGNETIC RESONANCE ANATOMY

Axial Images

Superior or proximal axial images (Fig. 7–9) demonstrate the anterior coronoid fossa and posterior olecranon fossa. Bright signal intensity fat within these fossa represent the anterior and posterior fat pads. The brachialis muscle is identified anteriorly, whereas the triceps muscle and tendon are located posterior to the distal humerus and olecranon. The low to intermediate signal intensity ulnar

nerve lies directly posterior to the medial epicondyle. The median nerve lies between the pronator teres and brachialis muscles anteriorly. Superficial and deep branches of the radial nerve are situated between the brachialis and brachioradialis muscles. Anterior to the brachialis muscle, the course of the biceps tendon can be followed. The distinctive medial flange of the trochlea and the prominence of the medial epicondyle are seen at the level of the distal humerus in the superior aspect of the elbow joint.

The thin, low signal intensity band of the medial collateral ligament is located distal to the medial epicondyle. The common extensor tendon, low in signal intensity, flanks the elbow lateral to the capitellum. The thin dark line of the bicipital aponeurosis may be seen anterior to and between the brachial artery and biceps tendon. The lateral collateral and annular ligaments are found at the level of the distal capitellum and proximal to the radial head. At the level of the radial head, the biceps tendon dives deep to insert into the posterior border of the tuberosity of the radius. The bicipital aponeurosis traverses the deep fascia of the forearm to insert on the medial aspect of the forearm (*i.e.,* proximal ulna).

The superior or proximal radioulnar joint is shown on axial images through the radial head. The radial head should be positioned within the concave semilunar notch of the ulna. The thin annular ligament, which secures the head of the radius, is of low signal intensity and can be differentiated from the intermediate signal intensity articular cartilage of the radial head.

A transverse line of low to intermediate signal intensity in the articular surface of the radial head represents a partial volume artifact, not a fracture. This can be confirmed by imaging the contralateral elbow.

The insertion of the biceps tendon on the radius and the brachialis tendon on the anterior surface of the coronoid process of ulna are seen distal to the proximal radioulnar joint. The brachial artery is seen as an area of signal void medial to the biceps and superficial to the brachialis muscles. Immediately distal to the elbow joint, the brachial artery divides into radial and ulnar branches.

Sagittal Images

Two of the three joints of the elbow, the trochlear–ulnar and the capitellar–radial head articulations, are defined on medial and lateral sagittal images, respectively (Fig. 7–10).[10] The conjoined insertion of the triceps muscle demonstrates low signal intensity at its attachment to the posterosuperior surface of the olecranon. The anconeus muscle, which extends from the medial epicondyle to the posterolateral olecranon, can be seen on either sagittal or axial images. The biceps and brachialis muscle

(text continues on page 657)

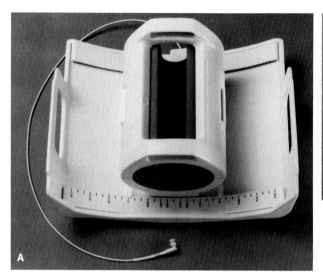

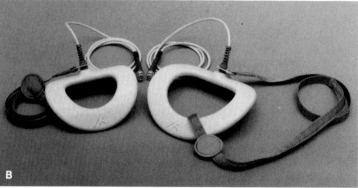

FIGURE 7–1. (**A**) An extremity coil can be adapted for use in imaging the elbow and the proximal radioulnar joint. (**B**) Shoulder coils are used in patients unable to extend the elbow for proper positioning in the knee coil.

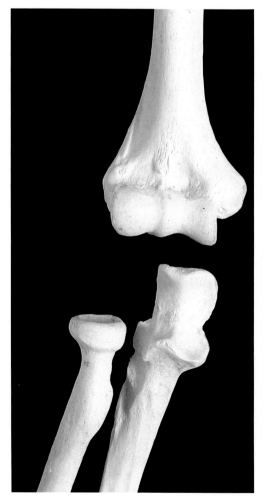

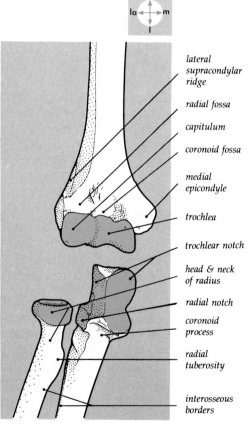

lateral
supracondylar
ridge

radial fossa

capitulum

coronoid fossa

medial
epicondyle

trochlea

trochlear notch

head & neck
of radius

radial notch

coronoid
process

radial
tuberosity

interosseous
borders

FIGURE 7–2. The bones that form the elbow and proximal radioulnar joints.

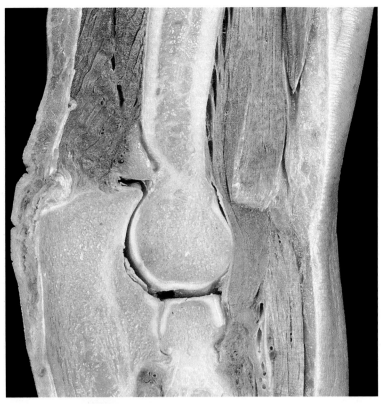

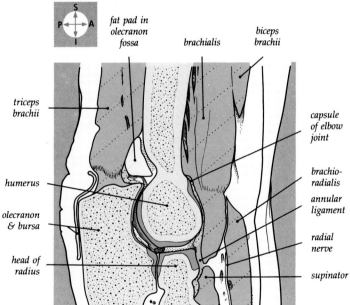

FIGURE 7–3. An oblique longitudinal section of the extended elbow and proximal radioulnar joints shows the articular surfaces and relations of the joints.

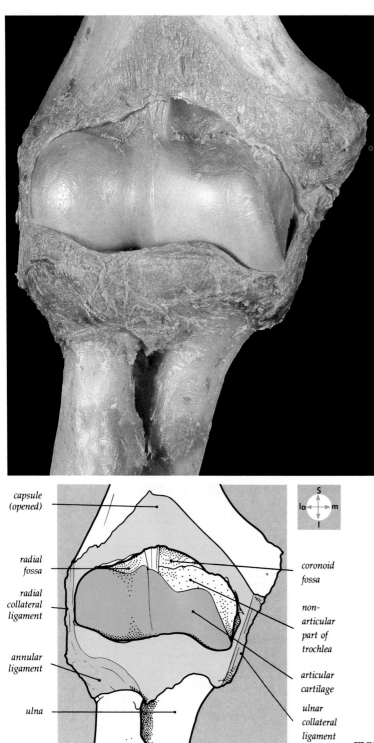

capsule (opened)

radial fossa

radial collateral ligament

annular ligament

ulna

coronoid fossa

non-articular part of trochlea

articular cartilage

ulnar collateral ligament

FIGURE 7–4. The anterior aspect of the elbow joint. The capsule has been opened to expose the interior of the joint.

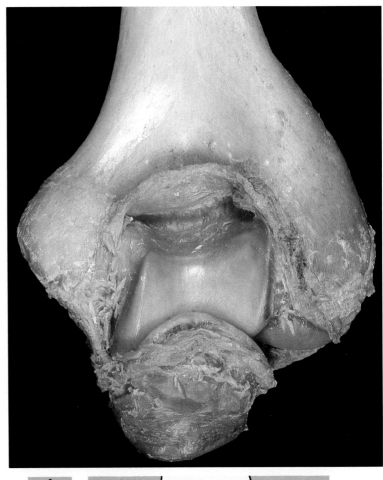

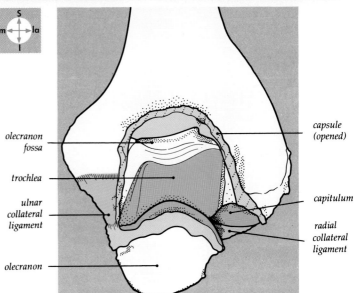

FIGURE 7–5. The posterior aspect of the flexed elbow joint. The capsule has been opened to reveal the olecranon fossa.

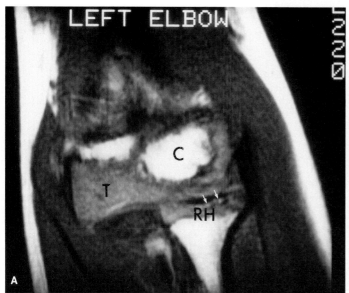

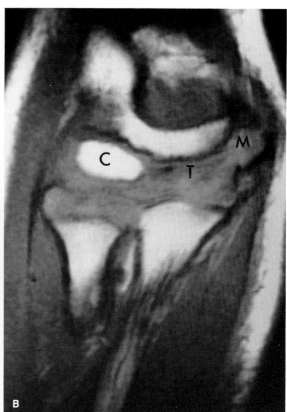

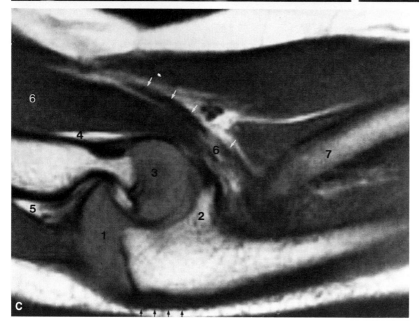

FIGURE 7–6. Epiphyseal maturation. (**A**) On a T1-weighted image of the left elbow in a 5-year-old child, ossification of the capitellum (C) and early appearance of the radial head (RH) ossification center (*arrows*) can be seen. The trochlear center is still a cartilage template of intermediate signal intensity (T). (**B**) On a T1-weighted image of the right elbow in a 2-year-old child, the ossification center of the capitellum (C) is demonstrated. The radial head, trochlea (T), and medial epicondyle (M) are of cartilage composition. (**C**) Normal parasagittal anatomy and epiphyseal centers in the elbow are shown: cartilaginous olecranon apophysis (1), coronal process (2), cartilaginous trochlea (3), anterior fat pad (4), posterior fat pad (5), biceps (6), and proximal radius (7). The biceps tendon (*white arrows*) and the triceps tendon (*black arrows*) are also seen. (TR, 500 msec; TE, 20 msec.)

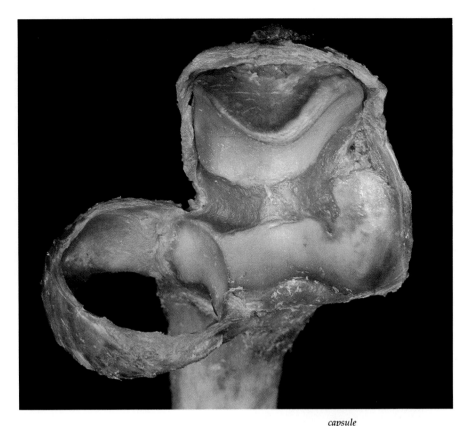

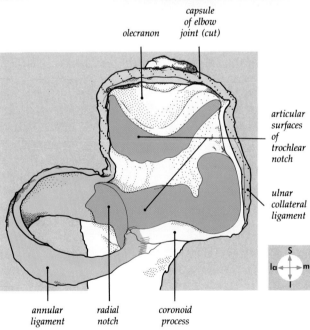

FIGURE 7-7. An anterior view of the proximal end of the ulna with the attached annular ligament shows the articular surfaces of the trochlear and radial notches.

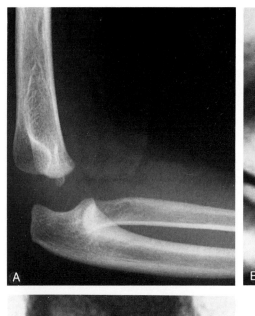

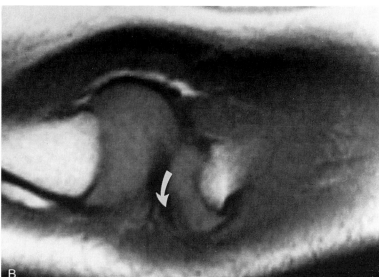

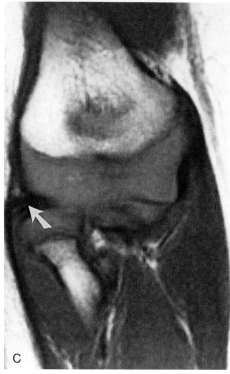

FIGURE 7–8. Elbow subluxation. (**A**) A lateral radiograph of the elbow without alignment of the radial shaft and capitellar ossification center. The corresponding T1-weighted MR images demonstrate (**B**) posterior subluxation (*curved arrow*) on the sagittal image and (**C**) lateral subluxation (*straight arrow*) on the coronal image. Epiphyseal cartilage of the distal humerus and radial head demonstrate intermediate signal intensity. (**B, C:** TR, 600 msec; TE, 20 msec.)

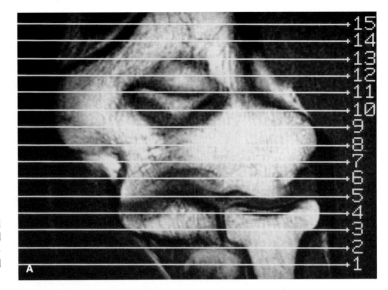

FIGURE 7–9. Normal axial MR anatomy. (**A**) This coronal localizer was used to graphically prescribe axial T1-weighted image locations from (**B**) proximal to (P) distal. Image locations correspond to prescriptions 15 through 1 as indicated on the localizer.

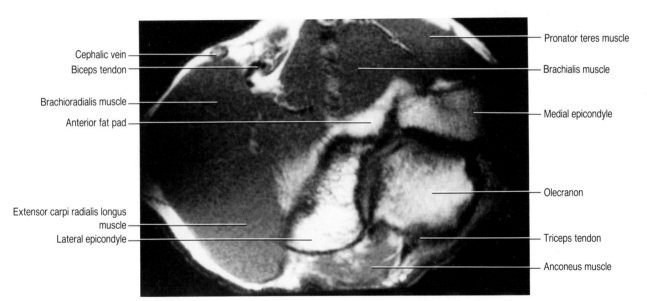

Cephalic vein

Biceps tendon

Brachioradialis muscle

Anterior fat pad

Extensor carpi radialis longus muscle

Lateral epicondyle

Pronator teres muscle

Brachialis muscle

Medial epicondyle

Olecranon

Triceps tendon

Anconeus muscle

FIGURE 7–9B.

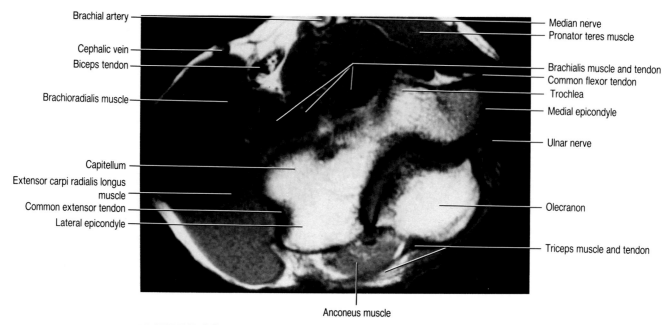

Brachial artery

Cephalic vein

Biceps tendon

Brachioradialis muscle

Capitellum

Extensor carpi radialis longus muscle

Common extensor tendon

Lateral epicondyle

Median nerve

Pronator teres muscle

Brachialis muscle and tendon

Common flexor tendon

Trochlea

Medial epicondyle

Ulnar nerve

Olecranon

Triceps muscle and tendon

Anconeus muscle

FIGURE 7–9C.

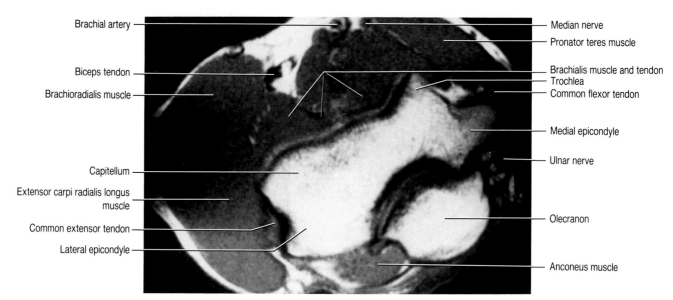

Brachial artery

Biceps tendon

Brachioradialis muscle

Capitellum

Extensor carpi radialis longus muscle

Common extensor tendon

Lateral epicondyle

Median nerve

Pronator teres muscle

Brachialis muscle and tendon

Trochlea

Common flexor tendon

Medial epicondyle

Ulnar nerve

Olecranon

Anconeus muscle

FIGURE 7–9D.

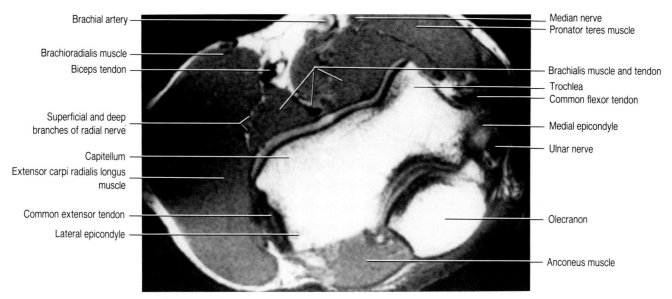

Brachial artery —
Brachioradialis muscle —
Biceps tendon —

Superficial and deep branches of radial nerve —
Capitellum —
Extensor carpi radialis longus muscle —
Common extensor tendon —
Lateral epicondyle —

Median nerve
Pronator teres muscle
Brachialis muscle and tendon
Trochlea
Common flexor tendon
Medial epicondyle
Ulnar nerve
Olecranon
Anconeus muscle

FIGURE 7–9E.

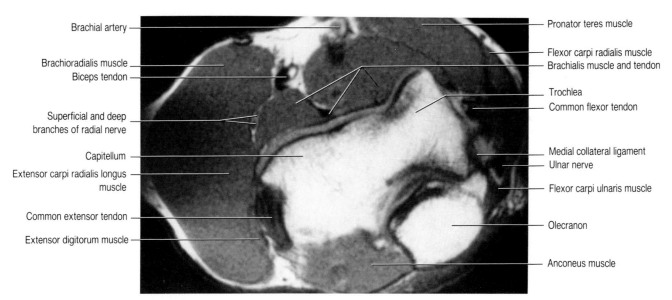

Brachial artery —
Brachioradialis muscle —
Biceps tendon —

Superficial and deep branches of radial nerve —
Capitellum —
Extensor carpi radialis longus muscle —
Common extensor tendon —
Extensor digitorum muscle —

Pronator teres muscle
Flexor carpi radialis muscle
Brachialis muscle and tendon
Trochlea
Common flexor tendon
Medial collateral ligament
Ulnar nerve
Flexor carpi ulnaris muscle
Olecranon
Anconeus muscle

FIGURE 7–9F.

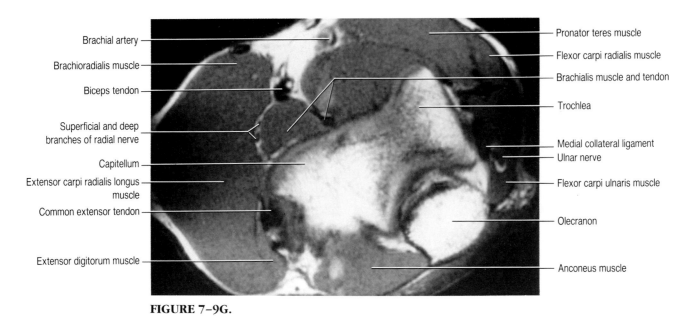

FIGURE 7–9G.

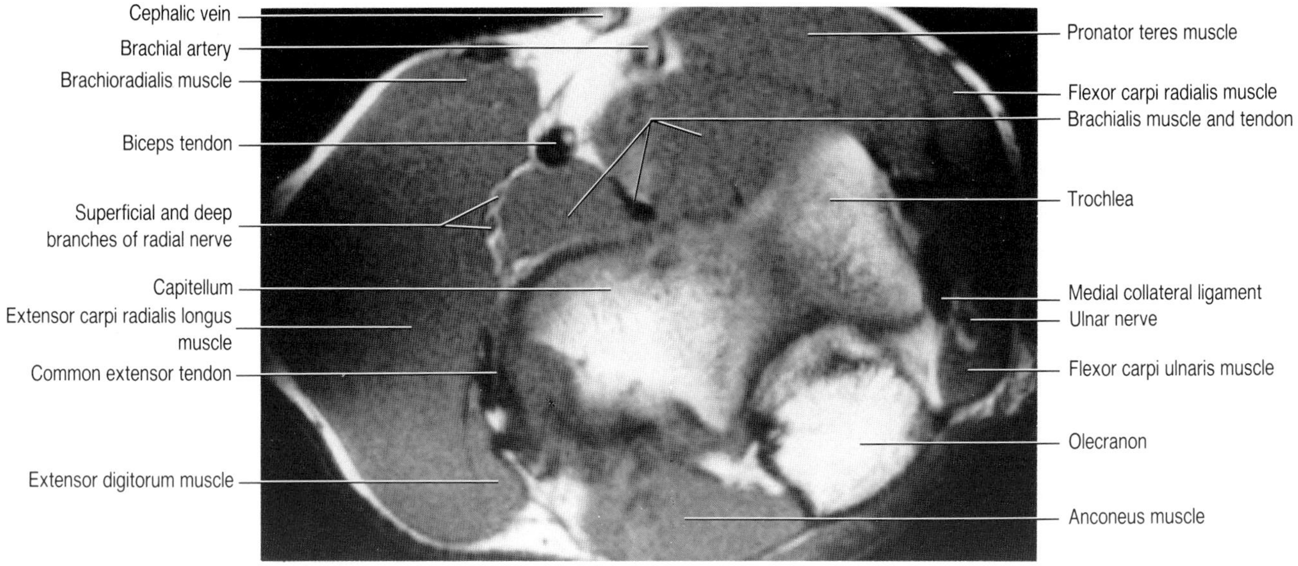

FIGURE 7–9H.

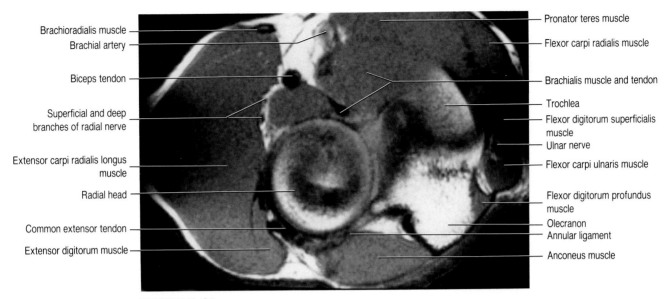

Brachioradialis muscle —
Brachial artery —

Biceps tendon —

Superficial and deep branches of radial nerve —

Extensor carpi radialis longus muscle —

Radial head —

Common extensor tendon —

Extensor digitorum muscle —

Pronator teres muscle —
Flexor carpi radialis muscle —

Brachialis muscle and tendon —
Trochlea —
Flexor digitorum superficialis muscle —
Ulnar nerve —
Flexor carpi ulnaris muscle —

Flexor digitorum profundus muscle —
Olecranon —
Annular ligament —

Anconeus muscle —

FIGURE 7–9I.

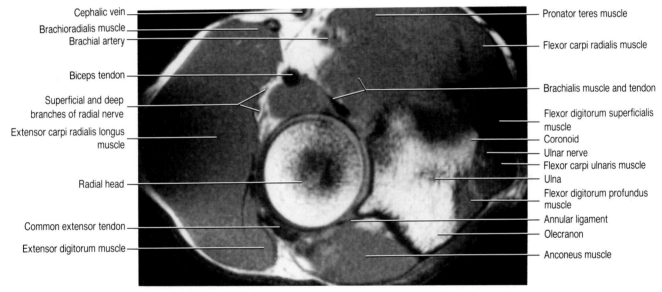

Cephalic vein —
Brachioradialis muscle —
Brachial artery —

Biceps tendon —

Superficial and deep branches of radial nerve —

Extensor carpi radialis longus muscle —

Radial head —

Common extensor tendon —

Extensor digitorum muscle —

Pronator teres muscle —

Flexor carpi radialis muscle —

Brachialis muscle and tendon —

Flexor digitorum superficialis muscle —
Coronoid —
Ulnar nerve —
Flexor carpi ulnaris muscle —
Ulna —
Flexor digitorum profundus muscle —
Annular ligament —
Olecranon —

Anconeus muscle —

FIGURE 7–9J.

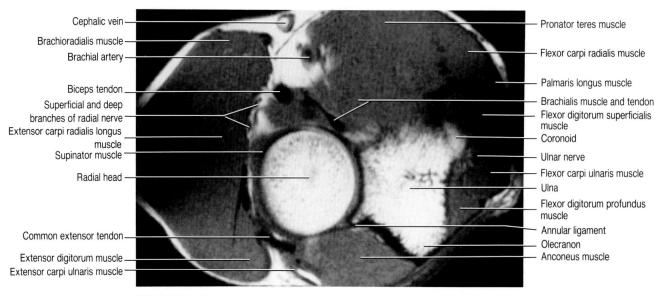

Cephalic vein

Brachioradialis muscle

Brachial artery

Biceps tendon

Superficial and deep branches of radial nerve

Extensor carpi radialis longus muscle

Supinator muscle

Radial head

Common extensor tendon

Extensor digitorum muscle

Extensor carpi ulnaris muscle

Pronator teres muscle

Flexor carpi radialis muscle

Palmaris longus muscle

Brachialis muscle and tendon

Flexor digitorum superficialis muscle

Coronoid

Ulnar nerve

Flexor carpi ulnaris muscle

Ulna

Flexor digitorum profundus muscle

Annular ligament

Olecranon

Anconeus muscle

FIGURE 7–9K.

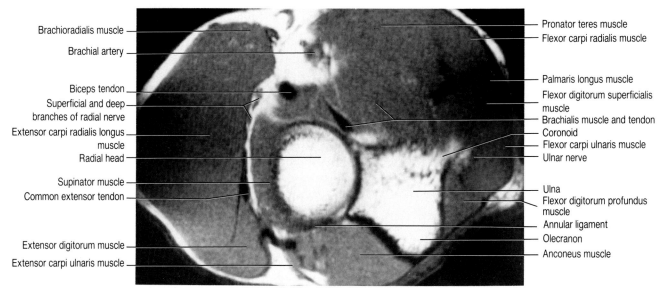

Brachioradialis muscle

Brachial artery

Biceps tendon

Superficial and deep branches of radial nerve

Extensor carpi radialis longus muscle

Radial head

Supinator muscle

Common extensor tendon

Extensor digitorum muscle

Extensor carpi ulnaris muscle

Pronator teres muscle

Flexor carpi radialis muscle

Palmaris longus muscle

Flexor digitorum superficialis muscle

Brachialis muscle and tendon

Coronoid

Flexor carpi ulnaris muscle

Ulnar nerve

Ulna

Flexor digitorum profundus muscle

Annular ligament

Olecranon

Anconeus muscle

FIGURE 7–9L.

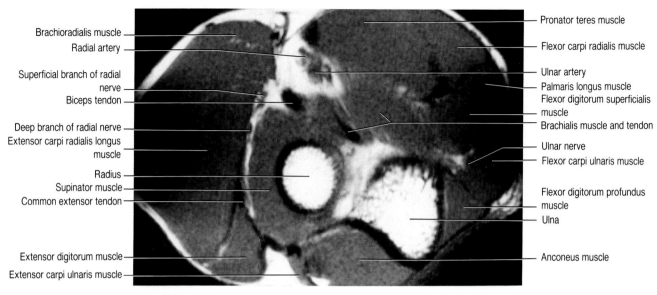

Brachioradialis muscle

Radial artery

Superficial branch of radial nerve

Biceps tendon

Deep branch of radial nerve

Extensor carpi radialis longus muscle

Radius

Supinator muscle

Common extensor tendon

Extensor digitorum muscle

Extensor carpi ulnaris muscle

Pronator teres muscle

Flexor carpi radialis muscle

Ulnar artery

Palmaris longus muscle

Flexor digitorum superficialis muscle

Brachialis muscle and tendon

Ulnar nerve

Flexor carpi ulnaris muscle

Flexor digitorum profundus muscle

Ulna

Anconeus muscle

FIGURE 7–9M.

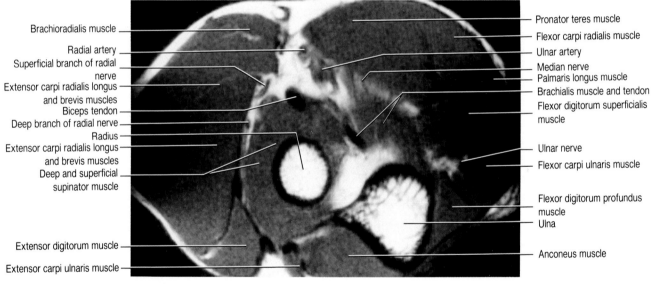

Brachioradialis muscle

Radial artery

Superficial branch of radial nerve

Extensor carpi radialis longus and brevis muscles

Biceps tendon

Deep branch of radial nerve

Radius

Extensor carpi radialis longus and brevis muscles

Deep and superficial supinator muscle

Extensor digitorum muscle

Extensor carpi ulnaris muscle

Pronator teres muscle

Flexor carpi radialis muscle

Ulnar artery

Median nerve

Palmaris longus muscle

Brachialis muscle and tendon

Flexor digitorum superficialis muscle

Ulnar nerve

Flexor carpi ulnaris muscle

Flexor digitorum profundus muscle

Ulna

Anconeus muscle

FIGURE 7–9N.

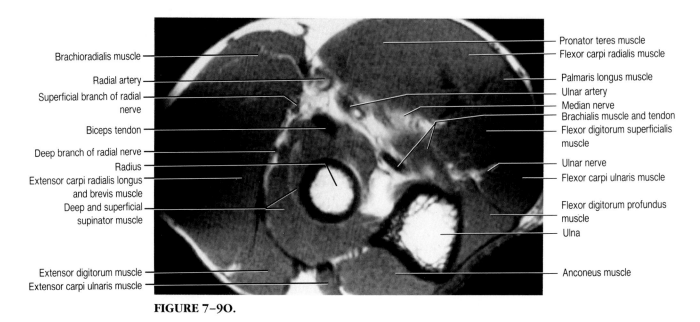

Brachioradialis muscle

Radial artery

Superficial branch of radial nerve

Biceps tendon

Deep branch of radial nerve

Radius

Extensor carpi radialis longus and brevis muscle

Deep and superficial supinator muscle

Extensor digitorum muscle

Extensor carpi ulnaris muscle

Pronator teres muscle

Flexor carpi radialis muscle

Palmaris longus muscle

Ulnar artery

Median nerve

Brachialis muscle and tendon

Flexor digitorum superficialis muscle

Ulnar nerve

Flexor carpi ulnaris muscle

Flexor digitorum profundus muscle

Ulna

Anconeus muscle

FIGURE 7–9O.

Brachioradialis muscle

Radial artery

Superficial branch of radial nerve

Biceps tendon

Deep branch of radial nerve

Extensor carpi radialis longus and brevis muscle

Deep and superficial supinator muscle

Radius

Extensor digitorum muscle

Extensor carpi ulnaris muscle

Pronator teres muscle

Flexor carpi radialis muscle

Palmaris longus muscle

Ulnar artery

Median nerve

Flexor digitorum superficialis muscle

Brachialis muscle and tendon

Ulnar nerve

Flexor carpi ulnaris muscle

Flexor digitorum profundus muscle

Ulna

Anconeus muscle

FIGURE 7–9P.

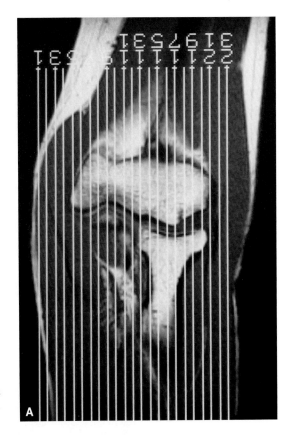

FIGURE 7–10. Normal sagittal MR anatomy. (**A**) This coronal localizer was used to graphically prescribe sagittal T1-weighted image locations from (**B**) medial to (**L**) lateral.

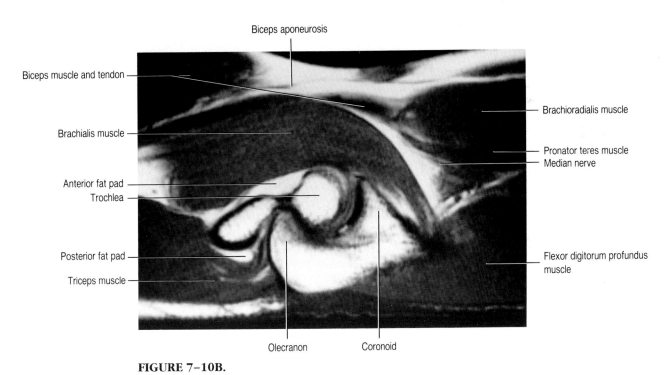

Biceps aponeurosis

Biceps muscle and tendon

Brachioradialis muscle

Brachialis muscle

Pronator teres muscle
Median nerve

Anterior fat pad
Trochlea

Posterior fat pad

Flexor digitorum profundus muscle

Triceps muscle

Olecranon   Coronoid

FIGURE 7–10B.

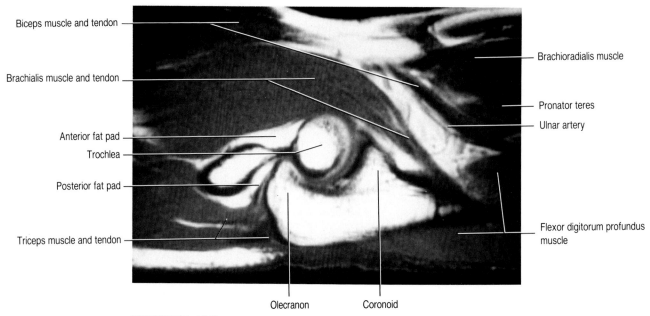

Biceps muscle and tendon

Brachialis muscle and tendon

Anterior fat pad

Trochlea

Posterior fat pad

Triceps muscle and tendon

Brachioradialis muscle

Pronator teres

Ulnar artery

Flexor digitorum profundus muscle

Olecranon   Coronoid

FIGURE 7–10C.

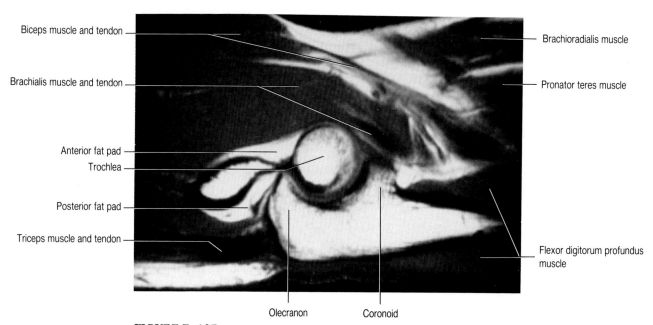

Biceps muscle and tendon

Brachialis muscle and tendon

Anterior fat pad

Trochlea

Posterior fat pad

Triceps muscle and tendon

Brachioradialis muscle

Pronator teres muscle

Flexor digitorum profundus muscle

Olecranon   Coronoid

FIGURE 7–10D.

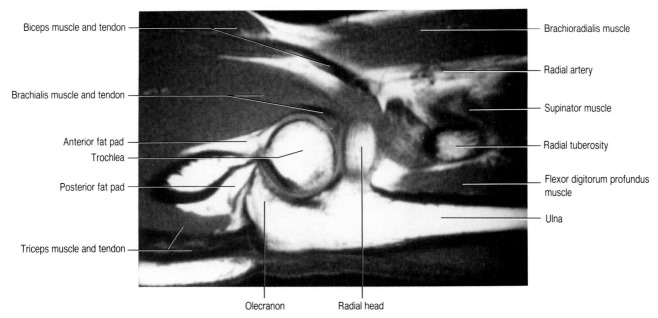

Biceps muscle and tendon

Brachialis muscle and tendon

Anterior fat pad

Trochlea

Posterior fat pad

Triceps muscle and tendon

Brachioradialis muscle

Radial artery

Supinator muscle

Radial tuberosity

Flexor digitorum profundus muscle

Ulna

Olecranon

Radial head

FIGURE 7–10E.

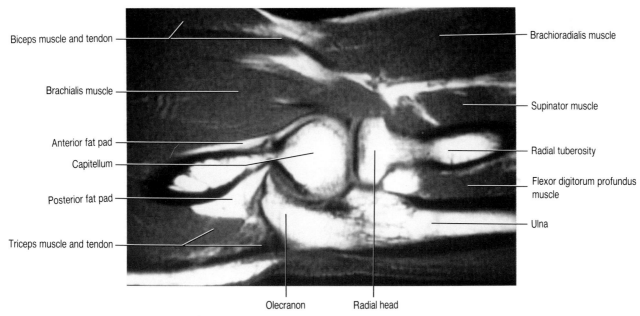

Biceps muscle and tendon

Brachialis muscle

Anterior fat pad

Capitellum

Posterior fat pad

Triceps muscle and tendon

Brachioradialis muscle

Supinator muscle

Radial tuberosity

Flexor digitorum profundus muscle

Ulna

Olecranon

Radial head

FIGURE 7–10F.

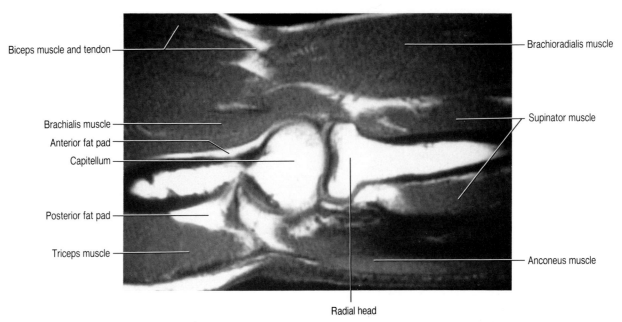

Biceps muscle and tendon —
Brachioradialis muscle
Brachialis muscle —
Supinator muscle
Anterior fat pad —
Capitellum —
Posterior fat pad —
Triceps muscle —
Anconeus muscle
Radial head

FIGURE 7–10G.

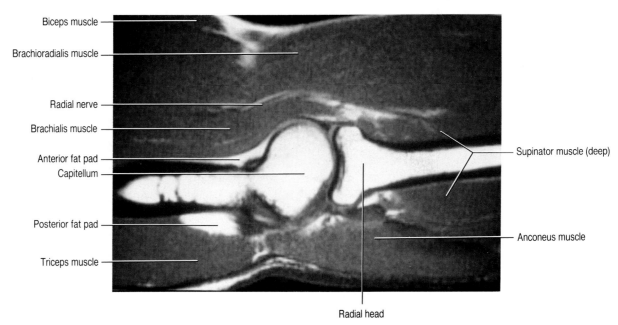

Biceps muscle —
Brachioradialis muscle —
Radial nerve —
Brachialis muscle —
Anterior fat pad —
Supinator muscle (deep)
Capitellum —
Posterior fat pad —
Triceps muscle —
Anconeus muscle
Radial head

FIGURE 7–10H.

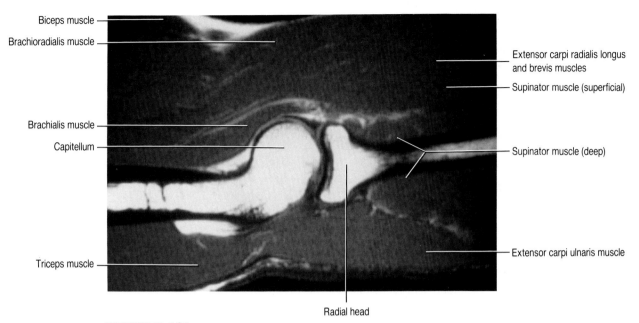

Biceps muscle

Brachioradialis muscle

Extensor carpi radialis longus
and brevis muscles

Supinator muscle (superficial)

Brachialis muscle

Capitellum

Supinator muscle (deep)

Extensor carpi ulnaris muscle

Triceps muscle

Radial head

FIGURE 7–10I.

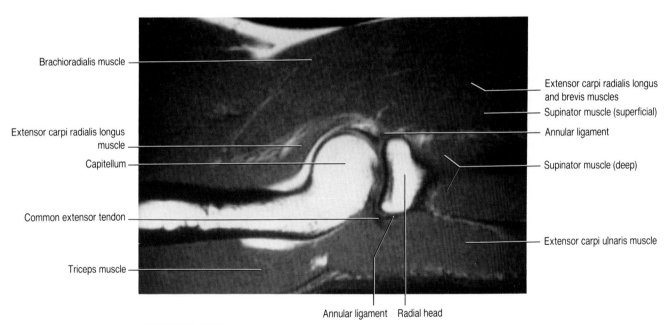

Brachioradialis muscle

Extensor carpi radialis longus
and brevis muscles

Supinator muscle (superficial)

Annular ligament

Extensor carpi radialis longus
muscle

Capitellum

Supinator muscle (deep)

Common extensor tendon

Extensor carpi ulnaris muscle

Triceps muscle

Annular ligament   Radial head

FIGURE 7–10J.

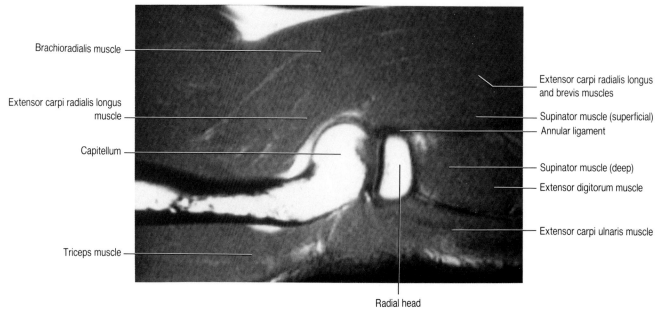

Brachioradialis muscle

Extensor carpi radialis longus
and brevis muscles

Extensor carpi radialis longus
muscle

Supinator muscle (superficial)

Annular ligament

Capitellum

Supinator muscle (deep)

Extensor digitorum muscle

Extensor carpi ulnaris muscle

Triceps muscle

Radial head

FIGURE 7–10K.

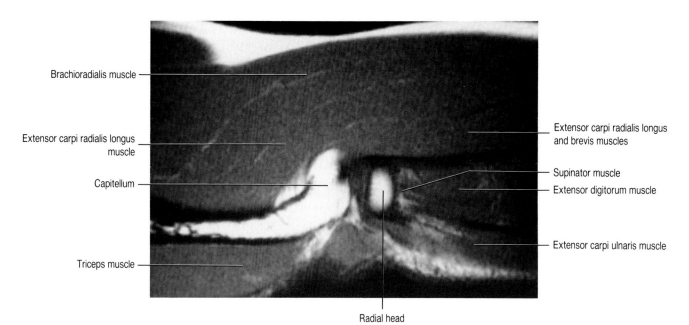

Brachioradialis muscle

Extensor carpi radialis longus
and brevis muscles

Extensor carpi radialis longus
muscle

Supinator muscle

Extensor digitorum muscle

Capitellum

Extensor carpi ulnaris muscle

Triceps muscle

Radial head

FIGURE 7–10L.

groups are visible in the long axis on sagittal images. The biceps tendon, superior to the muscle proper, is particularly well delineated on sagittal images. The anterior and posterior fat pads are shown as high signal intensity bands, proximal to the trochlea and in the coronoid and olecranon fossae, respectively. The hyaline articular cartilage of the radial-head–capitellum articulation and the trochlear–olecranon joints is displayed with intermediate signal intensity on sagittal images through the elbow. In the immature skeleton, cartilage thickness is especially prominent in the unfused apophysis.

Coronal Images

The trochlear–ulnar and capitellar–radial-head joints can be seen on the same coronal image through the elbow (Fig. 7–11). The intermediate signal intensity articular cartilage and the low signal intensity medial and lateral collateral ligaments are also well defined in the coronal plane. The anatomy of the radial head and physeal plates or scars is also shown in this plane of section. The pronator teres and extensor carpi radialis muscles flank the medial and lateral articulations of the elbow, respectively. Posteriorly, the olecranon fossa may be bordered by a semicircular region of low signal intensity. On midjoint coronal images, the biceps and supinator muscles are inferior to the capitellum and radial head. The ulnar nerve, as it courses posterior and distal to the medial epicondyle of the humerus, demonstrates intermediate signal intensity and can be differentiated from the adjacent flexor carpi ulnaris muscle by the high signal intensity of the surrounding perineural fat.

PATHOLOGY OF THE ELBOW JOINT

Osteochondrosis of the capitellum, or Panner's disease, involves the immature skeleton, whereas osteochondritis dissecans occurs after ossification of the capitellum is completed in adolescence or adulthood.

Osteochondrosis

Capitellar osteochondrosis usually affects males between 5 and 10 years of age and is frequently associated with a history of trauma.[11] When associated with overuse in the adolescent thrower, this condition is referred to as "little league elbow."[12] In young baseball pitchers, the process of throwing produces severe valgus stress and extensor thrust. Tenderness of the medial joint line, swelling, and limitation of joint motion occur. Occasionally, there is bilateral involvement.

Conventional radiographs demonstrate fissuring, fragmentation, and sclerosis of the capitellum. Repetitive traction placed on an open medial epicondylar epiphysis causes decreased capitellar size and accelerated growth of the medial epicondyle. Abnormal morphology of the radial head may be secondary to reactive hyperemia, although revascularization and reconstruction of the capitellum usually occur with conservative treatment. Removal of loose bodies is necessary to prevent joint degeneration.

The normally thick articular cartilage surface and the morphology of the capitellar epiphysis is well delineated on MR scans. On T1-weighted images, the capitellum demonstrates low signal intensity (Fig. 7–12). Peripheral irregularity is present, and the ossific nucleus is smaller than normal. Early degeneration or maturational changes are reflected by changes in marrow signal intensity in the radial head articulation. The detection of osteochondral fragments requires thin sections in all three planes. Associated joint effusion and revascularization are best monitored by MR imaging.

Osteochondritis Dissecans

Osteochondritis dissecans usually occurs in adolescents and may be related to acute or chronic repetitive trauma.[13] Early in its course, the disease may be silent or asymptomatic. Subchondral bone is primarily affected, with initial preservation of the underlying articular cartilage surface that receives its nutrition through the synovium. Infarction and softening of subchondral bone secondary to fracture may lead to separation of the articular cartilage. There is often discoloration, fibrillation, or a cartilage flap overhanging an excavated crater.

The anterior and posterior aspects of the supratrochlear fossa are common locations for loose bodies. The development of a loose body may result in spontaneous locking with pain and joint effusion.

Magnetic resonance examination confirms enlargement of the posterolateral radial head, premature physeal fusion, and a funnel-shaped metaphysis. Cartilaginous and marrow-containing osteocartilaginous loose bodies can be identified on T1- and T2-weighted images. Sagittal MR images are useful for showing flattening of the capitellum or irregularities of the radial head. T2*-weighted images are useful for identifying fluid signal intensity and outlining deep craters and osteochondral fragments (Fig. 7–13).

Surgical treatment is indicated in advanced disease with joint locking and degenerative arthritis.[14] Minimizing incongruities between the radial head and capitellum and the removal of joint fragments reduces disease progression.

Overuse Syndromes

Lateral Epicondylitis

Lateral epicondylitis, commonly known as tennis elbow, refers to a syndrome of pain overlying the radiohumeral articulation.[9,12,15] Although it is designated lateral epicondylitis, its origin is still unclear. The syndrome of pain and tenderness over the lateral epicondyle is common in tennis players, carpenters, and those whose occupation requires frequent rotatory forearm motion. Pain is elicited with forearm supination and active dorsiflexion of the wrist. The etiology is thought to involve tearing of extensor tendon fibers at the lateral epicondyle. One theory attributes the syndrome to chronic repetitive trauma with fibroangiomatous hyperplasia of the extensor carpi radialis brevis.

Although conventional radiography is usually negative, calcification overlying the extensor origin, roughening or periostitis of underlying bone, or medial epicondylar avulsion may be present (Fig. 7–14). Axial or coronal MR imaging with T2, T2*, or STIR protocols may identify edema and thickening of the common extensor tendon (Fig. 7–15). The low signal intensity contour of the underlying cortex and the normally homogeneous signal from the adjacent subchondral marrow should be evaluated for changes indicative of traumatic avulsion.

Initial treatment is conservative (*i.e.,* rest, nonsteroidal antiinflammatory drugs). Surgical release of the extensor aponeurosis from the lateral epicondyle is reserved for chronic cases.

Medial Epicondylitis

Overuse and microtears of the common flexor pronator muscle group result in medial epicondylitis.[12,16] Forceful flexion, such as that seen in baseball pitchers, produces stress in the common flexor origin. As in lateral epicondylitis, treatment consists of conservative management.

Cubital Tunnel Syndrome

Cubital tunnel syndrome involves compression of the ulnar nerve at the elbow joint. The compression may be caused by trauma to the ulnar nerve due to ulnar neuritis, chronic repetitive blunt trauma, fracture, cubitus valgus deformity, arthritis, recurrent subluxation or dislocation of the nerve, or muscle compression.[17] The cubital tunnel—the site of ulnar nerve compression at the elbow—consists of an aponeurotic arcade or arch between the origins of two heads of the flexor carpi ulnaris. The flexor carpi ulnaris form the roof of the cubital tunnel; the floor is formed by the medial capsule. In flexion, the cubital tunnel space is diminished.

Compression of the ulnar nerve at the elbow joint must be differentiated from ulnar nerve injuries at the wrist. Ulnar nerve compression at the wrist does not cause sensory impairment of the dorsal cutaneous nerve that originates from the parent ulnar nerve distal to the elbow joints. Patients with ulnar nerve compression may present with both sensory and motor deficits.

I have evaluated one patient who presented with pain and paresthesia along the ulnar distribution. On T2*-weighted axial images performed at the level of the medial epicondyle, the ulnar nerve was enlarged and edematous, and it demonstrated high signal intensity (Fig. 7–16). The ulnar nerve normally demonstrates intermediate signal intensity on T2- and T2*-weighted images. Subsequent electrodiagnostic studies confirmed slowing of conduction of the ulnar nerve at the elbow. Additionally, a compressive osteophyte about the ulnar groove can be excluded with MR studies. Subluxations of the ulnar nerve may occur without symptoms unless associated with trauma.

Although minimal nerve irritation usually resolves spontaneously, chronic involvement requires surgical decompression and transposition of the nerve.[18]

Biceps Tendon Rupture

Forced flexion against strong resistance may produce a partial tear or rupture of the biceps tendon (Fig. 7–17).[9,19] Adjacent to its insertion on the bicipital tuberosity, the biceps brachii originates from the supraglenoid tubercle of the scapula (*i.e.,* long head) and the tip of the coracoid process of the scapula (*i.e.,* short head). The biceps tendon inserts at the tuberosity of the radius, through the bicipital aponeurosis. The biceps functions as a supinator and flexor of the elbow joint. Clinical signs of tearing of the biceps tendon include weakness of active flexion of the elbow and supination of the forearm. Tense antecubital fascia may minimize swelling despite localized tenderness. Proximal retraction of the biceps tendon during active flexion produces a mass or bulbous swelling in the upper arm.

The site of rupture and degree of proximal retraction of the biceps tendon are best seen on volar coronal, sagittal, or axial MR T1- and T2- or T2*-weighted images (Fig. 7–18). Associated degenerative thickening and increased tendon signal intensity are best demonstrated on T2*-weighted sagittal images. Axial images must extend distal to the proximal radioulnar joint to adequately display the biceps tendon insertion along the ulnar aspect of the radius (Fig. 7–19). The anterior ulnar insertion of the brachialis should not be mistaken for an intact biceps tendon. Images more proximal to the brachialis insertion may show an absence of the biceps tendon anterior to

(text continues on page 670)

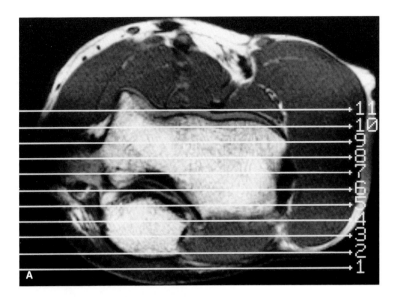

FIGURE 7–11. Normal coronal MR anatomy. (**A**) This axial localizer was used to graphically prescribe coronal T1-weighted image locations from (**B**) posterior to (**K**) anterior. Image locations correspond to prescriptions 2 through 11, as indicated on the localizer.

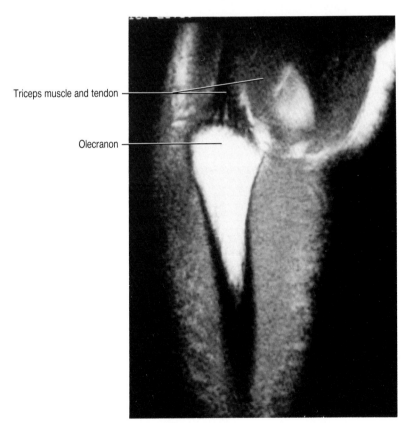

Triceps muscle and tendon

Olecranon

FIGURE 7–11B.

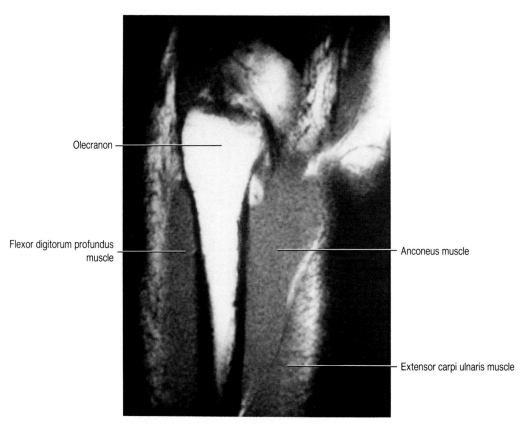

Olecranon

Flexor digitorum profundus muscle

Anconeus muscle

Extensor carpi ulnaris muscle

FIGURE 7–11C.

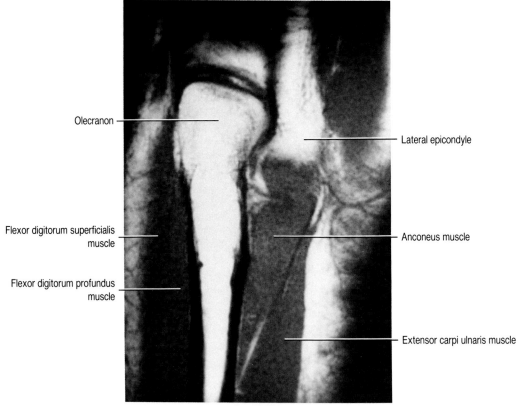

Olecranon

Lateral epicondyle

Flexor digitorum superficialis muscle

Flexor digitorum profundus muscle

Anconeus muscle

Extensor carpi ulnaris muscle

FIGURE 7–11D.

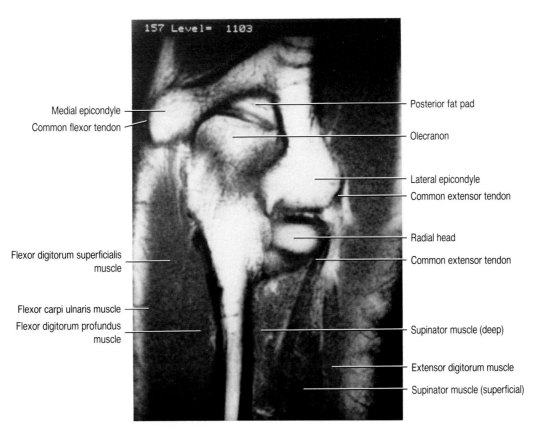

FIGURE 7–11E.

Medial epicondyle
Common flexor tendon

Flexor digitorum superficialis muscle

Flexor carpi ulnaris muscle
Flexor digitorum profundus muscle

Posterior fat pad

Olecranon

Lateral epicondyle
Common extensor tendon

Radial head
Common extensor tendon

Supinator muscle (deep)

Extensor digitorum muscle
Supinator muscle (superficial)

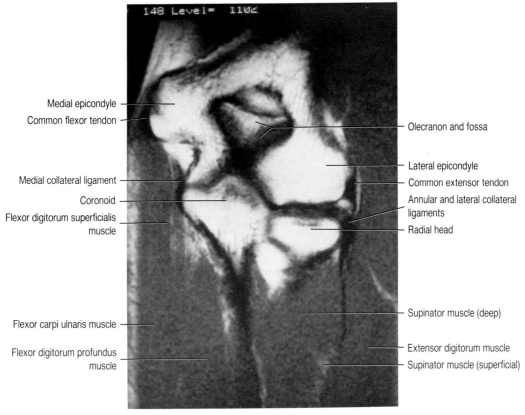

FIGURE 7–11F.

Medial epicondyle
Common flexor tendon

Medial collateral ligament
Coronoid
Flexor digitorum superficialis muscle

Flexor carpi ulnaris muscle

Flexor digitorum profundus muscle

Olecranon and fossa

Lateral epicondyle
Common extensor tendon
Annular and lateral collateral ligaments
Radial head

Supinator muscle (deep)

Extensor digitorum muscle
Supinator muscle (superficial)

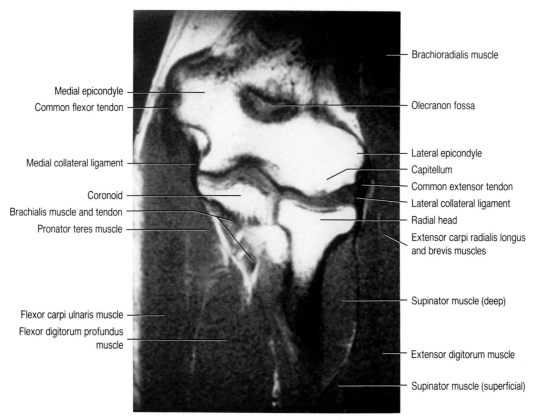

Brachioradialis muscle

Medial epicondyle

Common flexor tendon

Olecranon fossa

Medial collateral ligament

Lateral epicondyle

Capitellum

Common extensor tendon

Coronoid

Lateral collateral ligament

Brachialis muscle and tendon

Radial head

Pronator teres muscle

Extensor carpi radialis longus and brevis muscles

Supinator muscle (deep)

Flexor carpi ulnaris muscle

Flexor digitorum profundus muscle

Extensor digitorum muscle

Supinator muscle (superficial)

FIGURE 7–11G.

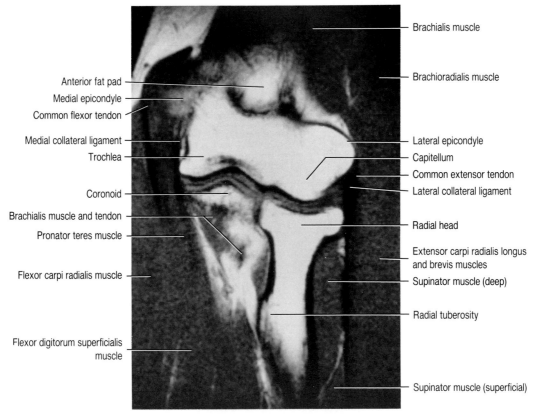

Brachialis muscle

Anterior fat pad

Medial epicondyle

Brachioradialis muscle

Common flexor tendon

Medial collateral ligament

Lateral epicondyle

Trochlea

Capitellum

Common extensor tendon

Coronoid

Lateral collateral ligament

Brachialis muscle and tendon

Radial head

Pronator teres muscle

Flexor carpi radialis muscle

Extensor carpi radialis longus and brevis muscles

Supinator muscle (deep)

Radial tuberosity

Flexor digitorum superficialis muscle

Supinator muscle (superficial)

FIGURE 7–11H.

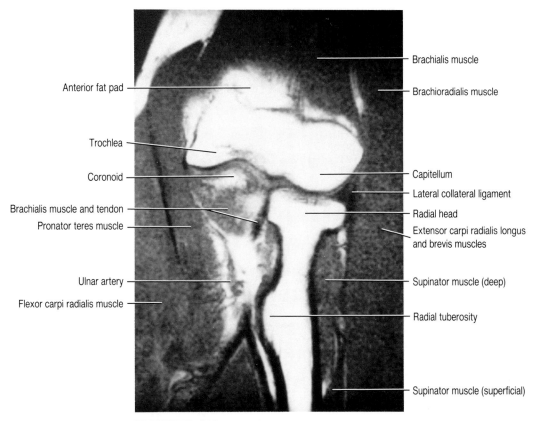

Anterior fat pad

Trochlea

Coronoid

Brachialis muscle and tendon
Pronator teres muscle

Ulnar artery

Flexor carpi radialis muscle

Brachialis muscle

Brachioradialis muscle

Capitellum
Lateral collateral ligament
Radial head
Extensor carpi radialis longus
and brevis muscles

Supinator muscle (deep)

Radial tuberosity

Supinator muscle (superficial)

FIGURE 7–11I.

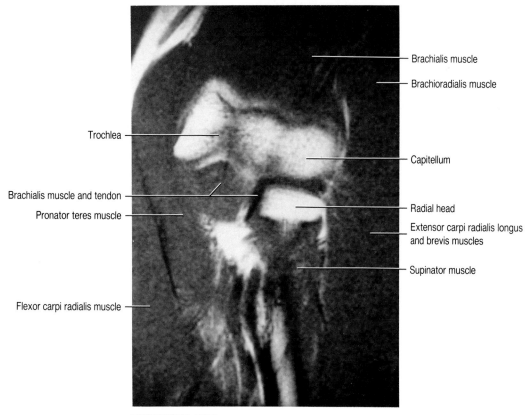

Trochlea

Brachialis muscle and tendon
Pronator teres muscle

Flexor carpi radialis muscle

Brachialis muscle

Brachioradialis muscle

Capitellum

Radial head

Extensor carpi radialis longus
and brevis muscles

Supinator muscle

FIGURE 7–11J.

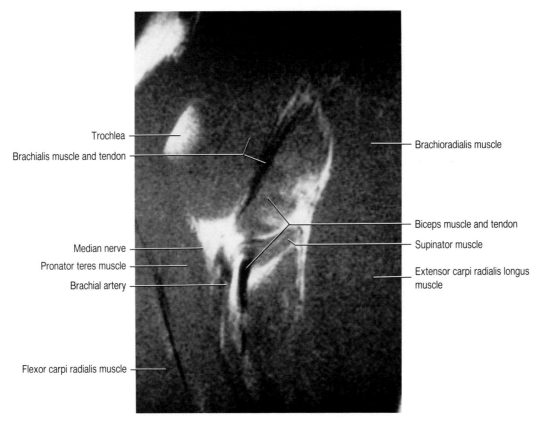

Trochlea

Brachialis muscle and tendon

Median nerve

Pronator teres muscle

Brachial artery

Flexor carpi radialis muscle

Brachioradialis muscle

Biceps muscle and tendon

Supinator muscle

Extensor carpi radialis longus muscle

FIGURE 7–11K.

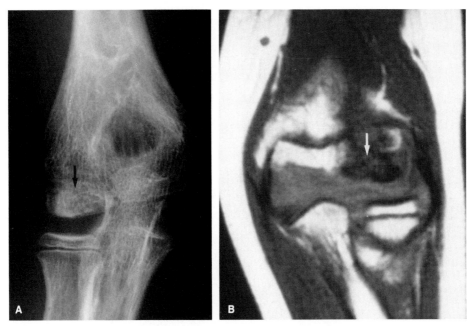

FIGURE 7–12. Panner's disease is seen in adolescent pitchers and has been related to valgus stress of the elbow. (**A**) Sclerosis of the capitellar ossification center (*arrow*) can be seen on a plain film radiograph. (**B**) A T1-weighted coronal image displays low signal intensity sclerosis (*arrow*) and subtle flattening of the capitellum. (TR, 600 msec; TE, 20 msec.) (**C**) A T1-weighted sagittal image shows a low signal intensity capitellum (*arrows*). (TR, 500 msec; TE, 20 msec.) (**D**) On a sagittal T2*-weighted image, a subchondral cyst (*large arrow*) and flattening of the epiphysis (*small arrows*) are revealed. (TR, 400 msec; TE, 20 msec; flip angle, 25°.) (**E**) An axial T1-weighted image displays a sclerotic capitellum (*large arrow*) and thickness of the overlying articular cartilage (C; *small arrows*). (TR, 500 msec; TE, 20 msec.)

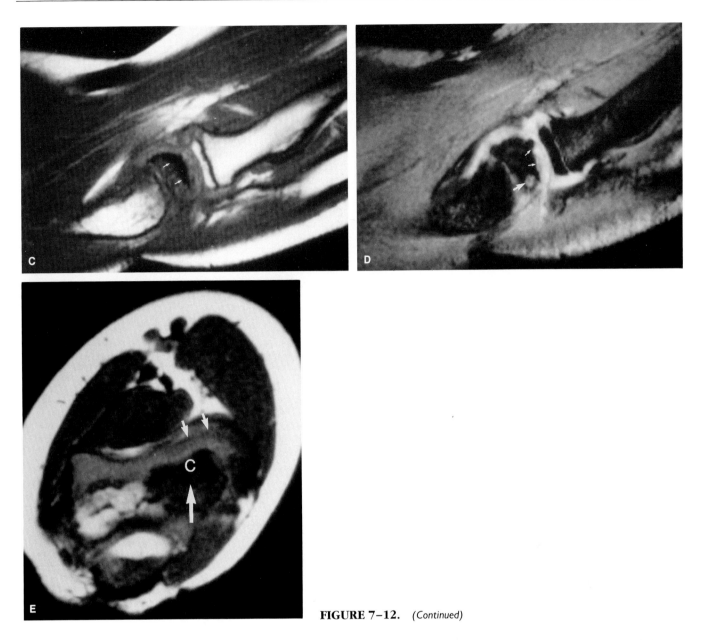

FIGURE 7–12. *(Continued)*

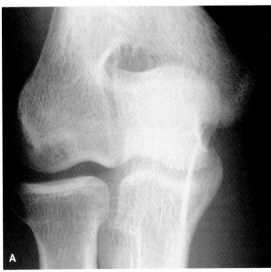

FIGURE 7–13. Osteochondritis dissecans. (**A**) A lesion of the capitellum is radiolucent in a 17-year-old adolescent with completed ossification. (**B**) A coronal T1-weighted image reveals a low signal intensity necrotic focus (*black arrows*) and intermediate signal intensity articular cartilage (*white arrows*). (TR, 600 msec; TE, 20 msec.) (**C**) On an axial T2*-weighted image, fragment loosening with subchondral hyperintense fluid (*white arrows*) and anterior projection of the involved osteochondral fragment (*black arrows*) are seen. (TR, 400 msec; TE, 20 msec; flip angle, 25°.)

(continued)

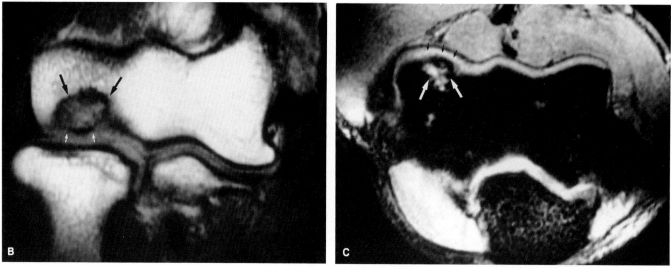

FIGURE 7–13. *(Continued)*

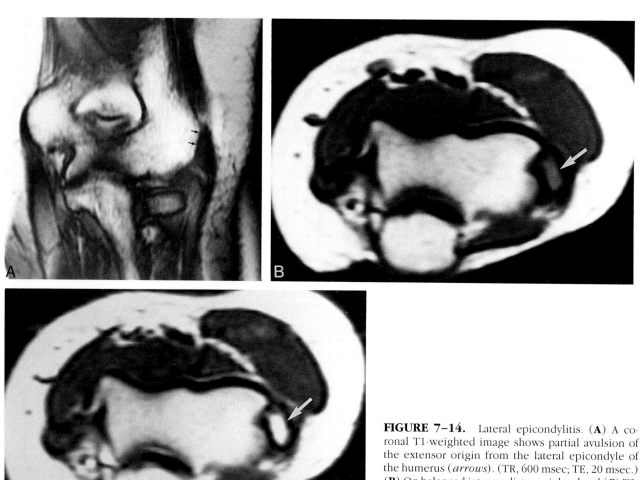

FIGURE 7–14. Lateral epicondylitis. (**A**) A coronal T1-weighted image shows partial avulsion of the extensor origin from the lateral epicondyle of the humerus (*arrows*). (TR, 600 msec; TE, 20 msec.) (**B**) On balanced intermediate-weighted and (**C**) T2-weighted images, edema (*arrows*) in the extensor tendon origin demonstrates intermediate signal intensity and high signal intensity, respectively. (TR, 1500 msec; TE, 20, 70 msec.)

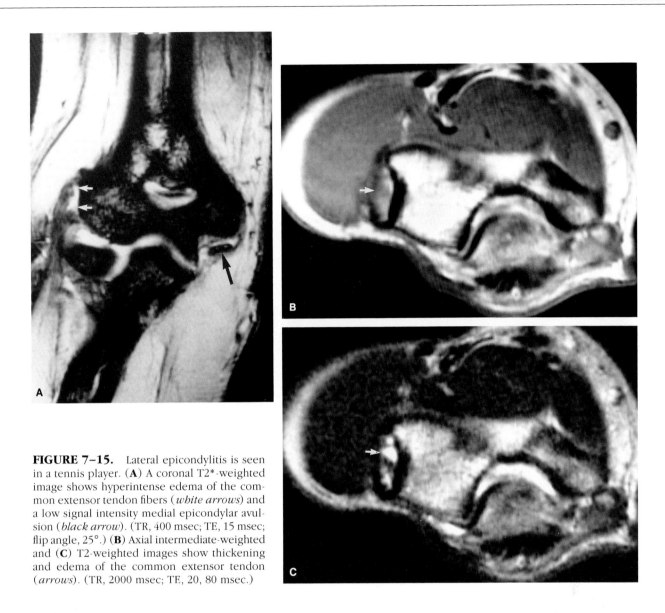

FIGURE 7–15. Lateral epicondylitis is seen in a tennis player. (**A**) A coronal T2*-weighted image shows hyperintense edema of the common extensor tendon fibers (*white arrows*) and a low signal intensity medial epicondylar avulsion (*black arrow*). (TR, 400 msec; TE, 15 msec; flip angle, 25°.) (**B**) Axial intermediate-weighted and (**C**) T2-weighted images show thickening and edema of the common extensor tendon (*arrows*). (TR, 2000 msec; TE, 20, 80 msec.)

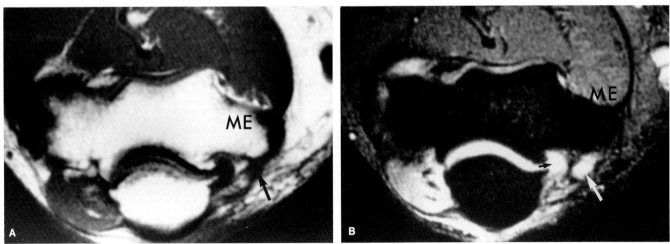

FIGURE 7–16. Cubital tunnel syndrome. An edematous ulnar nerve (*large arrows*) demonstrates (**A**) low signal intensity in a T1-weighted image and is (**B**) hyperintense on a T2*-weighted image. A small elbow joint effusion is seen lateral to the nerve (*small arrow*). (ME, medial epicondyle; **A:** TR, 500 msec; TE, 20 msec; **B:** TR, 400 msec; TE, 20 msec; flip angle, 25°.)

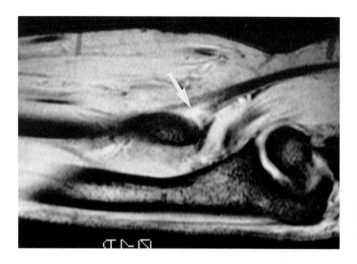

FIGURE 7–17. A partial tear of the biceps tendon attachment to the tuberosity of the radius appears as an area of increased signal intensity without tendinous gap or retraction (*arrow*) on a T2*-weighted image. (TR, 400 msec; TE, 20 msec; flip angle, 25°.)

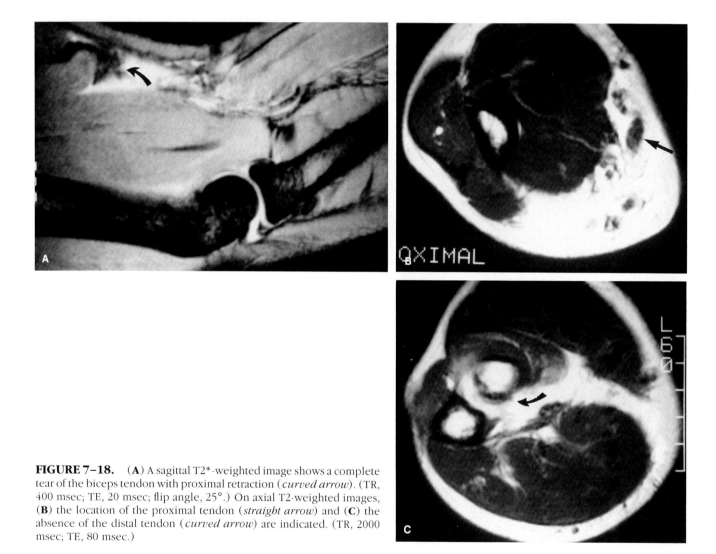

FIGURE 7–18. (**A**) A sagittal T2*-weighted image shows a complete tear of the biceps tendon with proximal retraction (*curved arrow*). (TR, 400 msec; TE, 20 msec; flip angle, 25°.) On axial T2-weighted images, (**B**) the location of the proximal tendon (*straight arrow*) and (**C**) the absence of the distal tendon (*curved arrow*) are indicated. (TR, 2000 msec; TE, 80 msec.)

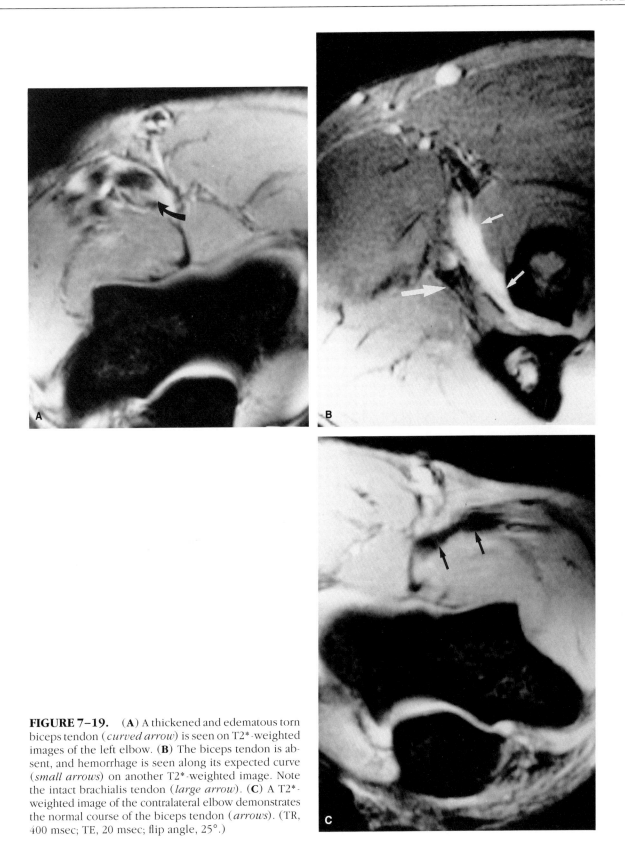

FIGURE 7–19. (**A**) A thickened and edematous torn biceps tendon (*curved arrow*) is seen on T2*-weighted images of the left elbow. (**B**) The biceps tendon is absent, and hemorrhage is seen along its expected curve (*small arrows*) on another T2*-weighted image. Note the intact brachialis tendon (*large arrow*). (**C**) A T2*-weighted image of the contralateral elbow demonstrates the normal course of the biceps tendon (*arrows*). (TR, 400 msec; TE, 20 msec; flip angle, 25°.)

the brachialis muscle in association with proximal tendon retraction. T2-weighted or T2*-weighted images highlight areas of tendon edema or hemorrhage. The biceps is visible and demonstrates redundancy as the tendon retracts into the upper arm. After repair, the biceps tendon can be seen sutured directly to the brachialis insertion. Significant trauma may produce brachialis muscle hemorrhage in partially torn muscle fibers (Fig. 7–20). Triceps avulsion from its olecranon insertion less common than tears of the biceps tendon, and is usually secondary to forced extension against resistance.

Radial Head Fractures

Fractures involving the radial head are secondary to indirect or direct trauma. A fall on an outstretched arm transmits a longitudinal force along the axis of the radius, driving it against the capitellum. The addition of a valgus force vector against the elbow may result in an associated capitellar injury. In the Mason classification, a type 1 radial head fracture is nondisplaced; a type 2 fracture is a marginal fracture with displacement; a type 3 fracture is a comminuted fracture involving the entire radial head; and a type 4 injury involves dislocation of the ulnohumeral joint.[20] The presence of a posterior fat pad and localized pain over the radial head are pathognomonic of radial head fracture. In the presence of an intraarticular free fragment (*i.e.,* loose body) proximal to the radial head, should exclude a diagnosis of associated capitellar fracture. Myositis ossificans is a known complication of type 4 injuries. Most fractures of the radial head are vertically oriented and involve its lateral aspect.

Nondisplaced or minimally displaced (*i.e.,* less than 2 mm) type 1 fractures may be difficult to identify without oblique or radial head radiographs; absence of the posterior fat pad cannot be used to exclude a fracture (Fig. 7–21). Fracture morphology, displacement, angulation, and volume or area of involvement are best delineated on T1-weighted axial, coronal, and sagittal images and on 3D image displays (Fig. 7–22). T2, T2*, or STIR protocols are used to increase the signal intensity of associated effusions or marrow hemorrhage. Displacement of the anterior and posterior fat pads is directly visible in the sagittal plane (see Fig. 7–21). The presence of associated capitellar contusion, fracture, and free fragments can also be evaluated on these scans.

Open reduction and internal fixation or excision, especially in the presence of comminution, are recommended for treatment of radial head fractures that demonstrate depression greater than 3 mm, angulation greater than 30°, or involvement of greater than one-third of the surface area of the radial head. Emphasis has also been placed on preserving the radial head by the reconstruction of displaced fragments.

Epicondylar Fractures

Avulsion fractures of the epicondyle are uncommon after closure of the physis, especially as an isolated injury.[12] In the immature skeleton, medial epicondyle avulsion fractures are associated with posterior dislocation of the elbow prior to fusion of its ossification center with the medial condyle. A lateral epicondylar fracture is extremely rare.

Magnetic resonance examination of the pediatric elbow is valuable in demonstrating the articular cartilage surface and the anatomy of the medial epicondyle in the early stages of ossification. Displacement of the medial epicondyle or a step-off from the normal contour of the thick articular cartilage epiphysis is diagnostic of fracture (Fig. 7–23). Magnetic resonance should also be used to identify a trapped medial epicondyle that is displaced into the joint.

Olecranon Bursitis

Two bursae are related to the insertion of the triceps tendon. The anterior and more superior subtriceps bursa lies between the triceps tendon and the superior surface of the olecranon. The larger and more important olecranon bursa is located between the skin and the extensor or dorsal surface of the olecranon. Olecranon bursal distention and inflammation may result from trauma, infection, rheumatoid arthritis, or gout. Inflammation of the olecranon bursa may present with decreased range of motion at the elbow and localized tenderness.

Magnetic resonance imaging in the sagittal and axial planes best depicts bursal distention. The signal intensity of inflamed bursae is higher on T2*-weighted and STIR images than on corresponding conventional T2-weighted images (Fig. 7–24). Despite characteristic uniform high signal intensity, however, aspiration may not yield a productive fluid tap. The distended bursa produces a crescent contour, with an anterior convexity posterior to the lateral epicondyle, the anconeus muscle, the olecranon, and the medial epicondyle.

Arthritis

Osteoarthritis

Humeroulnar compartment osteoarthritis (Fig. 7–25) is uncommon compared with radiocapitular osteoarthritis (Fig. 7–26), which may develop subsequent to a radial head fracture. The differential diagnosis for elbow osteoarthritis includes the spondyloarthropathies, gout and pseudogout, and septic arthritis.[21] Computed tomography

(text continues on page 682)

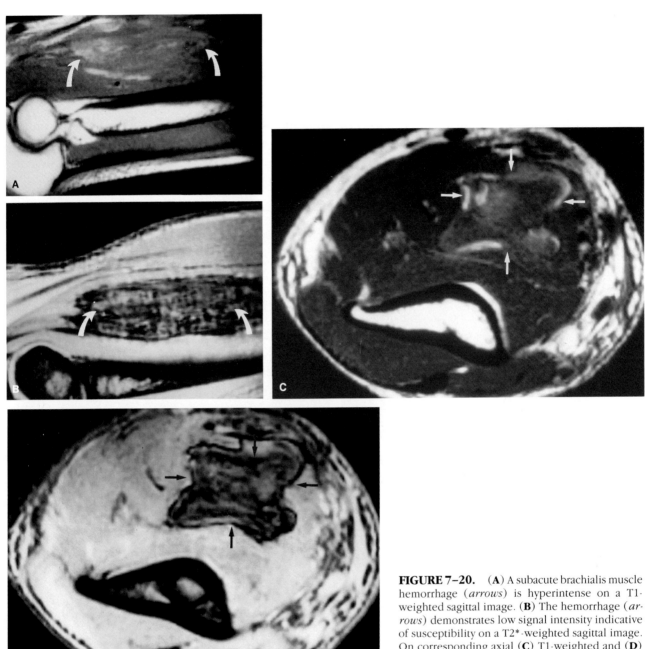

FIGURE 7–20. (**A**) A subacute brachialis muscle hemorrhage (*arrows*) is hyperintense on a T1-weighted sagittal image. (**B**) The hemorrhage (*arrows*) demonstrates low signal intensity indicative of susceptibility on a T2*-weighted sagittal image. On corresponding axial (**C**) T1-weighted and (**D**) T2*-weighted images, the hemorrhage (*arrows*) is seen in partially torn brachialis muscle fibers.

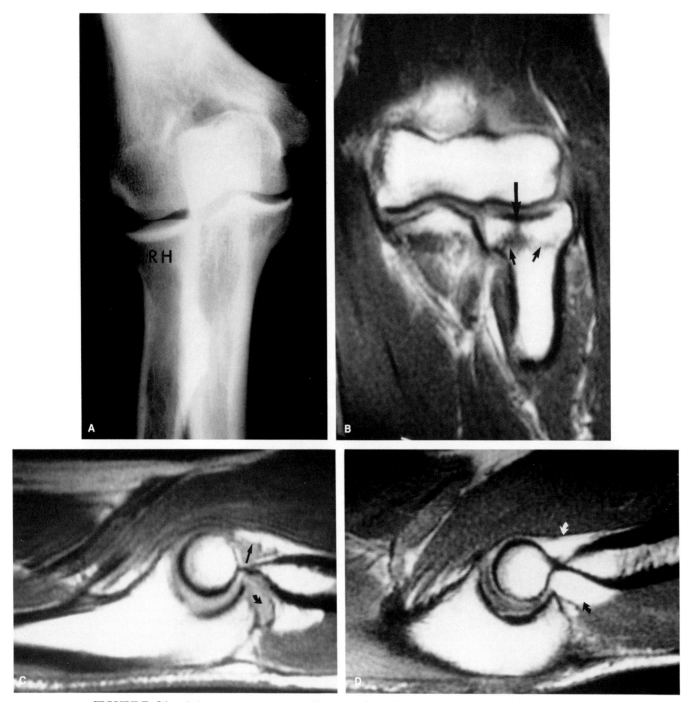

FIGURE 7–21. (**A**) An anteroposterior radiograph of the elbow is unremarkable. (**B**) A T1-weighted coronal image reveals a nondisplaced radial head fracture (*small arrows*) with intraarticular extension (*large arrow*). (**C**) A T1-weighted sagittal image shows displaced anterior (*straight arrow*) and posterior (*curved arrow*) fat pads secondary to hemorrhagic effusion. (**D**) A T1-weighted sagittal image in a normal elbow provides a comparison for the location of anterior (*curved white arrow*) and posterior (*curved black arrow*) fat pads. (TR, 600 msec; TE, 20 msec.)

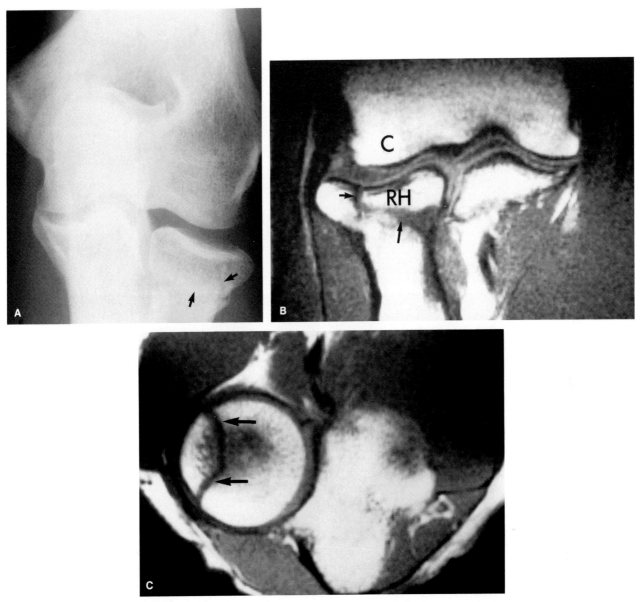

FIGURE 7–22. (**A**) A nondisplaced marginal type 1 radial head fracture (*arrow*) is demonstrable on a plain film radiograph. T1-weighted (**B**) coronal, (**C**) axial, and (**D**) sagittal images best demonstrate fracture morphology and intraarticular extension (*large arrows*). A linear, low signal intensity segment parallel with the long axis of the radium represents the demarcation of the radial tuberosity and not a fracture (*small arrows*). (C, capitellum; RH, radial head.) (**E, F**) Corresponding 3D CT images show the surface morphology of the fracture (*arrows*). (C, capitellum; R, radius; T, trochlea.) *(continued)*

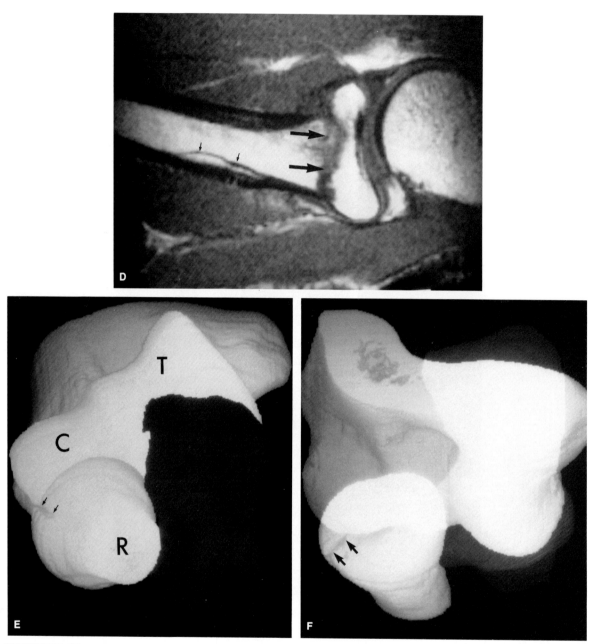

FIGURE 7–22. (Continued)

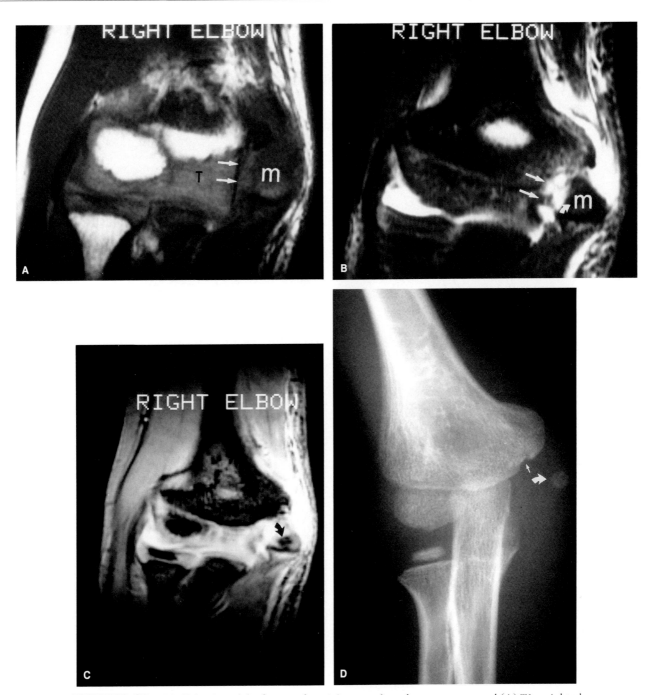

FIGURE 7–23. Medial epicondylar fracture (*straight arrows*) can be seen on coronal (**A**) T1-weighted and (**B**) short TI inversion recovery (STIR) images. The medially displaced epicondyle is best depicted on a STIR sequence (*curved arrow*). (**A:** TR, 600 msec; TE, 20 msec; **B:** TR, 2000 msec; TI, 160 msec, TE, 43 msec.) (**C**) A coronal T2*-weighted image reveals a medially displaced small ossification center (*curved arrows*) confirmed on (**D**) an anteroposterior radiograph. The radiograph also shows a local cortical defect at the fracture site (*small arrow*). The radiograph cannot demonstrate the cartilage fracturing displayed on coronal MR images. (m = medial epicondyle) (**C:** TR, 400 msec; TE, 15 msec; flip angle, 20°.)

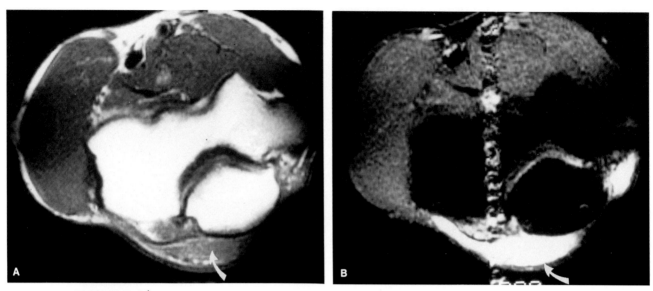

FIGURE 7–24. Olecranon bursitis. Inflammation and distention of the olecranon bursa (*arrow*) demonstrates (**A**) low signal intensity on an axial T1-weighted image and is (**B**) hyperintense on an axial short TI inversion recovery image. (**A:** TR, 600 msec; TE, 20 msec; **B:** TR, 2000 msec; TI, 160 msec; TE, 43 msec.)

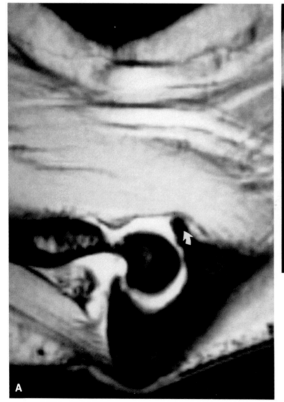

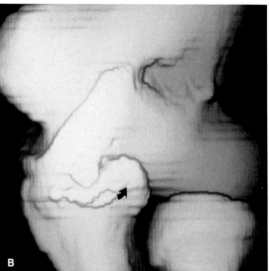

FIGURE 7–25. Osteoarthritis of the humeroulnar joint. A coronoid process osteophyte (*curved arrow*) is seen on (**A**) sagittal T2*-weighted and (**B**) coronal 3D CT images.

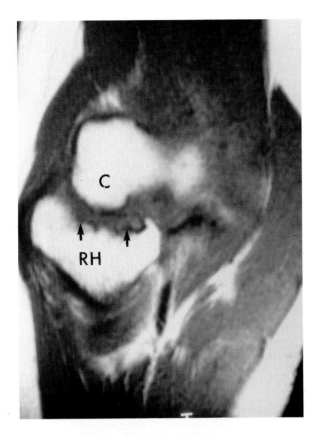

FIGURE 7–26. Low signal intensity subchondral sclerosis (*arrows*) and denuded articular cartilage in the radial head (RH) are seen on a coronal T1-weighted image of osteoarthritis of the humerodistal joint. (C, capitellum.)

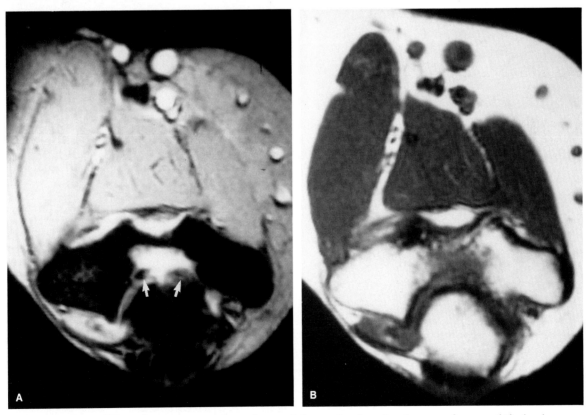

FIGURE 7–27. Olecranon osteophytes (*arrows*) that project into the olecranon fossa are (**A**) clearly demonstrated on an axial T2*-weighted image and (**B**) poorly seen on the corresponding axial T1-weighted image. Effusion within the elbow joint is seen. (**A:** TR, 400 msec; TE, 15 msec; flip angle, 20°; **B:** TR, 600 msec; TE, 20 msec.)

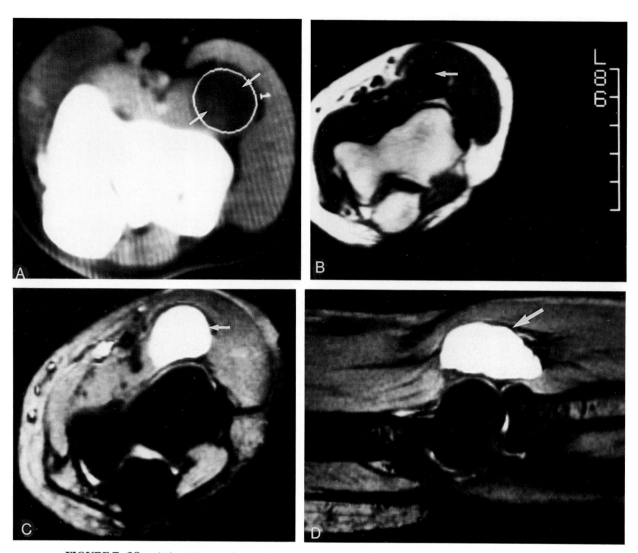

FIGURE 7–28. (**A**) A CT scan shows a juxtaarticular synovial cyst about the elbow as a low attenuation lesion deep to the brachioradialis (*arrows*). (**B**) The corresponding axial T1-weighted image shows the cyst (*arrow*) as isointense with adjacent muscle tissue. (TR, 600 msec; TE, 20 msec.) T2*-weighted (**C**) axial and (**D**) sagittal images show the cyst as a focus of uniform high signal intensity (*arrows*). (TR, 400 msec; TE, 20 msec; flip angle, 30°.)

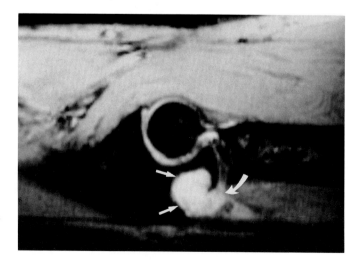

FIGURE 7–29. A subchondral cyst of the olecranon (*straight arrows*) with a cortical extension (*curved arrow*) is seen on a T2*-weighted sagittal image.

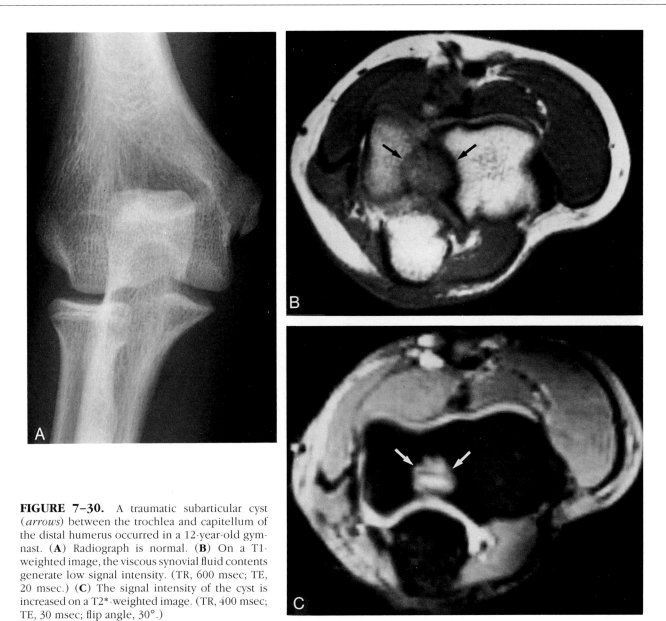

FIGURE 7–30. A traumatic subarticular cyst (*arrows*) between the trochlea and capitellum of the distal humerus occurred in a 12-year-old gymnast. (**A**) Radiograph is normal. (**B**) On a T1-weighted image, the viscous synovial fluid contents generate low signal intensity. (TR, 600 msec; TE, 20 msec.) (**C**) The signal intensity of the cyst is increased on a T2*-weighted image. (TR, 400 msec; TE, 30 msec; flip angle, 30°.)

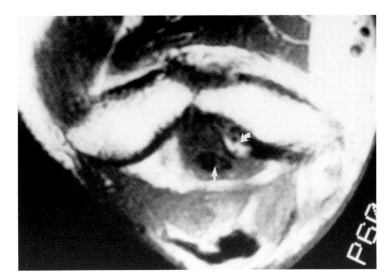

FIGURE 7–31. A loose body (*straight arrow*) and an osteophyte (*curved arrow*) are seen in the olecranon fossa on axial (**A**) T1-weighted and (**B**) T2*-weighted images. High signal intensity effusion is displayed in both the coronoid and olecranon fossae on the T2*-weighted image. The osteophyte demonstrates marrow signal intensity on the T1-weighted image. (**C**) The corresponding 3D CT image spatially displays the location of the loose body (*straight arrow*) and the posterior projecting osteophyte (*curved arrow*). (L, lateral epicondyle; M, medial epicondyle; O, olecranon.)

(continued)

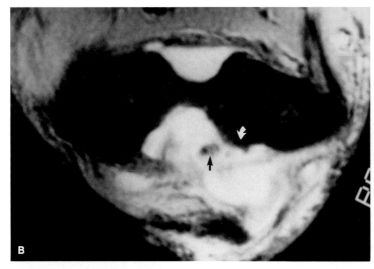

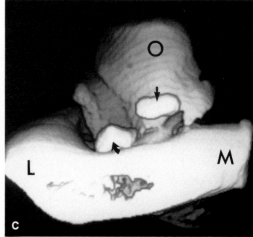

FIGURE 7–31. *(Continued)*

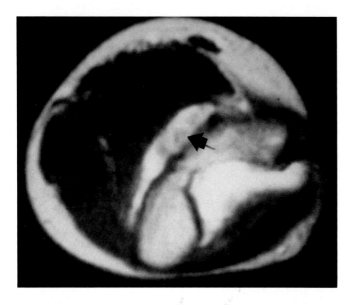

FIGURE 7–32. Multiple cartilaginous loose bodies in the coronoid fossa demonstrate intermediate signal intensity on a T1-weighted image. The corresponding radiographs (not shown) were negative. (TR, 600 msec; TE, 20 msec.)

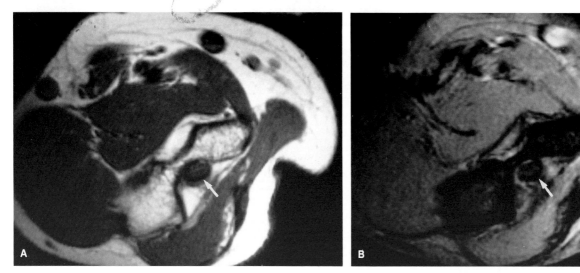

FIGURE 7–33. A large loose body (*arrows*) in the olecranon fossa demonstrates low signal intensity on axial (**A**) T1-weighted and (**B**) T2*-weighted images. (**A:** TR, 600 msec; TE, 20 msec; **B:** TR, 400 msec; TE, 20 msec; flip angle, 25°.)

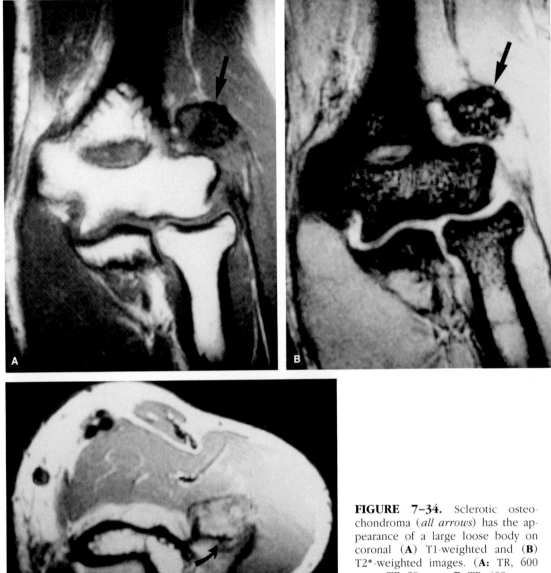

FIGURE 7–34. Sclerotic osteochondroma (*all arrows*) has the appearance of a large loose body on coronal (**A**) T1-weighted and (**B**) T2*-weighted images. (**A:** TR, 600 msec; TE, 20 msec; **B:** TR, 400 msec; TE, 20 msec; flip angle, 25°.) (**C**) The corresponding axial T1-weighted image shows continuity of the marrow and cortex with the humerus. (TR, 600 msec; TE, 20 msec.)

may prove to be more accurate than MR in characterizing roughened joint surfaces, osteophyte anatomy, and osteocartilaginous loose bodies characteristic of osteoarthritis. Assessment of articular cartilage surfaces, however, requires MR imaging. Osteophytes (Fig. 7–27), synovial cysts (Fig. 7–28), and subchondral cysts (Figs. 7–29 and 7–30) are best defined on T2- or T2*-weighted images.

Rheumatoid Arthritis

The elbow is frequently involved in rheumatoid arthritis. A positive fat-pad sign representing effusion and erosions of the distal humerus, radial head, and coronoid are associated with synovial inflammation.[22] Joint-space narrowing may be more prominent in the humeroulnar compartment, although the entire elbow joint may demonstrate loss of joint space.[21]

Loose Bodies

Intraarticular cartilaginous or osteocartilaginous loose bodies are found in association with osteochondritis dissecans, osteochondral fractures, and synovial osteochondromatosis. Computed tomography scans at 1.5 mm with coronal and sagittal reformations provide the greatest detail in identifying osteocartilaginous loose bodies and osteophytic spurs (Fig. 7–31). Reformatted scans are necessary to more accurately differentiate loose bodies from partial voluming of osteophytes. With MR imaging, it is possible to identify cartilaginous fragments not seen on CT or obscured on CT arthrography (Fig. 7–32). The olecranon and coronoid fossae are common locations for these loose bodies. In interpreting T2*-weighted images, it should be remembered that hypertrophied synovium and fat adjacent to irritated synovium may simulate the appearance of a low signal intensity loose body. Therefore, conventional T2-weighted images may be valuable in improving the accuracy of detecting free fragments. Loose bodies or free fragments frequently do not demonstrate fat marrow signal intensity (Fig. 7–33). Osteophytic projections or osteochondromas may be mistaken for loose bodies if not followed to their site of origin (Fig. 7–34).

REFERENCES

1. Franklin PD, et al. Computed tomography of the normal and traumatized elbow. J Comput Assist Tomogr 1988;12:817.
2. Hindman BW, et al. Supracondylar fractures of the humerus: prediction of the cubitus varus deformity with CT. Radiology 1988;168:513.
3. Greenberg DA. Anatomy of pathology of the pediatric elbow using magnetic resonance imaging. Contemp Orthop 1989;19:345.
4. Berquist TH. MR imaging of the elbow and wrist. Top Magn Reson Imaging 1989;1:15.
5. Middleton WD, Macrander S, Kneeland JB, et al. MR imaging of the normal elbow: anatomic correlation. AJR 1987;149:543.
6. Pitt MJ, Speer DP. Imaging of the elbow with an emphasis on trauma. Radiol Clin North Am 1990;28:293.
7. McMinn RMH. Last's anatomy: regional and applied. 8th ed. Edinburgh: Churchill-Livingston, 1990:84.
8. Williams PL. Gray's anatomy. 37th ed. Edinburgh: Churchill-Livingston, 1989:505.
9. Turek SL. Orthopaedics. Philadelphia: JB Lippincott, 1984:967.
10. Bunnell DH, Risher DA, Bassett LA, et al. Elbow joint: normal anatomy on MR images. Radiology 1987;165:527.
11. Margles SW. Avascular necrosis in the upper extremity. In: Dee R, ed. Principles of orthopaedic practice. New York: McGraw-Hill, 1989;781.
12. Sampson S, et al. Traumatic injury to the upper extremity. In: Dee R, ed. Principles of orthopaedic practice. New York: McGraw-Hill, 1989:536.
13. Pappas AM. Osteochondritis dissecans. Clin Orthop 1981;158:59.
14. Tivnon MC, Anzel SH, Waugh TR. Surgical management of osteochondritis dissecans of the capitellum. Am J Sports Med 1976;4:121.
15. Nirsch RP. Tennis elbow. Orthop Clin North Am 1973;43:787.
16. Deharen KE, Evarts CM. Throwing injuries of the elbow in athletes. Orthop Clin North Am 1973;1:801.
17. Hurst LC. Peripheral nerve injuries and entrapment. In: Dee R, ed. Principles of orthopaedic practice. New York: McGraw-Hill, 1989:678.
18. Craven PR, Green DP. Cubital tunnel syndrome. Treatment by medial epicondylectomy. J Bone Joint Surg [Am] 1980;62:986.
19. Baker BE, Bierwagen D. Rupture of the distal tendon of the biceps brachii. J Bone Joint Surg [Am] 1985;67:414.
20. Mason ML. Some observations on fractures of the head of the radius with a review of one hundred cases. Br J Surg 1954;43:123.
21. Dee R. Rheumatological and degenerative disorders of the elbow. In: Dee R, ed. Principles of orthopaedic practice. New York: McGraw-Hill, 1989:635.
22. Quinton DN, Rinlay D, Butterworth R. Elbow fat pad sign: brief report. [abstr] Radiology 1988;168:294.

The Wrist and Hand

Magnetic resonance (MR) imaging of the wrist and hand, to identify both normal anatomy and pathology, has become a subject of increased attention at hand and radiologic society meetings. For the first time, MR makes it possible for the radiologist to accomplish accurate, noninvasive imaging of specific ligamentous injuries, rendering the vague diagnosis of wrist sprain obsolete. As new data on the biomechanics of the carpus is collected, applications are developed for kinematic imaging. As techniques for dynamic MR imaging of the carpus advance, these methods may well become the standard for evaluating instability from a physiologic viewpoint. This "instability" can be best defined as the inability of two bones or groups of bones to maintain a normal physiologic relationship.

STATUS OF IMAGING TECHNIQUES

Standard Radiography

Standard radiographic evaluation of the wrist and hand is restricted primarily to demonstrating the osseous structures. With the localization of certain pathologic processes, select views, such as the scaphoid and carpal tunnel views, may provide additional information. The scaphoid fat stripe, which can be identified radial to the scaphoid, and the pronator quadratus line, which is frequently obscured by fracture, are shown in posteroanterior and lateral radiographic views, respectively. The usefulness of the scaphoid fat stripe in diagnosing acute scaphoid fractures has been challenged. The static bony relationships of the radius, lunate, and capitate can be measured in longitudinal axes in a lateral radiograph.

Arthrography

Wrist arthrography has been used to evaluate the integrity of the triangular fibrocartilage (TFC) and the scapholunate (SL) and lunotriquetral (LT) interosseous ligaments.[1-4] The three-compartment (*i.e.,* triple injection) arthrogram, in which contrast is introduced into the radiocarpal, distal radioulnar, and midcarpal joints, is considered the standard technique.[5,6] Although arthrographic findings correlate quite well with ulnar-sided wrist pain, the technique is far less effective for radial-sided problems. Manaster found that, although 88% of patients with ulnar pain had LT perforations, only 26% of patients with SL dissociation had SL perforations.[7] Thus, arthrography does not appear to be useful in assessing the physiologic integrity of the interosseous ligaments on the radial side of the wrist. Another limitation is that, because of the nature of the technique, it is impossible to differentiate small, pinhole perforations from those that are large and biomechanically significant. Anatomic studies of aging wrists have shown that degenerative perforations of both the interosseous ligaments and the triangular fibrocartilage complex (TFCC) are quite common in people older than 35 years of age;[8,9] therefore, arthrography is less diagnostically useful for these patients.

Computed Tomography

Computed tomography (CT) has limited application in the wrist. Primarily, it is used to evaluate the carpal tunnel and the nonosseous structures about the wrist and hand (Fig. 8–1). Although subtle differences in closely related soft-tissue attenuation values cannot be optimally resolved with CT, it is an excellent modality for defining the location and extent of carpal bone fractures and complex intraarticular fractures of the distal radius.[10,11] Reformatted coronal and sagittal scans, direct coronal scans, and three-dimensional (3D) CT renderings are useful for evaluating fractures and for displaying fracture morphology displacement, nonunion, and alignment through specific anatomic areas (*e.g.,* the hook of the hamate).[12,13] Small chip fractures and loose bodies may be identified in thin section (*i.e.,* 1.5-mm) CT scans.

Ultrasound and Miscellaneous Techniques

Ultrasound has been used to study the gross motion of the tendons in the carpal tunnel during flexion.[14] Videofluoroscopy and cine CT studies of wrist motion may provide indirect evidence of pathology in tendons, ligaments, and cartilage, without direct imaging or arthroscopy of these structures.

Magnetic Resonance Imaging

Magnetic resonance imaging of the wrist provides the high spatial and contrast resolution of soft-tissue and osseous components needed for evaluation of the small and complex anatomy of the wrist and hand.[15-26] Supporting muscles, ligaments, tendons, tendon sheaths, vessels, nerves, and marrow are demonstrated on MR images with excellent spatial resolution using small fields of view (FOVs) and uniform signal intensity penetration. Magnetic resonance has the potential to replace conventional wrist arthrography in diagnosing tears involving the intercarpal ligaments and the TFCC. Multiplanar images permit direct anatomic and pathologic discrimination in axial, coronal, sagittal, and oblique planes without the delayed reconstructions or reformatting required for CT. Sagittal MR images display bone and ligamentous anatomy in a selective "tomographiclike" section, without the overlapping of carpal bones seen in lateral radiographs. This facilitates a more accurate assessment of carpal instabilities. Three-dimensional Fourier transform (3DFT) volume imaging allows for single-plane acquisition with retrospective reformatting of other orthogonal or nonorthogonal oblique planar images. Kinematic imaging in coronal and sagittal orientations provides information regarding carpal bone motion and synchrony with supporting ligamentous structures.

Magnetic resonance is presently used in the evaluation of trauma (*i.e.,* fracture), avascular necrosis (AVN), and Kienböck's disease (KD), as well as the TFC and carpal tunnel. In addition, the status of articular cartilage and the cortical and subchondral bone response in arthritis can be assessed and categorized.

MAGNETIC RESONANCE IMAGING TECHNIQUES

The wrist and hand are imaged using a dedicated circumferential design send–receive coil to optimize the signal-to-noise ratio (SNR) and obtain high-resolution images (Fig. 8–2). With this coil design, the patient's arm may be positioned at his or her side. When high spatial resolution images requiring smaller FOVs are necessary for the opposite wrist or hand, separate acquisitions can be performed in the area of suspected pathology and a comparison of normal and abnormal anatomy can be made. Anatomic symmetry of both extremities can be demonstrated in the same FOV by placing both hands in a large diameter coil. Proper positioning requires alignment of the long axis of the distal radius and central metacarpal axis with the wrist in neutral position. Oblique prescriptions are not required to produce orthogonal images with this colinear alignment of the distal radius and carpus. Radial or ulnar deviation and dorsal or volar angulation should be avoided to maintain consistent alignment of the carpus. The wrist is studied in pronation, with the fingers held in extension.

In the axial plane, T1-weighted images, used as the initial localizer, are acquired with a repetition time (TR) of 500 msec and an echo time (TE) of 20 msec. Four-millimeter sections are obtained at a 256 × 256 (*i.e.,* 192) acquisition matrix, using an 8- to 10-cm FOV. Either T2*-weighted or short TI inversion recovery (STIR) axial images may be substituted for T1-weighted images when tenosynovitis, ganglia, carpal tunnel syndrome, or neoplasms are suspected. Gradient-echo axial images through the phalanges optimally differentiate between the flexor digitorum superficialis and profundus tendons. Coronal T1-weighted 3-mm images are acquired without an interslice gap and with an 8- to 10-cm FOV, a TR of 400 to 500 msec, and a TE of 15 to 20 msec. This protocol provides adequate dorsal to volar wrist coverage. Multiplanar T2*-weighted images, including the image locator, are obtained in the coronal plane, which best displays the anatomy of the TFC and SL and lunotriquetral liga-

ments. Multiple signal averages may be necessary to optimize the SNR when using gradient-echo techniques. T2*-weighted protocols use a TR of 55 to 85 msec, a TE of 20 to 25 msec, and a θ flip angle of 25°. Longer TRs (*i.e.,* 400 msec) are used to obtain multiple slice locations. T1-weighted sagittal images are performed with a TR of 400 to 500 msec and a TE of 15 to 20 msec, in 3-mm sections with a 1-mm interslice gap, and with a 10-cm FOV.

Conventional T2-weighted images may be substituted for T2*-weighted images in the axial plane, although image quality is usually poor in second-echo images when using 8- to 10-cm FOVs. T2*-weighted coronal images produce superior contrast between the intercarpal ligaments and the TFCC. Three-dimensional FT volume acquisitions, which use gradient-echo protocols, are not limited by slice thickness and can be used to reformat anatomy in other planes of section at FOVs less than 16 cm. In 3DFT volume imaging, the imaging time and the SNR are proportional to the number of slices, the TR, and the number of excitations. Scan time also increases when imaging with a high acquisition matrix (*i.e.,* 256 or 512). Coupled 3-in circular surface coils positioned in a kinematic wrist device have been used with gradient-echo protocols to track distal and carpal row motion with radial and ulnar deviation of the wrist. This information is displayed in a cine loop format and can be recorded on video or photographed.

Dorsiflexion and palmarflexion motions are best studied in the sagittal plane and require either greater degrees of freedom from the surface coil or pivoting of the coil to accommodate the increased range of motion. Image quality considerations need to be balanced in designing a surface coil with an increased diameter or anatomic coverage. Separate axial imaging sequences in positions of pronation and supination may be useful in the evaluation of subluxation patterns in the distal radioulnar joint (DRUJ). Developments in hyperscan technology may facilitate true dynamic joint imaging, which would be able to more accurately describe carpal translations and impingements in various instability patterns.

FUNCTIONAL ANATOMY OF THE WRIST

Osseous Structures

The osseous elements of the wrist consist of the distal radius and ulna, the proximal and distal carpal rows, and the bases of the metacarpals. There are three major compartments of the wrist as defined by arthrographic studies:

1. The radiocarpal compartment
2. The midcarpal compartment
3. The DRUJ compartment.

Distal Radioulnar Joint

On its medial side, the distal radius forms a shallow depression for articulation with the ulnar head (Fig. 8–3). The sigmoid notch acts as a seat for the rotating pole of the distal ulna and provides some bony stability to the DRUJ. The DRUJ is inclined 20° distally and ulnarly; this angle of inclination is thought to be important in maintaining forearm rotation. The stabilizing ligaments for the joint include the TFC and the dorsal and volar capsular ligaments, which are often poorly defined tissues (Fig. 8–4). The TFC connects the ulna and radius at their most distal edges. It runs from the ulnarmost edge of the lunate facet and sigmoid notch to the base of the ulnar styloid, where it inserts into a small depression in the distal ulna known as the fovea. The ulnar insertion consists of two limbs, one distal and one proximal. However, traumatic loss of the soft-tissue stabilizers of the DRUJ, primarily the TFCC, may cause subluxation of the radius on the fixed unit of the ulna.[27]

Radiocarpal Joint

The radiocarpal joint is defined by the TFC and the distal radial surface proximally, and the triquetrum and scaphoid distally. The distal articular surfaces of the radius and ulna are usually at the same level (*i.e.,* neutral ulnar variance) at the site of the radiolunate articulation. The distal radius forms two facets that articulate with the scaphoid and lunate of the proximal carpal row (see Figs. 8–3 and 8–4). This articulation of the proximal pole of the scaphoid in the scaphoid fossa is quite congruent; even a small degree of malpositioning of the scaphoid may cause rotatory subluxation, such as that which accompanies a scapholunate advanced collapse (SLAC) wrist as described by Watson.[28] The lunate facet commonly becomes incongruent following distal radius fractures.

Lister's tubercle, the most prominent dorsal radial ridge, separates the extensor pollicis longus tendon (ulnar side) from the extensor carpi radialis and brevis tendons (radial side). This is the site where bone spurs form and attrition ruptures occur in rheumatoid arthritis.

Carpus

The proximal carpal row consists of the scaphoid, the lunate, and the triquetrum (Figs. 8–5 and 8–6). It is thought that, with a congenital bipartite scaphoid, the proximal row should include only the proximal pole of the scaphoid. The distal pole should be thought of as a component of the distal row. The scaphoid, lunate, and triquetrum are linked by strong interosseous ligaments that work together to form a flexible socket or acetabulum that cradles the distal row. Occasionally, anatomic imperfections in this socket lead to arthritic degeneration. The lunate may have a medial facet which measures 1 to 6 mm in diameter. This facet is present in approximately two-thirds of cadaver hands studied, and 44% of these had arthritic degeneration of the proximal pole of the hamate. Hamate arthritis was not seen unless the medial facet was present on the lunate.[29] The distal carpal row consists of the trapezium, the trapezoid, the capitate, and the hamate (see Figs. 8–5 and 8–6).

Ligamentous Anatomy

Much of the interest in and appreciation of the ligamentous anatomy of the wrist derives from the advent of wrist arthroscopy. Arthroscopy allows direct examination of the ligaments of the wrist and testing of their physiologic integrity. All arthroscopic portals are, of necessity, dorsally placed, making examination of the volar ligaments especially easy. As a result, the dorsal ligaments initially received less attention, although many investigators are now studying their biomechanics. Definition of pathologic conditions naturally followed elucidation of the ligamentous anatomy, and new treatment procedures were devised.[30]

Traditionally, the ligaments of the wrist have been classified into intrinsic and extrinsic groups (Table 8–1).[31] The extrinsic ligaments extend from the radius, ulna, and metacarpals; and the intrinsic ligaments originate and insert within the carpus. In general, the role of the intrinsic ligaments is to maintain the relationship between the individual carpal bones, whereas the extrinsic ligaments are important in the relationship of the carpus as a whole to the distal radius and ulna as well as the bases of the metacarpals. Many investigators object to this classification scheme because it is possible for imbalances of the extrinsic ligaments to cause carpal instability, a condition that was formerly thought to occur only through dysfunction of the intrinsic ligaments. However, this scheme remains useful, if only as an anatomic guide.

Extrinsic Ligaments

Radiocarpal Ligaments. The volar extrinsic ligaments are the most constant and the strongest of the extrinsic ligaments. Several mechanically important ligaments originate from the region of the radial styloid and distal radius, including the radial collateral ligament and the palmar radiocarpal ligament. The latter consists of the radioscaphocapitate (RSC) ligament, the long radiolunate (LRL) ligament, the radioscapholunate (RSL) ligament, and the short radiolunate (SRL) ligament (Fig. 8–7).

Although the radial collateral ligament is not a true

TABLE 8–1.

Extrinsic and intrinsic ligaments of the wrist

RADIOCARPAL (RADIAL ORIGIN)	ULNOCARPAL (TFCC LIGAMENTS)	DORSAL
Extrinsic Ligaments		
Radial collateral ligament	Dorsal radioulnar ligament	Dorsal radioscapholunotriquetral ligament
Palmar radiocarpal ligament	Volar radioulnar ligament	Scaphotriquetral ligament
Radioscaphocapitate ligament	Ulnolunate ligament	
Long radiolunate ligament	Ulnotriquetral ligament	
Short radiolunate ligament	Ulnar collateral ligament	
Radioscapholunate ligament	Meniscus homologue	
Radiolunate ligament or ligament of Testut		
Radioscaphoid ligament or ligament of Kuenz		
Intrinsic Ligaments		
Scapholunate ligament		
Lunotriquetral ligament		
Deltoid or arcuate ligaments		
Trapezium–trapezoid ligament		
Trapezoid–capitate ligament		
Capitate–hamate ligament		

TFCC, triangular fibrocartilage complex.

collateral ligament because ulnar and radial deviation are normal motion arcs in the wrist, and, by definition, a collateral ligament resists only pathologic or abnormal motion, it has been shown to be mechanically significant and to play a role in the mechanism of midwaist scaphoid fractures by compressing the bone along its longitudinal axis.[32] This ligament originates on the tip of the styloid and inserts into the radial surface of the scaphoid at its waist.

The RSC ligament is a very stout ligament that is readily identifiable through the arthroscope. It originates from the radial styloid and has a minor insertion into the radial aspect of the waist of the scaphoid. The bulk of the fibers continue in an ulnodistal direction and merge with the fibers of the TFCC palmar to the head of the capitate to form a supporting sling. As the fibers cross the proximal pole of the scaphoid, there is a fold of synovium that separates them from the bone.[33] In this position, the ligament can be interposed between the fragments of a scaphoid fracture and contribute to nonunion.

Progressing ulnarly, the LRL ligament is the next ligament that originates from the radius. This strong ligament stabilizes the proximal carpal row on the radius and should be differentiated from the RSL ligament (*i.e.,* ligaments of Testut and Kuenz). The LRL ligament originates from the palmar lip of the radius and courses ulnodistally, parallel with the RSC ligament, to insert into the radial aspect of the palmar surface of the lunate.

The SRL ligament was described by Berger and Landsmeer.[33] This ligament originates from the radius in the region of the lunate facet and inserts distally into the palmar surface of the lunate. At its insertion, its fibers merge with those of the LRL ligament. The RSL ligament is interposed dorsally between the LRL and the SRL ligaments (Fig. 8–8). This structure was first described in detail by Testut, and the RSL ligament is often called by his name (*i.e.,* ligament of Testut).[34] From his work on fetal wrists, Landsmeer described a vascular pedicle which supplied the RSL ligament.[35] It has since been shown that this structure is a neurovascular umbilical cord that may provide a clinically significant blood supply to the proximal pole of the scaphoid via the SL interosseous ligament and a sensory or proprioceptive pathway to the SL joint.[36] The RSL ligament has been studied extensively, and it has been shown to contain the most elastic tissue of any ligament in the wrist. It does not appear to provide any mechanical support to the carpus.

By virtue of their orientation and mechanical properties, the radiocarpal ligaments maintain the carpus within its radial articulation. Loss of these ligaments allows the carpus to move down the inclined plane of the distal radius and undergo ulnar translation. This condition is not uncommon in rheumatoid arthritis, where synovitic degeneration of these soft-tissue supporting structures occurs. With ulnar translation the distance between the radial styloid and the scaphoid increases and the scaphoid and lunate are displaced from their articular fossae. The lunate comes to rest where it articulates with the distal ulna, and the scaphoid becomes perched on the ridge between its own articular the lunate fossae. This incongruent loading leads to degeneration of the cartilaginous surfaces and ulnolunate impingement. Overexuberant surgical resection of the radial styloid can destroy the origin of these ligaments and cause this type of instability.

Ulnocarpal Ligaments. The ulnar portion of the extrinsic volar ligaments of the wrist is formed by the TFCC (Figs. 8–9 and 8–10). The TFCC consists of the TFC proper (the articular disc) and the dorsal and volar radioulnar ligaments, (discussed previously), the meniscus homologue, and the ulnolunate and the ulnotriquetral ligaments. The term TFCC was coined to describe all of the ligamentous and cartilaginous structures that were thought to play a role in suspending the distal radius and the ulnar carpus from the distal ulna.[37] As noted above, the study of the biomechanics of the structures of the TFCC is in its infancy, but there are clinical and laboratory data to support their role in maintaining both the stability of the DRUJ and the stability of the carpus as a whole (preventing pronosupination of the carpus). The TFCC also contributes to stability within the carpus by preventing carpal instabilities, nondissociative (CIND).

Dorsal Ligaments. Although the palmar radiocarpal ligaments have attracted a great deal of attention in the past, new insights into the biomechanics of the wrist have focused interest on the dorsal ligaments. The dorsal ligaments do not exist as discrete anatomic entities and they vary considerably from subject to subject. Two major components can be discerned (Figs. 8–11 and 8–12). The first is the dorsal radioscapholunotriquetral (RSLT), a thickening of the dorsal capsule that courses from the dorsal lip of the radius to insert on the dorsal surface of the scaphoid, lunate, and triquetrum. This ligament acts as a checkrein on the proximal carpal row and prevents it from assuming a position of excessive volarflexion. Biomechanical studies have shown that, in the final stage of ulnar-sided perilunate instability, it is the RSLT ligament that is injured.[38] Laxity of the RSLT ligament has been implicated in palmar midcarpal instability patterns in which the lunate is allowed to go into volarflexion, which leads to instability. The second major component of the dorsal ligamentous structure is the scaphotriquetral ligament. This is a transversely oriented thickening of the dorsal capsular fibers. It runs from the scaphoid to the triquetrum.

Intrinsic Interosseous Ligaments

Scapholunate and Lunotriquetral Ligaments.
The interosseous ligaments are of paramount importance in maintaining the biomechanical relationship among the carpal bones, especially those of the proximal row (Fig. 8–13). For the proximal carpal row to function properly, the bones must be associated or linked together, and the interosseous ligaments provide this flexible linkage. The SL and LT ligaments are comparable in strength to the anterior cruciate ligament of the knee. They connect the bones at the level of the proximal articular surface and consist of thick dorsal and volar components with thinner membranous portions in between. Most commonly perforations occur in the thin, membranous portions and may not be mechanically significant.

The SL and LT ligaments extend from the dorsal to the volar synovial surfaces and completely separate the radiocarpal and midcarpal compartments. The SL ligament can be directly palpated dorsally, or it can be evaluated by the scaphoid stress test—a provocative clinical maneuver to determine the degree of mobility and the symptom level secondary to this mobility. The LT-ligament interspace can also be directly palpated dorsally, and it too can be mechanically stressed by the LT ballottement test. In this test, the triquetrum is held between the thumb and index finger of one hand and the lunate is held in the other hand. Excessive pain or motion when AP forces are placed on the bones indicates a positive result.

Arcuate Ligaments. More distally, there are a set of ligaments that stabilize the distal row on the proximal row. These have been referred to as the deltoid[39] and arcuate ligaments.[40] The ulnar arcuate ligament extends from the volar surface of the lunate and triquetrum to the neck of the capitate, and plays a role in preventing the proximal row from volarflexion (Fig. 8–14). Progressing radially, the substance of this structure becomes quite thin in the region of the capitolunate articulation. The radial limb (*i.e.,* radial arcuate ligament) of this V-shaped ligament runs from the capitate to the distal pole of the scaphoid. The thin tissue between the limbs of the arcuate or deltoid ligament is known as the space of Poirier. This weak area in the ligamentous floor of the carpus may function as a trap door through which the lunate or capitate may dislocate. The particular functions of these ligaments with respect to midcarpal instabilities will be discussed below.

Distal Carpal Row Interosseous Ligaments. Within the distal row, the trapezius and trapezium, trapezoid and capitate, and capitate and hamate are connected by interosseous ligaments. In contradistinction to the interosseous ligaments of the proximal row, these ligaments do not extend from the dorsal to volar surface; thus there is normally communication between the midcarpal space and the carpometacarpal joints.

Tendons of the Wrist and Hand

Palm of the Hand

The flexor retinaculum and palmar aponeurosis represent thickened deep fascia of the wrist (Figs. 8–15, 8–16, and 8–17). The superficial palmaris longus tendon is fused to the midline of the flexor retinaculum and expands distally into the palmar aponeurosis. Guyon's canal, a site of potential compression of the ulnar nerve, is formed by an ulnar extension of the flexor retinaculum superficial to the ulnar nerve and artery.

The concave volar surface of the carpus and the flexor retinaculum form the anatomic boundaries of the carpal tunnel for passage of the long flexor tendons of the fingers and thumb (Fig. 8–18). The four flexor digitorum superficialis tendons are arranged in two rows, with the tendons to the third (*i.e.*, middle) and fourth (*i.e.*, ring) digits superficial to the tendons for the second (*i.e.*, index) and fifth (*i.e.*, little) digits (Fig. 8–19). After entering their respective fibrous flexor sheaths, the tendons of the flexor digitorum superficialis divide into two halves opposite the proximal phalanx and partially decussate around the flexor digitorum profundus tendons. Distal to the site of perforation by the flexor digitorum profundus, the superficialis tendons pass deep to the flexor digitorum profundus and send slips to attach to the sides of the middle phalanx. The tendons of the flexor digitorum profundus are arranged in the same plane and pass deep to the flexor digitorum superficialis (Fig. 8–20). The tendons of the flexor digitorum profundus attach distally to the base of the terminal phalanx and change from a deep to a superficial location at the partial decussation of the superficialis at the level of the middle phalanx (Fig. 8–21).

Dorsum of the Hand

The extensor digitorum tendons extend across the metacarpophalangeal (MP) joints and contribute to the posterior capsule of this joint, then they broaden out onto the dorsum of the proximal phalanx (Figs. 8–22 and 8–23). The extensor expansion represents the joining of the extensor tendons and posterior fascia. The extensor tendons and expansion divide into a central slip that inserts into the base of the middle phalanx and two lateral or marginal slips that diverge around the central slip and then converge to insert into the base of the distal phalanx. The interosseous and lumbrical tendons insert onto the dorsal extensor expansion from each of its sides and from its lateral side, respectively.

Ligamentous Support of the Digits

The MP, proximal interphalangeal (PIP), and distal interphalangeal joints are reinforced by palmar and paired collateral ligaments. The palmar ligament, or fibrocartilaginous volar plate, is located between and connected to the collateral ligaments. The palmar ligament blends with the deep transverse metacarpal ligament in the second to fifth MP joints.

NORMAL MAGNETIC RESONANCE ANATOMY OF THE WRIST AND HAND

Axial Images

In the axial plane (Fig. 8–24), the flexor digitorum superficialis and profundus tendons are seen as tubular low signal intensity structures with invested synovial sheaths. In proximal sections, the flexor pollicis longus is seen deep to the median nerve. Distally, it is flanked by the adductor pollicis medially and by the thenar muscles laterally toward the thumb. At the level of the DRUJ, the volar distal radioulnar ligament is identified as a thin, low signal intensity band, deep to the flexor digitorum profundus tendons and Parona's space. The position of the distal ulna in relation to the sigmoid notch is determined at this level. The TFCC is displayed on the ulnar aspect of the ulnar styloid. The curve of the ulnolunate ligament is demonstrated at the level of the proximal lunate and distal radius, where it follows the contour of the ulnar and volar aspect of the lunate. The palmaris longus tendon is superficial to the medial nerve. The thin low signal intensity flexor retinaculum spans the palmar border of the carpal tunnel. Its distal attachments to the hook of the lunate and tubercle of the trapezium are more reliably defined than the proximal attachments to the tubercles of the pisiform and scaphoid. The separate extensor tendons of the extensor carpi ulnaris, extensor digiti minimi, extensor digitorum and indicis, extensor carpi radialis brevis, extensor pollicis longus, and extensor carpi radialis longus are displayed from the ulnar to the radial dorsal aspect of the wrist. The LT, SL, and radiolunate (*i.e.*, ligament of Testut) portions of the RSL are usually demonstrated on the volar aspect of the proximal carpal row. The arcuate ligament is seen volar to the capitate and deep to the flexor tendons. The radial collateral ligament is closely applied to the radial surface of the scaphoid. The palmaris longus tendon is superficial to the median nerve and the flexor retinaculum. The two central tendons of the superficial flexor group are located superiorly within the carpal tunnel before they fan out to their insertions on the middle phalanx. Definition of the four separate tendons of the flexor profundus group is possible in axial planar images. In axial sections through the distal carpal tunnel, the lumbrical muscle origins are seen deep to the flexor tendons and dem-

(text continues on page 712)

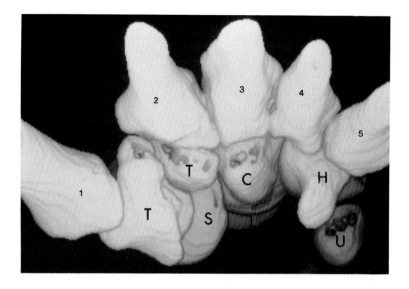

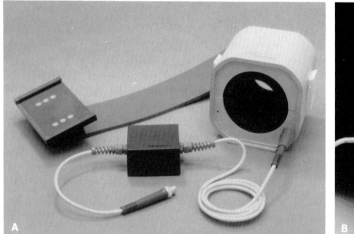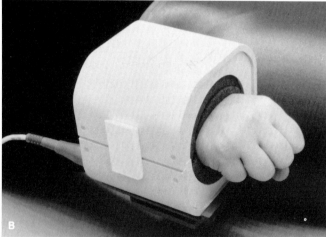

FIGURE 8–1. A 3D CT image of the osseous anatomy of the carpal tunnel shows the metacarpals, labeled 1 through 5. (C, capitate; H, hamate; S, scaphoid; T, trapezium proximal to 1st metacarpal; T, trapezoid proximal to 2nd metacarpal; U, ulna.)

FIGURE 8–2. (**A**) A dedicated send–receive wrist coil. (**B**) The coil is correctly positioned at a patient's side; however, normally the wrist is studied with the fingers relaxed and held in extension.

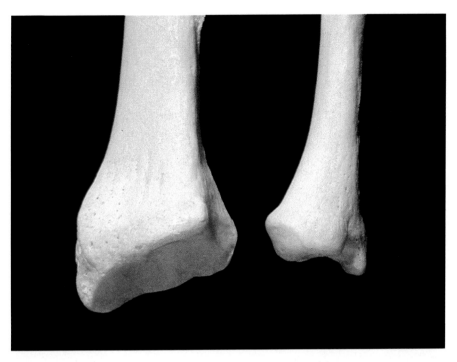

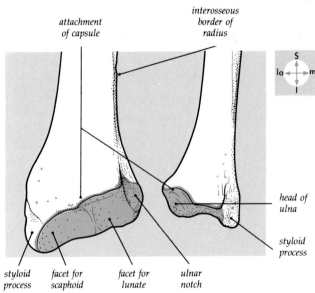

FIGURE 8–3. An anterior view of the distal ends of the radius and ulna. The bones have been separated to reveal the ulnar notch.

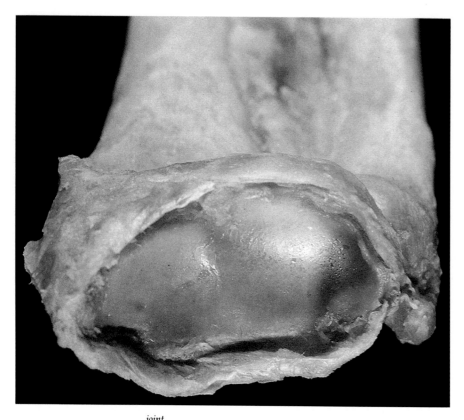

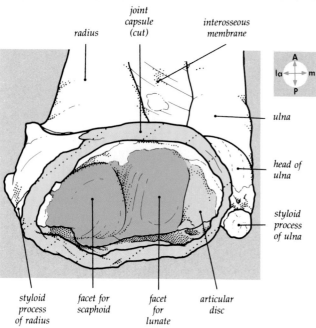

FIGURE 8–4. The articular surface of the distal end of the radius and the adjacent triangular cartilage are exposed by removal of the carpal bones.

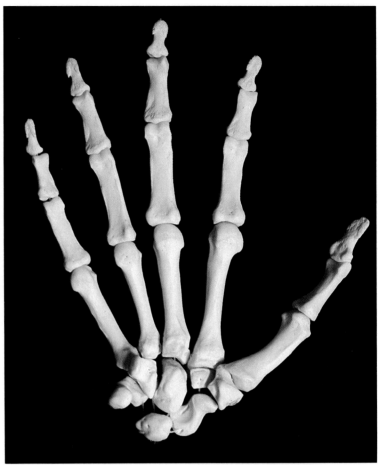

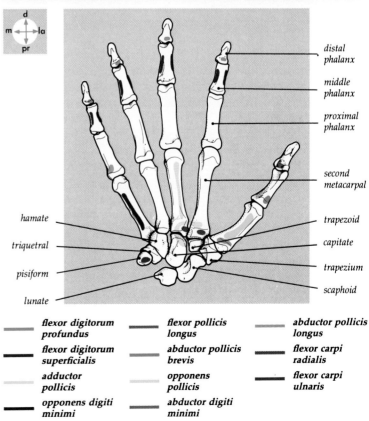

distal
phalanx

middle
phalanx

proximal
phalanx

second
metacarpal

trapezoid

capitate

trapezium

scaphoid

hamate

triquetral

pisiform

lunate

flexor digitorum profundus	flexor pollicis longus	abductor pollicis longus
flexor digitorum superficialis	abductor pollicis brevis	flexor carpi radialis
adductor pollicis	opponens pollicis	flexor carpi ulnaris
opponens digiti minimi	abductor digiti minimi	

FIGURE 8–5. The bones of the hand. Adjacent bones, particularly in the carpus, have been slightly separated to reveal their articular surfaces.

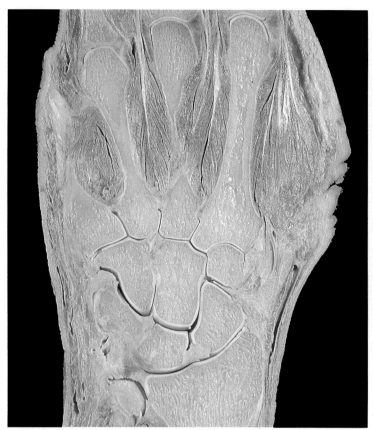

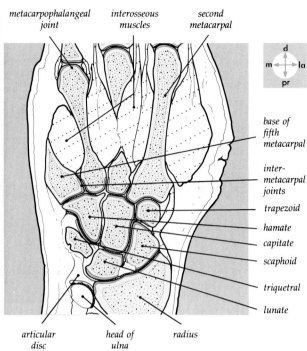

metacarpophalangeal joint · interosseous muscles · second metacarpal

d · m · la · pr

base of fifth metacarpal

inter-metacarpal joints

trapezoid

hamate

capitate

scaphoid

triquetral

lunate

articular disc · head of ulna · radius

FIGURE 8–6. A coronal section of the hand shows the joints of the carpal region. The thumb and little finger are anterior to the plane of section.

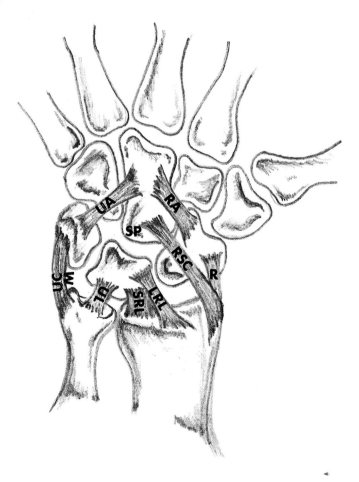

FIGURE 8–7. The volar intrinsic and extrinsic carpal ligaments. **Extrinsic ligaments.** Radiocarpal (radial origin): LRL, long radiolunate ligament; R, radial collateral ligament; RSC, radioscapho-capitate ligament; SRL, short radiolunate ligament. Ulnocarpal: M, meniscal homologue; UC, ulnar collateral ligament; UL, ulnolunate ligament. The dorsal and volar radioulnar ligaments, the ulnotriquetral ligament, and the radioscapholunate ligament are not shown. **Intrinsic ligaments.** Arcuate ligaments: RA, radial arcuate ligament; SP, space of Poirier; UA, ulnar arcuate ligament. The scapholunate ligament and lunotriquetral ligament are not shown.

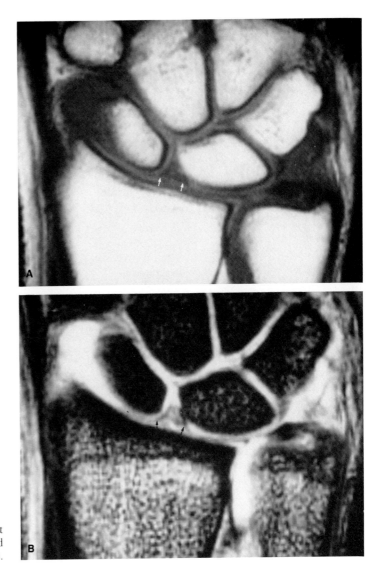

FIGURE 8–8. Anatomy of the radioscapholunate ligament (*arrows*) on coronal (**A**) T1-weighted and (**B**) T2*-weighted images. Note the attachment of the ligament to the distal radius.

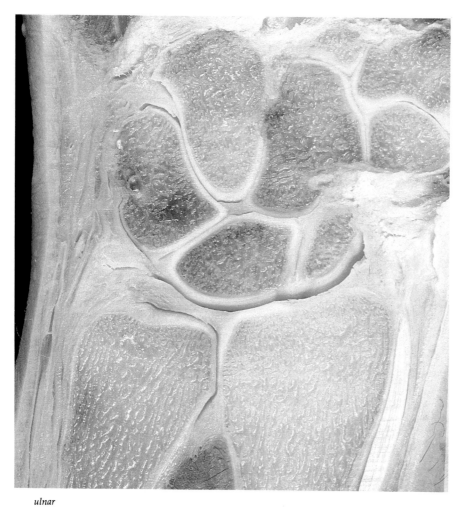

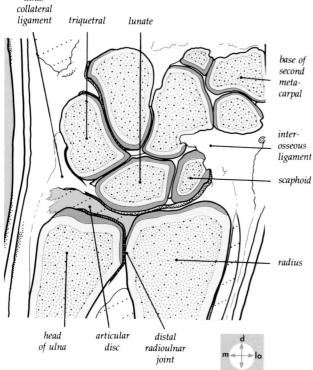

FIGURE 8–9. A coronal section of the wrist joint shows the articular surfaces and triangular cartilage.

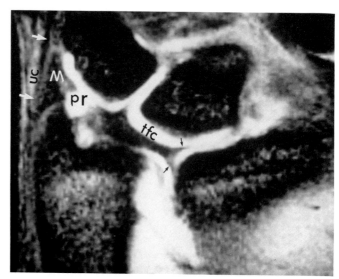

FIGURE 8–10. A T2*-weighted image shows the triangular fibrocartilage complex. (*black arrows,* radial attachments of triangular fibrocartilage; *white arrows,* UC, ulnar collateral ligament; M, meniscus homologue; pr, prestyloid recess; tfc, triangular fibrocartilage.)

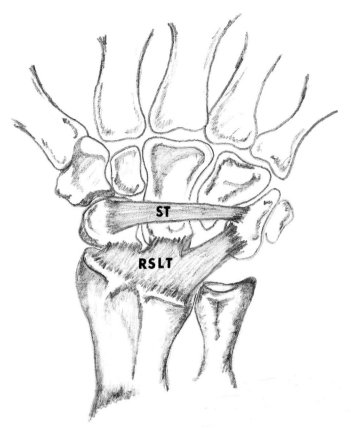

FIGURE 8–11. The dorsal intrinsic and extrinsic ligaments. (RSLT, dorsal radioscapholunotriquetral ligament; ST, scaphotriquetral ligament.)

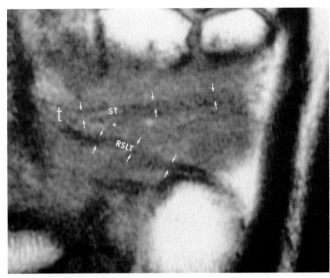

FIGURE 8–12. The dorsal ligaments of the wrist include the dorsal radioscapholunotriquetral ligament (RSLT, *diagonally oriented white arrows*) and the scaphotriquetral ligament (ST, *transversely oriented white arrows*), as seen in this T1-weighted coronal image. (T, triquetrum.)

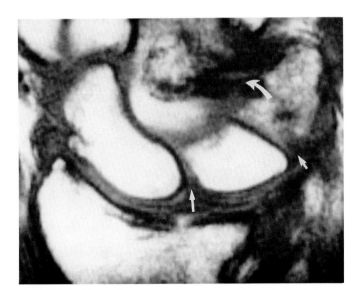

FIGURE 8–13. The intrinsic ligaments of the wrist include the scapholunate interosseous ligament (*long straight white arrow*), the lunotriquetral ligament (*short straight white arrow*), and the ulnar limb of the arcuate ligament (*curved white arrow*).

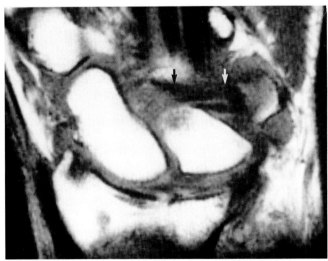

FIGURE 8–14. A T1-weighted 3-mm coronal image shows the ulnar limb of the arcuate ligament with its attachments to the volar capitate (*black arrow*) and triquetrum (*white arrow*).

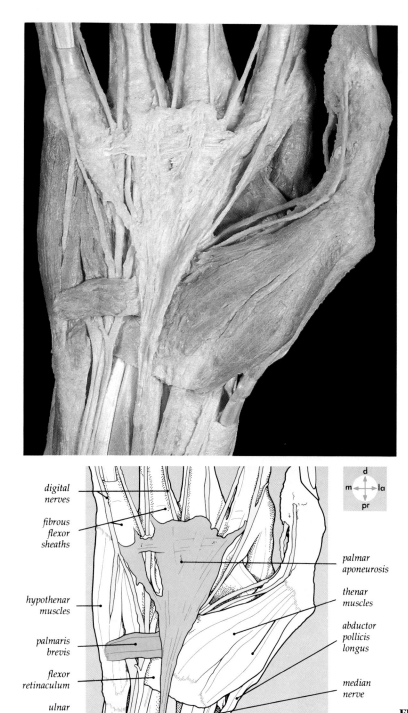

digital
nerves

fibrous
flexor
sheaths

hypothenar
muscles

palmaris
brevis

flexor
retinaculum

ulnar
nerve &
artery

d

m ⟷ la

pr

palmar
aponeurosis

thenar
muscles

abductor
pollicis
longus

median
nerve

tendon of
palmaris
longus

FIGURE 8–15. The palmar aponeurosis is revealed by removing the skin and superficial fascia. The investing fascia has been removed proximal to the flexor retinaculum.

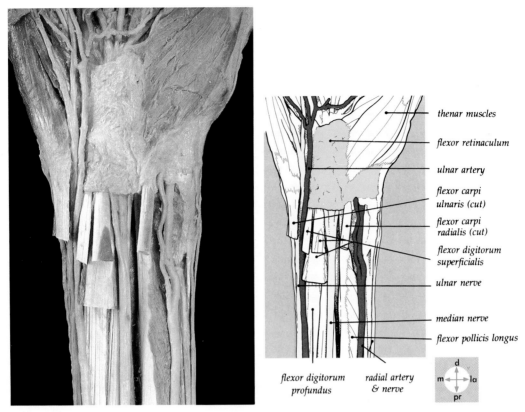

FIGURE 8–16. The flexor retinaculum and its superficial relations and structures are seen entering the carpal tunnel.

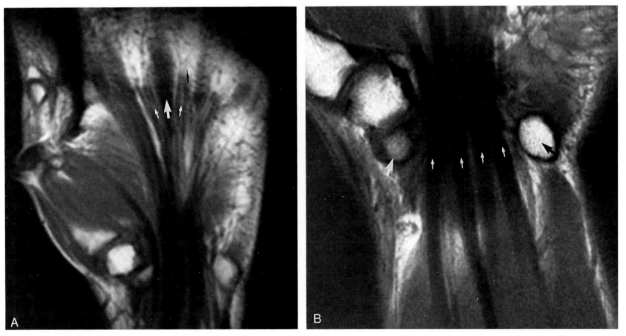

FIGURE 8–17. Volar coronal anatomy. (**A**) A T1-weighted coronal image shows the normal low signal intensity tendon (*large arrow*) and intermediate signal intensity palmar aponeurosis (*small arrows*) distal to the carpal tunnel. (**B**) At a deeper level, a T1-weighted coronal image shows the low signal intensity flexor tendons (*small white arrows*) passing through carpal tunnel. The trapezium (*large white arrow*) and pisiform (*black arrow*) are also seen.

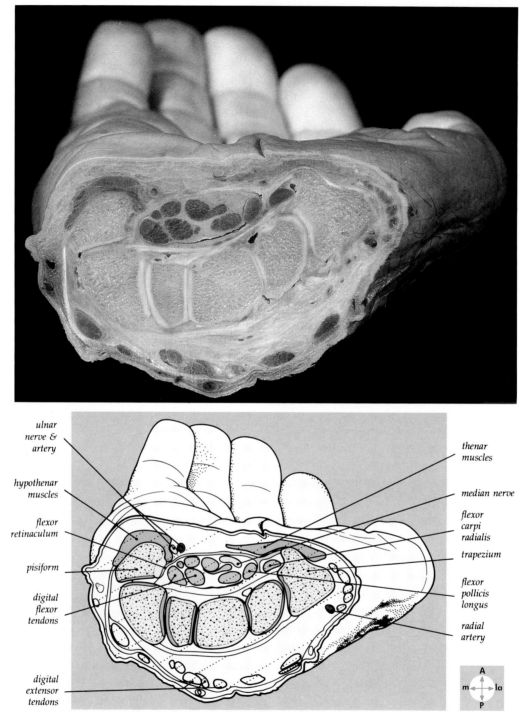

FIGURE 8–18. A transverse section through the carpus shows the carpal tunnel and its contents.

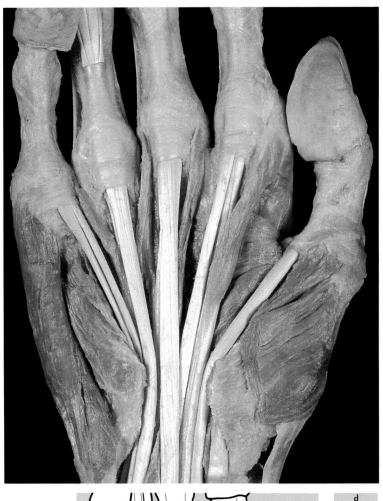

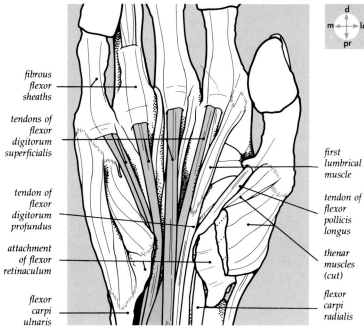

fibrous
flexor
sheaths

tendons of
flexor
digitorum
superficialis

tendon of
flexor
digitorum
profundus

attachment
of flexor
retinaculum

flexor
carpi
ulnaris

first
lumbrical
muscle

tendon of
flexor
pollicis
longus

thenar
muscles
(cut)

flexor
carpi
radialis

FIGURE 8–19. The palmar aponeurosis, flexor retinaculum, investing fascia, and palmar vessels and nerves
have been removed to reveal the tendons of the flexor
digitorum superficialis in the palm.

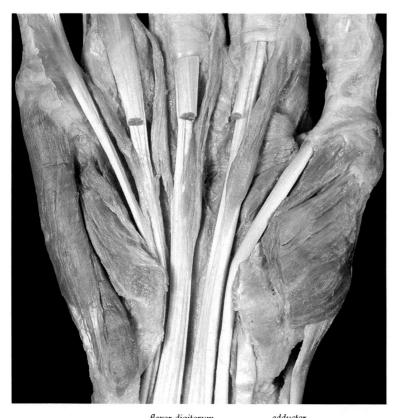

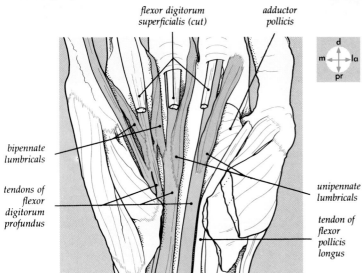

flexor digitorum superficialis (cut)

adductor pollicis

bipennate lumbricals

tendons of flexor digitorum profundus

unipennate lumbricals

tendon of flexor pollicis longus

FIGURE 8–20. Removal of the tendons of the flexor digitorum superficialis reveals the attachments of the lumbrical muscles to the tendons of the flexor digitorum profundus.

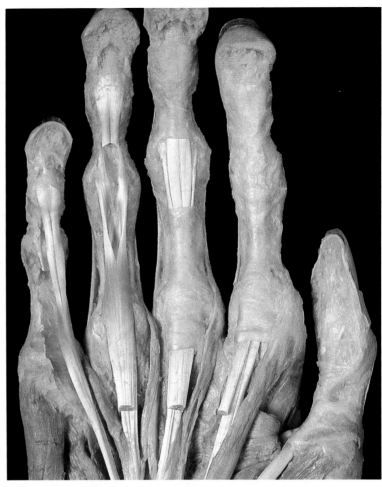

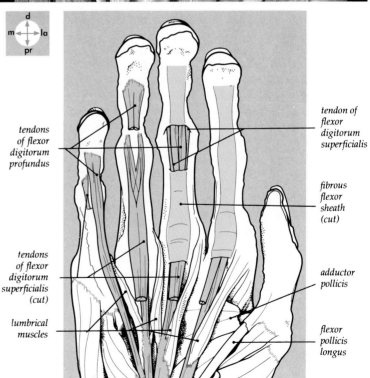

tendons
of flexor
digitorum
profundus

tendon of
flexor
digitorum
superficialis

fibrous
flexor
sheath
(cut)

tendons
of flexor
digitorum
superficialis
(cut)

lumbrical
muscles

adductor
pollicis

flexor
pollicis
longus

FIGURE 8–21. Partial cutting away of the digital fibrous flexor sheath of the middle finger exposes the tendons of flexor digitorum superficialis and profundus, revealing the phalangeal attachments in the ring and little fingers.

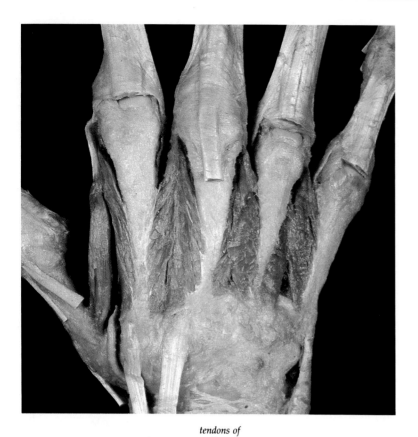

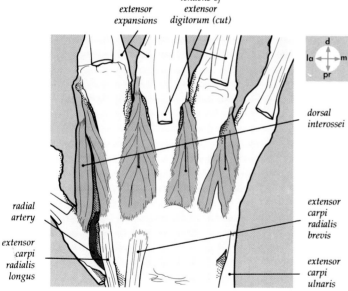

extensor expansions

tendons of extensor digitorum (cut)

dorsal interossei

radial artery

extensor carpi radialis longus

extensor carpi radialis brevis

extensor carpi ulnaris

FIGURE 8–22. The dorsal interossei is exposed by removing the deep fascia and the tendons of the extensor digitorum.

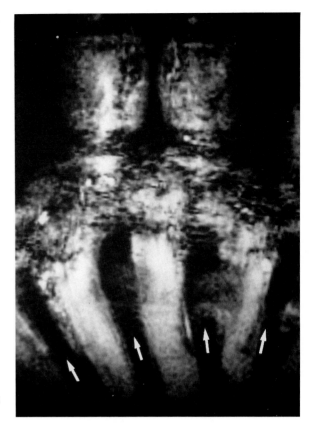

FIGURE 8–23. The low signal intensity tendons of the extensor digitorum (*white arrows*) are seen on a T2*-weighted dorsal coronal image.

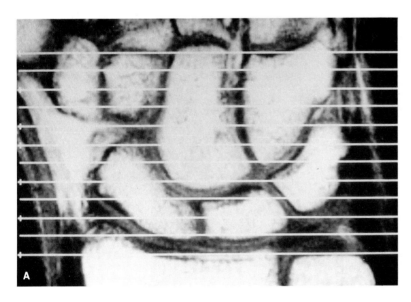

FIGURE 8–24. Normal axial MR anatomy. (**A**) This T1-weighted coronal localizer was used to graphically prescribe axial image locations from (**B**) proximal to (**M**) distal. Images were made at 12 different locations.

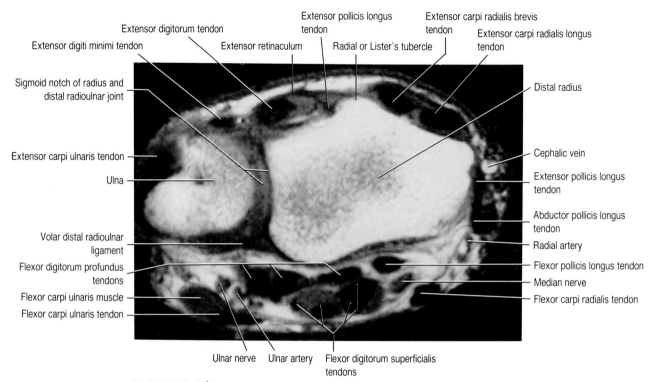

FIGURE 8–24B.

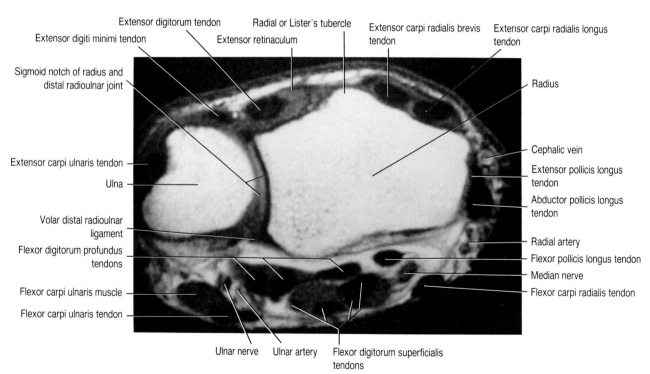

FIGURE 8–24C.

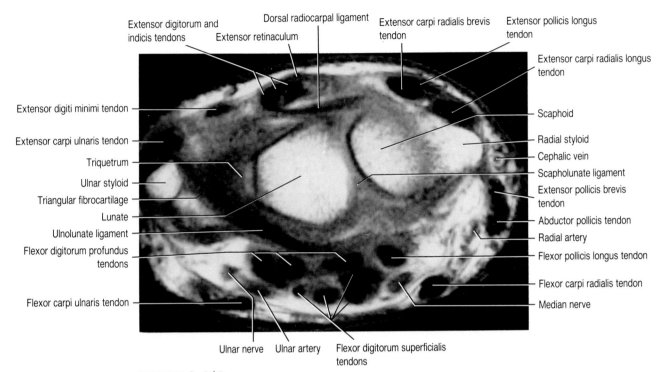

Extensor digitorum and indicis tendons
Extensor retinaculum
Dorsal radiocarpal ligament
Extensor carpi radialis brevis tendon
Extensor pollicis longus tendon
Extensor carpi radialis longus tendon
Extensor digiti minimi tendon
Extensor carpi ulnaris tendon
Triquetrum
Ulnar styloid
Triangular fibrocartilage
Lunate
Ulnolunate ligament
Flexor digitorum profundus tendons
Flexor carpi ulnaris tendon
Scaphoid
Radial styloid
Cephalic vein
Scapholunate ligament
Extensor pollicis brevis tendon
Abductor pollicis tendon
Radial artery
Flexor pollicis longus tendon
Flexor carpi radialis tendon
Median nerve
Ulnar nerve
Ulnar artery
Flexor digitorum superficialis tendons

FIGURE 8–24D.

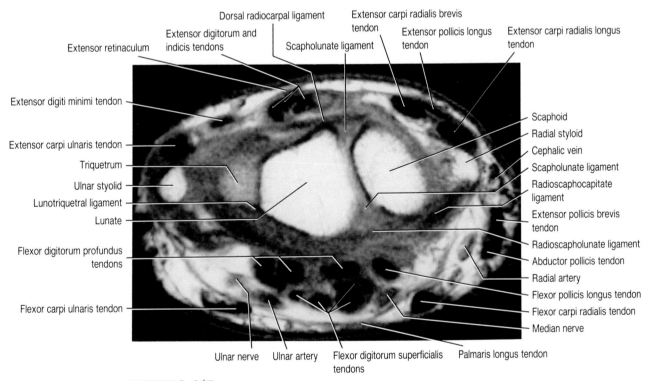

Dorsal radiocarpal ligament
Extensor digitorum and indicis tendons
Scapholunate ligament
Extensor carpi radialis brevis tendon
Extensor pollicis longus tendon
Extensor carpi radialis longus tendon
Extensor retinaculum
Extensor digiti minimi tendon
Extensor carpi ulnaris tendon
Triquetrum
Ulnar styolid
Lunotriquetral ligament
Lunate
Flexor digitorum profundus tendons
Flexor carpi ulnaris tendon
Scaphoid
Radial styloid
Cephalic vein
Scapholunate ligament
Radioscaphocapitate ligament
Extensor pollicis brevis tendon
Radioscapholunate ligament
Abductor pollicis tendon
Radial artery
Flexor pollicis longus tendon
Flexor carpi radialis tendon
Median nerve
Ulnar nerve
Ulnar artery
Flexor digitorum superficialis tendons
Palmaris longus tendon

FIGURE 8–24E.

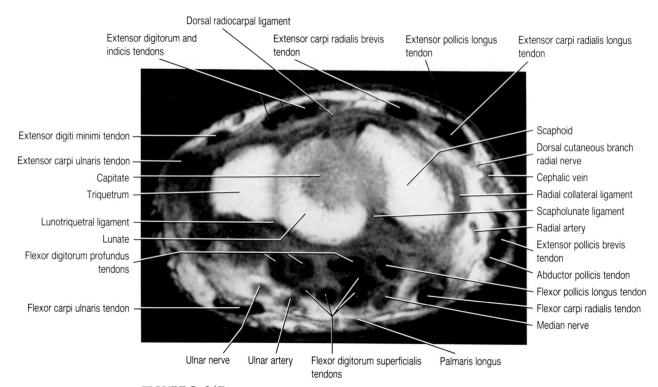

Dorsal radiocarpal ligament

Extensor digitorum and indicis tendons

Extensor carpi radialis brevis tendon

Extensor pollicis longus tendon

Extensor carpi radialis longus tendon

Extensor digiti minimi tendon

Extensor carpi ulnaris tendon

Capitate

Triquetrum

Lunotriquetral ligament

Lunate

Flexor digitorum profundus tendons

Flexor carpi ulnaris tendon

Scaphoid

Dorsal cutaneous branch radial nerve

Cephalic vein

Radial collateral ligament

Scapholunate ligament

Radial artery

Extensor pollicis brevis tendon

Abductor pollicis tendon

Flexor pollicis longus tendon

Flexor carpi radialis tendon

Median nerve

Ulnar nerve

Ulnar artery

Flexor digitorum superficialis tendons

Palmaris longus

FIGURE 8–24F.

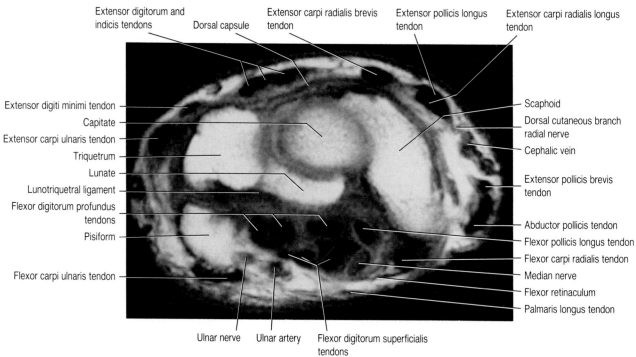

Extensor digitorum and indicis tendons

Dorsal capsule

Extensor carpi radialis brevis tendon

Extensor pollicis longus tendon

Extensor carpi radialis longus tendon

Extensor digiti minimi tendon

Capitate

Extensor carpi ulnaris tendon

Triquetrum

Lunate

Lunotriquetral ligament

Flexor digitorum profundus tendons

Pisiform

Flexor carpi ulnaris tendon

Scaphoid

Dorsal cutaneous branch radial nerve

Cephalic vein

Extensor pollicis brevis tendon

Abductor pollicis tendon

Flexor pollicis longus tendon

Flexor carpi radialis tendon

Median nerve

Flexor retinaculum

Palmaris longus tendon

Ulnar nerve

Ulnar artery

Flexor digitorum superficialis tendons

FIGURE 8–24G.

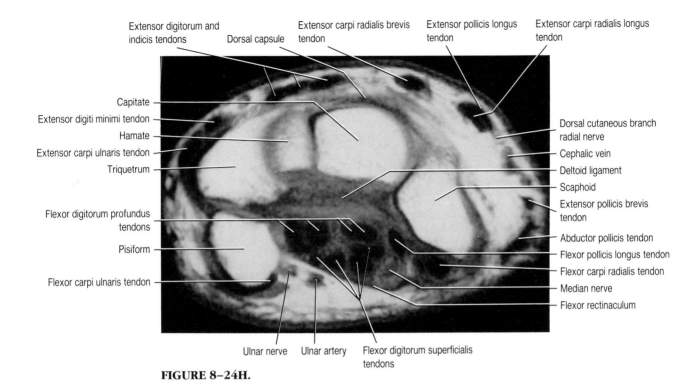

FIGURE 8–24H.

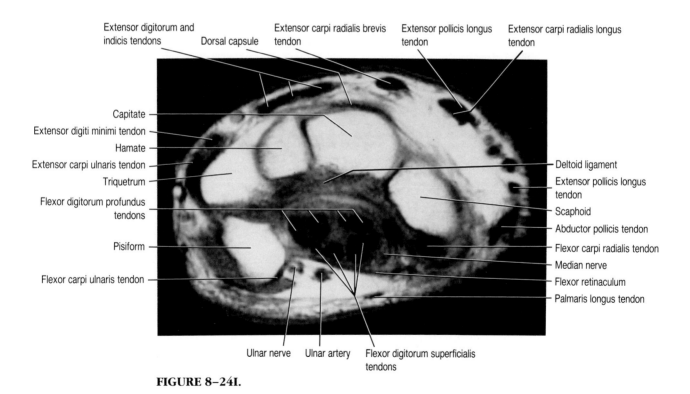

FIGURE 8–24I.

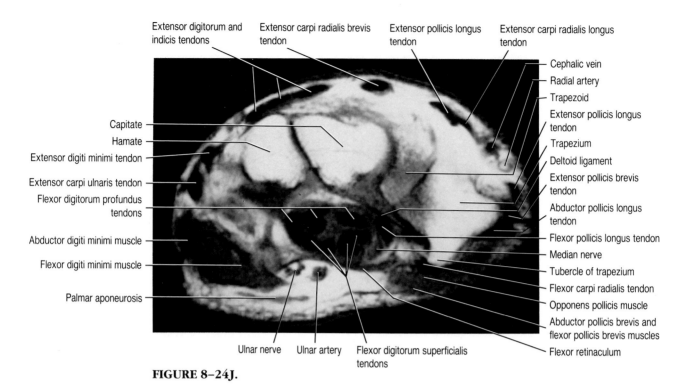

Extensor digitorum and indicis tendons — Extensor carpi radialis brevis tendon — Extensor pollicis longus tendon — Extensor carpi radialis longus tendon

Capitate
Hamate
Extensor digiti minimi tendon
Extensor carpi ulnaris tendon
Flexor digitorum profundus tendons
Abductor digiti minimi muscle
Flexor digiti minimi muscle
Palmar aponeurosis

Cephalic vein
Radial artery
Trapezoid
Extensor pollicis longus tendon
Trapezium
Deltoid ligament
Extensor pollicis brevis tendon
Abductor pollicis longus tendon
Flexor pollicis longus tendon
Median nerve
Tubercle of trapezium
Flexor carpi radialis tendon
Opponens pollicis muscle
Abductor pollicis brevis and flexor pollicis brevis muscles
Flexor retinaculum

Ulnar nerve   Ulnar artery   Flexor digitorum superficialis tendons

FIGURE 8–24J.

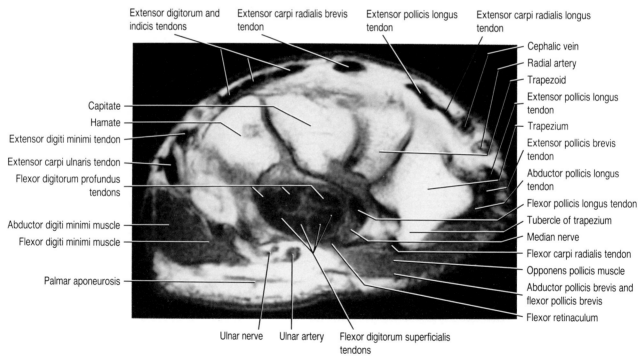

Extensor digitorum and indicis tendons — Extensor carpi radialis brevis tendon — Extensor pollicis longus tendon — Extensor carpi radialis longus tendon

Capitate
Hamate
Extensor digiti minimi tendon
Extensor carpi ulnaris tendon
Flexor digitorum profundus tendons
Abductor digiti minimi muscle
Flexor digiti minimi muscle
Palmar aponeurosis

Cephalic vein
Radial artery
Trapezoid
Extensor pollicis longus tendon
Trapezium
Extensor pollicis brevis tendon
Abductor pollicis longus tendon
Flexor pollicis longus tendon
Tubercle of trapezium
Median nerve
Flexor carpi radialis tendon
Opponens pollicis muscle
Abductor pollicis brevis and flexor pollicis brevis
Flexor retinaculum

Ulnar nerve   Ulnar artery   Flexor digitorum superficialis tendons

FIGURE 8–24K.

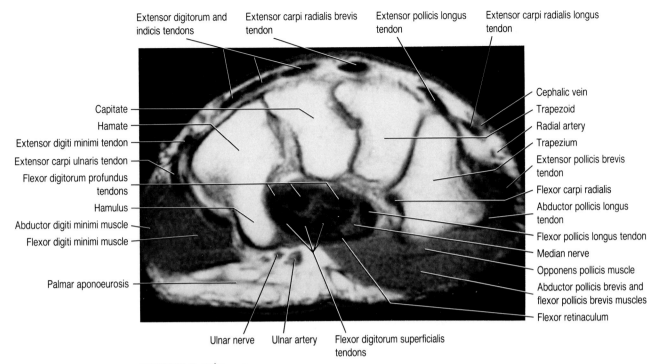

Extensor digitorum and indicis tendons

Extensor carpi radialis brevis tendon

Extensor pollicis longus tendon

Extensor carpi radialis longus tendon

Capitate

Hamate

Extensor digiti minimi tendon

Extensor carpi ulnaris tendon

Flexor digitorum profundus tendons

Hamulus

Abductor digiti minimi muscle

Flexor digiti minimi muscle

Palmar aponoeurosis

Cephalic vein

Trapezoid

Radial artery

Trapezium

Extensor pollicis brevis tendon

Flexor carpi radialis

Abductor pollicis longus tendon

Flexor pollicis longus tendon

Median nerve

Opponens pollicis muscle

Abductor pollicis brevis and flexor pollicis brevis muscles

Flexor retinaculum

Ulnar nerve

Ulnar artery

Flexor digitorum superficialis tendons

FIGURE 8–24L.

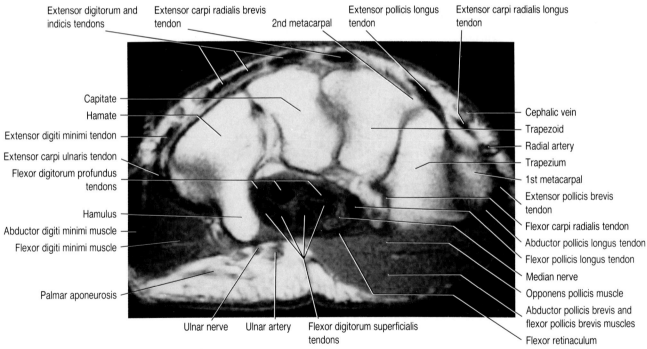

Extensor digitorum and indicis tendons

Extensor carpi radialis brevis tendon

2nd metacarpal

Extensor pollicis longus tendon

Extensor carpi radialis longus tendon

Capitate

Hamate

Extensor digiti minimi tendon

Extensor carpi ulnaris tendon

Flexor digitorum profundus tendons

Hamulus

Abductor digiti minimi muscle

Flexor digiti minimi muscle

Palmar aponeurosis

Cephalic vein

Trapezoid

Radial artery

Trapezium

1st metacarpal

Extensor pollicis brevis tendon

Flexor carpi radialis tendon

Abductor pollicis longus tendon

Flexor pollicis longus tendon

Median nerve

Opponens pollicis muscle

Abductor pollicis brevis and flexor pollicis brevis muscles

Flexor retinaculum

Ulnar nerve

Ulnar artery

Flexor digitorum superficialis tendons

FIGURE 8–24M.

onstrate intermediate signal intensity. The median nerve can be identified in the superficial radial aspect of the carpal tunnel, displaying intermediate signal intensity. In axial images through the midmetacarpals, the flexor tendons are seen anterior to the palmar interossei muscles, whereas the dorsal interossei are identified lying between the metacarpal bones.

Blood vessels display low signal intensity, except in venous structures demonstrated by even-echo rephasing or paradoxical enhancement secondary to slow flow. With gradient-echo techniques, both arterial and venous structures demonstrate high signal intensity.

Sagittal Images

The sagittal imaging plane (Fig. 8–25) is routine in wrist protocols and especially useful in the evaluation of static instability patterns and wrist shortening (*i.e.,* proximal migration of capitate) and in viewing the volar to dorsal aspects of the TFC. Kienböck's fracture and fracture deformity (*i.e.,* humpback scaphoid) are seen in sagittal images, complementary to coronal or axial images. The abductor pollicis longus and extensor pollicis brevis tendons can be seen in radial sagittal images. The scaphoid is identified in sagittal sections through the trapezium and, more dorsally, the trapezoid. The low signal intensity RSC ligament is represented by fibers seen along the volar aspect of the scaphoid between the volar distal radius and the distal pole of the scaphoid. The extensor pollicis longus tendon is dorsal to the radioscaphoid articulation. The pronator quadratus muscle extends along the volar surface of the radial metaphysis and distal diaphysis. The low signal intensity tendon of the flexor carpi radialis is draped volarly over the distal pole of the scaphoid. The long axis (*i.e.,* vertical orientation) of the flexor pollicis longus tendon is seen at the ulnar aspect of the scaphoid. The capitate, lunate, and radius are colinearly aligned in sagittal images through the third metacarpal axis.

The radial limb of the deltoid or arcuate ligament extends proximally from the volar aspect of the capitate to the scaphoid. In the sagittal plane, the deltoid ligament may appear to connect to the volar distal surface of the lunate. The radiolunate ligament is located between the volar lunate surface and the distal radius at the radiolunate articulation, deep to the flexor digitorum profundus tendon. The ulnolunate ligament is radial to the TFC. The flexor digitorum superficialis and profundus tendons are best seen volar to the capitate and lunate. The flexor retinaculum is a thin dark line superficial to the flexor digitorum superficialis. The ulnar limb of the arcuate ligament is seen volar to the radial aspect of the triquetrum and the ulnar aspect of the lunate, ulnar to the plane of section through the capitate. The fourth metacarpal, the hook of the hamate, and the triquetrum are seen in the same sagittal section at the most ulnar aspect of the lunate or the radial aspect of the ulna. The LT interosseous ligament is also seen at this level. The TFCC is located between the lunate and the ulna and has a concave distal surface. In ulnar sagittal images, the flexor carpi ulnaris extends in a volar direction to insert on the pisiform. The pisohamate and pisometacarpal ligaments attach to the hook of the hamate and the base of the fifth metacarpal, respectively. The intermediate signal intensity ulnar nerve is deep to the flexor carpi ulnaris. The ulnar collateral ligament component of the TFCC extends between the triquetrum and ulna, as can be seen in ulnar sagittal images out of the plane of the TFC. The thick extensor carpi ulnaris tendon is seen as a groove in the posterior aspect of the distal ulna. In peripheral ulnar sagittal sections, it can be seen to extend dorsal to the triquetrum and insert into the base of the fifth metacarpal.

Coronal Images

Coronal plane images (Fig. 8–26) are important in understanding the relationship between cartilage and ligamentous structures of the wrist. Three-dimensional FT volume imaging is more reliable for identification of the volar extrinsic ligaments of the wrist than T2*-weighted techniques with thicker (3-mm or greater) sections. On volar images, the flexor retinaculum is seen superficial to the flexor tendons as a transverse band. En face, the low signal intensity bands of the flexor digitorum tendons are seen passing through the carpal tunnel between the hook of the hamate and the trapezium. The intermediate signal intensity median nerve may also be discerned in this plane of section. The pisohamate and pisometacarpal ligaments are shown in sections at the level of the hook of the hamate and pisiform. The abductor pollicis longus and extensor pollicis brevis tendons border the volar radial aspect of the wrist in sections through the volar surfaces of the scaphoid and lunate. The TFC is seen as a curvilinear bow-tie band of low, homogeneous signal intensity. The band extends horizontally to the base of the ulnar styloid process from the ulnar surface of the distal radius. The meniscal homologue has an intermediate signal intensity on T1- and T2*-weighted images. The LRL is represented by obliquely directed fibers extending from the volar radius to the lunate, volar to the proximal pole of the scaphoid. The distal radioulnar joint and compartment are separated from the radiocarpal compartment by the TFC. The interosseous SL and LT are routinely visualized on 3-mm coronal T1- and T2*-weighted images. The extensor carpi ulnaris tendon borders the ulnar aspect of the wrist on the same coronal sections that display the TFC and interosseous ligaments. The radial collateral ligament may be partially visualized located between the scaphoid and radial styloid. The articular cartilage surfaces of the carpal bones are of intermediate signal intensity on T1-weighted images and increase in signal intensity on T2*-weighted images. On dorsal images through the corpus, the interosseous ligaments of the distal carpal row can be defined. Dorsally, the obliquely oriented extensor digiti minimi tendon on the ulnar side of the triquetrum and the extensor carpi radialis longus tendon are seen. Lister's tubercle, which contains fatty marrow, is situated between and separates the ulnar aspect of the extensor pollicis longus from the radial aspect extensor carpi radialis brevis. The dorsal interossei muscles are demonstrated between the metacarpal shafts.

NORMAL MAGNETIC RESONANCE ANATOMY OF THE FINGERS

Axial Images

Sections through the MP joint (Fig. 8–27) show the flexor digitorum superficialis and profundus tendons as a low signal intensity (*i.e.,* dark) structure, with poor differentiation between the deep profundus and the more volar superficialis. The extensor expansion can be seen dorsolaterally. The four lumbrical muscles that arise from the flexor digitorum profundus attach to the radial aspect of the extensor expansion. The interosseous tendons insert volarlaterally onto the extensor expansions and the bases of the proximal phalanges. The low to intermediate signal intensity palmar digital artery and the intermediate signal intensity palmar nerve are better visualized than the dorsal neurovascular structures. The intermediate signal intensity palmar ligament (*i.e.,* volar plate) is seen between the MP joint and the flexor tendons. The fibrocartilaginous volar plate extends from the base of the proximal phalanx to the metacarpal head. The thin, intermediate signal intensity transverse metacarpal ligaments connect the volar plates of the second through the fifth MP joints. The collateral ligaments are seen lateral to the MP joints and are composed of two parts—a weaker, fanlike more proximal part and a stronger, cord-like distal part.

At the level of the PIP joint (Figs. 8–28 and 8–29), the flexor digitorum superficialis tendon, after having split at the level of the midproximal phalanx, reunites and is deep to (*i.e.,* flanks) the flexor digitorum profundus tendon. The proximal and distal interphalangeal joints have palmar ligamentous (*i.e.,* volar plate) and collateral ligamentous anatomy similar to that of the MP joints.

Sagittal Images

Differentiation between the flexor digitorum superficialis and the profundus is best seen at the mid and proximal aspect of the proximal phalanx before the superficialis divides (Figs. 8–30 and 8–31). The central band of the extensor tendon and volar plate are identified on the distal and volar aspects of the PIP joints. The volar plate is also easily identified at the level of the MP and distal interphalangeal joints. The dorsal extensor expansion is parallel with and blends with the dorsal, low signal intensity cortex of the proximal phalanx.

Coronal Images

The parts of the collateral ligament are seen along the sides of the MP and interphalangeal joints (Fig. 8–32). The lateral bands of the extensor tendon and interosseous tendons are parallel with the proximal phalangeal diaphysis and demonstrate intermediate signal intensity. In the coronal plane, imaging of the collateral ligaments, the flexor digitorum, and the extensor tendons requires thin section (*i.e.,* 3-mm or less) imaging (Fig. 8–33).

CARPAL INSTABILITIES

The terms stability and instability, as used in reference to conditions affecting the carpus, must be rigidly defined. Stability refers to the ability of two structures to maintain a normal relationship under applied physiologic loading. Similarly, two structures are said to be unstable if they cannot maintain this normal relationship under physiologic loading conditions. Carpal instabilities thus represent deviations from the normal spatial relationships of the carpal bones to each other and their surrounding structures such as the radius, the ulna, and the metacarpals. Since the wrist, like the hip, is virtually always under some load condition, this definition includes instabilities that are seen on routine radiographs as well as those seen on motion studies.

Magnetic resonance offers the advantage of revealing associated carpal ligament disruptions when characterizing instabilities in any specified plane of section. Fixed instabilities seen on routine radiographs and coronal or sagittal MR images are often referred to as static, and those that are only revealed by provocative maneuvers in motion studies are referred to as dynamic. Kinematic MR imaging represents a series of static evaluations displayed in a cine loop without true dynamic motion.

In many cases, the difference between a dynamic and static instability is a matter of the degree of the pathology of the structures that maintain the spatial relationship between the bones. A static instability that is present at all times implies contracture of the soft-tissue constraints. This condition may not be amenable to surgical repair; treatment may require arthrodeses to overcome these

(text continues on page 729)

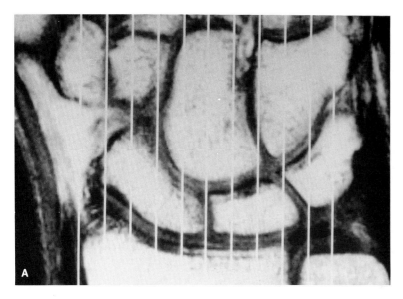

FIGURE 8–25. Normal sagittal MR anatomy. (**A**) This T1-weighted coronal localizer was used to prescribe sagittal image locations from the (**B**) radial to (**L**) ulnar aspect of the wrist.

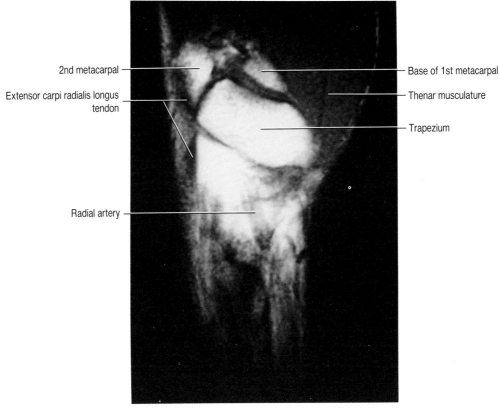

2nd metacarpal

Extensor carpi radialis longus tendon

Radial artery

Base of 1st metacarpal

Thenar musculature

Trapezium

FIGURE 8–25B.

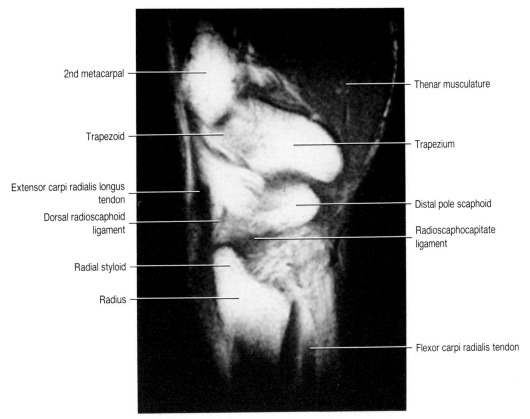

2nd metacarpal

Trapezoid

Extensor carpi radialis longus tendon

Dorsal radioscaphoid ligament

Radial styloid

Radius

Thenar musculature

Trapezium

Distal pole scaphoid

Radioscaphocapitate ligament

Flexor carpi radialis tendon

FIGURE 8–25C.

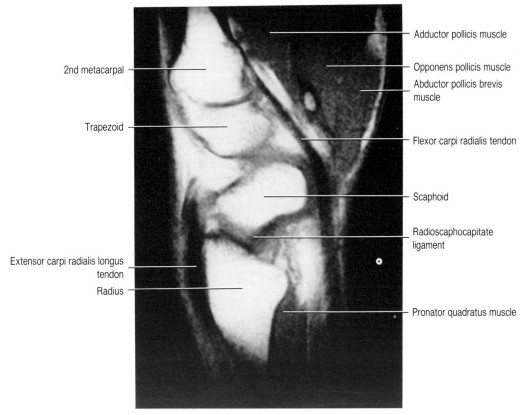

2nd metacarpal

Trapezoid

Extensor carpi radialis longus tendon

Radius

Adductor pollicis muscle

Opponens pollicis muscle

Abductor pollicis brevis muscle

Flexor carpi radialis tendon

Scaphoid

Radioscaphocapitate ligament

Pronator quadratus muscle

FIGURE 8–25D.

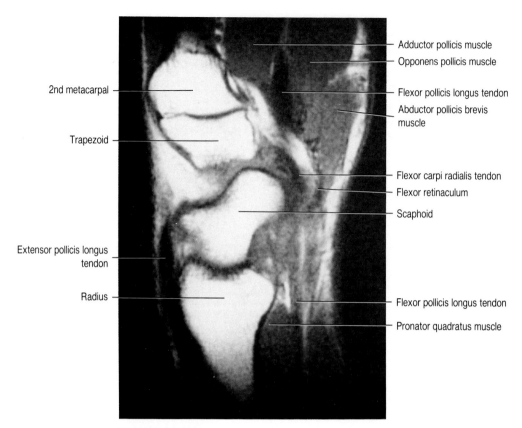

2nd metacarpal

Trapezoid

Extensor pollicis longus
tendon

Radius

Adductor pollicis muscle

Opponens pollicis muscle

Flexor pollicis longus tendon

Abductor pollicis brevis
muscle

Flexor carpi radialis tendon

Flexor retinaculum

Scaphoid

Flexor pollicis longus tendon

Pronator quadratus muscle

FIGURE 8–25E.

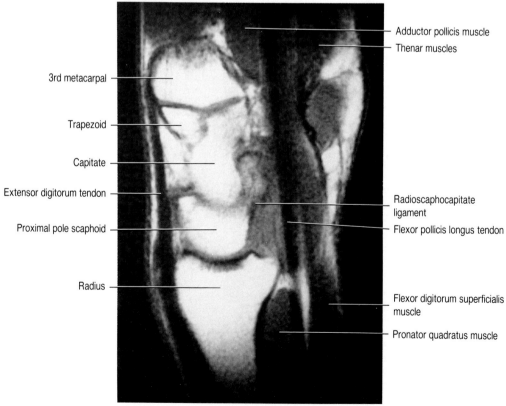

3rd metacarpal

Trapezoid

Capitate

Extensor digitorum tendon

Proximal pole scaphoid

Radius

Adductor pollicis muscle

Thenar muscles

Radioscaphocapitate
ligament

Flexor pollicis longus tendon

Flexor digitorum superficialis
muscle

Pronator quadratus muscle

FIGURE 8–25F.

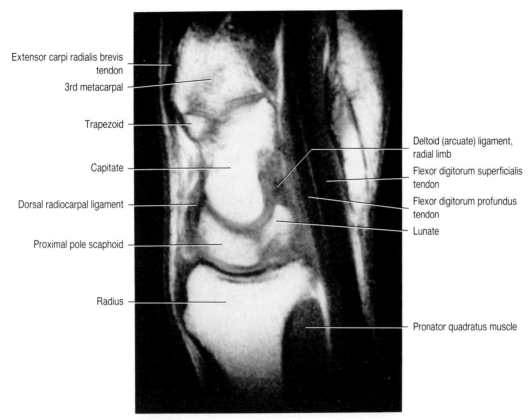

Extensor carpi radialis brevis tendon

3rd metacarpal

Trapezoid

Capitate

Dorsal radiocarpal ligament

Proximal pole scaphoid

Radius

Deltoid (arcuate) ligament, radial limb

Flexor digitorum superficialis tendon

Flexor digitorum profundus tendon

Lunate

Pronator quadratus muscle

FIGURE 8–25G.

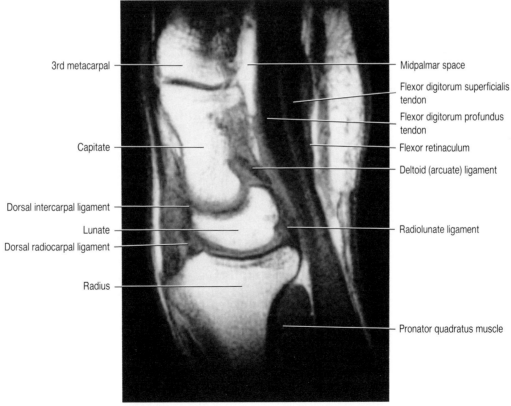

3rd metacarpal

Capitate

Dorsal intercarpal ligament

Lunate

Dorsal radiocarpal ligament

Radius

Midpalmar space

Flexor digitorum superficialis tendon

Flexor digitorum profundus tendon

Flexor retinaculum

Deltoid (arcuate) ligament

Radiolunate ligament

Pronator quadratus muscle

FIGURE 8–25H.

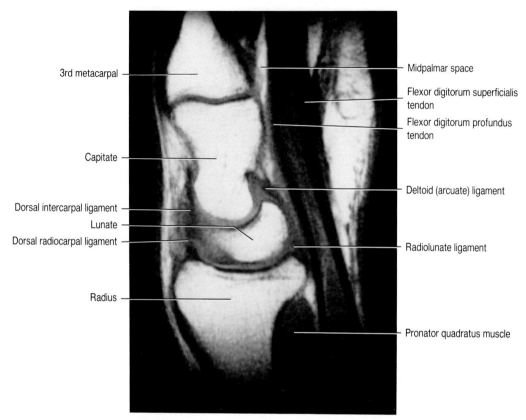

3rd metacarpal

Capitate

Dorsal intercarpal ligament

Lunate

Dorsal radiocarpal ligament

Radius

Midpalmar space

Flexor digitorum superficialis tendon

Flexor digitorum profundus tendon

Deltoid (arcuate) ligament

Radiolunate ligament

Pronator quadratus muscle

FIGURE 8–25I.

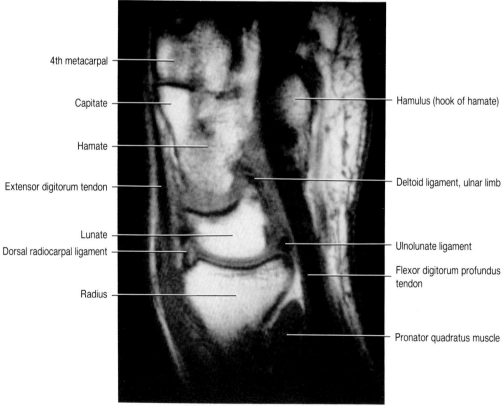

4th metacarpal

Capitate

Hamate

Extensor digitorum tendon

Lunate

Dorsal radiocarpal ligament

Radius

Hamulus (hook of hamate)

Deltoid ligament, ulnar limb

Ulnolunate ligament

Flexor digitorum profundus tendon

Pronator quadratus muscle

FIGURE 8–25J.

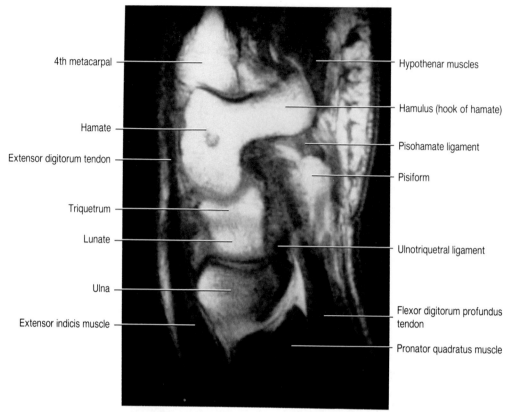

4th metacarpal — Hypothenar muscles

Hamate — Hamulus (hook of hamate)

Extensor digitorum tendon — Pisohamate ligament

Pisiform

Triquetrum — Ulnotriquetral ligament

Lunate

Ulna — Flexor digitorum profundus tendon

Extensor indicis muscle — Pronator quadratus muscle

FIGURE 8–25K.

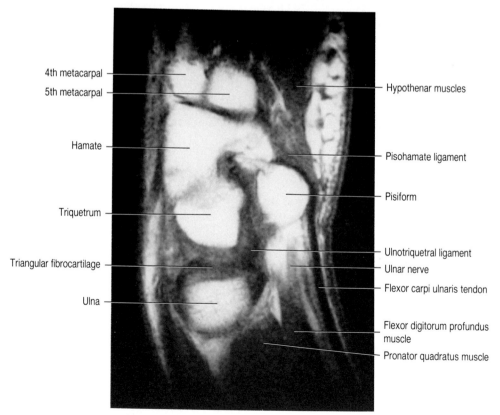

4th metacarpal — Hypothenar muscles

5th metacarpal

Hamate — Pisohamate ligament

Pisiform

Triquetrum — Ulnotriquetral ligament

Ulnar nerve

Triangular fibrocartilage — Flexor carpi ulnaris tendon

Ulna — Flexor digitorum profundus muscle

Pronator quadratus muscle

FIGURE 8–25L.

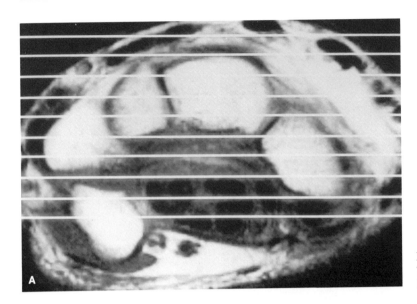

FIGURE 8–26. Normal coronal MR anatomy. (**A**) This T1-weighted axial localizer was used to prescribe coronal image locations from (**B**) dorsal to (**K**) volar.

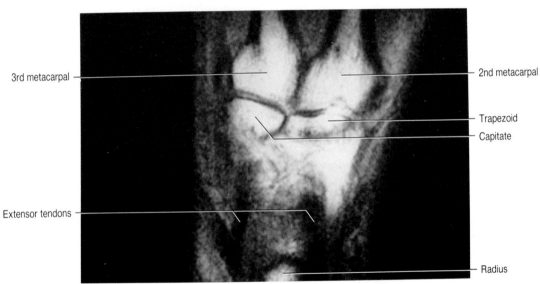

3rd metacarpal

2nd metacarpal

Trapezoid

Capitate

Extensor tendons

Radius

FIGURE 8–26B.

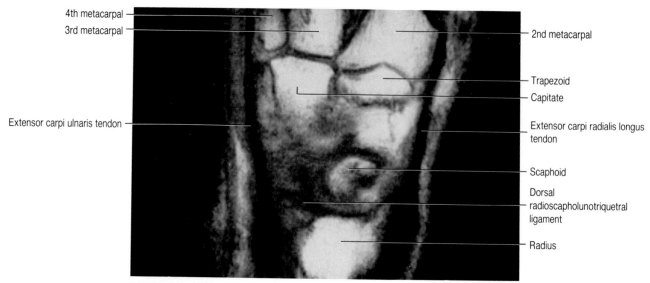

4th metacarpal
3rd metacarpal
2nd metacarpal
Trapezoid
Capitate
Extensor carpi ulnaris tendon
Extensor carpi radialis longus tendon
Scaphoid
Dorsal radioscapholunotriquetral ligament
Radius

FIGURE 8–26C.

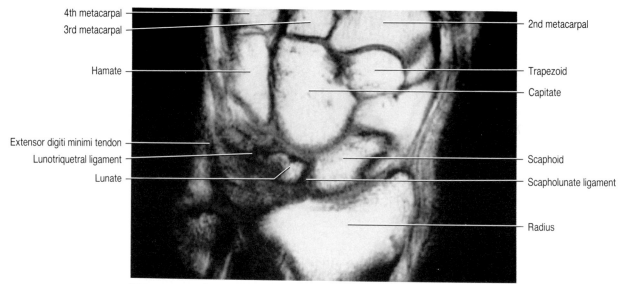

4th metacarpal
3rd metacarpal
Hamate
2nd metacarpal
Trapezoid
Capitate
Extensor digiti minimi tendon
Lunotriquetral ligament
Lunate
Scaphoid
Scapholunate ligament
Radius

FIGURE 8–26D.

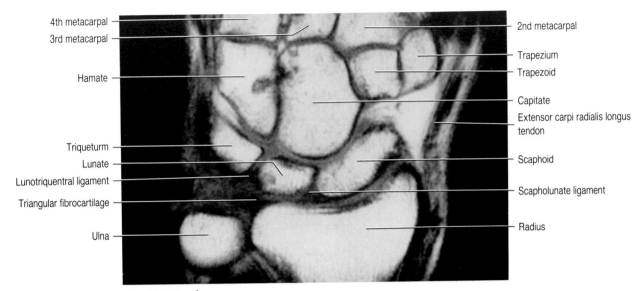

4th metacarpal
3rd metacarpal
Hamate
Triqueturm
Lunate
Lunotriquentral ligament
Triangular fibrocartilage
Ulna

2nd metacarpal
Trapezium
Trapezoid
Capitate
Extensor carpi radialis longus tendon
Scaphoid
Scapholunate ligament
Radius

FIGURE 8–26E.

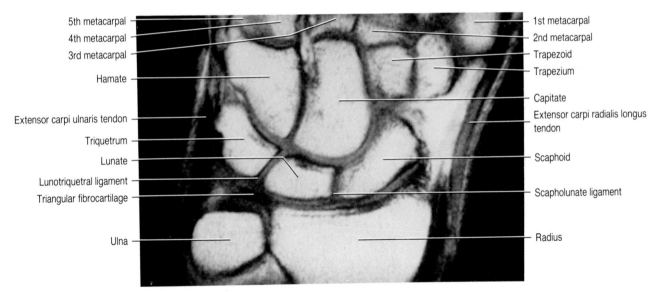

5th metacarpal
4th metacarpal
3rd metacarpal
Hamate
Extensor carpi ulnaris tendon
Triquetrum
Lunate
Lunotriquetral ligament
Triangular fibrocartilage
Ulna

1st metacarpal
2nd metacarpal
Trapezoid
Trapezium
Capitate
Extensor carpi radialis longus tendon
Scaphoid
Scapholunate ligament
Radius

FIGURE 8–26F.

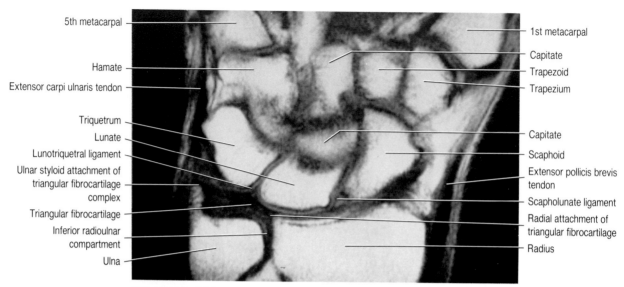

5th metacarpal

Hamate

Extensor carpi ulnaris tendon

Triquetrum

Lunate

Lunotriquetral ligament

Ulnar styloid attachment of
triangular fibrocartilage
complex

Triangular fibrocartilage

Inferior radioulnar
compartment

Ulna

1st metacarpal

Capitate

Trapezoid

Trapezium

Capitate

Scaphoid

Extensor pollicis brevis
tendon

Scapholunate ligament

Radial attachment of
triangular fibrocartilage

Radius

FIGURE 8–26G.

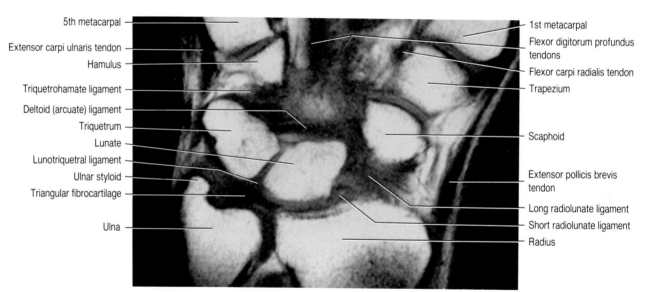

5th metacarpal

Extensor carpi ulnaris tendon

Hamulus

Triquetrohamate ligament

Deltoid (arcuate) ligament

Triquetrum

Lunate

Lunotriquetral ligament

Ulnar styloid

Triangular fibrocartilage

Ulna

1st metacarpal

Flexor digitorum profundus
tendons

Flexor carpi radialis tendon

Trapezium

Scaphoid

Extensor pollicis brevis
tendon

Long radiolunate ligament

Short radiolunate ligament

Radius

FIGURE 8–26H.

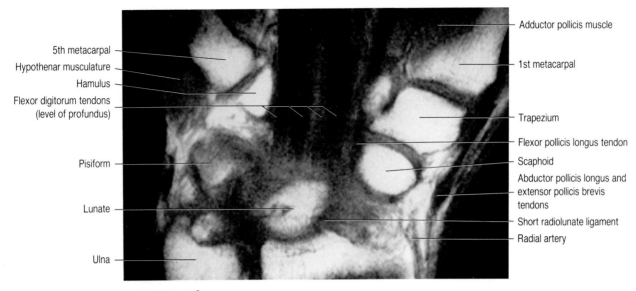

FIGURE 8–26I.

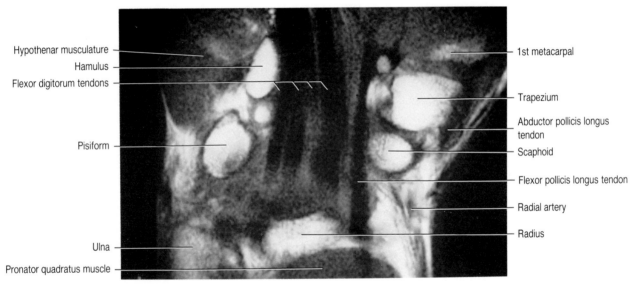

FIGURE 8–26J.

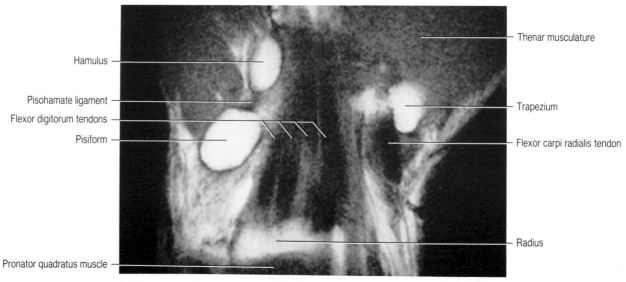

Hamulus

Pisohamate ligament

Flexor digitorum tendons

Pisiform

Pronator quadratus muscle

Thenar musculature

Trapezium

Flexor carpi radialis tendon

Radius

FIGURE 8–26K.

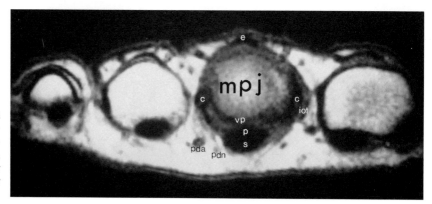

FIGURE 8–27. Axial anatomy as seen through the metacarpophalangeal joint. (c, collateral ligament; e, extensor digitorum tendon; iot, interosseous tendon; mpj, metacarpophalangeal joint; p, flexor digitorum profundus tendon; pda, palmar digital artery; pdn, palmar digital nerve; s, flexor digitorum superficialis tendon; vp, volar plate.)

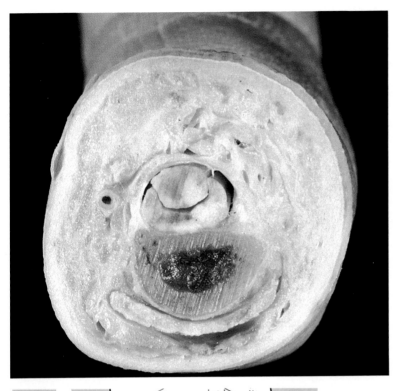

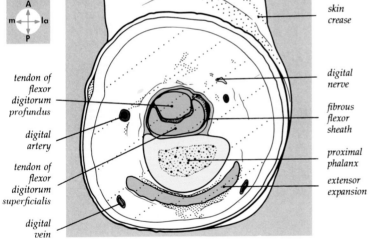

skin
crease

digital
nerve

fibrous
flexor
sheath

proximal
phalanx

extensor
expansion

tendon of
flexor
digitorum
profundus

digital
artery

tendon of
flexor
digitorum
superficialis

digital
vein

FIGURE 8–28. A transverse section through the index finger at the level of the proximal phalanx.

FIGURE 8–29. Axial anatomy as seen through the proximal interphalangeal joint. (c, collateral ligament; e, extensor expansion; p, flexor digitorum profundus tendon; pip, proximal interphalangeal joint; s, flexor digitorum superficialis tendon.)

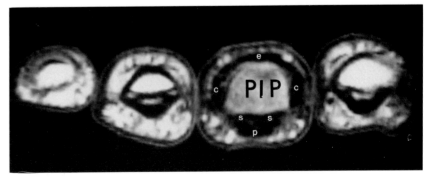

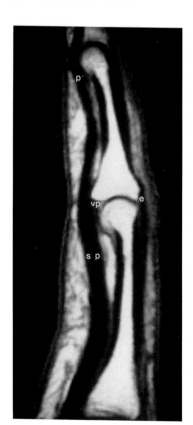

FIGURE 8–30. A sagittal section of a finger shows the capsules and the relations of the joints.

nail plate

distal phalanx

articular cartilage

d

P ⟷ A

pr

articular cartilage

tendon of flexor digitorum profundus

tendon of flexor digitorum super-ficialis

proximal phalanx

extensor expansion

head of metacarpal

FIGURE 8–31. Sagittal finger anatomy. (e, central band of extensor tendon; p, flexor digitorum profundus tendon; s, flexor digitorum superficialis tendon; vp, volar plate.)

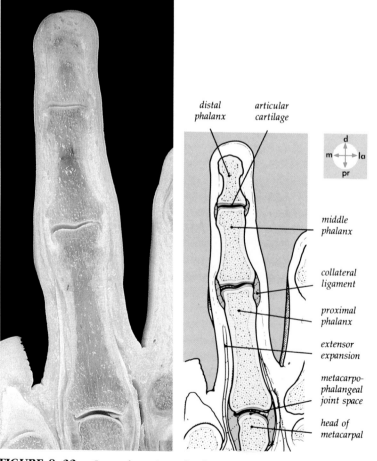

distal phalanx

articular cartilage

d

m ⟷ la

pr

middle phalanx

collateral ligament

proximal phalanx

extensor expansion

metacarpo-phalangeal joint space

head of metacarpal

FIGURE 8–32. Coronal section of a finger. The interphalangeal and metacarpophalangeal joint spaces are exaggerated by slight extension of the specimen.

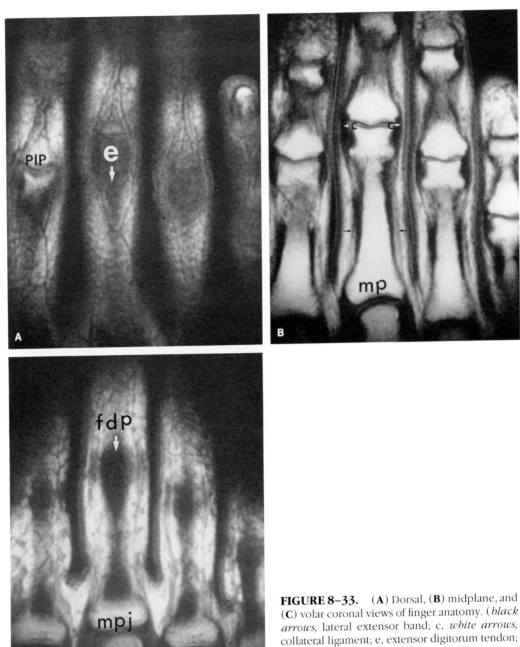

FIGURE 8–33. (**A**) Dorsal, (**B**) midplane, and (**C**) volar coronal views of finger anatomy. (*black arrows*, lateral extensor band; c, *white arrows*, collateral ligament; e, extensor digitorum tendon; fdp, flexor digitorum profundus tendon; mp or mpj, metacarpophalangeal joint; pip, proximal interphalangeal joint.)

forces. On the other hand, a dynamic instability that is revealed only by a provocative maneuver may be due to a relatively minor ligament tear or laxity that can be repaired with a soft-tissue procedure and allows preservation of joint motion.

Stable and Unstable Equilibrium in the Wrist

The normal spatial relationships of the individual components of the wrist (*e.g.,* carpal bones, radius, ulna, metacarpals) can be thought of as an example of a stable equilibrium condition. By definition, a stable equilibrium exists when any displacement of a body from its position will result in a restoring force that tends to return the body to its equilibrium position. When all of the supporting constraints of the wrist are normal and intact, any load within physiologic limits may change the spatial relationship of the components, but there will be a simultaneous increase in the tension within these constraining structures that counteracts the deforming force and tends to return the components to their normal spatial relationship. Neutral, dorsiflexion, and palmarflexion motions can be used as an example of the different colinear relationships among the capitate, lunate, and radius (Figs. 8–34 through 8–36).

Conversely, an unstable equilibrium exists when any displacement of a body from its position results in a force that tends to push the body further from the equilibrium position.[41] This condition is present in the wrist when the constraining structures become incompetent. Constraining or supporting structures about the wrist include not only the ligamentous structures discussed above, but also the tendons that cross the joint, as well as the geometry of the carpal bones and their surrounding articular surfaces. The tendency for the wrist to assume a condition of unstable equilibrium when the constraining structures are damaged can be seen as an extension of the normal motions of the carpal bones. To understand these motions, the wrist can be thought of as a flexible spacer interposed between the hand (*i.e.,* metacarpals) and the distal radius/ulna. The purpose of this deformable spacer is to maintain a constant position between the base of the third metacarpal and the articular surface of the radius. This theory is supported by the fact that, with radial or ulnar deviation, the carpal height index does not change from its value as measured in a neutral position.[42] This index or ratio is defined as the carpal height measured from the distal capitate surface to the proximal lunate surface, divided by the length of the third metacarpal. In normal individuals, the value is 0.54 ± 0.03.

In order for this ratio to remain constant with radial and ulnar deviation, there must be a change in the dimensions of the ulnar and radial borders of the flexible spacer between the metacarpals and distal radius. Since the bones of the distal carpal row are rigidly held in place by their ligamentous restraints, they do not move; the normal motions of the three bones of the proximal row must account for these changes in the dimensions of the radial and ulnar borders of the wrist.

With radial deviation, the radial border must shorten; this is accomplished by rotation of the scaphoid into a flexed position (Fig. 8–37). The ulnar border is lengthened as the triquetrum slides out from beneath the hamate. On plain radiographs or coronal MR images in this position, the scaphoid is foreshortened and the joint space is evident between the hamate and triquetrum; no superimposition of these bones occurs. The lunate is linked or associated with the scaphoid and triquetrum through the interosseous ligaments, which are displayed as homogeneous low signal intensity structures on coronal MR images. The SL ligament has a triangular morphology, whereas the LT ligament is more linear in shape. Lunate motion is thus a reflection of this proximal carpal row linkage as well as the compressive forces placed on it by the capitate. At extreme radial deviation the summation of these forces produces slight volarflexion of the lunate. Since a condition of stable equilibrium exists, the bones of the proximal row return to their neutral position when the radial-deviating force is removed.

With ulnar deviation, the radial side of the flexible spacer must lengthen and the ulnar side must shorten. Therefore, the scaphoid becomes more horizontal or extended to lengthen the radial side and the triquetrum slides beneath the hamate to shorten the ulnar side. Posteroanterior radiographs show an elongated scaphoid and superimposition of the hamate on the triquetrum. Coronal MR images demonstrate the triquetral movement in an ulnar direction on the slope of the hamate (Fig. 8–38). Palmar movement of the triquetrum in relationship to the hamate results in the palmar position of the lunate axis relative to the capitate. Compressive forces transmitted by the capitate produce dorsal rotation or dorsiflexion of the lunate. Associated volar shift of the lunate maintains colinear alignment of the capitate and radius. During lunate dorsiflexion, there is elevation of the distal pole of the scaphoid (*i.e.,* scaphoid extension).

Interosseous Ligament Pathology

If an injury to these constraints occurs, such as a tear of the SL ligament, the linkage between the scaphoid and lunate is removed and these bones are dissociated. A SL ligament tear, however, may exist without a static instability (Fig. 8–39). The lunate is no longer under the influence of the scaphoid and instead follows the triquetrum, and the loading force of the capitate is not opposed by torque transmitted through the SL ligament from the flexed scaphoid. Similarly, the lunate no longer exerts

(text continues on page 734)

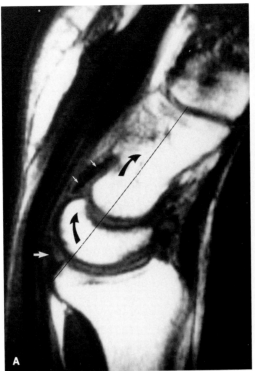 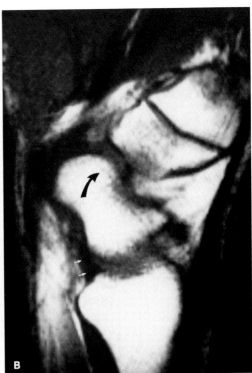

FIGURE 8–34. (**A**) In wrist dorsiflexion, colinear alignment (*long thin black line*) of the dorsiflexed capitate and lunate (*curved arrows*) takes place. The deltoid or arcuate ligament (*small white arrows*) and the radiolunate component of radioscapholunate ligament (*large white arrow*) are indicated. Dorsiflexion occurs primarily at the radiocarpal joint. (**B**) In wrist dorsiflexion, the radio-scaphocapitate ligament (*small white arrows*) tightens, locking motion between the proximal and distal carpal rows and creates a sling across the waist of the scaphoid, dorsiflexing both the scaphoid (*curved arrow*) and capitate.

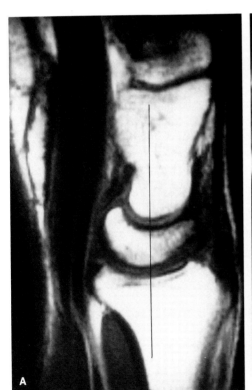 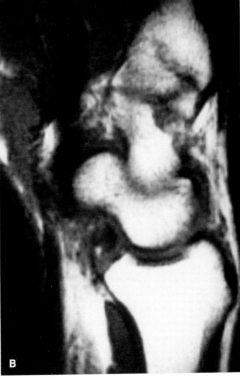

FIGURE 8–35. (**A**) With the wrist in neutral position, normal colinear alignment of the capitate, lunate, and radius takes place (*black line*). The normal capitolunate angle is between 0° and 30°. (**B**) The normal position of the scaphoid without dorsiflexion or palmar flexion shows the normal scapholunate angle to be between 30° and 60°.

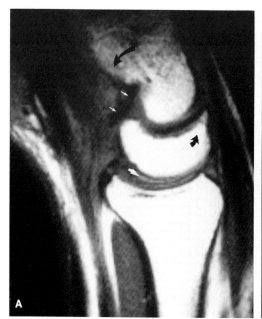

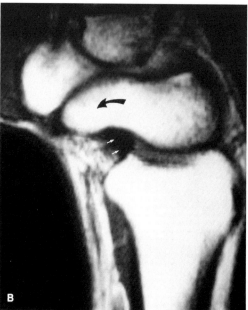

FIGURE 8–36. (**A**) Palmar flexion occurs primarily at the midcarpal articulation. Palmar flexion of the capitate (*long curved arrow*) and some palmar flexion of the lunate (*short curved arrow*) takes place. The arcuate or deltoid ligament is more lax (*small white arrows*). (*Large white arrow,* radiolunate articulation.) (**B**) Flexion of the scaphoid (*curved arrow*) shows a lax radioscaphocapitate ligament (*straight arrows*).

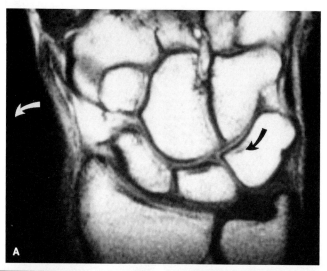

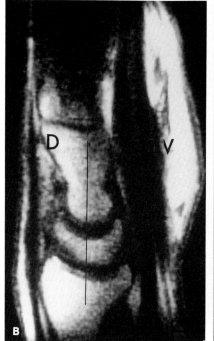

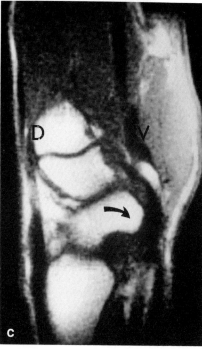

FIGURE 8–37. (**A**) Radial deviation of the wrist (*curved white arrow*) produces radial and dorsal translation of the triquetrum relative to the slope of the hamate (*curved black arrow*). (**B**) Colinear alignment of the capitate and lunate (*straight line*). There may be mild palmar flexion of the lunate in extreme radial deviation. (**C**) Palmar flexion of the scaphoid (*curved black arrow*). (D, dorsal; V, volar.)

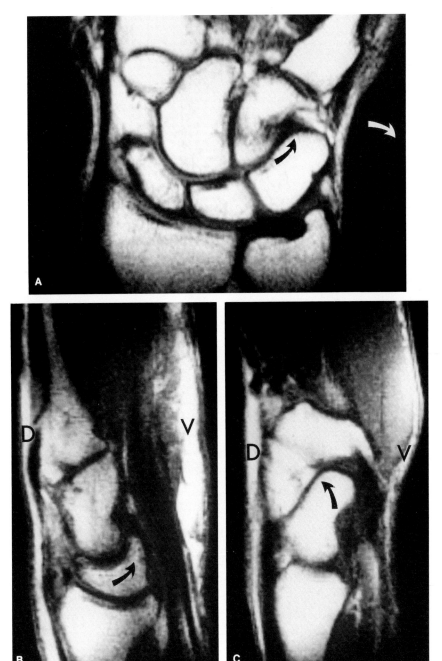

FIGURE 8–38. (**A**) Ulnar deviation of the wrist (*curved white arrow*) produces ulnar translation of the triquetrum relative to the slope of the hamate (*curved black arrow*). (**B**) Dorsiflexion of the lunate (*i.e.,* dorsal tilt) with associated volar shift (*curved arrow*) allows the capitate to remain colinear with the radius. In contrast, dorsal intercalated segmental instability (DISI) is characterized by dorsal tilting of the lunate without an associated volar shift. Thus, DISI results in dorsal displacement of the capitate relative to the radius and no colinear relationship between the capitate and radius. (**C**) Elevation (*i.e.,* extension) of the distal pole of the scaphoid (*curved arrow*). (D, dorsal; V, volar.)

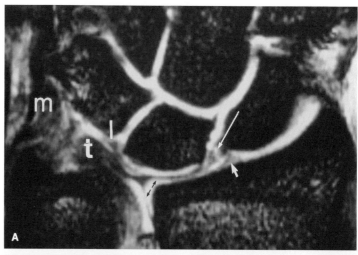

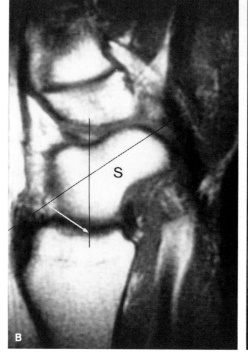

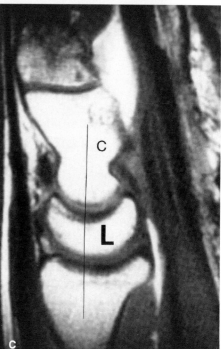

FIGURE 8–39. (**A**) A T2*-weighted coronal image demonstrates a vertical high signal intensity tear of the scapholunate ligament (*long white arrow*) without static carpal instability. A proximal portion of the radial scapholunate (*short white arrow*), the lunotriquetral ligament (l), the meniscus homologue (m), and the triangular fibrocartilage (t) with its radial attachments (*black arrows*) are shown. There is positive ulnar variance with an intact triangular fibrocartilage. (**B**) The normal scapholunate angle (*double-headed arrow*) is shown. (S, scaphoid.) (**C**) Colinear (*i.e.,* coaxial) alignment of the capitate (C), lunate (L), and radius, with normal capitolunate angle. There is no instability pattern.

force on the scaphoid, and there is less opposing force to its flexion.

In this situation, radial deviation produces an exaggeration of the normal motions of the bones of the proximal row. With SL interosseous ligament disruption, the scaphoid becomes more flexed in relation to the lunate, and the SL angle, normally less than 30° to 60°, increases to more than 70° (Fig. 8–40). The SL angle is determined from two sagittal images to demonstrate the separate lunate and scaphoid axes, which are not shown together in the same sagittal image. The lunate, free of the influence of the scaphoid, tips into a dorsiflexed position in relation to the axis of the capitate. As the scaphoid flexes, a gap appears between the scaphoid and the lunate, and, in time, the capitate will fall into this gap, contributing to a reduction in carpal height.

Rotatory subluxation of the scaphoid, which begins as an SL dissociation, has been described. In its final stages, as the lunate is dorsiflexed, a dorsal intercalated segment instability (DISI) pattern is established (see Fig. 8–40; Fig 8–41). On lateral radiographs, there is 10° or more of lunate dorsiflexion relative to the radius. On sagittal MR images, dorsal tilting of the lunate is associated with proximal migration of the capitate and loss of colinear alignment of the capitate, lunate, and radius. The capitolunate angle, normally 0° to 30°, can be directly measured on sagittal images and may be increased in dorsiflexion ligamentous instability.

Disruption of the SL ligament is shown on T2*-weighted images as either complete ligamentous disruption or as a discrete area of linear bright signal intensity in a partial or complete tear (Fig. 8–42). In complete tears, synovial fluid communication between the radiocarpal and midcarpal compartments may be identified (Fig. 8–43). Associated stretching (*i.e.,* redundancy) or tearing of the radiolunate ligament and the RSC ligament is shown in sagittal images. A loss of linkage (*i.e.,* dissociation) between the triquetrum and the lunate—due to a tear of the LT ligament—allows the lunate to follow the scaphoid (Fig. 8–44). Under this influence, volarflexion of the lunate occurs and gives rise to a volar intercalated segment instability pattern (VISI) (Fig. 8–45). Volar intercalated segment instability may be defined as a carpal instability characterized by proximal and volar migration of the bones of the distal row, associated with flexion of the lunate. Sagittal MR images characterize the palmar tilting of the lunate and scaphoid. The SL angle is decreased to less than 30°, and the capitolunate angle may measure up to 30°. Disruption of the LT ligament is frequently identified by its absence on T2*-weighted coronal images.

Magnetic Resonance Diagnosis

In evaluating SL interosseous ligament pathology, MR was shown to have a sensitivity rate of 93%, specificity of 83%, and accuracy of 90% when compared with arthrography.[22] In the diagnosis of ligament tears, with arthroscopy as the gold standard, MR was 86% sensitive, 100% specific, and 95% accurate. In the diagnosis of LT interosseous ligament tears, MR was 56% sensitive, 100% specific and 90% accurate compared with arthrography,[22] and 50% sensitive, 100% specific, and 80% accurate when compared with arthroscopy. The LT ligament is less substantial than the SL ligament; therefore, 3DFT coronal images may be needed to improve the sensitivity of diagnosis. Osseous widening of the LT articulation is uncommon in comparison to SL ligament dissociations, which may make the detection of LT ligament pathology more difficult, especially in the presence of an effusion or synovitis. Thin section axial images may further improve the identification of both SL and LT ligament pathology.

Classification

There are numerous classification schemes for instabilities of the carpus. This is partly due to the fact that the understanding of the biomechanics and treatment of these conditions is rapidly changing. The most useful classification reflects the anatomy and pathophysiology of the condition and indicates treatment.

Amadio has suggested four characteristics to be described in classification of carpal instabilities:

1. Severity
2. Direction of displacement
3. Location of injury
4. Type of injury.[43]

Severity can be categorized as the following:

- dynamic
- static subluxation
- static dislocation.

The direction of displacement may be DISI, VISI, or translation (*e.g.,* ulnar, radial, distal, proximal). Proximal or distal displacements are represented by axial carpal dislocations.[44] These are rare traumatic injuries, usually associated with a crush or blast mechanism. There is a longitudinal transarticular derangement of both the carpal and metacarpal transverse arches, with complete loss of the normal relationship between the two columns of the carpus. The radiologic hallmarks are an abnormal widening of any joint between the bones of the distal carpal row, a disruption of Gilula arc III defined by the proximal articular surfaces of the bones of the distal row, and an abnormal gap between the bases of two adjacent metacarpals.[44a] The location can be proximal, distal, radial, ulnar, dorsal, volar, radiocarpal, or midcarpal.

(text continues on page 738)

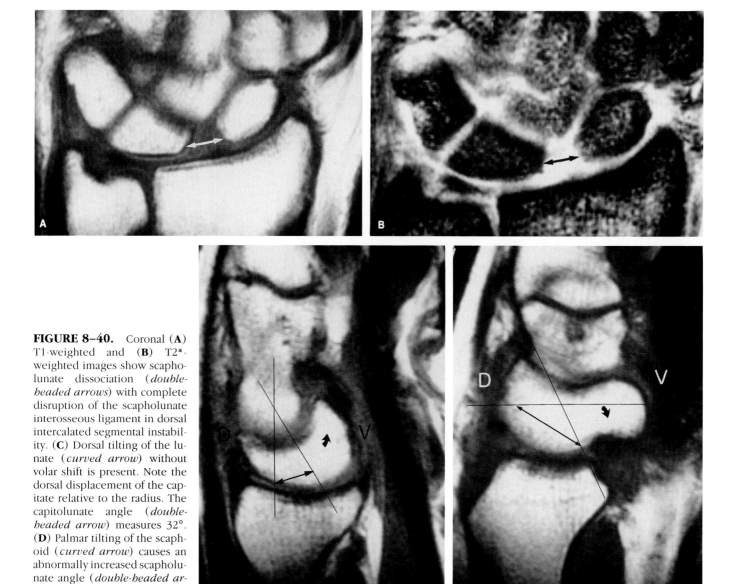

FIGURE 8–40. Coronal (**A**) T1-weighted and (**B**) T2*-weighted images show scapholunate dissociation (*double-headed arrows*) with complete disruption of the scapholunate interosseous ligament in dorsal intercalated segmental instability. (**C**) Dorsal tilting of the lunate (*curved arrow*) without volar shift is present. Note the dorsal displacement of the capitate relative to the radius. The capitolunate angle (*double-headed arrow*) measures 32°. (**D**) Palmar tilting of the scaphoid (*curved arrow*) causes an abnormally increased scapholunate angle (*double-headed arrow*) of 124°. (D, dorsal; V, volar.)

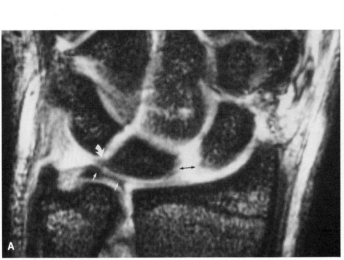
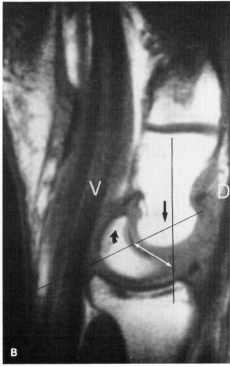

FIGURE 8–41. Dorsal intercalated segmental instability (DISI). (**A**) A coronal T2*-weighted image shows complete disruption of the scapholunate ligament in scapholunate dissociation with a scapholunate interval of greater than 2 mm (*double-headed arrow*). The lunotriquetral ligament (*curved arrow*) and triangular fibrocartilage (*small white arrows*) are intact. (**B**) A corresponding T1-weighted sagittal image demonstrates DISI with dorsal tilting of the lunate (*curved arrow*), and dorsal displacement and proximal migration of the capitate (*straight black arrow*) resulting in wrist shortening. The capitolunate angle (*double-headed arrow*) is abnormally increased to 66°. (V, volar.)

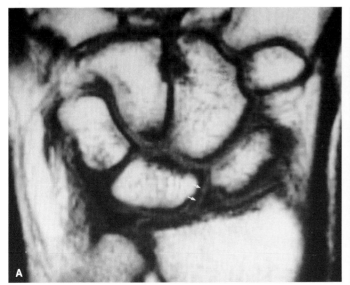
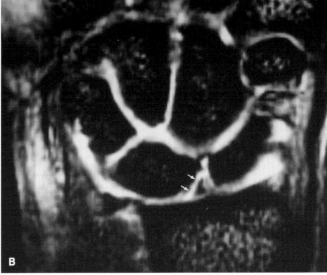

FIGURE 8–42. Direct linear extension of synovial fluid (*arrows*) across the lunate attachment of the scapholunate interosseous ligament is seen on coronal (**A**) T1-weighted and (**B**) T2*-weighted images. This is an isolated scapholunate ligament tear without an instability pattern.

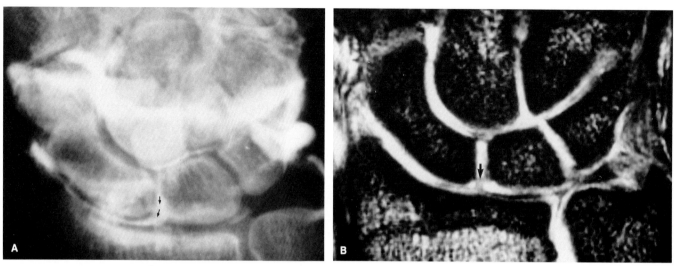

FIGURE 8–43. Scapholunate ligament tear. (**A**) Midcarpal arthrogram injection shows extension of contrast into the radiocarpal compartment (*arrows*) by crossing the scapholunate interval. There is no widening of the scapholunate interval and no rotatory subluxation or malpositioning of the scaphoid. (**B**) The corresponding T2*-weighted coronal image shows the abnormal morphology of a disrupted scapholunate interosseous ligament (*arrow*).

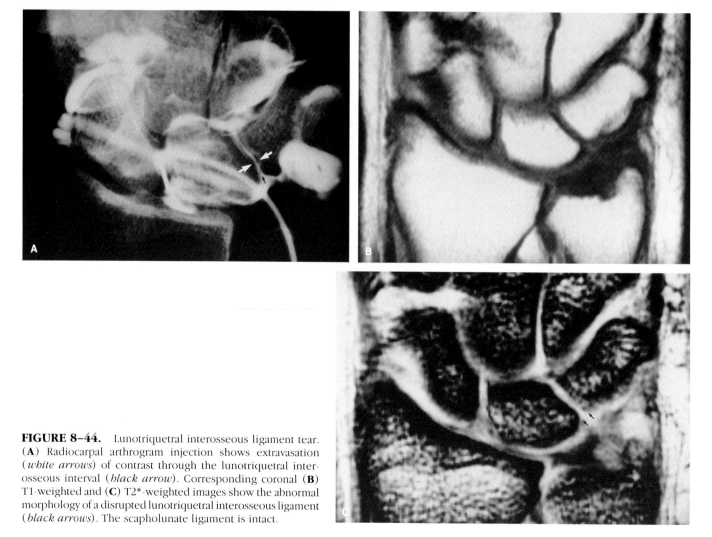

FIGURE 8–44. Lunotriquetral interosseous ligament tear. (**A**) Radiocarpal arthrogram injection shows extravasation (*white arrows*) of contrast through the lunotriquetral interosseous interval (*black arrow*). Corresponding coronal (**B**) T1-weighted and (**C**) T2*-weighted images show the abnormal morphology of a disrupted lunotriquetral interosseous ligament (*black arrows*). The scapholunate ligament is intact.

There are three major types of injuries.

1. Those affecting intracapsular intercarpal ligaments, as described in the examples above, are referred to as carpal instabilities, dissociative (CID).
2. Those involving the capsular ligaments with no dissociation of the carpal bones themselves are referred to as CIND.
3. Those complex injuries that involve both dissociative and nondissociative elements are referred to as the carpal instabilities complex.

Carpal instabilities, dissociative may be diagnosed if there is radiographic or arthroscopic evidence of dissociation between rows as well as within rows. Disruption affects both the intercarpal and the capsular wrist ligaments. In the dissociated form of DISI (CID-DISI), there is extension of the scaphoid and lunate, whereas in the interosseous ligaments, extension does not occur. The same holds true for VISI. In CID, there is flexion of the scaphoid and triquetrum; in CIND, there is no flexion of these bones.

Midcarpal Instabilities

Midcarpal instabilities are recognized more frequently, and there is greater experience with MR imaging of these wrist injuries. In palmar midcarpal subluxation, first studied by Lichtman, patients present with palmar subluxation at the midcarpal joint and a painful clunk with ulnar deviation of the wrist (see Fig. 8–45). Lichtman found that this instability is due mainly to laxity of the ulnar arm of the volar arcuate ligament.[45] There is also evidence of increased ligamentous laxity in these patients, and sagittal MR images show palmarflexion of the lunate, as in a VISI pattern. In ulnar deviation, the excessive volar tilt of the lunate allows the head of the capitate to sublux volarly into the space of Poirier. With radial deviation, the lunate dorsiflexes, and there is relocation of the capitate. This type of instability is classified as dynamic CIND, since there is no dissociation of the carpal bones. The intensity of the clunk and the pain increase with loading of the capitolunate joint such as that which occurs when the fist is clenched. Lichtman has further observed that dorsally directed pressure on the pisiform will eliminate this subluxation. He has designed dynamic splints that apply this directional force and successfully relieve the symptoms. This dorsally directed pressure on the pisiform can also be used to diagnose this condition.

The pathology in CIND of this type is related to the intrinsic ligaments of the carpus, but there are also extrinsic causes for midcarpal instability of CIND. Taleisnik and Watson have described these extrinsic causes in conjunction with malunited fractures of the distal radius.[46] In these cases, there is dorsal angulation of the distal radial articular surface that results in dorsiflexion of the lunate and dorsal subluxation of the midcarpal row. This instability can be treated with an osteotomy of the distal radius to restore its normal volar tilt.

Another type of CIND, involving the radiocarpal and ulnocarpal joints, occurs more proximally, and ulnar translation of the carpus is commonly seen in rheumatoid arthritis. Normally, the volar radiocarpal ligaments, which originate from the region of the radial styloid, act as guy to keep the carpus (*i.e.,* scaphoid and lunate) well seated in their fossae in the distal radius. In rheumatoid arthritis, however, destructive synovitis weakens the RSC and RL ligaments, and the carpus begins to migrate down the inclined plane of the distal radius in an ulnar direction. The distance between the radial styloid and scaphoid increases, as can be seen in posteroanterior radiographs or coronal plane images. Resection of the distal ulna (*i.e.,* Darrach procedure) results in loss of the buttressing effect of the ulna and increased ulnar translation.[47] Post-traumatic ulnar translocation of the carpus has also been described.[48]

Proximally occurring cases of CIND can also be seen with dorsal or volar displacements. Patients with malunited dorsal or volar intraarticular fractures lose the stability that the bony contour of the distal radius provides. This allows the proximal row to slip dorsally or volarly depending on whether the malunited fracture is dorsal or volar.

Treatment

Treatment for most of the carpal instabilities described above remains extremely controversial. This is especially true of CID. In general, the goal of most surgical approaches has been to restore the anatomy and biomechanics of the injured part of the carpus.

Carpal Instability, Nondissociative

In the extrinsic forms of CIND caused by malunited fractures of the distal radius, surgical correction of the instability is aimed at restoring the anatomy of the radius. Unfortunately, the injured soft-tissue constraints seen in CIND with ulnar translation in rheumatoid arthritis cannot be reconstructed surgically. Reduction of the carpus and radiolunate fusion has been successful in preventing recurrence of ulnar translation. The lunate, when fused to the radius, acts as a doorstop and prevents the carpus from sliding down the inclined plane of the radius.

Carpal instability, nondissociative, associated with dorsal midcarpal instability secondary to a malunited distal radius fracture with dorsal tilt of the articular surface, can be treated with an osteotomy of the distal radius, which restores normal volar angulation.

Carpal instability, nondissociative, with palmar midcarpal instability, presents a more difficult problem. The pathology is excessive volar tilt of the lunate caused by

laxity of the ulnar arm of the volar arcuate ligament. Lichtman has devised a soft-tissue reconstruction that consists of tightening the volar arcuate and dorsal radiolunate ligaments to correct the excessive VISI of the lunate. This procedure has been successful in a small number of patients. A more reliable operation is the four corner fusion. This is an intercarpal fusion of the lunate-triquetrum-capitate-hamate. Although some range of motion is lost with this procedure, it has been quite successful in eliminating the clunk as the subluxing joint is fused.

Carpal Instability, Dissociative

There is little agreement on the treatment of the various forms of CID. In many cases, these conditions remain unsolved problems—scapholunate dissociation is an excellent example. Early cases of ligament rupture without rotatory subluxation can usually be satisfactorily treated by pinning the SL interval and performing open suture repair of the torn ligament, followed by immobilization.[49] Accurate reduction is necessary to align the ligament fibers for optimal healing. Once rotation of the scaphoid is accomplished, the proximal pole must be reduced in relation to the lunate and a procedure performed to hold it firmly in place. Ligament reconstructions similar in concept to those devised to substitute for the anterior cruciate in the knee have met with uniformly poor results.[50] When the scaphoid rotates or flexes, its proximal pole becomes incongruent in the radial fossa. Several methods use intercarpal fusions to insure that the proximal pole remains congruent in the scaphoid fossa of the radius. Watson has used triscaphe (*i.e.,* scaphoid-trapezoid-trapezius) arthrodesis with great success.[51] Others have performed scaphocapitate fusions with similar results. An alternative to intercarpal fusion is dorsal capsulodesis.[52] In this procedure, a strip of the dorsal capsule of the wrist is left attached proximally to the radius on one end and the other is inserted into the distal pole of the scaphoid. By pulling dorsally on the distal pole, the scaphoid is held in a horizontal, reduced position. If possible, the SL ligament should be repaired.

Lunotriquetral Dissociations

The treatment of LT dissociations can be approached in two ways. If there is no VISI and positive ulnar variance is present, ulnar shortening unloads the LT interval and provides excellent symptomatic relief. The torn LT ligament should be repaired if possible. Lunotriquetral intercarpal fusion is also an option, although meticulous technique is required to avoid pseudoarthrosis. Lunotriquetral fusion is an attractive concept because this is the most common carpal coalition. These coalitions are usually asymptomatic and are often diagnosed in radiographs taken for other reasons. However, achieving a stable LT fusion has proven difficult, and most series show significant rates of nonunion (*i.e.,* up to 40%). Newer techniques with larger bone grafts and compression fixation devices have improved the success of this procedure. We have had 100% success in achieving fusion using the Herbert bone screw with precompression of the fusion site.

DISTAL RADIOULNAR JOINT

The ulna articulates with the distal radius through the sigmoid or ulnar notch.[53] The distal or inferior radioulnar compartment extends proximally as far as the synovium-lined recessus sacciformis. The distal ulna is wrapped in the extensor retinaculum but is not directly attached to it. The extensor carpi ulnaris tendon is deep to the extensor retinaculum and has subsheath attachment to the distal ulna. The articular disc, or TFC, is composed of collagen and elastic fibers, is triangular in shape, and bridges the distal ends of the radius and ulna. The volar aspect of the TFC has strong attachments to the lunato-triquetral and ulnotriquetral ligaments and a weaker attachment to the ulnolunate ligament. There is 150° of forearm rotation at the DRUJ, with rotation of the distal radius around the ulnar head. In pronation and supination, the ulnar head moves dorsally and palmarly, respectively, in the sigmoid notch (Fig. 8–46). Contact between the ulnar head and the sigmoid notch is greatest during forearm midrotation and least in maximum pronation or supination. These are the positions most commonly used in imaging the wrist with a dedicated wrist coil. Relative to the distal radius, distal movement of the ulnar head in pronation and proximal movement of the ulnar head during supination occurs. The distribution of load across the wrist is 82% through the distal radius and 18% through the distal ulna. The TFCC supports a portion of the ulnar forces that are unloaded in complete excision of the distal ulna.[53] In ulnar deviation, there is increased ulnar load transmission.

Ulnar Variance

The concept of ulnar variance is critical in the management of distal radial fractures, in the pathogenesis of KD, and in TFC pathology. Ulnar variance refers to the relative lengths of the radius and ulna, and can be defined as the relative level of the distal end of the ulna to that of the radius. If the ulna is short, ulnar variance is considered negative (Fig. 8–47). If the ulna is long, the variance is referred to as positive (Fig. 8–48). Neutral ulnar variance occurs when the lengths of the radius and ulna are relatively equal. Radiographically, the relative lengths of

(text continues on page 742)

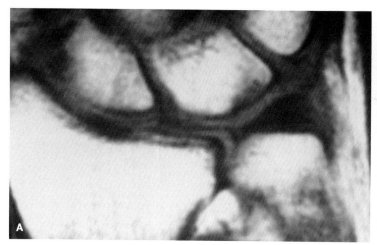

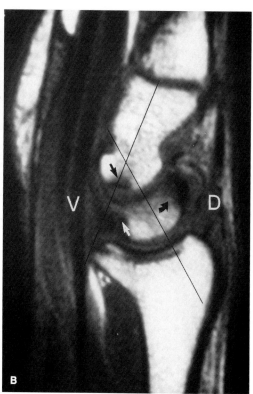

FIGURE 8–45. A volar intercalated segment instability pattern is apparent in clinical midcarpal instability. (**A**) A coronal T1-weighted image reveals subchondral sclerosis of the proximal ulnar aspect of the lunate in a patient who presented with clinical midcarpal instability. (**B**) A corresponding sagittal T1-weighted image shows the volar tilt of the lunate (*curved black arrow*), increased capitolunate angle, and subchondral sclerosis of the opposing surfaces of the capitate (*straight black arrow*) and lunate (*white arrow*). The ulnar arm of the arcuate ligament was not visible in this midcarpal instability. MR imaging was the first modality able to document degeneration of the proximal pole of the capitate in subluxation of the capitate on the lunate.

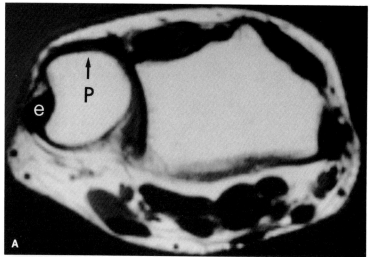

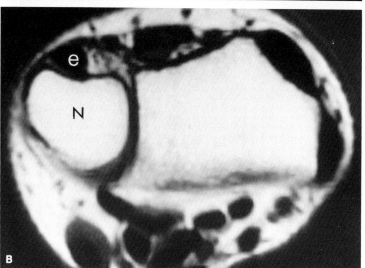

FIGURE 8–46. Normal biomechanics of the distal radioulnar joint. (**A**) Mild dorsal shift (*arrow*) of the ulna relative to the sigmoid notch of the distal radius in full pronation (p) is normal. The extensor carpi ulnaris tendon (e) is located within its groove in the medial distal aspect of the ulna. (**B**) The neutral position (N) of the wrist reveals a symmetric relationship between the position of the distal ulna and sigmoid notch relative to dorsal or volar directions. The extensor carpi ulnaris tendon is seen dorsally, within its ulnar groove. (**C**) Mild volar shift (*arrow*) of the ulna in full wrist supination (s) is normal. The extensor carpi ulnaris tendon (e) may be located within its ulnar groove or subluxed medially in extreme supination.

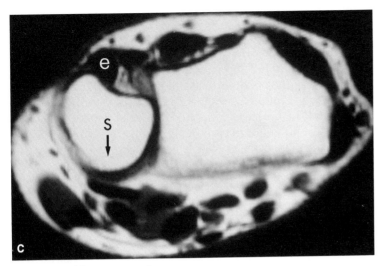

FIGURE 8–46. *(Continued)*

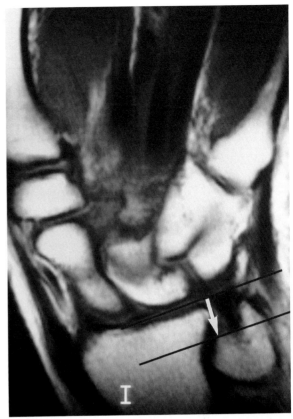

FIGURE 8–47. Negative ulnar variance with the articular surface of the ulna projecting proximal to the articular surface of the radius (*arrow*). Note the secondary deformity of the triangular fibrocartilage. There is an increase in the normal 80% of axial loading forces are supported by the radius, with relative ulnar shortening.

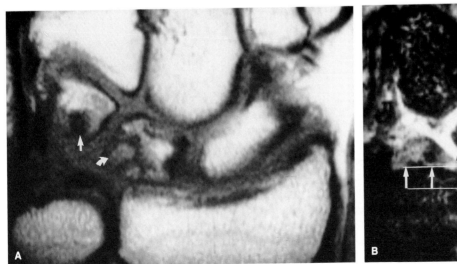

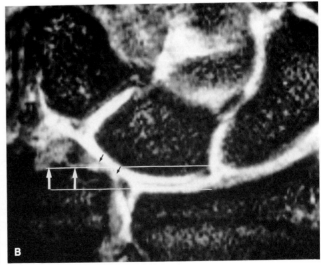

FIGURE 8–48. Ulnolunate impingement syndrome. (**A**) A T1-weighted coronal image shows low signal intensity subchondral degenerative sclerosis involving the ulnar aspect of the lunate (*straight arrow*) and triquetrum (*curved arrow*). (**B**) Positive ulnar variance (*white arrows*), triangular fibrocartilage perforations (*black arrows*), and a torn lunotriquetral ligament are features of ulnolunate (*i.e.,* ulnocarpal) impingement syndrome.

the radius and ulna are measured from the centers of their distal articular surfaces. There are three commonly used methods for measuring ulnar variance—all are similarly accurate and reliable.[54] It should be noted that wrist position is an important determinant of ulnar variance. Supination causes relative ulnar shortening, and pronation causes lengthening.[55] For this reason, it is critical that ulnar variance be determined with the forearm and wrist in 0° of pronation and supination.

Ulnolunate Impingement Syndrome

The syndrome of ulnolunate impingement occurs when there is excessive positive ulnar variance (see Fig. 8–48).[53] In this condition, there is a painful compression of the distal ulna on the medial surface of the lunate. It is not unusual to see full-thickness defects of the cartilage of the lunate as well as tears of the TFC. In extreme cases of excessive ulnar length—common in patients with rheumatoid arthritis—dorsal subluxation of the ulna occurs, and supination is blocked. Severe dorsal subluxation with supination of the carpus is common. Attritional ruptures of the extensor tendons of the fourth and fifth compartments often occur due to erosion caused by this prominent ulna.

Magnetic Resonance Findings

With the exception of positive ulnar variants or a prominent ulnar styloid, plain radiographs in patients with ulnolunate (*i.e.,* ulnocarpal) impingement are unremarkable. Bone scintigraphy may show nonspecific uptake in the ulnolunate region. Magnetic resonance imaging shows central perforations of the TFC in association with neutral or positive ulnar variance (see Fig. 8–48; Fig 8–49); these tears occur between contact surfaces of the lunate and ulna. With MR, it is also possible to detect the earliest changes of subchondral sclerosis on the ulnar aspect of the lunate. Sclerotic changes demonstrate low signal intensity on T1-, T2- and T2*-weighted images. The cyst demonstrates low or low to intermediate signal intensity on T2*-weighted images. Coronal images reveal the initial degenerative changes in the articular cartilage surfaces of the distal ulna or proximal lunate surfaces. These degenerative changes are indicated by either attenuation of articular cartilage or irregularity or denuding of the articular cartilage surface. Another feature of the ulnolunate impingement syndrome that can be documented on coronal and sagittal MR images is lunatotriquetral ligament disruption and resultant instability. Treatment with TFCC debridement and ulnar shortening may be necessary to relieve pain and halt progression of impingement.

Instability of the Distal Radioulnar Joint

Both CT and MR imaging of both wrists in both full pronation and full supination have been shown to be useful in the diagnosis of distal radioulnar subluxation.[56,57] A new technique to evaluate instability at this joint uses a frame that places a calibrated degree of stress on the distal ulna and radius in conjunction with CT.[58] The controlled load placed on the joint is supposed to simulate the physiology of dynamic subluxation, a condition that is difficult to diagnose. Useful quantitation of the degree of subluxation may also be possible with this technique.

The advantage of MR axial imaging in maximum pronation and supination is the identification of the relative positions of the distal radius and ulna with soft-tissue contrast information (Fig. 8–50). Axial images display the condition of the dorsal and volar radioulnar ligaments, and volar radioulnar ligament tears may be associated with dorsal instability of the DRUJ. The normal volar distal radioulnar ligament is maximally taut when the wrist is studied in pronation. TFCC tears or distal radial fractures may lead to DRUJ instability with subluxation, and the TFC can be assessed during the same examination with MR imaging in the coronal plane. Compared with CT, MR is more accurate in the characterization of associated effusions of the DRUJ, which are a secondary sign of TFC pathology. Axial and sagittal images are useful in demonstrating displacement of the distal ulna in relationship to the TFCC.

TRIANGULAR FIBROCARTILAGE COMPLEX

Gross Anatomy

The TFCC, which includes the dorsal and volar radioulnar ligaments, the ulnar collateral ligaments, the meniscus homologue, the articular disc or TFC, and the extensor carpi ulnaris sheath, is classified as part of the ulnocarpal extrinsic ligamentous group. It stabilizes the DRUJ and ulnocarpal articulation. The dorsal and volar radioulnar ligaments reinforce the peripheral margins of the TFC, which is thinned centrally and thickened peripherally. The thickened ulnar collateral fibers that are distal to the TFC comprise the meniscus homologue. These fibers then insert distally into the triquetrum, the hamate, and the base of the fifth metacarpal. The ulnolunate ligament originates on the anterior border of the TFC and inserts on the lunate. The TFC has a biconcave morphology and articulates with the distal ulna and triquetrum in the proximal carpal row. With a strong radial attachment of the TFC, ligaments that have or share TFC attachment function to connect the volar aspect of the carpus to the radius.

Arthroscopic Evaluation

Anatomy

The TFCC arises from the medial surface of the radius at the level of the articular cartilage. Its origin is flush with the radial articular surface, and the only way to differentiate these structures arthroscopically is by palpation with a probe. As noted above, the TFCC courses toward the base of the ulnar styloid to insert into the fovea. The articular disc is continuous with the volar ulnocarpal ligaments as well as the dorsal capsular structures. There is a strong dorsal insertion into the undersurface of the sheath of the extensor carpi ulnaris tendon. More radially, the articular disc of the TFCC is suspended from the dorsal capsular structures of the wrist.

Pathology

The TFCC is under tension when all of the suspensory insertions around its periphery are intact. When there is a problem, ballottement under arthroscopy produces a resiliency that has been called the "trampoline effect." Separation of the peripheral insertions of the TFCC, especially at the fovea or radius, result in a loss of this suspensatory trampoline effect.[59]

The central portion, or centrum, of the TFCC is thin and is the most common site of tears. The dorsal and volar portions of the TFCC are thicker than the central portion; they have been referred to as the dorsal and volar limbi by Ekenstam.[27] Whereas the thin central portion can be excised if torn, much like the meniscus of the knee, the limbi should be preserved because they appear to play an important mechanical role in the stability of the DRUJ. On average, the limbi are 4 to 5 mm thick.[60] Tears of the centrum can be associated with a variety of causes. Perforations from excessive loading in patents with positive or neutral ulnar variance and ulnocarpal impingement syndromes are common. As noted above, these patients may present with findings indicative of cartilage degeneration of the distal ulna and medial lunate. Some patients with ulnocarpal impingement present with a triad of symptoms, including positive or neutral ulnar variance, TFCC perforations, and LT instability. An ulnar unloading procedure, such as ulnar shortening, relieves the pressure on the LT ligament and allows the symptoms to subside. With extreme instability or cartilage degeneration between the lunate and triquetrum, fusion of the LT joint may be necessary in addition to the ulnar shortening.[60]

Studies of the vascular anatomy of the articular disc have shown that, similar to the meniscus of the knee, only the peripheral 15% to 20% of the disc is vascularized. The central portion is avascular.[61] Therefore, although there is a potential for surgical repair of peripheral lesions, central lesions cannot be expected to heal and should be treated by excision. Reinsertion of peripheral ulnar avulsions of the TFCC that resulted restoration of the biomechanical function of the structure and symptomatic relief has been reported.[59]

The TFC is continuous with the volar ulnolunate and ulnotriquetral ligaments, and these structures provide a strong insertion into the carpus. Tears of these ligaments have been implicated as a cause of ulnar wrist pain. These lesions can be depicted in MR studies, and there are reports of successful treatment with arthroscopic debridement.[62]

Magnetic Resonance Evaluation

Anatomy

Both the distal and the proximal surfaces of the TFC are depicted with MR; this information is not available through wrist arthroscopy or single compartment radiocarpal arthrography (Fig. 8–51). On coronal plane T1-, T2-, or T2*-weighted images, the TFC is depicted as a biconcave disc of homogeneous low signal intensity. The tendon of the extensor carpi ulnaris is seen on the radial aspect of the ulnar styloid process. Coronal plane images of the TFC disc demonstrate the lateral attachment to the ulnar aspect of the distal radius with separate superior and inferior radial attachments. The inferior radial attachment is not seen in arthroscopic evaluation restricted to the radiocarpal surface of the TFC.

The contours of the TFC (*i.e.,* proximal and distal surfaces) and ulnar variance are best assessed in coronal images. The distribution of force across the radial plate is increased by negative ulnar variance and is reduced by positive ulnar variance. The TFC is thus an important contributor in the stabilization of the medial aspect of the radiocarpal joint. Disruption of the TFC is associated with DRUJ subluxation during pronation.

On axial images, the TFC is shaped like an equilateral triangle. The apex of the TFCC converges on the ulnar styloid, with the base of the triangle attached on the superior margin of the distal radial sigmoid notch. Sagittal images show the TFC in sections through the triquetrum. In this plane, the TFC has discoid morphology as seen from anterior to posterior. The TFC is located immediately distal to the dome of the ulna, and is thinned centrally with broader volar and distal margins (*i.e.,* peripheral thickening). This peripheral thickening is composed

(text continues on page 746)

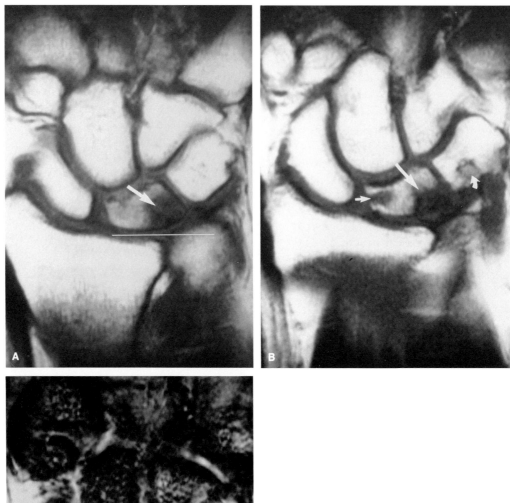

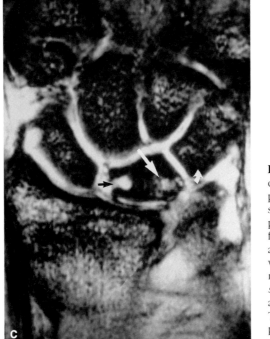

FIGURE 8–49. Ulnolunate impingement syndrome. (**A**) A coronal T1-weighted image shows predominant low signal intensity subchondral sclerosis (*arrow*) affecting the proximal ulnar aspect of the lunate. This sclerosis may be mistaken for Kienböck's disease. Mild positive ulnar variance (*white line*) is present. Coronal (**B**) T1-weighted and (**C**) T2*-weighted images show more extensive subchondral cystic changes (*small straight arrows*), sclerosis (*large straight arrows*), and triquetral involvement (*curved arrows*). There is degeneration of the distal ulnar and proximal lunate articular cartilage surfaces, as well as disruption of the triangular fibrocartilage.

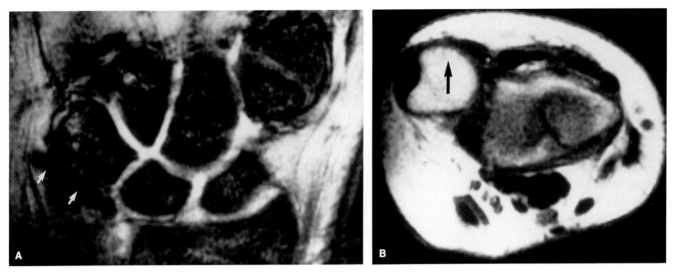

FIGURE 8–50. Postoperative repair of the triangular fibrocartilage. (**A**) A T2*-weighted coronal image shows residual dorsal instability (*arrows*) of the distal radioulnar joint. (**B**) A T1-weighted axial image shows associated detachment of the volar radioulnar ligament from its ulnar insertion (*arrow*). Dorsal displacement of the ulna is best depicted in the axial image.

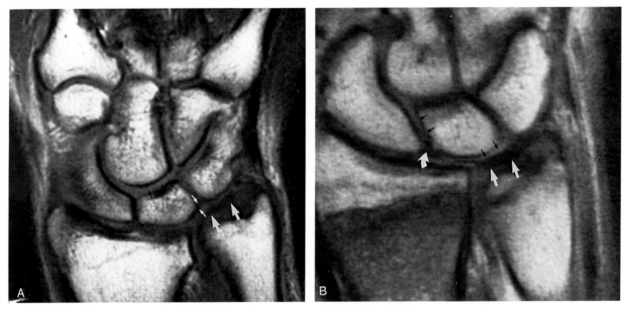

FIGURE 8–51. Coronal T1-weighted images with (**A**) a 10-cm field of view (FOV) and (**B**) an 8-cm FOV of normal wrists show intact low signal intensity triangular fibrocartilage (*large white arrows*) and intermediate signal intensity hyaline articular cartilage of the carpal bones (*black arrows*). The scapholunate (*curved white arrow*) and lunotriquetral (*small white arrows*) interosseous ligaments are identified.

of lamellar collagen and gives rise to the dorsal and volar radioulnar ligaments. The ulnocarpal ligament arises from the volar distal surface of the TFC.

Pathology

Magnetic resonance imaging of the TFCC reveals many tears that previously went undetected.[63] These include intrasubstance (*i.e.,* horizontal) tears and peripheral lesions of the insertions of the TFCC that do not show contrast leakage (Figs. 8–52 and 8–53).

Central perforations of the TFC are unusual in the first two decades of life. By the fifth decade of life, however, symptomatic perforations can be identified in 40% of TFC studies, and by the sixth decade, perforations are found in 50% of patients studied.[8,64] This finding may explain the poor correlation between clinical findings of wrist pain and communication of contrast across the TFC seen in radiocarpal arthrograms. The fact that radiocarpal compartment communication with the inferior radioulnar compartment is found more frequently in anatomic dissections than with arthrographic injection can be explained by the existence of partial tears and unidirectional flap tears.

The thin layer of hyaline articular cartilage proximal to the radial attachment of the TFC along the ulnar aspect of the distal radius is seen on MR images as bright signal intensity on T2*-weighted images and should not be mistaken for fluid communication with the inferior radioulnar joint or detachment of the radial aspect of the TFC (Fig. 8–54). Intrasubstance degeneration of the TFC is best depicted on T2*-weighted images, and appears as regions of increased signal intensity without extension to the superior or inferior margins of the TFC. The meniscus homologue demonstrates greater signal intensity than the TFC on T2*-weighted images. Partial tears in this area may be more difficult to identify due to the increased signal intensity and inhomogeneity of the meniscal homologue. Tears of the TFC may occur either as an isolated injury or in association with subluxations of the DRUJ or perilunate dislocations. Patients with TFC pathology often present with pain, clicking, or both on the ulnar aspect of the wrist. An unstable flap of tissue from a torn TFC causes catching on the ulnar aspect of the wrist, especially when loaded in extension or ulnar deviation (Fig. 8–55). TFC tears, demonstrated by discontinuity or fragmentation, are most commonly located near or adjacent to the radial attachment (Figs. 8–56 and 8–57).[65] Contour irregularities, especially with associated regions of increased signal intensity, can be identified on T1-, T2-, and T2*-weighted images. Tears on the radial aspect of the TFC frequently have a dorsal-to-volar orientation extending to both its proximal and distal surfaces (Fig 8–58).

Associated synovitis presents as a localized fluid collection or radiocarpal joint effusion on T2- or T2*-weighted images and may be associated with chondromalacia of the lunate, triquetrum, or ulna. In younger populations, there is a higher incidence of tears on the ulnar aspect of the TFC (Fig. 8–59). Peripheral tears are usually secondary to traumatic avulsion, whereas central perforations may be associated with findings of TFC degeneration (Fig. 8–60).[66] These degenerative changes of the TFC include increased signal intensity on T1- and T2*-weighted images and thinning or attenuation of the articular disc. Whereas deformity of the TFC is common in patients with negative ulnar variance, TFC tears are associated with positive ulnar variance.

Magnetic resonance is valuable in assessing postoperative TFC repairs and associated distal joint instability (Fig. 8–61). Magnetic resonance accuracy for detecting TFC tears is reported to be 95% when compared with arthrography and 89% compared with arthroscopy and arthrotomy.[22,63]

Treatment

The significance of TFCC lesions must be evaluated as a part of the whole clinical presentation. As noted above, Mikic found that beyond age 35, asymptomatic tears become more and more common.[8] In many cases, a TFCC lesion is not actually responsible for the patient's symptoms, but is rather a clue to the pathologic process. In these cases, treatment modalities are not directed at the TFCC tear itself, but at the underlying pathology. For example, in the patient with positive ulnar variance and a TFCC tear, treatment is aimed at relieving the overloading of the distal ulna rather than merely repairing or debriding the tear. Frequently, there is severe painful chondromalacia of the distal ulna.

Triangular fibrocartilage complex resection and debridement have been the treatments of choice for a flap tear of the TFCC—similar to that of the meniscus of the knee—that causes pain; these treatments also are indicated if there is instability of the DRUJ due to the TFCC injury. If repair is not possible, then the structure should be augmented. We use an intraarticular ligament reconstruction to augment tears of the dorsal limbus of the TFCC that lead to DRUJ instability. There are data, however, that indicate that no resection of the TFCC is mechanically benign, even though the avascular, thin centrum of the disc was thought by many to be mechanically insignificant, and the mechanics for stabilizing the DRUJ were thought to be primarily derived from the intact dorsal and volar limbi. Adams has reported that although the dorsal and volar limbi of the TFCC provide the final restraints to DRUJ dislocation, the centrum is an important component for normal motion.[67] Resection of the centrum was found to alter the mechanics of the DRUJ and the remainder of the TFCC.[67] These findings suggest that the TFCC should not be resected with impunity, and that methods of reconstruction need to be studied more carefully.

The meniscus homologue is a structure that consists of a fold of fibrous tissue interposed between the tip of the ulnar styloid and the triquetrum. This is an evolutionary remnant of the early primate wrist, in which weight bearing was facilitated by an elongated ulnar styloid that articulated, through a free meniscus, with the triquetrum.[68] Occasionally, a free meniscus or an abnormally long ulnar styloid tipped with articular cartilage that impinges against the triquetrum can be seen in humans. Triquetral impingement of the ulnar styloid results in cartilage degeneration of the triquetrum. This impingement can be treated with a limited ulnar styloidectomy. The meniscus homologue forms the entrance to the prestyloid recess seen in arthrographic examination of the wrist.

FRACTURES OF THE DISTAL RADIUS AND CARPUS

Conventional radiography is limited in the detection of nondisplaced or partially displaced fractures of the carpus and distal radius. Trispiral tomography depends on correct planar positioning, or carpal fractures may be underdiagnosed. Early bone scintigraphy, performed within 72 hours of an acute fracture, may be negative or equivocal. Computed tomography using thin (1.5-mm) sections in either direct coronal or axial planes with reformatting and 3D rendering is the most accurate modality for identifying fractures and for characterizing morphology and associated comminution or displacement. Chip fractures have been detected by CT in patients with negative MR studies. Fracture extent and adjacent marrow hyperemia are well seen in MR images. In subacute and chronic fractures, sclerosis demonstrates low signal intensity on T1-weighted images. The temporal stage of a fracture (*e.g.*, acute, subacute, chronic) and its location determine the optimal diagnostic imaging plane (*e.g.*, coronal, axial, sagittal). Magnetic resonance shows associated ligamentous injury in isolated or multiple carpal bone trauma. If initial imaging is inadequate, delayed diagnosis and treatment may lead to poor anatomic reduction and function.

Distal Radius Fractures

There are several systems for classifying fractures of the distal radius, but the Frykman classification has received the most attention.[69] This system differentiates fractures based on whether they are intraarticular or extraarticular and on the degree to which they involve the DRUJ. Melone has proposed a system for classifying articular frac-

tures of the distal radius which depends on the degree and direction of displacement of the articular fragments (Figs. 8–62 and 8–63).[70] This system is clinically useful because it indicates when open reduction is necessary to achieve accurate anatomical reduction (see Fig. 8–62). In routine lateral radiographs, the normal palmar tilt of the articular surface of the distal radius is 10° to 14°. On posteroanterior radiographs, the inclination of the radial articular surface forms an angle of 23° with the long axis of forearm. These angles must be accurately restored with fracture reduction. If the palmar tilt is not anatomically correct, the patient will have a limited range of motion in flexion and may develop an intercalated instability pattern of the carpus. Loss of the angle of inclination leads to increased loading of the radial articular surface and arthritic degeneration.[71]

Colles' Fractures

Colles' fractures occur secondary to a fall on the outstretched hand, with a pronated forearm in dorsiflexion. The fracture commonly occurs in adult females older than 50 years of age. The fracture line occurs within 2 to 3 cm of the articular surface of the distal radius (Figs. 8–64 and 8–65). The distal fracture segment may demonstrate dorsal displacement, angulation, or both. Medial or lateral displacement may also be present. The transmission of force across the transverse carpal ligament may result in an associated ulnar styloid fracture.

With MR, it is possible to assess the articular surface of the distal radius and to document precise angular deformities in sagittal, axial, and coronal planes. The median and ulnar nerves, which may be involved at the time of injury, are best seen on axial MR images.

Die Punch Fractures

In a die punch fracture, the lunate impacts the distal radius, splitting its fossa in both the coronal and sagittal planes and depressing the articular surface, much like a tibial plateau fracture (Fig. 8–66).[72,73] It is critical to restore the articular surface to anatomic continuity following this injury to prevent the development of late traumatic arthritis.

Recent clinical studies have shown that over 90% of young adult patients with incongruity (defined as more than 2 mm of displacement) develop arthritis.[74] Since the die punch lesion is a common cause of incongruity, surgeons have increased their efforts to reestablish normal articular anatomy following these injuries. Newer surgical techniques which show some promise include arthroscopic percutaneous pinning and reduction. Once the depressed articular fragments are reduced, they can be augmented with buttressing bone grafts placed via an extraarticular approach.

(text continues on page 756)

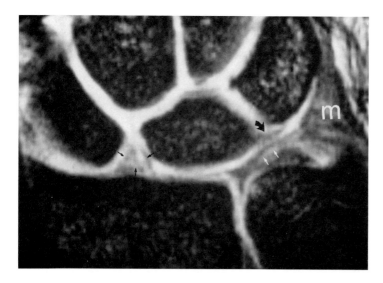

FIGURE 8–52. An intrasubstance tear (*white arrows*) of the triangular fibrocartilage is present without surface discontinuity. The radioscapholunate ligament (*straight black arrows*), the lunotriquetral ligament (*curved black arrow*) and the meniscus homologue (m) are also seen on a T2*-weighted coronal image.

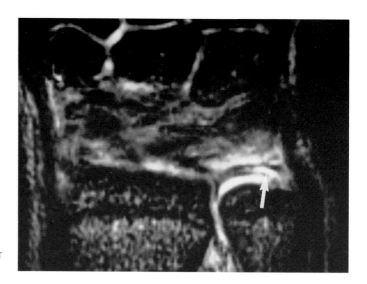

FIGURE 8–53. A dorsal surface tear (*arrow*) of the triangular fibrocartilage is seen on a T2*-weighted coronal image.

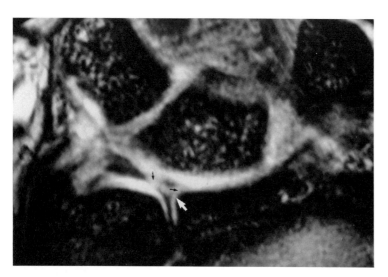

FIGURE 8–54. A T2*-weighted coronal image shows a high signal intensity linear triangular fibrocartilage tear with distal surface and radial extension (*black arrows*). Note the normal high signal intensity hyaline articular cartilage at the ulnar aspect of the distal radius (*white arrow*).

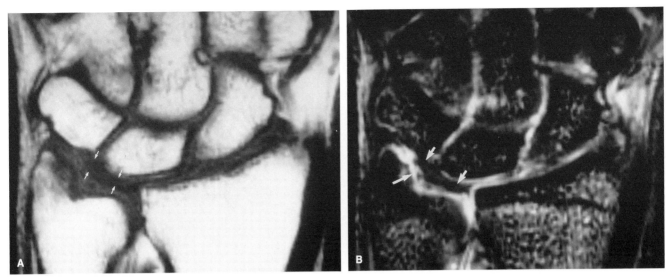

FIGURE 8–55. Coronal (**A**) T1-weighted and (**B**) T2*-weighted images show a complete tear of the ulnar attachment of the triangular fibrocartilage, which is adherent to the proximal aspect of the triquetrum and lunate (*small arrows*). There is direct communication of joint fluid between the radiocarpal and inferior radioulnar joint (*large arrows*).

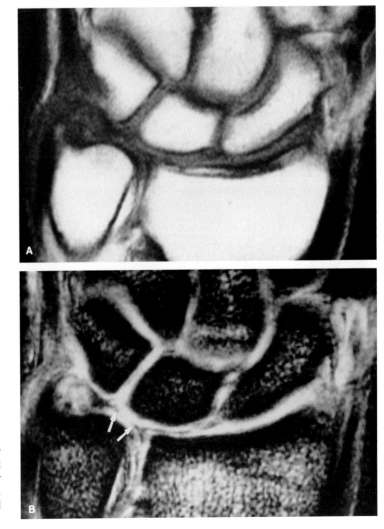

FIGURE 8–56. A large central disruption of the triangular fibrocartilage (*arrows*) is seen on coronal (**A**) T1-weighted and (**B**) T2*-weighted images. This degree of discontinuity is not characteristic of a degenerative central perforation. Morphology of the tear is best depicted on the T2*-weighted image.

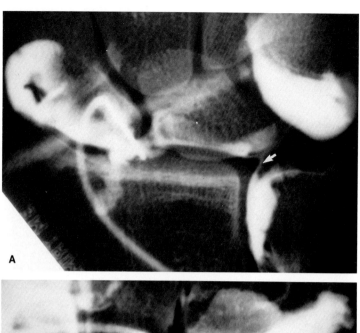

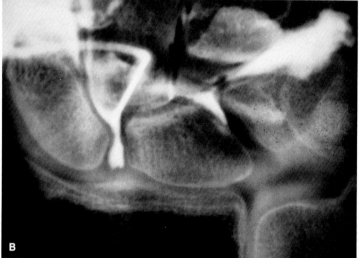

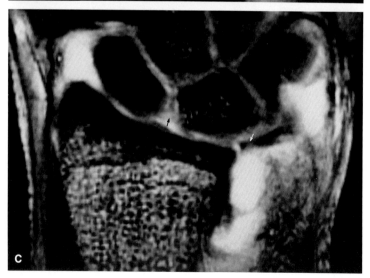

FIGURE 8–57. Triangular fibrocartilage (TFC) tear. (**A**) A radiocarpal arthrogram injection of a patient with a triangular fibrocartilage tear reveals extension of contrast into the inferior radioulnar joint (*arrow*). (**B**) A separate midcarpal injection confirms that the scapholunate interval is intact. (**C**) The corresponding T2*-weighted coronal image demonstrates the oblique path of fluid across the TFC to communicate with the inferior radioulnar compartment (*white arrow*). The intact scapholunate is shown (*black arrow*).

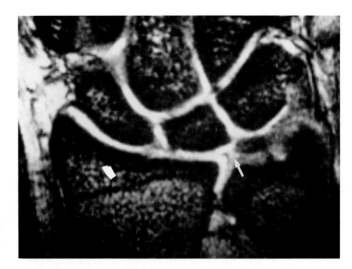

FIGURE 8–58. A T2*-weighted coronal image shows a vertical tear located near the radial attachment of the triangular fibrocartilage (*arrow*). This is a common tear pattern that usually extends in a dorsal to volar direction.

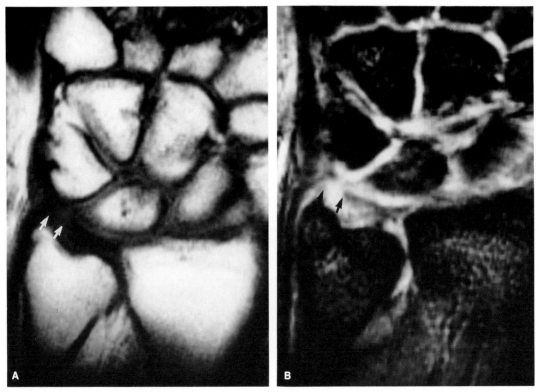

FIGURE 8–59. Avulsion of the triangular fibrocartilage from its attachment to the fovea of the ulna (*arrows*) is seen on coronal (**A**) T1-weighted and (**B**) T2*-weighted images.

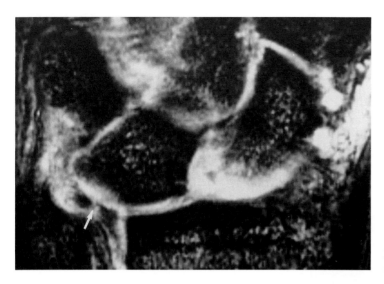

FIGURE 8–60. A central vertical tear (*arrow*) of the triangular fibrocartilage is seen on a T2*-weighted coronal image.

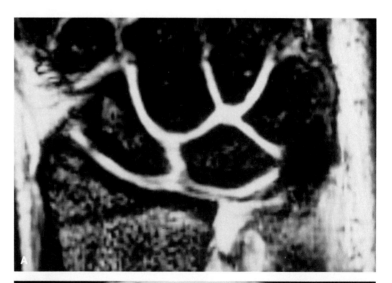

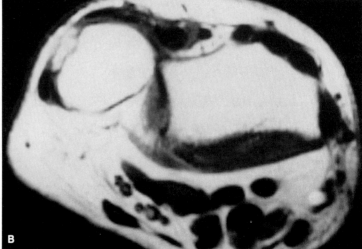

FIGURE 8–61. Postoperative repair of the ulnar aspect of the triangular fibrocartilage. (**A**) A T2*-weighted coronal image shows a postoperative artifact (*arrow*). (**B**) A T1-weighted axial image shows dorsal instability of the distal radioulnar joint, with dorsal displacement of the distal ulna (*straight arrow*). Note the intact dorsal radioulnar ligament (*curved arrow*) and the absence of the volar radioulnar ligament (*open arrow*).

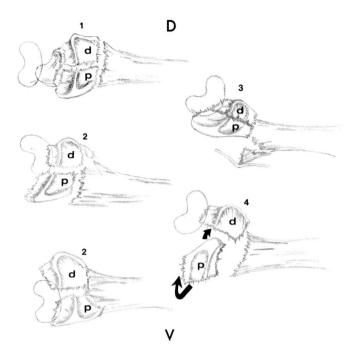

FIGURE 8–62. The Melone classification of distal radius articular fractures. The displacement of the medial complex, which consists of medial fragments and ligamentous attachments to the ulnar styloid and carpus, is the basis for classifying four types of articular fractures. (**1**) In a type 1 fracture, the medial complex may be displaced or not, with stable reduction and congruity of the joint surface. (**2**) In a type 2 fracture, there is comminution and the fracture is unstable. The medial complex is posteriorly or anteriorly displaced. (**3**) In a type 3 fracture, the medial complex is displaced, and a spike fragment from comminuted radial shaft is present. (**4**) In a type 4 fracture, separation or rotation of the dorsal and palmar medial fragments occurs, with severe disruption of the distal radial articular surface. (*small and large curved arrows,* rotation of distal and palmar medial fragments; D, dorsal; d, dorsal medial fragment; p, palmar medial fragment; V, volar.)

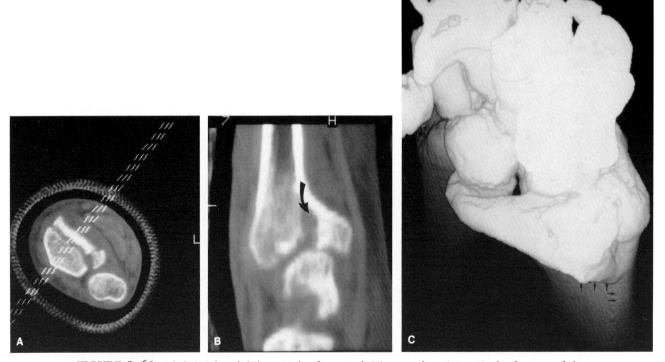

FIGURE 8–63. (**A**) Axial and (**B**) sagittal reformatted CT scans show intraarticular fracture of the distal radius with anterior displacement (*curved arrow*) of the palmar articular surface. This is a Melone type 2 fracture, or reverse Barton's fracture, involving the volar and not the dorsal lip of the radius. (**C**) The corresponding 3D CT shows an intraarticular fracture of the palmar articular surface or volar lip of the radius (*arrows*).

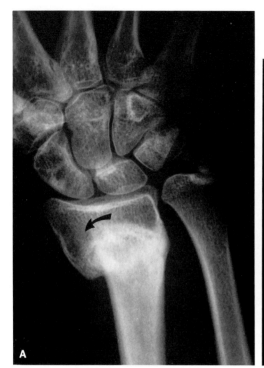

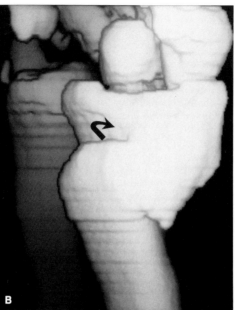

FIGURE 8–64. Colles' fracture. (**A**) An anteroposterior radiograph shows nonarticular distal radius and ulnar styloid fractures. Lateral displacement of the distal radius fracture fragment is present (*arrow*), with associated radial shortening. (**B**) The corresponding 3D CT image reveals dorsal impaction with apex volar angulation (*arrow*).

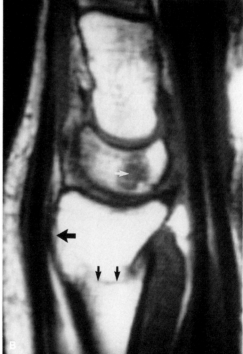

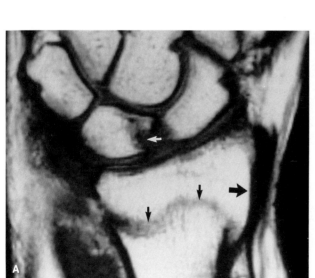

FIGURE 8–65. (**A**) A T1-weighted coronal image shows a postreduction Colles' fracture (*small black arrows*) with lateral displacement (*large black arrow*). Subchondral cystic erosion is present in the radial aspect of the lunate (*white arrow*). (**B**) A T1-weighted sagittal image shows dorsal displacement (*large black arrow*) with angulation of the distal fracture fragment. The fracture site (*small black arrows*) and lunate cystic erosion (*white arrow*) are also shown.

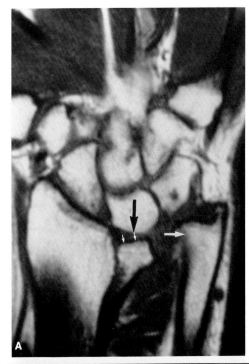

FIGURE 8–66. Die punch fracture. Coronal (**A**) T1-weighted and (**B**) 2D CT reformatted images show splitting and depression of the lunate fossa (*small white arrows*) of the distal radius, with proximal migration of the lunate (*black arrows*). Associated diastasis (*large white arrows*) of the distal radioulnar joint is present, with complete disruption of the triangular fibrocartilage complex. (**C**) The corresponding 3D coronal CT image shows an intraarticular fracture (*vertical arrow*) and distal radioulnar joint diastasis (*horizontal arrow*).

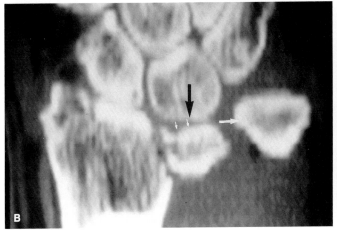

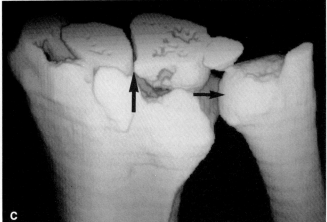

Carpal Fractures

Scaphoid Fractures

Scaphoid fractures are the most common fractures involving the carpus.[75] Fracture of the scaphoid is frequently associated with dorsiflexion loading and a radial deviation mechanism. A conventional radiographic diagnostic series includes posteroanterior, ulnar deviation, oblique, and lateral radiographs. Repeat studies after a 2 to 3 week delay may be necessary if plain film radiographs are negative. Negative bone scintigraphy may require repeat studies 48 hours after the initial injury. Patients with trauma to the scaphoid often present with pain over the anatomical snuff box.

Fractures with a gap of 1 mm or less of diastasis are considered stable. Unstable scaphoid fractures may have a nonunion rate of up to 50% with closed treatment. Seventy percent of scaphoid fractures involve the middle one-third, or waist, of the scaphoid (Fig. 8–67), and these fractures have an increased risk for delayed union and AVN. Twenty percent of scaphoid fractures involve the proximal one-third of the scaphoid, and 10% involve the distal one-third (Fig. 8–68). The blood supply of the scaphoid is primarily through the distal pole, entering via the dorsal ridge from branches of the radial artery. Thus, with fractures through the waist of the scaphoid, blood supply to the proximal pole is poor; this accounts for the AVN and delayed healing. Other complications of scaphoid fractures include deformity, carpal instability, secondary osteoarthritis, carpal tunnel syndrome, and sympathetic dystrophy (Fig. 8–69).

On MR imaging studies of scaphoid fractures, the low signal intensity fracture line is clearly displayed and may persist, contrasting with the surrounding bright signal intensity of marrow during healing (Fig. 8–70). The identification of extension to cortical bone is necessary to accurately differentiate acute from chronic fractures, and it allows MR to be more sensitive than CT or conventional radiography in evaluating the progress of subacute or chronic fractures.

Sagittal images demonstrate the abnormal morphology of the scaphoid, secondary to fracture fragmentation or suboptimal healing (*i.e.,* humpback deformity). This foreshortening of the scaphoid may lead to a DISI instability (Fig. 8–71). Herbert screws are imaged with minimal artifact. The articular cartilage surface of the scaphoid and the congruity of adjacent coronal surfaces should be assessed. T2*-weighted images are not as sensitive to the range of contrast as conventional T1-weighted images and may not identify a nonacute, nondisplaced fracture. Gradient-echo images are, however, useful in demonstrating the integrity of the adjacent SL ligament. The volar capsule (the RSC ligament and radiolunotriquetral ligament) is shown on sagittal images, and adjacent synovitis or edema of ligamentous structures may be identified on T1- or T2*-weighted images at the level of the scaphoid. Short TI inversion recovery imaging is more sensitive to hyperemia in the proximal pole or in bone adjacent to the fracture site which may be misdiagnosed as sclerosis, necrosis, or both on conventional T1-, T2-, or T2*-weighted images.

Triquetrum Fractures

Fractures of the triquetrum represent the second most common fracture of the carpus.[75] Correct positioning in lateral and pronated oblique projections is usually required to identify fractures of the triquetrum in standard radiography. Computed tomography examination of the triquetrum is not limited by overlapping of proximal and distal carpal rows, which may obscure identification of a fracture line. Triquetral fractures include chip fractures that involve the dorsal surface and occur secondary to an avulsion injury at the insertional site of the ulnotriquetral ligament, or trauma to the wrist positioned in hyperextension and ulnar deviation (Fig. 8–72). Fracture through the body of the triquetrum is less common. Triquetral body fractures may be associated with perilunate dislocations.

Multiple fracture lines and acute fracture through the triquetrum may obscure fracture morphology secondary to reactive hyperemia of subchondral bone (Fig. 8–73). T1-weighted images in the axial, coronal, and sagittal imaging planes identify low signal intensity in the area of the fracture. In our experience, CT has been more useful in displaying cortical detail and fracture morphology.

Lunate Fractures

Fracture of the lunate is an uncommon injury that usually occurs secondary to a fall with the wrist in dorsiflexion.[75] Acute fractures of the lunate associated with KD may be related to single or multiple episodes of compression forces. However, fracture of the lunate is more commonly seen during the advanced stages of KD, as a pathologic fracture through areas of necrotic bone. Associated perilunate dislocation with ligamentous trauma should be evaluated.

Pisiform Fractures

The pisiform is a sesamoid bone within the flexor carpi ulnaris tendon.[75] Pisiform fracture is caused by direct or blunt trauma, such as that which occurs when the heel of the hand is used as a hammer. It appears as a comminuted or simple fracture. Pisotriquetral arthritis may develop secondary to pisiform fracture. Sagittal and axial T1-weighted images display a larger surface area of the pisiform bone, minimizing the partial voluming that may complicate coronal images.

Hamate Fractures

Fractures of the hamate, which account for approximately 2% of carpal fractures,[75] may involve either the body or the hook (*i.e.,* the hamulus).[76] Fracture of the hook of the hamate may involve an avulsion injury of the transverse carpal ligament. Direct trauma to the volar aspect of the wrist, the most common mechanism of injury, usually occurs in activities that require a grasping movement, such as holding a bat, club, or racket. Conventional radiographic imaging is often negative for hamate fracture; diagnosis may require the use of a carpal tunnel projection. For MR studies, T1-weighted axial and sagittal images are best suited for display of the anatomy of the hook of the hamate and for identification of a hamate fracture (Fig. 8–74). Thin (1.5-mm) CT scans, however, more accurately identify the extent and location of fractures of the hamate, especially the hook of the hamate. The proximity of the ulnar nerve to the hamate may contribute to the presentation of ulnar wrist pain in patients sustaining hamate trauma.

Capitate Fractures

Fractures of the capitate, which account for 1% to 3% of carpal bone fractures,[75] are similar to scaphoid fractures in that the blood supply of the capitate extends through the waist of the capitate, making the proximal pole susceptible to AVN. Capitate fractures are caused by either direct trauma or forced dorsiflexion, and may be associated with perilunate dislocation (Fig. 8–75). The most frequent site of fracture involves the waist or neck of the capitate. Sagittal MR images are helpful in assessing rotation at the fracture site.

Trapezium and Trapezoid Fractures

Fractures of the trapezium involve either the body or margin of the trapezium.[75] The trapezoid is the least commonly fractured bone of the carpus.

AVASCULAR NECROSIS OF THE SCAPHOID

Avascular necrosis of the scaphoid is primarily a post-traumatic injury that occurs secondary to proximal pole or waist fractures that endanger the dominant blood supply of the scaphoid (Fig. 8–76). In 30% of cases, there is sclerosis of the proximal pole related to osteopenia and

hyperemia of adjacent non-necrotic bone. By the time sclerosis, resorption, and collapse are evident in plain film radiographs, however, the disease is in an advanced state. Avascular necrosis of the scaphoid may also occur in the absence of fracture, and is then referred to as Preiser's disease (Fig. 8–77).

The application of MR imaging to the detection and evaluation of AVN is facilitated by the bright signal intensity contrast generated from the normal fatty marrow content of the carpal bones. Magnetic resonance has been reported to be as sensitive as bone scintigraphy in the detection of AVN, and to possess even greater specificity in diagnosis.[77–82] On T1-weighted (*i.e.,* short TR/TE) sequences, MR sensitivity rates for the detection of decreased marrow signal associated with AVN are 87.5%. With the addition of T2-weighted sequences, specificity is reported to be 100%.

The most common MR appearance of AVN of the scaphoid is low signal intensity in the proximal pole on both T1- and T2-weighted images (Fig. 8–78). In diffuse marrow necrosis, low signal intensity marrow may not be restricted to the proximal pole. T2-weighted images may demonstrate localized fluid accumulation and limited marrow edema of the proximal pole. Reactive marrow hyperemia of the distal pole may be confused with diffuse changes of necrosis (Fig. 8–79). Short TI inversion recovery images can be used to document increased hyperemia of the distal pole marrow, which may not be appreciated on conventional T1-, T2-, or T2*-weighted images. Accurate assessment of vascularity may be limited to gradient-echo sequences. Corticocancellous graft or silastic prosthetic replacement are treatments prescribed for scaphoid nonunion with a nonviable proximal fragment.

KIENBÖCK'S DISEASE

Kienböck's disease is a condition marked by AVN of the lunate. The onset of KD, which can be quite insidious, peaks between the ages of 20 and 40 years. There is a 2:1 male-to-female ratio. Although uncommon, bilaterality does occur. Initially, patients note dorsal tenderness about the lunate and may develop stiffness due to synovitis. The synovitis and inflammation may affect surrounding structures, and one patient presented with acute carpal tunnel syndrome as the first indication of KD. Patients also complain of weakness and decreased grip strength. Kienböck's disease is a great dissembler, and a number of other conditions should be considered. Any history of trauma should be carefully elicited. The differential diagnosis includes dorsal ganglion cysts, rheumatoid arthritis, degenerative or post-traumatic arthritis,

(text continues on page 770)

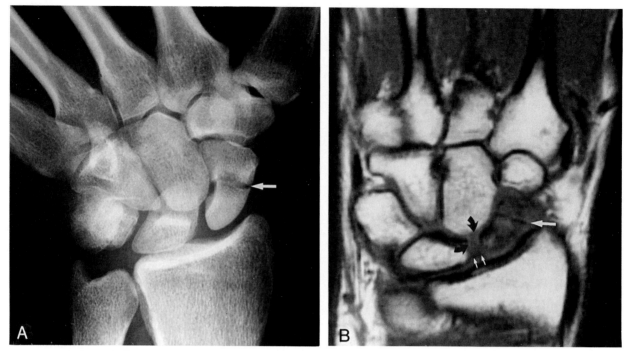

FIGURE 8–67. (**A**) A scaphoid waist fracture (*arrow*) with avascular necrosis is present on an anteroposterior radiograph. No sclerosis is demonstrated in the proximal or distal fragments. (**B**) On the corresponding T1-weighted coronal image, the proximal pole necrotic marrow demonstrates lower signal intensity, and the remaining hyperemic marrow demonstrates intermediate to low signal intensity. The low signal intensity scapholunate ligament (*small white arrows*) and fluid in the widened scapholunate space (*curved arrows*) are also seen. The fracture site (*large white arrow*) is also shown.

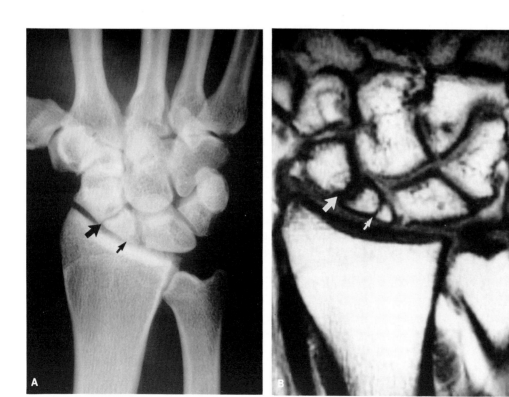

FIGURE 8–68. (**A**) An anteroposterior radiograph shows a scaphoid waist fracture (*large arrow*). No additional fractures are seen in the proximal pole segment (*small arrow*). (**B**) On a T1-weighted coronal image, two distinct fracture lines are revealed. The scaphoid waist fracture extends to both the proximal and distal cortices (*large arrow*). A second fracture of the proximal pole does not extend to cortical bone; it represents the healing stage of trabecular bone (*small arrow*).

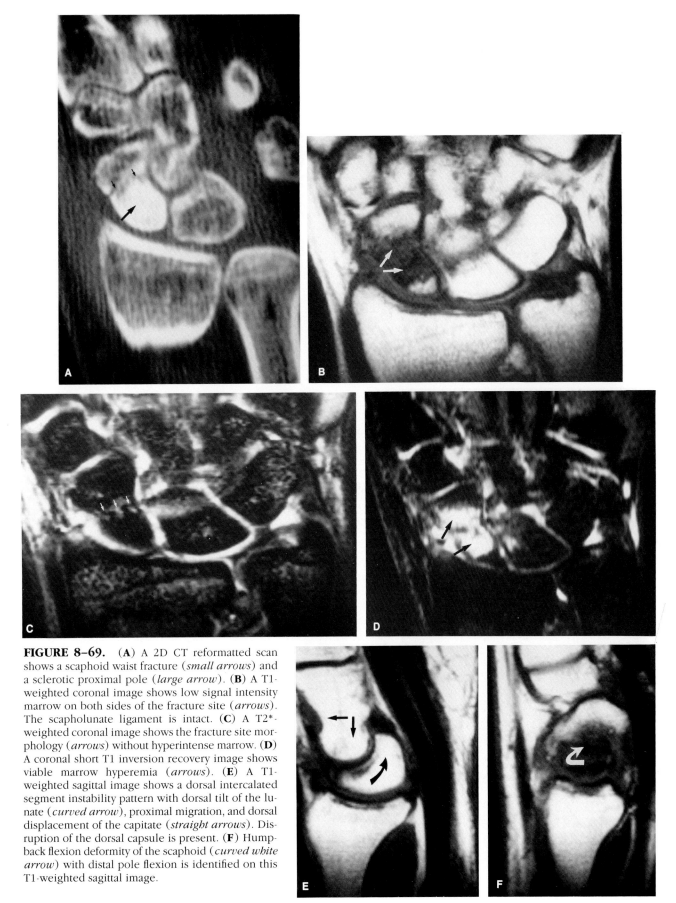

FIGURE 8–69. (**A**) A 2D CT reformatted scan shows a scaphoid waist fracture (*small arrows*) and a sclerotic proximal pole (*large arrow*). (**B**) A T1-weighted coronal image shows low signal intensity marrow on both sides of the fracture site (*arrows*). The scapholunate ligament is intact. (**C**) A T2*-weighted coronal image shows the fracture site morphology (*arrows*) without hyperintense marrow. (**D**) A coronal short T1 inversion recovery image shows viable marrow hyperemia (*arrows*). (**E**) A T1-weighted sagittal image shows a dorsal intercalated segment instability pattern with dorsal tilt of the lunate (*curved arrow*), proximal migration, and dorsal displacement of the capitate (*straight arrows*). Disruption of the dorsal capsule is present. (**F**) Hump-back flexion deformity of the scaphoid (*curved white arrow*) with distal pole flexion is identified on this T1-weighted sagittal image.

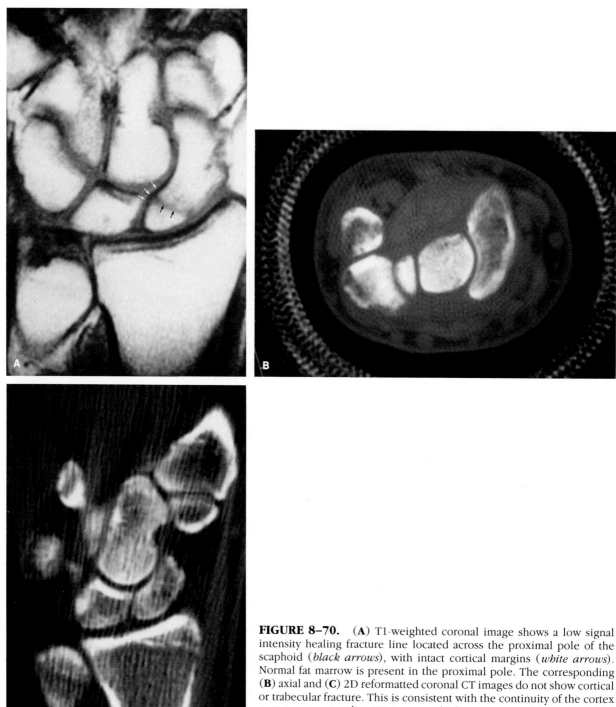

FIGURE 8–70. (**A**) T1-weighted coronal image shows a low signal intensity healing fracture line located across the proximal pole of the scaphoid (*black arrows*), with intact cortical margins (*white arrows*). Normal fat marrow is present in the proximal pole. The corresponding (**B**) axial and (**C**) 2D reformatted coronal CT images do not show cortical or trabecular fracture. This is consistent with the continuity of the cortex seen on corresponding MR images, which are more sensitive in the initial and healing stages of scaphoid fractures. Small chip fractures of other carpal bones, however, are still best evaluated with thin section CT.

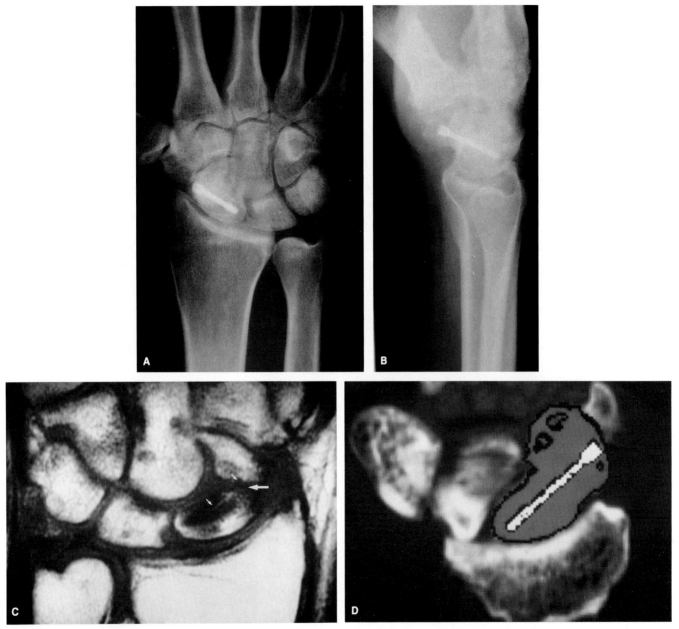

FIGURE 8–71. Scaphoid fracture with dorsal intercalated segment instability (DISI). (**A**) Anteroposterior and (**B**) lateral radiographs show a scaphoid waist fracture fixed with titanium screw. (**C**) A T1-weighted coronal image shows minimal artifact adjacent to the screw (*small arrows*). A low signal intensity fracture line (*large arrow*) is seen in the middle one-third of the scaphoid, without development of avascular necrosis of the proximal pole. (**D**) A 2D CT reformatted image shows the morphology of the titanium screw. (**E**) A 3D CT rendering of the foreshortened scaphoid (*curved arrows*) is displayed in a 2D CT reformatted background. (**F**) A T1-weighted sagittal image illustrates the humpback scaphoid deformity characterized by flexion of the distal pole (*curved arrow*) relative to the fracture line (*straight arrow*) and proximal pole. The radioscaphocapitate ligament is not seen, and there is localized synovitis in its expected location. (**G**) A T1-weighted sagittal image demonstrates DISI secondary to the humpback deformity, and wrist shortening without scapholunate interosseous ligament tear. The dorsal tilt of the lunate (*curved arrow*) and increased capitolunate angle (*double-headed arrow*) are indicated. The capitate is dorsally displaced relative to the radius, as is characteristically seen in DISI instabilities. (D, dorsal; V, volar). *(continued)*

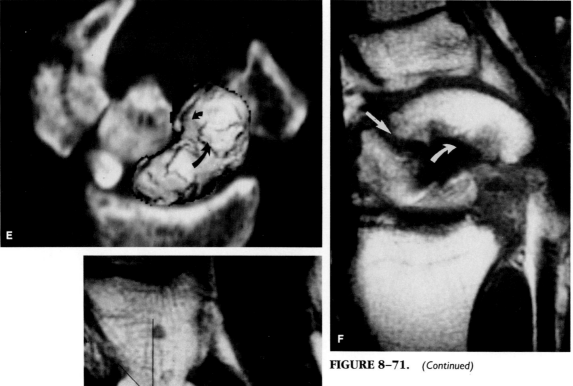

FIGURE 8–71. *(Continued)*

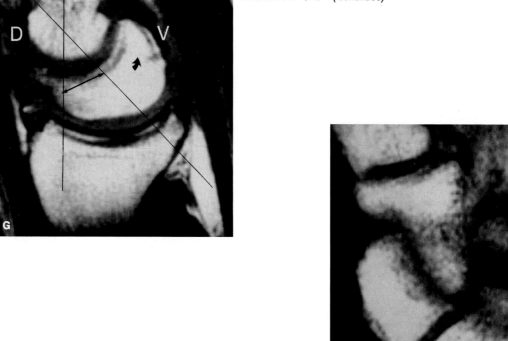

FIGURE 8–72. (**A**) T1-weighted coronal MR image is negative for triquetrum fracture. Coronal (**B**) 2D reformatted and (**C**) 3D CT reveal small chip fractures involving the proximal ulnar aspect of the triquetrum (*arrow*).

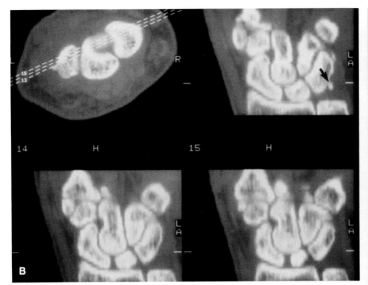

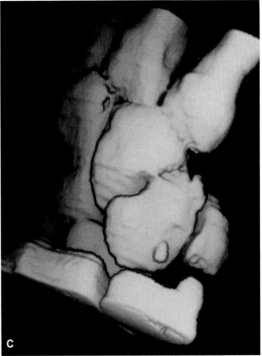

FIGURE 8–72. *(Continued)*

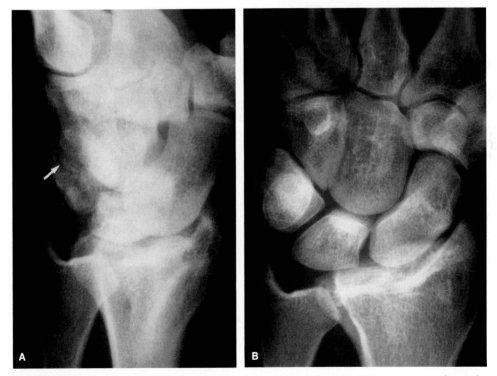

FIGURE 8–73. (**A**) An oblique radiograph shows a dorsal fracture of the triquetrum (*arrow*) (**B**) that was not seen in standard AP projection. (**C**) On a T1-weighted coronal image, marrow hyperemia and hemorrhage (*arrow*) demonstrate low signal intensity; (**D**) in a T2*-weighted coronal image, marrow hyperemia and hemorrhage (*arrow*) demonstrate hyperintensity. (**E**) On a direct axial CT image, a complete dorsal fracture is seen (*arrow*). (**F**) A reformatted coronal CT image shows trabecular bone disruption (*arrows*) that corresponds to the area of marrow hemorrhage seen on the T1- and T2*-weighted MR images. *(continued)*

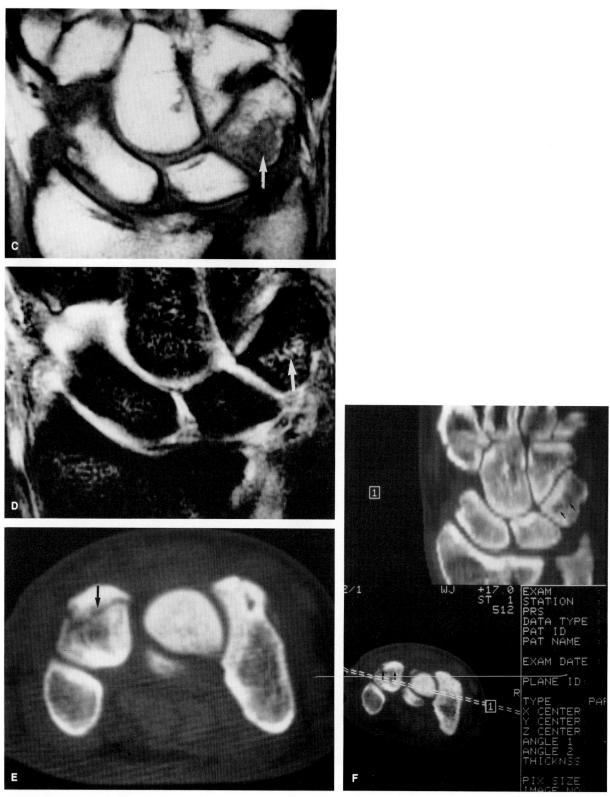

FIGURE 8–73. *(Continued)*

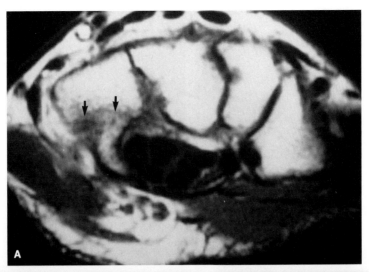

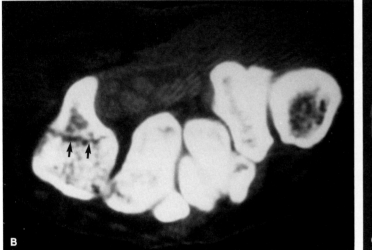

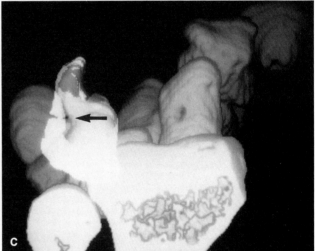

FIGURE 8–74. Hamate fracture. (**A**) A T1-weighted axial image shows a low signal intensity transition (*arrows*) between a fractured hook of the hamate and normal fat marrow signal intensity. Guyon's canal is also seen. Corresponding axial (**B**) CT and (**C**) 3D CT images of the carpal tunnel show a transverse nondisplaced fracture (*arrows*) with greater cortical edge detail. MR, however, allows imaging of Guyon's canal and assessment of the ulnar neurovascular structures, which may be secondarily compromised. Fractures of the hook of the hamate are more common than body fractures and may be overlooked on clinical exam or standard radiographs because a carpal tunnel view is required for their identification.

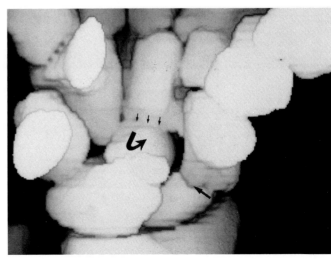

FIGURE 8–75. 3D CT image demonstrates transscaphoid (*large straight arrow*), transcapitate (*small straight arrows*), and perilunate dislocation with 90° rotation of the proximal capitate fragment (*curved arrow*).

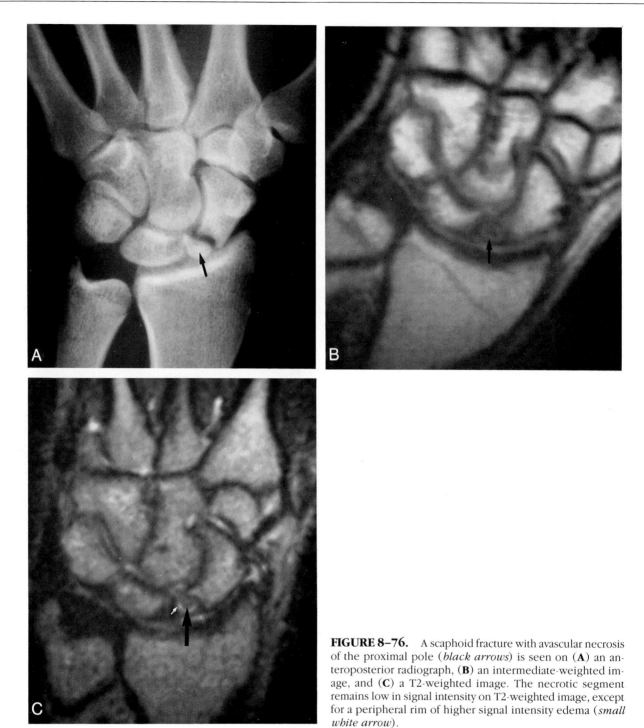

FIGURE 8–76. A scaphoid fracture with avascular necrosis of the proximal pole (*black arrows*) is seen on (**A**) an anteroposterior radiograph, (**B**) an intermediate-weighted image, and (**C**) a T2-weighted image. The necrotic segment remains low in signal intensity on T2-weighted image, except for a peripheral rim of higher signal intensity edema (*small white arrow*).

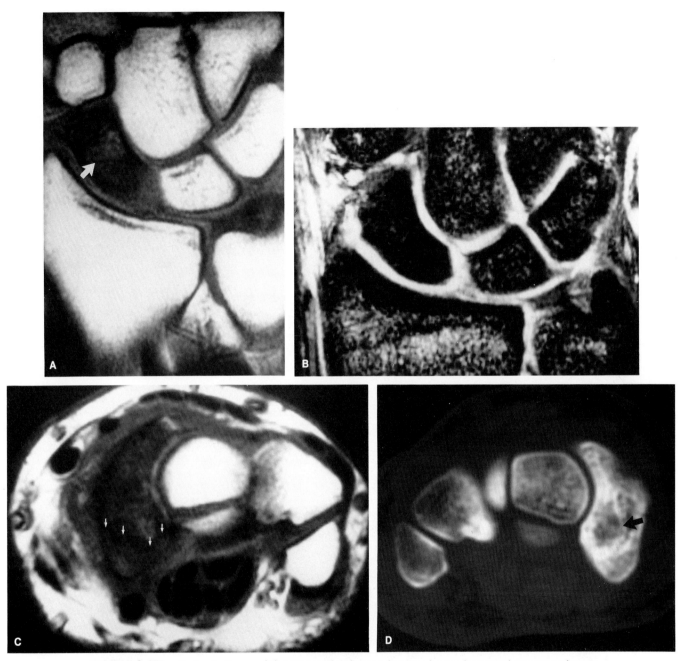

FIGURE 8–77. Preiser's disease. (**A**) A T1-weighted coronal image shows a low signal intensity sclerotic scaphoid (*arrow*) without an identifiable fracture site. (**B**) A T2*-weighted coronal image does not show increased signal intensity. (**C**) A T1-weighted axial image and (**D**) an axial CT scan show stress fracture morphology (*arrows*). (**E**) A T1-weighted sagittal image shows rotatory subluxation and palmar tilt of the scaphoid (*long white line*) with an edematous, lax radioscaphocapitate ligament (*open arrow*). (**F**) A 3D CT image shows normal surface morphology of the scaphoid. *(continued)*

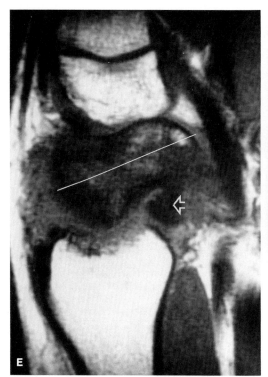

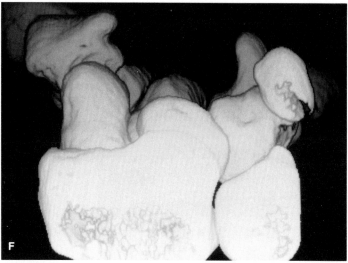

FIGURE 8–77. *(Continued)*

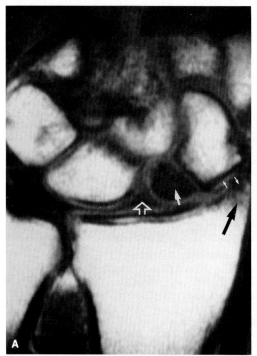

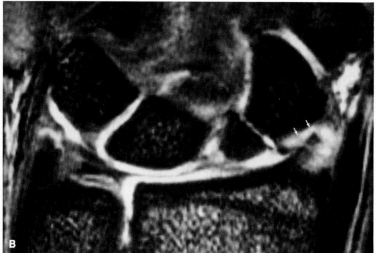

FIGURE 8–78. Avascular necrosis (AVN) of the scaphoid, with early scapholunate advanced collapse (SLAC) wrist. (**A**) A low signal intensity "corner sign" of radial styloid subchondral sclerosis (*black arrow*) is seen in the presence of scaphoid nonunion and AVN of the proximal pole (*large white arrow*) on a T1-weighted coronal image. There is mild narrowing of the radioscaphoid articulation with respect to the distal pole (*small white arrows*). The scapholunate interosseous ligament is intact (*open arrow*). (**B**) Attenuated articular cartilage is seen in the proximal aspect of the distal pole of the scaphoid in early SLAC degeneration (*arrows*) on a T2*-weighted coronal image. The radiolunate joint is characteristically unaffected. (**C**) A 3D CT image shows the fracture site (*solid arrow*) and narrowing of the radioscaphoid articulation at the level of the distal pole of the scaphoid (*open arrow*).

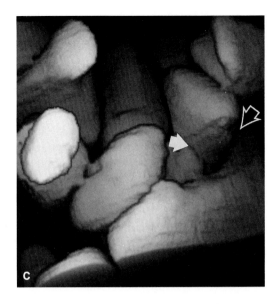

FIGURE 8–78. *(Continued)*

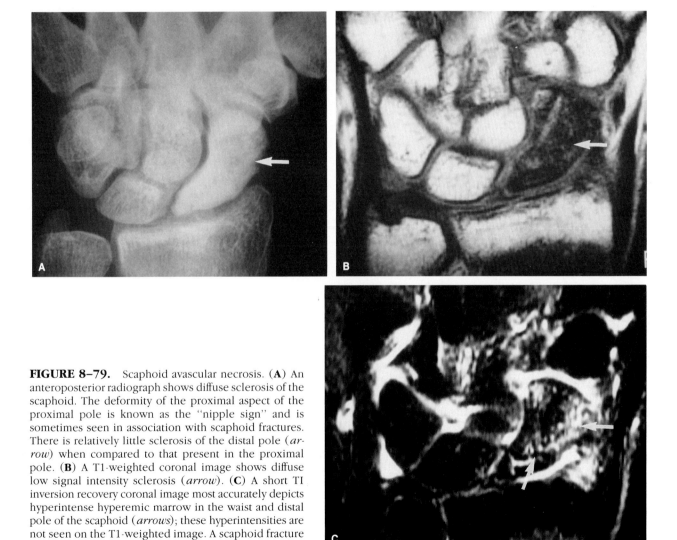

FIGURE 8–79. Scaphoid avascular necrosis. (**A**) An anteroposterior radiograph shows diffuse sclerosis of the scaphoid. The deformity of the proximal aspect of the proximal pole is known as the "nipple sign" and is sometimes seen in association with scaphoid fractures. There is relatively little sclerosis of the distal pole (*arrow*) when compared to that present in the proximal pole. (**B**) A T1-weighted coronal image shows diffuse low signal intensity sclerosis (*arrow*). (**C**) A short TI inversion recovery coronal image most accurately depicts hyperintense hyperemic marrow in the waist and distal pole of the scaphoid (*arrows*); these hyperintensities are not seen on the T1-weighted image. A scaphoid fracture is not identified.

synovitis of the wrist from any cause, acute fractures, carpal instabilities, and ulnar impingement syndrome. It is critical that KD be suspected when evaluating dorsally located central wrist pain.

Although the imaging of KD is discussed in detail (see Magnetic Resonance Findings), a few comments are in order concerning the early presentation of the disease. In stage I of KD, plain film radiographs are normal; before MR imaging became available, the standard test at this stage was the three-phase [99m]TC-MDP study.[83] When there is abnormal uptake of technetium, especially in the third or delayed phase, a CT scan should be performed to assess trabecular bone morphology and to identify fractures. The three-phase technetium study is extremely sensitive, but does not provide detail about physiologic changes in the marrow, which can seen on MR scans. Magnetic resonance is potentially the best first imaging examination to be done after routine radiographs (Fig. 8–80). Magnetic resonance not only allows assessment of the lunate, but also facilitates ruling out or adding other diagnoses in the differential. Magnetic resonance studies may reveal occult ganglion cysts as well as inflammatory arthritides with synovitis.

Etiology

In 1928, Hulten noted a correlation between negative ulnar variance and the occurrence of KD.[84] He found that 78% of patients with KD had a relatively short ulna, whereas only 23% of patients with normal wrists had negative ulnar variance.[84] Despite his primitive radiographic techniques and measurement methods, this correlation has withstood the test of time. It should be noted that the association between a short ulna and KD is not absolute. Although exceedingly uncommon, KD may also occur in patients with neutral or positive ulnar variance. The significance of negative ulnar variance is that it subjects the lunate to an increased mechanical load compared with that associated with neutral or positive ulnar variance.

As noted above, the relative lengths of the ulna and radius vary with the forearm position; it is critical that measurements be made with the forearm in neutral pronosupination. There is no evidence that Hulten was aware of this, and he did not control the forearm position. When forearm position is carefully controlled, there is virtually no difference in accuracy among the several methods available for measuring variance; Gelberman and colleagues have developed a simple method which requires no special tools.[85] In this technique, a line is extended perpendicularly from the most proximal portion of the distal radial articular surface. This point can be found by carefully inspecting posteroanterior radiographs for the three sclerotic lines that represent different portions of the articular surface. The most distal line is

the dorsal lip of the radius. The middle line, because of the normal volar tilt of the distal radius articular surface, is the volar lip of the radius. The most proximal line is the most proximal portion of the articular surface, and this is where the perpendicular line should originate. The distance between this line and the distal articular surface of the ulna is then measured.

The theory that acute fractures and trauma play a role in the etiology of this progressive disease dates as far back as 1843,[86,87] and the anatomy of the vascular supply of the lunate places it at risk for the development of AVN. Gelberman and colleagues found that all lunates could be classified into three types based on their intraosseous microvascular anatomy.[88] The extraosseous blood supply was found to be abundant, and AVN could not be ascribed to interruption of these vessels at a single pole of the lunate. However, the subchondral bone adjacent to the radial articular surface was found to be relatively avascular, and this is the area where collapse is most commonly seen. Gelberman and colleagues concluded that AVN is secondary to disruption of the intraosseous blood vessels caused by repeated trauma with compression fractures.

Treatment

The treatment of KD is a subject of great debate among hand surgeons. No single surgeon or center has been able to develop a large enough experience with all stages of the disease to provide truly definitive treatment recommendations, because this condition is relatively rare. As a result, many types of procedures are recommended in the literature. In general, treatment modalities have been tailored to the stage of disease. Early stages—marked by the absence of changes in articular cartilage, minimal collapse of the lunate, and permanent carpal instability patterns—have been treated with procedures designed to unload and revascularize the lunate. Later stages with established instability patterns and degenerative arthritis must be treated with arthrodeses and salvage procedures. As noted below, the change in therapeutic strategy occurs with the transition from stage IIIA to stage IIIB of KD.

Staging

The clinical and radiographic characteristics of KD vary according to the stage of the disease.[89] The staging classification devised by Lichtman has the most clinical relevance.[90]

Stage I

In stage I of KD, plain radiographs are normal, with the possible exception of evidence of a linear or compression fracture in the lunate. Ulnar variance should be noted. The initial treatment after diagnosis is immobilization and nonsteroidal antiinflammatory drugs (NSAIDs). If there is no improvement with this treatment, then surgical intervention should be considered. A halfway step to an open surgical procedure is the placement of an external fixation device with distraction to unload the lunate. Although this may help, it is impossible to keep such an appliance in place for more than 3 months, which is insufficient time to allow revascularization. If the patient has negative ulnar variance, then radial shortening is frequently advocated to unload the lunate. Although ulnar lengthening is equally effective, it is technically more demanding. Surgical intervention in stage I is rarely indicated, and all patients should receive a trial of conservative therapy. It should be emphasized that, until advent of MR, identification of stage I was exceedingly rare; therefore, there is very little data to assess the efficacy of treatment at this stage of the disease. Magnetic resonance can be used to document healing during cast immobilization.

Stage II

In stage II, a change in the density of the lunate occurs. It appears to be quite sclerotic compared with the other bones of the carpus, although it has not undergone any changes in its architecture. There is no significant carpal instability, but there may be a slight degree of collapse of the radial side of the lunate. At this stage, conservative therapy is not effective, and unloading, revascularization, or both procedures are necessary. This is probably the optimal time for performing a revascularization procedure. Computed tomography scans to assess bone detail should always be made prior to surgery, because a potentially repairable fracture could be identified in this way.

There are two approaches to revascularization. One entails transferring a vascularized bone graft to the lunate, and Braun has successfully used a portion of radial bone vascularized by a pedicle of pronator quadratus muscle for this transfer.[91] Revascularization with the transplantation of a vascular pedicle into the lunate was first reported in 1979 and is gaining in popularity.[92] In this procedure, the second intermetacarpal artery with its vena comitantes (VC) is passed through a dorsal-to-volar hole in the lunate. Recent studies verify that, as long as the VC is present, the artery remains patent. Several centers are beginning to report good results with this procedure. Unloading procedures can be combined with revascularization. Radial shortening or ulnar lengthening are options in the negative ulnar variance wrist. In the patient with neutral or positive ulnar variance, Almquist has recently introduced the technique of shortening the capitate by osteotomy to unload the lunate.[93] He has shown that shortening by 2 to 4 mm reduces the load on the lunate significantly and produces a good clinical result.

Intercarpal fusions have also been shown to unload the lunate. Triscaphe (*i.e.,* scaphoid-trapezoid-trapezium) and scaphocapitate fusions both appear to be effective.

Stage III

Kienböck's disease is considered to be in stage III when there is collapse of the entire lunate. Stage III is further subdivided into stages IIIA and IIIB. In stage IIIB there is a lunate collapse with fixed scaphoid rotation and proximal migration of the capitate (*i.e.,* CID). There is also a decrease in the carpal height ratio. In stage IIIA there is a lunate collapse, but scaphoid rotation is not fixed. There may be dynamic rotatory subluxation, but this can be treated by surgical reconstruction.

Unloading procedures may still be effective in stage IIIA. If a triscaphe (STT) or scaphocapitate (SC) fusion is done, the scaphoid fragments can be excised and the space left empty. This stage was formerly treated by lunate excision and replacement with a silicone prosthesis, but recent reviews of these patients have shown poor results and the frequent occurrence of silicone synovitis.[94] This procedure and use of the prosthesis are no longer indicated.

In patients with positive ulnar variance, capitate shortening, with or without revascularization with a vascular pedicle, can be used to unload and revascularize the lunate. Radial shortening is substituted for capitate shortening in the patient with negative ulnar variance.

During revascularization, every attempt should be made to reconstruct the lunate. When the dorsal cortex is entered, the collapsed articular surface can be elevated and buttressed with a bone graft. The vascular pedicle is then inserted.

In stage IIIB, there is a fixed rotation of the scaphoid which must be corrected. Careful assessment of the scaphoid fossa is important in these patients, and MR has been shown to be of use. Thinning of the cartilage and arthritic changes of the radial styloid can be imaged preoperatively. With fixed rotation of the scaphoid, there is noncongruous loading of the scaphoid fossa. This situation is identical to that in SLAC wrist, discussed previously.

If the cartilage is intact, the procedure of choice fixes the scaphoid in a normal anatomic position with congruous loading of the scaphoid fossa and simultaneously unloads the lunate. An STT or SC fusion, with careful attention to reducing the scaphoid, will accomplish this. The collapsed lunate should be excised in most cases.

Stage IV

Stage IV of KD has all the findings of stage III, with the addition of generalized arthritic changes throughout the carpus. At this point, the disease process is advanced, and some type of salvage procedure is necessary. If the articular cartilage in the lunate fossa of the distal radius and the proximal pole of the capitate are both in acceptable condition, then a proximal row carpectomy can be performed. Because of the tenuous vascular supply of the lunate, there is usually degeneration in the lunate fossa, although occasionally the distal articular surface of the lunate remains serviceable. In these cases, a RSL fusion may preserve motion at the intercarpal joint. This is not common, however, and arthritic degeneration is usually so advanced throughout the carpus that there is no choice but to perform a panarthrodesis of the wrist. Although there is a total loss of wrist motion, the patient is usually quite happy because of the pain relief.

Magnetic Resonance Findings

Magnetic resonance findings in KD can also be grouped according to the stage of disease.[82]

Stage I

As mentioned, conventional radiographs are usually normal in stage I, although an associated fracture line or compression fracture may be present. At this early stage, radiographs are both sensitive and nonspecific for the diagnosis of KD. Bone scintigraphy may be helpful, but is poor in differentiating fractures, osteochondral lesions, erosions, and the spectrum of degenerative changes which present as subchondral sclerosis. Magnetic resonance offers comparable or greater sensitivity and improved specificity compared with that available in radiographs (Fig. 8–81). With MR, it is possible to characterize the extent of necrosis and the morphology of marrow involvement, as well as the overall morphology of the lunate cortical surfaces, including articular cartilage. Focal or diffuse low signal intensity is seen on T1-weighted images in affected areas of marrow involvement. Coronal plane images best display the largest anterior-to-posterior surface area of involvement. The addition of sagittal or axial images provides more accurate assessment of the volume of marrow involvement. On T2*-weighted images, the lunate demonstrates uniform low signal intensity. Normal lunate marrow or recovering marrow vascularity usually displays a central region of mildly increased signal intensity or inhomogeneity in gradient-echo images. Short TI inversion recovery sequences are more sensitive to hyperemia or vascular dilation and demonstrate increased signal intensity restricted to the lunate. In contrast, T2*-weighted images are likely to demonstrate faint vascular signal intensity from all carpal bones, especially the scaphoid and lunate in the noninjured carpus.

In early KD, T1-weighted images show unaffected marrow with the high signal intensity of fat, isointense with the other carpal bones of the wrist. The distribution of low signal intensity necrosis may be restricted to a portion of the volar or dorsal coronal plane or may demonstrate an eccentric or central region of involvement. Radiocarpal joint effusions or more localized synovitis demonstrate bright signal intensity on T2-weighted, T2*-weighted, and STIR sequences.

Interval MR imaging can be used to show the progression of KD or to document healing with the return of normal marrow signal intensity in stage I disease (see Fig. 8–81; Fig. 8–82). The relative osteopenia of the remaining carpus is not seen using MR techniques.

Stage II

In stage II, plain film radiographs show sclerosis of the lunate which demonstrates low signal intensity on T1-weighted MR images. Short TI inversion recovery images demonstrate areas of increased signal intensity in patients who show sclerosis in corresponding radiographs. Generally, although morphology and size are preserved, decreased height of the radial aspect of the lunate may be seen in late stage II disease (Fig. 8–83).

Stage III

The lunate undergoes distal-to-proximal collapse in the coronal plane and elongation in the sagittal plane in stage III KD (Fig. 8–84). There is reciprocal proximal migration of the capitate. The absence or presence of SL disassociation with rotatory subluxation of the scaphoid divides patients into stage IIIA and IIIB, respectively. Rotation of the scaphoid may be accompanied by ulnar deviation of the triquetrum. With scaphoid rotation, the inability to see the entire long axis of the scaphoid in a single coronal image is the MR equivalent of the radiographic "ring" sign in conventional anteroposterior radiographic projections.

Stage IV

Stage IV is characterized by degenerative arthrosis of the lunate and carpus. There are no regions of increased signal intensity on T2*-weighted or STIR images in this advanced stage of disease. Lunate collapse can be defined in all three orthogonal planes with MR imaging. With splaying of the volar and dorsal poles of the lunate there is extrinsic effacement and convex bowing of the flexor tendons in the sagittal plane. This may contribute to symptoms of carpal tunnel syndrome, especially if there is associated proximal migration of the flexor retinaculum with wrist shortening. Fragmented portions of the lunate are usually identified with low signal intensity on T1- and T2*-weighted images. Thin section (1.5-mm) CT scans provide more accurate assessment of cortical fragmentation. Kienböck's disease of the lunate has also been associated with Madelung's deformity, a developmental anomaly involving the distal radius and carpus (Fig. 8–85).

CARPAL TUNNEL SYNDROME

The impairment of motor and/or sensory function of the median nerve as it transgresses the carpal tunnel (*i.e.,* carpal tunnel syndrome) may be caused by fractures and dislocations about the wrist, by intraneural hemorrhage, by infection, by infiltrative disease, and by various soft-tissue injuries. Carpal tunnel syndrome is most often found in patients between 30 and 60 years of age; it has a female-to-male ratio of between 3 to 5:1; and up to 50% of cases are bilateral.[95] The clinical presentation includes pain and numbness with increased nocturnal pain and/or burning. There is anesthesia in the thumb, index, and middle fingers and in the radial one-half of the ring finger. Sensory findings range from minimal hyperesthesia to complete anesthesia. Muscle atrophy and loss of function are late findings, although the abductor pollicis brevis muscle may show earlier involvement. A positive Tinel's sign (*i.e.,* tingling in the digits supplied by the median nerve), indicates nerve entrapment. Phalen's test, tourniquet compression, or direct compression can also be used to elicit signs of median nerve entrapment. A prolonged sensory conduction or distal motor latency test provide more quantitative information. Electrodiagnostic tests in patients with carpal tunnel syndrome are reported to be 85% to 90% accurate, with a false-negative rate of 10% to 15%.

Anatomy

An understanding of the anatomy of the carpal tunnel is important in understanding the pathophysiology of this syndrome. The carpus has a concave, bony contour on its flexor surface and is covered by the flexor retinaculum. The bony carpus thus forms the floor and walls of the carpal tunnel, with the rigid flexor retinaculum representing its roof. The flexor retinaculum, or transverse carpal ligament, attaches to the tubercle of the scaphoid and ridge of the trapezium and to the ulnar aspect of the hook of the hamate and pisiform. The long flexors of the fingers and thumb pass through the carpal tunnel. The separate flexor digitorum superficialis tendons are arranged in two separate rows, with the middle and ring finger volar to the index and little finger. The flexor digitorum profundus tendons are arranged in the same coronal plane; the tendon to the index finger is separated from the adjacent three profundus tendons. All eight flexor tendons are invested in a common synovial sheath. The flexor pollicis longus tendon, invested in its own synovial sheath, is located on the radial aspect of the flexor tendons within the carpal tunnel. The median nerve is deep to the flexor retinaculum and is seen on the lateral side of the flexor digitorum superficialis between the flexor tendon of the middle finger and the flexor carpi radialis. The proximal fibers of the volar carpal ligament contribute to the roof of the carpal tunnel. This contribution is not as significant as that of the thicker flexor retinaculum.

In dorsiflexion and palmarflexion of the wrist, the median nerve is forced against the transverse carpal ligament. This is compounded by friction forces between the median nerve tendons and the transverse carpal ligament during flexion and extension, with up to 20-mm excursion of the median nerve.

The median nerve is round or oval at the level of the distal radius; it becomes elliptical in shape at the pisiform and hamate. The position and morphology of the median nerve are altered during flexion and extension. With the wrist in a neutral position, the median nerve is seen anterior to the flexor digitorum superficialis tendon of the index finger or posterolaterally between the flexor digitorum tendon of the index finger and the flexor pollicis longus tendon. In wrist extension, the median nerve assumes a more anterior position, deep to the flexor retinaculum and superficial to the flexor digitorum superficialis tendon of the index finger. In wrist flexion, the median nerve can be found anterior to the flexor retinaculum or between the flexor digitorum superficialis tendons of the index finger and thumb or middle and ring fingers. In the flexed position, there is flattening of the elliptical shape of the median nerve. Alteration of morphology is less significant in wrist extension.

Etiology

In carpal tunnel syndrome, wick catheter measurements show increased pressures in the carpal canal (*i.e.,* 32 mmHg compared with 2.5 mmHg in asymptomatic patients).[95] Pressure changes may also be recorded in extremes of dorsiflexion and palmarflexion. Computed tomography studies of patients with carpal tunnel syndrome show a decreased cross-sectional area of the carpal canal. Processes that can cause decreased volume or space within the carpal canal include tenosynovitis of the flexor tendons, Colles' fracture, and fracture–dislocation of the carpal bone and carpometacarpal joints. These processes may also cause post-traumatic scarring, fibrosis, or both within the carpal tunnel. Inflammatory processes contributing to decreased volume within the carpal tunnel include rheumatoid arthritis, gout, pseudogout, amyloid deposition, and granulomatous infectious processes. All of these can produce a proliferative tenosynovitis with hyperplastic synovium. Tumors of the median nerve (*e.g.,* neurilemomas, fibromas, hematomas) as well as tumors extrinsic to the median nerve (*e.g.,* ganglia, lipomas, hemangiomas) produce space-occupying encroachment of the carpal canal.[95] Disorders that produce a volumetric increase within the carpal tunnel include acromegaly, hypothyroidism, pregnancy, the postmenopausal condition, diabetes mellitus, and lupus erythematosus. These systemic processes may increase extracapsular fluid retention and produce soft-tissue swelling. Developmental etiologies responsible for carpal tunnel syndrome include a persistent median artery, hypertrophied lumbricals, anomalous muscles, and a distal position of the flexor digitorum superficialis muscle.

Carpal tunnel syndrome can thus be produced by compression or swelling of the median nerve in synovial sheaths. In the differential diagnosis of carpal tunnel syndrome, it is important to exclude median nerve damage at a more proximal level. In the case of median nerve damage, the palmocutaneous branch of the median nerve may be affected by weakness of the corresponding flexor muscles of the forearm, including the flexor pollicis longus tendon. This is in contrast with carpal tunnel syndrome, in which the terminal phalanx of the thumb demonstrates normal flexion without motor impairment. Although the median nerve is composed of both sensory and motor nerve fibers, the sensory fibers predominate at the level of the carpal tunnel, explaining the initial findings of sensory deficit with numbness or paresthesias of the thumb, index finger, and middle one-half ring finger. As the disease progresses, there is wasting and weakness of the thenar muscles, with decreased opposition of the thumb, and anesthesia of the three and one-half digits on the thumb or radial side of the hand. There is no anesthesia of the thenar eminence, which is supplied by the cutaneous branch of the median nerve.

Treatment

Initial treatment of carpal tunnel syndrome is conservative and includes splints, NSAIDs, corticosteroids, or a combination of these.[95] Patients who receive the greatest short-term relief with corticosteroid injections have better results with surgical decompression.

Surgical decompression is recommended when there is progressive sensory loss and muscle atrophy plus weakness. The flexor retinaculum, or transverse carpal ligament, is usually divided on its ulnar aspect with complete release. This release may extend proximally into the volar carpal ligament, with an epineurotomy for thickened or scarred epineurium. Surgical treatment of carpal tunnel syndrome may be complicated by reflex sympathetic dystrophy, scar formation, damage to the branches of the median ulnar nerve, tenosynovitis, flexor tendon adhesions, or bow-stringing of the tendons.

Magnetic Resonance Findings

The ability to display the cross-sectional anatomy of the median nerve and adjacent structures on axial MR images and to trace the flexor tendons on coronal plane images makes MR valuable in characterizing normal anatomy and

pathology in the carpal tunnel.[96-100] Early detection of the cause of carpal tunnel syndrome requires soft-tissue discrimination not possible with standard radiographs or CT. Axial and coronal MR imaging of the wrist have shown potential for evaluating patients with a clinical presentation of median nerve deficits.

Axial MR images demonstrate bowing of the flexor retinaculum in patients with flexor tenosynovitis, and inflamed synovium and tendon sheaths demonstrate low signal intensity on T1-weighted images and increased signal intensity on T2-weighted, T2*-weighted, and STIR sequences (Fig. 8–86).

Changes in the median nerve are present regardless of the etiology of carpal tunnel syndrome (Fig. 8–87).[98] These findings include the following:

Diffuse swelling or segmental enlargement of the median nerve, best evaluated at the level of the pisiform
Flattening of the median nerve, best demonstrated at the level of the hamate
Palmar bowing of the flexor retinaculum, assessed at the level of the hamate[99]
Increased signal intensity within the median nerve on T2-weighted images (Figs. 8–88 and 8–89).

Comparison with the contralateral wrist may be misleading, because involvement is bilateral in one-half to two-thirds of patients with carpal tunnel syndrome.

Alterations in median nerve signal intensity are nonspecific, and may represent edema or demyelination within neural fibers. Signal intensity may be decreased when fibrosis is the primary median nerve pathology. Compression and flattening of the median nerve may be demonstrated at the level of the hamate along with bowing of the flexor retinaculum. Ratios of swelling can be calculated by dividing the cross-sectional area of the median nerve at the level of the pisiform and the hamate by the cross-sectional area of the median nerve at the level of the distal radius.[97,98] Significant differences, with doubling of ratios of swelling, have been shown in patients with carpal tunnel syndrome, despite the subjective flattening of the median nerve at the lateral and distal carpus. Ratios of flattening have been used to document statistically significant flattening of the median nerve at the level of the hamate.[98,99] The median nerve may display enlargement or dilation at the level of the pisiform, and compression with flattening at the level of the hook of the hamate.

Increased signal intensity of the median nerve, best demonstrated on gradient-echo axial or STIR images, may be accompanied by an increase in its cross-sectional diameter. Degenerative arthritis and instabilities in advanced arthrosis may cause a decrease in cross-sectional area of the carpal tunnel and produce symptoms of carpal tunnel disease. Attempts to use MR to measure the diameter of the median nerve, however, require further study. Magnetic resonance is most useful in characterizing space-occupying lesions, whether tenosynovitis, ganglia, lipomas, or granulomatous infections (Fig. 8–90).

Enlargement or swelling of the median nerve proximal to the carpal tunnel, referred to as a pseudoneuroma, has also been documented with MR. This condition may actually be associated with constriction of the median nerve within the carpal tunnel, distal to the point of swelling.

Chronic induration after transverse carpal ligament release is seen on MR scans as an area of neural constriction. Residual hyperintensity of the median nerve within the carpal tunnel may be identified with incomplete release of the flexor retinaculum (Fig. 8–91). Release of the transverse carpal ligament from the hook of the hamate may cause the flexor tendons or contents of the carpal canal to demonstrate a greater volar convexity because of the loss of the normal roof support of the flexor retinaculum. Widening of the fat stripe is normally seen posterior to the flexor digitorum profundus tendons postoperatively. In addition to incomplete release of the flexor retinaculum, MR changes in failed postoperative carpal tunnel surgery include excessive fat within the carpal tunnel, neuromas, and persistent neuritis.

ARTHRITIS

Conventional radiography has been the cornerstone of evaluation and follow-up of arthritides involving the hand, wrist, and elbow. The superior soft-tissue discrimination achieved by MR imaging, however, has proven useful in evaluating patients in both the initial and advanced stages of arthritis. Magnetic resonance imaging achieves noninvasive, accurate delineation of hyaline articular cartilage, ligaments, tendons, and synovium as distinct from cortical bone (Fig. 8–92).[101–103] Alterations in joint morphology or structure can be identified with MR studies before changes can be seen in standard radiographs. Although MR should neither replace radiography nor be used in every patient receiving rheumatologic evaluation, it can, in selected cases, offer specific information that may modify the patient's diagnosis or treatment.

Degenerative Arthritis

Joint-space narrowing, loss of articular cartilage, subchondral sclerosis, and cyst formation characterize degenerative patterns of the carpus (Fig. 8–93). The SLAC wrist develops from incongruent loading and degeneration across the radioscaphoid articulation, related to malalignment of the scaphoid.[104] The SLAC wrist represents the most common form of degenerative arthritis, and is associated with the gradual collapse and loss of ligamentous support. Scapholunate advanced collapse degeneration may occur with carpal collapse, including that caused by scaphoid nonunion and KD. The earliest

changes seen in the SLAC wrist involve spiking at the junction of the articular and nonarticular surfaces on the radial side of the scaphoid, sharpening at the radial styloid tip, and loss of cartilage. Early cartilage loss can be seen clearly on MR scans, and the low signal intensity initial changes in subchondral sclerosis of the radial styloid appear on MR images prior to any visible changes in conventional radiographs (Fig. 8–94). Later in the disease, there is narrowing of the radioscaphoid joint, and the capitolunate joint begins to degenerate. Once the articular space between the capitate and lunate is lost, the hamate impinges against the lunate and degeneration also occurs at this site.

Triscaphe arthritis is the second most frequent form of degenerative arthritis and involves the scaphoid, trapezium and trapezoid articulation.[104] Isolated scaphotrapezial involvement is more common than isolated scaphotrapezoidal involvement. A SLAC wrist may occur in combination with triscaphe degenerative arthritis. Other locations of degenerative arthritis include degeneration between the distal ulna and the lunate, and the LT joints.[104]

Rheumatoid Arthritis

Small joint involvement of the wrist in rheumatoid arthritis characteristically involves the carpus and the MP and PIP joints.[105] Soft-tissue swelling includes joint effusion, edema, and tenosynovitis (Fig. 8–95). Swan-neck and boutonniere deformities are frequent, and, in advanced disease, there are subluxations, dislocations, ulnar deviation in the MP joints, and radial deviation in the radiocarpal articulation. Destructive changes include "main en lorgnette" (*i.e.,* telescoping of the fingers), ulnar erosions, and SL dissociation.

Gadolinium contrast has been used in MR imaging to selectively enhance pannus tissue in synovitis involving the DRUJ; the ulnar styloid process; the radiocarpal, intercarpal, and MP joints; and the flexor and extensor tendons. Synovial involvement of ligamentous structures frequently affects the ulnolunate and ulnotriquetral ligaments, TFCC, radial and ulnar joint ulnocarpal meniscal homologue, ulnar collateral ligament, RSC ligament, RSL, LRL, and SRL.[106] The differential diagnosis of rupture of the extensor tendon at the wrist includes MP synovitis, posterior interosseous nerve palsy from rheumatoid disease of the elbow, and extensor tendon pathology overlying the metacarpal heads. With MR, it is possible to identify rupture of the extensor pollicis longus tendon, which may be difficult to assess clinically if the function of the thumb is intact.[106] Triangular fibrocartilage tears, dorsal displacement of the ulna, carpal tunnel pathology, and SL dissociation are also assessed on routine coronal, axial, and sagittal studies (Fig. 8–96).

(text continues on page 788)

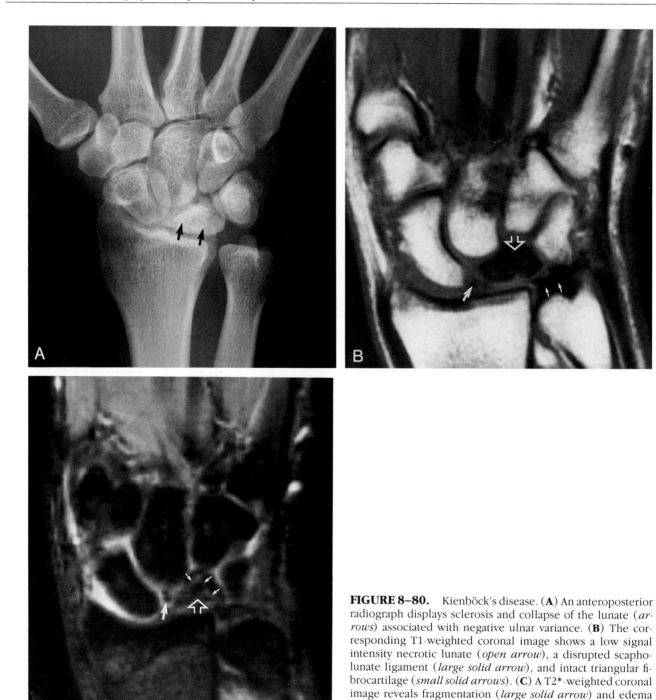

FIGURE 8–80. Kienböck's disease. (**A**) An anteroposterior radiograph displays sclerosis and collapse of the lunate (*arrows*) associated with negative ulnar variance. (**B**) The corresponding T1-weighted coronal image shows a low signal intensity necrotic lunate (*open arrow*), a disrupted scapholunate ligament (*large solid arrow*), and intact triangular fibrocartilage (*small solid arrows*). (**C**) A T2*-weighted coronal image reveals fragmentation (*large solid arrow*) and edema (*small solid arrows*) associated with a necrotic lunate (*open arrow*).

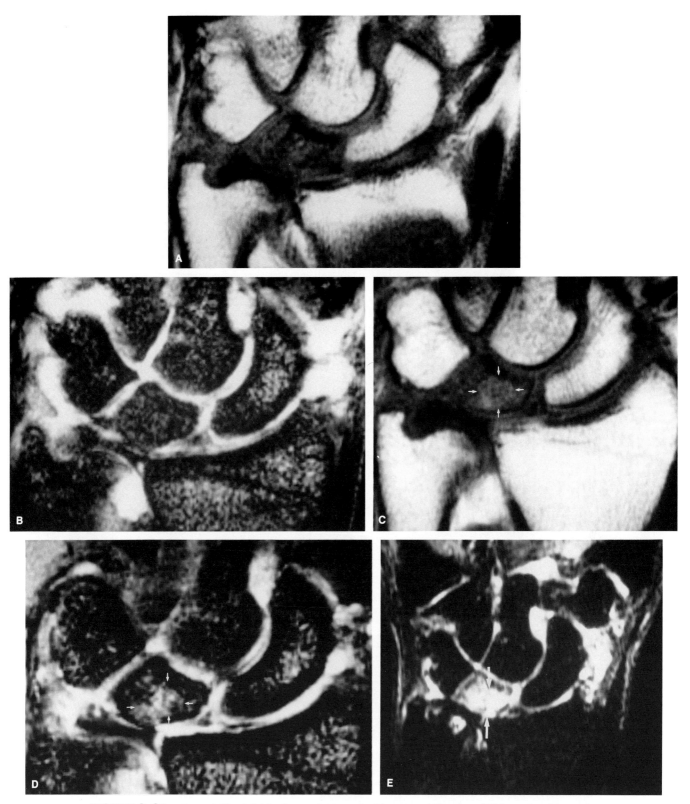

FIGURE 8–81. Stage 1 Kienböck's disease is treated with cast mobilization. (**A**) Low signal intensity replacement of lunate fat marrow is seen on a T1-weighted coronal image. (**B**) Uniform low signal intensity lunate marrow is present on the corresponding T2*-weighted coronal image. (**C**) Six months after the initial diagnosis, central fat marrow signal intensity (*arrows*) is seen on a T1-weighted coronal image. The corresponding (**D**) T2*-weighted and (**E**) short TI inversion recovery (STIR) images show lunate hyperintensity (*arrows*). The STIR image is more sensitive to marrow hyperemia.

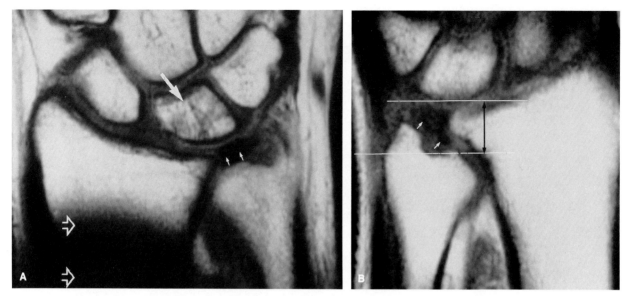

FIGURE 8–82. (**A**) Recovering fat marrow signal intensity (*large arrow*) is present after treatment of stage I Kienböck's disease of the right wrist. The lunate and triangular fibrocartilage (*small arrows*) are normal. A low signal intensity postoperative artifact secondary to radial shortening is present (*open arrows*). (**B**) The untreated left wrist shows severe negative ulnar variance (*black, double-headed arrow*) and deformed but intact triangular fibrocartilage (*white arrows*). The lunate marrow is unaffected.

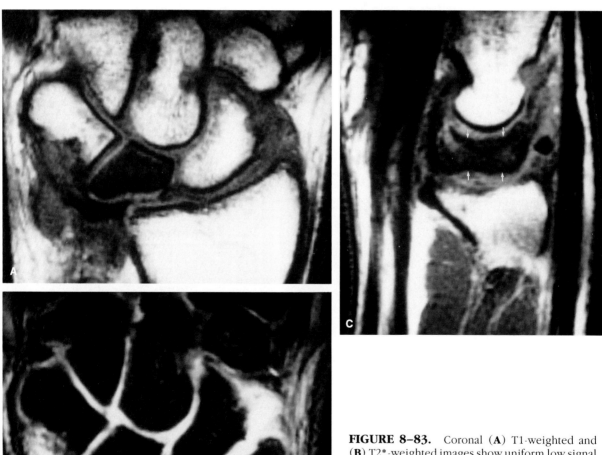

FIGURE 8–83. Coronal (**A**) T1-weighted and (**B**) T2*-weighted images show uniform low signal intensity lunate marrow in stage II Kienböck's disease. Associated negative ulnar variance is present, but no proximal migration of the capitate has occurred. (**C**) A T1-weighted sagittal image shows a mild loss of lunate height (*arrows*) and elongation of the lunate that were not revealed in corresponding coronal images. Abnormal morphology of the dorsal radiocarpal ligament is present.

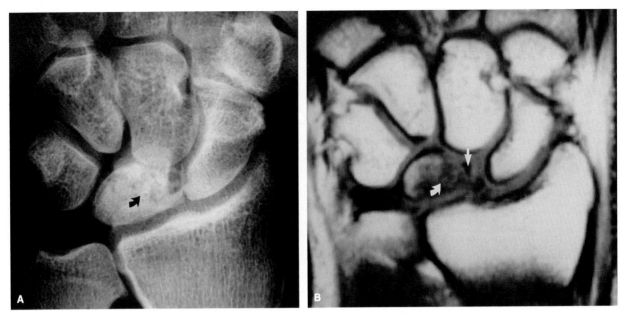

FIGURE 8–84. (**A**) An anteroposterior radiograph shows lunate collapse (*curved arrow*) and proximal migration of the capitate in stage III Kienböck's disease. (**B**) A T1-weighted coronal image better depicts necrotic marrow (*curved arrow*) and lunate collapse in the radial border (*straight arrow*).

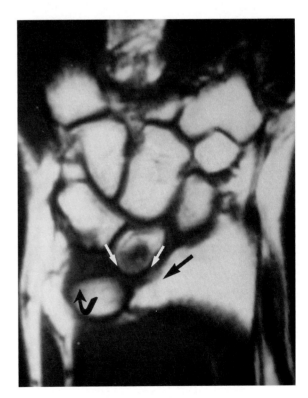

FIGURE 8–85. A T1-weighted coronal image shows medial angulation of the distal radial articular surface (*straight black arrow*), dorsal subluxation of the ulna (*curved black arrow*), and triangular configuration of the carpus with the lunate at the apex (*white arrows*), all of which constitute Madelung's deformity. Associated Kienböck's disease is shown as central low signal intensity marrow.

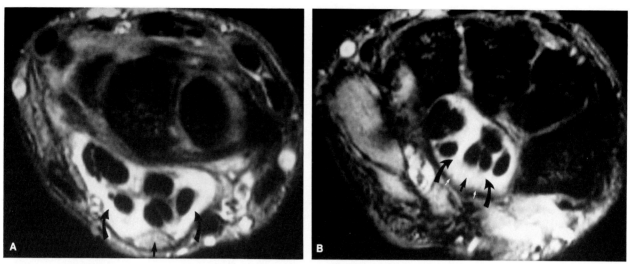

FIGURE 8–86. In carpal tunnel syndrome, T2*-weighted axial images show (**A**) severe, high signal intensity flexor tenosynovitis (*curved arrows*), swelling of the median nerve proximal to the carpal tunnel (*straight arrow*), and (**B**) hyperintense synovitis (*curved black arrow*) and median nerve (*straight black arrow*). The flexor retinaculum is bowed (*white arrows*).

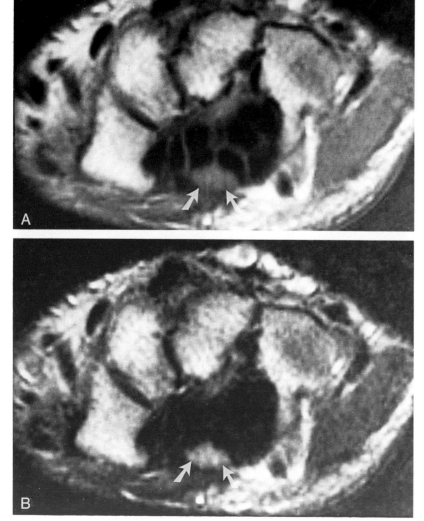

FIGURE 8–87. In carpal tunnel syndrome, an enlarged and edematous median nerve (*arrows*) demonstrates (**A**) intermediate signal intensity on intermediate-weighted images and (**B**) high signal intensity on T2-weighted images.

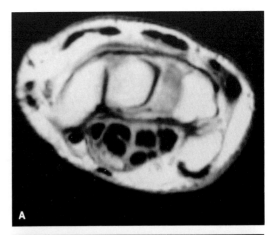

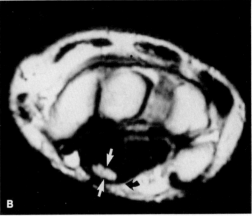

FIGURE 8–88. Carpal tunnel syndrome shown at the level of the pisiform on axial (**A**) intermediate-weighted and (**B**) T2-weighted images. On the T2-weighted image, the median nerve is hyperintense (*straight white arrows*) and the flexor retinaculum is bowed (*curved black arrow*).

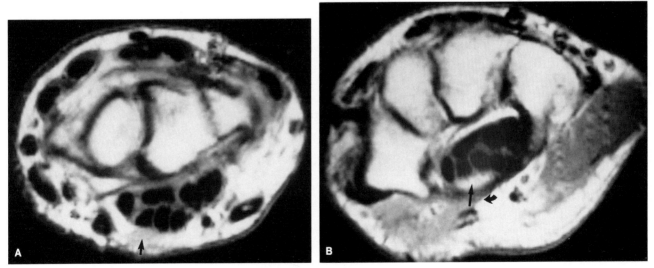

FIGURE 8–89. Carpal tunnel syndrome as seen on intermediate-weighted axial images. (**A**) Proximal to the carpal tunnel, the median nerve demonstrates intermediate signal intensity (*arrow*). (**B**) At the level of the hamate, the median nerve demonstrates high signal intensity (*straight arrow*). Convex bowing of the flexor retinaculum (*curved arrow*) and mild flexor tendon tenosynovitis are also present.

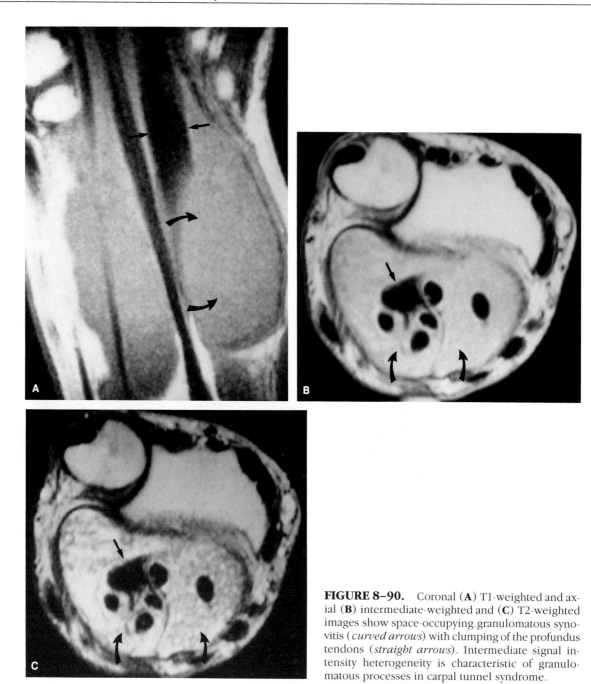

FIGURE 8–90. Coronal (**A**) T1-weighted and axial (**B**) intermediate-weighted and (**C**) T2-weighted images show space-occupying granulomatous synovitis (*curved arrows*) with clumping of the profundus tendons (*straight arrows*). Intermediate signal intensity heterogeneity is characteristic of granulomatous processes in carpal tunnel syndrome.

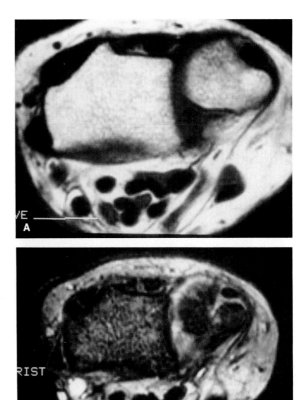

FIGURE 8–91. (A) A T1-weighted image shows the wrist after flexor retinaculum release. (B) Persistent hyperintensity of median nerve proximal to carpal tunnel is seen after flexor retinaculum release on a T2*-weighted axial image.

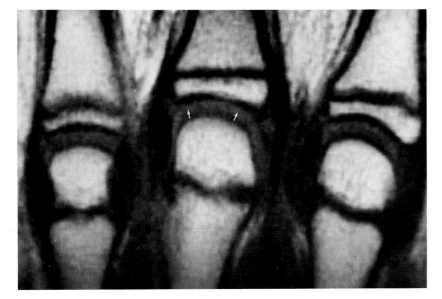

FIGURE 8–92. A T1-weighted coronal image shows the intermediate signal intensity of normal-thickness metacarpophalangeal joint hyaline articular cartilage (*arrows*).

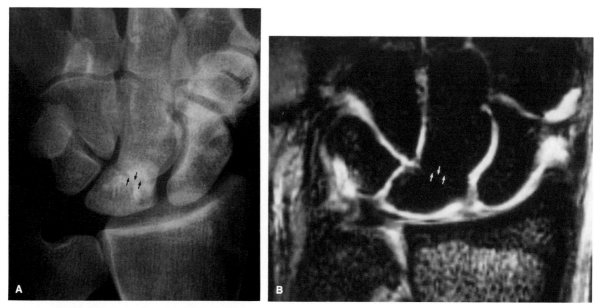

FIGURE 8–93. (**A**) An anteroposterior radiograph and (**B**) a T2*-weighted coronal image show degenerative changes at the capitolunate joint including loss of joint space (*arrows*) and hyaline articular cartilage.

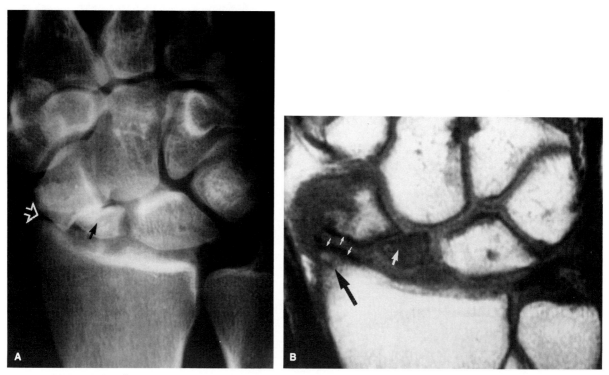

FIGURE 8–94. Scapholunate advanced collapse (SLAC) wrist. (**A**) An anteroposterior radiograph shows nonunion of a scaphoid fracture with degenerative joint-space narrowing between the distal pole of the scaphoid and radius (*open arrow*). Sclerosis is present in avascular necrosis (AVN) of the proximal pole (*solid arrow*). Coronal (**B**) T1-weighted and (**C**) T2*-weighted images of SLAC wrist reveal degeneration at the radioscaphoid joint (*open arrow*) and subchondral low signal intensity sclerosis in the radiostyloscaphoid area. Denuded articular cartilage (*small white arrows*) extends proximally only to the level of the nonunion. The proximal pole of the scaphoid functions as a second lunate with preserved articular cartilage. (**B**) Note the low signal intensity "corner sign" of the radial styloid, which is characteristic of early SLAC degeneration (*large black arrow*). AVN of the proximal pole is indicated (*large white arrow*). Increased loading of the capitolunate joint is associated with loss of radioscaphoid cartilage.

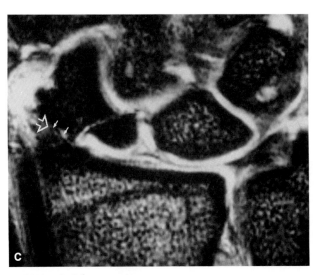

FIGURE 8–94. *(Continued)*

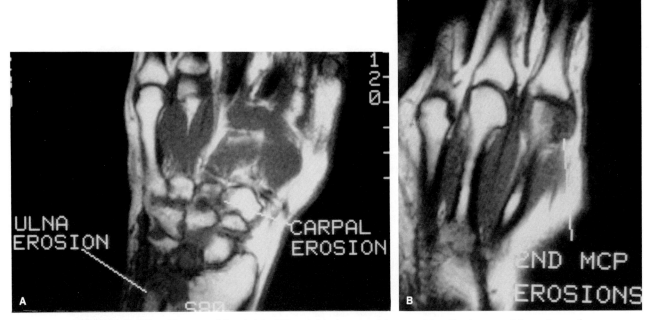

FIGURE 8–95. Rheumatoid arthritis. T1-weighted coronal images identify rheumatoid erosions of (**A**) the ulnar styloid and carpus and (**B**) the 2nd metacarpal. (**C, D**) The corresponding 3D MR renderings map out pannus formation (pink) and inferior distal radioulnar joint effusion (blue). The interosseous muscles are shown between the metacarpal bones. (**E**) Unenhanced and (**F**) enhanced T1-weighted coronal images in a different patient demonstrate the application of intravenous gadolinium used to selectively enhance and differentiate pannus from fluid in a patient with severe radiocarpal disease. (F, low signal intensity fluid; S, enhanced hyperintense synovium.) *(continued)*

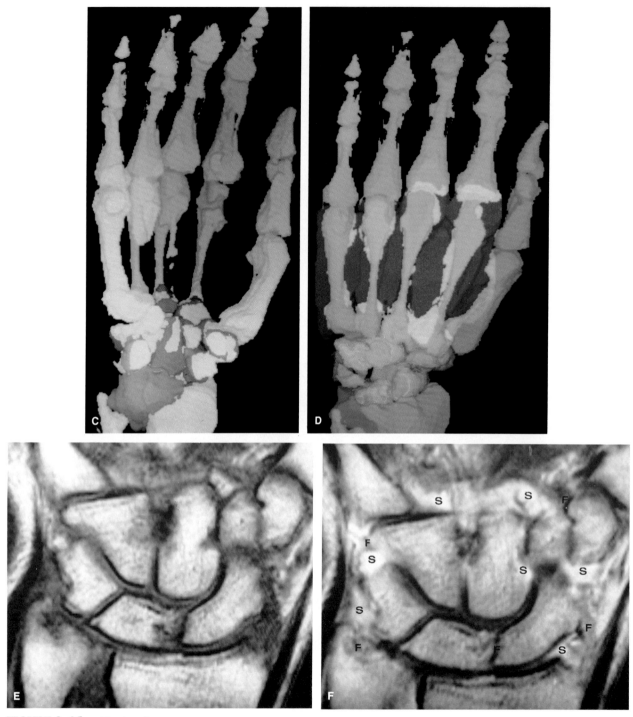

FIGURE 8–95. *(Continued)*

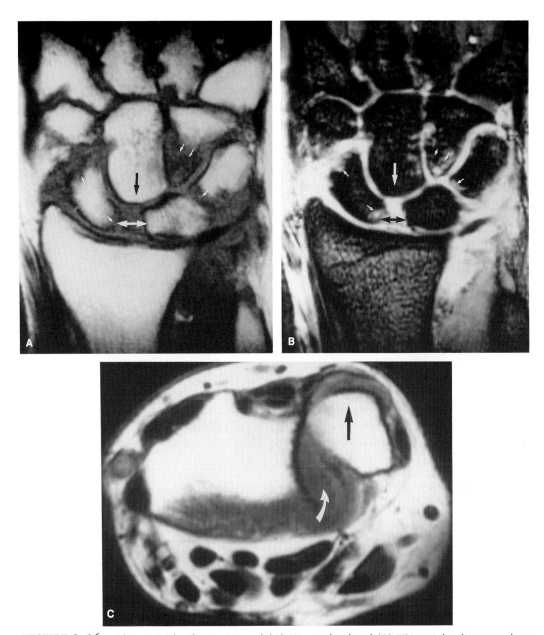

FIGURE 8–96. Rheumatoid arthritis. Coronal (**A**) T1-weighted and (**B**) T2*-weighted images show rheumatoid changes of scapholunate dissociation (*double headed arrows*), proximal migration of the capitate (*large single arrow*), and multiple erosions involving the scaphoid, triquetrum, and hamate (*small white arrows*). Erosions of the intermetacarpal joints are also present. Note that the carpus has begun to migrate toward the ulna, and the distance between the radial styloid and the scaphoid is increased. (**C**) An axial T1-weighted image shows dorsal subluxation of the ulna (*straight arrow*) and distal radioulnar joint effusion and pannus (*curved arrow*).

In patients with chronic rheumatoid disease, both plain film radiography and MR studies document the subluxations and erosions affecting the phalanges, carpals, metacarpals, and ulnar styloid (Fig. 8–97). The changes are more pronounced on MR images. Both T1 and T2 tissue relaxation times are prolonged in acute inflammation with edema and in joint effusion; therefore, both conditions demonstrate low signal intensity on T1-weighted images and high signal intensity on T2-weighted images. Inflammatory edema may also extend into the subcutaneous tissues. In contrast, chronically inflamed tissue remains low in signal intensity on both T1- and T2-weighted images. In more advanced rheumatoid disease, pannus formation can be identified and demonstrates low to intermediate signal intensity on both T1- and T2-weighted images. Adjacent areas of fluid collection demonstrate increased signal intensity on T2-weighted acquisitions. Although the signal intensity of localized edematous or inflammatory tissue may be similar to that of synovial fluid, noninflammatory effusions in the wrist do not, when imaged on T2-weighted sequences, display an irregular pattern or focal distribution at multiple sites.

Cystic carpal erosions are better delineated on MR images than on corresponding anteroposterior radiographs. In a series of four patients with rheumatoid arthritis with wrist involvement, destruction of cartilage and joint arthrosis were distinctly seen on T1-weighted images. Marrow changes (*e.g.,* subchondral sclerosis), present on both sides of the joint or carpal articulation, helped to differentiate arthrosis from intramedullary edema.

In patients with juvenile rheumatoid arthritis with wrist involvement, early fluid collections along tendon sheaths, subarticular erosions, and cysts, as well as attenuated intercarpal articular cartilage, were detected on MR images but were not revealed on conventional radiographs. Subluxations and areas of bone destruction were equally evident on both MR images and on plain film radiographs.

Magnetic resonance has the potential to become an important adjunct in diagnosing and monitoring patients with rheumatoid disease. Further studies with larger patient populations and comparisons with conventional radiographic studies are required before standard indications can be implemented in rheumatoid patients. Magnetic resonance may also prove to be valuable in monitoring a patient's response to drug therapy, including remitative agents such as methotrexate or gold in juvenile and adult rheumatoid disease.

Miscellaneous Arthritides

In evaluating nonrheumatoid arthritic disease, we have had the opportunity to evaluate patients with psoriatic arthritis, Lyme disease, intraosseous sarcoid, hemophilia, calcium pyrophosphate deposition disease, and the more commonly found osteoarthritis (Fig. 8–98).

Magnetic resonance studies in psoriatic arthritis demonstrate destruction of the TFC with pancompartmental joint-space narrowing, erosions, SL ligament disruption, and subchondral low signal intensity sclerosis in the carpus (Fig. 8–99). Synovitis of the flexor carpi radialis tendon, the inferior radioulnar compartment, intermediate signal intensity inflammatory tissue, and dorsal subluxation of the distal ulna can be identified on T1- and T2-weighted axial images. The integrity of an artificial silastic interphalangeal joint replacement can be assessed on coronal images and is seen as an area of low signal intensity without artifact. The site of fusion of the interphalangeal articulation of the thumb may be degraded by residual metallic artifact, despite prior surgical removal of fixation pins. In diffuse soft-tissue swelling of a single digit secondary to psoriatic arthritis MR may be successful in excluding the diagnosis of osteomyelitis (Fig. 8–100).

Magnetic resonance studies of Lyme arthritis of the wrist reveal information not available on conventional radiographs. Pockets of fluid collection, characterized by high signal intensity on T2-weighted images, can be detected, and a scalloped contour of fluid interface can be demonstrated adjacent to inflamed synovium (Fig. 8–101). Joint deformities or cartilaginous erosions are not usually detected.

The hand is a predominant site of involvement in patients who have the relatively rare disorder of skeletal sarcoidosis. In one case studied, conventional radiographs demonstrated lytic changes characteristic of sarcoid in both the middle and distal phalanges. Although MR images did not provide any additional diagnostic formation, the extent of soft-tissue granulomatous proliferation in the cystic defects and areas of cortical destruction were more accurately demonstrated on coronal and axial MR images (Figs. 8–102 and 8–103). The noncaseating, granulomatous tissue typical of sarcoidosis demonstrates low to intermediate signal intensity on T1-weighted sequences and high signal intensity on T2-weighted images.

In hemophilia, acute hemorrhage into the soft tissue may be seen with a fluid–fluid level. Higher signal intensity serum will layer above hemorrhagic sediment. More subacute or chronic hemorrhage demonstrates hemosiderin (*i.e.,* dark) signal intensity on T1-, T2-, or T2*-weighted images.

We have studied one patient with calcium pyrophosphate deposition disease. On T1-weighted images, areas of intraarticular calcification were not satisfactorily demonstrated when compared with high-quality magnification radiographs. T2 and T2* weighting and photography at high contrast settings may prove useful in identifying areas of calcified crystalline depositions. Subchondral carpal sclerosis, erosions, and intraosseous cysts are better characterized on MR images than conventional radiographs (Fig. 8–104). Thin (1.5-mm) section CT scans show greater detail of the peripheral outline of the cystic bony involvement (Fig. 8–105).

OTHER ABNORMALITIES OF THE SYNOVIUM

In addition to changes seen in arthritis, other abnormalities of the synovium, such as synovial cysts, ganglia, tenosynovitis, and capsular synovitis, have been characterized on MR images of the hand, wrist, and elbow.

Ganglions

Cystic swellings overlying a joint or tendon sheath are referred to as ganglions, and are thought to be secondary to protrusions of synovial tissue (Fig. 8–106).[107–109] On MR images, ganglions generate uniform low signal intensity on T1-weighted images and high signal intensity on T2-weighted images. Fibrous septations may cause loculation of the ganglion. Even with infiltration or edema of adjacent tissues, these lesions are well demarcated on MR. Intercarpal communication of a ganglion is more frequent than communication with the radiocarpal joint.

Magnetic resonance is used to identify the joint or tendon of origin and to exclude other soft-tissue masses, such as neoplasms, when an accurate preoperative clinical assessment is difficult and wrist arthrography is not satisfactory (Figs. 8–107 through 8–109). Wrist ganglions may be associated with the flexor tendon and the dorsal joint or extensor surface (Fig. 8–110). The neck or tail of the ganglion frequently can be discerned on MR images.

Pigmented villonodular synovitis of the tendon (*i.e.,* giant cell tumor of the tendon sheath) presents as an extraarticular soft-tissue swelling which may be mistaken for a ganglion. Low to intermediate signal intensity on T1- and T2-weighted images is characteristic (Fig. 8–111).

Tenosynovitis and Capsular Effusion

Tenosynovitis and capsular synovitis may occur together as part of the spectrum of rheumatoid disease, or they may exist as isolated conditions with a traumatic or infectious etiology (Figs. 8–112 and 8–113). Thickening, swelling, or fluid associated with an irritated synovial tendon sheath may be demonstrated on MR images. An edematous sheath appears as a rim of increased signal intensity on T2-weighted images. Both flexion and extensor tenosynovitis may occur without a history of infection. Carpal distention may be evident in the small

interphalangeal or metacarpal joints when small amounts of synovial fluid accumulate.

PATHOLOGY OF THE FINGER

Ligament Pathology

Ligamentous injuries of the fingers and thumb include disruptions of the collateral ligaments frequently involving the MP and PIP joints.[108] The PIP joint is a relatively rigid hinge joint and is therefore susceptible to injury through transmission of lateral and torque stress. Volar plate injuries, which are caused by hyperextension, may result in hyperextension or flexion deformities of the joint. Initial treatment for these injuries is short-term splinting in 25° to 30° of flexion.

Ulnar Collateral Ligament Tears of the Thumb

Ulnar collateral ligament tears, sometimes called gamekeeper's thumb, involves disruption of the ulnar collateral ligament of the first MP joint and is frequently associated with a proximal phalanx base fracture.[108] This injury may produce instability with abduction stress and is commonly seen in ski-pole, football, hockey, wrestling, and baseball injuries. Ulnar collateral ligament pathology involves a partial tear, usually at its distal attachment to the proximal phalanx. Complete ulnar collateral ligament tears result in MP joint instability, with 20° greater laxity than the contralateral thumb. T1-, T2-, or T2*-weighted coronal MR images demonstrate edema, thickening, disruption, displacement, or entrapment of the ulnar collateral ligament (Fig. 8–114).[109] The thumb should be positioned so that the radial collateral ligament is included in the imaging plane. The adductor pollicis aponeurosis may be interposed between the disrupted portions of the ulnar collateral ligament; therefore, surgical repair is indicated.

Tendon Injuries

Magnetic resonance imaging has been used to identify the anatomy, site, and specific flexor tendon involved in primary tendon tears or postsurgical retears (Figs. 8–115 through 8–119). The differential diagnosis of tendon injury includes motor nerve injuries, which impair active motion but in which the viscoelastic muscle tendon unit remains intact; extensor tendon injuries; flexor extensor tenosynovitis; and rupture. These conditions, which are often clinically difficult to diagnose on clinical examination, can be evaluated and examined for subluxation,

(text continues on page 805)

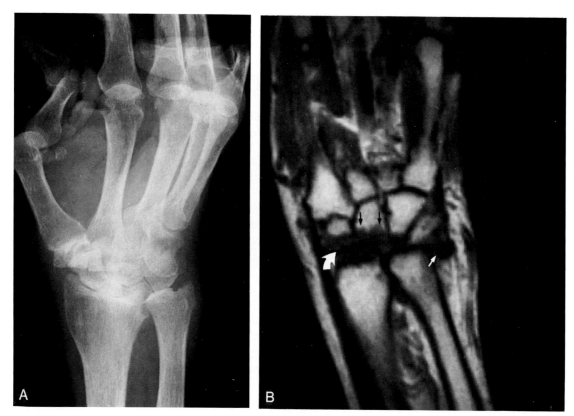

FIGURE 8–97. (**A**) An anteroposterior radiograph of the hand of an adult with rheumatoid arthritis demonstrates carpal erosions, collapse, subluxation, and marginal erosion changes. (**B**) The corresponding T1-weighted coronal image identifies capitate erosion (*small black arrows*), low signal intensity fluid and pannus at the ulnar styloid (*small white arrow*), and radiocarpal compartment (*curved arrow*). The scaphoid and lunate are difficult to identify because they also demonstrate low signal intensity.

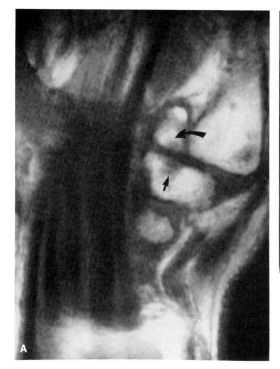

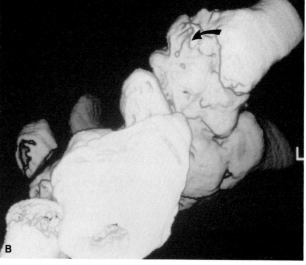

FIGURE 8–98. (**A**) T1-weighted coronal image and (**B**) 3D CT image illustrate degenerative osteophytosis of the 1st carpal metacarpal joint (*curved arrow*) in a patient with osteoarthritis. Low signal intensity subchondral sclerosis of the trapezium is indicated (*straight arrow*).

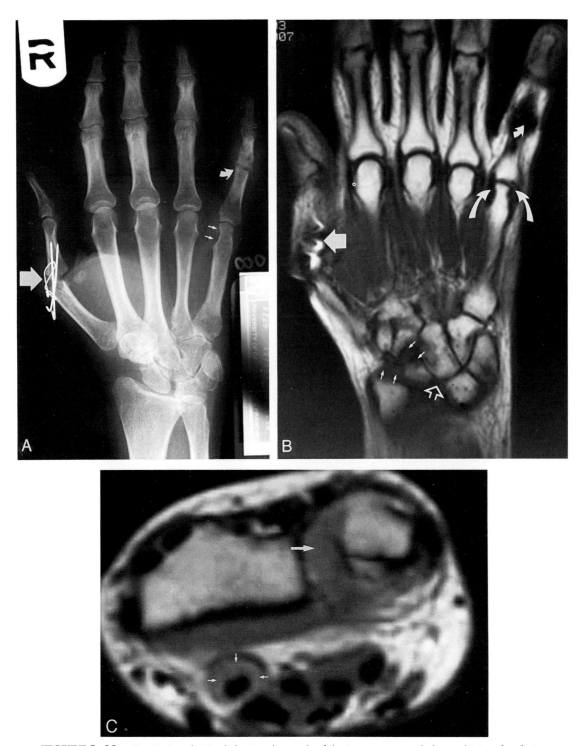

FIGURE 8–99. Psoriatic arthritis. (**A**) AP radiograph of the 1st metacarpophalangeal joint after fusion for subluxation (*large straight arrow*). Erosion of the 5th metacarpal head (*small straight arrows*) and a proximal interphalangeal joint silastic implant (*curved arrow*) are shown. Diffuse carpal joint-space narrowing is evident. (**B**) The corresponding T1-weighted coronal image shows a 1st metacarpophalangeal metallic artifact (*large straight solid arrow*), a low signal intensity silastic joint implant (*small curved arrow*), proximal interphalangeal joint erosions and fibrous tissue (*large curved arrow*), scapholunate dissociation (*open arrow*), and subchondral sclerosis of the scaphoid (*small arrows*). Axial images depicting tenosynovitis of a flexor tendon (*small arrows*) and fluid collecting in the radioulnar space (*large arrow*) as (**C**) low signal intensity on T1-weighted image, and as (**D**) high signal intensity on T2-weighted image. (**E**) A distal axial T2-weighted image of the wrist shows dorsal ulnar subluxation (*curved arrow*) with associated joint effusion (*straight solid black arrows*) and intermediate intensity synovial hypertrophy (*open arrow*). Erosions of the distal radius are identified (*straight solid white arrows*). *(continued)*

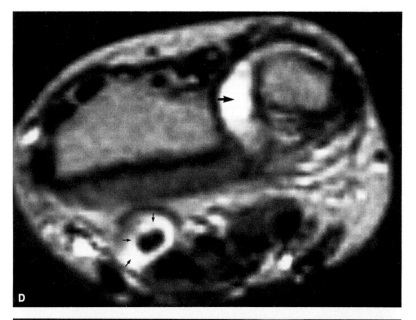

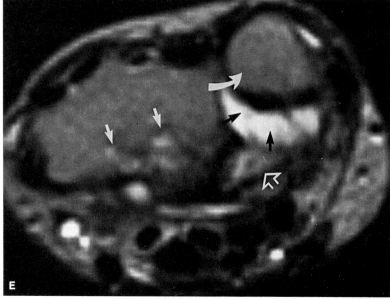

FIGURE 8–99. *(Continued)*

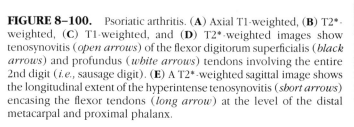

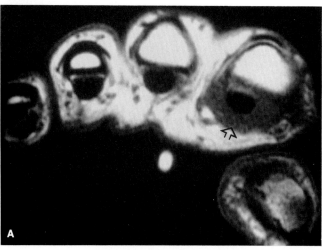

FIGURE 8–100. Psoriatic arthritis. (**A**) Axial T1-weighted, (**B**) T2*-weighted, (**C**) T1-weighted, and (**D**) T2*-weighted images show tenosynovitis (*open arrows*) of the flexor digitorum superficialis (*black arrows*) and profundus (*white arrows*) tendons involving the entire 2nd digit (*i.e.,* sausage digit). (**E**) A T2*-weighted sagittal image shows the longitudinal extent of the hyperintense tenosynovitis (*short arrows*) encasing the flexor tendons (*long arrow*) at the level of the distal metacarpal and proximal phalanx.

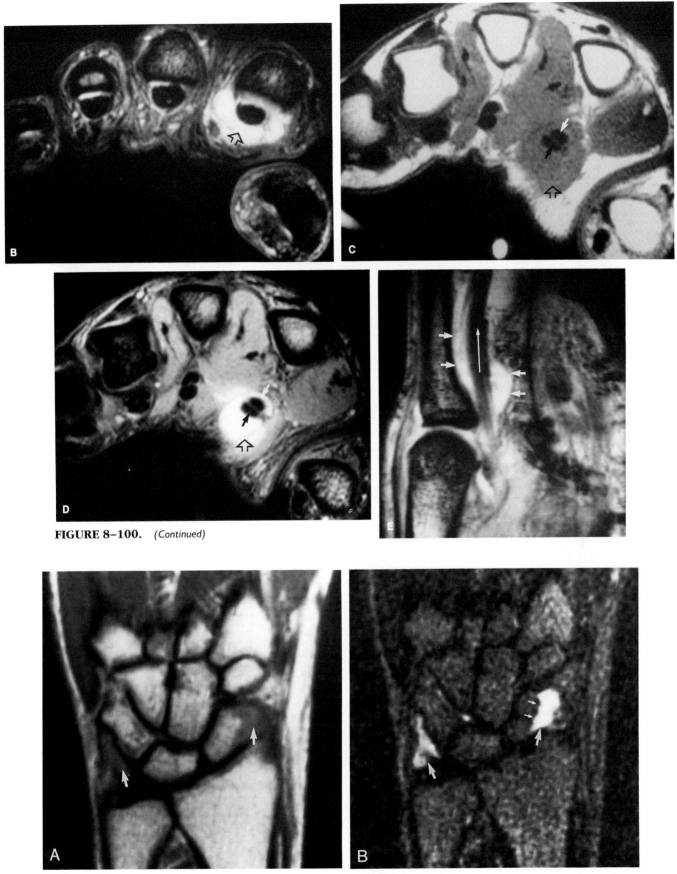

FIGURE 8–100. (Continued)

FIGURE 8–101.   Synovitis of the wrist with focal fluid pockets (*large arrows*) demonstrates (**A**) low signal intensity on a T1-weighted coronal image and (**B**) high signal intensity on a T2-weighted coronal image. The irregular or corrugated contour of the fluid represents contact with inflamed synovium (*small arrows*).

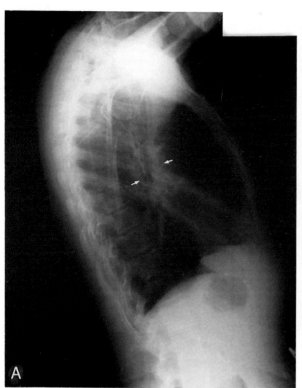

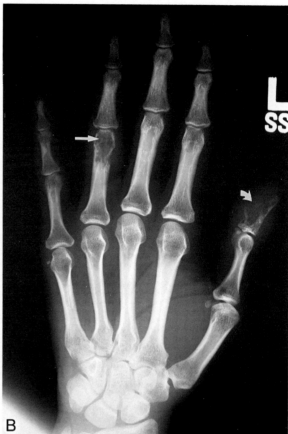

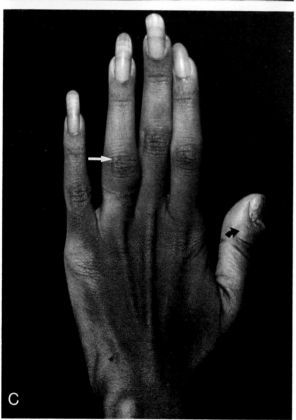

FIGURE 8–102. Skeletal sarcoid. (**A**) A lateral chest radiograph shows hilar lymphadenopathy (*arrows*). (**B**) An anteroposterior radiograph shows lytic lesions of the sarcoid in the proximal phalanx of the 4th digit (*straight arrow*) and the distal phalanx of the thumb (*curved arrow*). (**C**) A gross photograph shows soft-tissue swelling of the 4th proximal interphalangeal joint (*straight arrow*). Characteristic nail changes and swelling are seen in the thumb (*curved arrow*).

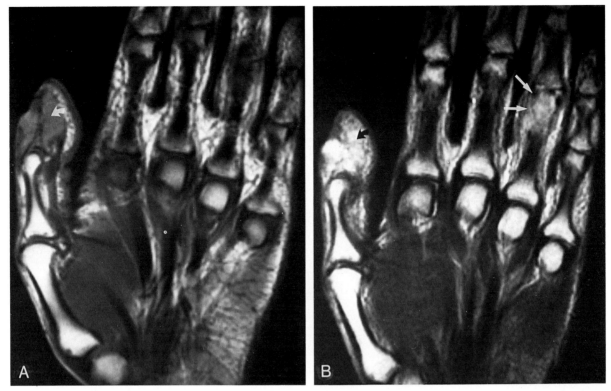

FIGURE 8-103. Skeletal sarcoid. (**A**) A T1-weighted coronal image shows an intermediate signal intensity soft-tissue mass (*curved arrow*) and cortical destruction. (**B**) A T2-weighted coronal image shows high signal intensity granulomatous tissue in the distal phalanx of the thumb (*curved arrow*) and proximal phalanx of the ring finger (*straight arrows*).

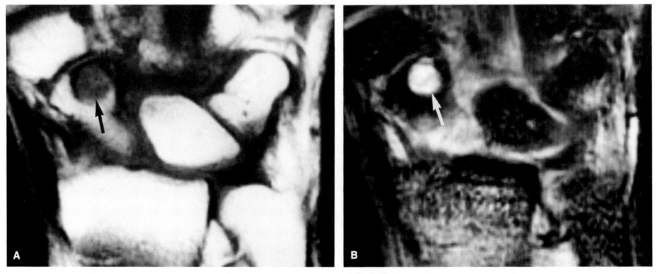

FIGURE 8-104. An intraosseous cyst (*arrows*) of the distal pole of the scaphoid demonstrates (**A**) low signal intensity on a coronal T1-weighted image and (**B**) high signal intensity on a T2*-weighted image.

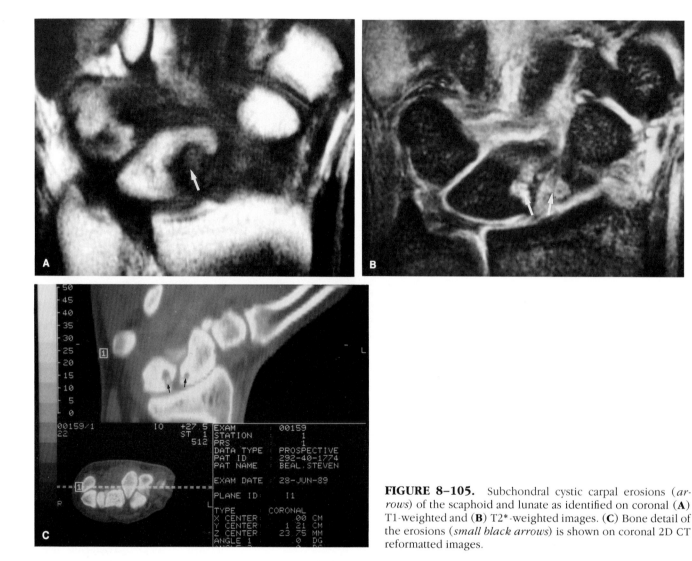

FIGURE 8–105. Subchondral cystic carpal erosions (*arrows*) of the scaphoid and lunate as identified on coronal (**A**) T1-weighted and (**B**) T2*-weighted images. (**C**) Bone detail of the erosions (*small black arrows*) is shown on coronal 2D CT reformatted images.

FIGURE 8–106. Coronal (**A**) T1-weighted and (**B**) T2*-weighted images and axial (**C**) T1-weighted and (**D**) T2*-weighted images show a viscous, cystic, synovial-fluid–filled volar ganglion (*solid arrows*) of the 2nd digit flexor tendons (*open arrows*).

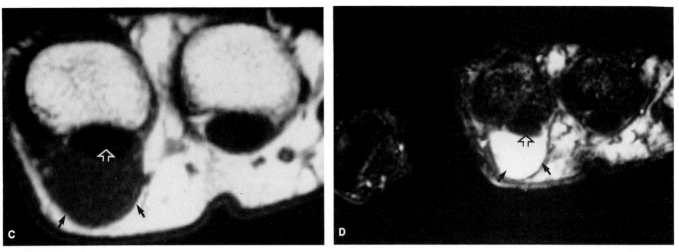

FIGURE 8–106. *(Continued)*

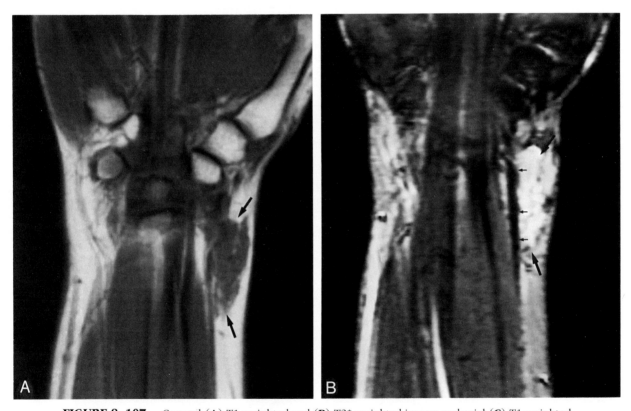

FIGURE 8–107. Coronal (**A**) T1-weighted and (**B**) T2*-weighted images and axial (**C**) T1-weighted and (**D**) T2-weighted images show a synovial ganglion (*large arrows*) associated with the flexor carpi radialis tendon (*small arrows*). The relationship of the cyst (*curved arrows*) to the flexor tendon (*short arrows*) is shown in the axial plane. Mucinous synovial contents demonstrate low signal intensity on T1-weighted images and high signal intensity on T2-weighted images. *(continued)*

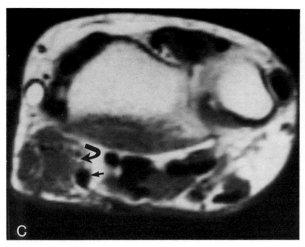

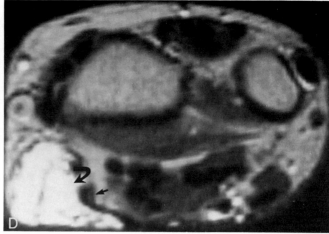

FIGURE 8–107. *(Continued)*

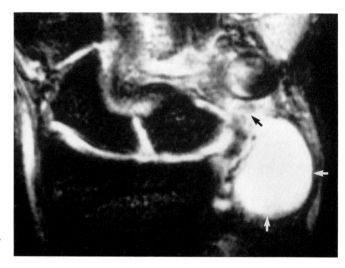

FIGURE 8–108. A large cystic ganglion (*white arrows*) projects from the ulnar aspect of a torn triangular fibrocartilage (*black arrow*).

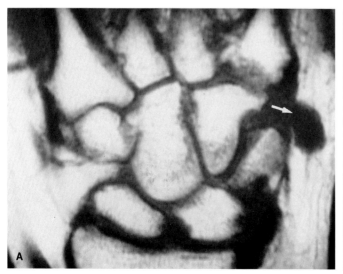

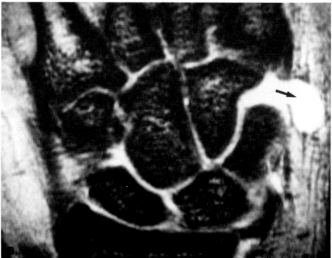

FIGURE 8–109. A cystic ganglion (*arrows*) communicates with the hamate triquetral joint. The lesion demonstrates (**A**) low signal intensity on a T1-weighted coronal image and is (**B**) hyperintense on a T2*-weighted coronal image.

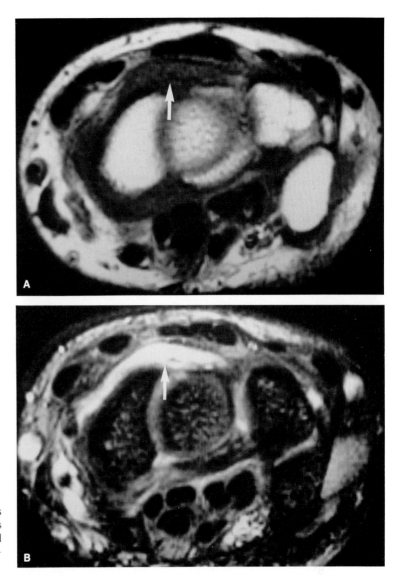

FIGURE 8–110. A dorsal ganglion (*arrows*) projects over the scaphoid and capitate. The lesion demonstrates (**A**) uniform low signal intensity on an axial T1-weighted image and (**B**) high signal intensity on an axial T2*-weighted image.

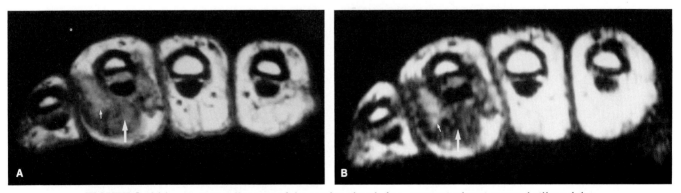

FIGURE 8–111. A giant cell tumor of the tendon sheath (*i.e.,* extraarticular pigmented villonodular synovitis; *large arrows*) demonstrates low signal intensity on axial (**A**) intermediate-weighted and (**B**) T2-weighted images. Minimal fluid signal intensity (*short arrows*) is seen.

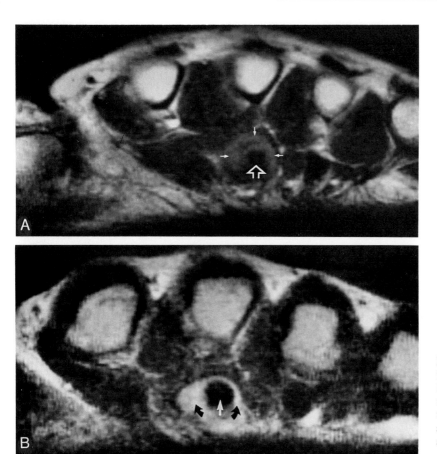

FIGURE 8–112. Peritendinous edema in flexor tendon tenosynovitis. The fluid demonstrates (**A**) low signal intensity (*small white arrows*) on an intermediate-weighted image and (**B**) high signal intensity (*curved black arrows*) on a T2-weighted axial image. The flexor tendon demonstrates low signal intensity on both images (*large white arrow and open arrow*).

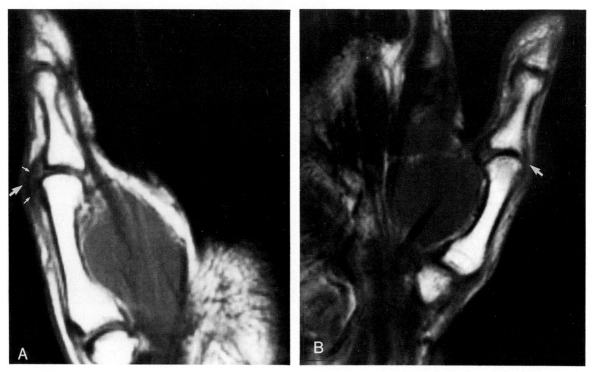

FIGURE 8–113. (**A**) Capsular synovitis with bowing of overlying extensor tendon in the 1st metacarpal phalangeal joint (*large and small arrows*) is seen on a T1-weighted coronal image. (**B**) The corresponding normal contralateral metacarpophalangeal joint (*arrow*) is shown for comparison.

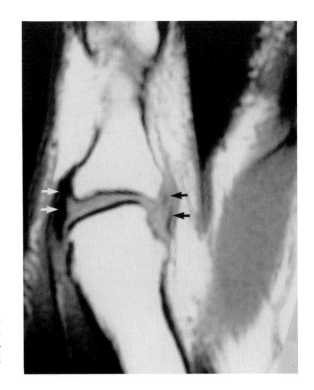

FIGURE 8–114. Gamekeeper's thumb with disruption of the ulnar collateral ligament (*black arrows*) is shown on a T1-weighted coronal image. An intact, low signal intensity radial collateral ligament is shown (*white arrows*). MR can be used to evaluate for entrapment of the ulnar collateral ligament.

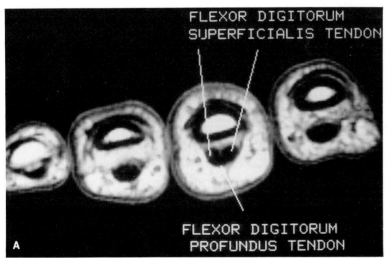

FLEXOR DIGITORUM
SUPERFICIALIS TENDON

FLEXOR DIGITORUM
PROFUNDUS TENDON

A

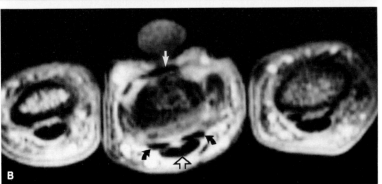

B

FIGURE 8–115. (**A**) A T1-weighted axial image shows the flexor tendon anatomy at the level of the proximal middle phalanx. (**B**) A T2*-weighted axial image provides superior discrimination of the flexor digitorum superficialis slips (*curved black arrows*) from the flexor digitorum profundus tendon (*open arrow*). The extensor tendon is shown deep to the marker (*white arrow*).

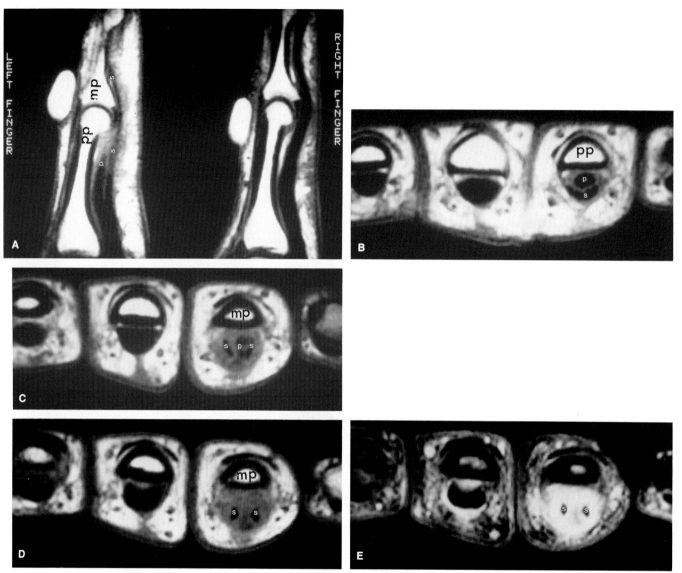

FIGURE 8–116.   An isolated flexor digitorum profundus tendon tear. (**A**) T1-weighted sagittal images show the retracted profundus tendon (p) over the left 4th digit at the level of the proximal phalanx (pp). The intact superficialis tendon (s) is shown where it attaches to the borders of the middle phalanx (mp). Morphology of the normal right finger flexor tendon is shown for comparison. (**B**) A T1-weighted axial image shows the intact flexor digitorum profundus (p) and superficialis (s) tendons at the level of the proximal phalanx (pp). Normally, the superficialis divides into two halves opposite the middle phalanx and passes deep to the profundus tendon, where it decussates and attaches to the middle phalanx. (**C**) A T1-weighted axial image shows the site of flexor digitorum profundus rupture (p) flanked by divided superficialis tendons (s) opposite the middle phalanx (mp). (**D**) A more distal axial T1-weighted image and (**E**) a T2*-weighted image through the middle phalanx (mp) show the absence of the profundus tendon. The flexor digitorum profundus tendon normally inserts onto the anterior aspect of the base of the distal phalanx. The flexor digitorum superficialis (s) divides normally.

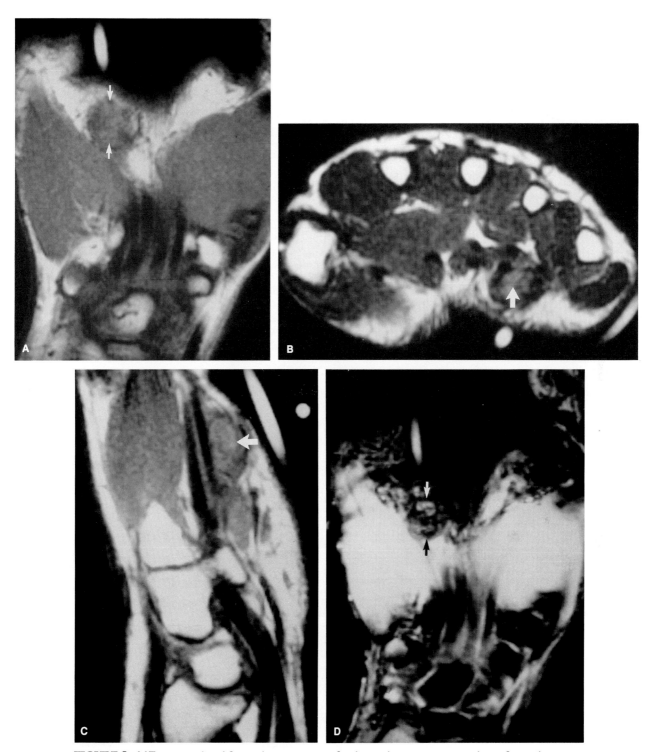

FIGURE 8–117. An isolated flexor digitorum superficialis tendon tear. A retracted torn flexor digitorum superficialis tendon (*arrows*) is shown on T1-weighted (**A**) coronal, (**B**) axial, and (**C**) sagittal images. The condensed tendon mimics a ganglion in morphology. (**D**) There is no increased signal intensity on the T2*-weighted coronal image, however.

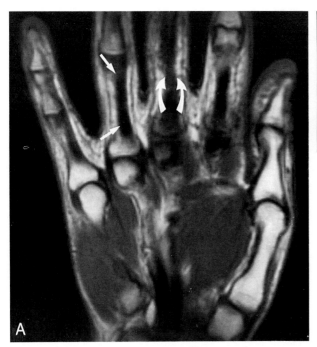

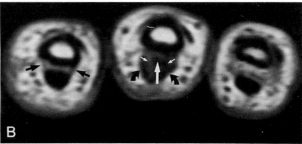

FIGURE 8–118. An intact flexor tendon is shown after repair. (**A**) A T1-weighted coronal image shows the attenuated low signal intensity flexor tendon at the site of primary surgical repair (*curved arrows*). The normal contour of the uninvolved flexor tendon is shown for comparison (*straight arrow*). (**B**) The corresponding axial image demonstrates the central low signal intensity flexor digitorum profundus (*large white arrow*) and the dividing tendons of the flexor digitorum superficialis (*curved black arrows*). Fibrous thickening of the tendon sheaths demonstrates intermediate signal intensity (*small white arrows*). The intact digital fibrous sheaths, which form the osteofibrous canal, support the flexor tendons (*straight black arrows*).

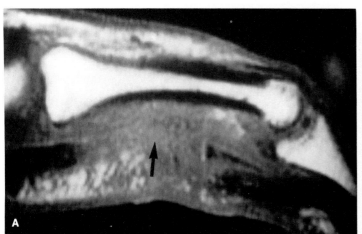

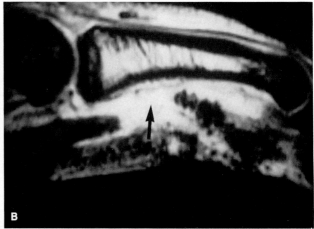

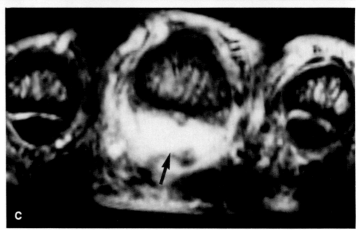

FIGURE 8–119. Complete disruption of the flexor digitorum superficialis and profundus tendons (*arrow*) are seen on (**A**) T1-weighted sagittal, (**B**) T2*-weighted, and (**C**) T2*-weighted axial images after primary tendon repair.

synovitis, or tears with MR studies. Chronic tenosynovitis may lead to tendon attrition and result in tear.

REFERENCES

1. Manaster BJ. Digital wrist arthrography: precision in determining the site of radiocarpal-midcarpal communication. AJR 1986;147: 563.

2. Braunstein EM, et al. Fluoroscopic and arthroscopic evaluation of carpal instability. AJR 1985;144:1259.

3. Tirman RM, et al. Midcarpal wrist arthrography for detection of tears of the scapholunate and lunatotriquetral ligaments. AJR 1985;144:107.

4. Hall FM. Wrist arthrography. Radiology 1990;175:585.

5. Palmer A. Arthrography of the wrist. J Hand Surg [Am] 1983;8: 15.

6. Zinberg E, et al. The triple injection wrist arthrogram. J Hand Surg [Am] 1988;13:803.

7. Manaster B, Mann R, Rubenstein S. Wrist pain: correlation of clinical and plain film findings with arthrographic results. J Hand Surg [Am] 1989;14(3):466.

8. Mikic Z. Age changes in triangular fibrocartilage of the wrist joint. J Anat 1978;126:367.

9. Mikic Z. Arthrography of the wrist joint. An experimental study. J Bone Joint Surg [Am] 1984;66:371.

10. Quinn SF, et al. Advanced imaging of the wrist. Radiographics 1989;9:229.

11. Hindman BW, et al. Occult fractures of the carpals and metacarpals demonstrated by CT. AJR 1989;153:529.

12. Pennes DR, et al. Direct coronal CT of the scaphoid bone. Radiology 1989;171:870.

13. Biondetti PR, et al. Three-dimensional surface reconstruction of the carpal bones from CT scans: transaxial versus coronal technique. Comput Med Imag Graph 1988;12:67.

14. DeFlaviis L, et al. High resolution ultrasonography of wrist ganglia. JCU 1987;15:17.

15. Weiss KL, et al. High field strength surface coil imaging of the hand and wrist. Part I, normal anatomy. Radiology 1986;160:143.

16. Baker LL, et al. High resolution magnetic resonance imaging of the wrist. Normal anatomy. Skeletal Radiol 1987;16:128.

17. Middleton WD, et al. High resolution surface coil imaging of the joints. Anatomic correlation. Radiographics, 1987;7:645.

18. Koenig H, et al. Wrist: preliminary report of high resolution MR imaging. Radiology 1986;160:463.

19. Mark S, et al. High resolution MR imaging of peripheral joints using a quadratus coil at 0.35T. ROFO 1987;146:397.

20. Fisher MR, et al. MR imaging using specialized coils. Radiology 1985;157:443.

21. Quinn SF, et al. Advanced imaging of the wrist. Radiographics 1989;9:229.

22. Zlatkin MB, et al. Chronic wrist pain: evaluation with high resolution MR imaging. Radiology 1989;173:723.

23. Greenan T, et al. Magnetic resonance imaging of the wrist. Semin US CT MR 1990;11:267.

24. Gundry CR, et al. Is MR better than arthrography for evaluating the ligaments of the wrist? In vitro study. AJR 1990;154(2):337.

25. Binkovitz LA, et al. Magnetic resonance imaging of the wrist: normal cross sectional imaging and selected abnormal cases. Radiographics 1988;8:1171.

26. Heuck A, et al. Possibilities of MR tomography of diseases of the hand and wrist. Radiologue 1989;29(2):53.

27. Ekenstam F: The distal radioulnar joint. Uppsala: Acta Universitatis Up Salvensis Uppsala Universitet, 1984.

28. Watson H, Ryu J. Degenerative disorders of the carpus. Orthop Clin North Am 1984;15:337-353.

29. Viegas S, et al. Medial (hamate) facet of the lunate. J Hand Surg [Am] 1990;15(4):565.

30. North E, Thomas S. An anatomic guide for arthroscopic visualization of the wrist capsular ligaments. J Hand Surg [Am] 1988;13: 815.

31. Cooney W, et al. Anatomy and mechanics of carpal instability. Surgical Rounds for Orthopaedics 1989;Sept:15-24, 1989.

32. Webster E, Chao E. An experimental approach to mechanism of scaphoid wrist fractures. J Hand Surg [Am] 1978;3:142.

33. Berger R, Landsmeer J. The palmar radiocarpal ligaments: a study of adult and fetal human wrist joints. J Hand Surg [Am] 1990;15(6): 847.

34. Testut, L. Traite d'anatomie humaine. Paris: Gaston Doin & Company, 1928:628.

35. Landsmeer J. Atlas of anatomy of the hand. New York: Churchill-Livingstone, 1976:11.

36. Berger R, et al. Radioscapholunate ligament: a gross anatomic and histologic study of fetal and adult wrists. J Hand Surg [Am] 1991;16(2):350.

37. Palmer A, Werner F. The triangular fibrocartilage complex of the wrist—anatomy and function. J Hand Surg [Am] 1981;6:153.

38. Viegas S, et al. Ulnar-sided perilunate instability: an anatomic and biomechanic study. J Hand Surg [Am] 1990;15(2):268.

39. Taleisnik J. The ligaments of the wrist. In: Taleisnik J. ed. The wrist. New York: Churchill-Livingstone, 1985:13.

40. Lichtman D, et al. Ulnar midcarpal instability—clinical and laboratory analysis. J Hand Surg [Am], 1981;6:515.

41. Resnick R, Halliday D. Physics. New York: Wiley & Sons, 1966.

42. Youm Y, et al. Kinematics of the wrist, part I—an experimental study of radial-ulnar deviation and flexion-extension. J Bone Joint Surg [Am] 1978;60:423.

43. Amadio P. Personal communication, 1990.

44. Garcia-Elias M, et al. Traumatic axial dislocations of the carpus. J Hand Surg [Am] 1989;14(3):446.

44a. Gilula LA. Carpal injuries: analytic approach and case exercises. AJR 1979;133:503.

45. Lichtman D, et al. Ulnar midcarpal instability: clinical and laboratory analysis. J Hand Surg [Am] 1981;9:350.

46. Taleisnik J, Watson H. Midcarpal instability caused by malunited fractures of the distal radius. J Hand Surg [Am] 1984;9:350.

47. Gainer B, Schaberg J. The rheumatoid wrist after resection of the distal ulna. J Hand Surg [Am] 1985;10:837.

48. Rayhack J, et al. Posttraumtic ulnar translocation of the carpus. J Hand Surg [Am] 1982;12:180.

49. Loeb T, et al. Traumatic carpal instability: putting the pieces together. Orthop Trans 1977;1:163.

50. Glickel S, Millender L. Results of ligamentous reconstruction for chronic intercarpal instability. Orthop Trans 1982;6:167.

51. Watson H, Mempton R. Limited wrist arthrodesis. Part I. J Hand Surg [Am] 1980;5:320.

52. Blatt G. Dorsal capsulodesis for rotatory subluxation of the carpal scaphoid. Presented at the Annual Meeting of the American Society for Surgery of the Hand, New Orleans, 1986.

53. Palmer AC: The distal radioulnar joint. In: Lichtman D, ed. The wrist and its disorders. Philadelphia: WB Saunders, 1988:220.

54. Steyers C, Blair W. Measuring ulnar variance: a comparison of techniques. J Hand Surg [Am] 1989:14:607.

55. Epner R, et al. Ulnar variance: the effect of wrist positioning and roentgen filming technique. J Hand Surg [Am] 1982;7:298.

56. Olerud C, et al. The congruence of the distal radioulnar joint. A magnetic resonance imaging study. Acta Orthop Scand 1988;59(2):183.

57. Wechsler R, et al. Computed tomography diagnosis of distal radioulnar subluxation. Skeletal Radiol 1987;16(1):1.

58. Pirela-Cruz M, et al. Stress computed tomography analysis of the distal radioulnar joint: a diagnostic tool for determining translational motion. J Hand Surg [Am] 1991;16(1):75.

59. Hermandsdorfer J, Kleinman W. Management of chronic peripheral tears of the triangular fibrocartilage complex. J Hand Surg [Am] 1991;16(2):340.

60. Pin P, et al. Management of chronic lunotriquetral ligament tears. J Hand Surg [Am] 1989;14(1):77.

61. Thiru R, et al. Arterial anatomy of the triangular fibrocartilage of the wrist and its surgical significance. J Hand Surg [Am] 1986;11(2):258.

62. Mooney J, Poehling G. Disruption of the ulnolunate ligament as a cause for chronic ulnar wrist pain. J Hand Surg [Am] 1991;16(2):347.

63. Golimbu CN, et al. Tears of the triangular fibrocartilage of the wrist: MR imaging. Radiology 1989;173:731.

64. Lewis OJ, et al. The anatomy of the wrist joint. J Anat 1970;106:539.

65. Weber ER. Wrist mechanics and its association with ligamentous instability. In: Lichtman D, ed. The wrist and its disorders. Philadelphia: WB Saunders, 1988:41.

66. Greenan T, et al. Magnetic resonance imaging of the wrist. Semin US CT MR 1990;11:267.

67. Adams B. Detrimental effects of resections in the articular disc of the TFCC. Transactions of the 37th Meeting of the ORS 1991;16:212.

68. Lewis O. The development of the human wrist joint during the fetal period. Anat Rec 1970;166:499.

69. Frykman, G. Fracture of the distal radius including sequelae. Shoulder-hand-finger syndrome, disturbance in the distal radioulnar joint, and impairment of nerve function: a clinical and experimental study. Acta Orthop Scand 1967;108(suppl):1.

70. Melone C Jr. Open treatment for displaced articular fractures of the distal radius. Clin Orthop 1986;202:103.

71. Werner F, Murphy D, Palmer A. Pressures in the distal radioulnar joint: effect of surgical procedures used for Kienböck's disease. J Orthop Res 1989;7(3):445.

72. Scheck M. Long term follow up of treatment for comminuted fractures of the distal end of the radius by transfixation with Kirschner wires and cast. J Bone Joint Surg [Am] 1962;44:337.

73. Stevens J. Compression fractures of the lower end of the radius. Ann Surg 1920;71:594.

74. Knirk J, Jupiter J. Intraarticular fractures of the distal end of the radius in young adults. J Bone Joint Surg [Am] 1986;68(5):647.

75. O'Brien ET. Acute fractures and dislocations of the carpus. In: Lichtman D, ed. The wrist and its disorders. Philadelphia: WB Saunders, 1988:129.

76. Gillespy T III, et al. Dorsal fractures of the hamate: radiographic appearance. AJR 1988;151:351.

77. Ruby LK, et al. Natural history of scaphoid nonunion. Radiology 1985;156:856.

78. Reinus WR, et al. Carpal avascular necrosis: MR imaging. Radiology 1986;160:689.

79. Weiss KL, et al. High field MR surface coil imaging of the hand and wrist. Normal anatomy. Skeletal Radiol 1987;16:128.

80. Baker LL, et al. High resolution magnetic resonance imaging of the wrist. Normal anatomy. Skeletal Radiol 1987;16:128.

81. Cristiani G, et al. Evaluation of ischaemic necrosis of carpal bones by magnetic resonance imaging. J Hand Surg [Br] 1990;15(2):249.

82. Desser TS, et al. Scaphoid fractures and Kienböck's disease of the lunate: MR imaging with histopathologic correlation. Magn Res Imag 1990;8:357.

83. Duong R, et al. Kienböck's disease: scintigraphic demonstration in correlation with clinical, radiographic and pathologic findings. Clin Nucl Med 1982;7:418.

84. Hulten O. Uber anatomische variationen der handgelenkknochen. Acta Radio Scand 1928;9:155.

85. Gelberman R, et al. Ulnar variance in Kienböck's disease. J Bone Joint Surg [Am] 1975;57:674-676.

86. Peste. Discussion. Bull Soc Anat 1943;18:169.

87. Beckenbaugh R, et al. Kienböck's disease: the natural history of Kienböck's disease and consideration of lunate fractures. Clin Orthop 1980;149:98.

88. Gelberman R, et al. The vascularity of the lunate bone and Kienböck's disease. J Hand Surg [Am] 1980;5:272.

89. Alexander AH, Lichtman D. Kienböck's disease. In: Lichtman D, ed. The wrist and its disorders. Philadelphia: WB Saunders, 1988:329.

90. Lichtman D, et al. Kienböck's disease—update on silicone replacement arthroplasty. J Hand Surg [Am] 1983;7:343.

91. Braun R. Pronator pedicle bone grafting in the forearm and proximal carpal row. Presented at 38th Annual Meeting of the American Society for Surgery of the Hand, March, 1983.

92. Hori Y, et al. Blood vessel transplantation to bone. J Hand Surg [Am] 1979;4:23.

93. Almquist E, et al. Capitate shortening as a treatment for early Kienböck's disease. Presented at the 45th Annual Meeting of the American Society for Surgery of the Hand, March, 1990.

94. Alexander A, et al. Lunate silicone replacement arthroplasty in Kienböck's disease: a long-term follow up. J Hand Surg [Am] 1990;15(3):401.

95. Coyle MP. Nerve entrapment syndromes in the upper extremity. In: Dee R, ed. Principles of orthopaedic practice. vol 1. New York: McGraw-Hill, 1989:672.

96. Middleton WD, et al. MR imaging of the carpal tunnel: normal anatomy and preliminary findings in the carpal tunnel syndrome. AJR 1987;148:307.

97. Mesgarzadah M, et al. Carpal tunnel: MR imaging. Part I. Normal anatomy. Radiology 1989;171(3):743.

98. Mesgarzadah M, et al. Carpal tunnel: MR imaging. Part II. Carpal tunnel syndrome. Radiology 1989;171(3):749.

99. Healy C, et al. Magnetic resonance imaging of the carpal tunnel. J Hand Surg [Br] 1990;15(2):243.

100. Zeiss J, et al. Anatomic relations between the median nerve and flexor tendons in the carpal tunnel: MR evaluation in normal volunteers. AJR 1989;153(3):533.

101. Yulish BS, et al. Juvenile rheumatoid arthritis: assessment with MR imaging. Radiology 1987;165:149.

102. Baker LL, et al. High resolution magnetic resonance imaging of the wrist. Normal anatomy. Skeletal Radiol 1987;16:128.

103. Meske S, et al. Rheumatoid arthritis lesions of the wrist examined by rapid gradient echo magnetic resonance imaging. Scand J Rheumatol 1990;19(3):235.

104. Watson KH. Degenerative disorders of the carpus. In: Lichtman D, ed. The wrist and its disorders. Philadelphia: WB Saunders, 1988:286.

105. Renner WR, et al. Early changes of rheumatoid arthritis in the hand and wrist. Radiol Clin North Am 1988;26:1185.

106. Ellstein JL, et al. Rheumatoid disorders of the hand and wrist. In: Dee R, ed. Principles of orthopaedic practice. vol 1. New York: McGraw-Hill, 1989:646.

107. Hollister AM, et al. The use of MRI in the diagnosis of an occult wrist ganglion cyst. Orthop Rev 1989;18(11):1210.

108. Feldman F, et al. Magnetic resonance imaging of para-articular and ectopic ganglia. Skeletal Radiol 1989;18(5):353.

109. Louis DS, et al. Magnetic resonance imaging of the collateral ligaments of the thumb. J Hand Surg [Am] 1989;14(4):739.

The Temporomandibular Joint

The primary interest in the temporomandibular joint (TMJ) is in the evaluation of internal disc derangements. Abnormalities in both position and morphology of the TMJ meniscus (*i.e.,* disc) have been implicated in myofascial pain syndromes and in biomechanical joint dysfunction. Young and middle-aged women are thought to represent a significant proportion of patients with TMJ abnormalities, mostly caused by bruxism (*i.e.,* grinding of the teeth). However, internal disc derangements may also result from direct trauma or indirect trauma (*e.g.,* prolonged dental procedures), or they may occur spontaneously. Internal derangements of the TMJ represent one component of craniofacial pain syndromes; other components include myofascial pain dysfunction, abnormalities of the cervical spine, and dental occlusion.

Clinical diagnosis and documentation of TMJ disorders are difficult, and patients may present with symptoms of dysfunction without objective joint disease. However, documentation of internal disc derangements is required by third-party payers before long-term treatment or surgical intervention is approved. Unfortunately, the articular disc cannot be seen by conventional radiography or computed tomography (CT), because these modalities rely on the assessment of osseous structures. Of the available imaging techniques, magnetic resonance (MR) imaging is rapidly becoming the procedure of choice to image the TMJ.

Computed tomography provides information that enables assessment of maxillofacial trauma; infection, including osteomyelitis; congenital abnormalities; and bony invasion by tumor. However, disc derangements cannot be appreciated by CT. Arthroscopy indirectly characterizes disc morphology, through either an inferior joint-space injection or dual-space contrast study; however, this is an invasive procedure. Arthrotomography relies on imaging contrast material coating the articular disc relative to the adjacent condyle, the glenoid fossa, and the eminence in closed-, partially open-, and open-mouth positions. With arthrography, the lower compartment of the TMJ is filled with contrast material to assess the position of the disc or, indirectly, the presence of a perforation.[1-7] Arthrography also is an invasive procedure with associated morbidity, and is limited in accuracy (*e.g.,* inability to inject contrast material into the lower joint compartment or injection into both compartments mimics disc perforation). Complications of arthrography include pain, prolonged discomfort, contrast extravasation into retrodiscal and pericapsular tissues, localized hemorrhage, and transient facial paralysis.

Computed tomography requires the use of ionizing radiation and only allows imaging of the TMJ disc through the use of reformatted sagittal images obtained from a series of transaxial joint scans.[8-13] The meniscus and bony anatomy are demonstrated in soft-tissue and bone algorithms. Computed tomography number highlighting for reformatting sagittal sections may not accurately differentiate the lateral pterygoid tendinous attachment from the articular disc, and is limited in evaluating a thinned or attenuated disc. Direct sagittal scanning has improved resolution over reformatting, and may replace it using the "identity" or "blink" mode for CT number highlighting. Proper angulation and patient positioning is required to minimize radiation to the orbit and lens.

Magnetic resonance imaging is rapidly replacing arthrography and CT as the examination of choice in evaluating the TMJ.[13-26] Magnetic resonance is noninvasive and provides direct sagittal images that not only display the TMJ meniscus, but also differentiate the cortex, marrow, hyaline cartilage, muscle, fluid, fibrous tissue, and adhesions. This inherent soft-tissue discrimination facilitates thin section acquisitions with specialized surface coils. The development of faster imaging techniques and dual-coil imaging has facilitated routine bilateral examinations with functional or kinematic positioning of the joint.[27,28] Magnetic resonance can also be used to study other disease processes affecting the TMJ (*e.g.,* trauma, arthritis, neoplasia) as well as to make postsurgical assessments.[29-35]

GROSS ANATOMY OF THE TEMPOROMANDIBULAR JOINT

The TMJ is a synovial diarthroidal joint located between the condyle of the mandible and mandibular fossa of the temporal bone (Fig. 9–1). The joint capsule is composed of loose connective tissue, which allows condylar translation, mandibular protrusion, retroaction, and side-to-side excursion.[36,37] The articular disc, or meniscus, partitions the joint into a large superior (*i.e.,* upper) joint space and an inferior (*i.e.,* lower) joint space. The mandibular condyle divides the inferior joint space into anterior and posterior recesses. The biconcave fibrous fibrocartilaginous disc measures 1 mm centrally, and thickens peripherally into two bands, the anterior and the posterior. The anterior band is 2 mm thick, and the larger posterior band is 2.8 mm thick. Small perforations in the thin, central portion of the disc are normal. However, there is no direct communication between the separate synovium-lined upper and lower compartments. In the closed-mouth position, the bow-tie– or sigmoid-shaped disc is positioned within the temporal fossa with the posterior band directly superior to the condylar head. The thin, central region of the disc is located between the temporal articular eminence and the anterior condylar head. The anterior band, with the attached superior head of the lateral pterygoid muscle, is located inferior to the articular eminence and anterior to the condylar head.

The posterior attachment of the disc (*i.e.,* the bilaminar zone) represents a neurovascular area consisting of fat, collagen, and elastic fibers.[38] The posterior–superior ligament of the bilaminar zone is composed of elastin and inserts into the tympanic bone of the glenoid fossa. The posterior–inferior ligament of the bilaminar zone

has a fibrous, nonelastic insertion into the posterior subcondylar area. Tearing or stretching of this ligament facilitates meniscal displacement.

The lateral pterygoid muscle, which controls mouth opening, consists of superior and inferior heads. The superior head is parallel with the inferior head and inserts onto the anterior joint capsule and condylar neck. The tendinous fibers of the superior head attach directly into the anterior band of the articular disc. The lateral pterygoid muscle produces anterior or forward rotation of the condylar head under the disc, and anterior translation of both the condylar head and the disc below the articular eminence. The medial pterygoid muscle, which is without any disc insertion, attaches onto the medial surface of the angle of the mandible and assists the lateral pterygoid in closing the jaw. The temporalis muscle has a tendinous insertion anteriorly onto the coronoid process of the mandible. The temporomandibular ligament bridges the posterior zygomatic arch and the lateral aspect of the condylar neck, reinforcing the lateral joint capsule. The sphenomandibular and stylomandibular ligaments are located medial and posterior to the TMJ, respectively.

IMAGING PROTOCOLS FOR THE TEMPOROMANDIBULAR JOINT

Direct sagittal images through the TMJ are acquired with the use of a small (3-in) diameter surface coil placed over the region of interest (Fig. 9–2). A high signal-to-noise ratio is achieved by using thin (3-mm) sections, a 12-cm field of view, a 256×256 acquisition matrix, and one to two excitations. Axial and coronal images, if obtained, are used as localizers for the sagittal plane acquisition. Oblique prescription lines, oriented in a anteromedial to posterolateral direction, are placed on the axial localizer. A bilateral surface coil set-up is used. Oblique images can also be prescribed from a coronal localizer, to properly elongate the mandibular condyle (Fig. 9–3).

A series of sagittal images can provide information about medial and lateral disc position without a separate coronal acquisition. Routine imaging is obtained using a T1-weighted protocol with a repetition time (TR) of 600 sec and echo time (TE) of 20 msec. The addition of a T2-weighted sequence can highlight joint effusions with bright signal intensity, but this doubles imaging time and is not routinely used. Partial flip-angle fast-scan techniques permit the acquisition of T2*-weighted images of the TMJ in a fraction of the time needed for conventional spin-echo techniques.[28] Using multiplanar gradient-echo software (MPGR; General Electric, Milwaukee, WI), we have used T2* gradient refocused images with a TR of 400 msec, TE of 15 to 25 msec, and a flip angle of 30°.

Gradient-echo three dimensional Fourier transform volume imaging provides thin section capability in bilateral examinations with the option to reformat images retrospectively in other imaging planes.[39] Gradient-echo techniques are also used in kinematic protocols, which use the Burnett mouth positioning device and display images in the simulated cine mode, to evaluate the TMJ throughout the spectrum of closed- to open-mouth positions.

Simultaneous, bilateral imaging of the TMJ will be possible with coil designs, in production, that will eliminate the need for separate unilateral studies (see Fig. 9–2).[40,41] Although many dentists find studies of only the affected or symptomatic side acceptable, others prefer to evaluate both sides routinely because of the known incidence of bilateral involvement in internal disc derangements.

There has been some controversy concerning the position of the mouth (*i.e.,* closed, partially open, or open) for optimal MR evaluation of TMJ disc displacements.[42] Advocates of the partially open-mouth position feel that the morphology of the TMJ meniscus is not as distorted in this position as it is in the closed-mouth position. In the closed-mouth position, the articular disc may become compressed between the articular eminence of the temporal bone and the condyle. In studies comparing closed- and partially open-mouth positions, it was found that up to one-third of patients inadvertently reduce the meniscus with partial mouth opening.[43,44] Therefore, we routinely evaluate the meniscus in the closed-mouth position. The TMJ is also routinely evaluated in a full open-mouth position to verify meniscal reductions. Although disc reduction is frequently evident on clinical examination, full open- and closed-mouth studies are needed to document meniscus position and degree of reduction in many cases of chronic meniscal derangements. If time permits only one acquisition, then closed-mouth imaging eliminates the possibility of a recaptured disc during forward translation of the condyle.

NORMAL MAGNETIC RESONANCE ANATOMY OF THE TEMPOROMANDIBULAR JOINT

Sagittal Images

The articular eminence of the temporal bone and the condyle of the mandible, the bony support of the TMJ, demonstrate the high signal intensity of fatty marrow (Fig. 9–4). Cortical bone, which is of low spin density (*i.e.,* dark signal intensity), displays a uniform surface on the condylar head, glenoid fossa, and articular eminence.

The TMJ meniscus (*i.e., disc*), is composed of type

I collagen, elastic fibers, and glycosaminoglycans.[36,38] It is positioned on the superior surface of the condyle. The disc demonstrates low or dark signal intensity on T1-, T2-, and T2*-weighted images, whereas synovium in the superior or inferior joint spaces demonstrates intermediate signal intensity.

The articular disc is composed of three parts: an anterior band, a thin intermediate zone, and a thicker posterior band (Fig. 9–5).[14–22] Although all three parts of the normal biconcave disc demonstrate low signal intensity, it is normal to see a central portion of intermediate signal intensity in the posterior band (Fig. 9–6). The anterior band, positioned in front of the condyle, is anchored to the superior head of the lateral pterygoid muscle, which demonstrates intermediate signal intensity, by tendinous fibers, which demonstrate low signal intensity. The oblique orientation of the lateral pterygoid tends to direct most meniscal displacements in an anteromedial path. The thin intermediate zone is located between the low signal intensity cortical surfaces of the articular eminence and condylar head. The intermediate zone, also referred to as the weight-bearing zone, maintains a consistent relationship to the condyle and temporal eminence during translation. The thick posterior band is attached to a vascularized bilaminar zone in the retrodiscal tissue complex, which is anchored to the temporal bone (Fig. 9–7). Within the bilaminar zone, a parallel band of low signal intensity may be distinguished, demarcating superior and inferior fibers of the bilaminar zone. The transition between the posterior band and the bilaminar-retrodiscal complex may be marked by a vertical line of intermediate signal intensity (Fig. 9–8).[45] In the closed-mouth position, the posterior band occupies a 12-o'clock position in relation to the condylar head. Mild asymmetry between the condylar positions of the articular disc is common (see Fig. 9–8). In the open-mouth position, with forward translation and posterior disc rotation, the posterior band may be seen just dorsal to the 12-o'clock position. The articular disc defines and separates the upper and lower joint compartments. Capsular signal intensity is difficult to differentiate from joint synovial tissue.

Coronal Images

Coronal plane images, which are less frequently used, best demonstrate the articular disc in the plane of section through the posterior band in the closed-mouth position.[46] Although coronal images do not adequately define the anatomy of the intermediate zone, they are preferred for demonstrating the medial and lateral boundaries of the joint capsule and the lateral supporting temporomandibular ligament. Images through the anterior TMJ display the lateral pterygoid muscle and the more inferior medial pterygoid muscle. The low signal intensity maxillary vessels encased in fat are identified lateral to the pterygoid muscles and medial to the mandible.

PATHOLOGY OF THE TEMPOROMANDIBULAR JOINT

Internal Derangement

Internal derangements of the TMJ may present with localized pain and tenderness, clicking, joint crepitus, and limited opening of the mouth. The location of the posterior band is used to define the location and degree of disc displacement.

Meniscal Displacement

Internal derangements usually involve anteromedial displacement of the meniscus relative to the condylar head and temporal fossa (Figs. 9–9 and 9–10).[14–22,47–49] Trauma, degeneration, ligamentous laxity, and retrodiscal rents can be contributing factors. Such an anteriorly positioned disc blocks normal forward translation of the condyle, and the patient may present clinically with limited jaw opening and deviation of the mandible toward the affected side.

Displacement of the posterior band may be partial or complete, depending on the relative position of the disc between the condyle and articular eminence and on the area of contact between the posterior band and the condyle. The posterior attachment or bilaminar zone also translates anteriorly and is subjected to increased loading between the condyle and articular eminence.

Secondary remodeling may alter the morphology and signal intensity of the abnormally located posterior band, causing enlargement of a portion of the posterior band with associated foreshortening of the intermediate zone (Fig. 9–11).[38,50] Flexion of the disc and remodeling may also be seen in the intermediate zone (Fig. 9–12). More advanced changes include fibrosis of the posterior attachment and loss of the normally distinct anterior and posterior band morphology. Displaced discs display surface irregularities, including fissuring, fibrillation, and fraying, all of which are easily identified on routine MR evaluation. Dystrophic calcification, neovascularization, and perforations may also be associated with internal disc derangements. When remodeling is insufficient to accommodate increased loading of the disc and posterior detachment, the result may be pain, additional disc deformity, and increased susceptibility to injury. The addition of a medial or lateral pull to an anteriorly displaced disc contributes to a more complex rotational displacement.

An opening click is usually associated with reduction of the thick posterior band recaptured by the condylar head in the open-mouth position (Figs. 9–13 and 9–14). This audible or palpable click is often associated with relief of pain as the condyle successfully passes under the posterior band (Fig. 9–15). Less frequently, a reciprocal click occurs during closure, as the posterior band redislocates, anterior to the condyle. The elastic fibers of the bilaminar zone are unable to retract the disc as the condyle moves posteriorly during closing of the mouth. With stretching of the bilaminar zone, the condyle pushes forward to augment the disc during anterior translation and does not pass under the posterior band, therefore, no click is produced (Fig. 9–16).

When the jaw is locked in the closed-mouth position (*i.e.,* closed-lock), the meniscus is displaced in both closed- and open-mouth positions, preventing anterior condylar motion (Fig. 9–17). In a closed-lock derangement, early deformations of the disc may be seen during partial mouth opening, which compresses the displaced disc (Fig. 9–18). Eventually, disc deformity is seen in the closed-mouth position, and is characterized by the loss of biconcavity, disc folding, perforation, and a further decrease in disc signal intensity secondary to fibrosis and dystrophic calcification. Thickening of the bilaminar zone directly over the condyle may mimic the appearance of a normal posterior band (Fig. 9–19). With more severe stretching of the bilaminar zone, there may be some degree of anterior condylar translation without contact with the anteriorly displaced disc, giving the clinical appearance of improved mouth opening. In the stage of derangement, however, advanced disc deformity and degeneration are present.

A grading system for characterizing disc displacements by morphology has been developed.[44,51,52] The normally positioned meniscus (*i.e.,* grade 0; Fig. 9–20) has a drumstick contour and may have a bull's-eye or target region of intermediate signal intensity in the posterior band. In grade 1 meniscal displacement, the meniscus maintains a normal morphology (Figs. 9–21 and 9–22). Abnormal disc morphology (*i.e.,* loss of the drumstick shape) represents a grade 2 displacement (Fig. 9–23). A grade 2 meniscus is most likely to be associated with degenerative joint disease, and may not be repairable at surgery. The higher grades of internal disc derangements appear to correlate not only with degenerative joint disease, but also with severity of pain, chronicity, and restriction of joint motion.

A more subjective evaluation of disc displacement includes the observation of decreased posterior band signal intensity relative to the anterior band and intermediate zone. These signal changes are seen in more advanced displacements, especially in association with degenerative joint disease. Magnetic resonance imaging thus provides the potential to both identify a displaced meniscus and to evaluate the severity of the derangement, and thus the possible response to therapy.

In addition to classification by grade, disc displacements may also be classified as acute, subacute, or chronic.[53] Acute displacement is characterized by recapture of the disc in the open-mouth position without alteration in disc size or morphology (Fig. 9–24). In subacute displacement, the displaced disc does not reduce with mouth opening and may show signs of deformity with folding or flexion atrophy of the anterior band and thickening of the posterior band (Fig. 9–25). In chronic disc displacement, disc perforation, adhesions, fibrosis, and degenerative joint disease may be present.

Scarring or adhesions within the TMJ demonstrate intermediate signal intensity on both T1- and T2-weighted images. In contrast, joint fluid is of high signal intensity on T2-weighted images. Engorged veins in the vascular pterygoid attachments may mimic upper and lower joint compartment fluid and result in a false-positive diagnosis of effusion.

Disc Perforations

Perforations of the meniscus are more difficult to identify on MR images than in arthrograms.[32] With arthrography, a small disc perforation may be demonstrated by communication of contrast material between the superior and inferior joint recesses. However, false-positive rates as high as 20% have been reported with arthrography. In addition, the majority of these perforations are associated with a dislocated meniscus that would be detected by MR.

Degenerative osseous changes associated with disc derangements include sclerosis and an uneven or attenuated cortical surface in the condylar head, articular eminence, and fossa. Flattening of the condylar head and anterior osteophytes are demonstrated in sagittal images (Fig. 9–26). The normally high signal intensity fatty marrow is replaced with low signal intensity external subchondral sclerosis on T1-, T2-, and T2*-weighted images. Advanced osteoarthritic changes include bony ankylosis, fibrous ankylosis, and avascular necrosis of the mandibular condyle. Fibrous tissue decreases the internal signal intensity of normal joint synovium.

Treatment

Conservative splint therapy is used to position the mandible and condyle more anteriorly to recapture the displaced meniscus and to relax the lateral pterygoid muscle which may be in spasm. Magnetic resonance studies can be performed both before and after splint application to assess the location of the TMJ meniscus and to measure condylar translation (Figs. 9–27 and 9–

28). There has been limited experience imaging patients undergoing an experimental arthroscopic procedure in which saline is injected into the lower joint recess to force reduction of a displaced disc (Fig. 9–29). Engorged veins in the vascular pterygoid attachment can mimic upper and lower joint compartment fluid and may result in a false-positive diagnosis of effusion (Fig. 9–30).

Postsurgical plication (Fig. 9–31) and proplast prosthetic replacements of the TMJ meniscus should preserve the same anatomic relationships to the condylar and articular eminences as the normal native disc, and they are evaluated using the same criteria.[54-56]

Trauma

In complex fractures about the mandible and TMJ, CT is useful in demonstrating osseous fragments and their degree of displacement.[32,57] In selected cases, MR imaging may provide additional information regarding soft-tissue injury and the integrity of the articular disc (Fig. 9–32). Since forces are transmitted through the condyle, internal derangement of the TMJ can occur in the absence of fractures. A direct mandibular blow may stretch the meniscus and cause lateral pterygoid spasm and anterior disc displacement. In children, TMJ trauma may result in disruption of the condylar growth center of the jaw.

Arthritis

In the adult, osteoarthritis may occur as a sequela to TMJ trauma and internal disc derangements.[32] The TMJ may also be affected in episodes of gout, rheumatoid arthritis, lupus, or the seronegative arthropathies such as psoriatic arthritis[58] and ankylosing spondylitis. In the presence of synovitis and articular destruction, the disc is vulnerable to perforation and displacement. Temporomandibular joint pain may be present in the absence of significant appendicular joint involvement.

In osteoarthritis, cortical and articular cartilage thinning, with flattening and deformity of the condylar head, is seen on MR images. Osteophytes, which are usually located anteriorly, joint-space narrowing, and erosions of both the temporal eminence and condyle are frequently seen in degenerative joint disease (Figs. 9–33 and 9–34). Extensive subchondral or bony sclerosis in the condylar head, neck, and articular eminence may be seen on both T1- and T2-weighted images as areas of diffuse low signal intensity (Fig. 9–35). Low signal intensity may also represent the development of avascular necrosis.[55] Joint effusions, articular erosions, and synovial proliferation are all identifiable on T1- and T2-weighted

(text continues on page 827)

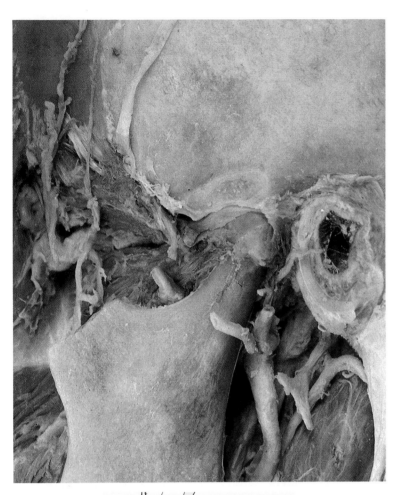

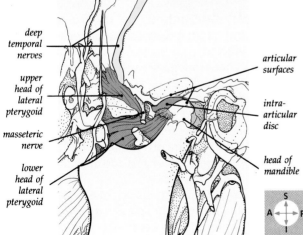

deep
temporal
nerves

upper
head of
lateral
pterygoid

masseteric
nerve

lower
head of
lateral
pterygoid

articular
surfaces

intra-
articular
disc

head of
mandible

FIGURE 9–1. The temporomandibular joint as opened by excision of the lateral part of its capsule.

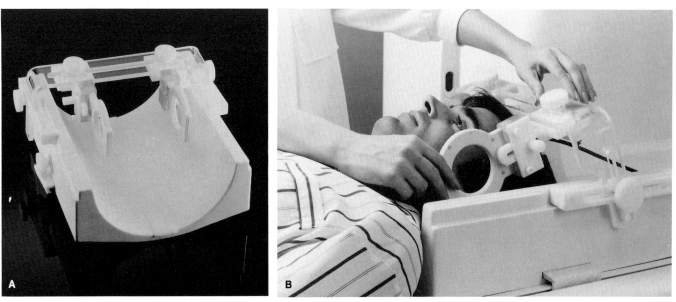

FIGURE 9–2. (**A**) Dual 3-in diameter surface coils and holder. (**B**) Proper patient positioning for use of the imaging coils.

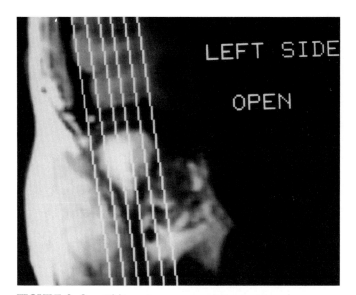

FIGURE 9–3. Oblique image prescriptions are made on a coronal localizer parallel with the mandibular condyle.

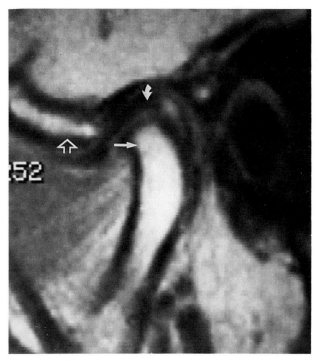

FIGURE 9–4. A T1-weighted sagittal image shows high signal intensity yellow marrow in the articular eminence (*open arrow*) and mandibular condyle (*straight arrow*). The posterior band is located in the expected position, superior to the condylar head (*curved arrow*). (TR, 1000 msec; TE, 40 msec.)

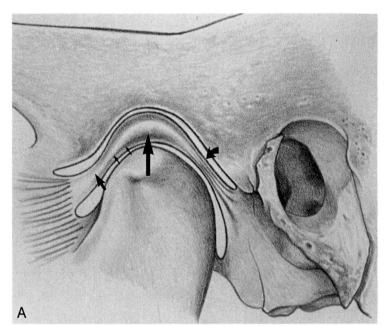

A

FIGURE 9–5. (**A**) In normal relationships of the temporomandibular joint meniscus to joint landmarks in the closed-mouth position, the posterior band (*large arrow*) is in the 12-o'clock position, superior to the condylar head; the intermediate zone (*small arrows*) is between the articular eminence and the condylar head; and the anterior band (*medium arrow*) is anterior to the condyle and attached to the lateral pterygoid muscle. The bilaminar attachment is seen posteriorly (*curved arrow*). (**B**) A gross anatomic section in the open-mouth position reveals the thick posterior band (*large arrow*), the thin intermediate zone (*small arrows*), and the anterior band (*medium arrow*).

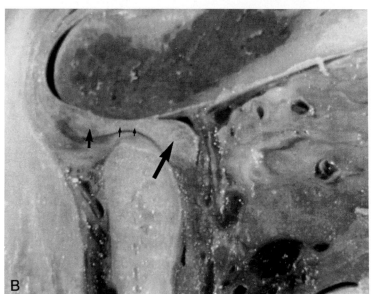

B

FIGURE 9–6. On a T1-weighted image, an intact temporomandibular joint meniscus appears as a central region of intermediate signal intensity in the posterior band (*vertical arrow*). The anterior band demonstrates uniform dark signal intensity (*horizontal arrow*). (TR, 600 msec; TE, 20 msec.)

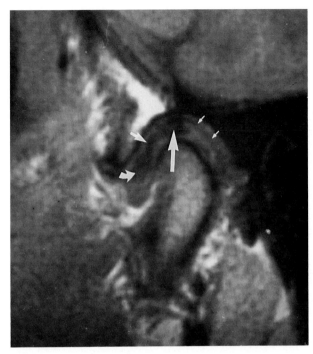

FIGURE 9–7. A T1-weighted image of normal meniscus anatomy shows the anterior band (*curved arrow*), intermediate zone (*medium straight arrow*), posterior band (*large straight arrow*), and a low signal intensity band within the bilaminar zone (*small straight arrows*). (TR, 600 msec; TE, 20 msec.)

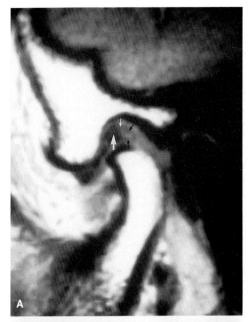

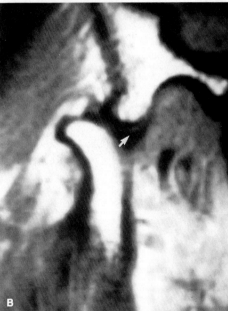

FIGURE 9–8. Disc anatomy. (**A**) The posterior band (*large white arrow*) is in the 11-o'clock position with the patient in the closed-mouth position. A vertical transition between the posterior band and the bilaminar zone can be seen (*small white arrow*). The locations of the superior and inferior bilaminar fibers are shown (*small black arrows*). (**B**) Normal anterior translation of the condyle relative to articular eminence occurs in the open-mouth (30-mm) position. The posterior band (*arrow*) can be seen.

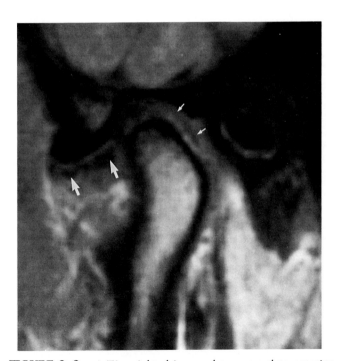

FIGURE 9–9. A T1-weighted image shows complete anterior displacement of the temporomandibular joint meniscus (*large arrows*). The anterior band, intermediate zone, and posterior band are all anterior to the condylar head. The retrodiscal bilaminar zone (*small arrows*) is seen. (TR, 600 msec; TE, 20 msec.)

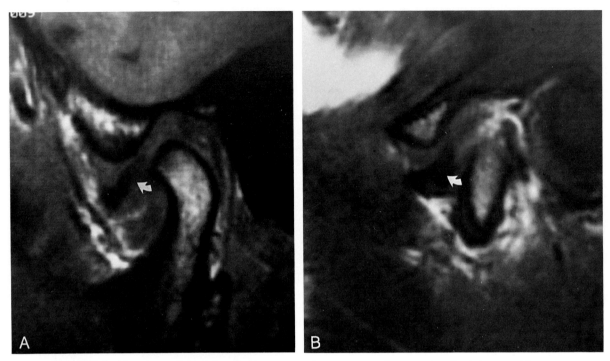

FIGURE 9–10. Anterolateral disc displacement is less common than anterior displacement. The meniscus (*curved arrows*) is located (**A**) anterior and (**B**) medial to the condylar head.

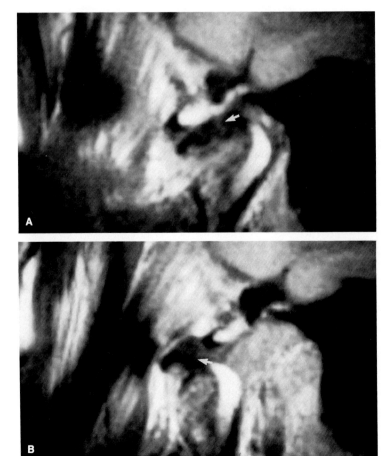

FIGURE 9–11. Anterior disc (*i.e.,* meniscus) displacement is seen in (**A**) closed- and (**B**) open-mouth positions. Secondary changes of disc remodeling with disc flexion, intermediate zone shortening, and enlargement of the posterior band (*arrows*) are present. Intermediate signal intensity in the area of the posterior band represents fibrosis, myxomatous change, and fluid.

The Temporomandibular Joint

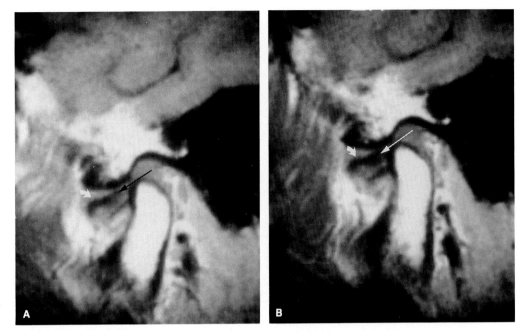

FIGURE 9–12. Remodeling of anterior disc displacement has occurred. Irreducible anterior disc displacement (*straight arrow*) is seen in (**A**) closed- and (**B**) open-mouth positions. Note the limitation of anterior translation relative to the articular eminence. Remodeling, foreshortening, and upward flexion of the intermediate zone (*curved arrow*) are present.

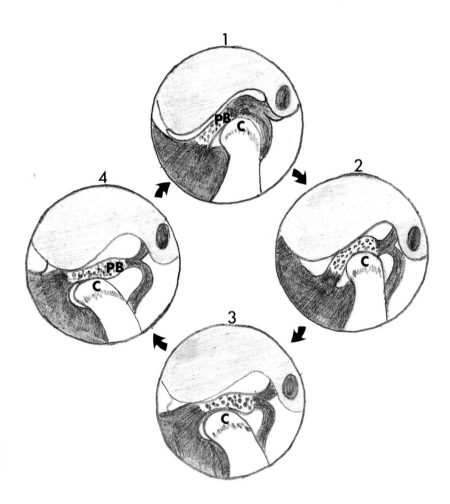

FIGURE 9–13. The progressive stages (1–4) of condylar translation, with anterior displaced disc (3) and recapture (4). (PB, posterior band; C, condylar head.)

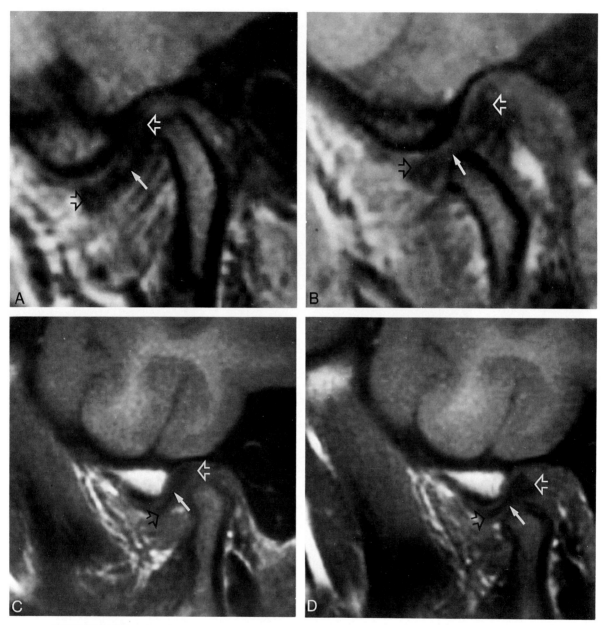

FIGURE 9–14. (**A, C**) Two examples of anterior displaced temporomandibular joint meniscus as seen in the closed-mouth position. (**B, D**) Recapture of the disc occurs in the open-mouth position. The anterior band (*open black arrow*), intermediate zone (*solid arrow*), and posterior band (*open white arrow*) are seen. In the closed-mouth position, the posterior band is anterior to the condylar head. In the open-mouth position with reduction, the posterior band is directly superior to the condylar head.

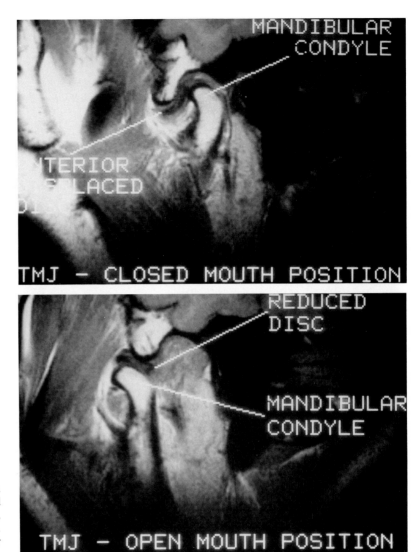

FIGURE 9–15. (**A**) Closed- and (**B**) open-mouth positions showing reduction of the anterior displaced disc. The bilaminar zone is in the 12-o'clock position, the expected normal location of the posterior band. There is adequate anterior translation of the condylar head.

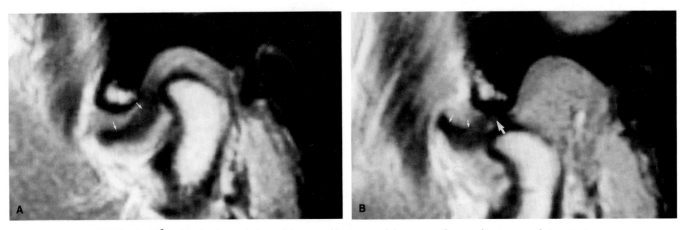

FIGURE 9–16. Blocked translation of the mandibular condyle occurred secondary to complete anterior disc displacement (*small arrows*), as seen in (**A**) closed- and (**B**) open-mouth positions. A portion of disc tissue (*large arrow*) is identified between the articular eminence and condylar head in the attempted open-mouth position. The bilaminar zone is stretched (*curved arrow*) and no opening click was present during mouth opening.

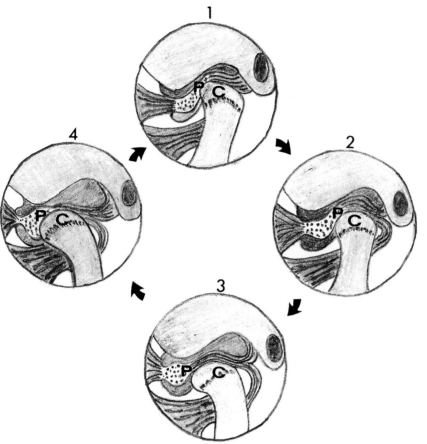

FIGURE 9–17. An anterior displaced disc is seen in (1) closed- and (4) open-mouth positions without recapture. Deformity of the disc occurs with progressive anterior translation (1–4). (P, posterior band; C, condylar head.)

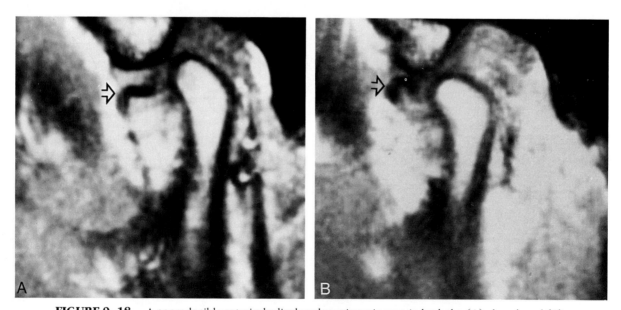

FIGURE 9–18. A nonreducible anteriorly displaced meniscus is seen in both the (**A**) closed- and (**B**) open-mouth positions. Limited condylar translation and deformity of the meniscus is demonstrated in the open-mouth image. Loss of normal biconcave disc morphology and irregular folding in the anterior portion (*i.e.,* intermediate zone; *arrow*) have taken place.

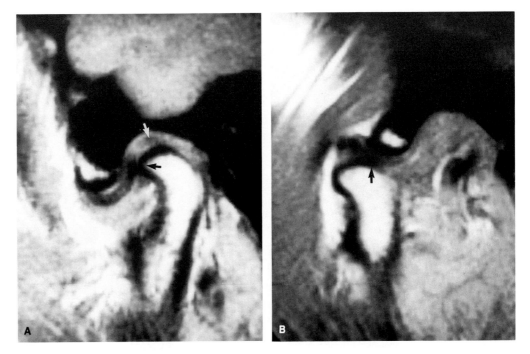

FIGURE 9–19. (**A**) An anteriorly displaced disc (*black arrow*) is seen in the closed-mouth position with early remodeling and thickening of the bilaminar zone (*white arrow*). (**B**) The disc is reduced in the open-mouth position (*arrow*).

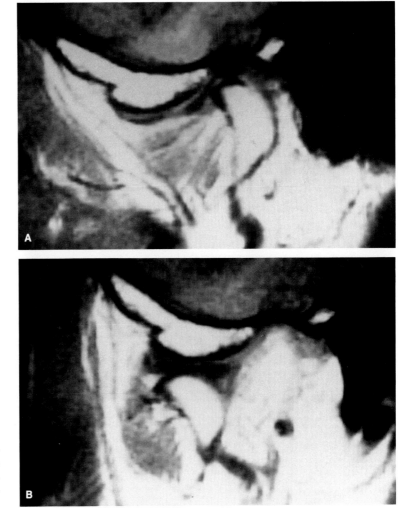

FIGURE 9–20. A grade zero disc shows normal morphology and position of the anterior band, the intermediate zone, and the posterior band in the (**A**) closed- and (**B**) open-mouth positions. Grading of disc displacement is independent of disc recapture.

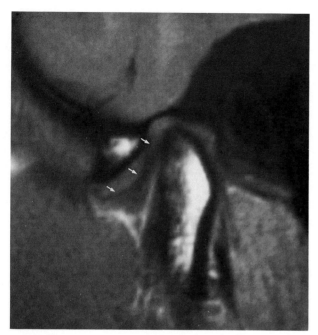

FIGURE 9–21. A T1-weighted image shows grade 1 displacement of the disc with intact morphology (*arrows*). (TR, 600 msec; TE, 20 msec.)

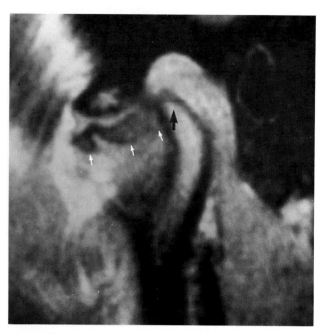

FIGURE 9–22. A grade 1 displacement of the disc (*white arrows*) may show grossly intact morphology, although the intermediate zone is flexed and foreshortened. The condylar head with overlying retrodiscal tissue (*black arrow*) is seen. Normal intermediate signal intensity is present in the posterior band.

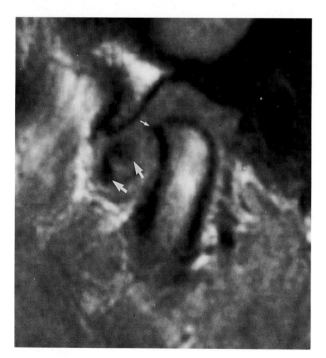

FIGURE 9–23. Grade 2 meniscal derangement with complete loss of normal morphology is seen on a T1-weighted image. The meniscus is redundantly compressed anterior to the condylar head (*large arrows*). Associated degenerative change is seen as a low signal intensity anterior osteophyte (*small arrow*). (TR, 600 msec; TE, 20 msec.)

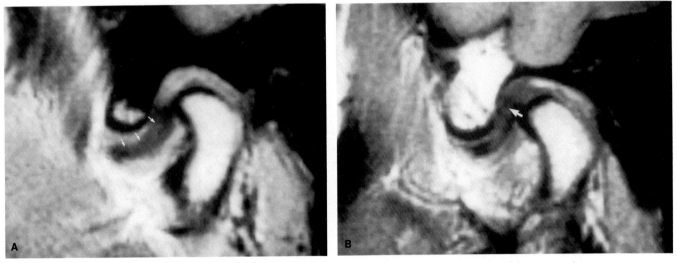

FIGURE 9–24. (**A**) Acute anterior disc displacement (*arrow*) is seen in closed-mouth centric occlusion, in which there is maximal intercuspation (*i.e.,* contact) between opposing occlusal surfaces (*arrows*). (**B**) The posterior band is in its normal location when the patient is in the open-mouth position. Normal disc morphology is maintained in closed- and open-mouth positions.

FIGURE 9–25. (**A**) Subacute anterior disc displacement (*arrows*) with mild folding of the intermediate zone is seen in the closed-mouth position. (**B**) The disc is not recaptured in the open-mouth position (*arrow*).

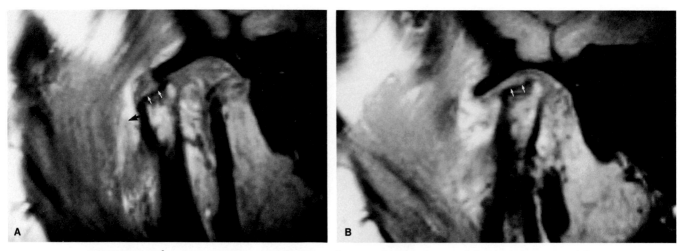

FIGURE 9–26.   Degenerative osteoarthritis results in an absent–macerated disc with flattening of the condylar head (*white arrows*) and subchondral low signal intensity sclerosis, as seen in the (**A**) closed- and (**B**) open-mouth positions. Anterior translation is unimpeded (*black arrow*) due to the absent disc.

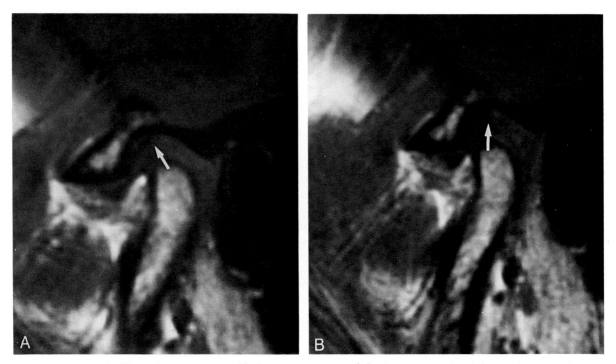

FIGURE 9–27.   The temporomandibular joint meniscus. (**A**) The posterior band (*arrows*) is seen anterior to the condylar head without the internal splint (*i.e.,* mild anterior displacement). (**B**) With insertion of the internal splint, the posterior band is positioned directly superior to the condylar head.

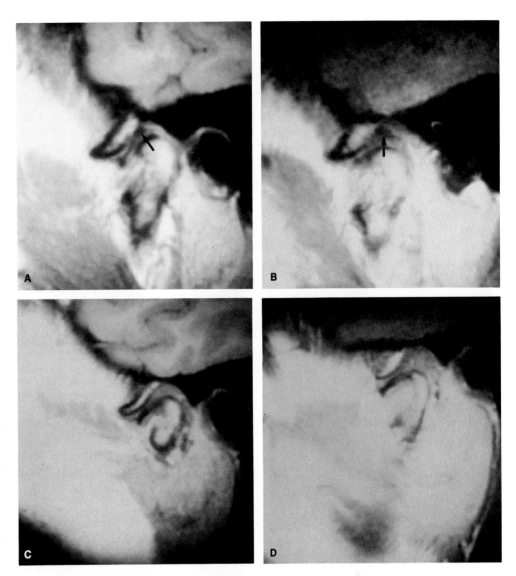

FIGURE 9–28. (**A**) The posterior band (*arrow*) is an anterior position in the left temporomandibular joint in a patient in the closed-mouth position without splint. (**B**) The posterior band (*arrow*) is relocated to the 12-o'clock position in the left temporomandibular joint after placement of an internal splint. In the right temporomandibular joint, the disc appears in an anterior position both (**C**) without and (**D**) with an internal splint.

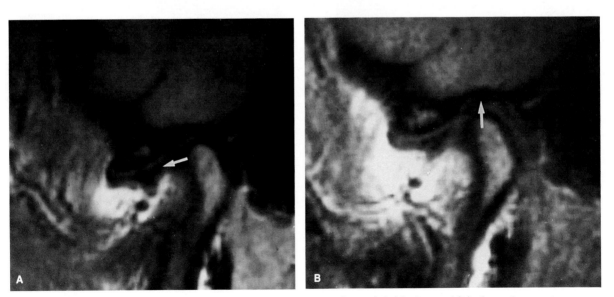

FIGURE 9–29. The temporomandibular joint meniscus (*arrow*) (**A**) before and (**B**) after arthroscopic saline reduction.

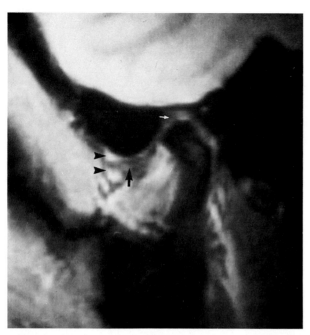

FIGURE 9–30. A T2*-weighted image produces high signal intensity in engorged veins (*black arrowheads*) in the lateral pterygoid attachment (*black arrow*) to the temporomandibular joint meniscus. The intact posterior band is seen superior to the condylar head between the 11- and 12-o'clock positions (*white arrow*). (TR, 400 msec; TE, 30 msec; flip angle, 30°.)

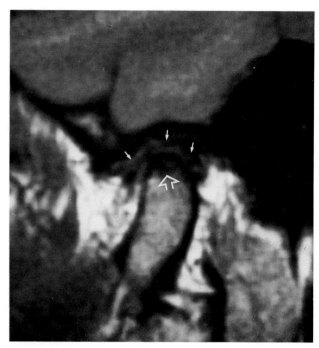

FIGURE 9–31. A focus of low signal intensity subchondral sclerosis is seen (*open arrow*) in an image of postsurgical primary plication of the temporomandibular joint meniscus in the normal position (*small arrows*).

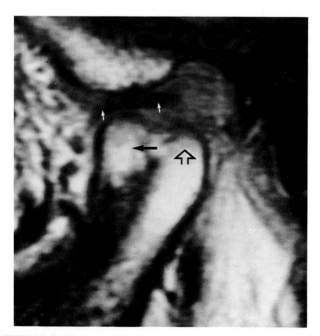

FIGURE 9–32. Pseudo-double-condyle is seen in post-traumatic fracture of the mandibular condyle with displacement of the articular head (*solid black arrow*) anterior to the condylar neck (*open black arrow*). The associated temporomandibular joint meniscus is seen (*white arrows*).

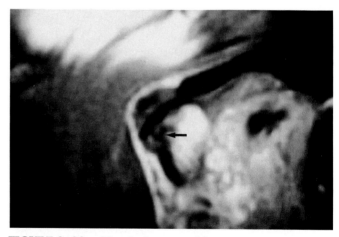

FIGURE 9–33. Mixed sclerosis and fat marrow signal intensity (*arrow*) are seen in a large anterior condylar osteophyte.

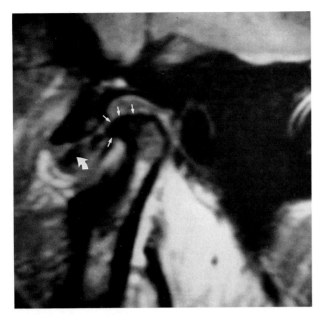

FIGURE 9–34. A large anterior osteophyte (*straight arrows*) demonstrates low signal intensity. Associated anterior meniscal displacement is also present (*curved arrow*).

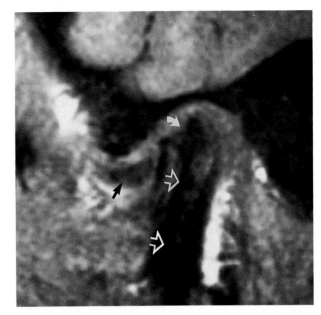

FIGURE 9–35. Degenerative sclerosis (*open arrows*) demonstrates low signal intensity in the mandibular condyle. The anterior displaced meniscus (*black arrow*) and articular head deformity (*curved arrow*) are shown.

images. On T2-weighted images, hyperplastic synovium and pannus demonstrate intermediate signal intensity, not the high signal intensity seen with associated fluid.

Rarely, the TMJ is involved with cartilaginous metaplasia in synovial chondromatosis.[31] Magnetic resonance images are characterized by small calcifications and an associated soft-tissue mass in the presence of synovial chondromatosis.

REFERENCES

1. Jacobs JM, Manaster BJ. Digital subtraction arthrography of the temporomandibular joint. AJR 1987;148:344.
2. Kaplan PA, et al. Inferior joint space arthrography of normal temporomandibular joints: reassessment of diagnostic criteria. Radiology 1986;159:585.
3. Kaplan PA, et al. Temporomandibular joint arthrography following surgical treatment of internal derangements. Radiology 1987;163:217.
4. Kaplan PA, et al. Temporomandibular joint arthrography of normal subjects: prevalence of pain with ionic versus nonionic contrast agents. Radiology 1985;156:825.
5. Katzberg RW, et al. Temporomandibular joint arthrography: comparison of morbidity with ionic and low osmolality contrast media. Radiology 1985;155:245.
6. Ross JB. Arthrography compared with MRI for TMJ intracapsular soft tissue diagnosis. TMJ Update 1989;7:31.
7. Duvoisin B, Klaus E, Schnyder P. Coronal radiographs and video-fluoroscopy improve the diagnostic quality of temporomandibular joint arthrography. AJR 1990;155:105.
8. Christiansen EL, et al. Correlative thin section temporomandibular joint anatomy and computed tomography. RadioGraphics 1986;6:703.
9. Christiansen EL, et al. CT number characteristics of malpositioned TMJ menisci: diagnosis with CT number highlighting (blink-mode). Invest Radiol 1987;22:315.
10. Larheim TA, Kolbenstvedt A. High resolution computed tomography of the osseous temporomandibular joint. Radiology 1985;157:573.
11. Swartz JD, et al. High-resolution computed tomography, part 5: evaluation of the temporomandibular joint. Radiology 1986;159:823.
12. Manco LG, et al. Internal derangements of the temporomandibular joint evaluated with direct sagittal CT: prospective study. Radiology 1985;157:407.
13. Helms CA, Kaplan P. Diagnostic imaging of the temporomandibular joint: recommendations for use of various techniques. AJR 1990;154:319-322.
14. Kneeland JB, et al. High-resolution MR imaging using loop-gap resonators. Radiology 1986;158:247.
15. Middleton WD, et al. High resolution surface coil magnetic resonance imaging of the joints: anatomic correlation. RadioGraphics 1987;7:645.
16. Helms CA, et al. Magnetic resonance imaging of internal derangement of the temporomandibular joint. Radiol Clin North Am 1986;24:189.
17. Harms SE, Wilf RM. Magnetic resonance imaging of the temporomandibular joint. RadioGraphics 1987;7:521.
18. Katzberg RW, et al. Normal and abnormal temporomandibular joint: MR imaging with surface coil. Radiology 1986;158:183.
19. Westesson P, et al. Temporomandibular joint: comparison of MR images with cryosectional anatomy. Radiology 1987;164:59.
20. Robers D, et al. Temporomandibular joint: magnetic resonance imaging. Radiology 1985;154:829.
21. Harms SE, et al. Temporomandibular joint: magnetic resonance imaging using surface coils. Radiology 1985;157:133.
22. Laurell KA, et al. Magnetic resonance imaging of the temporo-

mandibular joint, part I: literature review. J Prosthet Dent 1987;58:83.

23. Kaplan P, Helms C. Current status of temporomandibular joint imaging for the diagnosis of internal derangements. AJR 1989;152:697.

24. Hansson L, Westesson P, Katzberg RW, et al. MR imaging of the temporomandibular joint: comparison of images of autopsy specimens made at 0.3 T and 1.5 T with anatomic cryosections. AJR 1989;152.

25. Fulmer JM, Harms SE. The temporomandibular joint. Top Magn Reson Imag 1989;1(3):75.

26. Rao VM, Farole A, Karasick D. Temporomandibular joint dysfunction: correlation of MR imaging, arthrography, and arthroscopy. Radiology 1990;174:663.

27. Burnett KR, et al. Dynamic display of the temporomandibular joint meniscus by using "fast-scan" MR imaging. AJR 1987;149:959.

28. Stoller DW, et al. Fast MR improves imaging of the musculoskeletal system. Diagnostic Imaging 1988;:98.

29. Manco LG, DeLuke DM. CT diagnosis of synovial chondromatosis of the temporomandibular joint. AJR 1987;148:574.

30. Kneeland JB, et al. Failed temporomandibular joint prostheses: MR imaging. Radiology 1987;165:179.

31. Nokes ST, et al. Temporomandibular joint chondromatosis with intracranial extension: MR and CT contributions. AJR 1987;148:1173.

32. Murphy WA. The temporomandibular joint. In: Resnick D, Niwayama G, eds. Diagnosis of bone and joint disorders. 2nd ed. vol. 3. Philadelphia: WB Saunders, 1988.

33. Schellhas KP. Temporomandibular joint injuries. Radiology 1989;173:211.

34. Larheim TA, Smith HJ, Aspestrand F. Rheumatic disease of the temporomandibular joint: MR imaging and tomographic manifestations. Radiology 1990;175:527.

35. Schellhas KP, Wilkes C. Temporomandibular joint inflammation: comparison of MR fast scanning with T1- and T2-weighted imaging techniques. AJR 1989;153:93.

36. Shannon M, et al. MR of the normal temporomandibular joint. In: Palacios E, et al, eds. Magnetic resonance of the temporomandibular joint. Stuttgart/New York: Thieme, 1990:48.

37. Katzberg RW, Westesson P, Rallents RH, et al. Temporomandibular joint: MR assessment of rotational and sideways disc displacements. Radiology 1988;169:741.

38. Scapino RP. Histopathology of the disc and posterior displacement in disc displacement internal derangements of the TMJ. In: Palacios E, et al, eds. Magnetic resonance of the temporomandibular joint. Stuttgart/New York: Thieme, 1990:63.

39. Wilk RM, Harms SE. Temporomandibular joint: multislab, three-dimensional Fourier transform MR imaging. Radiology 1988;167:861.

40. Hardy CJ, et al. Simultaneous MR image acquisition with electronically decoupled surface receiver coils. Radiology 1987;165:91.

41. Harms SE, et al. Specialized receiver coils for bilateral MR imaging examinations of the temporomandibular joint. Radiology 1987;165:159.

42. Drace JE, Enzmann DR. Defining the normal temporomandibular joint: closed-, partially open-, and open-mouth MR imaging of asymptomatic subjects. Radiology 1990;177:67.

43. Drace J, Enzmann DR. MR imaging of the temporomandibular joint (TMJ): closed-, partially open-, and open-mouth views of the abnormal TMJ. Radiology 1987;165:149.

44. Helms CA, et al. Staging of internal derangements of the temporomandibular joint with MR imaging, and optimal mouth position for diagnosis. Radiology 1987;165:149.

45. Drace JE, Young SW, Enzmann DR. TMJ meniscus and bilaminar zone: MR imaging of the substructure—diagnostic landmarks and pitfalls of interpretation. Radiology 1990;177:73.

46. Schwaighofer BW, Tanaka TT, Klein MV, et al. MR imaging of the temporomandibular joint: a cadaver study of the value of coronal images. AJR 1990;154:1245.

47. Katzberg RW, et al. Magnetic resonance imaging of the temporomandibular joint meniscus. Oral Surg Oral Med Oral Pathol 1985;59:332.

48. Schellhas KP, et al. Temporomandibular joint: diagnosis of internal derangements using magnetic resonance imaging. Minn Med 1986;69:519.

49. Cirbus MT, et al. Magnetic resonance imaging in confirming internal derangement of the temporomandibular joint. J Prosthet Dent 1987;57:487.

50. Palacios E, et al. Internal derangement and other pathology in magnetic resonance imaging of the temporomandibular joint. In: Palacios E, et al, eds. Magnetic resonance of the temporomandibular joint. Stuttgart/New York: Thieme, 1990:75.

51. Helms CA, Doyle GW, Orwig D, et al. Staging of internal derangements of the TMJ with magnetic resonance imaging: preliminary observations. Journal of Craniomandibular Disorders 1989;3(2):93.

52. Helms CA, Kaban LB, McNeil C, et al. Temporomandibular joint: morphology and signal intensity characteristics of the disc at MR imaging. Radiology 1989;172:817.

53. Hasso AN, Christiansen EL, Alder ME. The temporomandibular joint. Radiol Clin N Amer 1989;27:301.

54. Kneeland JB, et al. MR imaging of a fractured temporomandibular disc prosthesis. J Comput Assist Tomogr 1987;11:199.

55. Schellhas KP, et al. Temporomandibular joint: MR imaging of internal derangements and postoperative changes. AJR 1988;150:381.

56. Schellhas KP, Wilkes CH, el Deeb M, et al. Permanent proplast temporomandibular joint implants: MR imaging of destructive complications. AJR 1988;15:731.

57. Katzberg RW, et al. Dislocation of jaws. Radiology 1985;154:556.

58. Kononen M. Radiographic changes in the condyle of the temporomandibular joint in psoriatic arthritis. Acta Radiol 1987;28:185.

Kinematic Magnetic Resonance Imaging

Although the application of static-view magnetic resonance (MR) imaging has been extremely beneficial for assessing abnormalities of the joints, patients frequently present with arthralgia associated with particular positions, movements, or forceful loading of the joint; the causes of these problems may not be identifiable in a routine MR examination. Therefore, in addition to determining the presence of an anatomic abnormality, it may be necessary to evaluate functional aspects of the joint using kinematic MR imaging.

Kinematics is the science of motion; the term is applied to the study of body movement without reference to force or mass.[1] Kinematic MR imaging involves evaluation of various interactions of the important soft tissue and bony anatomic features that comprise a joint, as well as the relative alignment of these structures through a specific range of motion.[2] Kinematic MR imaging provides the clinician with an augmented data base of anatomic and movement-related information.

Kinematic MR imaging protocols have been used most effectively to evaluate the temporomandibular and patellofemoral joints.[2-13] Studies to define the role of this diagnostic technique in assessment of the wrist and ankle have begun to appear.[14-16] This chapter reviews the application of kinematic MR imaging for these four joints, describes normal joint kinematics, and illustrates the use of this imaging technique for diagnosis or elucidation of various pathologic conditions.

THE TEMPOROMANDIBULAR JOINT

The inability of MR imaging to provide a functional assessment of jaw biomechanics and meniscocondylar coordination was initially seen as a limitation of this imaging technique for evaluating temporomandibular joint (TMJ) dysfunction. Therefore, one of the first applications of kinematic MR imaging was in assessment of the TMJ at different increments of mouth opening. This technique has proven to be extremely valuable in the examination of the TMJ.[3-7]

Kinematic Magnetic Resonance Protocol

Functional abnormalities that affect the TMJ are primarily associated with the position of the disc relative to the mandibular condyle. Kinematic MR images obtained with T1-weighted (*i.e.,* short echo time [TE], short repetition time [TR]) pulse sequences best depict the meniscocondylar orientations through the range of motion of this joint.[6,7] Partial flip angle or "fast-scan" pulse sequences have also been proposed for kinematic studies,[3] but these techniques have intrinsically poor spatial resolution and are more susceptible to artifacts.[6,7] Typically, the T1-weighted images obtained for kinematic MR study of the TMJ are of sufficiently high quality to demonstrate important anatomic features of the joint as well as provide functional assessment.[6]

The high incidence of bilateral abnormalities in patients with internal derangements of the TMJ makes it advisable to perform kinematic MR imaging on both joints to thoroughly examine patients with TMJ dysfunction. This is optimally accomplished with dual 3-in circular surface coils, which provide an adequate signal-to-noise ratio for imaging this small joint (Fig. 10–1). The use of dual surface coils also permits images to be obtained simultaneously from both the right and left TMJs so a direct comparison may be made between the two joints at the same relative degree of mouth opening. This is especially important for identifying motion-related abnormalities such as lateral deviation and asymmetrical movement.[5,6]

The mandibular condyle is positioned at oblique angles in both the sagittal and coronal planes.[17] Investigations have demonstrated that the best orientation for images of the TMJ is with reference to the long axis of the condylar head, because a significant number of both normal individuals and patients have abnormally configured condyles with respect to size, shape, and orientation.[17] Therefore, slice locations for kinematic MR imaging of the TMJ should be determined by the user and selected in planes that are perpendicular (*i.e.,* oblique sagittals) to the long axis of the condylar head, as viewed in an axial plane localizer scan (Fig. 10–2). This not only provides standardized and consistent information, but also decreases scan time, because only the slice locations from the anatomic regions of interest are obtained.

To obtain diagnostic information related to the movement of the TMJ, a nonferromagnetic positioning device (Medrad, Pittsburgh, PA; Fig. 10–3) is used to passively open the patient's mouth at predetermined increments. Magnetic resonance imaging is then performed at each position. Prior to kinematic MR imaging study, the range of motion for each patient is determined by having the patient open his or her mouth as wide as possible, with the positioning device in place, without forcing the joint or causing pain. This procedure is repeated three times, and the average range of motion is calculated for each patient. The increments of opening are then based on this information.

Two or three thin slice (≤3-mm) images are acquired through the TMJ in the oblique sagittal plane at the following mouth positions:

Closed mouth (*i.e.,* maximum intercuspation of the teeth).
Closed mouth with the positioning device in place. The distance the patient's mouth is opened at this increment is dependent on the length of the incisors.
Repeatedly at progressive increments of opening using 20% intervals of the range of motion until the full open-mouth position is attained.

Total imaging time for a kinematic MR study of the bilateral TMJs takes approximately 15 minutes using the following protocol:

- dual 3-in surface coils
- TR of 600 msec
- TE of 20 msec
- acquisition matrix of 128 × 256
- 10-cm field of view (FOV)
- 3-mm slice thickness
- 0.5-mm interslice gap
- 1 excitation (NEX)
- 6 slice locations—three through each condylar head
- 7 different increments.

Images may be viewed individually or displayed as a cine loop using commercially available software commonly found on MR scanners. For cine loop display, the slice locations (obtained through each TMJ at the same location) that best depict the meniscus, condyle, glenoid fossa, and articular eminence are selected and displayed at a user-controlled speed. The cine loop may be recorded on videotape and sent to the referring clinician.

Normal Kinematics

The normal anatomic features of the TMJ are reviewed in Chapter 9. When the mouth is closed, the meniscus is positioned such that the posterior band is in a 12-o'clock position (±10%) relative to the condylar head (Fig. 10–4).[18] As the mouth opens, the condyle rotates anteriorly and moves onto the intermediate zone of the meniscus. The condyle remains positioned on the intermediate zone as the mouth continues to open, and translates anteriorly until it reaches the base of the articular eminence or slightly anterior to this position. The appearance of this entire movement in kinematic MR imaging is that of rotation and then free gliding or smooth anterior translation of the condylar head (see Fig. 10–4).

Pathology

Kinematic MR imaging provides useful diagnostic information for a range of TMJ abnormalities of varying degrees of severity. The internal derangements best evaluated by kinematic MR imaging are usually anterior displacements of the meniscus. However, abnormal movements of the mandible are also easily identified.[4-7]

Anterior Displacement of the Meniscus With Reduction

In evaluating the TMJ with an anteriorly displaced meniscus, many clinicians believe that it is important to determine whether or not the meniscus resumes its normal orientation relative to the mandibular condyle with the mouth open (*i.e.,* reduction of an anteriorly displaced meniscus). By using kinematic MR imaging evaluation of the TMJ and viewing the joint at different increments between closed and fully opened positions of the mouth, it is possible to ascertain if there is reduction of the meniscus, and the relative position of the mandible at the point it occurs (Fig. 10–5). This information is helpful in the correct application of splint therapy, which is frequently used to treat anterior displacements of the meniscus.[19,20] If splint therapy is not properly applied, the internal derangement of the TMJ may progress or, at the least, may not be corrected.[19,20] Recapture of an anteriorly displaced meniscus may occur at any point in the range of motion of the TMJ. Anteriorly displaced menisci that reduce early are considered less severe than those that reduce late.

Anterior Displacement of the Meniscus Without Reduction

A more severe form of internal derangement of the TMJ is an anterior displacement of the meniscus that is not recaptured. In this case, kinematic MR imaging typically demonstrates a markedly displaced meniscus that becomes distorted during mouth-opening and is often associated with a limited range of motion of the joint as well as severe laxity of meniscal attachments and/or tears of associated soft-tissue structures (Fig. 10–6). Other joint abnormalities, such as osteophytes, adhesions, and degenerative arthritis (Fig. 10–7), may also be found with this more advanced stage of TMJ dysfunction. Treatment of anterior displacements of the menisci that do not reduce often requires surgery. Therefore, kinematic MR differentiation between the meniscus that is recaptured late and the meniscus that is not recaptured in the full open-mouth position is especially useful.

Asymmetrical Motion Abnormalities

Since the mandible has a bilateral articulation with the cranium, both TMJs should function synchronously; any disordered movement is regarded as an abnormality.[5,17] Kinematic MR imaging is extremely useful for identifying and characterizing the extent of any asymmetrical motion that may affect this joint.[5]

As mentioned above, in normal kinematic MR imaging of the TMJ, initial rotation of the condylar head takes place, followed by smooth translation. Asymmetrical motion may take the form of lateral deviations with opening and closing of the mouth, as well as other more peculiar movements. For example, there may be progressive anterior translation of one condyle while the other moves in a retrograde manner (Fig. 10–8). Asymmetric motion of the TMJ may be caused by muscle spasm, shortened or atrophic muscles, fibrous adhesions, fibrotic contractures, or by other mechanisms. In addition, associated displacements of the meniscus, as well as degenerative alterations in the bony anatomy, may or may not be present.

THE PATELLOFEMORAL JOINT

Abnormalities of the patellofemoral joint are a major cause of knee pain and occur as frequently as meniscal lesions.[21-23] Patellar malalignment and its associated sequelae is the primary pathologic entity that affects the patellofemoral joint. The diagnosis of patellofemoral incongruence by physical examination alone is extremely difficult, because the clinical signs may mimic other forms of internal derangements of the knee, and there is a high incidence of combined abnormalities.[21,23,24] In addition, patients whose symptoms persist after patellar realignment surgery present a particular diagnostic challenge.[2,12] Therefore, a kinematic MR imaging technique was developed and implemented to identify and characterize abnormal functional aspects of the patellofemoral joint. Since most abnormalities occur during the early degrees of flexion, and kinematic MR imaging is able to evaluate patellar alignment and tracking during these initial increments, it is considered to be an extremely sensitive and effective diagnostic method of examining the patellofemoral joint.

Kinematic Magnetic Resonance Protocol

Positioning for the kinematic MR study is accomplished with a patient-activated, nonferromagnetic device (Fig. 10–9), designed to allow simultaneous axial imaging of bilateral patellofemoral joints from extension to 30° of flexion at 5° increments. The patient is placed in a prone position on the device, with special care taken to position the lower extremities so that alignment is maintained. This positioning scheme does not inhibit rotational movements of the lower extremities during flexion of the patellofemoral joint, which is important because excessive internal or external rotation may be partially responsible for abnormal patellar alignment. The kinematics of the patellofemoral joint are comparable in the prone and supine positions (Fig. 10–10).

Using the body coil of the MR scanner, T1-weighted spin-echo axial images are obtained with the following protocol:

- TR of 500 ms
- TE of 20 msec
- 0.5 NEX
- 256 × 128 acquisition matrix
- 40-cm FOV
- 5-mm slice thickness
- 0.5-mm interslice gap
- 9 slice locations.

Using these imaging parameters, kinematic MR imaging of the patellofemoral joint usually takes 34 seconds per acquisition. These parameters provide good anatomic detail so that the relationship of the patella to the femoral trochlear groove can be assessed. In addition, the data acquisition time is kept to a minimum. Ultrafast imaging techniques allow for dynamic patellofemoral tracking with active knee flexion and extension (Fig. 10–11; see Future Directions).

After completion of the scan, the patient is instructed to adjust the handle on the positioning device to move to the next increment of joint flexion. In this manner, seven different flexion positions of the patellofemoral joint are acquired at several different slice locations through the joint. The total examination time using these parameters is approximately 15 minutes.

Slice locations obtained with the patellofemoral joint in the extended position are carefully inspected to assess the anatomic features of the joint. The images obtained during extension are also useful for identifying patella alta and patella baja, since the position of the patella, particularly its inferior pole, is clearly demonstrated relative to the femoral trochlear groove (Fig. 10–12).

For kinematic MR evaluation, patellar alignment is assessed, and the positions at which the patella articulates with the femoral trochlear groove or femoral trochlea are tracked. Three to four different slice locations through the femoral trochlear groove or femoral trochlea (depending on the position of the patella) at 5° to 30° of flexion are evaluated to thoroughly determine all kinematic aspects of the patellofemoral joint. Cine loop display is preferable to individual static images of patellar alignment and tracking. Cine loop display optimally demonstrates various patterns of patellar motion and provides the best qualitative information regarding the patellofemoral joint.[2,9–12,25]

Normal Kinematics

Several methods for quantitative assessment of the position of the patella relative to the femoral trochlear groove have been proposed over the years. Most of these methods, however, were developed to assess single-view plain film radiographs of the patellofemoral joint,[23,26–29] and for various reasons are not useful for kinematic MR imaging. Qualitative cine loop data often provide more important information, because kinematic studies show the overall pattern of patellar motion.[2,9–12,25] In addition, there is no consensus on the usefulness of any of the various quantitative measurements in the identification of patellar malalignment, and reports indicate that even minor patellofemoral incongruence, within "normal" limits, can produce clinical symptoms.[30] To further complicate the situation, many patellofemoral joints have associated anatomic abnormalities (*e.g.,* structural irregularities of the patella or femoral trochlear groove, patella alta, patella baja) that preclude accurate assessment of patellar alignment using quantification schemes because there are no consistent landmarks for proper performance of the congruency measurements.[2,9–12,25] Therefore, it is more appropriate and practical to use qualitative criteria to describe the patella relative to the femoral trochlear groove or femoral trochlea during flexion of the patellofemoral joint.

In addition to evaluating patellar alignment and tracking, assessment of the bony and soft-tissue anatomy may provide indications of the mechanisms responsible for patellofemoral joint abnormalities. The patella articulates with the femoral trochlear groove during knee flexion; therefore, the congruous formation of the patella and femoral trochlear surfaces is especially important, because it produces a mechanical restraint to abnormal alignment and tracking. Inspection of the shapes of the patella and femoral trochlear groove may provide additional evidence concerning the presence of a patellofemoral disorder (Fig. 10–13); however, the existence of pathologic morphology does not preclude normal patellar alignment and tracking.

A variety of patellar forms are compatible with normal patellofemoral joint function, while others tend to be associated with patellar malalignment or dislocation. In addition, patellofemoral instability may be present when the patellar shape is normal, but the femoral trochlear groove is abnormal, or when the patella is positioned either too high or too low relative to the femoral trochlear groove.[22,28,31,32] The most commonly found patellar configurations considered to be normal include the Wiberg type I and II shapes. In the Wiberg type I patellar shape (Fig. 10–14), the lateral and medial facets are symmetrical. In the Wiberg type II patellar shape (Fig. 10–15), the lateral facet is longer than the medial facet. In the Wiberg type III patellar shape (Fig. 10–16), the lateral facet is dominant, and the medial facet is significantly smaller. Other patellar forms believed to be dysplastic (Figs. 10–17 and 10–18) are commonly observed in conjunction with patellofemoral arthrosis, chondromalacia, and recurrent dislocation.[22,28,31]

(text continues on page 842)

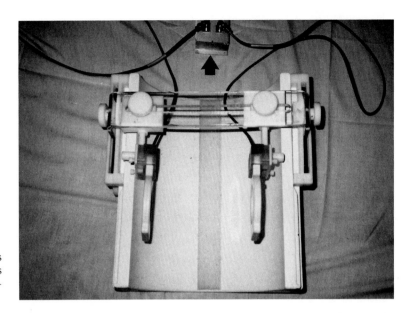

FIGURE 10–1. Dual 6.5-cm receive-only surface coils with a combiner box (*arrow*) are used for simultaneous high-resolution MR imaging of bilateral temporomandibular joints.

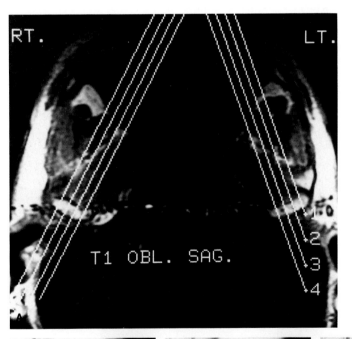

FIGURE 10–2. (**A**) An MR axial plane localizer is used to prescribe the oblique sagittal slice locations for kinematic MR imaging of the temporomandibular joint. The slice locations are selected in an orientation that is perpendicular to the long axis of the right and left condylar heads using graphic prescription software. (TR, 400 msec, TE, 20 msec; slice thickness, 5 mm.) (**B**) In an example of oblique sagittal plane images obtained for kinematic MR study of the temporomandibular joint, there is anterior displacement of the meniscus in the closed-mouth position (*arrow*). (**C, D**) In the subsequent images, reduction occurs during opening of the mouth as the condylar head moves onto the intermediate zone of the meniscus. (TR, 600 msec; TE, 20 msec; slice thickness, 3 mm.)

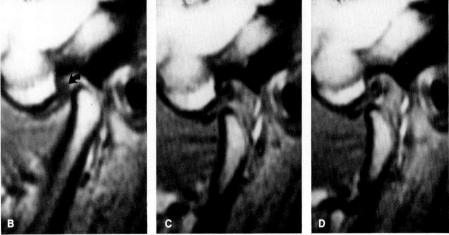

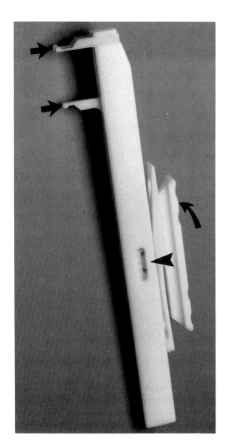

FIGURE 10–3. A special nonferromagnetic positioning device is used to open the patient's mouth at predetermined increments for kinematic MR imaging of the temporomandibular joint. A gauge (*arrowhead*) is used to determine the degree of mouth opening based on the distance between the disposable mouthpieces (*straight arrows*). Movement of the mouthpieces is controlled by pressing the patient-activated handle (*curved arrow*).

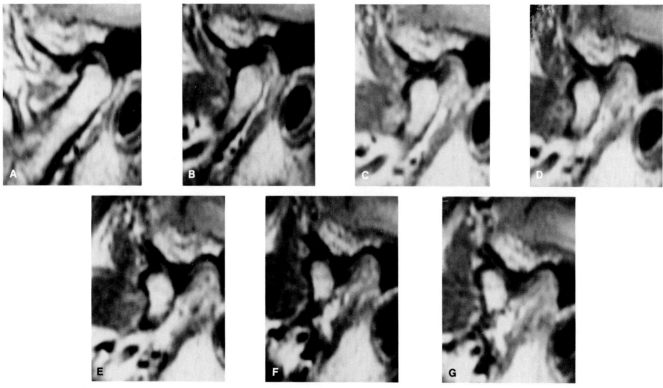

FIGURE 10–4. (**A**) In a kinematic study of the normal temporomandibular joint, the posterior band of the meniscus is in a 12-o'clock position relative to the condylar head in the closed-mouth position. (**B–G**) As the mouth progressively opens, the condyle moves onto the intermediate zone of the meniscus; this relative meniscocondylar relationship is maintained throughout the remaining range of motion of the joint as the condyle translates anteriorly. The range of motion in this subject was 48 mm; images were obtained in the oblique sagittal plane. (TR, 600 msec; TE, 20 msec; slice thickness, 3 mm.)

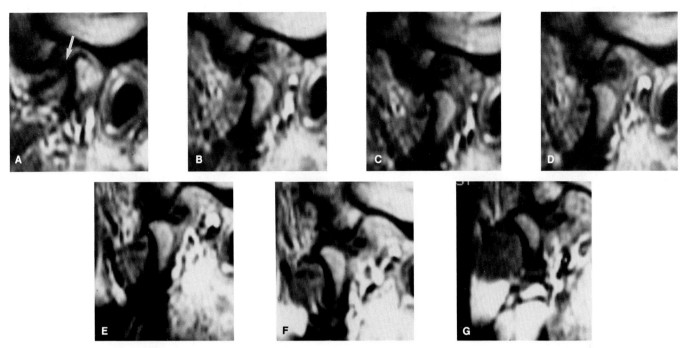

FIGURE 10-5. Anterior displacement of the meniscus with reduction. (**A**) The posterior band of the meniscus (*arrowhead*) is anteriorly displaced in the closed-mouth position. (**B–G**) As the mouth opens, the condylar head moves onto the intermediate zone of the meniscus and recaptures the meniscus. Images were obtained in the oblique sagittal plane. (TR, 600 msec; TE, 20 msec; slice thickness, 3 mm.)

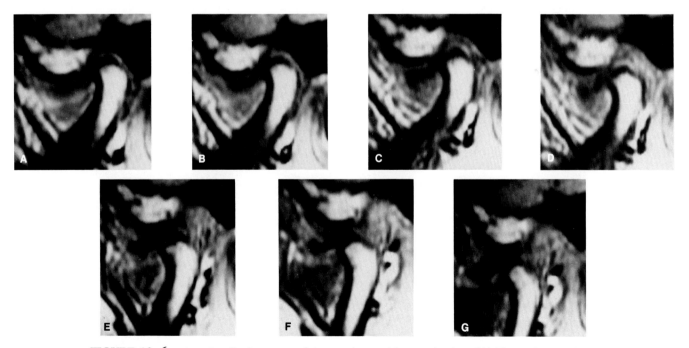

FIGURE 10-6. Anterior displacement of the meniscus without reduction. (**A**) The entire meniscus is anteriorly displaced relative to the condylar head in the closed-mouth position. (**B–G**) As the mouth opens, the condylar head translates anteriorly but does not recapture the meniscus. The meniscus remains in front of the condylar head during progressive positions of mouth opening. In addition, there is a limited range of motion of the joint. Images were obtained in the oblique sagittal plane. (TR, 600 msec; TE, 20 msec; slice thickness, 3 mm.)

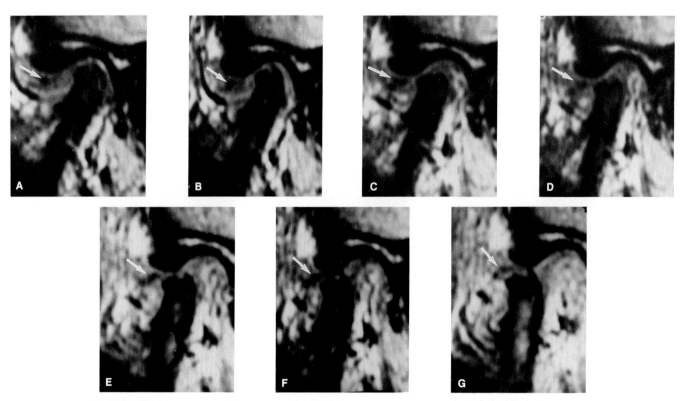

FIGURE 10–7. Anterior displacement of the meniscus without reduction and with advanced degenerative changes. (**A**) The entire meniscus (*arrow*) is anteriorly displaced in the closed-mouth position and appears to have lost its posterior attachment. (**B–G**) As the mouth opens, the condylar head translates anteriorly and the shape of the meniscus (*arrows*) appears to be distorted, as it remains in front of the condylar head. There is marked degeneration of the joint, and the bony anatomy is sclerotic. Images were obtained in the oblique sagittal plane. (TR, 600 msec; TE, 20 msec; slice thickness, 3 mm.)

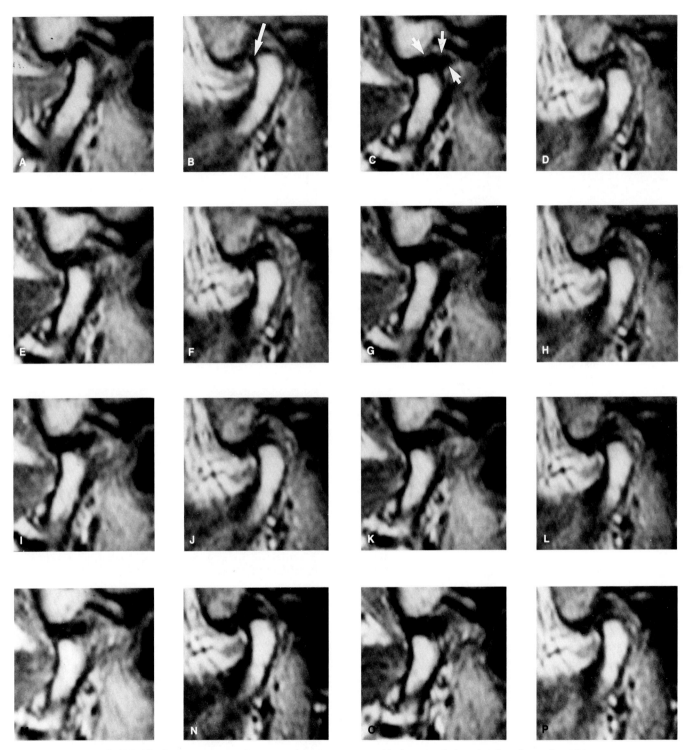

FIGURE 10–8. Asymmetrical motion of the temporomandibular joint. (**A**) In the closed-mouth position, the meniscus on the right temporomandibular joint is in a normal position; however, (**B**) a small spur is seen on the condyle (*arrow*) of the left temporomandibular joint and there is a slight anterior displacement of the meniscus. (**C, E, G, I, K, M, O**) During incremental opening of the mouth, the meniscus becomes slightly deformed during the initial phase of anterior movement of the condyle (*arrows*), and there is progressive anterior translation of the right condyle. (**D**) On the left temporomandibular joint, there is early recapture of the meniscus as the condyle translates anteriorly. (**D, F, H, J, L, N, P**) However, there is retrograde movement of the condyle as it moves back toward the glenoid. This patient had clinical evidence of lateral deviation of the mandible during opening of the mouth. Images were obtained in the oblique sagittal plane. (TR, 600 msec; TE, 20 msec; slice thickness, 3 mm.)

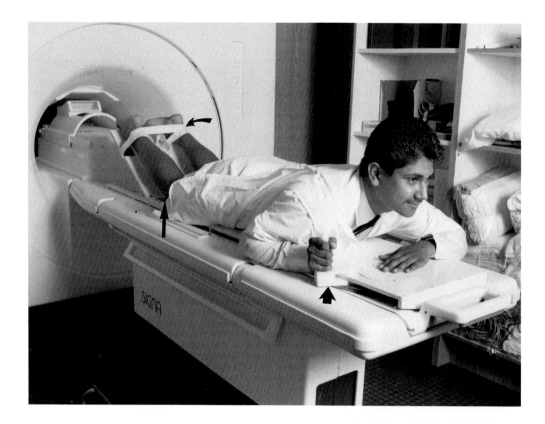

FIGURE 10–9. A nonferromagnetic positioning device is used for kinematic MR imaging of the patellofemoral joint. This device flexes the knees from extension through 30° of flexion at 5° increments using a patient-activated mechanism (*short straight arrow*). A gauge indicates the degree of flexion. A cut-out area permits uninhibited movement of patellofemoral joints (*long straight arrow*). A loosely applied strap is used to maintain the relative alignment of the lower extremities (*curved arrow*), while still allowing rotational movements of the lower extremities to occur during flexion.

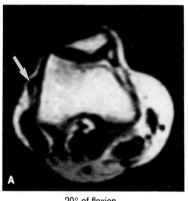
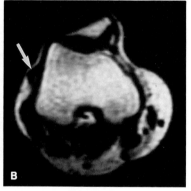

20° of flexion
Prone position

20° of flexion
Supine position

FIGURE 10–10. Medial subluxation is seen in axial images in a patient with persistent symptoms after a lateral retinacular release performed to correct lateral subluxation of the left patella. This patient was imaged in both prone and supine positions with the patellofemoral joints at 20° of flexion. Medial subluxation of the patella is noted in both instances, with slight laxity of the lateral retinaculum (*arrows*). (TR, 400 msec; TE, 20 msec; slice thickness, 5 mm.)

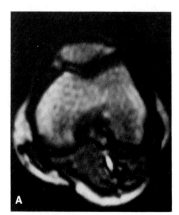
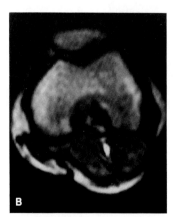
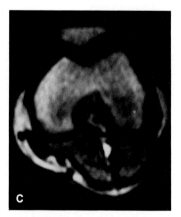

FIGURE 10–11. Six axial images were obtained in 9 seconds with ultrafast spoiled GRASS technique while the patient actively moved the knee joint from (**A**) extension through (**F**) approximately 40° of flexion. The patella is in the central position relative to the femoral trochlear groove, demonstrating normal patellar alignment. (TR, 8 msec; TE, 3 msec; slice thickness, 7 mm.)

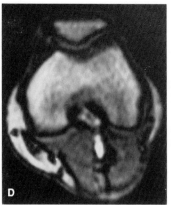

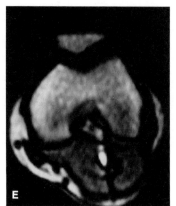

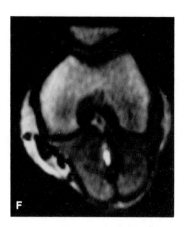

FIGURE 10–11. *(Continued)*

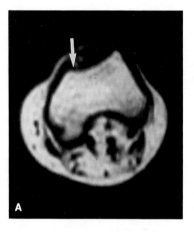

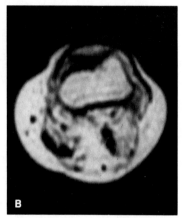

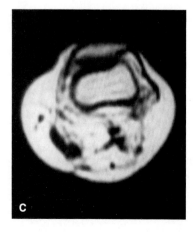

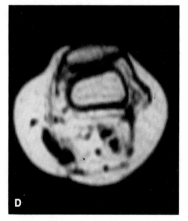

FIGURE 10–12. Sequential axial images demonstrate patella alta. (**A**) The patella is positioned well-above the femoral trochlear groove, which has a hypoplastic medial aspect (*arrow*). (**B–D**) In addition, the patella is poorly formed. (TR, 400 msec; TE, 20 msec; slice thickness, 5 mm.)

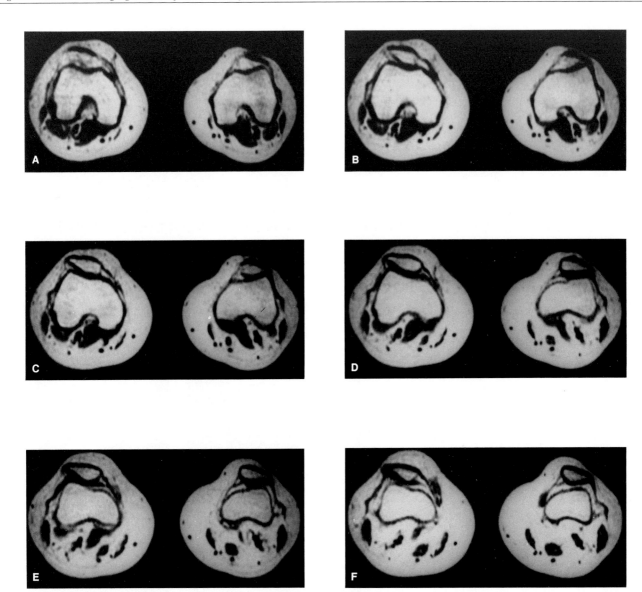

FIGURE 10–13. Sequential axial images taken through bilateral patellofemoral joints during extension are useful in showing the anatomic features of the patellofemoral joint, including the femoral trochlear grooves, femoral trochlea, and patellae, as well as the relative inferior–superior position of the patellae in relation to the femoral trochlear grooves. In this example, (**A**) both patellofemoral joints have relatively shallow femoral trochlear grooves, and (**B–F**) the patellae are misshapen. In addition, the inferior poles of the patellae are positioned above the femoral trochlear grooves, a condition known as bilateral patella alta. (TR, 400 msec; TE, 20 msec; slice thickness, 5 mm.)

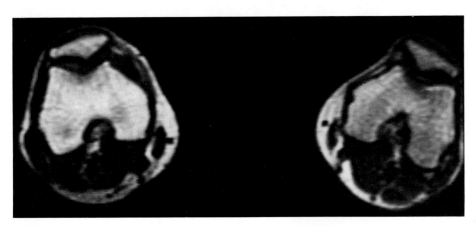

FIGURE 10–14. An axial image shows Wiberg type I patellar shapes. The lateral and medial patellar facets are symmetrical. (TR, 400 msec; TE, 20 msec; slice thickness, 5 mm.)

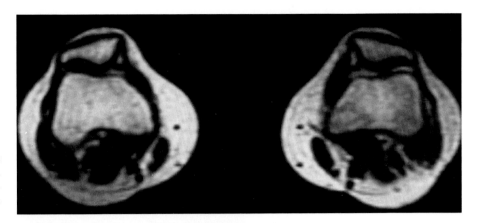

FIGURE 10–15. An axial image shows Wiberg Type II patellar shapes. The lateral patellar facets are longer than the medial patellar facets. (TR, 400 msec; TE, 20 msec; slice thickness, 5 mm.)

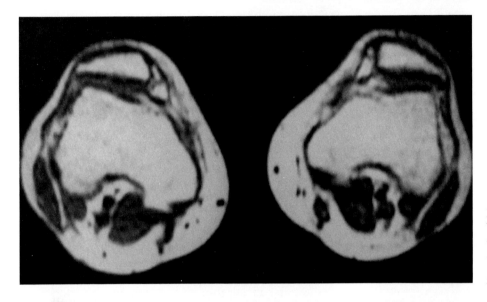

FIGURE 10–16. An axial image shows Wiberg Type III patellar shapes. The lateral patellar facets are dominant, with significantly smaller medial patellar facets. (TR, 400 msec; TE, 20 msec; slice thickness, 5 mm.)

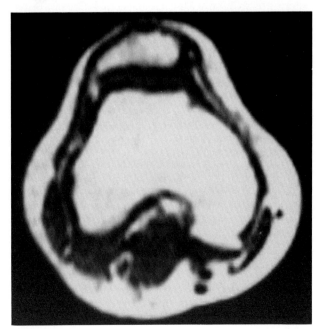

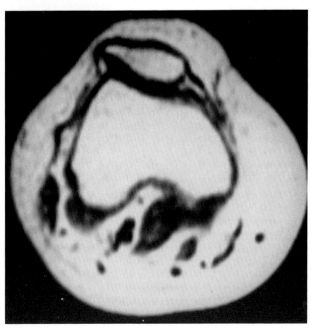

FIGURE 10–17. A dysplastic patella has no well-formed patellar ridge. The femoral trochlear groove is flattened. (TR, 400 msec; TE, 20 msec; slice thickness, 5 mm.)

FIGURE 10–18. A dysplastic patella has no well-formed patellar ridge. The medial aspect of the femoral trochlea is hypoplastic. (TR, 400 msec; TE, 20 msec; slice thickness, 5 mm.)

The normal femoral trochlear shape has well-defined medial and lateral facets that are either equal in size, or have a slightly larger lateral facet. Most importantly, the shape of the groove must conform to the shape of the patella for proper articulation,[22] and should provide a stable means of support to guide the patella during flexion of the joint. Abnormal shapes of the femoral trochlear groove are extremely variable insofar as the medial aspect, the lateral aspect, or both may be hypoplastic or dysplastic (see Figs. 10–17 and 10–18).

Patellar alignment and tracking is normal when the ridge of the patella is positioned in the femoral trochlear groove as it travels in a vertical plane during flexion of the knee, and no transverse displacement of the patella occurs.[1,2,9] This orientation causes the patella to appear centered in the femoral trochlear groove (Fig. 10–19). Any deviation from this normal pattern seen at one or more slice locations at 5° or more of flexion on the kinematic MR study is regarded as an abnormality.[1,2,9–12] In addition, if subluxation or displacement is seen with kinematic MR imaging, it is useful to know the following:

Is the patella further subluxated with increasing degrees of knee flexion?

Does the subluxation improve during knee flexion (*i.e.,* does the patella move into a more normal orientation relative to the femoral trochlear groove)?

Does the relative degree of subluxation remain the same during knee flexion?[2,9,12]

The normal movements of the patella during flexion are maintained by the interplay among static stabilizers (*e.g.,* patellar tendon, medial patellofemoral ligament, medial meniscal patellar ligament, lateral patellofemoral ligament, lateral meniscal patellar ligament, medial retinaculum, lateral retinaculum, fascia lata), dynamic stabilizers (*e.g.,* rectus femoris muscle, vastus medialis muscle, vastus lateralis muscle, vastus intermedius muscle), bony structures (*e.g.,* the shapes of the patella and the femoral trochlea groove in particular), and the alignment of the femur and tibia.[22,23,31] The disturbance of one or more of the above may be responsible for abnormal patellar tracking.[22,23,31]

Pathology

Lateral Subluxation of the Patella

Lateral subluxation of the patella (Figs. 10–20 through 10–26) is a form of patellar malalignment i n which the ridge of the patella is laterally displaced relative to the femoral trochlear groove or the centermost part of the femoral trochlea, and the lateral facet of the patella overlaps the lateral aspect of the femoral trochlear groove.[2,9,12,22,23,31] This is the most common form of abnormal patellar malalignment; it occurs with varying degrees of severity.[22,23,31] Large peripatellar effusions may also cause lateral subluxation, tilting, and other forms of displacement of the patella (see Fig. 10–26). A cartilage defect (see Figs. 10–25 and 10–26) is often found at the site of impact between the patella and the femoral trochlear groove as a result of the chronic pressure that develops from contact stress due to lateral subluxation of the patella.[22,33,34]

Kinematic MR demonstration of a redundant lateral retinaculum associated with lateral subluxation of the patella (see Figs. 10–22 and 10–23) is an especially important finding, because it indicates that surgical release of the lateral retinaculum, a procedure commonly performed in an attempt to realign a laterally displaced patella, will not be beneficial.[2,12] Abnormal lateral forces, possibly combined with insufficient medial stabilizing forces, are the likely cause of this particular form of lateral subluxation of the patella.[12]

Excessive Lateral Pressure Syndrome

Excessive lateral pressure syndrome (ELPS) was first described by Ficat.[22] This form of abnormal patellar alignment is a clinicoradiologic entity characterized clinically by patellofemoral pain and radiologically by tilting of the patella with functional patellar lateralization, usually onto a dominant lateral facet. Kinematic MR studies of patients with ELPS may also reveal a small degree of lateral subluxation of the patella during knee flexion (Fig. 10–27), as increasing tension from one or more overly taut soft–tissue structures (*e.g.,* lateral retinaculum, lateral patellofemoral ligament, lateral meniscal patellar ligament, fascia lata) progressively displace the patella. The patellar malalignment that occurs with ELPS has a tendency to worsen with increasing degrees of joint flexion; therefore, kinematic MR imaging is particularly well suited for identifying this abnormality.[2,9,12]

Medial Subluxation of the Patella

Medial subluxation of the patella (*i.e.,* patella ad entro) is distinguished by medial displacement of the patellar ridge relative to the femoral trochlear groove or the centermost part of the femoral trochlea.[2,9,12] Medial subluxation of the patella is often found in patients with persistent knee pain after surgical realignment procedures if there is overcompensation of the lateral subluxation.[12,35] It also occurs in a high percentage of patients following lateral retinacular release (Fig. 10–28).[12,35] Medial subluxation of the patella may also be observed in patients with no prior surgery (Figs. 10–29 and 10–30). As with other forms of abnormal patellar alignment, medial subluxation may cause localized pressure and be associated with cartilage defects of the medial patellar facet (Fig. 10–31). A variety of mechanisms, which may act separately or in combination, are thought to be responsible for medial subluxation of the patella. These include an insufficient lateral retinaculum, an overly taut medial retinaculum, abnormal patellofemoral anatomy, and unbalanced quadriceps.[2,12] Excessive internal rotation of the lower extremities is a common clinical finding in medial subluxation of the patella (Fig. 10–32).

It is particularly important to distinguish medial subluxation of the patella from lateral or tilting forms of patellar subluxation, because various surgical stabilization techniques (*e.g.,* medial transposition of the extensor mechanism and lateral retinacular release) can increase medial displacement and not only lead to failure of the procedure, but also exacerbate patient's symptoms. It is also important to remember that most physical rehabilitation techniques are implemented to correct lateral subluxation of the patella;[36] these techniques need to be modified for patients with medial subluxation (Fig. 10–33).

Lateral-to-Medial Subluxation of the Patella

Lateral-to-medial subluxation of the patella is a pattern of abnormal patellar tracking in which the patella is in a slight lateral subluxated position during the early increments of knee flexion, moves across the femoral trochlear groove or femoral trochlea as flexion continues, and displaces medially at higher increments of flexion (Fig. 10–34). This type of abnormal patellar tracking is commonly exhibited in the patellofemoral joint that tends to have patella alta, a poorly developed femoral trochlear groove, a misshapen patella, or a combination of these.[13] The actual mechanisms responsible for lateral-to-medial subluxation of the patella are complicated and not well understood.[2] Multiple disordered or uncoordinated forces apparently act on the patella to produce this unusual patellar movement. As with other patellar malalignment syndromes, kinematic MR imaging is particularly well suited to identify this unusual type of patellar tracking, because it shows the various motions and positions of the patella at several different increments of flexion of the joint.

THE WRIST

Kinematic MR imaging has only recently been applied to examination of the wrist;[2,15,16] its full potential in this application has yet to be realized. Despite limited experience, kinematic MR imaging of the wrist has been shown to be helpful in detecting subtle abnormalities of carpal motion, as well as other instability patterns[2,15,16] that are not easily evaluated by routine, high-resolution MR images of the wrist.[37–40] Kinematic MR imaging of the wrist offers several advantages over conventional wrist fluoroscopy; kinematic MR imaging can provide tomographic information and a direct means of viewing the interosseous ligaments.[2,15,16] In addition, elicitation of

pain associated with a specific movement of the wrist may be evaluated by kinematic MR methods in patients who are asymptomatic in a neutral position. Idiopathic pain syndromes related to motion are often not sufficiently characterized by static-view MR techniques, especially if transitory subluxations are present. Kinematic MR examination provides enhanced imaging of the muscles, tendons, ligaments, hyaline, and fibrocartilaginous structures during controlled motion; this factor may be useful in assessment of impingement or other abnormalities related to movement.[2,15,16]

Kinematic Magnetic Resonance Protocol

The relatively small size of the wrist makes it necessary to use either single or dual 3- or 5-in receive-only circular surface coils to obtain high-resolution images for kinematic MR study. This surface coil configuration may also be used to obtain high-resolution static MR views of the wrist. The surface coils are placed above, or above and below (if dual surface coils are used) the wrist. The wrist is placed in radial, neutral, and ulnar deviated positions. Several T1-weighted, spin-echo images are acquired in the coronal plane, with an 8- to 10-cm FOV.

A nonferromagnetic positioning device is used to incrementally position the wrist through this range of motion (Fig. 10–35). The patient is placed in a prone position with the elbow extended, and foam padding is placed at various sites under the axilla, arm, and elbow for support and comfort. As with other types of kinematic MR studies, either multiple static images or a cine loop format may be used to assess the acquired images. However, the cine loop display is best for demonstrating subtle instability patterns of the carpal bones.

Normal Kinematics

Coronal plane kinematic MR studies of normal motion of the wrist during radial, neutral, and ulnar deviation show the carpal bones, bordered by the radius and ulna, moving in a smooth, symmetrical manner (Fig. 10–36).[41,42] Any deviation from this symmetrical movement of the carpal bones is indicative of instability.

The normal carpal relationships have been classically described by Gilula[42] as three separate arcs. Arc I follows the main convex curvatures of the proximal surfaces of the scaphoid, lunate, and triquetrum carpal bones. Arc II outlines the distal concave curvatures of these three bones; and Arc III traces the main proximal curvatures of the hamate and capitate. Any disruption of these arcs is indicative of an abnormality at this site; these abnormalities may be caused by a torn ligament, laxity of the ligament, or a carpal bone fracture.[1,41,42]

Assessment of intercarpal spacing may also provide evidence of an abnormality.[1,41–44] Spacing should be evenly distributed between the carpal bones, without any significant or uneven intercarpal widening, proximal or distal movement, or anterior or posterior displacement of the carpal bones.[42] The normal intercarpal space is approximately 1 to 2 mm wide.[1,42] Increased joint space is suggestive of an abnormal ligament, increased joint fluid, synovial hypertrophy, or other form of pathology.[1,41–44] Decreased joint space may be caused by an abnormal ligament, loss of cartilage, carpal coalition, or dislocated or subluxated carpal bones.[1,41–44]

The presence of ulnar variance, whether positive or negative, should also be noted on kinematic MR study of the wrist, because it may provide an indication of the mechanism responsible for the abnormality. For example, positive ulnar variance has been associated with tears of the triangular fibrocartilage complex and articular erosions of the lunate and triquetrum. Alternatively, negative ulnar variance is often seen with Kienbock's disease or avascular necrosis of the lunate.

Pathology

Since kinematic MR imaging of the wrist is a relatively new technique, only a few cases are used to illustrate the applications of this diagnostic procedure. The full range of its capabilities in wrist evaluation is still being investigated.

Carpal Instability

Carpal bone instability is typically caused by a hyperextension impact injury.[42,43,45] The specific carpal site of the instability is dependent on the position of the hand (*i.e.,* whether it is flexed or extended, or in ulnar or radial deviation) at the time of contact.[42,43] Early detection and treatment of carpal bone dissociations are crucial for a satisfactory clinical outcome.[42,43,45] Conventional plain film x-rays, computed tomography, or static-view MR imaging may be inconclusive in identifying carpal bone instability because the abnormality may be so subtle that it escapes detection unless the wrist is manipulated so that asynchronous motion of the carpals, widening of the joint space, or both may be appreciated (Fig. 10–37). Kinematic MR imaging of the wrist provides an adequate depiction of the pathokinematic aspects of carpal instability.[15,16]

Motion-Related Impingement

Kinematic MR imaging of the wrist may also furnish additional useful diagnostic information related to bony and soft-tissue pathologic changes that occur in conjunc-

tion with motion-related impingement syndromes.[2] In positive ulnar variance, for example, kinematic MR imaging can not only identify the impingement during wrist movement, which is ulnar deviation in this case, but can also characterize the abnormalities; thus, this image modality can offer pertinent diagnostic information (Fig. 10–38).

THE ANKLE

Like kinematic MR imaging of the wrist, kinematic MR imaging of the ankle is a relatively new procedure,[2,14] and its role in the diagnostic assessment of this joint is still being defined. By using a combination of standard, high-resolution static MR imaging methods and kinematic MR imaging, a variety of pathologic conditions that affect this joint have been studied.[2,14] Initial data suggest that kinematic MR imaging helps provide a more thorough examination of the ankle, particularly in cases of functional abnormalities associated with bony subluxations or soft-tissue impingement.[2,14]

Kinematic Magnetic Resonance Protocol

The small size and complex anatomy of the ankle make high-resolution kinematic MR views essential for optimal examination of this joint.[14,46–50] Therefore, an apparatus that incorporates dual 5-in receive-only circular surface coils (Captain Plastic, Fountain Valley, CA) was developed for this procedure (Fig. 10–39). This device permits high-resolution MR imaging for both static and kinematic studies.

The patient is placed in a supine position, and the ankle is fixed to a nonferromagnetic positioning device with Velcro straps (see Fig. 10–39A). The kinematic MR study is performed with the ankle positioned in dorsiflexion and then progressively moved through a range of motion to plantarflexion, while sagittal T1-weighted, spin-echo images are acquired at each increment with a 10- to 14-cm FOV. Either static views or the cine loop format may be used to evaluate the multiple images obtained with this study.

Normal Kinematics

The ankle joint is involved in both weight-bearing and kinematic functions. The movement of this joint occurs primarily in the sagittal plane, which permits plantarflexion (*i.e.,* extension) and dorsiflexion (*i.e.,* flexion) of the foot as the talus rotates beneath the tibia and fibula (Fig. 10–40).[1,51]

(text continues on page 867)

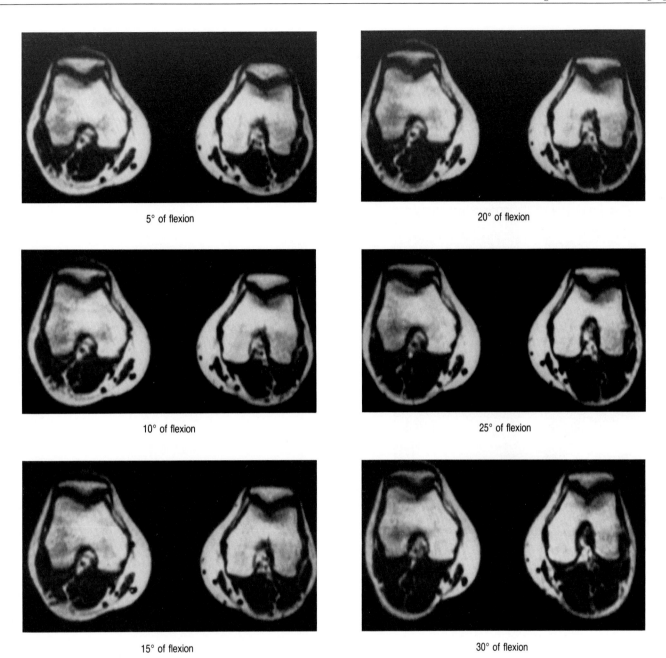

5° of flexion

20° of flexion

10° of flexion

25° of flexion

15° of flexion

30° of flexion

FIGURE 10–19. In a kinematic study of normal bilateral patellofemoral joints, the patellae, in centralized positions from 5° through 30° of flexion, are Wiberg type I shapes. The femoral trochlear grooves are well-formed, with equal medial and lateral aspects. Images were obtained in the axial plane. (TR, 400 msec; TE, 20 msec; slice thickness, 5 mm.)

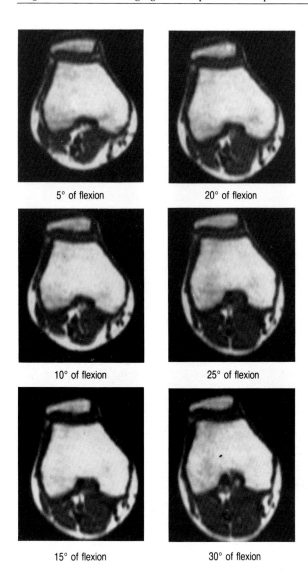

5° of flexion

20° of flexion

10° of flexion

25° of flexion

15° of flexion

30° of flexion

FIGURE 10–20. Axial images show slight lateral subluxation of the patella. The patella is dysplastic with no ridge and the femoral trochlear groove is flattened. The combination of these patellar and femoral trochlear groove shapes tends to be associated with patellofemoral instability, because no buttressing effect is provided by the bony anatomy. (TR, 400 msec; TE, 20 msec; slice thickness, 5 mm.)

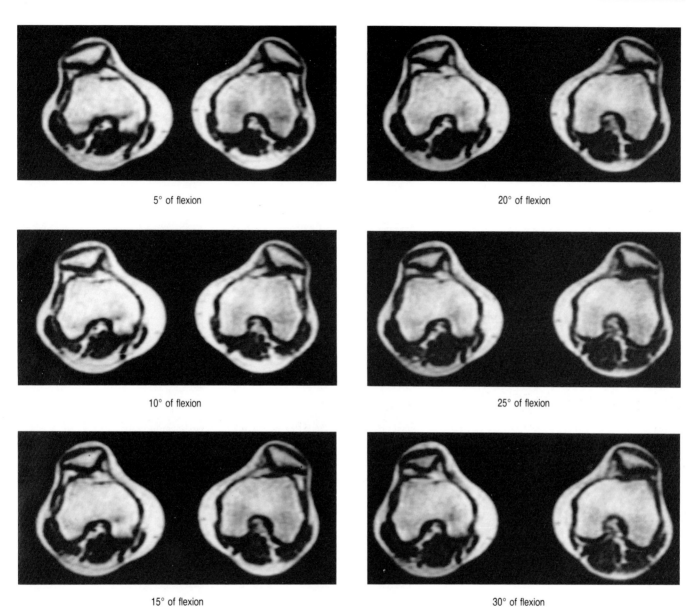

5° of flexion

20° of flexion

10° of flexion

25° of flexion

15° of flexion

30° of flexion

FIGURE 10–21. Bilateral lateral subluxation of both patellae and tilting of the left patella can be seen in axial images. The right patella centralizes by 20° of flexion, while there continues to be slight lateral subluxation and tilting of the left patella in up to 30° of flexion. The patellae are Wiberg type I shapes. The right femoral trochlear groove is flattened, and the left femoral trochlear groove is shallow. (TR, 400 msec; TE, 20 msec; slice thickness, 5 mm.)

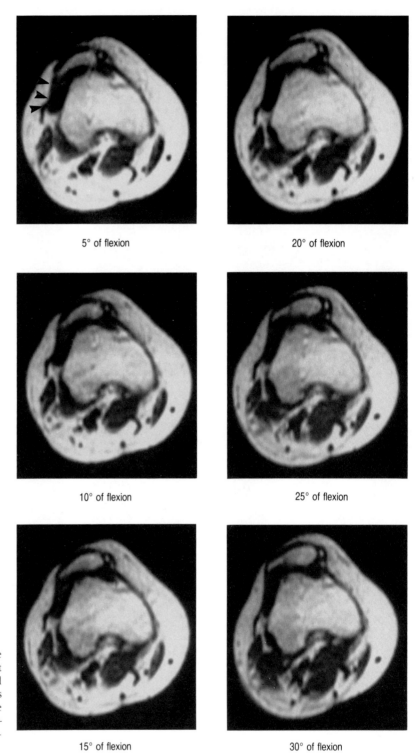

5° of flexion

20° of flexion

10° of flexion

25° of flexion

FIGURE 10–22. Severe lateral subluxation of the patella is seen in axial images in a symptomatic patient after a lateral retinacular release. The amount of lateral subluxation of the patella is constant and persists throughout the range of motion studied. Note the thickened appearance of the lateral retinaculum (*arrowheads*). (TR, 400 msec; TE, 20 msec; slice thickness, 5 mm.)

15° of flexion

30° of flexion

FIGURE 10–24. (**A**) A "skyline-view" plain film radiograph of the patellofemoral joint, obtained at approximately 35° of flexion, shows congruency between the patella and femoral trochlear groove. (**B**) An axial image obtained at 20° of flexion in the same patient shows lateral subluxation of the patella (*arrow*). Plain film radiographs obtained at patellofemoral joint flexion angles above 30° may not be helpful in the assessment of patellar malalignment, because, as the joint flexes, the patella is drawn deeper into the femoral trochlear groove by the extensor mechanism. This can cause a subluxated patella to move into a centralized position, obscuring patellar tracking and alignment abnormalities that occur during the early increments of flexion. (TR, 400 msec; TE, 20 msec; slice thickness, 5 mm.)

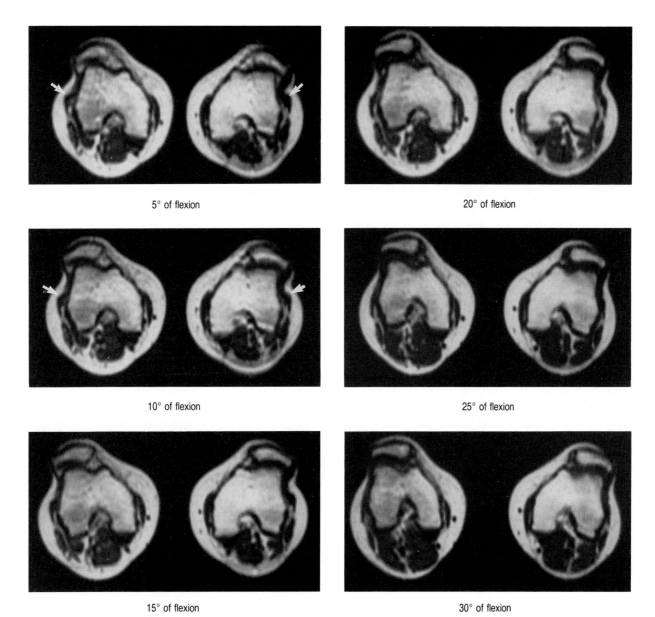

5° of flexion

20° of flexion

10° of flexion

25° of flexion

15° of flexion

30° of flexion

FIGURE 10–23. Axial images show bilateral lateral subluxation of the patellae with redundant lateral retinacula (*arrows*) noted at initial degrees of flexion. The presence of a redundant lateral retinaculum suggests that the lateral patellar subluxation is not caused by excessive force produced by exorbitant stretching of this particular soft-tissue structure. (TR, 400 msec; TE, 20 msec; slice thickness, 5 mm.)

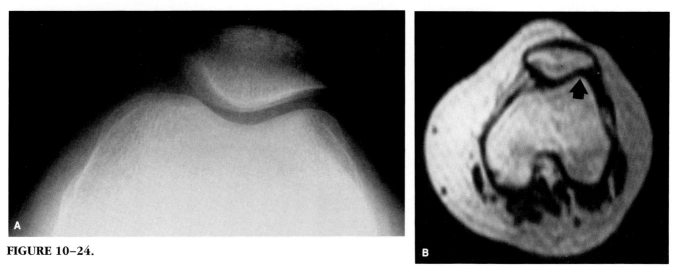

FIGURE 10–24.

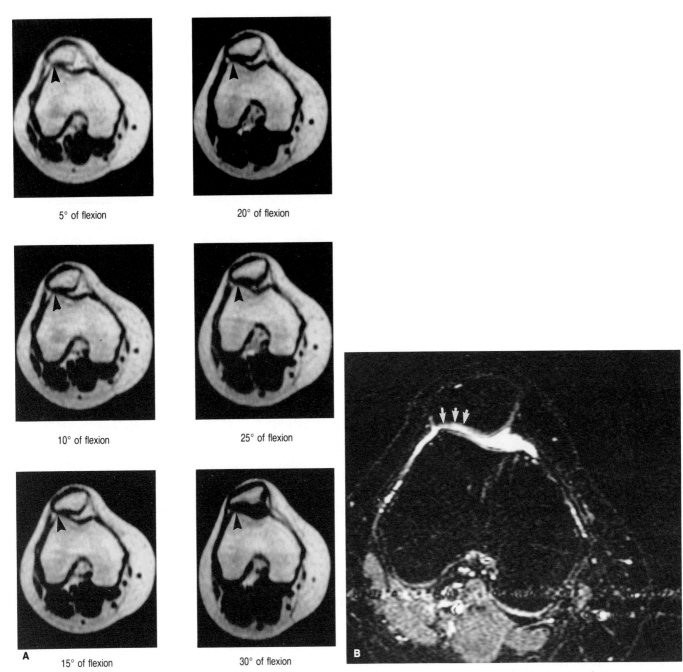

5° of flexion

20° of flexion

10° of flexion

25° of flexion

A   15° of flexion

30° of flexion

B

FIGURE 10–25. (**A**) Lateral tilting and subluxation of the patella are seen in axial images. Note the impact point between the lateral patellar facet and the femoral trochlear groove (*arrowheads*). (TR, 400 msec; TE, 20 msec; slice thickness, 5 mm.) (**B**) An axial image obtained using an extremity coil and short TI inversion recovery highlights articular cartilage. A cartilage defect (*white arrows*) that corresponds to the contact point observed in the kinematic study is noted on the lateral patellar facet.

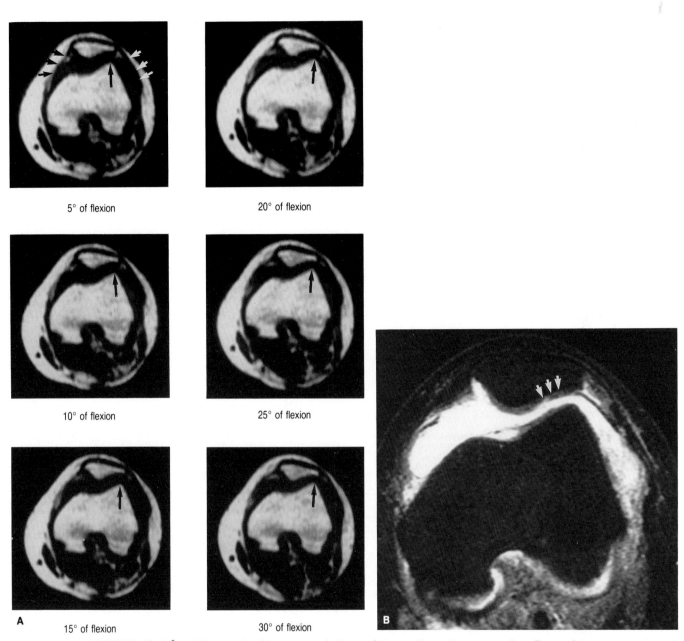

5° of flexion

20° of flexion

10° of flexion

25° of flexion

A

15° of flexion

30° of flexion

B

FIGURE 10–26. (**A**) Lateral subluxation and tilting of the patella with a peripatellar effusion (*short arrows*) are seen in axial images. Note the impact point between the lateral patellar facet and the femoral trochlear groove (*long arrows*). (TR, 400 msec; TE, 20 msec; slice thickness, 5 mm.) (**B**) An axial image obtained using an extremity coil and short TI inversion recovery shows the large peripatellar effusion and a cartilage defect that corresponds to the contact point observed in the kinematic study on the lateral patellar facet (*white arrows*).

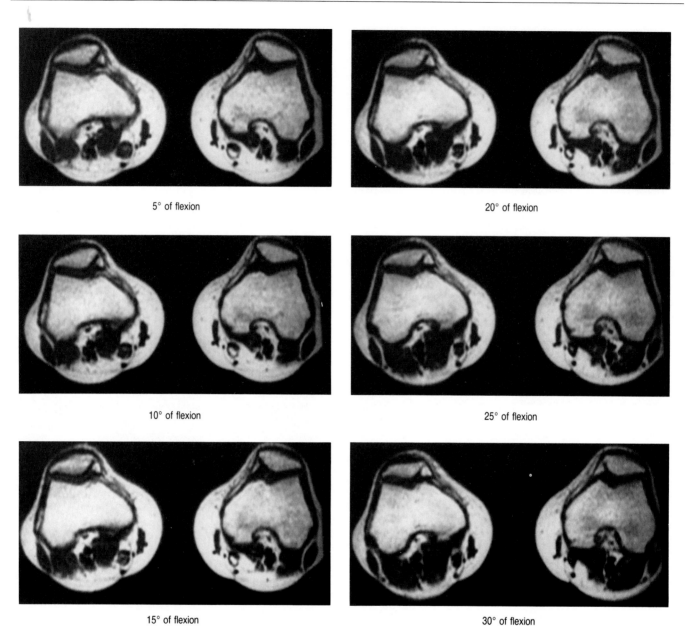

5° of flexion

20° of flexion

10° of flexion

25° of flexion

15° of flexion

30° of flexion

FIGURE 10–27. Excessive lateral pressure syndrome of the left patella is seen in axial images. Note that the lateral tilting of patella increases at the higher increments of flexion. In addition, there is a also slight lateral subluxation of the patella. (TR, 400 msec; TE, 20 msec; slice thickness, 5 mm.)

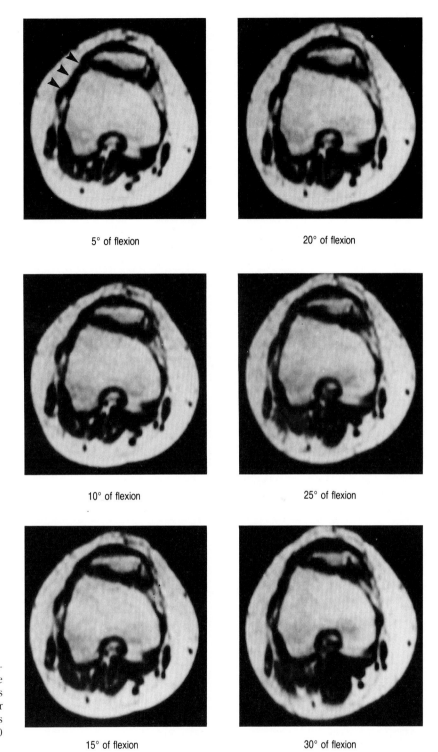

5° of flexion

20° of flexion

10° of flexion

25° of flexion

FIGURE 10–28. Medial subluxation of the patella in a patient with prior lateral retinacular release is seen in axial images. The lateral retinaculum is thickened (*arrowheads*). The femoral trochlear groove is flattened; it therefore cannot function as a buttressing structure for the patella. (TR, 400 msec; TE, 20 msec; slice thickness, 5 mm.)

15° of flexion

30° of flexion

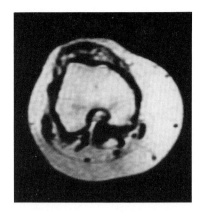

5° of flexion

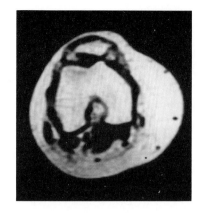

20° of flexion

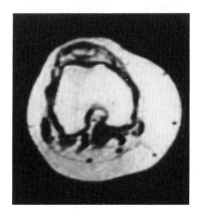

10° of flexion

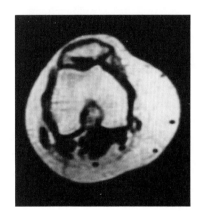

25° of flexion

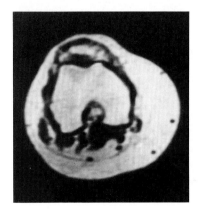

15° of flexion

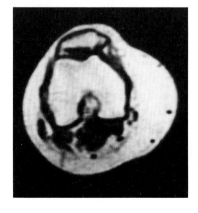

30° of flexion

FIGURE 10–29. Severe medial subluxation of the patella in a patient without prior surgery is seen in axial images. (TR, 400 msec; TE, 20 msec; slice thickness, 5 mm.)

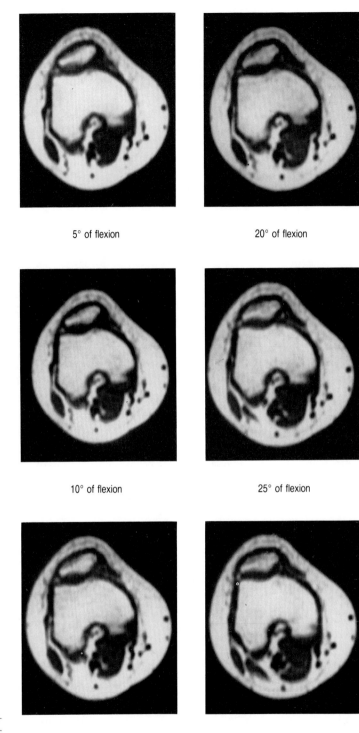

5° of flexion

20° of flexion

10° of flexion

25° of flexion

15° of flexion

30° of flexion

FIGURE 10–30. Medial subluxation of the patella that centralizes by 30° of flexion is seen in axial images. (TR, 400 msec; TE, 20 msec; slice thickness, 5 mm.)

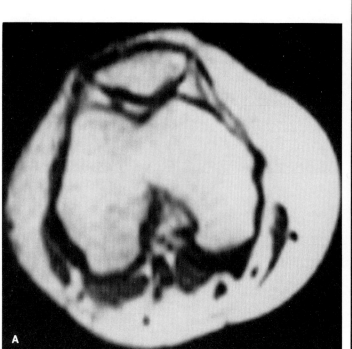

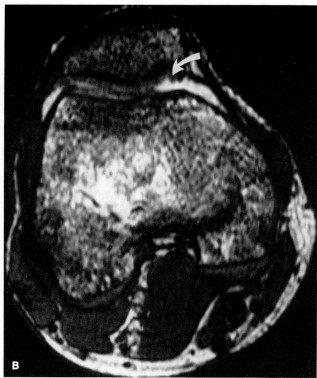

FIGURE 10–31. (**A**) An axial image obtained at 20° of flexion shows medial subluxation of the patella. (TR, 400 msec; TE, 20 msec; slice thickness, 5 mm.) (**B**) An axial image obtained using an extremity coil and 3D Fourier transform technique reveals a cartilage defect (*arrow*) that corresponds to the contact point observed in the kinematic study on the medial patellar facet. This image was obtained with the patient's knee in an extended position, therefore medial subluxation is not apparent. (TR, 60 msec; TE, 15 msec; flip angle, 30°; slice thickness, 1.5 mm.)

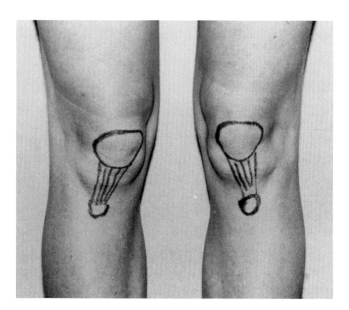

FIGURE 10–32. Bilateral internal rotation of the lower extremities is commonly found in association with medial subluxation of the patella.

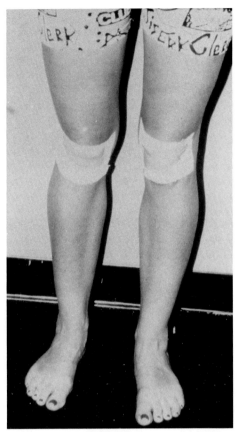

FIGURE 10–33. The McConnell taping technique is used to treat subluxation of the patella.

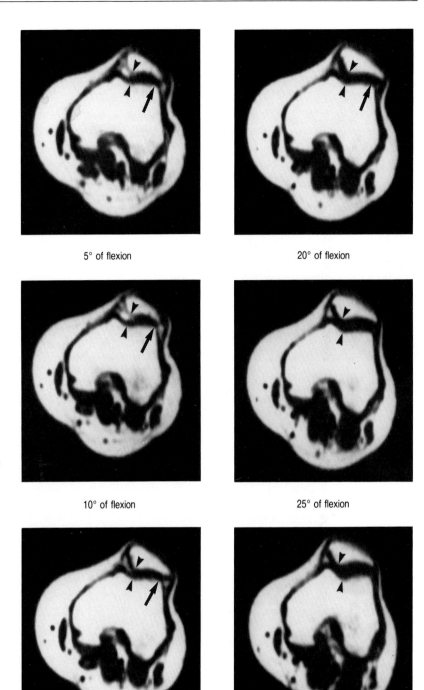

5° of flexion

20° of flexion

10° of flexion

25° of flexion

15° of flexion

30° of flexion

FIGURE 10–34. Slight lateral subluxation of the patella occurs at 5° through 20° of flexion (*long black arrows, alignment of arrowheads*). At 25° of flexion, the patella centralizes (*alignment of arrowheads*). At 30° of flexion, there is a slight medial subluxation of the patella (*alignment of arrowheads*). This kinematic pattern is indicative of lateral-to-medial subluxation of the patella. Images were obtained in the axial plane. (TR, 400 msec; TE, 20 msec; slice thickness, 5 mm.)

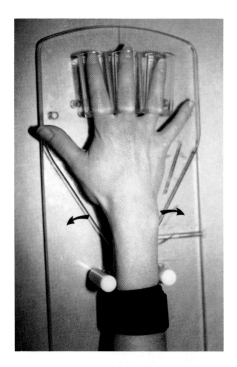

FIGURE 10–35. A special nonferromagnetic positioning device is used to position the wrist incrementally from ulnar, through neutral, through radial deviation (*curved arrows*) for kinematic MR examination.

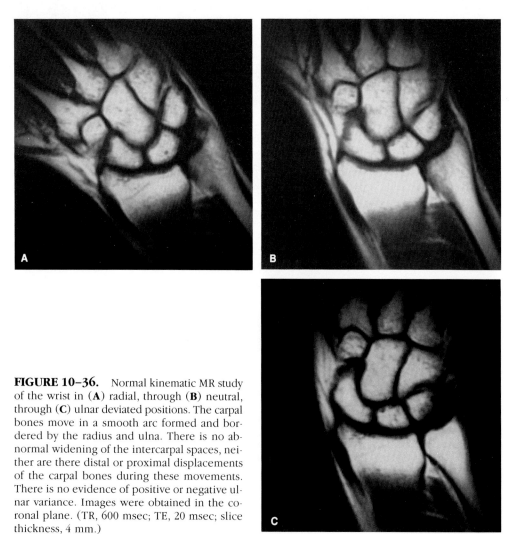

FIGURE 10–36. Normal kinematic MR study of the wrist in (**A**) radial, through (**B**) neutral, through (**C**) ulnar deviated positions. The carpal bones move in a smooth arc formed and bordered by the radius and ulna. There is no abnormal widening of the intercarpal spaces, neither are there distal or proximal displacements of the carpal bones during these movements. There is no evidence of positive or negative ulnar variance. Images were obtained in the coronal plane. (TR, 600 msec; TE, 20 msec; slice thickness, 4 mm.)

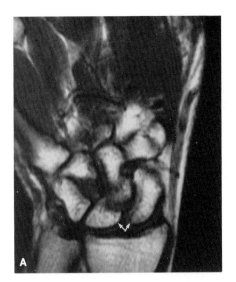

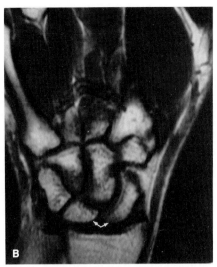

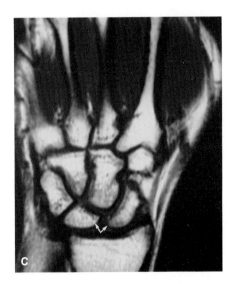

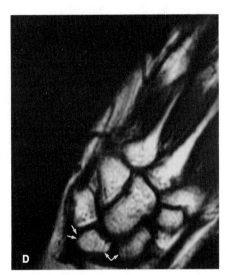

FIGURE 10–37. (**A–C**) In carpal instability, widening of the joint space between the scaphoid and lunate (*joined arrows*) occurs. (**D**) This widening is most apparent during radial deviation. In addition, the scaphoid is slightly displaced during radial deviation (*white arrows*). There is negative ulnar variance. Images were obtained in the coronal plane. (TR, 600 msec; TE, 20 msec; slice thickness, 4 mm.)

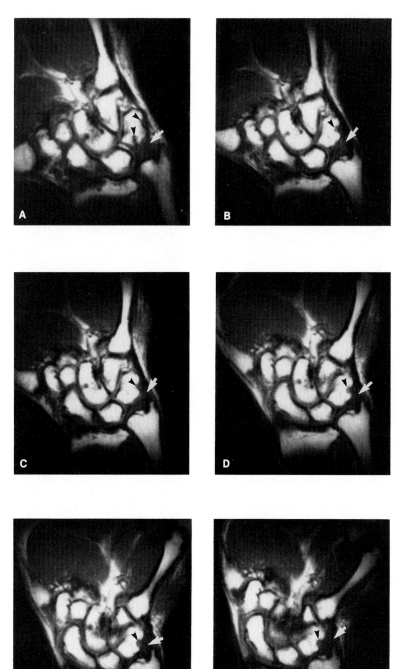

FIGURE 10–38. (**A–D**) Cystic degeneration is present in the triquetrum (*black arrowheads*). There is also positive ulnar variance. Signal changes are noted in the triangular fibrocartilage complex that are compatible with a tear (*white arrows*). (**E, F**) Impingement between the distal ulna and triquetrum occurs during ulnar deviation. Images were obtained in the coronal plane. (TR, 600 msec; TE, 20 msec; slice thickness, 4 mm.)

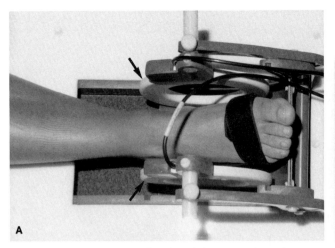

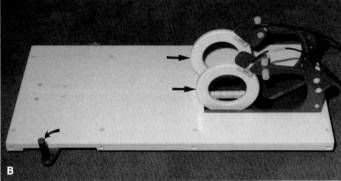

FIGURE 10–39. (**A**) A special nonferromagnetic positioning device is used to incrementally move the ankle from dorsiflexion through neutral and plantarflexion positions by means of a patient-activated mechanism (*curved arrow*). This device incorporates dual, 5-in, circular, receive-only surface coils (*straight arrows*); therefore high-resolution MR imaging and a kinematic MR study may be accomplished with the same device. (**B**) A close-up shows the features of the positioning device with ankle in place.

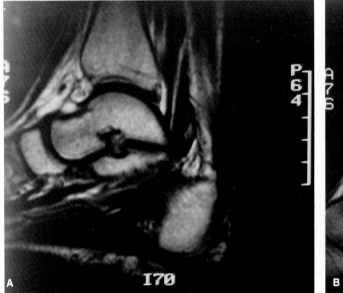

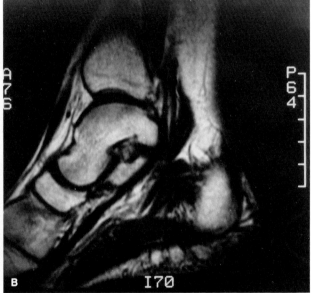

FIGURE 10–40. Normal kinematic MR study of the ankle. There is a smooth movement as the talus rotates from dorsiflexion through plantarflexion without anterior or posterior displacements. The bony and soft-tissue anatomy are normal. Images were obtained in the sagittal plane. (TR, 600 msec; TE, 20 msec; slice thickness, 4 mm.)   *(continued)*

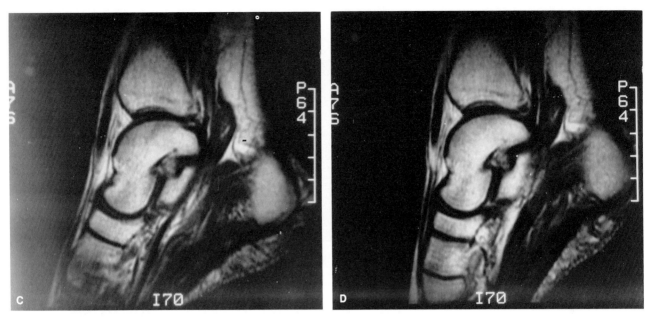

FIGURE 10–40. *(Continued)*

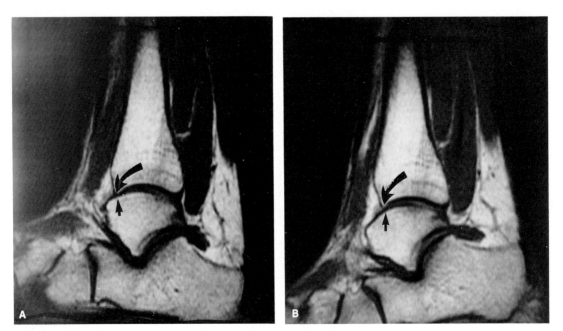

FIGURE 10–41. (**A, B**) Bony impingement (*arrows*) occurs between a small osteophyte on the tibia that impacts with the talus, primarily during dorsiflexion positioning of the ankle. There is also a slight anterior displacement of the talus relative to the tibia. (**C, D**) Bony impingement is not observed during plantar flexion of the ankle. Images were made in the sagittal plane. (TR, 600 msec; TE, 20 msec; slice thickness, 4 mm.)

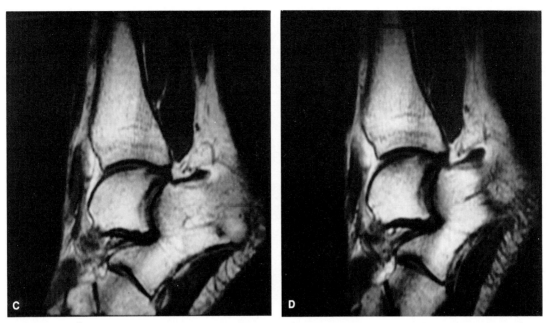

FIGURE 10–41. *(Continued)*

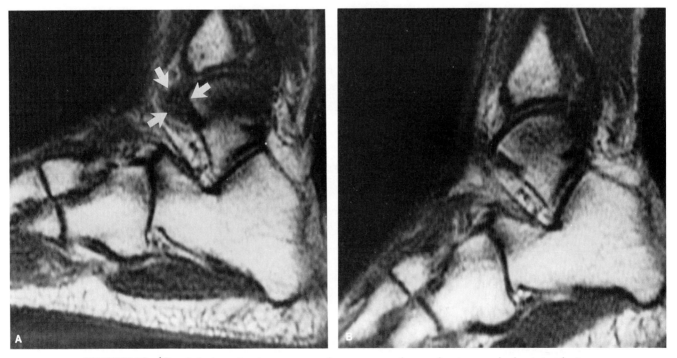

FIGURE 10–42. Soft-tissue impingement syndrome occurred secondary to capsular hypertrophy in a patient with chronic ankle sprains. (**A**) During dorsiflexion, there is evidence of thickening of soft tissues anterior to and in between the talus and fibula (*white arrows*). (**B**) These changes are not evident during plantar flexion of the ankle. (Sagittal plane images; (TR, 600 msec; TE, 20 msec; slice thickness, 4 mm.)

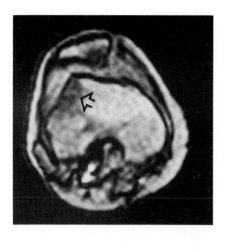
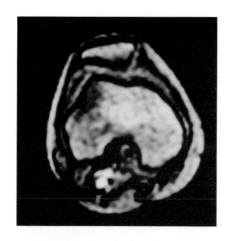
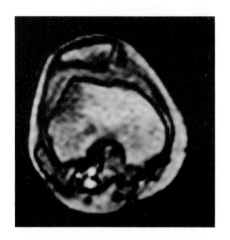
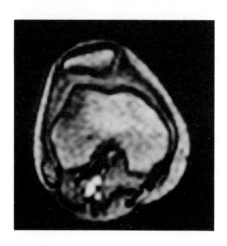
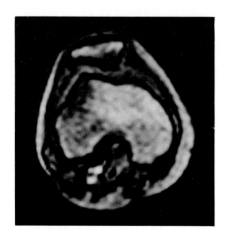
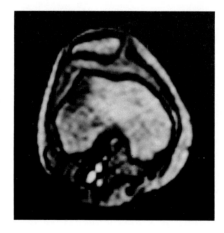

FIGURE 10–43. Lateral subluxation of the patella. There are areas of low signal intensity in the ridge of the patella and lateral aspect of the femoral condyle indicative of bone bruises (*open arrow*). This suggests a prior traumatic lateral dislocation of the patella. This kinematic MR study was performed using an ultrafast MR technique during active flexion of the patellofemoral joint. Images were obtained in the axial plane by ultrafast spoiled GRASS pulse sequence. (TR, 8 msec; TE, 3 msec; flip angle, 30°; slice thickness, 7 mm.)

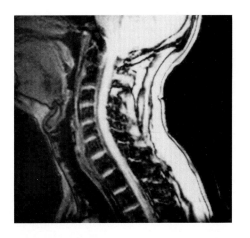
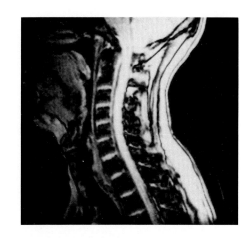

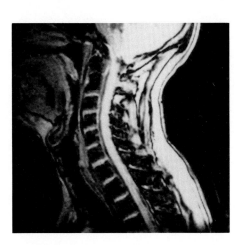
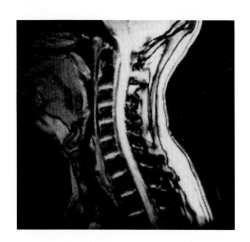

FIGURE 10–44. A kinematic MR study of the normal cervical spine shows normal movement and alignment of the cervical vertebra in the various positions. This series was performed using an ultrafast MR technique during active flexion and extension of the cervical spine. Images were obtained in the sagittal plane by ultrafast spoiled GRASS pulse sequence. (TR, 8 msec; TE, 3 msec; flip angles, 45°; slice thickness, 7 mm.)

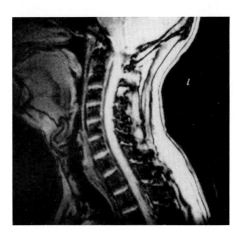
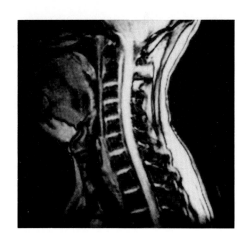

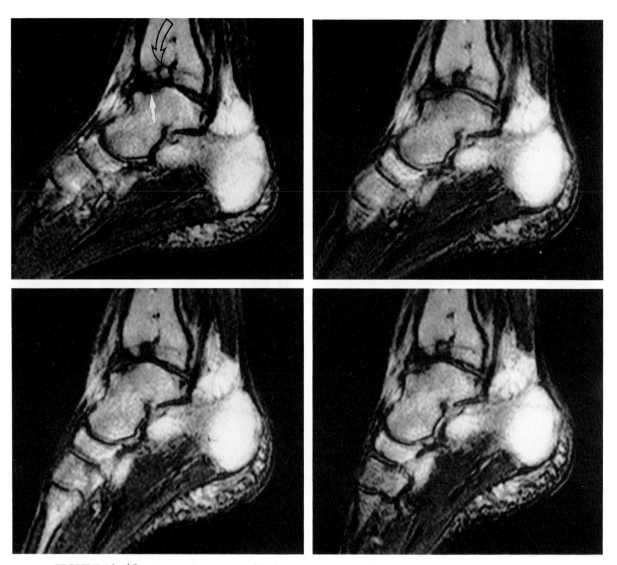

FIGURE 10–45. Severe destruction of the articular cartilage affects the talar dome (*white arrow*) and tibia (*open curved arrow*). Abnormal ankle kinematics are present, secondary to traumatic injury. This kinematic MR study was performed using an ultrafast technique during active dorsiflexion and plantarflexion of the ankle. Images were obtained in the sagittal plane by ultrafast spoiled GRASS pulse sequence. (TR, 8 msec; TE, 3 msec; flip angles, 60°; slice thickness, 5 mm.)

The stability of the ankle is preserved primarily by the configuration of the talus and its conformation to the shapes of the tibia and fibula.[1,51,52] Soft-tissue stabilizing structures include the anterior talofibular and calcaneofibular ligaments on the lateral aspect of the joint and the deltoid ligament on the medial side.[1,51,52] The musculotendinous structures that encompass the ankle are involved in stabilization of the joint to a lesser degree.

Abnormalities of the bony anatomy and alterations of the structural soft-tissue restraints markedly affect the stability of the ankle and cause significant malalignment of joint surfaces.[1] These changes are typically manifested as a loss of range of motion, particularly in dorsiflexion.[51-53] Furthermore, slight displacements of the tibiotalar or fibulotalar articulations can produce substantial changes in loading stress on the ankle and subsequent, severe pathologic conditions.[1,51,52]

Pathology

Due to limited experience with kinematic MR imaging of the ankle, the following examples represent only the potential usefulness of this diagnostic imaging technique. The full range of its usefulness is yet to be determined.

Motion-Related Impingement

Evaluation of patients with chronic ankle pain is difficult because there are a variety of possible mechanisms potentially responsible for the symptoms, including impingement of soft-tissue structures (Fig. 10–41), impingements of bony anatomy (Fig. 10–42), osteochondritis dissecans, avascular necrosis, or loose bodies. Kinematic MR imaging combined with high-resolution static-view MR imaging of the ankle provides information that permits differentiation among these various conditions.[2,14,46-50]

Bony or soft-tissue impingement syndromes that affect the ankle (see Fig. 10–42) typically cause pain and inhibit motion during dorsiflexion.[51-54] In the past, it was thought that impingement syndromes of the ankle were caused by osseous structures, such as an osteophyte on the anterior aspect of the tibia that impacts with the talus during dorsiflexion (see Fig. 10–42). However, soft-tissue impingement syndromes associated with plantar flexion inversion injuries of the ankle have since been described.[54] Following tears of the lateral ankle ligaments, usually the talofibular ligament, the calcaneofibular ligament, or both, the healing process may be accompanied by scarring and capsular hypertrophy in the anterolateral space. This can produce a soft-tissue impingement during dorsiflexion of the ankle.[2,54] In these cases, kinematic MR imaging of the ankle demonstrates impingement of the soft-tissue mass during movement of the ankle.

FUTURE DIRECTIONS

In the future, the use of echo planar and ultrafast MR imaging techniques will provide several benefits for kinematic MR studies of the joints.[55-59] The time required to perform these examinations will be significantly reduced, producing sufficient temporal resolution to allow images to be obtained during actual dynamic movement of the joints.[55-59] Kinematic MR imaging of the joints implemented in this manner will permit a more physiologic and functional examination to be achieved, because the contribution of the associated contracting muscles and related soft-tissue structures may be assessed.[55-59] In addition, sophisticated devices to passively position the joint incrementally through a range of motion will no longer be needed. However, simpler devices that guide the joint in a particular plane of movement will probably still be necessary. The development of kinematic MR imaging schemes and the criteria for evaluation of these studies have already been initiated.[55-60] Figures 10–43 through 10–45 show examples of kinematic MR studies of joints obtained with ultrafast MR imaging pulse sequences.

REFERENCES

1. Nordin M, Frankel VH. Basic biomechanics of the musculoskeletal system. 2nd ed. Philadelphia: Lea & Febiger, 1989.
2. Shellock FG, Mandelbaum B. Kinematic MRI of the joints. In: Mink JH, Deutsch AL, eds. MRI of the musculoskeletal system: a teaching file. New York: Raven Press, 1990.
3. Burnett KR, Davis CL, Read J. Dynamic display of the temporomandibular joint meniscus by using "fast-scan" MR imaging. AJR 1987;149:959.
4. Pressman BD, Shellock FG. Static and kinematic MR imaging of the TMJ. California Dental Association Journal 1988;August:32.
5. Pressman BD, Shellock FG, Tourje JE. Dual coil MR imaging of temporomandibular joints: value in assessment of asymmetrical motion abnormalities. [abstract] AJNR 1988.
6. Pressman BD, Shellock FG. The temporomandibular joint. In: Mink JH, Deutsch AL, eds. MRI of the musculoskeletal system: a teaching file. New York: Raven Press, 1990.
7. Shellock FG, Pressman BD. MR imaging of the temporomandibular joint: improvements in the imaging protocol. AJNR 1989;10:595.
8. Shellock FG, Deustch A, Mink JH, Fox JA. Identification of medial subluxation of the patella in a dancer using kinematic MRI of the patellofemoral joint: a case report. Kinesiology and Medicine for Dance 1991;13:1.
9. Shellock FG, Mink JH, Deutsch A, Fox JM. Evaluation of patellar tracking abnormalities using kinematic MR imaging: clinical experience in 130 patients. Radiology 1989;172:799.
10. Shellock FG, Mink JH, Deutsch A, Fox JM. Kinematic magnetic resonance imaging for evaluation of patellar tracking. The Physician and Sports Medicine 1989;17:99.
11. Shellock FG, Mink JH, Fox JM. Patellofemoral joint: kinematic MR imaging to assess tracking abnormalities. Radiology 1988;168:551.
12. Shellock FG, Mink JH, Deutsch A, Fox JM, Ferkel RD. Evaluation of patients with persistent symptoms after lateral retinacular release by kinematic magnetic resonance imaging of the patellofemoral joint. Arthroscopy 1990;6:226.

13. Shellock FG, Mink J, Fox JM, Ferkel R, Friedman M, Molnar T. Kinematic MRI evaluation of symptomatic patients following two or more patellar realignment surgeries. J Magn Reson Imag 1991; 1:175.

14. Shellock FG, Mink JH, Sullenberger P. High-resolution static and kinematic MRI of the ankle. Society of Magnetic Resonance in Medicine, Berkeley, Ninth Annual Meeting. Book of Abstracts. vol. 2. 1990:766.

15. Fulmer JM, Harms SE, Flamig DP, Guerdon G, Machek J, Dolinar J. High-resolution cine MR imaging of the wrist. Radiology 1989;173:26.

16. Bergey PD, Zlatkin MB, Dalinka M, Osterman AL, Machek J, Dolinar J. Dynamic MR imaging of the wrist: early results with a specially designed positioning device. Radiology 1989;173:26.

17. Helms CA, Katzberg RW, Dolwick MF. Internal derangements of the temporomandibular joint. San Francisco: University of California Printing Department, 1983.

18. Drace JE, Enzmann DR. Defining the normal temporomandibular joint: closed-, partially open-, and open mouth MR imaging of asymptomatic subjects. Radiology 1990;177:67.

19. Manzione JV, Tallents RF, Katzberg RW, Oster C, Miller TL. Arthrographically guided therapy for recapturing the temporomandibular joint meniscus. Oral Surg Oral Med Oral Pathol 1984;57:235.

20. Tallents RH, Katzberg RW, Miller TL, Manzione JV, Oster C. Arthrographically assisted splint therapy. J Prosthet Dent 1985;53:235.

21. Kummel BM. The diagnosis of patellofemoral derangements. Prim Care 1980;7:199.

22. Ficat RP, Hungerford DS. Disorders of the patello-femoral joint. Baltimore: Williams & Wilkins, 1977.

23. Wiberg G. Roentgenographic and anatomic studies on the femoropatellar joint, with special reference to chondromalacia patellae. Acta Orthop Scand 1941;12:319.

24. Martinez S, Korobkin M, Fondren FB, Hedlund LW, Goldner JL. Diagnosis of patellofemoral malalignment by computed tomography. J Comput Assist Tomogr 1983;7:1050-1053.

25. Stanford W, Phelan J, Kathol MH, et al. Patellofemoral joint motion: evaluation by ultrafast computed tomography. Skeletal Radiol 1988;17:487.

26. Laurin CA, Dussault R, Levesque HP. The tangential X-ray investigation of the patellofemoral joint: x-ray technique, diagnostic criteria and their interpretation. Clin Orthop 1979;144:16.

27. Merchant AC, Mercer RL, Jacobsen RH, Cool CR. Roentgenographic analysis of patellofemoral congruence. J Bone Joint Surg [Am] 1974;56:1391.

28. Carson WG, James SL, Larson RL, Singer KM, Winternitz WW. Patellofemoral disorders: physical and radiographic evaluation. Part II: radiographic examination. Clin Orthop 1984;185:178.

29. Schutzer SF, Ramsby GR, Fulkerson JP. Computed tomographic classification of patellofemoral joint pain patients. Orthop Clin North Am 1986;17:235.

30. Moller BN, Krebs B, Jurik AG. Patellofemoral incongruence in chondromalacia and instability of the patella. Acta Orth Scand 1986;57:232.

31. Larson RL. Subluxation-dislocation of the patella. In: Kennedy JC, ed. The injured adolescent knee. Baltimore: Williams & Wilkins, 1979:161.

32. MacNab L. Recurrent dislocation of the patella. J Bone Joint Surg [Am] 1952;34:957.

33. Insall J, Falvo KA, Wise DW. Patellar pain and incongruence. II: clinical application. Clin Orthop 1983;176:225.

34. Insall J. Chondromalacia patellae: patellar malalignment syndrome. Orthop Clin North Am 1979;10:117.

35. Hughston JC, Deese M. Medial subluxation of the patella as a complication of lateral release. Am J Sports Med 1988;16:383.

36. Dehaven KE, Solan WA, Mayer PJ. Chondromalacia patellae in athletes. Clinical presentation and conservative management. J Sports Med 1979;7:5.

37. Koenig H, Lucas D, Meissner R. The wrist: a preliminary report of high-resolution MR imaging. Radiology 1986;160:463.

38. Baker LL, Hajek PC, Bjorkengren A, et al. High-resolution magnetic resonance imaging of the wrist: normal anatomy. Skeletal Radiol 1987;16:128.

39. Weiss KL, Beltran J, Shamam OM, Stilla RF, Levey M. High-field MR surface-coil imaging of the hand and wrist. Part I. Normal anatomy. Radiology 1986;160:143.

40. Weiss KL, Beltran J, Shamam OM, Stilla RF, Levey M. High-field MR surface-coil imaging of the hand and wrist. Part II. Pathological correlations and clinical relevance. Radiology 1986;160:147.

41. Reicher MA, Kellerhouse LE. Normal wrist anatomy, biomechanics, basic imaging protocol, and normal multiplanar MRI of the wrist. In: Reicher MA, Kellerhouse LE, eds. MRI of the hand and wrist. Raven Press: New York, 1990.

42. Gilula LA. Carpal injuries: analytic approach and case exercises. AJR 1977;133:503.

43. Culver JE. Instabilities of the wrist. Clin Sports Med 1986;5:725.

44. Lichtman DM, Noble WH, Alexander CE. Dynamic triquetrolunate instability. J Hand Surg [Am] 1984;9:185.

45. Linscheid RL, Dobyns JH, Beabout JW, Bryan RS. Traumatic instability of the wrist. J Bone Joint Surg [Am] 1972;54:1612.

46. Kneeland JB, Macrandar S, Middleton WD, Cates JD, Jesmanowicz A, Hyde JS. MR imaging of the normal ankle: correlation with anatomic sections. AJR 1988;151:117.

47. Hajek PC, Baker LL, Bjorkengren A, Sartoris DJ, Neumann CH, Resnick D. High-resolution magnetic resonance imaging of the ankle: normal anatomy. Skeletal Radiol 1986;15:536.

48. Beltran J, Noto AM, Mosure JC, Shamam OM, Weiss KL, Zuelzer WA. Ankle: surface coil MR imaging at 1.5 T. Radiology 1986;161:203.

49. Sartoris DJ, Resnick D. Magnetic resonance imaging of tendons in the foot and ankle. J Foot Surg 1989;28:370.

50. Sierra A, Potchen EJ, Moore J, Smith HG. High-field magnetic-resonance imaging of aseptic necrosis of the talus. J Bone Joint Surg [Am] 1986;68:927.

51. Rodgers MM. Dynamic biomechanics of the normal foot and ankle during walking and running. Physical Therapy. 1988;68:1822.

52. Parlasca R, Shoh H, D'Ambrosia RD. Effects of ligamentous injury on ankle and subtalar joints: a kinematic study. Clin Orthop 1979;140:266.

53. Perlman M, Leveille D, DeLeonibus J, et al. Inversion lateral ankle trauma: differential diagnosis, review of the literature, and prospective study. J Foot Surg. 1987;26:95.

54. Bassett FH, Gates HS, Billys JB, Morris HB, Nikolaou PK. Talar impingement by anteroinferior tibiofibular ligament. J Bone Joint Surg [Am] 1990;72:55.

55. Shellock FG, Cohen MS, Brady T, Mink JH, Pfaff JM. Evaluation of patellar alignment and tracking: comparison between kinematic MRI and "true" dynamic imaging by hyperscan MRI. J Magn Reson Imag 1991; 1:148.

56. Shellock FG, Foo TKF, Mink JH. Dynamic imaging of the joints by ultrafast MRI techniques. European Congress of Radiology, Scientific Programme and Abstracts, 1991;S168.

57. Shellock FG, Foo TKF, Mink JH, Deutsch A, Kerr R, Myers S: MRI of the patellofemoral joint: comparison between passive positioning and active movement imaging techniques. Radiology 1991;181:179.

58. Shellock FG, Mink JH, Deutsch A, Kerr R, Foo TKF. Ultrafast MRI of the joints during active motion. J Magn Reson Imag 1992; 2 (p) 68.

59. Shellock FG, Foo TKF, Deutsch A, Mink JH. Patellofemoral joint: evaluation during active flexion with ultrafast spoiled GRASS MR imaging. Radiology 1991;180:581.

60. Shellock FG, Mink JH, Deutsch AL, Foo TKF. Kinematic MR imaging of the patellofemoral joint: comparison between passive positioning and active movement imaging techniques. Radiology 1992 (in press).

CHAPTER 11

David W. Stoller

The Spine

Accurate diagnosis and evaluation of the cervical, thoracic and lumbar spines are important in orthopaedics, rheumatology, neurology, and neurosurgery. At best, standard radiographs provide a limited interpretation of nonosseous events occurring in the discs, cord, cerebrospinal fluid (CSF), and ligaments; these structures are not directly seen in plain film radiographs). Myelography, an invasive procedure, provides an indirect evaluation of the disc by displaying the contour of the thecal sac and nerve root sleeves. Computed tomography (CT) is useful in delineating bone detail, and direct axial scans of the spine provide soft-tissue discrimination of the disc, nerve roots, and thecal sac.[1–6] Sagittal, coronal, or oblique views, however, cannot be directly acquired and require reformations (Fig. 11–1). Although CT is excellent for assessing postoperative pseudoarthrosis, fibrosis and scarring may be difficult to differentiate from disc material, especially in the absence of contrast enhancement.

Magnetic resonance (MR) imaging complements CT and myelography in the routine evaluation of the spine for degenerative disc disease, trauma, infection, neoplasia and intrinsic cord disease.[7–41] The intervertebral disc consists of the nucleus pulposus, the annulus fibrosis,

and the cartilaginous endplate (Figs. 11–2 and 11–3). With MR imaging, the separate components of the disc, including the nucleus pulposus and annulus fibrosus, can be distinguished and assessed in early degenerative disc disease. The disc–thecal-sac interface is defined without administration of a contrast agent; the structure of the cord is seen in contrast with surrounding CSF; and the dura and supporting ligaments of the spine are demonstrated in either sagittal or axial images (Figs. 11–4 and 11–5). The conus medullaris is displayed with superior contrast resolution in MR (Figs. 11–6 and 11–7). Magnetic resonance provides the unique advantage of direct marrow imaging in the study of patients with marrow infiltrative diseases, metastasis, infection, or reactive endplate changes.[42–57] The components of the atlantoaxial joint (Fig. 11–8) can be differentiated using MR in any of the three orthogonal planes (Fig. 11–9).

The cervical spine, cord, and paravertebral muscles are enclosed within the prevertebral fascia; their cross-sectional relationships are best displayed in axial images (Fig. 11–10). The spinal cord is surrounded by the dura, arachnoid, and pia mater (Fig. 11–11). Magnetic resonance imaging of the thoracic spine is obtained with fields of view (FOVs) that exclude unwanted information and artifact from mediastinal structures (Figs. 11–12 and 11–13).

Magnetic resonance imaging of the spine has advanced in parallel with the development of improved surface coils and software. Oblique imaging, cardiac gating, gradient-echo imaging, short TI inversion recovery (STIR) imaging, and enhancement with gadolinium contrast (Gd-DTPA; a paramagnetic contrast agent) have all been used to maximize the information obtained from MR images. Improved signal-to-noise ratios and excellent spatial and contrast resolution have made it possible to define spinal anatomy in direct sagittal, oblique, and axial planes with MR images obtained from circular and rectangular receive and quadrature coils (Figs. 11–14 and 11–15). A spine board can be used to move coils to specified locations in the thoracic or lumbar spine (Fig. 11–16). Three dimensional Fourier transform (3DFT) volume acquisitions, particularly when used in routine cervical spine studies, allow greater anatomic coverage with thin sections (Fig. 11–17).[58,59] These sequences permit retrospective reformatting of other imaging planes, including oblique images through the neural foramen. Kinematic flexion and extension sagittal images have been used in selected cases of instability and atlantoaxial subluxations (Fig. 11–18).

IMAGING PROTOCOLS FOR THE CERVICAL SPINE

The cervical spine is best studied with a custom-designed posterior or anterior quadrature cervical spine coil. Unless properly designed for anterior placement, greater respiratory artifact may be introduced in this position because of closer proximity of the coil to the trachea.

In the sagittal imaging plane, T1-weighted gradient echo images, which show low signal intensity CSF, are obtained with a repetition time (TR) of 400 to 500 msec, an echo time (TE) of 9 msec, and a flip angle of 110°. Thin (3- to 4-mm) sections, with or without an interslice gap of 1 mm, are acquired with a 20-cm FOV, a 256 × 192 acquisition matrix, and 4 signal averages or excitations (NEX). This protocol will show some degree of darkening of the vertebral bodies as a result of the T2* effect. Conventional T1-weighted sagittal images are acquired before and after Gd-DTPA administration using TRs of less than 600 msec. T2-weighted contrast in the sagittal plane is achieved using either T2 or effective T2 (*i.e.,* T2*) weighting, which minimize pulsation artifacts from CSF and cause flow-related enhancement of signal intensity. Gradient-echo or T2*-weighted images can be generated using a TR of 300 to 400 msec, TE of 15 msec, and a flip angle of 10°. With long spin-echo (SE) acquisition times (long TR/TE), CSF flow-related artifacts are more

common, but they can be reduced by gating the acquisition to the cardiac cycle using an electrocardiograph (ECG) or pulse trigger.[14,60]

Axial images are generated with a 3DFT T2*-weighted protocol using a TR of 35 msec, a TE of 15 msec, and a flip angle of 5°. A total of 64 images at 2 mm provides coverage from C1 through T1. Conventional T1-weighted images, if obtained, should be acquired with flow compensation to minimize vascular and CSF flow artifacts. Conventional T2-weighted images in the axial plane have poor signal-to-noise ratios and are degraded by motion artifact unless some form of cardiac gating is employed.

NORMAL MAGNETIC RESONANCE ANATOMY OF THE CERVICAL SPINE

Sagittal Images

T1-Weighted Images

In conventional T1-weighted sagittal images of the cervical spine, the yellow or fatty marrow of the vertebral bodies demonstrates bright signal intensity (Fig. 11–19). The noninjured cervical spine should exhibit a normal cervical lordotic curve, and C1 without a vertebral body can be identified by its anterior and posterior arches. The low signal intensity synchondrosis at the base of the odontoid may appear as a dark band, simulating a fracture. The basivertebral veins penetrate the midportion of the posterior cervical vertebral bodies and are connected to the epidural venous system. The short cervical pedicles connect the cervical vertebral body to the articular pillars. From the articular pillars, the posteromedially oriented lamina form the spinous process. As in the thoracic and lumbar spines, the superior articular process from the inferior cervical body projects anterior to the inferior articular process, which comes from the cervical vertebral body above. The foramina transversarium of the transverse processes of C2 through C6 contain the vertebral artery and small veins. The anterior–posterior diameter of the cervical canal is tapered from C1 to C3 and is relatively uniform thereafter (*i.e.,* from C3 through C7). The low signal intensity anterior and posterior longitudinal ligaments that connect the cervical vertebra are best seen in sagittal images.

On conventional T1-weighted spin-echo images, the fibrocartilaginous cervical discs are intermediate in signal intensity, and CSF, which is of low signal intensity, is seen in contrast with the higher signal intensity of the cord. On T1-weighted images, intervertebral discs are enhanced and demonstrate bright signal intensity, whereas the CSF remains of low signal intensity. On conventional T1-weighted images, differentiation of posterior cortical bone, longitudinal ligaments, and CSF is difficult because all generate low signal intensity on short TR/TE sequences. The ability to distinguish them is improved by using T1-weighted protocols, which more accurately define endplate and osteophyte anatomy.

The dorsal and ventral roots in the neural foramina are identified on peripheral sagittal images. These structures demonstrate intermediate signal intensity and are surrounded by high signal intensity foraminal fat. A 45° oblique sagittal image is also useful in displaying intervertebral foraminal anatomy in the cervical spine. On gradient-echo images, fat demonstrates intermediate signal intensity in the intervertebral foramina, and these sequences provide less contrast than corresponding T1-weighted images.

Intermediate signal intensity hyaline cartilage can be seen between the obliquely oriented inferior and superior articular facets (Fig. 11–20). The signal void of the anterior vertebral artery can be seen in parasagittal sections through the dorsal root ganglion and articular pillars. The subarachnoid space anterior and posterior to the cord are of equal dimensions. The ability to differentiate gray and white matter varies, depending on CSF pulsation and truncation artifacts. Truncation artifacts are seen as bands parallel with the cervical cord, and are related to FOV, TR/TE, and pixel size. Bright signal intensity from marrow is seen in both the anterior and posterior arches of C1 and in the body of C2. Signal intensity in the body of C2 is higher than that seen in the adjacent odontoid process, and there is a fat pad of high signal intensity directly superior to the odontoid.

T1-weighted gradient-echo images obtained with a TR of 400 to 500 msec, a TE of 9 msec, and a flip angle of 110° demonstrate high signal intensity discs, low signal intensity CSF, and high signal intensity cord (Fig. 11–21). This protocol is used to provide a more accurate characterization of the posterior disc margin from adjacent CSF and vertebral body endplates. Magnetic susceptibility is minimized at a TE of 9 msec.

T2-Weighted Images

On T2*-weighted images, the intervertebral discs and CSF demonstrate high signal intensity (Fig. 11–22).[41,60–62] When flip angles of less than 15° are used, the cord demonstrates low signal intensity (Fig. 11–23). Excellent cord–CSF contrast is also seen on conventional T2-weighted protocols (Fig. 11–24) High signal intensity subarachnoid CSF is seen anteriorly and posteriorly. Cerebrospinal fluid appears progressively darker with the use of higher flip angles. The marrow and cortex of the cervical vertebrae demonstrate low signal intensity on gradient-echo images, sharply delineating the spinal canal, impinging osteophytes, and the disc–thecal-sac interface. On heavily T2*-weighted images, however, discs

may not be as easily differentiated from osteophytes, and the posterior disc margin may be overestimated (Fig. 11–25). This can be avoided by comparison with corresponding T1-weighted images, in which the disc is brighter than the adjacent endplates or osteophytes. The basivertebral vein follows a horizontal course through the midvertebral body, and generates bright signal intensity. Facet cartilage, which is intermediate in signal intensity on conventional T1- and T2-weighted images, demonstrates high signal intensity on T2*-weighted images (Fig. 11–26).[63] Flowing arterial and venous blood display high signal intensity. Contrast between the nerve root and fat is diminished on T2- or T2*-weighted images, because fat demonstrates intermediate, not high signal intensity; therefore, the anatomy of the neural foramina is not accurately demonstrated in these images. The low signal intensity dura can be identified on T2*-weighted images, but it is not satisfactorily seen on corresponding conventional T1- or T2-weighted images. We have used STIR imaging techniques to evaluate metastatic disease by selectively nulling fatty marrow signal intensity. The additive effects of T1 and T2 contrast produce greater conspicuity than is possible with corresponding conventional T2- or T2*-weighted images.

Axial Images

T1-Weighted Images

On T1-weighted axial images, either conventional or spoiled gradient refocused acquisition in the steady state (GRASS), the intermediate signal intensity disc, the black CSF, and the higher signal intensity cord can be differentiated (Figs. 11–27 and 11–28). Differentiation of the nucleus pulposus and annulus, however, is not possible with short TR/TE sequences. The low signal intensity uncinate processes are located lateral to the disc margins, and the facet joints are demonstrated in their oblique orientation, with greater medial–lateral than superior–inferior dimensions. The low signal intensity transverse ligament extends posterior to the odontoid process of C2. The ventral and dorsal nerve roots form a triangle of intermediate signal intensity, with the anterolateral apex of the triangle, represented by the dorsal root ganglion, located proximal to the junction to the dorsal and ventral roots in the neural foramen. Anterior to the dorsal root ganglion, the low signal intensity vertebral artery can be seen. At the level of the cervical body, but not the intervertebral disc, high signal intensity neural foraminal fat may outline the intermediate signal intensity nerve roots and sheaths. Vertebrae C1 through C7 have spinal nerve roots which exit the intervertebral nerve root canals (*i.e.,* foramina) above the corresponding vertebral body level. Low signal intensity epidural veins are located posterior to the vertebral body and surround the vertebral artery in the venous plexus. The epidural venous plexus is enhanced following the administration of Gd-DTPA, especially along the anterolateral aspect of the spinal canal and neural foramen. Gray and white matter can be separately identified on T1-weighted axial images.

T2-Weighted Images

On T2*-weighted images, the intervertebral disc demonstrates high signal intensity generated from the nucleus pulposus (Figs. 11–29 and 11–30).[61] Annular fibers remain low in signal intensity. The anterior epidural venous plexus generates bright signal intensity, as do the vertebral arteries, allowing the low to intermediate signal intensity nerve roots and dorsal root ganglion to be seen. It may be difficult to distinguish the exiting nerve roots, because both the roots and neural foraminal fat are intermediate in signal intensity in these images. The thin line of the dural sac is identified anterior to the subarachnoid CSF. The common carotid artery and jugular vein, both of bright signal intensity, are defined anteromedially and posterolaterally, respectively, in axial planar images. Cortical bone and marrow both demonstrate low signal intensity in gradient-echo refocused images.

IMAGING PROTOCOLS FOR THE THORACIC AND LUMBAR SPINES

The thoracic and lumbar spines are imaged using a planar surface or quadrature coil with its long axis oriented parallel with the spine. This permits acquisition with an FOV approximating the anatomic region of interest. When the area of interest is restricted to one or two vertebral levels, a 5-in circular spine coil may be used to provide better signal-to-noise ratios. The region of interest can be changed without repositioning the patient if an external spine board housing the surface coil is used.

Sagittal images of the thoracic and lumbar spines are obtained with T1 and T2 or T2* weighting. Routine T1-weighted images are acquired with a TR of 600 msec, a TE of 15 to 20 msec, a 5-mm slice thickness, a 20- to 24-cm FOV, a 256 × 192 acquisition matrix, and 4 NEX. This sequence allows adequate coverage of the canal and neural foramina. Conventional T2-weighted images are acquired with a TR of 2000 msec, a TE of 20, 80 msec, a 256 × 192 acquisition matrix, and 2 NEX. Although less pronounced than that in the cervical spine, low signal intensity pulsatile CSF motion artifact, which occurs secondary to spin dephasing, may degrade image quality or obscure pathology in the thoracic space. Cardiac gating of studies in the upper thoracic spine minimizes the effects of flow. Aortic pulsation artifacts may also be problematic in thoracic spine studies that use long TR/TE sequences. Compared with conventional

spin-echo images, T2*-weighted images of the thoracic and lumbar spines minimize artifact from pulsatile CSF and generate increased signal-to-noise ratio and contrast. Gradient-echo sequences use a TR of 400 msec, a TE of 15 msec, and a flip angle of 30°. Although T2*-weighted contrast may be substituted for conventional T2 weighting, contrast properties are not equivalent. For instance, desiccated discs that demonstrate low signal intensity on T2-weighted images may remain isointense with intact intervertebral discs on T2*-weighted refocused images.

In the axial plane, T1-weighted images are obtained using a TR of 600 to 800 msec, a TE of 15 to 20 msec, 5-mm slice thickness, a 11-to 20-cm FOV, a 256 × 192 acquisition matrix, and 4 NEX. Less frequently, conventional T2-weighted axial sequence are obtained, using a TR of 2000 msec, a TE of 20, 80 msec, and a 256 × 192 acquisition matrix. Instead of this conventional T2 weighting, however, a T2*-weighted sequence is usually used to supplement the T1-weighted acquisition. T2* axial images are performed as stacked images in a 3DFT volume acquisition or as oblique prescriptions parallel with the intervertebral discs (Figs. 11–31 and 11–32). Infection and metastatic disease are evaluated with STIR protocols.

NORMAL MAGNETIC RESONANCE ANATOMY OF THE THORACIC AND LUMBAR SPINES

Sagittal Images

T1-Weighted Images

In the thoracic spine, the posterior subarachnoid space is larger than the subarachnoid space anterior to the cord (Fig. 11–33). Cerebrospinal fluid within the subarachnoid space demonstrates low signal intensity, in contrast to the brighter intermediate signal intensity of the cord, and the high signal intensity of the posterior epidural fat. Anterior epidural fat is prominent in the L5-S1 region. Yellow or fatty marrow and mixed elements of cancellous hematopoietic marrow within the vertebral bodies of the thoracic and lumbar spines demonstrate intermediate to high signal intensity, in contrast to the more intermediate signal intensity of intervertebral discs. A focal or diffuse increase in vertebral body marrow signal intensity with aging is attributed to a greater lipid or fatty component in vertebral body marrow stores. Nuclear annular differentiation is not precisely defined on T1-weighted images (Fig. 11–34). The cord demonstrates uniform intermediate signal intensity. The tapered conus medullaris, which is seen in sagittal images of the lumbar spine with a 24-cm FOV, terminates posteriorly at the

(text continues on page 891)

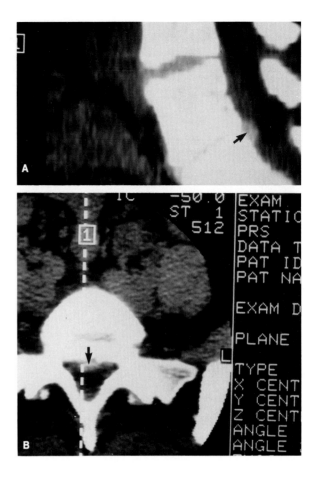

FIGURE 11-1. L5-S1 disc herniation (*arrow*) with soft-tissue density seen on (**A**) direct axial CT and (**B**) reformatted CT sagittal images.

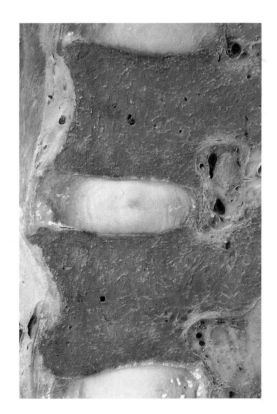

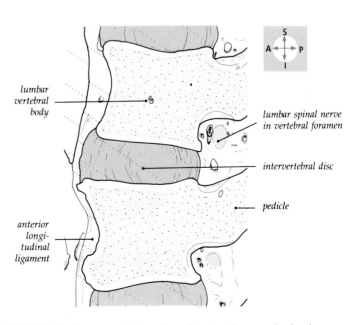

lumbar vertebral body

lumbar spinal nerve in vertebral foramen

intervertebral disc

pedicle

anterior longitudinal ligament

FIGURE 11-2. A sagittal section of the lumbar vertebral column.

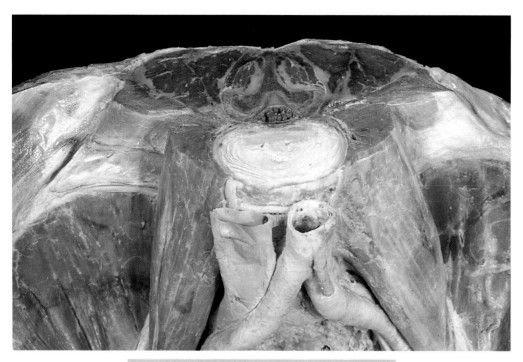

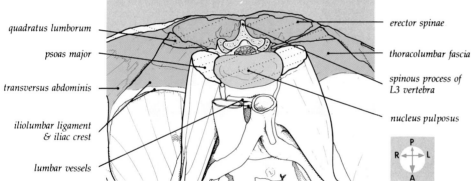

quadratus lumborum

psoas major

transversus abdominis

iliolumbar ligament
& iliac crest

lumbar vessels

erector spinae

thoracolumbar fascia

spinous process of
L3 vertebra

nucleus pulposus

FIGURE 11–3. An oblique view of a transverse section of the lumbar spine and muscles at the level of the disc between the third and fourth lumbar vertebrae.

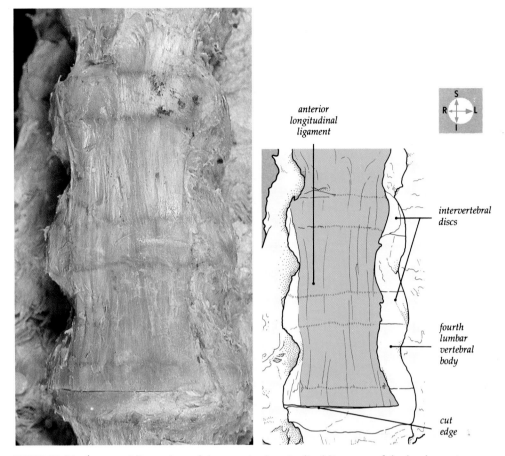

FIGURE 11–4. An oblique view of the anterior longitudinal ligament of the lumbar spine.

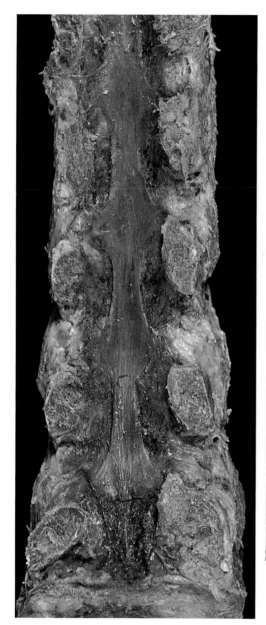

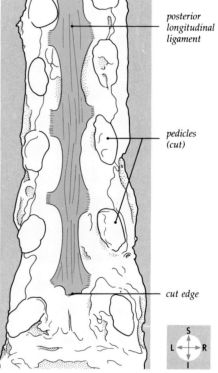

FIGURE 11–5. The posterior longitudinal ligament is exposed by removing the vertebral arches, meninges, and spinal cord.

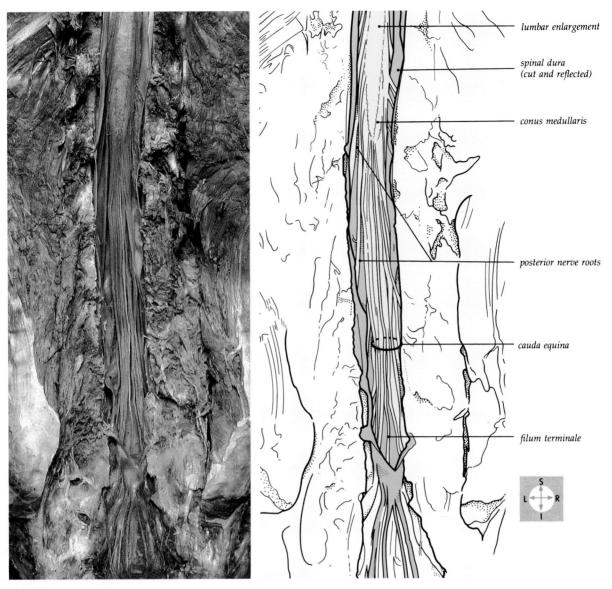

lumbar enlargement

spinal dura
(cut and reflected)

conus medullaris

posterior nerve roots

cauda equina

filum terminale

FIGURE 11–6. The spinal dura and arachnoid are opened posteriorly and reflected laterally, exposing the lumbar enlargement, conus medullaris, and cauda equina.

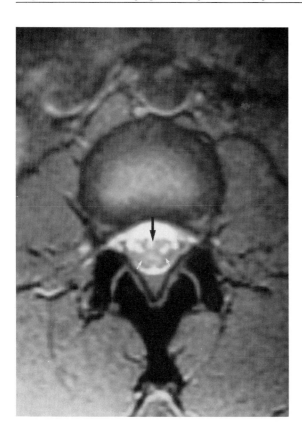

FIGURE 11–7. Normal morphology of the conus medullaris (*black arrow*) at the level of L1-2 is seen on a T2*-weighted axial image. The cauda equina (*white arrows*) are seen posterolaterally.

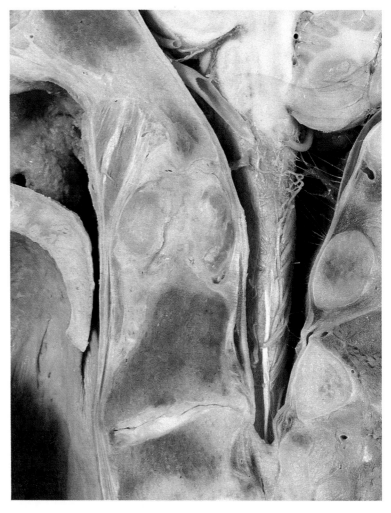

FIGURE 11–8. A near sagittal section through the median atlantoaxial joint.

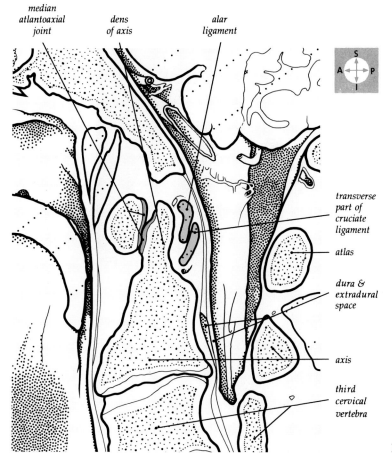

median atlantoaxial joint

dens of axis

alar ligament

transverse part of cruciate ligament

atlas

dura & extradural space

axis

third cervical vertebra

FIGURE 11–8. *(Continued)*

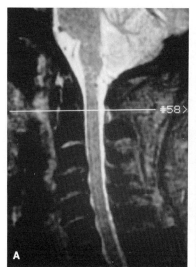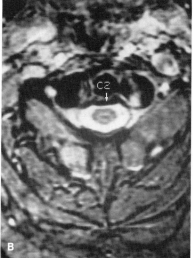

FIGURE 11–9. T2*-weighted (**A**) sagittal and (**B**) axial images at the level of the atlantoaxial joint. The low signal intensity intact transverse ligament is shown on the axial image (*arrow*).

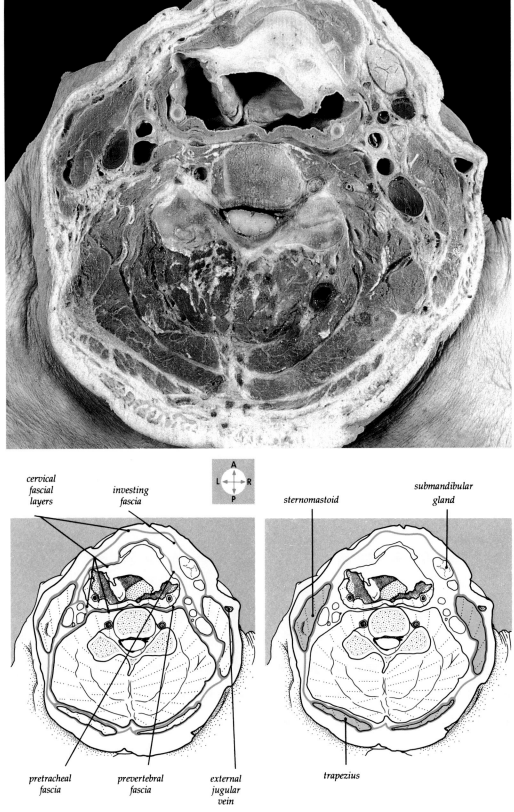

cervical
fascial
layers

investing
fascia

submandibular
gland

sternomastoid

pretracheal
fascia

prevertebral
fascia

external
jugular
vein

trapezius

FIGURE 11–10. A transverse section of the neck at the level of C4 shows the layers of cervical fascia. The layers are shown in separate diagrams.

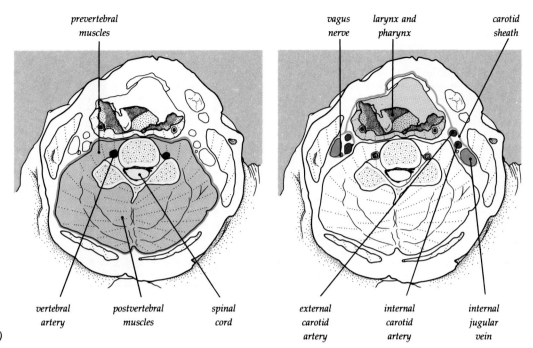

prevertebral
muscles

vagus
nerve

larynx and
pharynx

carotid
sheath

vertebral
artery

postvertebral
muscles

spinal
cord

external
carotid
artery

internal
carotid
artery

internal
jugular
vein

FIGURE 11–10. *(Continued)*

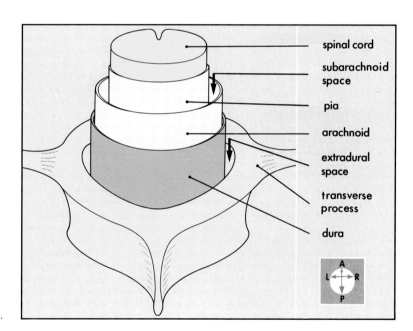

spinal cord

subarachnoid
space

pia

arachnoid

extradural
space

transverse
process

dura

FIGURE 11–11. The spinal meninges.

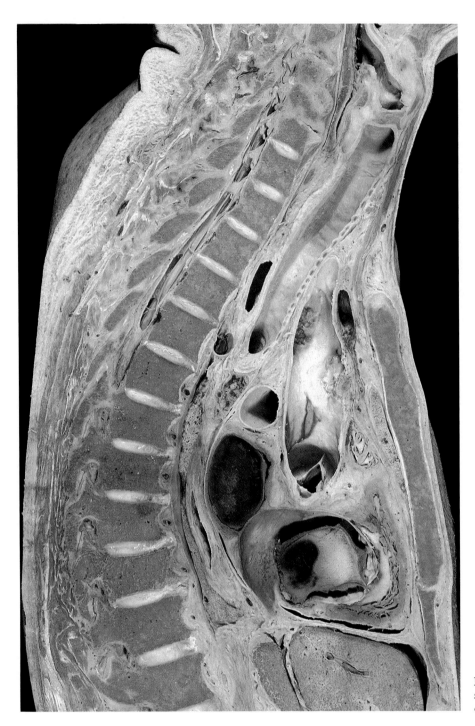

FIGURE 11–12. A near midline sagittal section through the thorax shows some mediastinal structures.

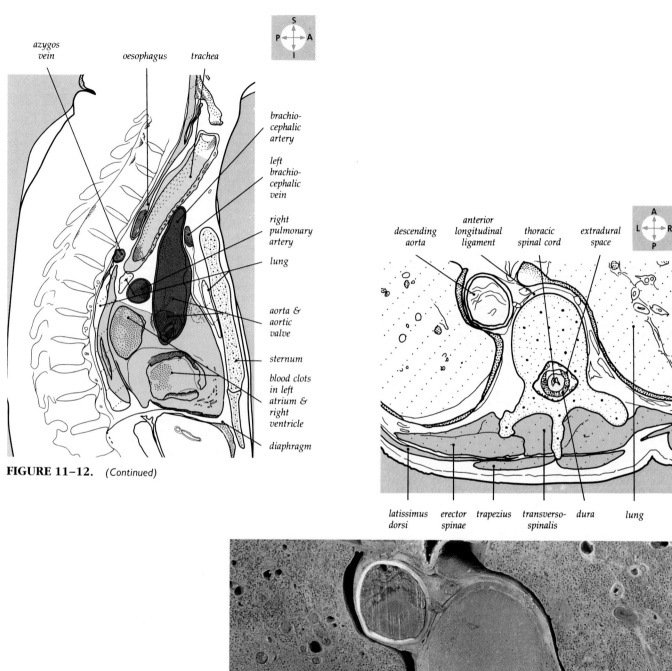

azygos vein

oesophagus

trachea

brachio-cephalic artery

left brachio-cephalic vein

right pulmonary artery

lung

aorta & aortic valve

sternum

blood clots in left atrium & right ventricle

diaphragm

FIGURE 11–12. *(Continued)*

descending aorta

anterior longitudinal ligament

thoracic spinal cord

extradural space

latissimus dorsi

erector spinae

trapezius

transverso-spinalis

dura

lung

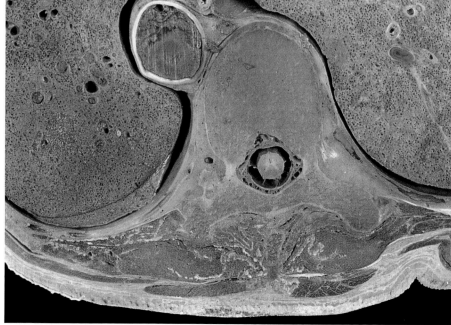

FIGURE 11–13. A transverse section at the level of the seventh thoracic vertebra shows the back muscles and contents of the vertebral foramen.

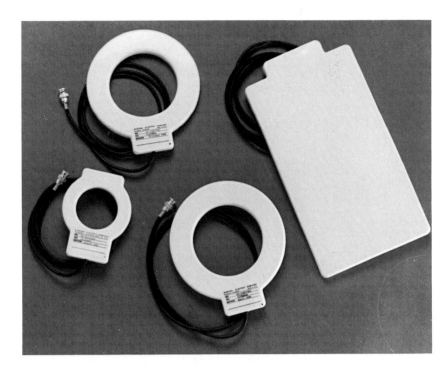

FIGURE 11–14. Circular and rectangular planar surface coils are used to image the thoracic and lumbar spine.

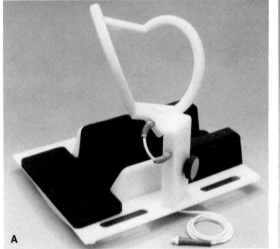

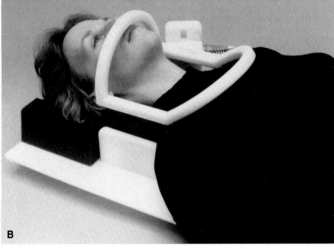

FIGURE 11–15. (**A**) A cervical quadrature spine coil. (**B**) Proper patient positioning for use of the coil.

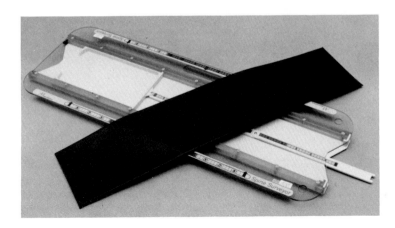

FIGURE 11–16. A spine board is used to position the spine coils.

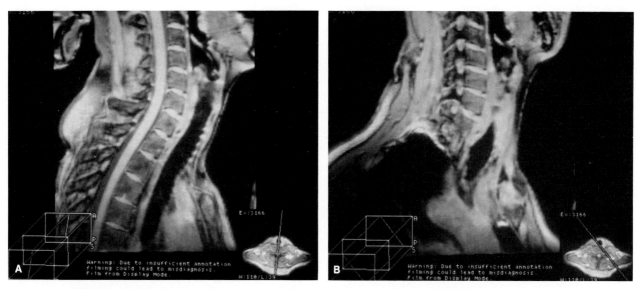

FIGURE 11–17. Three-dimensional Fourier transform volume axial images reformatted in the (**A**) midline and (**B**) sagittal oblique planes provide precise localization of the neural foramen (*i.e.,* intervertebral nerve root canal).

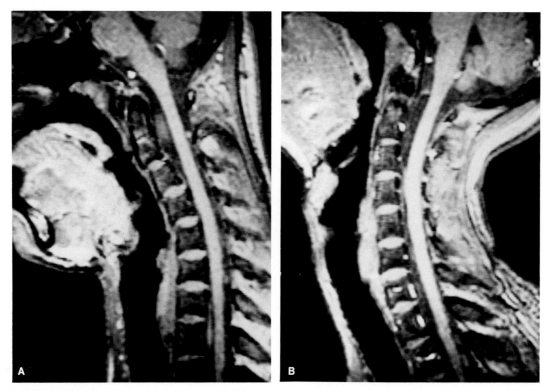

FIGURE 11–18. Normal (**A**) flexion and (**B**) extension of the cervical spine as seen on sagittal images.

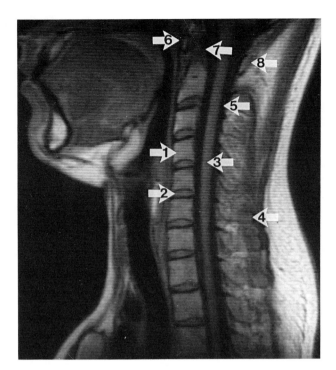

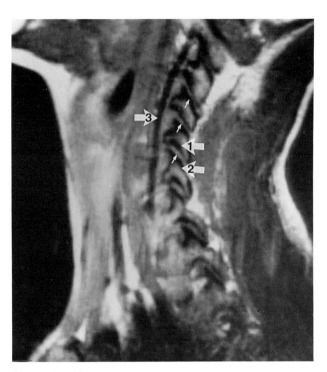

FIGURE 11–19. A T1-weighted image shows the midsagittal anatomy of the cervical spine. (1, bright marrow signal intensity vertebral body; 2, intermediate signal intensity disc; 3, spinal cord; 4, spinous process; 5, low signal intensity cerebrospinal fluid; 6, anterior arch of first cervical vertebra; 7, odontoid; 8, posterior arch of C1.)

FIGURE 11–20. A T1-weighted image shows the parasagittal anatomy of the cervical spine at the level of the facet joints. Intermediate signal intensity facet cartilage (*small arrows*) is identified. (1, superior articular facet; 2, inferior articular facet; 3, vertebral artery.)

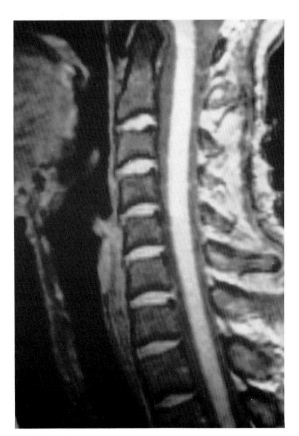

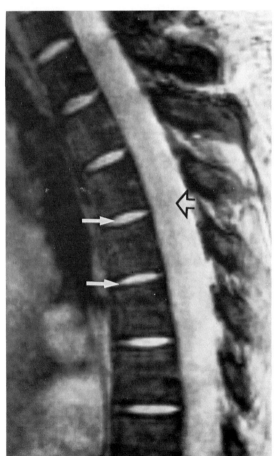

FIGURE 11–21. The disc–thecal-sac interface (*arrow*) is clearly defined on a multiplanar gradient-echo MR image with a TE of 9 msec and a flip angle of 110°.

FIGURE 11–22. High signal intensity discs (*solid arrows*) and cerebrospinal fluid (CSF; *open arrow*) are best imaged with T2*-weighted contrast. CSF–cord differentiation is poor in this image.

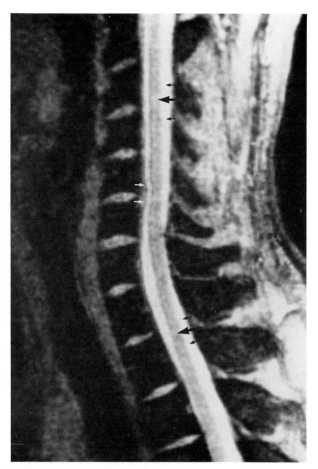

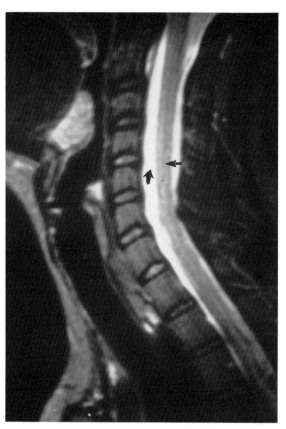

FIGURE 11–23. The low signal intensity cord (*large black arrows*) is clearly differentiated from bright signal intensity cerebrospinal fluid (*small black arrows*) on a T2*-weighted image. An extradural defect is seen as a minimal C5-6 disc bulge (*white arrows*).

FIGURE 11–24. The low signal intensity cord (*straight arrow*) and high signal intensity cerebrospinal fluid (*curved arrow*) can be seen on a conventional T2-weighted sagittal image.

FIGURE 11–25. (**A**) An accentuated posterior disc margin is difficult to differentiate from low signal intensity osteophytic ridging and annular fibers on a T2*-weighted image. (**B**) The corresponding 110° flip angle image more accurately distinguishes the vertebral endplates from the annulus.

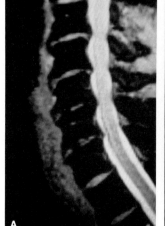
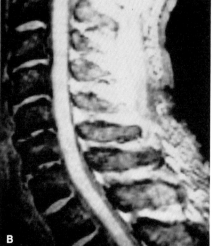

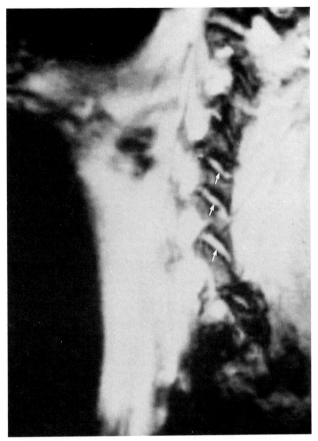

FIGURE 11–26. The facet articular cartilage of the apophyseal joint demonstrates high signal intensity (*arrows*) on a sagittal T2*-weighted image.

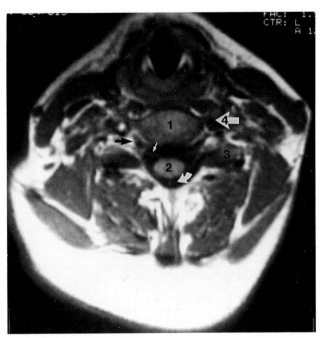

FIGURE 11–27. A T1-weighted axial image through cervical intervertebral disc shows the root sleeve (*black arrow*), ventral nerve root (*straight white arrow*), and cerebrospinal fluid (*curved white arrow*). (1, intervertebral disc; 2, spinal cord; 3, articular pillar; 4, vertebral artery.)

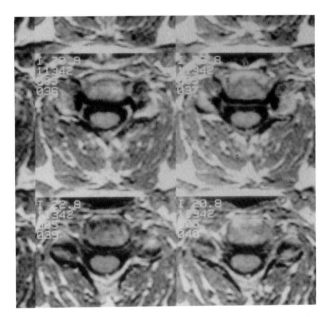

FIGURE 11–28. A volume spoiled GRASS protocol with a short TE (5 msec) and moderate flip angle (45°) produces T1-weighted contrast and eliminates T2 dependence. Cerebrospinal fluid is dark, the spinal cord is intermediate, and fat is bright in this sequence.

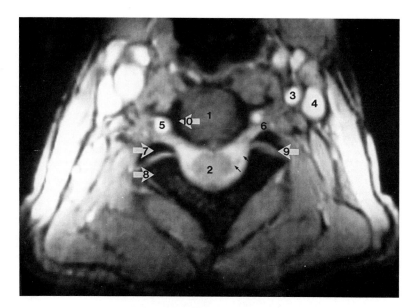

FIGURE 11–29. An axial T2*-weighted image at the midcervical level. (1, intervertebral disc; 2, spinal cord; 3, common carotid artery; 4, jugular vein; 5, vertebral artery; 6, dorsal root ganglion; 7, superior articular process; 8, inferior articular process; 9, facet cartilage; 10, uncinate process.)

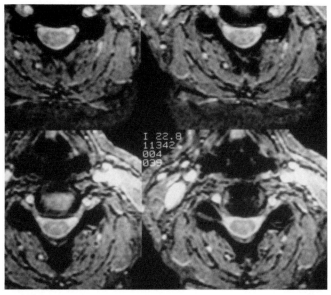

FIGURE 11–30. A protocol of 64 thin section (2 mm), contiguous, T2*-weighted 3D volume images produced with a TR of 35 msec, TE of 15 msec, and a flip angle of 5° produces a myelographic-like image with high signal intensity cerebrospinal fluid and low signal intensity spinal cord, vertebral bodies, and fat.

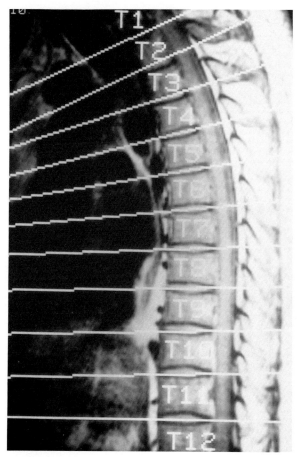

FIGURE 11–31. Thoracic disc axial prescriptions are graphically prescribed from a T1-weighted sagittal image.

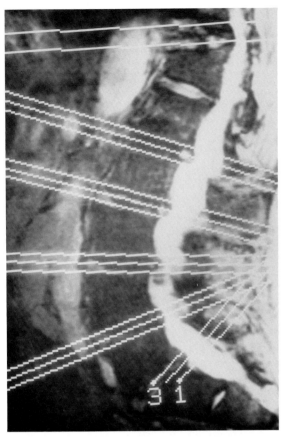

FIGURE 11–32. Axial lumbar disc locations are graphically prescribed from a T2*-weighted sagittal image.

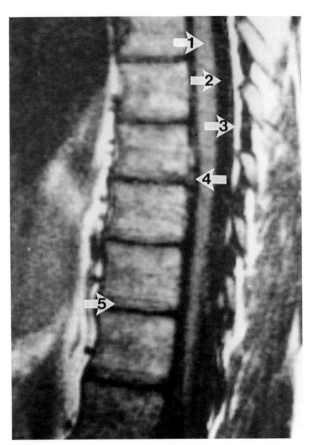

FIGURE 11–33. A T1-weighted sagittal image of thoracic spine. (1, spinal cord; 2, cerebrospinal fluid; 3, epidural fat; 4, thoracic disc herniation without cord compression; 5, intervertebral disc.)

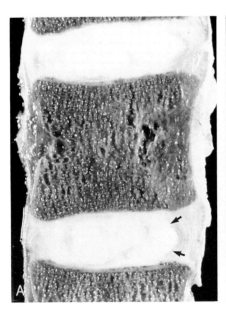

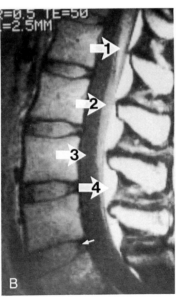

FIGURE 11–34. Lumbar spine. (**A**) A gross sagittal specimen of the lumbar spine demonstrates nuclear–annular separation (*arrows*). (**B**) A T1-weighted mid-sagittal image of the lumbar spine reveals annular fibers (*small arrow*). (1, conus medullaris; 2, cauda equina, 3, cerebrospinal fluid; 4, epidural fat.)

level of L1. The cauda equina is of lower signal intensity than the conus medullaris, secondary to greater surface contrast with surrounding CSF. The fibrous filum terminale may contain fat (5%) either focally or along its course as it extends from the conus to the distal thecal sac.[64] On T1-weighted images, anterior and posterior longitudinal ligaments are difficult to distinguish from low signal intensity cortical bone. The exiting nerve roots demonstrate intermediate signal intensity within the teardrop-shaped intervertebral foramina, and are surrounded by high signal intensity fat (Fig. 11–35). On parasagittal images, the low signal intensity radicular vein and intermediate signal intensity dorsal root are demarcated by abundant high signal intensity fat within the lumbar neutral foramina.

T2-Weighted Images

On T2-weighted images, the low signal intensity thoracic cord is seen in contrast to high signal intensity CSF. Thoracic and lumbar intervertebral discs demonstrate bright signal intensity on T2- and T2*-weighted images (Fig. 11–36), and epidural fat demonstrates intermediate signal intensity (Fig. 11–37). Vertebral body marrow demonstrates intermediate signal intensity on T2-weighted images and low signal intensity on T2*-weighted images. In T2-weighted images, the conus medullaris demonstrates lower signal intensity than the surrounding bright CSF. The nucleus pulposus and inner annular fibers display increased signal intensity on T2-weighted images, whereas peripheral annular fibers maintain low signal intensity. A low signal intensity band in the midportion of the intervertebral disc is thought to represent an invagination of annular fibers or fibrous tissue commonly seen in the adult spine. The basivertebral vein can be seen as a high signal intensity segment in the midposterior aspect of the vertebral body (Fig. 11–38). The low signal intensity fibrous posterior longitudinal ligament is adherent to the posterior annulus and posterior inferior and superior margins of the vertebral bodies. The anterior and posterior longitudinal ligaments may blend in with the adjacent cortex and annulus, which demonstrate low signal intensity on T1-, T2-, and T2*-weighted images.

Axial Images

T1-Weighted Images

In cross section, the thoracic cord demonstrates intermediate signal intensity, and the surrounding CSF demonstrates low signal intensity. High signal intensity from fatty marrow is seen in the vertebral body, pedicle, lamina, and transverse and spinous processes of the vertebrae. The low signal intensity intraforaminal vein can be seen anterior to the intermediate signal intensity dorsal root ganglion. The intermediate signal intensity dorsal

root ganglion, budding and exiting nerve roots are well defined and are surrounded by bright signal intensity fat (Fig. 11–39). Exiting nerve roots pass inferior to the pedicle of the corresponding vertebral body. Nerve roots within the thecal sac occupy a dependent position posteriorly following the crescentic or curved shape of the thecal sac. At lower lumbar vertebral levels, the nerve roots are fewer in number and become more dispersed within the CSF. A conjoined nerve root exists when two nerve roots exit from the same neural foramen. Nerve roots are often identified within the lower signal intensity thecal sac. Posterior epidural fat is identified behind the low signal intensity subarachnoid space. The basivertebral vein, retrovertebral plexus, and anterior epidural veins are displayed as low signal intensity structures. The ligamentum flavum parallels the inner surface of the lamina and demonstrates intermediate signal intensity.

T2-Weighted Images

An axial myelographic effect can be generated with gradient-echo refocused images in a fraction of the time required for conventional spin-echo techniques (Fig. 11–40). On T2-weighted images, the thoracic cord and lumbar cauda equina demonstrate low signal intensity, in contrast to the high signal intensity of the CSF (Figs. 11–41 and 11–42). Anterior signal void within the thecal sac is more frequent with long TR/TE sequences that accentuate CSF pulsation artifacts. Facet hyaline cartilage, which is 2 to 4 mm thick, demonstrates high signal intensity in gradient-echo images and intermediate signal intensity on conventional T2-weighted images. The ligamentum flavum has a high elastin content; therefore, it displays increased signal intensity on T2*-weighted images.

High signal intensity nuclear material, which is composed of well-hydrated collagen and protoglycans, and inner annular fibers can be distinguished from the low signal intensity outer collagen fibers of the annulus (Fig. 11–43). The transition between nucleus pulposus and annulus is not precise, but rather represents a spectrum from a hydrated gelatinous matrix in the nucleus pulposus to type II collagen in the inner annulus and type I collagen in the poorly hydrated peripheral annulus. Sharpey's fibers and the longitudinal ligaments attach the annulus to the vertebral endplates.

PATHOLOGY OF THE SPINE

In addition to the assessment of degenerative disc disease in the cervical spine, MR is useful in the evaluation of infection, trauma, and neoplasia involving osseous structures, soft tissue, and the cord.[7-45] Direct marrow imaging facilitates early detection in marrow replacement disorders (*e.g.,* leukemia, multiple myeloma, metastasis). Functional evaluation of atlantoaxial instability can be achieved by performing separate acquisitions with the patient positioned in flexion and extension.[65] Signal characteristics of cystic lesions (*e.g.,* syringomyelia, hydromyelia) are similar to those of CSF. Intramedullary lipomas demonstrate high signal intensity on T1-weighted images, intermediate to high signal intensity on T2-weighted images, and are dark in STIR sequences (Fig. 11-44). Lipomas can sometimes be confused with subacute hemorrhage, also bright on T1-weighted images, but hemorrhage shows increased signal intensity with long TR/TE (*i.e.,* T2-weighted) sequences. Detection of common intradural extramedullary tumors, such as neurofibromas[66] and meningiomas, may require the use of intravenous Gd-DTPA.

Degenerative Disc Disease

Cervical Spine

Disc Herniation. T1-weighted sagittal images display the subarachnoid disc and cervical cord outlines, allowing direct assessment of cord impingement (Fig. 11-45).[7-19,67] Early degenerative disc disease may be identified on conventional T2-weighted sagittal images and is characterized by loss of signal intensity in a desiccated intervertebral disc. Corresponding gradient-echo images are not as sensitive to changes in intradiscal signal intensity, and only in more advanced stages of degeneration are regions of low signal intensity from clefting, cavitation or complete desiccation demonstrated (Fig. 11-46). T2*-weighted sequences are useful in producing a myelographic CSF effect, important in assessing spinal canal stenosis and the disc–thecal-sac interface in herniations.[58,59] Gradient-echo techniques use a non-slice-selective acquisition without degradation or loss of signal intensity from pulsatile flow columns of CSF. With conventional spin-echo techniques, image quality is degraded by CSF flow artifact, and accuracy in interpreting extradural impressions (*e.g.,* disc herniations, osteophytosis) may be compromised. The absence of flow artifact, along with excellent differentiation between the cord and CSF, eliminates the need for cardiac gating in gradient-echo refocused imaging.

T1- and T2*-weighted gradient-echo images define the extent of most cervical disc herniations in the sagittal plane (Figs. 11-47 and 11-48).[68,69] Parasagittal and axial images are required to evaluate the lateral extension of a herniated disc (Figs. 11-49 and 11-50). Annular disc bulges may also demonstrate a posterior disc convexity in sagittal images (Fig. 11-51). However, the morphology of a contained herniation and the path of extruded disc material is more accurately demonstrated with axial plane images (Figs. 11-52 and 11-53). With 3DFT volume im-

aging at a slice thickness of 2 mm, cervical intervertebral discs are routinely sectioned at the level of the bright signal intensity nucleus pulposus. Increasing TE or decreasing the flip angle increases the contrast of the low signal intensity cord (Figs. 11-54 and 11-55). Cord compression and edema may be associated with larger disc protrusions. T1-weighted and T2*-weighted gradient-echo images demonstrate small disc herniations which might be missed on conventional T1-weighted spin-echo images because of the paucity of epidural and neural foraminal fat as contrast. A low signal intensity line or boundary between the herniated disc and cord represents the dura and the displaced posterior longitudinal ligament (Fig. 11-56). This dark interface may also be caused by a ridging osteophyte, by calcification, or by flow-related (*e.g.,* turbulence) artifact. The most common locations for cervical disc herniations are C5-6 and C6-7. They are usually midline or posterolateral, with the uncinate process offering some protection against lateral cervical herniations (Fig. 11-57).[70] When lateral disc herniations do occur, they can be seen in peripheral parasagittal and axial images. The superior inferior extension (*i.e.,* migration) of disc material is best demonstrated on T1- and T2*-weighted sagittal and axial T2*-weighted images (Figs. 11-58 and 11-59). This may be seen as a double dark line representing a herniated disc fragment crossing the posterior longitudinal ligament. I have not found it necessary to administer Gd-DTPA to enhance the epidural venous plexus in the diagnosis of more lateral herniations.

Without a corresponding T1-weighted gradient-echo image, it may not be possible to differentiate a posterior osteophyte from an annulus. The resultant magnetic susceptibility artifact on T2*-weighted sagittal images frequently causes overestimation of the degree of cervical disc herniation or stenosis (Fig. 11-60).

I have observed differences between flexion and extension in herniated disc morphology, and thus central canal stenosis (Fig. 11-61). Kinematic applications, however, have been more frequently used in assessing atlantoaxial subluxations.

Cervical Spinal Stenosis. A decrease in disc height and bulging of the peripheral annular fibers may contribute to spinal stenosis (Fig. 11-62). Associated osteophytes may project from the anterior (Fig. 11-63) and posterior (Fig. 11-64) vertebral body margins, and posterior osteophytes may be confused with low signal intensity annular bulges on heavily T2*-weighted images. Low signal intensity osteophytes and endplate sclerosis can be separated from high signal intensity discs on 110° flip angle gradient-echo images (Figs. 11-65 and 11-66). Intervertebral nerve root canal stenosis may be overestimated from magnetic-susceptibility artifact on T2*-weighted axial images (Fig 11-67). Enlarged osteophytes that compromise the subarachnoid space contribute to the development of cord myelopathy. Radiculopathy may result from impingement in the dural sac or root sleeve.[71] Neural foraminal stenosis and associated radiculopathy may also be caused by degenerative changes at the facet and uncinate (*e.g.,* uncinate process hypertrophy, uncovertebral spurs; Figs. 11–68 and 11–69).[72]

Degenerative facet arthrosis may result in vertebral body retrolisthesis, further compromising the anterior to posterior sagittal canal diameter.[73] Low signal intensity linear ossification of the posterior longitudinal ligament may also contribute to cord compression, especially when associated with congenital spinal stenosis or hypertrophic changes or spondylosis.[73,74]

Thoracic and Lumbar Spines

Disc Herniation

Classification. The term annular disc bulge should be reserved for a relatively symmetric or generalized extension of the posterior disc margin beyond the posterior borders of the adjacent vertebral body endplates (Fig. 11–70). This stage of disc degeneration represents stretching or increased laxity of the annulus without tearing of concentric annular fibers.[54]

Disc protrusions are characterized by a focal projection or asymmetry of the posterior disc margin beyond the posterior borders of the adjacent vertebral body endplates.[47] A disc protrusion is a contained disc herniation; herniated nuclear material extends through a tear of the inner annulus but does not extend through outermost annular fibers. Axial images are better than corresponding sagittal images for demonstrating the focal contour changes of the posterior disc margin in a protrusion. In sagittal images, an annular disc bulge and a protrusion may have similar morphology. Occasionally, annular fissuring or tears may be identified on T2-weighted or Gd-DTPA enhanced T1-weighted sagittal images (Fig. 11–71).

Although, by definition, a disc protrusion is a herniated disc, partial tearing of inner annular fibers cannot be reliably identified with either CT or MR. In an extruded disc, nuclear disc material extends through all layers of the annulus and produces an extradural mass that often indents the ventral aspect of the thecal sac (Fig. 11–72). Differentiation of a prominent disc protrusion from a small disc extrusion may not be possible in the absence of disrupted posterior annular fibers. Distinction between the two may be academic, however, in that both disc protrusions and extrusions are considered varying degrees of disc herniation. Extruded discs may extend superior or inferior to the intervertebral disc and are usually confined by the posterior longitudinal ligament.

A sequestered disc, or free fragment, represents disc material which is no longer in continuity with its parent intervertebral disc of origin, and may be found at another vertebral body level (Fig. 11–73). Intradural extrusion has also been reported.[38,40,75]

Magnetic Resonance Findings. The accuracy of MR in the assessment of thoracic and lumbar disc herniation has been reported to be equivalent to that for CT and myelography (Figs. 11–74 and 11–75).[32,34,76–79] The sagittal plane is sensitive in identifying the posterior disc margin, the annular complex, and the interface with the ventral aspect of the thecal sac. However, any sagittal plane findings should be confirmed in corresponding axial images for more accurate assessment of the degree of secondary central canal or neural foraminal stenoses and nerve root impingement.

On sagittal images, annular disc bulges have a low signal intensity intact posterior annular complex and may be associated with disc desiccation (Fig. 11–76). Conventional T2- and T2*-weighted images are useful in assessing intervertebral disc desiccation (Figs. 11–77 and 11–78). Desiccated disc material, which may be hyperintense on T2*-weighted images, is usually less intense than normally hydrated intervertebral discs at other levels. This greater sensitivity of conventional T2-weighted images to the detection of desiccation represents a potential limitation of gradient-echo protocols (Figs. 11–79 and 11–80). T2*-weighted images are particularly sensitive to disc calcifications and nitrogen gas in vacuum phenomena, secondary to magnetic susceptibility (Figs. 11–81 and 11–82).

Most disc protrusions or herniations demonstrate low signal intensity on T1- or T2-weighted images, although the converse is not true. Discs with normal morphology may be desiccated without associated herniation (Fig. 11–83). Annular fissures appear as focal areas of bright linear signal intensity within the posterior confines of the annulus on T2- or T2*-weighted sagittal images.[80,81] Disc herniations are subjectively categorized as mild, moderate, or severe. A mild disc herniation with superimposed spinal stenosis may produce more symptoms than a moderate disc herniation in a capacious canal. Disc–CSF differentiation may be difficult on T1-weighted images, because the posterior disc margin and thecal sac both demonstrate low signal intensity. Most herniated discs are depicted as degenerative or desiccated on conventional T2-weighted images, in contrast to T2*-weighted images. Lateral disc herniations can efface the bright signal intensity neural foraminal fat without compromising the thecal sac (Figs. 11–84 and 11–85). Gadolinium may improve imaging of lateral disc herniations by identifying the boundary between disc and exiting nerve root (Fig. 11–86). Large posterolateral disc herniations may compromise both the thecal sac and exiting nerve root. The sagittal imaging plane may be more sensitive in defining deformities of the thecal sac at the disc–thecal-sac interface, specifically, in demonstrating discontinuity of low signal intensity annular fibers (Fig. 11–87). T2-weighted images increase contrast discrimination between bright signal intensity CSF and low signal intensity annular fibers at the disc–thecal-sac boundary. Acute herniations may demonstrate increased signal intensity in both conventional T1- and T2-weighted images (Figs. 11–88 and 11–89). On gradient-echo images, the posterior annular fibers and longitudinal ligament demonstrate low signal intensity, facilitating differentiation of the disc and CSF. On gradient-echo images, the dura of the lumbar spine is depicted as a black line; it may be displaced in posterior disc herniations. Nuclear material extruded from the disc usually demonstrates low signal intensity on conventional T1- and T2-weighted images and high signal intensity in gradient-echo sequences (Figs. 11–90 and 11–91). Increases in the signal intensity of herniated nuclear material on T2- or T2*-weighted images, however, may be secondary to inflammation or to an increased water content in the extruded disc.[41,82] Axial images are important in evaluating neural foramina and nerve root effacement in cases of lateral and posterolateral disc herniations (Fig. 11–92). The path of the extruded nuclear material may be outlined on axial T2-weighted images due to a discogramlike effect (Fig. 11–93).

Separated disc material superior or inferior to the intervertebral disc level represent free fragments (Figs. 11–94 and 11–95). A low signal intensity (*i.e.*, dark) line between a sequestered disc fragment and the parent disc may be seen when penetration of the posterior longitudinal ligament has occurred; this is referred to as the double-fragment sign.[83] An intradural disc herniation demonstrates higher signal intensity than CSF on T1-weighted images. Gadolinium may be used to enhance granulation tissue around the peripheral border of a free fragment (Fig. 11–96). This is useful in excluding diagnoses such as neurofibroma, epidural fibrosis, and abscesses. After Gd-DTPA administration, the central portion of a free fragment or sequestered disc maintains low signal intensity, whereas the periphery is enhanced; this produces a bull's-eye appearance (Fig. 11–97). In the nonoperative spine, enhanced MR images have also been useful in identifying increased signal intensity in annular rents or tears, presumably due to the ingrowth of blood vessels, granulation tissue, or both, similar to that seen in Figure 11–98.[80] Calcified cysts of the facet joint may mimic a calcified free fragment (Fig. 11–99).

Surrounded by high signal intensity epidural fat, a conjoined nerve root is more clearly depicted in MR than in CT (Fig. 11–100). Schmorl's nodes represent extensions of herniations through vertebral body endplates and demonstrate increased signal intensity relative to adjacent subchondral bone on T2- and T2*-weighted images (Fig. 11–101). A limbus vertebra, identified as a defect in the anterior superior vertebral body endplate, is caused by the extension of a herniated disc through the rim apophysis.[81]

Thoracic disc herniations, which are less frequent than lumbar or cervical herniations, are usually identified in the midthoracic or lower-thoracic levels (see Figs. 11–74 and 11–75).[36,39] If no abnormality is found in sagittal images, oblique image prescriptions through all thoracic intervertebral discs are recommended to identify any small extradural defects.

Endplate Changes

Modic has characterized changes in vertebral body marrow signal intensity adjacent to the endplates of degenerative intervertebral discs.[47,53,55] In type I endplates, signal intensity is decreased on T1-weighted images and increased on T2- or T2*-weighted images (Fig. 11–102). This pattern is observed in 4% of MR studies for intervertebral disc disease and in 30% of patients after treatment with chymopapain. Type I endplate changes represent subchondral vascularized fibrous tissue associated with endplate fissuring and disruption. Type II endplate changes (Fig. 11–103) include fatty marrow endplate conversion, which demonstrates increased signal intensity in T1-weighted images, isointense to slightly hyperintense signal intensity on T2-weighted images, and isointense signal intensity on T2*-weighted images (Fig. 11–104). Type II changes are seen in approximately 16% of cases, and correlate with yellow marrow replacement and associated endplate degeneration or disruption. Type III endplate changes include sclerosis, which demonstrates low signal intensity on T1-, T2-, and T2*-weighted images (see Fig. 11–95). It is important not to mistake Gd-DTPA enhancement or increased signal intensity of areas of fibrovascular tissue in STIR images with endplate changes of osteomyelitis that cross the discovertebral junction.

Lumbar and Thoracic Spinal Stenosis

Spinal stenosis, acquired or congenital, may involve the central canal, the intervertebral foramen, or the lateral recess. In the lumbar spine, stenosis may be bony or secondary to soft-tissue (*i.e.*, disc) impingement (Figs. 11–105 through 11–107). Indentations of the thecal sac are caused by both disc and osteophytic impingement. Facet and ligamentum flavum hypertrophy contribute to neural foraminal and central canal stenosis (Figs. 11–108 and 11–109). The bright CSF-extradural interface on T2- and T2*-weighted images, makes these sequences preferable for assessment of canal dimensions. On T1-weighted images, there is a loss or decrease in bright signal intensity epidural fat, which makes these sequences preferable for identifying peripheral or neural

(text continues on page 934)

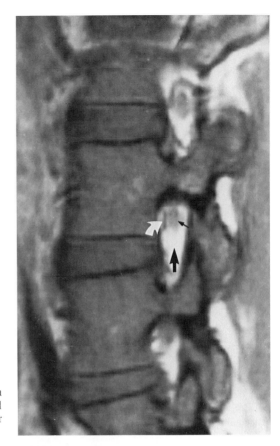

FIGURE 11–35. A parasagittal T1-weighted image of the intervertebral foramina shows high signal intensity epidural fat (*large black arrow*), intermediate signal intensity dorsal root ganglion (*small black arrow*), and low signal intensity radicular vein (*curved white arrow*).

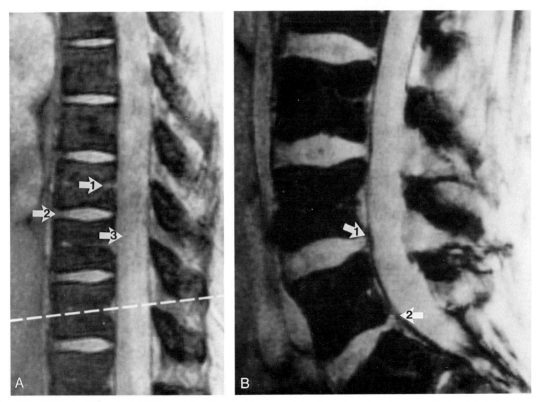

FIGURE 11–36. (**A**) A T2*-weighted sagittal image of the thoracic spine does not distinguish between high signal intensity cerebrospinal fluid (CSF) and cord. (1, basivertebral vein; 2, high signal intensity intervertebral disc; 3, CSF and cord.) (**B**) A T2*-weighted sagittal image of the lumbar spine. (1, low signal intensity annulus; 2, low signal intensity dural interface.)

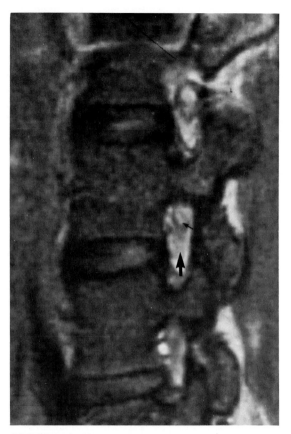

FIGURE 11–37. A conventional T2-weighted parasagittal image of the intervertebral foramina shows poor contrast between intermediate signal intensity neural foraminal fat (*large arrow*) and dorsal root ganglion (*small arrow*).

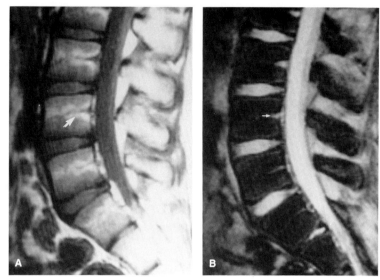

FIGURE 11–38. (**A**) High signal intensity fat (*arrow*) is associated with the basivertebral vein on a T1-weighted sagittal image. (**B**) The basivertebral vein (*arrow*) demonstrates increased signal intensity on a T2*-weighted sagittal image.

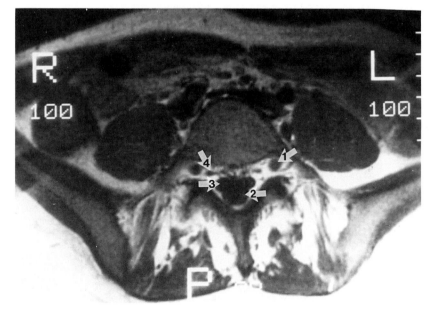

FIGURE 11–39. T1-weighted axial anatomy of the lumbar spine at the level of the superior neural foramina. (1, L5 nerve root sheath; 2, thecal sac; 3, budding S1 nerve root; 4, anterior epidural vein.)

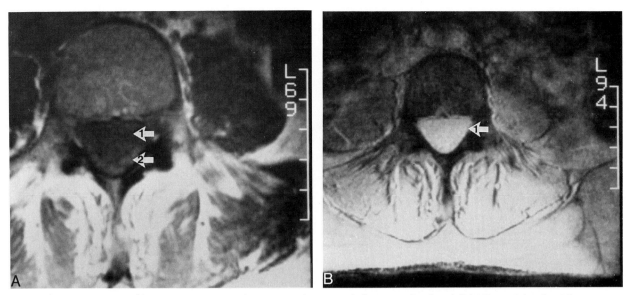

FIGURE 11–40. Axial myelographic contrast between (**A**) T1-weighted and (**B**) T2*-weighted axial images at midlumbar body level. The thecal sac demonstrates bright signal intensity in the T2*-weighted image. (1, thecal sac; 2, cauda equina.)

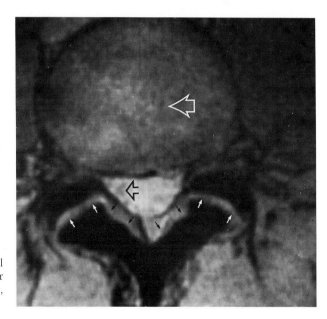

FIGURE 11–41. A T2*-weighted axial image of lumbar intervertebral disc shows the high signal intensity disc (*open white arrow*), articular cartilage (*solid white arrows*), ligamentum flavum (*solid black arrows*), and low signal intensity cauda equina (*open black arrow*).

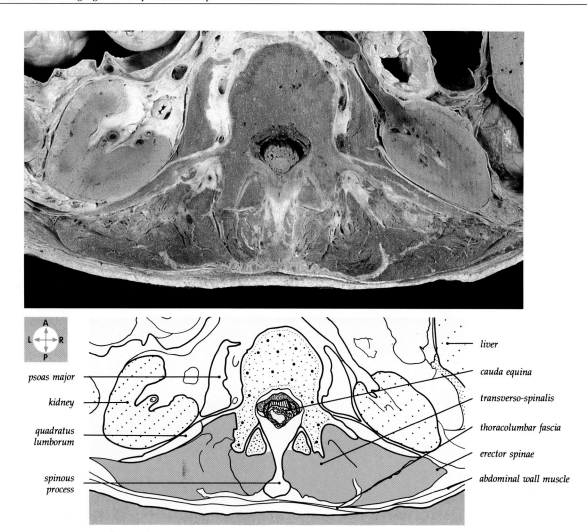

FIGURE 11–42.   A transverse section at the level of the second lumbar vertebra shows the back muscles and the contents of the vertebral foramen.

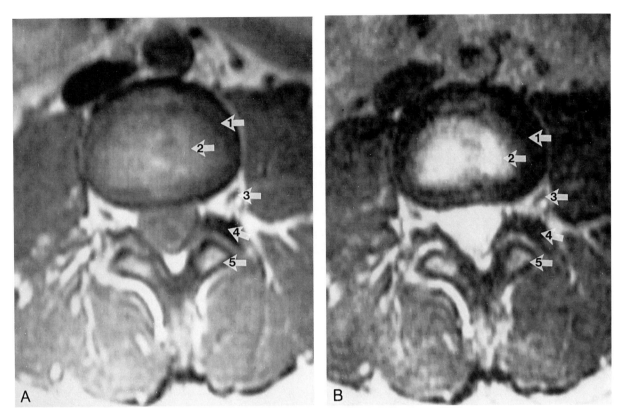

FIGURE 11–43. A conventional T2-weighted axial sequence at the intervertebral disc. (**A**) Intermediate-weighted and (**B**) T2-weighted axial images demonstrate increased signal intensity in the nucleus pulposus in T2-weighted contrast. (1, low signal intensity annular fibers; 2, nucleus pulposus; 3, exiting nerve root; 4, superior articular facet; 5, inferior articular facet.)

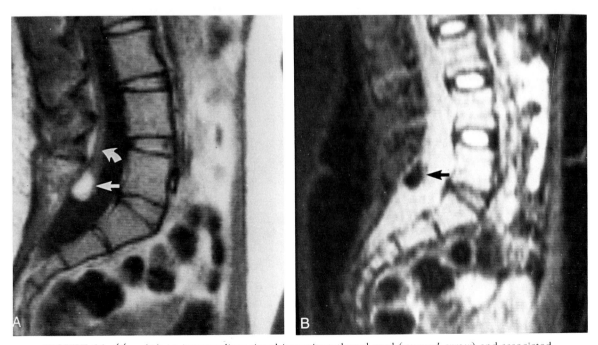

FIGURE 11–44. (**A**) An intermediate signal intensity tethered cord (*curved arrow*) and associated lipoma (*straight arrow*) are seen on (**A**) T1-weighted and (**B**) short TI inversion recovery (STIR) images. The lipoma demonstrates high signal intensity on the T1-weighted image and is dark on the STIR image. (**C**) The corresponding CT scan demonstrates low attenuation lipoma (*arrow*). (**D**) The lipoma demonstrates high signal intensity on a T1-weighted axial image. *(continued)*

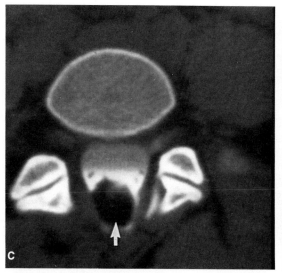

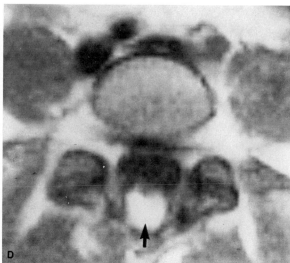

FIGURE 11–44. *(Continued)*

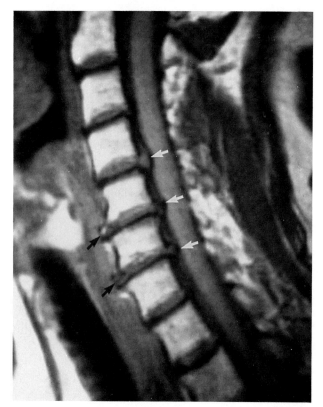

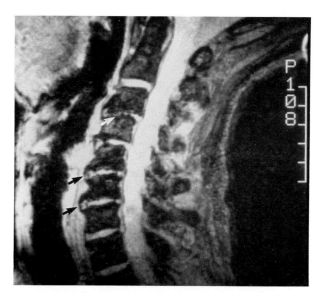

FIGURE 11–45. C3-4, C4-5, and C5-6 disc herniations (*white arrows*) compressing the spinal cord are seen on a T1-weighted sagittal image. Anterior disc bulges (*black arrows*) and loss of disc-space height are shown at levels C3-4 and C4-5.

FIGURE 11–46. Cervical osteophytosis is indicated by a degenerative cervical spine with osteophytes (*black arrows*) and an associated C3-4 disc (*white arrow*) on a T2*-weighted sagittal image.

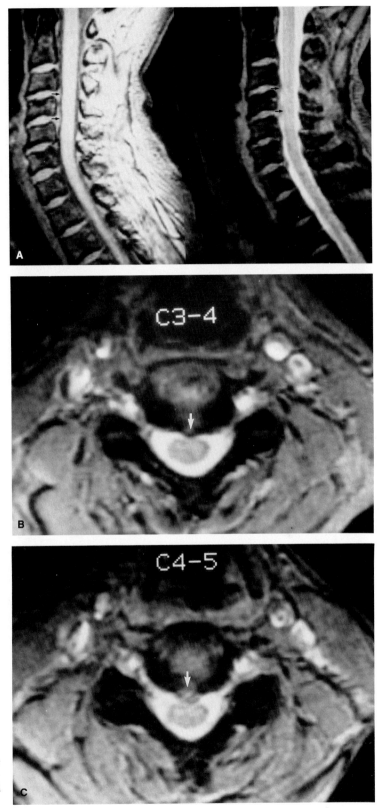

FIGURE 11–47. Mild C3-4 and moderate C4-5 midline cervical disc herniations (*arrows*) are seen on (**A**) gradient-echo sagittal and (**B, C**) 3D Fourier transform T2*-weighted axial images.

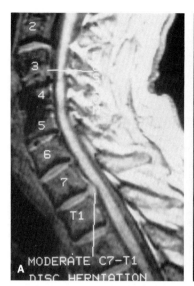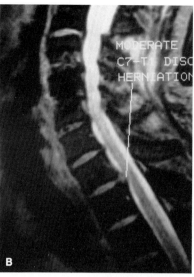

FIGURE 11–48. Moderate-to-severe C7-T1 herniation and anterior extradural defect after C3-C6 fusion is seen on (**A**) a gradient-echo image with 110° flip angle and (**B**) a T2*-weighted image.

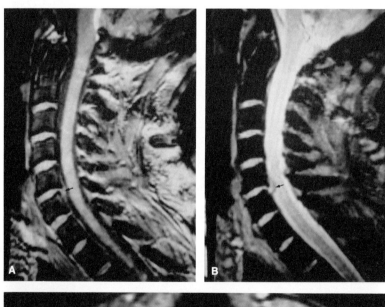

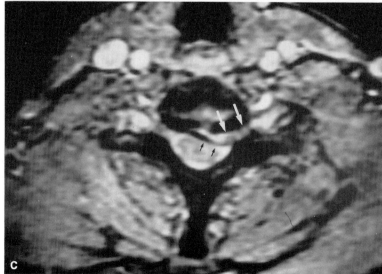

FIGURE 11–49. A C6-7 disc herniation with an anterior extradural defect on (**A**) a gradient-echo image with 110° flip angle and on (**B**) a T2*-weighted image. (**C**) Left paracentral–lateral herniation effaces the left ventrolateral cord (*black arrows*) and causes severe left neural (*i.e.,* intervertebral nerve root canal) stenosis (*white arrows*), as seen on a T2*-weighted axial image.

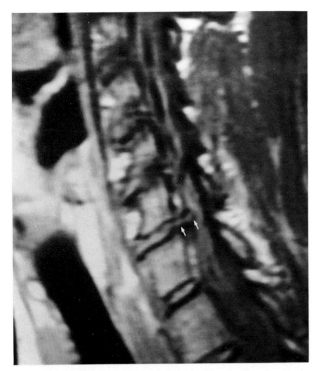

FIGURE 11–50. A lateral C6-7 disc herniation (*arrows*) is seen on T1-weighted parasagittal image.

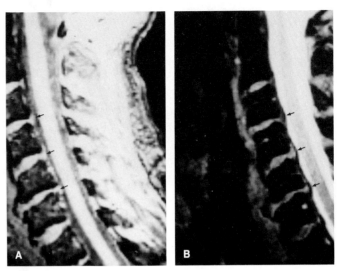

FIGURE 11–51. Annular bulging discs at C3-4, C4-5, and C5-6 with an intact posterior longitudinal ligament are seen on (**A**) a gradient-echo image with 110° flip angle and (**B**) a T2*-weighted sagittal image.

FIGURE 11–52. (**A**) A herniated disc (*arrow*) at the C5-6 level in midline is seen on a T2*-weighted sagittal image. (**B**) In left paracentral herniation, the disc is in contact with the ventral aspect of the cord. The posterior longitudinal ligament and dura demonstrate low signal intensity on a T2*-weighted axial image.

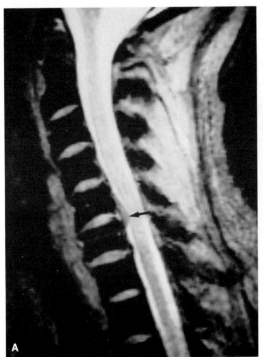

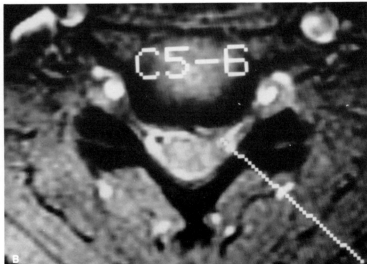

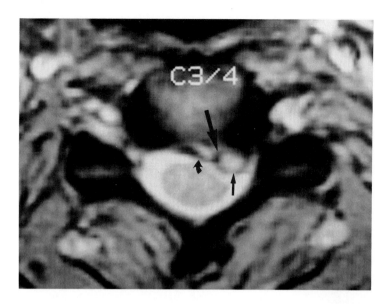

FIGURE 11–53. A severe left paracentral C3-4 herniation disc is seen on a T2*-weighted axial image. The herniated disc demonstrates high signal intensity (*large straight arrow*). A defect in the annulus and posterior longitudinal ligament (*curved arrow*) can be differentiated from the thin dark line between the disc and spinal cord that represents a contribution by the posterior longitudinal ligament and dura (*small straight arrow*).

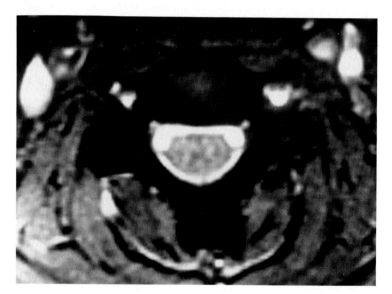

FIGURE 11–54. A TE of 25 msec and a flip angle of 10° improves the conspicuity of the low signal intensity cord on this T2*-weighted axial image.

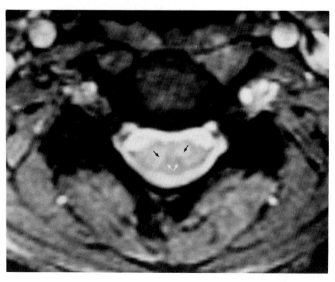

FIGURE 11–55. The white matter of the posterior columns (*white arrows*) demonstrate lower signal intensity than the gray matter of the cord (*black arrows*) on a T2*-weighted axial image.

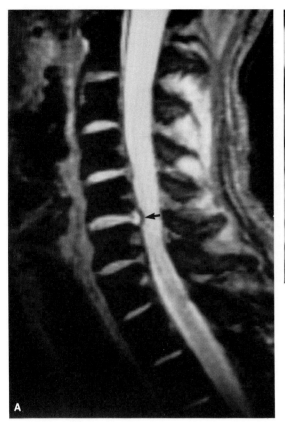

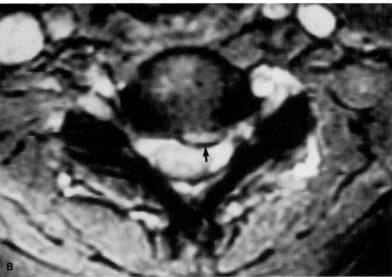

FIGURE 11–56. Moderate C5-6 herniation with a low signal intensity annular–dural interface (*arrow*) is seen on T2*-weighted (**A**) sagittal and (**B**) axial images.

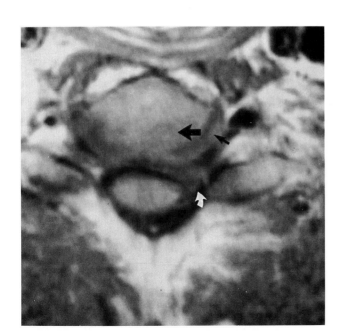

FIGURE 11–57. A T1-weighted axial image shows left lateral disc herniation (*curved white arrow*). The intervertebral disc (*large black arrow*) and uncinate process (*small black arrow*) are seen at this level.

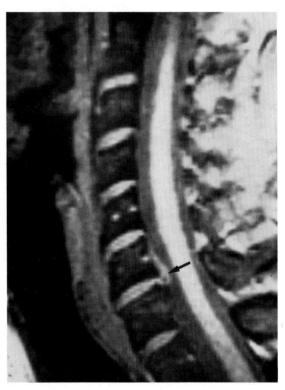

FIGURE 11–58. On a gradient-echo image with a flip angle of 110°, the superior extension of a C6-7 disc herniation demonstrates high signal intensity (*arrow*), in contrast to the low signal intensity of cerebrospinal fluid. The cervical cord is hyperintense.

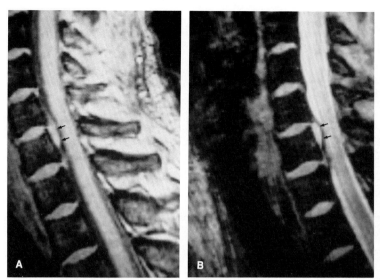

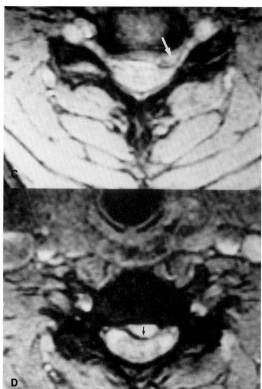

FIGURE 11–59. Severe herniation with inferior extrusion of disc material at C6-7 level (*arrows*) is seen on (**A**) a T1-weighted image at a flip angle of 110° and (**B**) a T2*-weighted sagittal image. (**C**) A severe left paracentral–lateral C6-7 herniation (*arrow*) with severe secondary left neural (*i.e.,* intervertebral) foraminal stenosis is seen on a T2*-weighted axial image. (**D**) An inferior extension of extruded disc (*arrow*) is shown at the level of the C7 vertebral body in another T2*-weighted axial image.

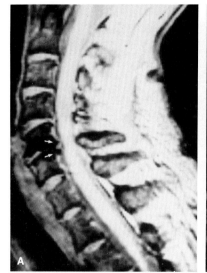

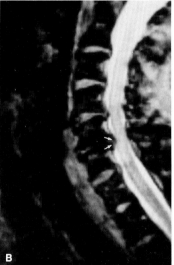

FIGURE 11–60. Vertebral osteophytes (*arrows*) are more accurately defined on (**A**) a gradient-echo image with a flip angle of 110° than on (**B**) a T2*-weighted image, where a magnetic-susceptibility artifact accentuates the degree of central canal stenosis.

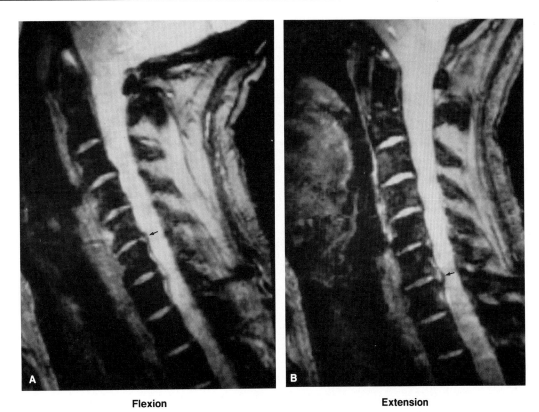

Flexion   **Extension**

FIGURE 11–61. C6-7 disc herniation is seen on (**A**) flexion and (**B**) extension on T2*-weighted images. In extension, the herniation is larger, and the central canal stenosis is greater.

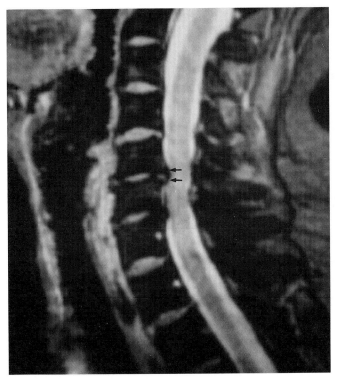

FIGURE 11–62. Posterior osteophytic ridging of the C5-6 level in association with degenerative loss of intervertebral disc-space height produces central canal stenosis. There is no disc herniation, as seen on a T2*-weighted sagittal image.

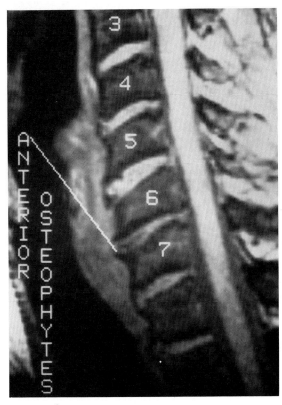

FIGURE 11–63. Anterior osteophytosis in continuity with corresponding vertebral bodies and distinct from the annulus is seen on a gradient-echo sagittal image with a flip angle of 110°.

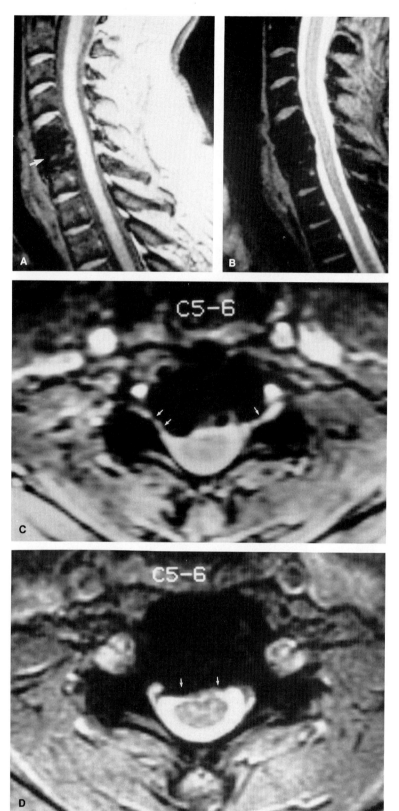

FIGURE 11–64. C5-6 fusion (*arrow*) is seen on (**A**) a gradient-echo sagittal image with a flip angle of 110° and (**B**) a T2*-weighted sagittal image (right). (**C**) Severe right (*double arrow*) and moderate left (*single arrow*) intervertebral nerve root canal (*i.e.,* neural foramen) stenosis is seen on a T2*-weighted axial image. (**D**) Moderate posterior osteophytic ridging (*arrows*) at the C5-6 fusion level effaces the anterior subarachnoid space on a T2*-weighted axial image.

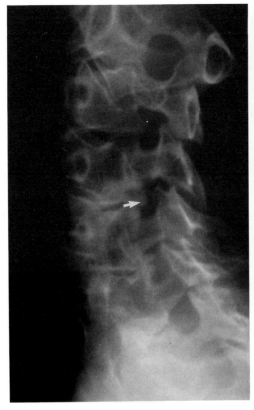
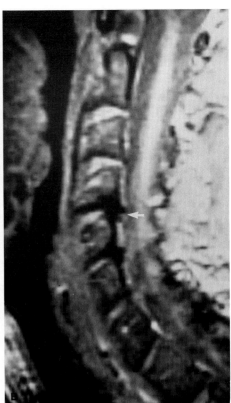

FIGURE 11–65. Stenosis of the left neural foramen (*i.e.,* intervertebral nerve root canal; *arrows*) on (**A**) an oblique radiograph and (**B**) the corresponding gradient-echo sagittal image. Low signal intensity osteophytic spurring is differentiated from the adjacent vertebral body marrow on the gradient-echo image.

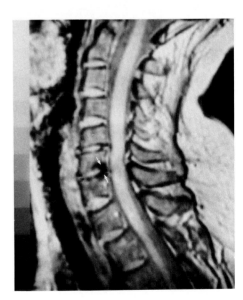

FIGURE 11–66. Low signal intensity posterior endplate sclerosis (*arrows*) is seen in a gradient-echo sagittal image with a flip angle of 110°.

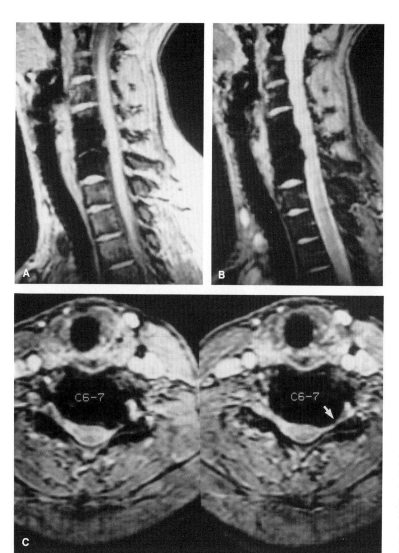

FIGURE 11–67. Postoperative changes at C5-C7 with increased magnetic-susceptibility artifact which is less severe on (**A**) a gradient-echo image with an TE of msec and a flip angle of 110° than on (**B**) a T2*-weighted sagittal image with an TE of 20 msec. (**C**) Magnetic susceptibility demonstrates accentuated severe left intervertebral nerve root canal stenosis (*arrow*) on the T2*-weighted axial image.

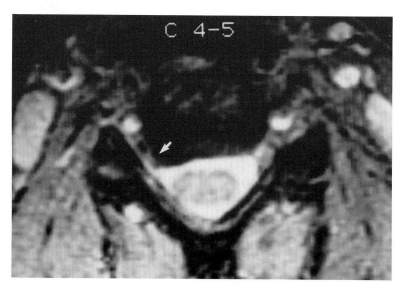

FIGURE 11–68. Moderate right neural foraminal (*i.e.,* intervertebral nerve root canal) stenosis secondary to degenerative uncinate hypertrophic spur (*arrow*) at the C4-5 level is seen on a T2*-weighted axial image.

FIGURE 11-69. (**A**) Left uncinate and facet hypertrophy (*arrows*) produces severe left neural (*i.e.,* intervertebral nerve root canal) foraminal stenosis. (**B**) The corresponding oblique radiograph confirms bony left C3-4 neural foraminal stenosis (*arrow*).

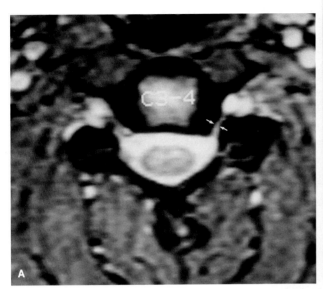

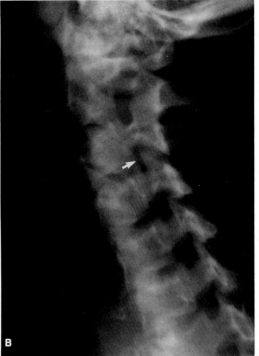

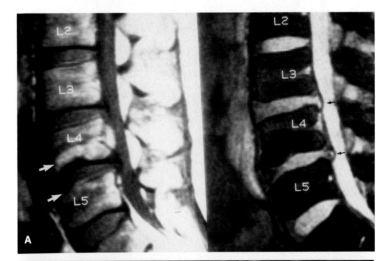

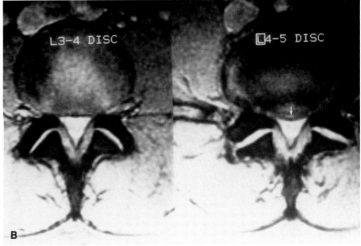

FIGURE 11-70. An L3-4 annular bulge (*arrow*) and mild L4-5 central disc protrusion (*arrow*) is seen on (**A**) T1-weighted (*left*) and T2*-weighted (*right*) sagittal images and on (**B**) T2*-weighted axial images. Yellow or fat marrow signal intensity of type II endplate change is shown on the T1-weighted sagittal image (*double arrow*). There is moderate central canal stenosis at L3-4 and moderate to severe central stenosis at L4-5. The L3-4 annular bulge shows no focal asymmetry of the posterior disc margin in the axial plane, whereas, at the L4-5 level, there is focal asymmetry of the posterior margin centrally (*arrow*).

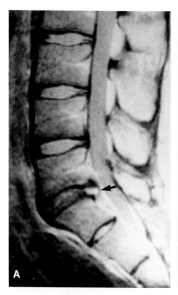

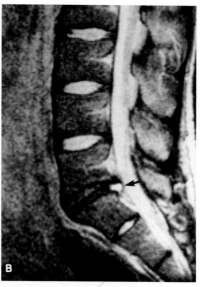

FIGURE 11–71. High signal intensity fissuring (*arrow*) in a posterior annular bulge is seen on (**A**) intermediate-weighted and (**B**) T2-weighted sagittal images.

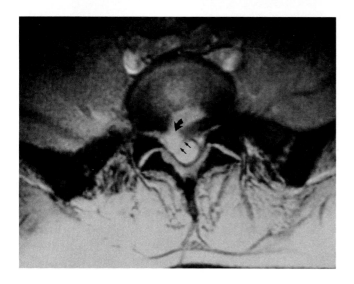

FIGURE 11–72. The path of extruded nuclear disc material is identified (*curved arrow*) in a right paracentral L5-S1 herniation. Indentation of the right ventral lateral aspect of the thecal sac (*small straight arrows*) has occurred.

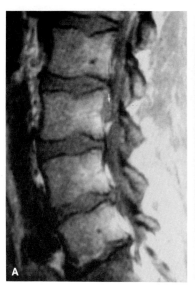

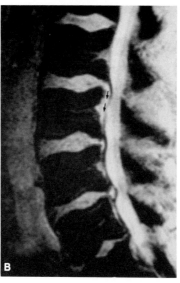

FIGURE 11–73. Disruption of the inferior aspect of the L2-3 annular complex is seen on (**A**) T1-weighted and (**B**) T2*-weighted sagittal images. Note the free fragment that has migrated posterior to the L3 vertebral body (*arrows*). (**C**) Soft-tissue signal intensity representing the sequestered disc is seen posterior to the L3 body (*arrow*) and displaces the thecal sac from right to left, as seen on a T1-weighted axial image.

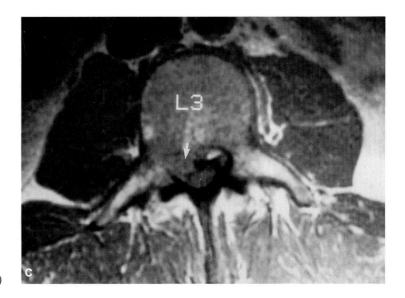

FIGURE 11–73. *(Continued)*

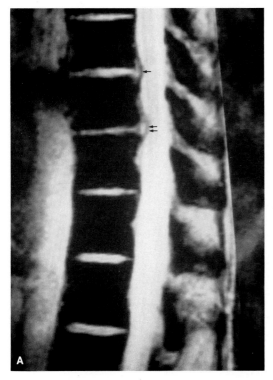

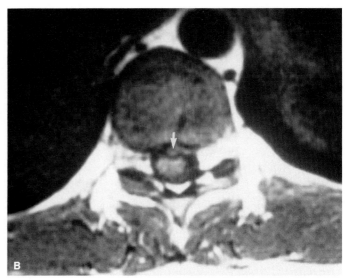

FIGURE 11–74. (**A**) Two level thoracic disc herniations (*arrows*) demonstrate the high signal intensity of extruded disc material on a T2*-weighted sagittal image. (**B**) Subligamentous herniation (*i.e.,* ruptured annulus fibrosis) produces a central extradural defect (*arrow*) on a T1-weighted axial image.

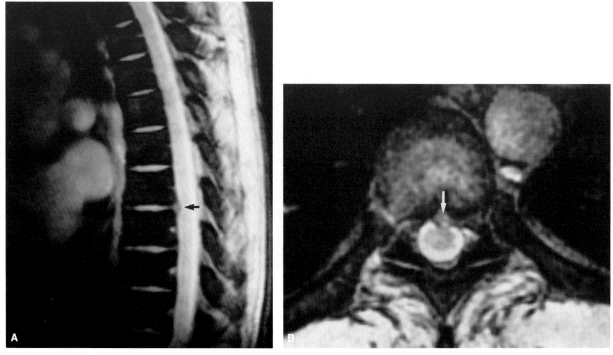

FIGURE 11–75. A moderate midthoracic disc herniation (*arrows*) is compressing the ventral cord as seen on T2*-weighted (**A**) sagittal and (**B**) axial images.

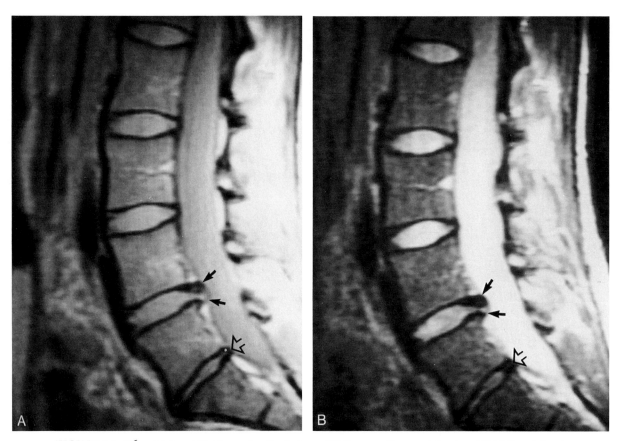

FIGURE 11–76. L4-5 and L5-S1 annular disc bulges. (**A**) Intermediate-weighted and (**B**) T2-weighted sagittal images demonstrate an isointense and low signal intensity desiccated L5-S1 lumbar disc, respectively (*open arrow*). Deformity of the anterior thecal sac secondary to the L4-5 annular bulge (*solid arrows*) is best seen on the T2-weighted image.

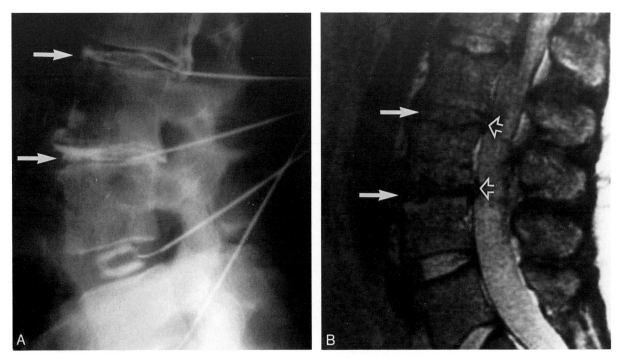

FIGURE 11–77. Desiccated and herniated L2-3 and L3-4 discs demonstrate (**A**) abnormal contrast distribution (*solid arrows*) in a lateral discogram and (**B**) loss of signal intensity (*solid arrows*) on a T2-weighted sagittal image. Disc bulges that are deforming the ventral aspect of the thecal sac are identified on the sagittal MR image (*open arrows*).

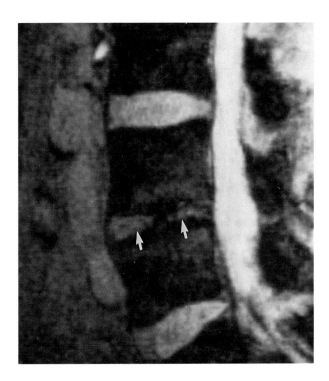

FIGURE 11–78. Severe intervertebral L4-5 disc desiccation (*arrows*) with loss of signal intensity and disc-space height is seen on a T2*-weighted sagittal image.

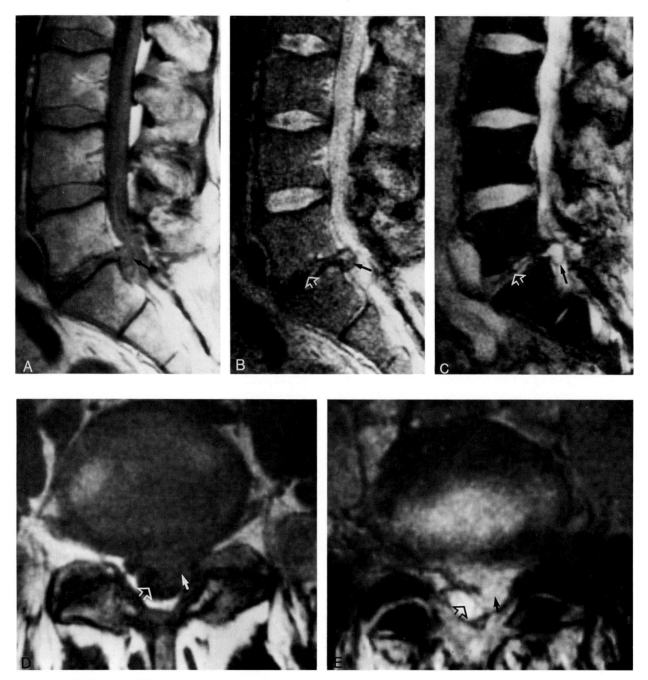

FIGURE 11–79. (**A**) T1-weighted, (**B**) T2-weighted, and (**C**) T2*-weighted images show herniated and extruded L5-S1 nuclear material (*black arrow*). The intervertebral disc contents (*open arrow*) remain low in signal intensity on conventional T2-weighted sequences. On T2*-weighted contrast, nuclear material generates high signal intensity, whereas the adjacent desiccated disc demonstrates signal inhomogeneity and low signal intensity clefting (*open arrow*). The corresponding (**D**) T1-weighted and (**E**) T2*-weighted axial images provide superior contrast definition of the herniated nuclear material (*solid arrow*) and deformed thecal sac (*open arrow*).

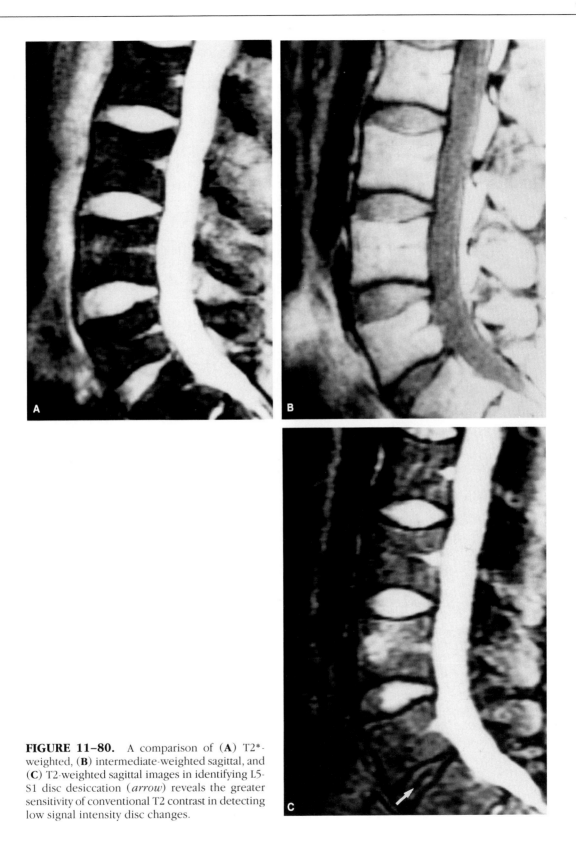

FIGURE 11–80. A comparison of (**A**) T2*-weighted, (**B**) intermediate-weighted sagittal, and (**C**) T2-weighted sagittal images in identifying L5-S1 disc desiccation (*arrow*) reveals the greater sensitivity of conventional T2 contrast in detecting low signal intensity disc changes.

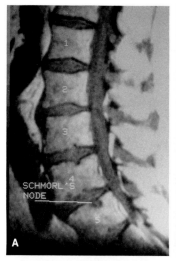

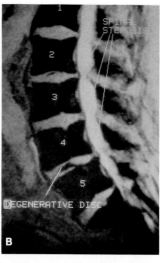

FIGURE 11–81. (**A**) Schmorl's node superior endplate L5 and (**B**) low signal intensity degenerative L4-5 vacuum phenomena. Central stenosis is best displayed on T2*-weighted contrast, where high signal intensity cerebrospinal fluid and the posterior annular complex are shown.

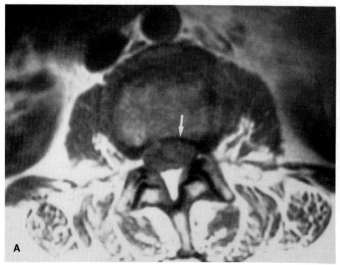

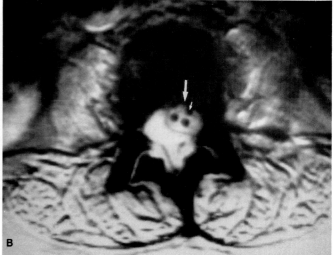

FIGURE 11–82. The low signal intensity susceptibility effects of calcium (*small arrow*) in a sequestered disc (*large arrow*) are seen on (**A**) T1-weighted and (**B**) T2*-weighted axial images.

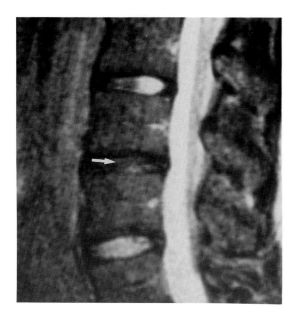

FIGURE 11–83. A desiccated L3-4 disc (*arrow*) without associated herniation shows mild narrowing of the intervertebral disc space on a T2-weighted sagittal image.

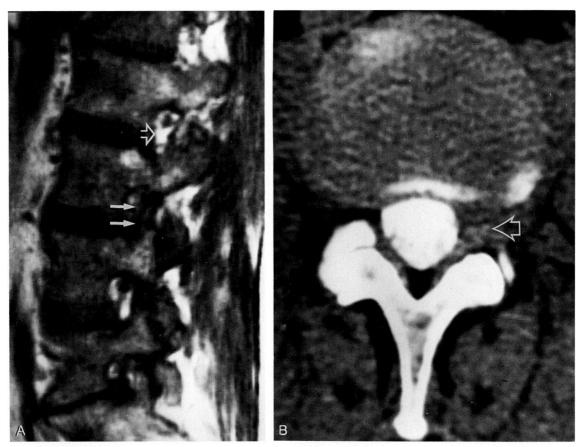

FIGURE 11–84. Lateral disc herniation. (**A**) Foraminal fat in the L3-4 intervertebral foramina (*solid arrows*) is absent, as seen on a T1-weighted parasagittal image. The intact L2-3 disc demonstrates normal high signal intensity foraminal fat for comparison (*open arrow*). (**B**) The corresponding axial CT shows left lateral disc material encroaching on the intervertebral foramina, with resultant stenosis (*open arrow*).

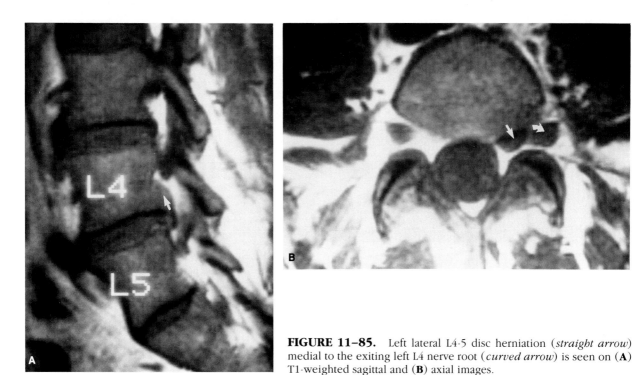

FIGURE 11–85. Left lateral L4-5 disc herniation (*straight arrow*) medial to the exiting left L4 nerve root (*curved arrow*) is seen on (**A**) T1-weighted sagittal and (**B**) axial images.

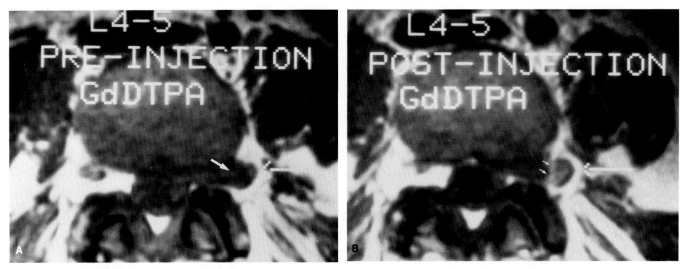

FIGURE 11–86. (**A**) The disc (*white arrow*) and enlarged L4 nerve root (*black arrow*) demonstrate intermediate tissue signal intensity on a T1-weighted axial image. (**B**) A Gd-DTPA enhanced T1-weighted axial image more accurately defines the high signal intensity granulation tissue interface (*arrows*) between the lateral herniation and nerve root.

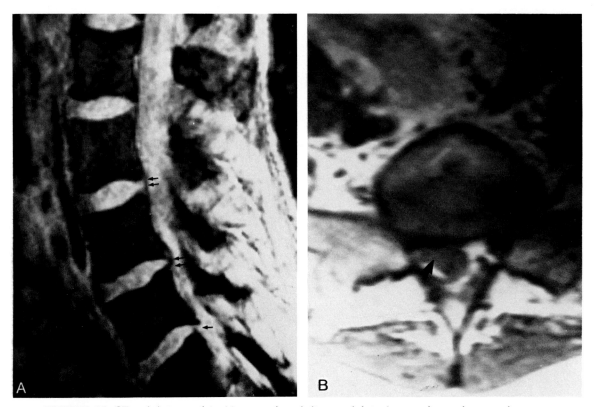

FIGURE 11–87. (**A**) Intact (*double arrows*) and disrupted (*single arrow*) annular complexes are seen on T2*-weighted refocused image. (**B**) The corresponding T1-weighted axial image shows left posterolateral disc herniation (*arrow*).

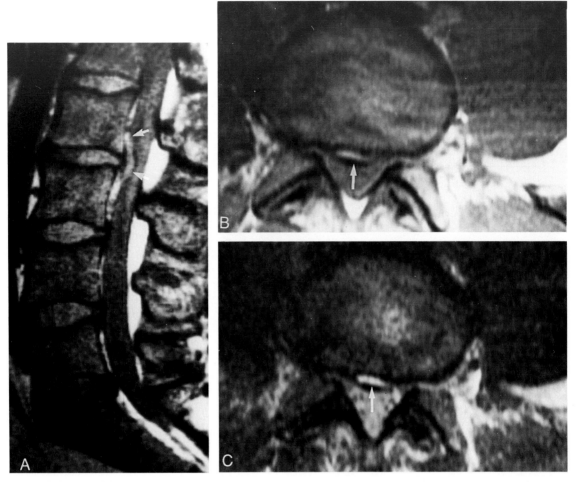

FIGURE 11–88. (**A**) A conventional T2-weighted sagittal image shows high signal intensity nuclear extrusion (*arrows*). In another patient, acute L4-5 central disc herniation (*arrows*) demonstrates high signal intensity on (**B**) T1-weighted and (**C**) T2-weighted axial images.

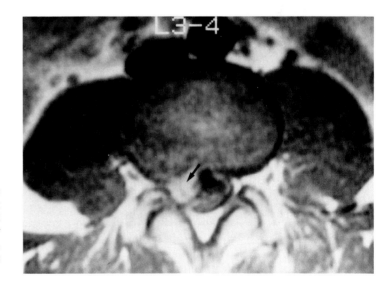

FIGURE 11–89. Extruded nuclear material through the ruptured annulus occurs in acute right paracentral L3-4 disc herniation (*arrow*). Disc material demonstrates increased signal intensity on a T1-weighted axial image. Hyperintensity of nuclear disc material on T1-weighted protocols, however, is uncommon. The right lateral aspect of the thecal sac is compressed.

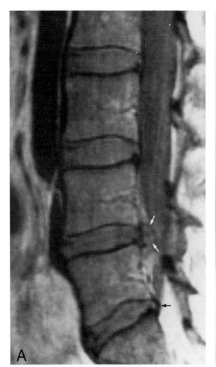 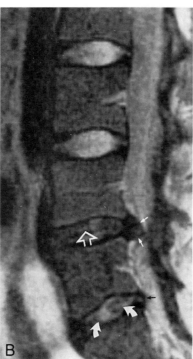

FIGURE 11–90. (**A**) T1-weighted and (**B**) T2-weighted sagittal images show mild L5-S1 (*black arrow*) and severe L4-5 (*solid straight white arrows*) lumbar disc herniations. Signal is still present in early L5-S1 disc desiccation (*curved arrows*), but no signal is observed in the L4-5 intervertebral disc (*open arrow*) on the T2-weighted sequence.

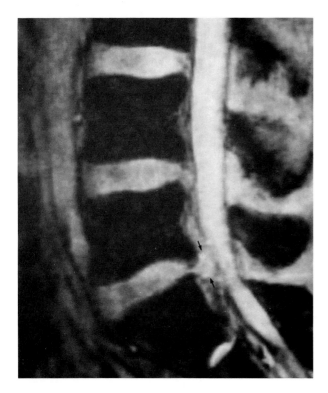

FIGURE 11–91. Nuclear herniation (*arrows*) is isointense with the intervertebral disc at L5-S1 with T2*-weighted technique.

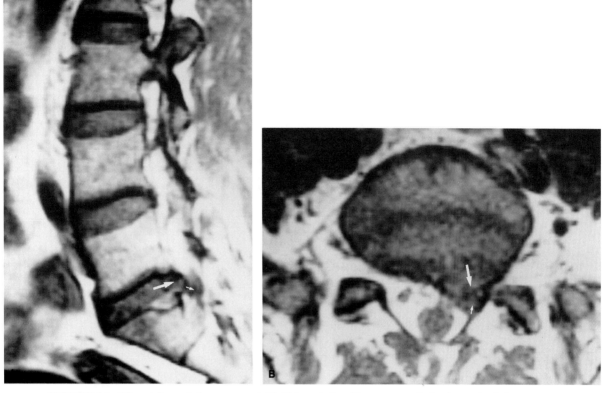

FIGURE 11–92. A large left paracentral L5-S1 herniation (*large arrows*) displaces the left S1 nerve root (*small arrows*) on T1-weighted (**A**) sagittal and (**B**) axial images. The left S1 nerve root is secondarily enlarged.

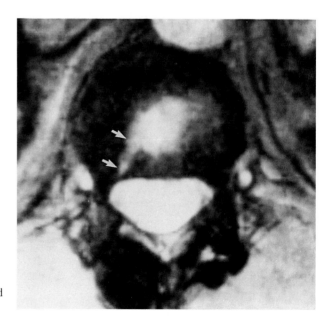

FIGURE 11–93. A discogramlike effect shows the path of extruded nuclear material (*arrows*) on a T2*-weighted axial image.

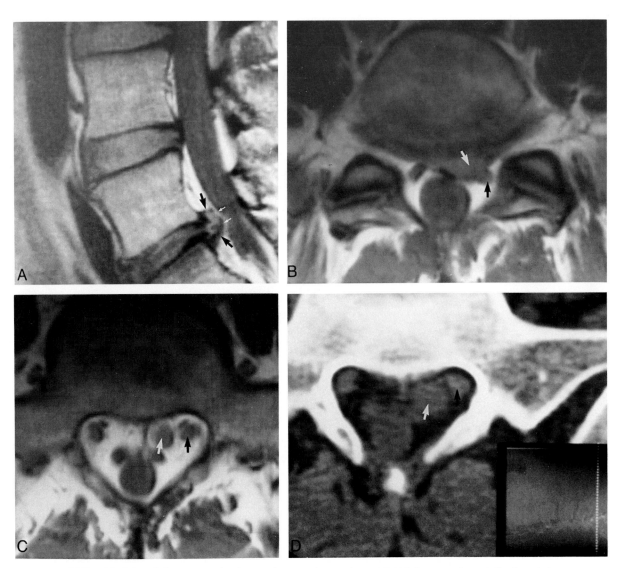

FIGURE 11–94. (**A**) A T1-weighted sagittal image shows a large L5-S1 left posterolateral disc herniation effacing the epidural fat (*black arrows*) and deforming the anterior aspect of the thecal sac (*white arrows*). (**B**) A T1-weighted axial image at L5-S1 intervertebral disc level shows the herniated disc (*white arrow*) and involved left S1 nerve root (*black arrow*). At a more inferior level, (**C**) a T1-weighted axial MR image and (**D**) an axial CT scan show a free disc fragment (*white arrow*) and adjacent intact left S1 nerve root (*black arrow*).

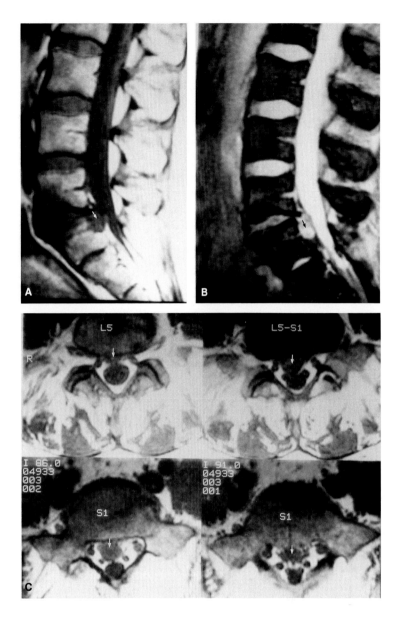

FIGURE 11-95. A herniated disc at L5-S1 with inferior migration (*arrow*) is present posterior to the S1 vertebral body. Disc herniation demonstrates (**A**) low signal intensity on a T1-weighted sagittal image and is (**B**) hyperintense on a T2*-weighted image. Associated type III marrow sclerosis is present and demonstrates low signal intensity on T1- and T2*-weighted images. (**C**) Inferior extension of the herniated disc is shown on consecutive T1-weighted axial images.

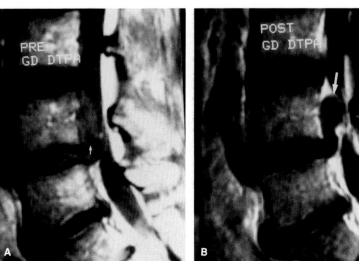

FIGURE 11-96. T1-weighted sagittal images of a sequestered L4-5 disc (*arrows*) (**A**) before and (**B**) after Gd-DTPA administration show high signal intensity granulation tissue in the post-Gd-DTPA images. (**C**) An enhanced T1-weighted axial image shows the enhanced margin of a sequestered disc (*black arrows*) and secondary compression and displacement of the thecal sac. *(continued)*

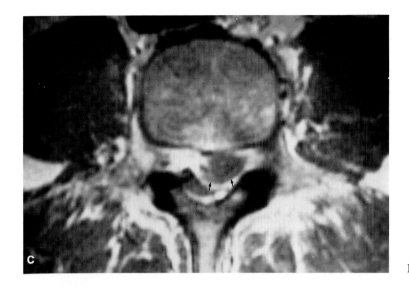

FIGURE 11–96. *(Continued)*

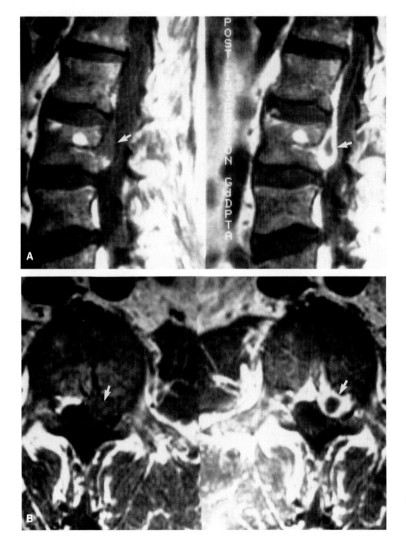

FIGURE 11–97. T1-weighted (**A**) sagittal and (**B**) axial images of an L2-3 free disc fragment (*arrows*) before (*left*) and after (*right*) Gd-DTPA administration. The hyperintense peripheral enhancement reveals an inflammatory reaction in granulation tissue.

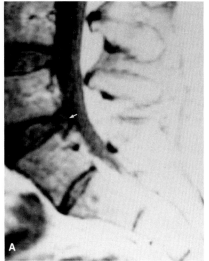
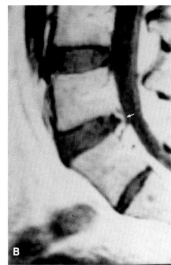

FIGURE 11–98. Enhancement of the posterior complex (*arrow*) of the L4-5 disc represents the development of granulation tissue, a hypervascular area of annular disruption, or both on T1-weighted sagittal images (**A**) before and (**B**) after GD-DTPA administration.

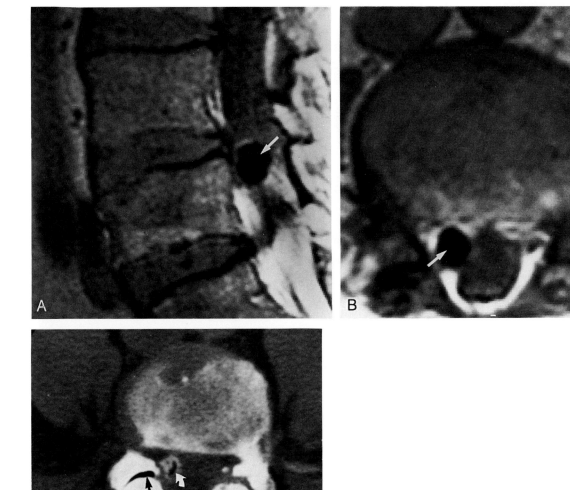

FIGURE 11–99. A dark signal intensity circular structure (*arrows*) is seen on (**A**) T1-weighted sagittal and (**B**) axial images. (**C**) The corresponding axial CT image shows air in the left facet joint (*straight arrow*) and a contiguous calcified apophyseal joint cyst (*curved arrow*).

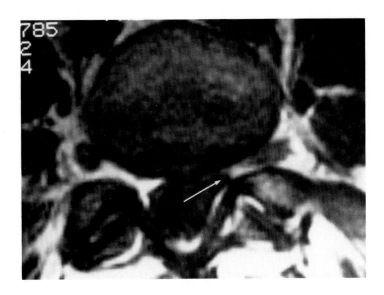

FIGURE 11–100. The L5-S1 left conjoined nerve root (*arrow*) branches off asymmetrically from the thecal sac. The normal right L5 nerve root has exited the intervertebral nerve root canal at this level, as seen on a T1-weighted axial image.

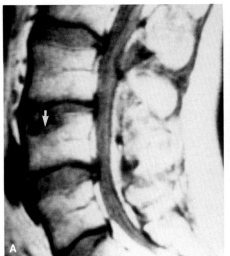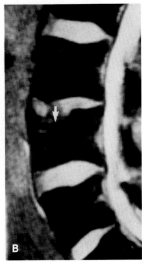

FIGURE 11–101. Schmorl's node (*arrows*) involves the superior endplate of L4 on (**A**) T1-weighted and (**B**) T2*-weighted images. Extension of the disc through the superior endplate is best displayed in gradient-echo contrast as an area of high signal intensity.

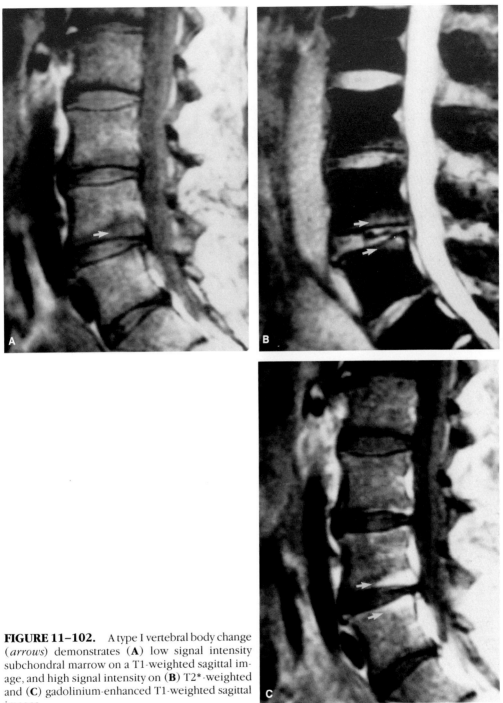

FIGURE 11–102. A type I vertebral body change (*arrows*) demonstrates (**A**) low signal intensity subchondral marrow on a T1-weighted sagittal image, and high signal intensity on (**B**) T2*-weighted and (**C**) gadolinium-enhanced T1-weighted sagittal images.

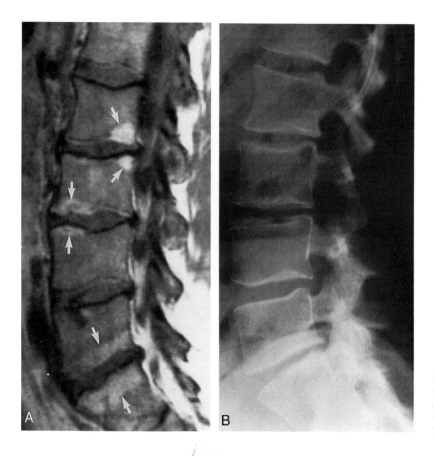

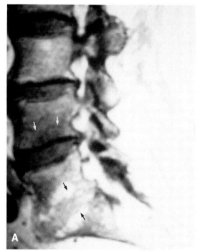

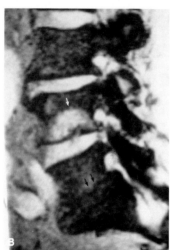

FIGURE 11–103. Type II endplate change in degenerative disease. (**A**) A T1-weighted sagittal image shows focal areas of endplate yellow marrow development (*arrows*) in a degenerative spine. (**B**) A conventional radiograph is provided for comparison.

FIGURE 11–104. Type I (*white arrows*) and type II (*black arrows*) marrow endplate changes are seen on (**A**) T1-weighted and (**B**) T2*-weighted sagittal images. Type I marrow change demonstrates low signal intensity with a T1-weighted protocol and high signal intensity with a T2*-weighted protocol. Type II marrow changes demonstrate increased signal intensity on the T1-weighted image and are isointense on the T2*-weighted image.

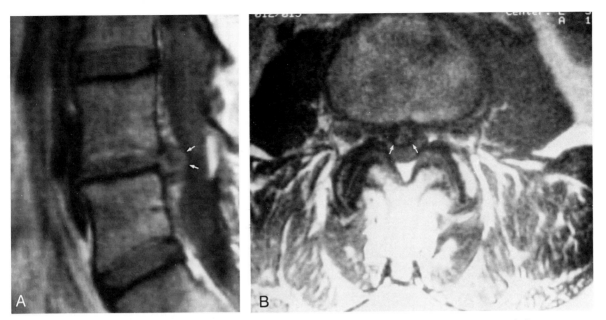

FIGURE 11–105. Central spinal stenosis was caused by severe posterior disc herniation. (**A**) A T1-weighted sagittal image shows a recurrent disc (*arrows*) after a percutaneous nuclectomy. (**B**) A T1-weighted axial image shows spontaneous central herniation (*arrows*) in a different patient.

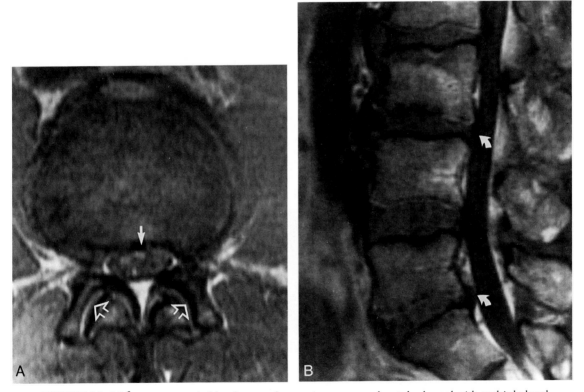

FIGURE 11–106. In congenital lumbar canal stenosis, a narrowed vertebral canal with multiple level disc bulges (*curved arrows*), vertebral bony encroachment, hypertrophied articular facets (*open arrows*), and a small thecal sac (*straight solid arrow*) is shown on T1-weighted (**A**) axial and (**B**) sagittal images and on (**C**) a T2*-weighted gradient refocused sagittal image. *(continued)*

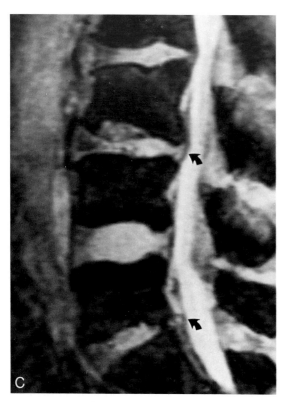

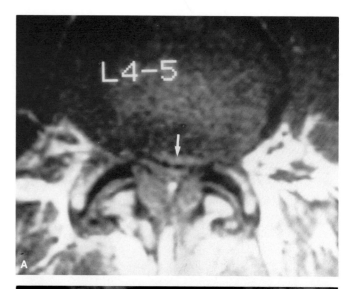

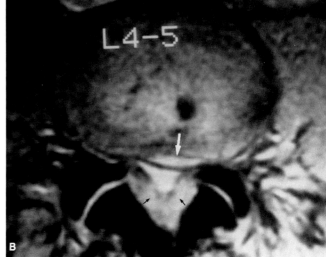

FIGURE 11–106. *(Continued)*

FIGURE 11–107. Moderate left paracentral L4-5 herniation with secondary central canal stenosis. The herniated portion of the disc (*white arrow*) demonstrates (**A**) intermediate signal intensity on a T1-weighted axial image and (**B**) high signal intensity on a T2*-weighted axial image. The ligamentum flavum (*black arrows*) is thickened.

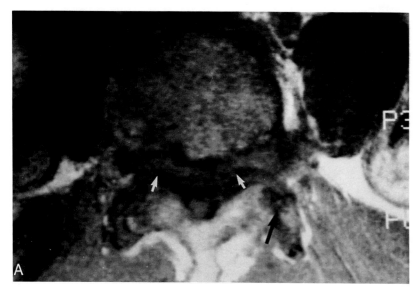

FIGURE 11–108. Central canal and neural foraminal stenosis. A broad-based disc bulge (*white arrows*) and degenerative facets (*black arrows*) contribute to central and neural foraminal stenosis as seen on (**A**) a T1-weighted axial MR image and on (**B**) an axial CT scan.

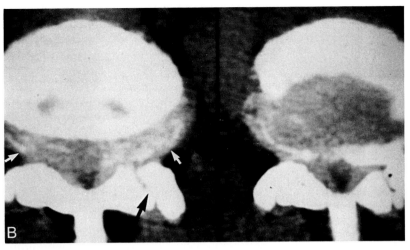

FIGURE 11–108. *(Continued)*

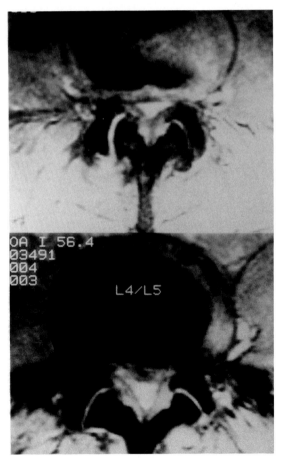

FIGURE 11–109. Degenerative facet arthrosis and disc bulging contribute to central canal stenosis at the L4-5 disc level, as seen on T2*-weighted axial images.

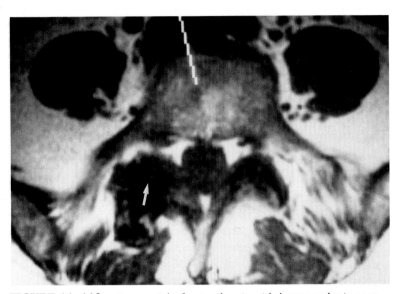

FIGURE 11–110. Severe right facet arthrosis with hypertrophy is seen on a T1-weighted axial image (*arrow*).

foraminal stenosis. Central canal stenosis is common from L2-3 through L4-5, and is frequently characterized by annular disc bulging and facet hypertrophy as components of degenerative disc disease.[83] Loss of bright signal intensity articular cartilage is seen through the facet joints on axial T2*-weighted images. Sclerosis of the facet joint demonstrates low signal intensity on T1-weighted images (Fig. 11–110). Facet effusions, synovial cysts, subchondral cysts, vacuum facets caused by gas formation, osteophyte overgrowth, and joint-space narrowing all contribute to the process of facet arthrosis. Synovial cysts may be unilateral or bilateral and may cause posterior thecal sac compression (Fig. 11–111).[84]

Thoracic spinal stenosis may result from spinal trauma from a retropulsed vertebral body fragment which compromises the usually spacious thoracic canal.[47]

Postoperative Spine

Computed tomography plays an important role in assessing bony detail in the postoperative spine, especially in evaluating pseudoarthrosis in lumbar spine fusions.[85] Magnetic resonance imaging, however, is also useful in characterizing endplate and associated marrow changes.[53,55]

Stable fusions of the lumbar spine are frequently associated with fatty marrow conversion of the endplates at the corresponding vertebral levels (*i.e.,* type II endplate changes) (Fig. 11–112).[86] This yellow or fatty marrow conversion demonstrates increased signal intensity on T1-weighted images and becomes isointense with adjacent marrow on T2-weighted images. Focal fatty marrow conversion may also be seen in patients with degenerated discs.[53]

Magnetic resonance imaging has also been used to assess postoperative changes after fusion, laminectomy, chymopapain, and percutaneous nuclectomy.[86–94] The sensitivity and specificity of MR is equal to intravenous contrast CT in distinguishing recurrent disc herniations from scar or fibrosis (Fig. 11–113). Scar tissue or epidural fibrosis demonstrates low to intermediate signal intensity on T1-weighted images and intermediate to increased signal intensity on T2-weighted images. In Gd-DTPA–enhanced images, epidural fibrosis surrounding a nerve root along the posterior disc margin or surgical bed demonstrates increased signal intensity (Figs. 11–114 and 11–115).[95] Disc herniations, both protrusions and extrusions, demonstrate a mass effect and do not increase in signal intensity after Gd-DTPA administration (Fig. 11–116). The normal postoperative disc margin will be enhanced by Gd-DTPA whether scar tissue is present or not (Fig. 11–117).

Gadolinium-enhanced imaging of the postoperative spine has also been performed with fat-suppression techniques, which may obviate the need for precontrast scanning.[83] In differentiating between recurrent disc herniations and scar tissue, the contrast between bright signal intensity fibrosis and adjacent low signal intensity disc and CSF is superior to that seen on conventional T2-weighted or gradient-echo techniques (Fig. 11–118). On gradient-echo images, herniated disc material may appear isointense or hyperintense relative to adjacent fibrosis or scar. When interpreting MR studies of the spine with a metallic artifact, the increased sensitivity to magnetic susceptibility with gradient-echo imaging must be taken into account.

Clumping and irregular separation of the nerve roots are characteristic of arachnoiditis,[96] which often requires T2-weighted axial images to display the distortion of the thecal sac and nerve roots (Fig. 11–119). Arachnoiditis is grouped into several MR categories based on the morphology of the separate nerve roots. Group 1 consists of central conglomerations of nerve roots within the thecal sac. In group 2, the nerve roots are clumped peripherally to the meninges, producing an empty thecal sac. In group 3, MR images show an increased soft-tissue signal intensity occupying the thecal sac with no discrimination of nerve roots. With Gd-DTPA administration, the cauda equina is enhanced.

In the normal postoperative spine, enhancement of a decompressed nerve root, located proximal to the affected root and extending toward the conus medullaris, may occur within the first six months postsurgery. This enhancement may occur in the absence of arachnoiditis.[97]

A postoperative fluid collection (*i.e.,* pseudomeningocele) has signal characteristics analogous to CSF; they both demonstrate low signal intensity on T1-weighted images and high signal intensity on T2-weighted images (Fig. 11–120).

Focal collections of Pantopaque in the thecal sac have a characteristic appearance in MR; they display high signal intensity on T1-weighted images and low signal intensity on T2-weighted images (Fig. 11–121).[98] Lipomas also show increased signal intensity on T1-weighted images and may be confused with residual Pantopaque. Lipomas, however, show associated spinal dysraphism or nulled fat signal intensity on STIR sequences, which helps to distinguish between the two.[99]

On conventional T1- or T2*-weighted axial or lateral parasagittal images, laminectomy and laminotomy defects with loss of continuity of corresponding cortical bone and marrow are shown (Fig. 11–122). Soft-tissue edema, which demonstrates intermediate signal intensity on T1-weighted images and is hyperintense on T2-weighted images, may persist up to six months postoperatively, until it is replaced by scar tissue. In the immediate postoperative period, edema may be enhanced after Gd-DTPA administration prior to formation of epidural fibrosis. In the postoperative cervical spine, bony stenosis and herniations of adjacent disc levels are evaluated (Fig. 11–123).

Spondylolisthesis

Spondylolisthesis may be either lytic or degenerative.[100,101] In lytic spondylolisthesis, anterior displacement of one vertebra onto another occurs secondary to bilateral fractures or defects in the pars interarticularis (Fig. 11–124). There is forward displacement of the superior vertebral body, and the posterior joints and neural arch are aligned with the posterior elements of the inferior vertebral body.[102] Peripheral parasagittal images, particularly T2*-weighted images acquired without an interslice gap, demonstrate the defects in the pars interarticularis (Fig. 11–125). The anteroposterior diameter of the spinal canal is characteristically enlarged in the presence of vertebral body displacement. Hypertrophic bone at the proximal side of the defect produces lateral recess stenosis. The vertebral canal is decompressed; therefore, neural foraminal stenosis may occur without central canal stenosis (Fig. 11–126). The posterior aspects or margins of the two involved vertebra may be seen in the same axial image. Axial images at the level of the spondylitic defect demonstrate low signal intensity sclerosis, fragmentation, or a discontinuity in the region of the pars defect. An associated disc herniation increases compression of the exiting nerve root.

In degenerative spondylolisthesis, there is forward displacement of the superior vertebral body secondary to medial superior facet erosion of the inferior vertebral body. This facet erosion allows forward movement of the inferior articular facet of the superior vertebral body (Fig. 11–127). In the absence of a pars defect, which would decompress the central canal, narrowing of the anteroposterior diameter of the spinal canal occurs, causing severe central spinal stenosis in addition to lateral recess stenosis, neural foraminal stenosis, or both (Fig. 11–128). The contours of the thecal sac have an hourglass or constricted outline. Neural foraminal and pars anatomy in lytic or degenerative spondylolisthesis is accurately displayed in CT scans. Posterior displacement or retrolisthesis of an involved vertebral body relative to an inferior level is also a manifestation of degenerative disc disease or facet arthrosis.[103]

Fractures

Magnetic resonance has been used to assess traumatic and nontraumatic vertebral body fractures.[77,103–107] In traumatic fractures, retropulsed fracture fragments can be identified relative to the cord, thecal sac, and neural foramina (Figs. 11–129 through 11–131). In acute and subacute stages, hemorrhage or edema demonstrate low signal intensity on T1-weighted images and high signal intensity on T2-weighted, T2*-weighted, or STIR images. A chronic fracture does not demonstrate increased signal intensity on long TR/TE sequences (Fig. 11–132).

On T1-weighted images, osteoporotic or nontraumatic compression fractures may be characterized by low signal intensity bands that are parallel with the endplates and demonstrate an increase in signal intensity on T2-weighted images (Figs. 11–133 and 11–134). Osteoporotic fractures frequently are wedge-shaped, with relative preservation of posterior vertebral body height (Fig. 11–135). In some cases, compression fractures cannot be differentiated from metastatic disease, although associated convexity or bulging of the posterior vertebral body margin suggests neoplastic disease and a pathologic fracture (Fig. 11–136). On T2-weighted images, the branching pattern of the high signal intensity basivertebral plexus may simulate fracture. When the etiology of the fracture is unclear, Gd-DTPA administration causes enhancement of neoplastic or metastatic tissue within a pathologic fracture (Fig. 11–137). Magnetic resonance evaluations of cord trauma have identified changes of post-traumatic myelopathy, including myelomalacia, which demonstrates low signal intensity T1-weighted images, is isointense in intermediate-weighted images, and is hyperintense on T2-weighted images (Fig. 11–138).

Infection

Magnetic resonance imaging is more sensitive in the detection of vertebral osteomyelitis than either conventional radiography or CT.[108–110] Magnetic resonance specificity is also superior to corresponding nuclear scintigraphic studies. On T1-weighted images, infection of vertebral bodies and adjacent intervertebral disc spaces is seen as areas of low signal intensity (Fig. 11–139). On T2-weighted images, high signal intensity is observed crossing the involved bone and disc space, with irregularity of cortical margins (Figs. 11–140 and 11–141). In advanced stages of infection such as tuberculous spondylitis, a soft-tissue mass, of low signal intensity on T1- and of high signal intensity on T2-weighted images, is frequently observed (Fig. 11–142).[111] Unlike neoplastic disease, infection is associated with loss of disc space height and the low signal intensity intranuclear cleft normally seen on T2-weighted images.

Epidural abscesses containing pus or granulation tissue, most commonly caused by *Staphylococcus aureus*, are best demonstrated on T2*-weighted or STIR images (Fig. 11–143). Gadolinium enhancement defines the peripheral outline of infected fluid.

Multiple Sclerosis

Mixed intracranial and spinal cord involvement with multiple sclerosis is more common than isolated spinal disease.[112] In the cervical spine, dual echo (*i.e.*, TE of 15 msec and 30 msec) T2*-weighted and STIR images can be used to identify areas of demyelination. Gadolinium-enhanced images have been found to be sensitive in identifying more active areas of plaque development in the cervical and thoracic cords (Fig. 11–144). Multiple-sclerosis plaques have a linear or elongated morphology and affect single or multiple levels. Localized swelling of the cord may be seen in more acute inflammatory stages of the disease.

Spinal Tumors

Intramedullary neoplasms include gliomas (*e.g.*, ependymoma, astrocytoma, oligodendroglioma, medulloblastoma); hemangioblastomas, which are uncommon; lipomas; dermoids; epidermoids; and rarely, metastatic disease. Extramedullary intradural lesions include meningiomas (Fig. 11–145); nerve sheath tumors (*i.e.*, neurofibromas; Fig. 11–146); embryonal lesions (*e.g.*, epidermoids, dermoids, lipomas); and metastases. Extradural tumors consist of primary and metastatic tumors with osseous, soft-tissue, and neural elements represented by both benign and malignant processes.[113–115]

Hemangiomas, aneurysmal bone cysts, and chordomas have characteristic MR findings. Hemangiomas demonstrate increased signal intensity on T1- and T2-weighted images, in part related to adipose elements. Vertebral hemangiomas with a content that is predominantly fat represent a more inactive form, whereas more vascular hemangiomas, which demonstrate lower signal intensity on T1-weighted images, are frequently more aggressive and are associated with compression fractures.[116] Focal fatty marrow deposition does not display increased signal intensity on T2-weighted images, and is dark in fat-suppression or STIR protocols. Aneurysmal bone cysts are blood filled and expansile and demonstrate inhomogeneous signal intensity on T1 and T2-weighted images due to paramagnetic influence. Chordomas are aggressive lesions related to notochord remnants located in the sacrococcygeal and basisphenoid regions. On T1-weighted images, they range from hypointense to isointense, and are hyperintense on T2-weighted images.

Hematoma

The longitudinal extent of subdural and epidural hematomas is best evaluated on sagittal T1-, T2-, or T2*-weighted images. Axial images are preferred in differentiating epidural from subdural involvement. Epidural hematomas are biconcave and produce extrinsic cord compression. Subdural hematomas are crescent-shaped, with a convex outer border and a concave inner border. Gadolinium contrast enhanced images may be required to define the peripheral margins of the hematoma.

Lipoma of the Filum Terminale

The fibrous filum terminale extends from the conus to the distal thecal sac and contains fat elements in 4% to 6% of normal individuals (Figs. 11–147 and 11–148).[63] Associated cord tethering must be evaluated.[117] Intradural lipomas have a relatively fusiform morphology and may cause expansion of the filum. Extradural filum lipomas, however, are more diffuse. Lipomas of the conus medullaris may coexist with lipoma of the filum.

Metastatic and Marrow Disease

On MR images, fatty or yellow marrow demonstrates high signal intensity and hematopoietic or red marrow demonstrates low signal intensity in both normal and pathologic states.[118–124] T1- and T2-weighted spin-echo imaging, T2*-weighted imaging, and STIR sequences have complementary roles in showing the replacement of normal marrow in primary, metastatic, and infiltrative disease processes.[46–52,125] Magnetic resonance is also useful in identifying benign processes that may mimic malignancy in conventional radiography.

Most metastatic tumors are characterized by long T1 and T2 values; therefore, there is good contrast discrimination between normal adult marrow and marrow infiltrated by metastatic processes.[126] On STIR images, signal from normal yellow marrow is suppressed, and T1 and T2 prolongation effects are additive. Metastatic lesions from carcinoma of the breast, prostate, lung, colon, and testes, from Ewing's sarcoma, and from multiple myeloma demonstrate increased signal intensity on conventional T2-weighted images, on T2*-weighted images, and in STIR images, even in cases where nuclear scintigraphy was equivocal (Fig. 11–149). Blastic lesions generally demonstrate low signal intensity, regardless of the pulsing parameters. On STIR images, however, increased signal intensity metastatic foci within a blastic reaction have been observed.[127] Epidural involvement with posterior cortical disruption is best seen on T2, T2*, STIR, or Gd-DTPA–enhanced studies.[128,129] After Gd-DTPA administration, neoplastic tissue demonstrates increased signal intensity on short TR/TE sequences as a result of T1 and T2 shortening, and adjacent CSF remains dark.[113] This precisely defines the boundary between the tumor and thecal sac, which is not possible with conventional T2 weighting or even with STIR im-

(text continues on page 962)

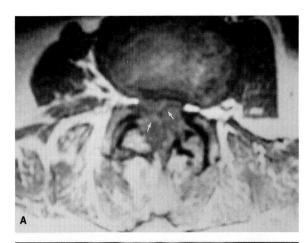

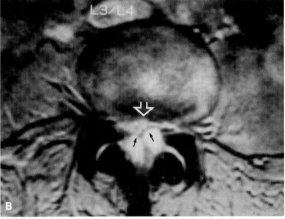

FIGURE 11–111. Bilateral synovial cysts (*solid arrows*) of the L3-4 facet joints result in severe central canal stenosis (*open arrow*). Gelatinous cysts demonstrate (**A**) low signal intensity on a T1-weighted image and (**B**) high signal intensity on a T2*-weighted image.

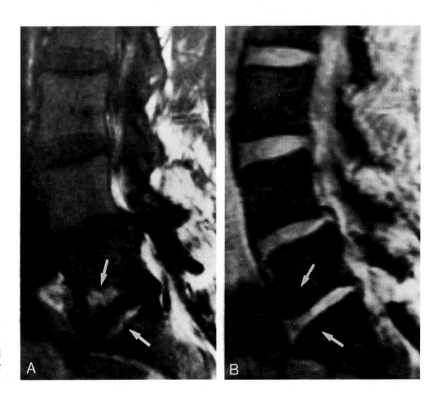

FIGURE 11–112. In stable lumbar fusion, L5-S1 yellow marrow conversion (*arrows*) demonstrates (**A**) bright signal intensity on a T1-weighted image and is (**B**) isointense with adjacent marrow on a T2*-weighted image.

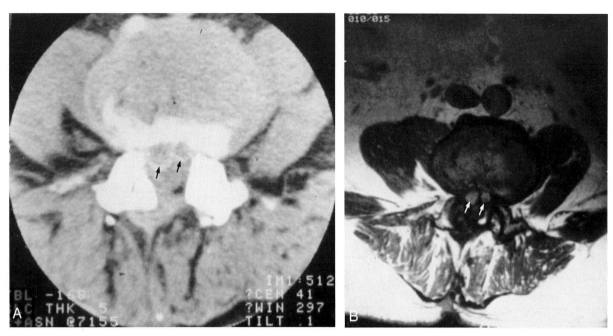

FIGURE 11–113. (**A**) A postcontrast CT scan and (**B**) a T1-weighted axial image show a bilobed recurrent disc (*arrows*) in a postlumbar laminectomy patient. MR provides superior soft-tissue contrast without the need for administration of contrast media.

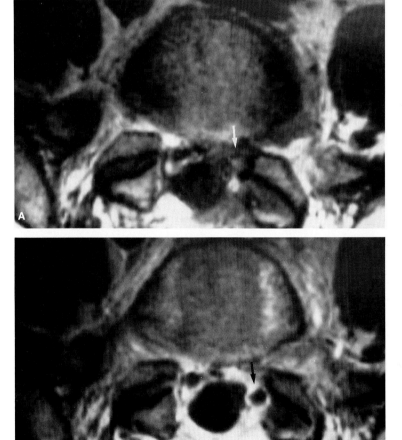

FIGURE 11–114. Gadolinium-enhanced postoperative fibrosis. (**A**) On an unenhanced T1-weighted axial image, a recurrent disc cannot be differentiated from scar tissue (*arrow*). The left S1 root is not defined. (**B**) An enhanced image shows a high signal intensity scar (*arrow*) with a posteriorly displaced left S1 nerve root. A laminectomy defect is present posteriorly. There is no recurrent disc herniation.

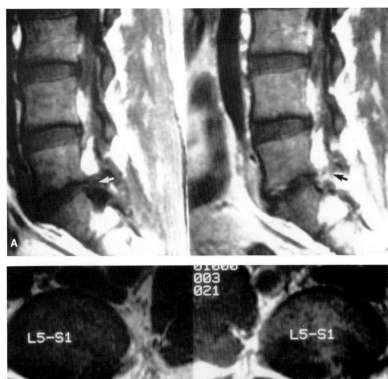

FIGURE 11–115. Epidural fibrosis (*arrows*) adjacent to enlarged left S1 nerve root is seen on T1-weighted (**A**) sagittal and (**B**) axial images, before (*left*) and after (*right*) Gd-DTPA administration. The epidural fibrosis is seen best on the enhanced images.

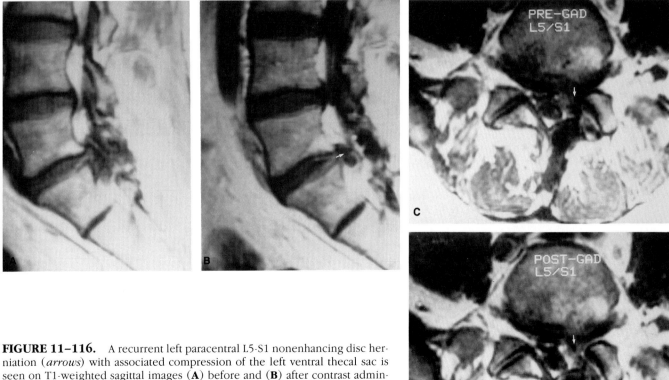

FIGURE 11–116. A recurrent left paracentral L5-S1 nonenhancing disc herniation (*arrows*) with associated compression of the left ventral thecal sac is seen on T1-weighted sagittal images (**A**) before and (**B**) after contrast administration and on T1-weighted axial images (**C**) before and (**D**) after contrast administration.

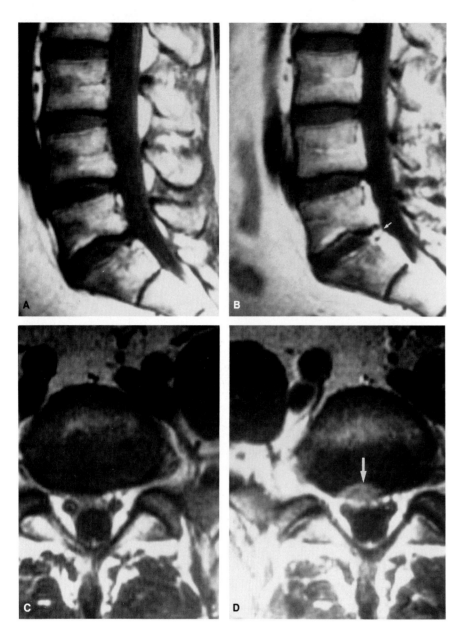

FIGURE 11-117. Postoperative enhancement of the posterior margin of the L5-S1 disc (*arrows*) is seen on (**A**) unenhanced and (**B**) enhanced T1-weighted sagittal images. Type II endplate change is identified. Fibrosis and posterior disc margin demonstrate (**C**) low signal intensity on an unenhanced T1-weighted axial image and (**D**) high signal intensity on an enhanced T1-weighted axial image.

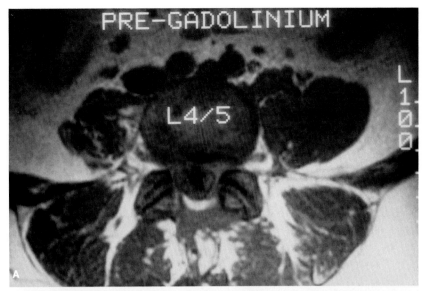

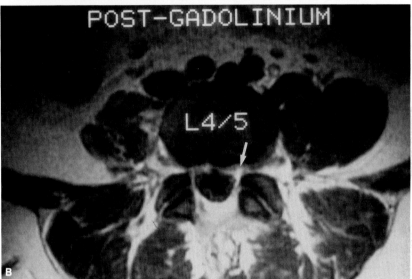

FIGURE 11–118. T1-weighted axial images (**A**) before and (**B**) after Gd-DTPA enhancement after laminectomy and discectomy of the L4-5 disc. The enhanced image demonstrates hyperintense epidural fibrosis (*arrow*) and normal thecal sac contours.

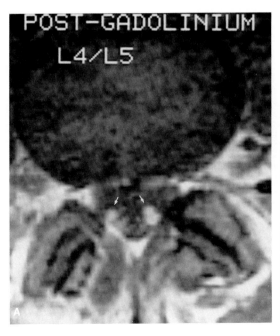

FIGURE 11–119. Arachnoiditis (*arrows*), with asymmetric high signal intensity peripheral clumping of nerve roots within the distal thecal sac, is seen on enhanced T1-weighted axial images at the (**A**) L4-5 and (**B**) L5 levels.

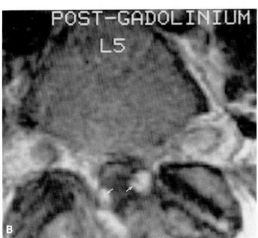

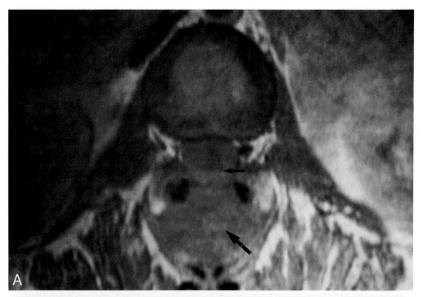

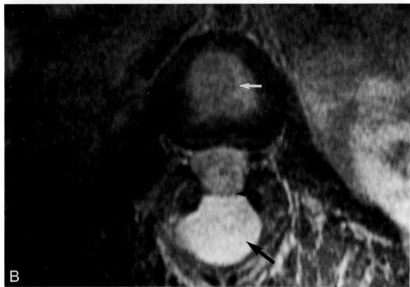

FIGURE 11–120. Postoperative pseudomeningocele (*large black arrows*) demonstrates (**A**) low signal intensity on an intermediate-weighted image and (**B**) high signal intensity on a T2-weighted image. Thecal-sac–fluid interface (*small black arrows*) and the bright signal intensity nucleus pulposus (*white arrow*) are best seen on the T2-weighted image.

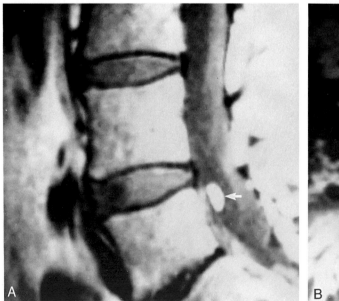

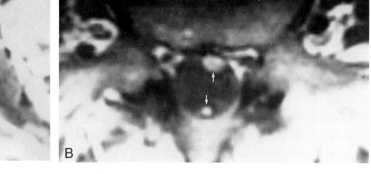

FIGURE 11–121.

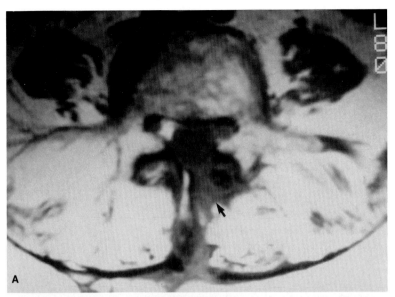

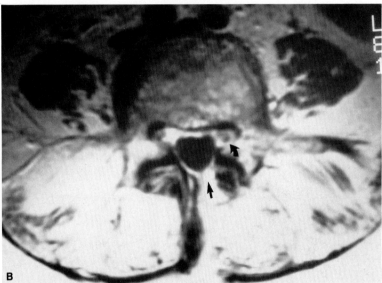

FIGURE 11–122. A left hemilaminectomy (*straight arrows*) defect with enhancing epidural fibrosis surrounding left L5 nerve root (*curved arrow*) is seen on T1-weighted axial images (**A**) before and (**B**) after contrast administration.

FIGURE 11–121. High signal intensity Pantopaque (*arrows*) is seen on T1-weighted (**A**) sagittal and (**B**) axial images.

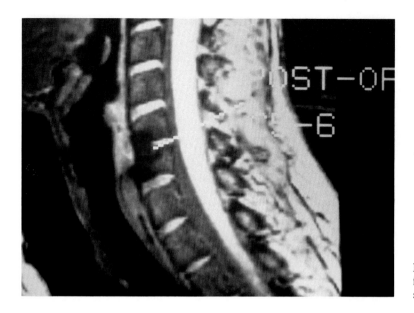

FIGURE 11–123. Uncomplicated anterior interbody fusion of C5-6, without central stenosis or herniation, is seen on a gradient-echo sagittal image.

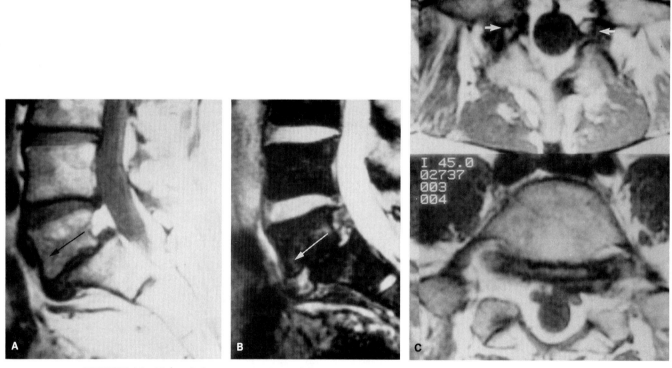

FIGURE 11–124. (**A**) T1-weighted and (**B**) T2*-weighted sagittal images show grade 1 lytic spondylolisthesis with forward displacement of L5 on S1 (*arrow*). (**C**) T1-weighted axial images show bilateral pars defects (*arrows*), which result in elongation of the anteroposterior dimension of the spinal cord (*top*).

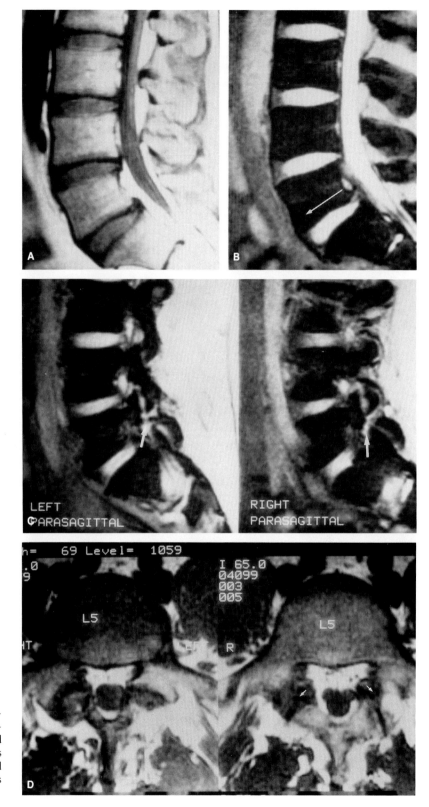

FIGURE 11–125. (**A**) T1-weighted and (**B**) T2*-weighted sagittal images show grade 1 lytic spondylolisthesis of L5 on S1 (*arrows*). (**C**) T2*-weighted sagittal images show bilateral defects or fractures (*arrows*) of the pars interarticularis. (**D**) T1-weighted axial images show sclerotic low signal intensity pars defects (*arrows*).

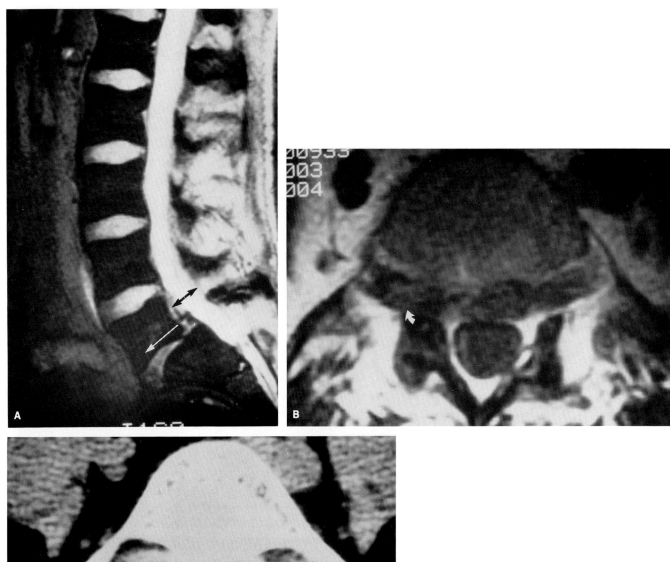

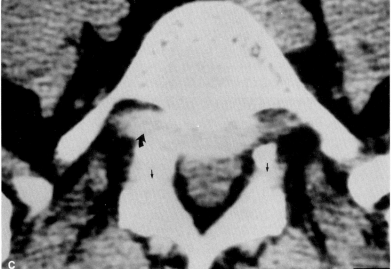

FIGURE 11–126. (**A**) A T2*-weighted sagittal image shows grade 1 lytic spondylolisthesis with forward movement of the L5 on S1 vertebral body (*white arrow*). The increase in anterior-to-posterior central canal diameter (*black arrows*) is characteristic. The corresponding (**B**) T1-weighted axial and (**C**) axial CT images show pars defects or fractures (*straight arrows*). There is severe right neural foraminal stenosis (*curved arrows*).

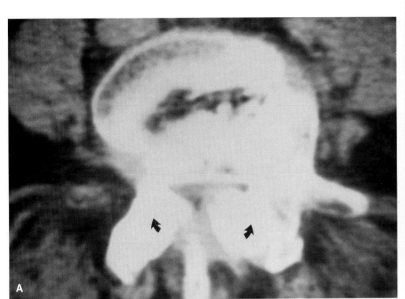

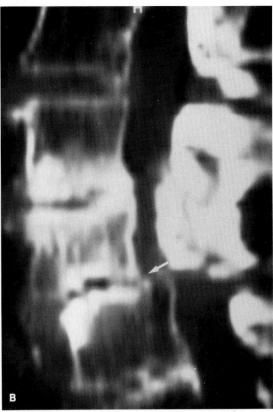

FIGURE 11–127. Degenerative spondylolisthesis at the L4-5 vertebral level with an intact pars inter-articularis and degenerative facet joints (*curved arrows*) are seen on (**A**) axial CT and (**B**) sagittal re-formatted CT images. There is associated severe central canal stenosis with narrowing of the anterior-to-posterior diameter of the spinal canal (*straight arrow*).

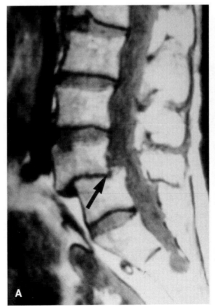

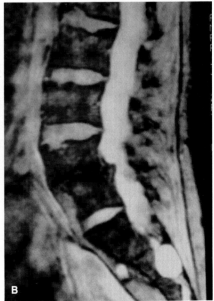

FIGURE 11–128. Degenerative spondylo-listhesis of L4 on L5 (*arrow*) with severe sec-ondary central canal stenosis is seen on (**A**) T1-weighted and (**B**) T2*-weighted sagittal images.

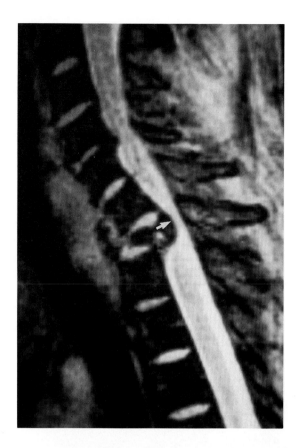

FIGURE 11–129. A C7 burst fracture (*arrow*) with secondary cord compression is seen on a T2*-weighted sagittal image.

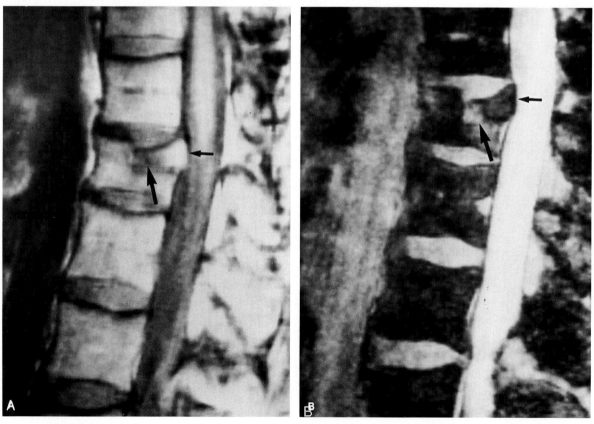

FIGURE 11–130. A post-traumatic L1 vertebral body fracture (*large arrows*) demonstrates (**A**) low signal intensity hemorrhagic marrow on a T1-weighted image and (**B**) increased signal intensity on a T2*-weighted image. A retropulsed fracture segment (*small arrows*) can be seen pressing on the thecal sac.

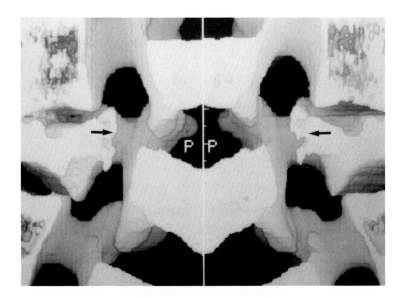

FIGURE 11–131. Three-dimensional CT images show a lumbar vertebral body burst fracture (*arrows*) with retropulsion of posterior fragment compromising the central canal.

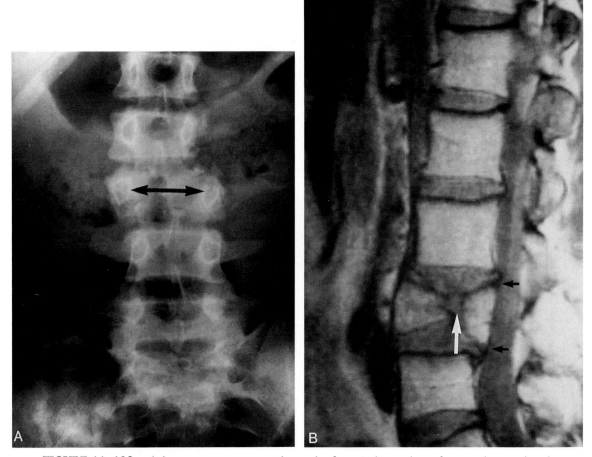

FIGURE 11–132. (**A**) An anteroposterior radiograph of an L3 chronic burst fracture shows splayed pedicles (*double-headed arrow*). (**B**) T1-weighted and (**C**) T2-weighted sagittal images reveal the fracture site (*white arrows*) and deformity of the anterior thecal sac (*black arrows*). No marrow edema is associated with this chronic fracture.

(continued)

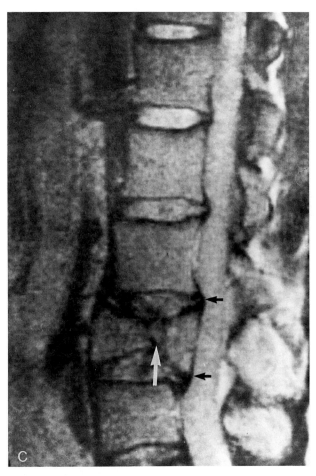

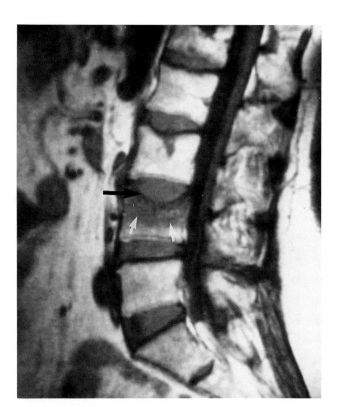

FIGURE 11–133. A low signal intensity band of marrow edema (*white arrows*) is seen in association with an L4 osteoporotic compression fracture (*black arrow*) on a T1-weighted sagittal image.

FIGURE 11–132. (*Continued*)

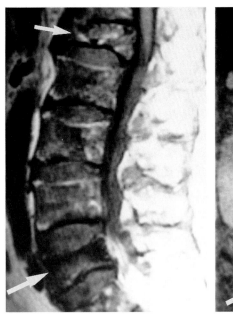

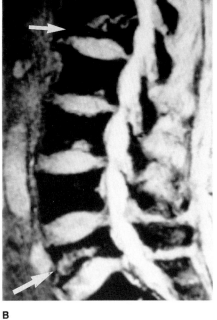

A   **B**

FIGURE 11–134. Osteoporotic compression fractures (*arrows*) of the L1 and L5 vertebral bodies are seen on (**A**) T1-weighted and (**B**) T2*-weighted sagittal images. The chronic L1 fracture has a wedge shaped morphology. The subacute L5 fracture is associated with central hemorrhage.

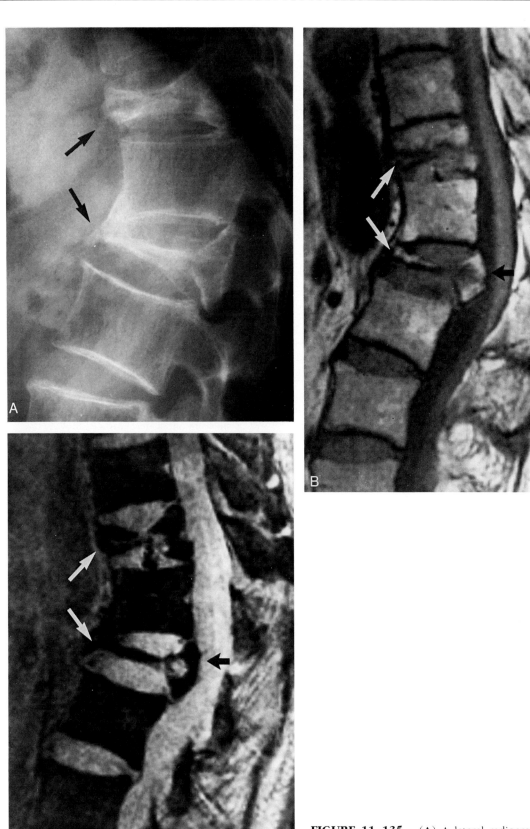

FIGURE 11–135. (**A**) A lateral radiograph shows multiple osteoporotic vertebral body wedge compression fractures (*arrows*). The corresponding (**B**) T1-weighted and (**C**) T2*-weighted images reveal the compression fractures (*white arrows*) and deformity of the thecal sac (*black arrows*).

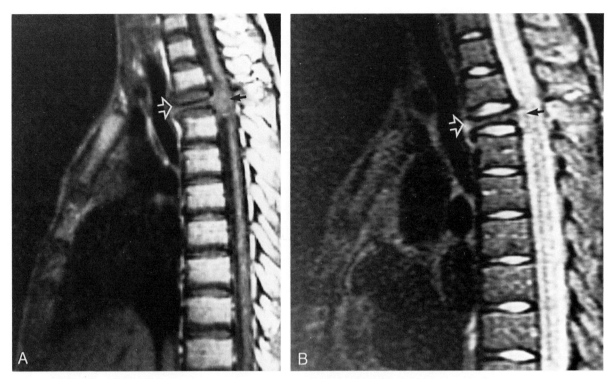

FIGURE 11–136. Pathologic fracture. (**A**) T1-weighted and (**B**) T2-weighted sagittal images show thoracic vertebral body collapse (*open arrow*) with posterior convexity (*solid arrow*) and soft-tissue mass in a patient with non-Hodgkin's lymphoma. The soft-tissue component demonstrates increased signal intensity, isointense with cerebrospinal fluid, on the T2-weighted image.

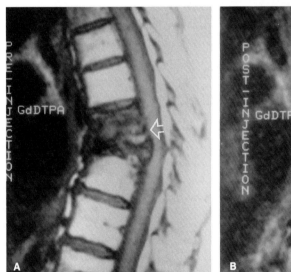

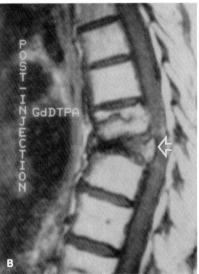

FIGURE 11–137. Pathologic fracture secondary to metastatic lung cancer is seen (**A**) before and (**B**) after Gd-DTPA injection on T1-weighted sagittal images. Note the posterior convexity of the involved vertebral cortex and its hyperintensity postinjection.

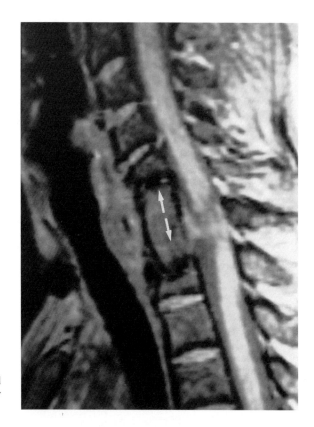

FIGURE 11–138. Cord myelomalacia as a complication of severe cord compression from a fracture flexion dislocation injury. Treatment was by cervical fusion (*white arrows*).

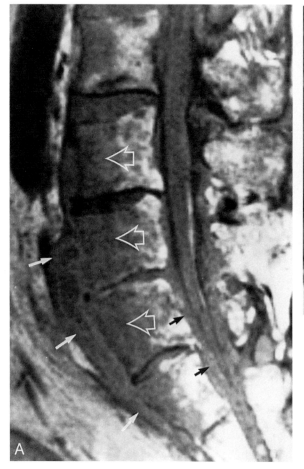

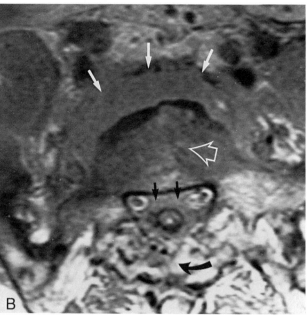

FIGURE 11–139. *Escherichia coli* osteomyelitis. T1-weighted (**A**) sagittal and (**B**) axial images show a low signal intensity *E. coli* abscess anterior to the L4 through S2 vertebral bodies (*solid white arrows*). There is adjacent cortical and cancellous destruction. Low signal intensity marrow involvement (*open white arrows*) and epidural spread (*straight black arrows*) are shown. Old posterior fusion mass is shown in the axial image (*curved black arrow*).

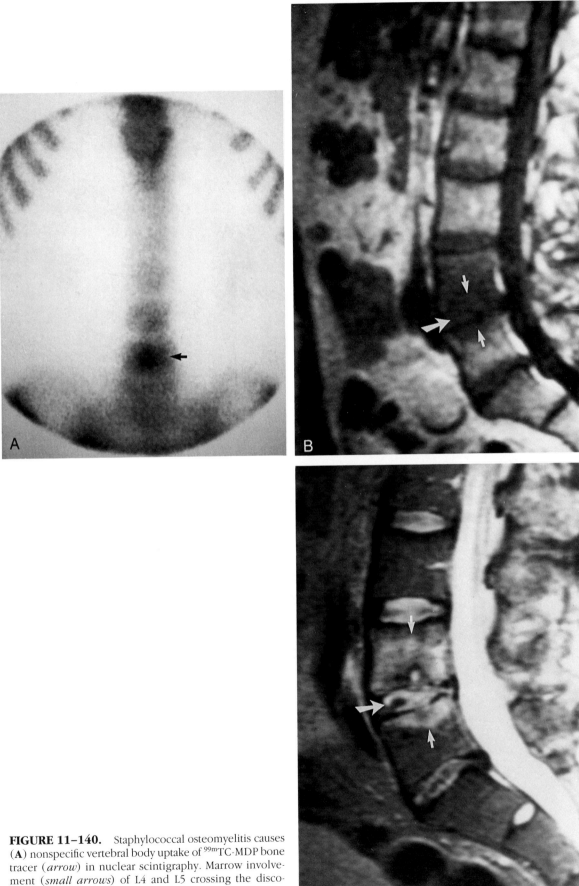

FIGURE 11–140. Staphylococcal osteomyelitis causes (**A**) nonspecific vertebral body uptake of ^{99m}TC-MDP bone tracer (*arrow*) in nuclear scintigraphy. Marrow involvement (*small arrows*) of L4 and L5 crossing the discovertebral junction (*large arrows*) demonstrates (**B**) low signal intensity on a T1-weighted image and (**C**) high signal intensity on a T2-weighted image.

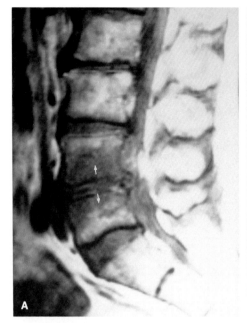 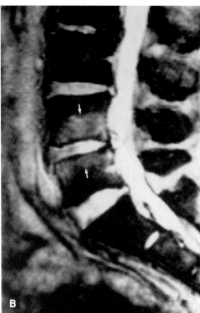

FIGURE 11–141. Discovertebral osteomyelitis (*arrow*) with marrow edema involves approximately 50% of the vertebral bodies, as seen on (**A**) T1-weighted and (**B**) T2*-weighted sagittal images. Marrow infiltration demonstrates low signal intensity on T1-weighted contrast and is hyperintense on T2-weighted contrast. Edematous change in epidural fat is present.

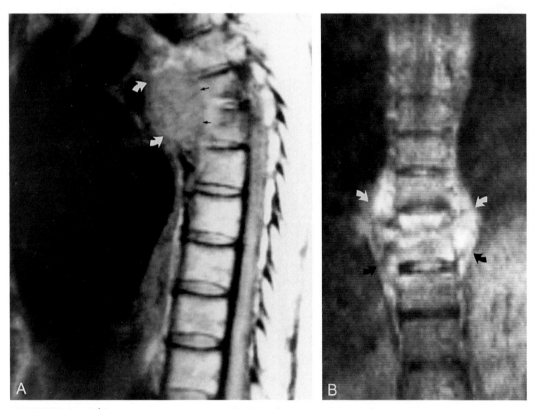

FIGURE 11–142. Two separate cases of tuberculous spondylitis infection of the thoracic spine. A paraspinal mass (*white arrows*) demonstrates (**A**) intermediate signal intensity on T1-weighted sagittal image and (**B**) high signal intensity on T2-weighted image. Erosion of the adjacent vertebral body (*black arrows*) can be seen on the T1-weighted image.

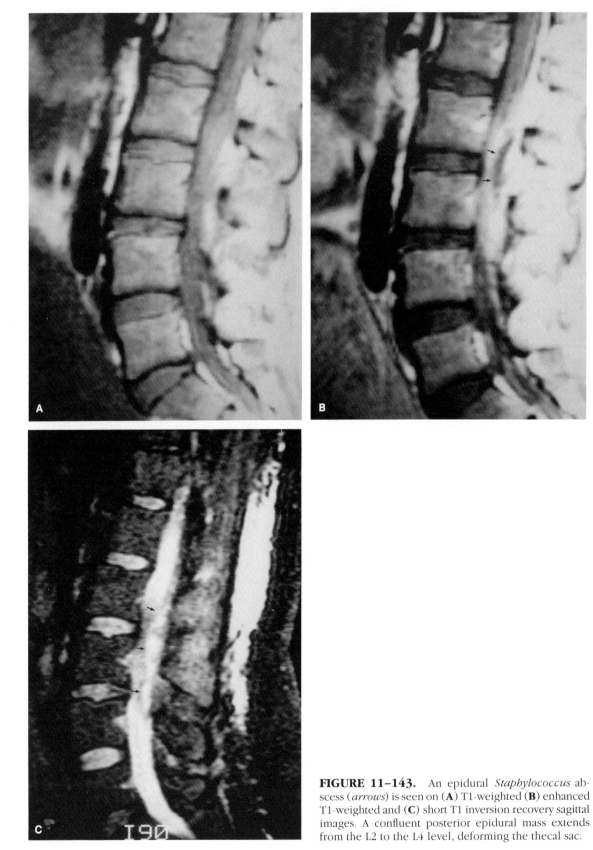

FIGURE 11–143. An epidural *Staphylococcus* abscess (*arrows*) is seen on (**A**) T1-weighted (**B**) enhanced T1-weighted and (**C**) short T1 inversion recovery sagittal images. A confluent posterior epidural mass extends from the L2 to the L4 level, deforming the thecal sac.

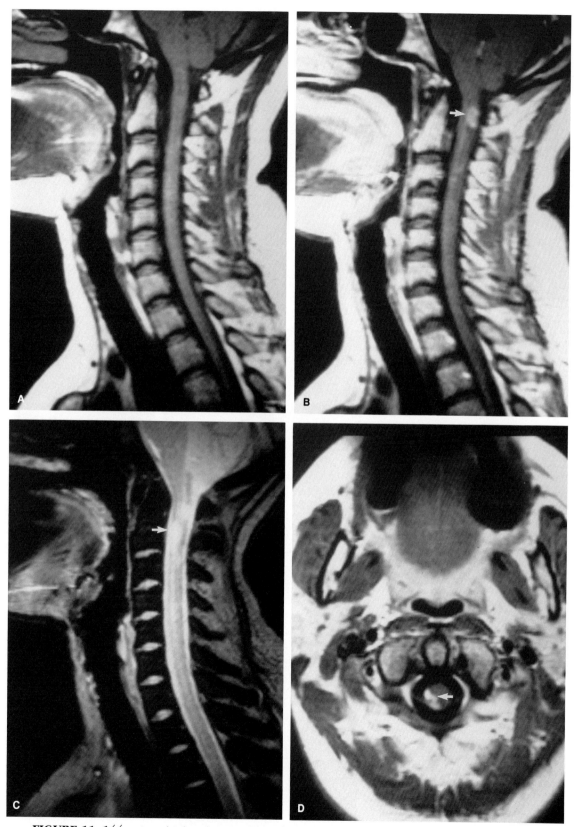

FIGURE 11–144. A multiple sclerosis plaque (*arrows*) demonstrates (**A**) low signal intensity or is isointense on a T1-weighted sagittal image and (**B**) is hyperintense on a Gd-DTPA–enhanced T1-weighted sagittal image. (**C**) The high signal intensity plaque is poorly differentiated from the cord on a T2*-weighted sagittal image. (**D**) The corresponding enhanced T1-weighted axial image shows the left lateral localization of the demyelinating plaque.

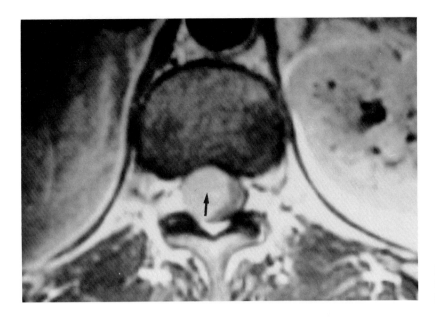

FIGURE 11–145. An extramedullary intradural meningioma (*arrow*) demonstrates increased signal intensity on an enhanced T1-weighted axial image.

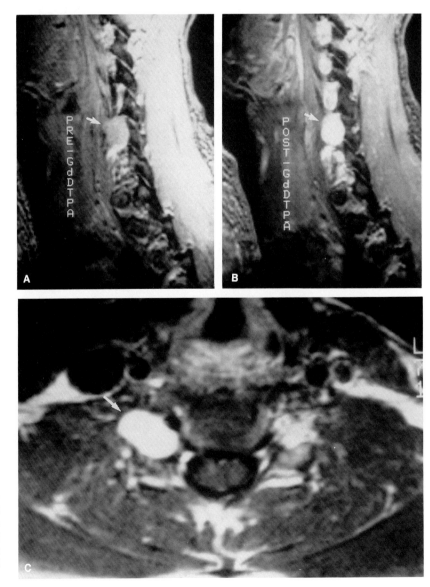

FIGURE 11–146. Right parasagittal C5-6 neurofibroma (*arrows*) is seen (**A**) before and (**B**) after intravenous Gd-DTPA administration. (**C**) An hyperintense dumbbell-shaped neurofibroma (*arrow*) extends through the right intervertebral nerve root canal, as seen on an enhanced T1-weighted axial image.

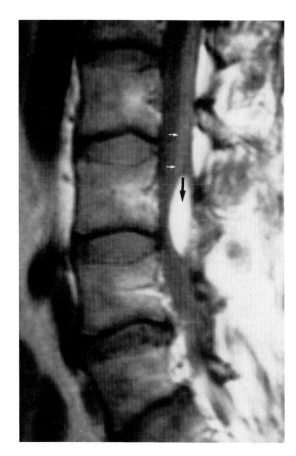

FIGURE 11–147. A T1-weighted sagittal image shows an intradural fusiform high signal intensity lipoma (*black arrow*) of the filum terminale (*white arrows*). The lipoma tapers superiorly and inferiorly. In tight filum terminale syndrome, the filum measures more than 2 mm in diameter.

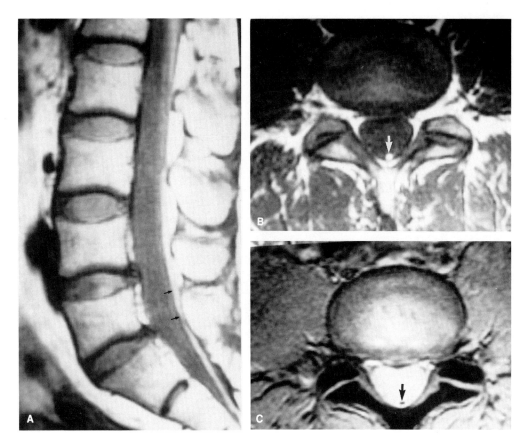

FIGURE 11–148. (**A**) Fat (*arrow*) in the filum terminale demonstrates high signal intensity on a T1-weighted sagittal image. (**B**) On a T1-weighted axial image, fat demonstrates high signal intensity. (**C**) On a T2*-weighted axial image, fat demonstrates low signal intensity.

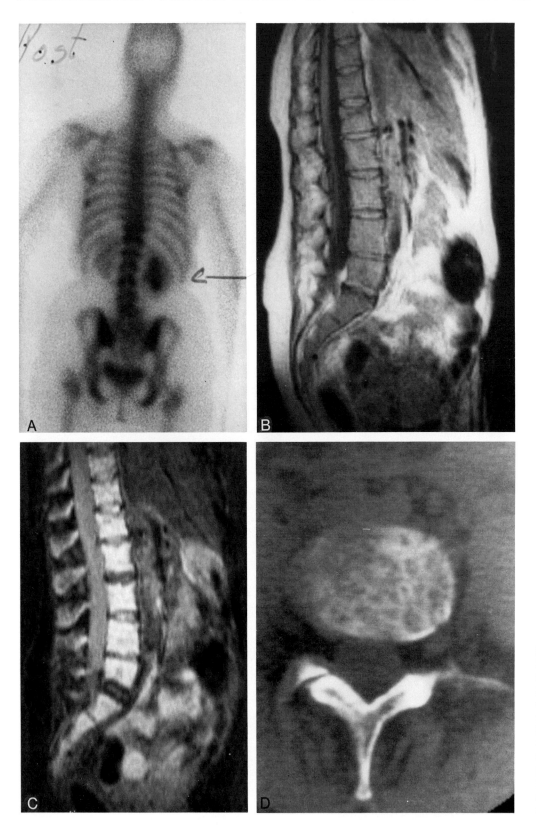

FIGURE 11–149. (**A**) A bone scan was unremarkable in a patient with aggressive metastatic breast carcinoma. (**B**) T1-weighted and (**C**) short TI inversion recovery images show low and high signal intensity, respectively, from diffuse marrow involvement of the entire thoracic and lumbar spines. (**D**) The corresponding axial CT scan confirms the lytic destruction of cancellous cortical bone.

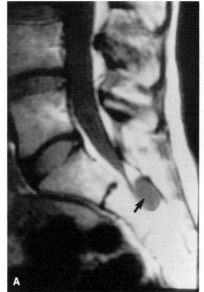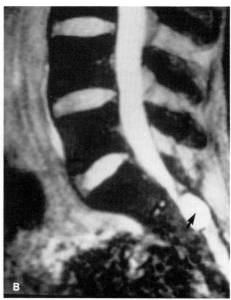

FIGURE 11–150. A Tarlov cerebrospinal fluid cyst (*i.e.,* meningeal cyst with nerve roots) is present at the S2 level (*arrow*), as seen on (**A**) T1-weighted and (**B**) T2*-weighted sagittal images. These cysts are normal variations and are rarely symptomatic.

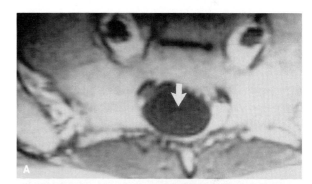

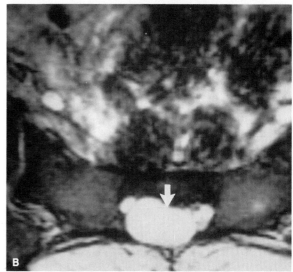

FIGURE 11–151. An extradural meningeal cyst (*arrows*) at the sacral level demonstrates (**A**) low signal intensity on a T1-weighted axial image and (**B**) high signal intensity on a T2*-weighted axial image. There is pressure erosion of the adjacent sacral cortex. This cyst does not involve nerve roots and represents a dural diverticula in continuity with the thecal sac.

ages, in which the CSF and tumor both demonstrate bright signal intensity.

Magnetic resonance is also sensitive in detecting replacement of marrow-fat with tumor cell populations that have T1 values significantly longer than those of normal yellow marrow.[123,127] Marrow infiltrates from leukemia and lymphoma can be successfully identified on STIR sequences as areas of bright signal intensity within a black or gray background of nulled fat signal from uninvolved marrow. In the spine and pelvis, lymphomatous involvement of marrow may be patchy or nodular, and MR localization prior to biopsy can reduce the amount of false-negatives from sampling error.

Fatty replacement of affected marrow in patients undergoing radiation and chemotherapy can be demonstrated on T1, T2, and STIR sequences.[130] Normal red or hematopoietic elements in the spine demonstrate gray contrast on STIR sequences, whereas fatty or yellow marrow replacement is seen as areas of dark nulled signal.

Extramedullary cysts of the meninges may present with adjacent bone erosion secondary to chronic local CSF pressure and without the more aggressive bone destruction of metastatic disease. Meningeal cysts may present with (Fig. 11–150) or without (Fig. 11–151) nerve root involvement.

REFERENCES

1. Dixon AK, Bannon RP. Computed tomography of the postoperative lumbar spine: the need for, and optimal dose of, intravenous contrast media. Br J Radiol 1987;60:215.
2. Braun IF, et al. Contrast enhancement in CT differentiation between recurrent disc herniation and postoperative scar: prospective study. AJNR 1985;6:607.
3. Zinreich SJ, et al. CT myelography for outpatients: an inpatient/outpatient pilot study to assess methodology. Radiology 1985;157:387.
4. Helms, CA, et al. CT of the lumbar spine: normal variants and pitfalls. RadioGraphics 1987;7:447.
5. Weiss T, et al. CT of the postoperative lumbar spine: value of intravenous contrast. Neuroradiology 1986;28:241.
6. Zinreich SJ, et al. Three-dimensional CT imaging in post-surgical "failed back" syndrome. J Comput Assist Tomogr 1990;14:574.
7. Mills DG. Imaging of the cervical spine. Proceedings of the MR Clinical Symposium. vol. 3. no. 5. Milwaukee: GE Medical Systems, 1987.
8. Berger PE, et al. High resolution surface coil magnetic resonance imaging of the spine: normal and pathologic anatomy. RadioGraphics 1986;6:573.
9. Smoker WRK, et al. MRI versus conventional radiologic examination in the evaluation of the craniovertebral and cervicomedullary junction. RadioGraphics 1986;6:953.
10. Maravilla KR, et al. Magnetic resonance demonstration of multiple sclerosis plaques in the cervical cord. AJNR 1984;5:685.
11. Kulkarni MV, et al. Acute spinal cord injury: MR imaging at 1.5T. Radiology 1987;164:837.
12. Modic MT, et al. Cervical radiculopathy: value of oblique MR imaging. Radiology 1987;163:227.
13. Rubin JB, Enzmann DR. Optimizing conventional MR imaging of the spine. Radiology 1987;163:777.
14. Enzmann DR, et al. Cervical spine MR imaging: generating high-signal CSF in sagittal and axial images. Radiology 1987;163:233.
15. Modic MT, et al. Magnetic resonance imaging of the cervical spine: technical and clinical observations. AJNR 1984;5:15.
16. Flannigan BD, et al. MR imaging of the cervical spine; neurovascular anatomy. AJR 1987;148:785.
17. Burnett KR, et al. MRI evaluation of the cervical spine at high field strength. Applied Radiol 1985.
18. Yu S, et al. Facet joint menisci of the cervical spine: correlative MR imaging and cryomicrotomy study. Radiology 1987;164:79.
19. Teresi LM, et al. Asymptomatic degenerative disc disease and spondylosis of the cervical spine: MR imaging. Radiology 1987;164:83.
20. Ross JS, et al. Thoracic disc herniation: MR imaging. Radiology 1987;165:511.
21. Modic MR, et al. Magnetic resonance imaging of intervertebral disc disease: clinical and pulse sequence considerations. Radiology 1984;152:103.
22. Grenier N, et al. Degenerative lumbar disc disease: pitfalls and usefulness of MR imaging in detection of vacuum phenomenon. Radiology 1987;164:861.
23. Ramsey RG. MRI's reputation grows in herniated disc evaluation. Diagnostic Imaging 1987:120.
24. Pech L, Haughton VM. Lumbar intervertebral disc: correlative MR and anatomic study. Radiology 1985;156:699.
25. Chafetz NI, et al. Recognition of lumbar disc herniation with NMR. AJR 1983;141:1153.
26. Schellinger D, et al. Facet joint disorders and their role in the production of back pain and sciatica. RadioGraphics, 1987;7:923.
27. Grenier N, et al. Normal and degenerative posterior spinal structures: MR imaging. Radiology 1987;165:517.
28. Ross JS, et al. Lumbar spine: postoperative assessment with surface-coil MR imaging. Radiology 1987;164:851.
29. Nokes SR, et al. Childhood scoliosis: MR imaging. Radiology 1987;164:791.
30. Heithoff KBN. Spontaneous lumbar epidural hematoma. Proceedings of the MR Clinical Symposium. vol. 3. no. 3. Milwaukee: GE Medical Systems, 1987.
31. Glenn WV, et al. Magnetic resonance imaging of the lumbar spine: nerve root canals, disc abnormalities, anatomic correlations and case examples. Milwaukee: GE Medical Systems, 1986.
32. Haughton VM. MR imaging of the spine. Radiology 1988;166:297.
33. Krause D, et al. Lumbar disc herniation: value of oblique magnetic resonance imaging sections. Neuroradiology 1988;15:305.
34. Winter DDB, et al. CT and MR lateral disc herniation: typical appearance and pitfalls of interpretation. Canad Assoc Radiol 1989;40:256.
35. Osborn AG, et al. CT/MR spectrum of far lateral and anterior lumbosacral disc herniations. AJNR 1988;9:775.
36. Williams MP, et al. Thoracic disc herniation: MR imaging. Radiology 1988;167:874.
37. Yu S, et al. Anulus fibrosus in bulging intervertebral discs. Radiology 1988;169:761.
38. Masaryk TJ, et al. High-resolution MR imaging of sequestered lumbar intervertebral discs. AJNR 1988;9:351.
39. Williams MP, et al. Significance of thoracic disc herniation demonstrated by MR imaging. J Comput Assist Tomogr 1989;13:211.
40. Schellinger D, et al. Disc fragment migration. Radiology 1990;175:831.
41. Murayama S, et al. Diagnosis of herniated intervertebral discs with MR imaging: a comparison of gradient-refocused-echo and spin-echo pulse sequences. AJNR 1990;11:17.

42. Porter BA. MR may become routine for imaging bone marrow. Diagnostic Imaging 1987.

43. Porter BA, et al. Magnetic resonance imaging of bone marrow disorders. Radiol Clin North Am 1986;24:269.

44. Kaplan PA, et al. Bone marrow patterns in aplastic anemia: observations with 1.5T MR Imaging. Radiology 1987;164:441.

45. McKinstry CS, et al. Bone marrow in leukemia and aplastic anemia: MR imaging before, during and after treatment. Radiology 1987;162:701.

46. Vogler JB III, et al. Bone marrow imaging. Radiology 1988;168:679.

47. Modic MT, et al. Degenerative disorders of the spine. In: Modic M, Masaryk T, Ross J, eds. Magnetic resonance imaging of the spine. Chicago: Year Book, 1989:75.

48. Pennes DR, et al. Bone marrow imaging. Radiology 1989;170:894.

49. Stevens SK, et al. Early and late bone marrow changes after irradiation. AJR 1990;154:745.

50. Rosenthal DI, et al. Fatty replacement of spinal bone marrow due to radiation: demonstration by dual energy quantitative CT and MR imaging. J Comput Assist Tomogr 1989;13:463.

51. Carmody RF, et al. Spinal cord compression due to metastatic disease: diagnosis with MR imaging versus myelography. Radiology 1989;173:225.

52. Avrahami E, et al. Early MR demonstration of spinal metastases in patients with normal radiographs and CT and radionuclide bone scans. J Comput Assist Tomogr 1989;13:598.

53. Modic TJ, et al. Degenerative disc disease: assessment of changes in vertebral body marrow with MR imaging. Radiology 1988;166:193.

54. Modic MT, et al. Imaging of degenerative disc disease. Radiology 1988;168:177.

55. Saywell WR, et al. Demonstration of vertebral body end plate veins by magnetic resonance imaging. Br J Radiol 1989;62:290.

56. Modic MT. Intervertebral disc: normal age-related changes in MR signal intensity. Radiology 1990;177:332.

57. Sether LA, et al. Intervertebral disc: normal age related changes in MR signal intensity. Radiology 1990;177:385.

58. Russell EJ. Cervical disc disease. Radiology 1990;177:313-325.

59. Tsuruda JS, et al. Three-dimensional gradient-recalled MR imaging as a screening tool for the diagnosis of cervical radiculopathy. AJNR 1989;10:1263.

60. Stoller DW, Genant HK. MRI helps characterize disorders of the spine. Diagnostic Imaging 1987;9:128.

61. Enzmann DR, Rubin JB. Cervical spine: MR imaging with a partial flip angle, gradient refocused pulse sequence, part 1: general considerations and disc disease. Radiology 1988;166:467.

62. Stoller DW, Genant HK. Fast imaging of the spine. In: Genant HK, ed. Spine update. San Francisco: Radiology Research and Education Foundation, 1987:47.

63. Xu GL, et al. Lumbar facet joint capsule: appearance at MR imaging and CT. Radiology 1990;177:415.

64. Okumura R, et al. Fatty filum terminale: Assessment with MR imaging. J Comput Assist Tomogr 1990;14:571.

65. Reynolds H, et al. Cervical rheumatoid arthritis: value of flexion and extension views in imaging. Radiology 1987;164:215.

66. Burk DL, et al. Spinal and paraspinal neurofibromatosis: surface coil MR imaging at 1.5T. Radiology 1987;162:797.

67. Flannigan BD, et al. MR imaging of the lumbar spine: anatomic correlations and the effects of technical variations. AJNR 1987;8:27.

68. Enzmann DR, et al. Cervical spine: MR imaging with a partial flip angle, gradient-refocused pulse sequence: part I. General considerations and disc disease. Radiology 1988;166:467.

69. Enzmann DR, et al. Cervical spine: MR imaging with a partial flip angle, gradient-refocused pulse sequence: part II. Spinal cord disease. Radiology 1988;166:473.

70. Nakstad PH, et al. MRI in cervical disc herniation. Neuroradiology 1989;31:382.

71. Czervionke LF, et al. Cervical neural foramina: correlative anatomic and MR imaging study. Radiology 1988;169:753.

72. Fletcher G, et al. Age-related changes in the cervical facet joints: studies with cryomicrotomy, MR and CT. AJR 1990;154:817.

73. Yamashita Y, et al. Spinal cord compression due to ossification of ligaments: MR imaging. Radiology 1990;175:843.

74. Harsh GR III, et al. Cervical spine stenosis secondary to ossification of the posterior longitudinal ligament. J Neurosurg 1987;67:349.

75. Holtras S, et al. MR imaging of intradural disc herniation. J Comput Assist Tomogr 1989;11:353.

76. Reicher MA, et al. MR imaging of the lumbar spine: anatomic correlations and the effects of technical variations. AJR 1986;147:891.

77. Modic MR, et al. Magnetic resonance imaging of the spine. Radiol Clin North Am 1986;24:229.

78. Edelman RR, et al. High resolution MRI: imaging anatomy of the lumbosacral spine. Magn Reson Imaging 1986;4:515.

79. Berger PE, et al. High resolution surface coil magnetic resonance imaging of the spine: normal and pathologic anatomy. RadioGraphics 1986;6:573.

80. Ross JS, et al. Tears of the anulus fibrosus: assessment with Gd-DTPA-enhanced MR imaging. AJR 1990;154:159.

81. Yu S, et al. Tears of the anulus fibrosus: correlation between MR and pathologic findings in cadavers. AJNR 1988;9:367.

82. Glickstein MF, et al. Magnetic resonance demonstration of hyperintense herniated discs and extruded disc fragments. Skeletal Radiol 1989;18:527.

83. Czervionke LF, et al. Degenerative disease of the spine. In: Atlas SW, ed. Magnetic resonance imaging of the brain and spine. New York: Raven, 1991:795.

84. Liu SS, et al. Synovial cysts of the lumbosacral spine: diagnosis by MR imaging. AJNR 1989;10:1239.

85. Stoller DW, et al. Applications of computed tomography in the musculoskeletal system. Current Orthopaedics 1987;1:219.

86. Lang P, et al. Magnetic resonance imaging in the assessment of functional lumbar spinal stability. [abstract] Sixth Annual Meeting and Exhibition of the Society of Magnetic Resonance in Medicine. New York City, August 17-21, 1987:149.

87. Huckman MS, et al. Chemonucleation and changes observed on lumbar MR scan: preliminary report. AJNR 1987;8:1.

88. Onik G, et al. Percutaneous lumbar discectomy using a new aspiration probe. AJNR 1985;6:290.

89. Ross JS, et al. Postoperative lumbar spine. Semin Roentgenol 1988;23:125.

90. Hueftle MG, et al. Lumbar spine: postoperative MR imaging with Gd-DTPA. Radiology 1988;167:817.

91. Sotiropoulous S, et al. Differentiation between postoperative scar and recurrent disc herniation: prospective comparison of MR, CT and contrast-enhanced CT. AJNR 1989;10:639.

92. Ross JS, et al. Gadolinium-DTPA-enhanced MR imaging of the postoperative lumbar spine: time course and mechanism of enhancement. AJNR 1989;10:37.

93. Ross JS, et al. MR imaging of the postoperative lumbar spine: assessment with gadopentetate dimeglumine. AJNR 1990;11:771.

94. Djukic S, et al. Magnetic resonance imaging of the postoperative lumbar spine. Radiol Clin North Am 1990;28:341.

95. Ross JS, et al. MR enhancement of epidural fibrosis by Gd-DTPA: biodistribution and mechanism. Radiology 1987;165:142.

96. Ross, JS, et al. MR imaging of lumbar arachnoiditis. AJR 1987;149:1025.

97. Boden SD, Davis DO, Dina TS, et al. Contrast-enhanced MR imaging performed after successful lumbar disc surgery: prospective study. Radiology 1992;182(1):59.

98. Hackney, DB, et al. MR characteristics of iophendylate (Pantopaque). J Comput Assist Tomogr 1986;10:401.

99. Altman NR, Altman DH. MR imaging of spinal dysraphism. AJNR 1987;8:533.

100. Johnson DW, et al. MR imaging of the pars interarticularis. AJR 1989;152:327.

101. Grenier N, et al. Isthmic spondylolysis of the lumbar spine: MR imaging at 1.5 T. Radiology 1989;170:489-493.

102. Gado MB. The spine. In: Lee JK, et al, eds. Computed body tomography with MRI correlation. 2nd ed. New York: Raven, 1989:991.

103. Sartoris, DJ, et al. Vertebral-body collapse in focal diffuse disease: patterns of pathologic processes. Radiology, 1986;160:479.

104. Kaplan, PA, et al. Osteoporosis with vertebral compression fractures, retropulsed fragments, and neurologic compromise. Radiology 1987;165:533.

105. Yuh WTC, et al. Vertebral compression fractures: distinction between benign and malignant causes with MR imaging. Radiology 1989;172:215.

106. Wiener SN, et al. Comparison of magnetic resonance imaging and radionuclide bone imaging of vertebral fractures. Clin Nucl Med 1990;14:666.

107. Baker LL, et al. Benign versus pathologic compression fractures of vertebral bodies: assessment with conventional spin-echo, chemical shift, and STIR MR imaging. Radiology 1990;174:495.

108. Modic MT, et al. Vertebral osteomyelitis: assessment using MR. Radiology 1985;157:157.

109. Appel B, et al. MRI of the spine and spinal cord: infectious and inflammatory pathology. Neuroradiology 1988;15:325.

110. Smith AS, et al. MR imaging characteristics of tuberculous spondylitis vs. vertebral osteomyelitis. AJR 1989;153:399.

111. deRoss A, et al. MRI of tuberculous spondylitis. AJR 1986;146:79.

112. Edwards M. White matter disease. In: Atlas SW, ed. Magnetic resonance imaging of the brain and spine. New York: Raven, 1991:467.

113. Parizel PM, et al. Gd-DTPA-enhanced MR imaging of the spine tumors. AJNR 1989;10:249.

114. Valk J. Gd-DTPA in MR of spinal lesions. AJNR 1988;9:345.

115. Takemoto K, et al. MR imaging of intraspinal tumors—capability in histologic differentiation and compartmentalization of extramedullary tumors. Neuroradiololgy 1988;30:303.

116. Laredo, DJ, et al. Vertebral hemangiomas: fat content as a sign of aggressiveness. Radiology 1990;177:467.

117. Raghaven N, et al. MR imaging in the tethered spinal cord syndrome. AJNR 1989;10:27.

118. Sugimura K, et al. Bone marrow disease of the spine: differentiation with T1 and T2 relaxation times in MR imaging. Radiology 1987;165:541.

119. Daffner RH, et al. MRI in the detection of malignant infiltration of bone marrow. AJR 1986;146:353.

120. Kricun ME. Red-yellow marrow conversion: its effect on the location of some solitary bone lesions. Skeletal Radiol 1985;14:10.

121. Hajek PC, et al. Focal fat deposition in axial bone marrow: MR characteristics. Radiology 1987;162:245.

122. Weaver GR, Sandler MP. Increased sensitivity of magnetic resonance imaging compared to radionuclide bone scintigraphy in the detection of lymphoma of the spine. Clin Nucl Med 1987;12:333.

123. Olson D, et al. Magnetic resonance imaging of the bone marrow in patients with leukemia, aplastic anemia and lymphoma. Invest Radiol 1986.

124. Beltran J, et al. Tumors of the osseous spine: staging with MR imaging versus CT. Radiology 1987;162:565.

125. Ross JS, et al. Vertebral hemangiomas: MR imaging. Radiology, 1988;165:165.

126. Sarpel S, et al. Early diagnosis of spinal-epidural metastasis by magnetic resonance imaging. Radiology 1987;164:887.

127. Porter BA, et al. Low field STIR imaging of marrow malignancies. Radiology 1987;165:275.

128. Emory TH, et al. Comparison of Gd-DTPA MR imaging and radionuclide bone scans (WIP). Radiology 1987;165:342.

129. Berry I, et al. Gd-DTPA enhancement of cerebral and spinal tumors on MR imaging. Radiology 1987;165P38.

130. Ramsey RG, Zacharias CE. MR imaging of the spine after radiation therapy: easily recognizable effects, JNR 1985;6:247.

C H A P T E R 12

David. W. Stoller
Bruce A. Porter
Terri M. Steinkirchner

Marrow Imaging

Conventional radiographic techniques, insensitive to many marrow infiltrations and tumors, are limited in providing accurate bone marrow characterization. Frequently, there is significant trabecular or cancellous destruction before disease progression is detected on standard radiographs. Computed tomography (CT), although accurate for detecting gross metastatic disease of the spine, is of limited use in imaging primary and metastatic marrow neoplasms in the rest of the skeleton. Changes in the CT attenuation value of medullary bone can be nonspecific and do not occur until pathology is well established. Radionuclide bone scanning, the standard method for screening the skeleton for metastatic disease, is relatively insensitive to certain marrow neo-

plasms, such as leukemia, lymphoma, and myeloma. Very aggressive metastatic tumors may be false-negative on radionuclide scans. Marrow studies with radiolabeled colloids, which have shown promise in research studies, have not become routine in clinical oncology.

Unlike these modalities, magnetic resonance (MR) imaging has the major benefit of imaging bone marrow directly. Multiplanar MR imaging provides the excellent spatial and contrast resolution necessary to differentiate the signal intensities of fatty (*i.e.,* yellow) marrow elements from hematopoietic (*i.e.,* red) marrow elements. Magnetic resonance imaging may thus become the diagnostic gold standard for diseases that involve or target the bone marrow.

NORMAL BONE MARROW

The normal distribution and MR appearance of bone marrow changes with age.[1-4] An understanding of these variations is important in examining MR patterns in appendicular skeletal locations and determining whether they are potential disease processes or normal variations of marrow. The general status of marrow in adults is best assessed on MR images in the coronal plane of the pelvis, unless symptoms indicate disease elsewhere.

Structure, Function, and Development

The bone marrow is the site of production of circulating blood elements (*i.e.,* granulocytes, erythrocytes, monocytes, platelets, uncommitted lymphocytes). Sustained cellular production is dependent on stem cells, which exhibit properties of both continuous self-replication and differentiation into specific cell lines. The tremendous flexibility of stem cells in the production of blood cellular elements is related to their proliferative activity, which is dependent on the microenvironment (*i.e.,* cell-to-cell interaction) and on humoral feedback.[5,6]

The marrow cavity is divided into compartments by plates of bony trabeculae. Red marrow (*i.e.,* hematopoietic marrow) is hematopoietically active bone marrow located within the spaces defined by the trabeculae. It is semifluid in consistency and is composed of the various hematopoietic stem cells and their progeny in assorted stages of granulocytic, erythrocytic, and megakaryocytic development. Uncommitted lymphocytes, as well as lymphoid nodules, are also present in the red marrow. The hematopoietic cellular elements are supported by reticulum cells and fat cells. Red marrow contains approximately 40% water, 40% fat and 20% protein.[7] The vascular system consists of centrally located nutrient arteries that send out branches that terminate in capillary beds within the bone. Postcapillary venules reenter the marrow cavity and coalesce to form venous sinuses. Hematopoietic cell production follows the vascular arrangement, forming active hematopoietic islands between the sinusoids. Bone marrow lacks lymphatic channels.[8,9]

Hematopoietically inactive marrow, or marrow not involved in blood cell production, is referred to as yellow marrow. Yellow marrow is predominantly fat; thus, it is sometimes called fatty marrow. It contains approximately 15% water, 80% fat, and 5% protein.

Red to Yellow Marrow Conversion

Hematopoiesis begins in utero, at approximately 19 gestational days, within the yolk sac. By week 16 of gestation, the main sites of fetal hematopoiesis are the liver

and spleen. After week 24 of gestation, marrow becomes the main organ of hematopoiesis. At birth, active hematopoiesis (*i.e.,* red marrow) is present throughout the entire skeleton. Normal physiological conversion of red to yellow marrow occurs during growth in a predictable and orderly fashion,[10] and is complete by 25 years of age, when the adult pattern is established.

The cellularity of red marrow varies with age and site. In the newborn, red marrow cellularity approaches 100%. In the adult, fat cells generally occupy approximately 50% of the active red marrow (Fig. 12–1), but the cellularity of marrow varies with the site. For example, at 50 years of age, the average cellularity is 75% in the vertebrae, 60% in the sternum, and 50% in the iliac crests.[9,10] In the adult, red marrow is primarily concentrated in the appendicular and axial (*i.e.,* spine) skeleton. The prevalence of fatty marrow within the spine increases with advancing age. In osteoporosis, fat replacement is associated with loss of cancellous (*i.e.,* trabecular) bone. Early in the normal ossification process, yellow marrow replaces the hyaline cartilage template in the epiphysis and apophysis.

Reconversion of Yellow to Red Marrow

Reconversion of yellow to red marrow occurs in the reverse order to that seen in the normal, physiologically maturing skeleton, starting in the axial skeleton and proceeding in a proximal-to-distal direction in the appendicular skeleton. Hematopoiesis occurs in the proximal metaphysis in the premature skeleton; therefore, reconversion of long bones occurs first in the proximal metaphysis and then in the distal metaphysis. The process of reconversion of red to yellow marrow is triggered by the body's demand for increased hematopoiesis, which may be caused by stress, anemia, or marrow replacement. The extent of reconversion depends on the duration and severity of the initiating cause. More extensive reconversion is seen in long-standing chronic anemias such as sickle-cell anemia or thalassemia major.[11] This process favors sites of residual red marrow stores.

Magnetic Resonance Appearance

Hydrogen protons in yellow marrow exist in hydrophobic side groups with short T1 relaxation times.[12,13] The bright signal intensity of yellow marrow reflects the shortened T1 relaxation time of fat. The differences in signal intensities of yellow and red marrow result primarily from differences in the proportional amounts of water and fat; the proportions are approximately equal in red marrow, but significantly more fat (80%) exists in yellow marrow.[3] The role of protein, which constitutes 40% of red marrow and 5% of yellow marrow, in modifying signal intensity is less clear, because protein may exist in either a bound state with long TI relaxation times or in solution with short T1 relaxation times.[12,14]

Therefore, on T1-weighted and conventional T2-weighted images, yellow marrow demonstrates the bright signal intensity of fat. On heavily T2*-weighted contrast images, yellow marrow appears dark or is of decreased signal intensity. This effect is unrelated to the low signal intensity of yellow marrow on short TI inversion recovery (STIR) images, in which signal from fat is nulled. Red marrow demonstrates low signal intensity on T1-weighted images, reflecting its increased water content, and intermediate signal intensity with progressive T2 weighting. Red and yellow marrow contrast differences become less distinct on heavily T2-weighted protocols with repetition times (TR) greater than 2500 msec.

With suppression of the signal from fat on STIR images, areas of red marrow demonstrate higher signal intensity than areas of yellow marrow. Separation of red and yellow marrow is most difficult on T2*-weighted images, where red marrow stores may actually demonstrate decreased signal intensity relative to adjacent yellow or fatty marrow.

In the newborn there are no yellow marrow stores, and red marrow signal intensity is equal to or less than that of muscle (Fig. 12–2). On T1-weighted sequences, articular cartilage in epiphyseal centers images with low signal intensity, similar to red marrow. On conventional T2-weighted sequences, articular cartilage is intermediate in signal intensity, but demonstrates an increase in signal intensity on T2*-weighted sequences, which are sensitive to imaging articular cartilage (Fig. 12–3).

As discussed above, the maturing skeleton undergoes a process of red to yellow marrow conversion beginning in the hands and feet, and progressing to the peripheral and then central skeleton.[1,3] In the long bones of the appendicular skeleton, red marrow conversion occurs first in the diaphysis and progresses to the distal and then proximal metaphysis (Figs. 12–4, 12–5, and 12–6).[15] In the adult, the proximal two-thirds of the femur and humerus contain a higher concentration of red marrow stores, accounting for the appearance in T1-weighted images of low signal intensity inhomogeneity against a background matrix of fatty marrow of bright signal intensity. Uniform fatty marrow within the long bones of the humerus or femur without any red marrow inhomogeneity is within the spectrum of normal findings.

MARROW IMAGING TECHNIQUES

Spin-Echo Imaging

Since both benign and malignant disorders that target the marrow have long T1 and T2 values and high proton density, imaging protocols for marrow characterization use T1-weighted spin-echo (SE) sequences. T2-weighted SE sequences have less contrast in the range of commonly used TRs (*i.e.*, approximately 2000 msec), and long TR and TE times (*i.e.*, TR values between 2000 and 3000 msec; TE values greater than 80 msec) would be necessary to optimize contrast. Many lesions become isointense with marrow on intermediate-weighted sequences; therefore, T1-weighted images with TR values between 400 and 700 msec and short TEs less than 30 msec are required.

Lower contrast, as well as artifacts caused by moving high signal intensity fat, may degrade the diagnostic quality of conventional T1- and T2-weighted SE images. Conventional MR imaging may also be of limited value when contrast is intrinsically low due to small differences in signal between tumors and adjacent fat, especially on long TR/TE sequences. The clinical usefulness of marrow MR imaging can be substantially expanded by combining T1-weighted SE and STIR sequences.

Short TI Inversion Recovery Imaging

The STIR technique is highly T1-weighted. The initial excitation pulse, 180°, is followed by a standard SE pulse sequence at inversion times (TI) after the initial 180° pulse (Fig. 12–7). The manner in which this pulse sequence becomes a T1-weighted sequence is shown in Figure 12–8. The strength of the signal that is returned from the SE sequence is proportional to the absolute magnitude of the Z component of the bulk magnetization vector at the instant of the 90° pulse; therefore, a TI can be determined for which fat, which has a short TI, will not emit a signal.

This type of inversion recovery technique (with a short TI) was initially used to eliminate the subcutaneous fat signal responsible for motion and breathing artifacts. It suppresses the signal from normal medullary fat, which allows the signal emanating from abnormal tissues to be more easily detected; therefore, it has proven to be highly sensitive for diseases within the medullary space of bone. The clinical advantages arise from the following STIR characteristics:

- additive T1 and T2 contrast
- marked suppression of the high signal from fat
- twice the magnetization range of SE sequences.

These characteristics produce extraordinarily high contrast that makes the lesion more conspicuous, but preserve the low signal-to-noise ratio. By selecting TI times that occur at the null point during the recovery of signal after an inverting 180° radiofrequency (RF) pulse, the signal from structures of known T1 relaxation times can be selectively suppressed.

The STIR sequence described above suppresses the signal from fat, which is the predominant component of marrow in normal adults. T1 is prolonged in most pathologic conditions affecting the marrow, and the T1 of marrow fat is short; therefore, there is extreme contrast on STIR images, a considerable advantage over routine SE imaging. On STIR images, fat is black, combinations of red and yellow marrow are light gray (*i.e.,* intermediate), and most marrow tumors are bright white. Although red marrow demonstrates increased signal intensity on STIR images, most pathologic conditions involving marrow replacement or infiltration generate greater signal intensities. Fibrous tissue, calcification, and hemosiderin deposits are low in signal intensity, whereas fluid, edema, or recent hemorrhage are all bright. Muscle remains intermediate in signal intensity. STIR sequences reflect age-dependent differences in the percentage of hematopoietic marrow.

Gradient–Echo Recall Imaging

Gradient-echo recall techniques (*i.e.,* T2*-weighted images) have become increasingly popular, primarily because of their ability to increase the rate of data acquisition and decrease scan times. A standard gradient recall sequence is shown in Figure 12–9. The initial excitation pulse is an RF pulse that typically possesses a flip angle of less than 90°. If a 90° flip angle is used, the Z component of the bulk magnetization vector is zero after the excitation pulse (Fig. 12–10), and a period of time on the order of T1 is needed for the Z component of the bulk magnetization vector to recover and to allow a second pulse sequence to generate significant signal. If the excitation pulse is less than 90°, however, the Z component of the bulk magnetization vector is not decreased to zero, and the subsequent excitation pulse can be separated from the first by a TR significantly less than T1 (see Fig. 12–10). In addition, the resultant signal is maximized by using free induction decay for data acquisition, instead of a standard SE with its associated long TE and signal drop-off. To balance phase shifts from the read-out frequency gradient so that all phase shifts are only those specifically introduced by the phase and encoding gradients, the initial read-out gradient is negative and cancels phase shifts introduced by the positive component of the frequency-encoded gradient during acquisition of the signal. Between the negative and positive gradient, a reversal occurs; thus, the term gradient reversal techniques is used (see Fig. 12–9). By using partial flip angles, TR values can be markedly shortened. As image acquisition time is directly proportional to the value of TR, marked time savings over SE techniques can be attained. However, because the contrast parameters sampled by the gradient-echo technique are predominantly T2*, the high contrast between soft tissues normally obtained by SE techniques is not routinely seen on gradient-echo images. It is possible to select parameters to provide contrast that is somewhat similar to standard SE imaging (Table 12–1).

Gradient-echo techniques are sensitive to magnetic-field inhomogeneities, chemical-shift frequencies, and magnetic susceptibility; therefore, they are prone to motion and distortion artifacts of tissue interfaces with different magnetic susceptibilities. Advantages of gradient-echo techniques, including effective T2 weighting, high resolution, and adequate signal-to-noise ratio without need for interslice spacing, however, make this a useful complement to T1 SE imaging. In addition, three dimensional Fourier transform volume acquisitions, which allow up to 120 images to a slice thickness of 0.7 mm, can be retrospectively reformatted. Susceptibility effects can be used to identify calcium or areas of hemorrhage.

The low signal intensity contrast of T2*-weighted images is not secondary to fat suppression, as with STIR images; therefore, many marrow neoplasms or infiltrative disease processes do not demonstrate increased signal intensity when compared with corresponding STIR images. Red marrow stores do not demonstrate increased signal intensity on T2*-gradient images, and may be difficult to differentiate from fatty marrow. A high proportion of trabecular bone in areas such as the epiphysis may

TABLE 12–1

Repetition- and echo-time pulse parameters for variously weighted images

	T1-WEIGHTED	MIXED	T2*-WEIGHTED	PROTON-DENSITY–WEIGHTED
TR (msec)	200–400	20–50	200–400	200–400
TE (msec)	12–15	12–15	30–60	12–15
Θ (degrees)	45–90	30–60	5–20	5–20

TE, echo time; TR, repetition time; Θ, flip angle.
(Wehrli FW, Shaw D, Kneeland B. Signal-to-noise, resolution, and contrast. In: Principles, methodology and applications of biomedical magnetic resonance imaging. New York: VCH Publishers, 1987.)

further modify gradient-echo contrast (decreasing effective transverse relaxation times), resulting in decreased signal intensity in these areas.[16]

Chemical-Shift Imaging

Chemical-shift imaging is used to produce images that emphasize either the water or fat component of marrow by temporal separation of their respective returning MR signals.[17] Red and yellow marrow differentiation is thus possible on T1-weighted images. Differences in resonant frequencies of fat and water protons (3.5 ppm or 75-150 Hz) allow for temporal dephasing after RF pulse excitation. This property is used to develop water and fat images by emphasizing in-phase or out-of-phase tissue properties, thus suppressing fat or water signal.

Magnetic Resonance Survey Evaluation

The protocol for an MR survey examination for marrow evaluation uses T1-weighted coronal images of the pelvis and proximal femurs, which are adult sites of red marrow concentration. These images are acquired with large (40-cm) fields of view to include assessment of lumbosacral spine marrow. Transcoronal STIR images are obtained to null fat signal and identify abnormal T1 or T1 prolongation. T2*-weighted images may be used when thin slices or multiplanar imaging is required in a limited period of time.

Axial T1-weighted, T2*-weighted, or STIR images may be obtained at specific sites of suspected pathologic processes and are important in determining cross-sectional marrow involvement. T1-weighted images are particularly valuable in evaluating blastic processes, which are low in signal on STIR and T2*-weighted images. Gadolinium-enhanced axial images may improve the visibility of lesions, especially in cases with soft-tissue or cord involvement. Sagittal T1-weighted and STIR images are routinely acquired to evaluate suspected spinal malignancies.

BONE MARROW PATHOLOGY

Malignant Disorders

Leukemia

Acute Leukemias. Acute leukemias are the twentieth most common cause of cancer deaths at all ages, and, as a group, they are the most common malignant disease in childhood. This aggressive group of disorders arises at the primitive stem cell level and is usually classified as either lymphocytic or myelogenous in type, based on cytologic features of the blast cell. Further classification of the leukemic blasts, based on immunologic markers, cytogenetics, and electron microscopy, provides useful prognostic and therapeutic information. Eighty percent of patients with acute lymphocytic (*i.e.,* lymphoblastic) leukemia are children, and 90% of patients with acute myelogenous leukemia are adults.[18,19]

The majority of acute leukemias arise de novo, although they may represent the final progression of a preexisting preleukemic state (*e.g.,* myelodysplasia) or the end stage of a chronic myeloproliferative disorder such as chronic myelogenous leukemia. The distinguishing feature of the acute phase is the uncontrolled growth of poorly differentiated blast cells. These cells rapidly accumulate in the marrow, suppressing the normal marrow elements and resulting in the commonly observed clinical symptoms of fatigue, weakness, infections, and hemorrhage.

Marrow involvement in acute leukemia is typically diffuse and is characterized by monotonous infiltration of immature cells in a hypercellular marrow (Fig. 12-11). In occasional cases of myeloblastic leukemia, particularly in very old patients, the marrow is normocellular or even hypocellular.[10] Leukemic expansion in the marrow may elicit symptoms of skeletal tenderness or swelling of the larger joints.[7]

Clinical Assessment. Clinical assessment of leukemia involves posterior iliac crest aspiration for biopsies and analysis of peripheral blood smears. Peripheral disturbances in hematopoiesis is often nonspecific and frequently occurs prior to significant increases in marrow blast cells. At present, the use of MR imaging in childhood leukemias is limited, but this may change because of the potential of MR imaging for monitoring the course of relapse and the complications of treatment in these patients.

Acute leukemia in relapse may present with focal or irregular areas of infiltration, which may represent surviving rests of treated tumor cells. This appearance is more patchy and irregularly marginated than that usually seen with focal metastatic disease.

Magnetic Resonance Appearance. In both children and adults, leukemic marrow involvement is homogeneous, diffuse, and symmetric (Fig. 12-12). Focal infiltration is more commonly seen in myelogenous leukemia (Fig. 12-13). On T1-weighted images, leukemic hypercellularity is seen as low signal intensity replacement of higher signal intensity marrow fat (Fig. 12-14). Due to the greater proportion of hematopoietic marrow in children, there is an overlap in the appearance of normal low signal intensity cellular hematopoietic marrow and

(text continues on page 976)

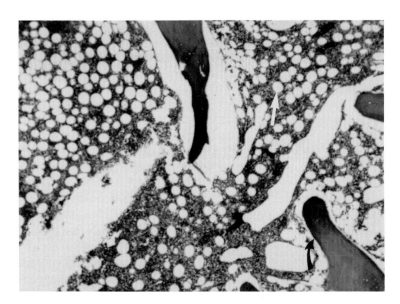

FIGURE 12–1. Normal bone marrow in a 51-year-old man consists of a 50:50 cell-to-fat ratio. Fat (*straight arrow*) is seen as white, round spaces surrounded by hematopoietic cells. The marrow is compartmentalized by trabecular bone (*curved arrow*). (H & E stain; original magnification ×100.)

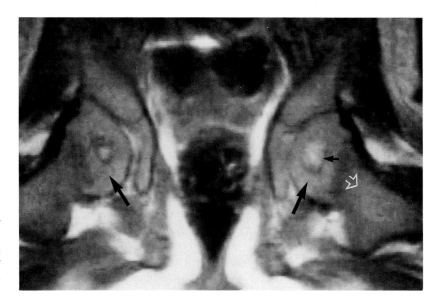

FIGURE 12–2. Intermediate signal intensity epiphyseal cartilage (*large arrows*) with a high signal intensity ossific nucleus (*small arrow*) is seen on a T1-weighted coronal image. Red marrow demonstrates low signal intensity (*open arrow*). (TR, 600 msec; TE, 20 msec.)

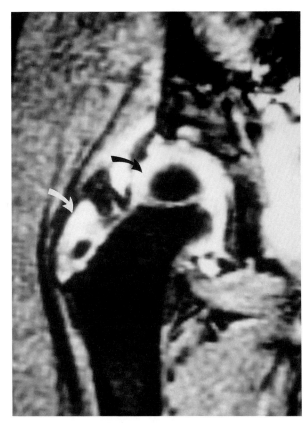

FIGURE 12–3. High signal intensity cartilage in the greater trochanter (*white arrow*) and femoral epiphyses (*black arrow*) can be seen on a T2*-weighted coronal image. (TR, 400 msec; TE, 20 msec; flip angle, 25°.)

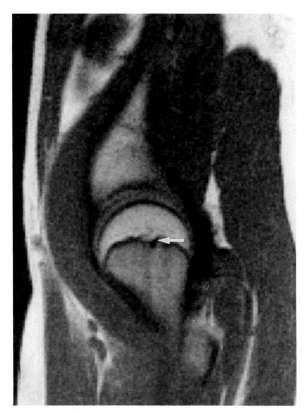

FIGURE 12–4. The low signal intensity physeal plate separates the bright signal intensity metaphyseal red marrow (*arrow*), as seen on a T1-weighted sagittal image. (TR, 600 msec; TE, 20 msec.)

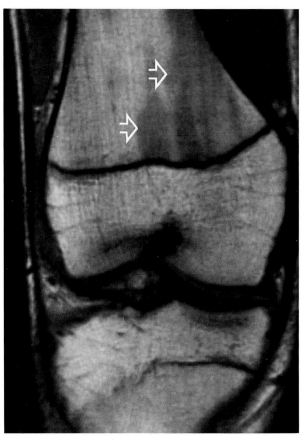

FIGURE 12–5. Residual metaphyseal red marrow in a child is seen as patchy regions of low signal intensity (*open arrows*) on a T1-weighted coronal image. (TR, 600 msec; TE, 20 msec.)

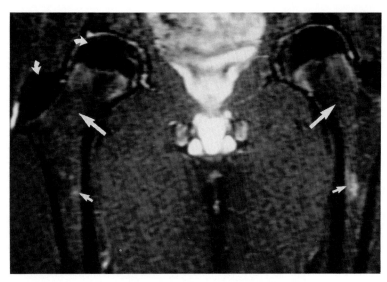

FIGURE 12–6. A coronal short TI inversion recovery image shows normal hematopoietic intermediate signal intensity in the femurs (*large straight arrows*) and dark fat marrow in the epiphyseal centers and greater trochanter in a 15-year-old boy. Note the early replacement of hematopoietic marrow by fat marrow in the diaphyses (*small straight arrows*).

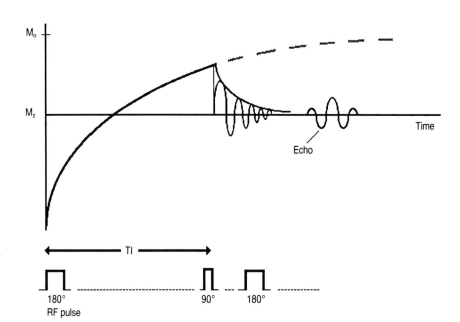

FIGURE 12–7. The inversion recovery pulse sequence is initiated by a 180° radiofrequency (RF) excitation pulse. After a time interval (TI), a 90° pulse followed by a 180° refocusing pulse is used to create a standard spin echo that is sampled for image acquisition.

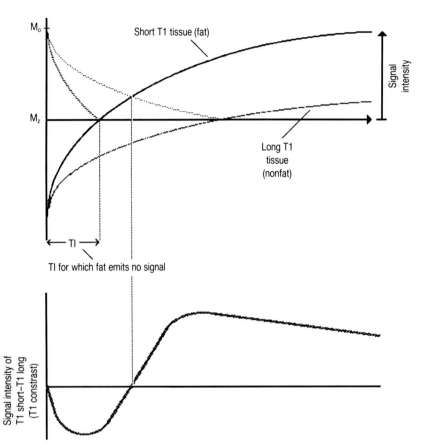

FIGURE 12–8. On T1 contrast using inversion recovery pulse sequences, the strength of the signal intensity with standard inversion recovery pulse sequences is proportional to the absolute value of the Z component of the bulk magnetization vector at the time of signal sampling that is an imaging time (TI) a variable amount of milliseconds after the initial 180° excitation pulse. A short TI can be chosen so that tissues such as fat, with short repetition-time (TR) values, will have a Z component of the bulk magnetization vector near zero at the time of tissue sampling. At this value, fat emits no signal, whereas surrounding tissues with longer TR emit a signal. This can be used to suppress unwanted fat signal when it overwhelms signal from abnormal surrounding tissue in bone marrow disease, or when it is responsible for unwanted motion artifacts.

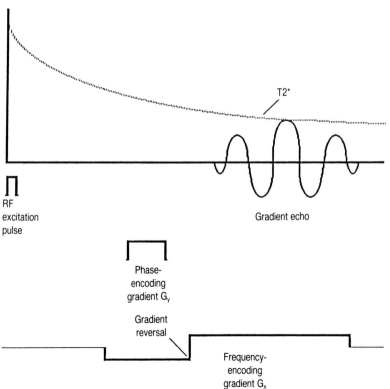

FIGURE 12–9. A highly schematic pulse sequence diagram of a theoretic gradient-echo pulse sequence known as the gradient recall sequence. The sequence is initiated by a radiofrequency (RF) pulse that is typically less than 90°. The pulse is followed by a dephasing gradient that is inverted, which rephases the nuclei during data acquisition. The technique allows a phase-encoded gradient as well as a frequency-encoded gradient to be applied during sampling, so that all necessary information to calculate a 2D image using the 2D Fourier transform method can be obtained during the course of a free induction decay.

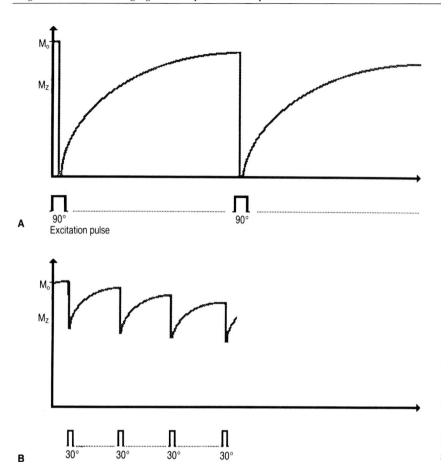

FIGURE 12–10. Small flip angle excitation pulses. After a standard 90° excitation pulse, the Z component of the bulk magnetization vector is zero. (**A**) Time on the order of T1 is required for the Z component of bulk magnetization to recover, so that a second excitation pulse can generate sufficient signal. (**B**) Smaller excitation pulses, such as a 30° pulse, do not decrease the Z component of bulk magnetization vector to zero, and additional excitation pulses can be used with TR values substantially less than T1.

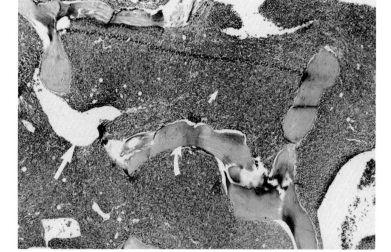

FIGURE 12–11. Acute lymphocytic leukemia. Bone marrow exhibits 100% cellularity consisting of a monotonous population of blast cells (*small arrow*). Fat cells are essentially absent. The vascular sinuses are dilated (*large arrow*), and the trabecular bone is indicated (*curved arrow*). (H & E stain; original magnification ×100.)

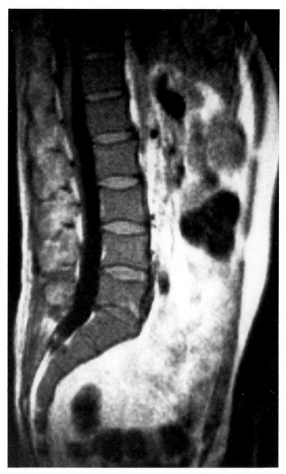

FIGURE 12–12. Diffuse low signal intensity leukemic infiltration of marrow occurs in acute lymphocytic leukemia, as seen on this T1-weighted sagittal image. (TR, 600 msec; TE, 20 msec.)

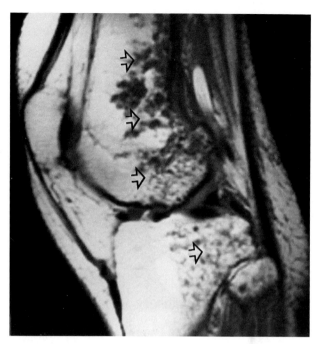

FIGURE 12–13. Low signal intensity leukemic infiltrates (*open arrows*) extending into the epiphysis are seen on a T1-weighted sagittal image. Extension of marrow infiltration crossing the physis is pathologic for acute myelogenous leukemia. (TR, 600 msec; TE, 20 msec.)

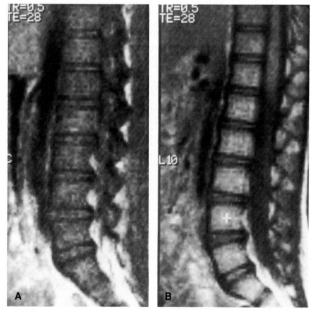

FIGURE 12–14. (**A**) In a patient with acute lymphocytic leukemia, marrow infiltration demonstrates low signal intensity on a T1-weighted sagittal image. (**B**) The spine of a normal age-matched control demonstrates high signal intensity from fatty marrow on a T1-weighted sagittal image. (TR, 500 msec; TE, 28 msec.)

low to intermediate intensity hypercellular leukemic marrow. Quantitative measurements of T1 relaxation times, still under investigation, have shown prolongation in patients with leukemia and leukemia in relapse.[20-23] These assessments, however, are not specific for the diagnosis of leukemia. Prolongation of T1 relaxation time is also seen in metastatic rhabdomyosarcoma and neuroblastoma. Normal bone marrow has a T1 relaxation time of 350 to 650 msec. At initial diagnosis of leukemia or in leukemia in relapse, T1 relaxation times of 750 msec have been identified. Further studies are needed to confirm the clinical significance of differences in T1 values among initial diagnosis, remission, and relapse.[24]

Conventional T2-weighted images may show increases in signal intensity. Unlike the situation with metastatic disease, however, T2-weighted images may not be sensitive to leukemia hypercellularity. Quantitative measurement of T2 relaxation times in leukemias has not shown any significant difference from control marrow.

T2*-weighted images, in which T1 and T2 contrast are not additive, are more limited in the evaluation of infiltrative processes of bone marrow. Larger areas or deposits of leukemic involvement may demonstrate hyperintensity on T2*-weighted images, but similarly affected regions may be less conspicuous (Fig. 12-15).

Chemical-shift imaging has also been used to identify pathologic marrow. Relative changes in the fat fraction show the greatest potential for understanding changes in bone marrow signal intensity and changes occurring with relapse.[21,25] Chemical-shift imaging may be more applicable in adult patients, because of the greater difference in the fat and water fraction of bone marrow.

Short TI inversion recovery imaging techniques offer superior contrast for demonstrating increased signal intensity in leukemic marrow, exceeding that displayed by normal hematopoietic cells. Nulling of fat signal intensity facilitates the detection of both focal and diffuse leukemic infiltrates.

Postchemotherapy. Patients with acute leukemia or chronic myelogenous leukemia in blast crisis are treated aggressively with myelotoxic drugs. This treatment results in cellular depletion (*i.e.,* hypoplasia) of the marrow, accompanied by edema and fibrin deposition. Total depletion of the marrow may require a month or less, depending on the particular chemotherapeutic scheduling and sensitivity of the leukemic cells. As leukemic depletion progresses, fat cells (*i.e.,* yellow marrow) regenerate. Normally, this phase of hypoplasia is followed by regeneration of hematopoietic elements (*i.e.,* red marrow). Occasionally, however, extensive fibrosis may develop postchemotherapy (Figs. 12-16 and 12-17). The fibrosis can be focal or wide spread, and may be accompanied by bone formation.[26,27]

Chemotherapy produces a spectrum of MR changes in normal and pathologic marrow, including leukemia and metastatic disease. Marrow hypoplasia is characterized by the appearance of fatty marrow, which demonstrates high signal intensity on T1-weighted images and intermediate signal intensity on T2-weighted images. Marrow fibrosis demonstrates low signal intensity on T1- and T2-weighted images. Reconversion of normal fatty marrow to hematopoietic marrow is seen as areas of decreased signal intensity on T1-weighted images and intermediate to mildly increased signal intensity on STIR images. When reconversion exists adjacent to an area of signal intensity from fat in treated marrow tumor, there is a reversal of the initial imaging signal intensity characteristics from pretreatment bone marrow to postchemotherapy marrow (Fig. 12-18). Marrow edema imaged immediately postchemotherapy may falsely exaggerate the course of disease progression. Follow-up examination can be performed to document a more accurate baseline.

Chronic Leukemias. In contrast to the acute leukemias, the malignant cell line in the chronic leukemias has a limited capacity for differentiation and function in the initial stages of the disease process. As the disease progresses, thrombocytopenia and granulocytopenia develop as they do in patients with acute leukemia. Compared with acute leukemias, the chronic leukemias are characterized by a long course with prolonged survival. Chemotherapy, which is used aggressively in acute myelogenous leukemia and produces significant bone marrow hypoplasia or aplasia, has a secondary role in the chronic leukemias, which tend to have a more indolent course.

Chronic Lymphocytic Leukemia. Chronic lymphocytic leukemia represents the most common form of leukemia in the United States; it is twice as common as chronic myelogenous leukemia. Ninety percent of patients with chronic lymphocytic leukemia are older than 50 years of age, and the disease shows a male predilection.[28] Lymph node involvement is present in the majority of patients. Chronic lymphocytic leukemia is characterized by abnormal clones of immunologically incompetent lymphocytes. Patients may be asymptomatic or the disease may be stable at the time of diagnosis; in this case, treatment with alkylating agents is withheld. Although bone marrow examination is not required to establish the diagnosis, examination reveals a hypercellular marrow with morphologically mature lymphocytes.

Myeloproliferative Disorders. The myeloproliferative disorders, a form of chronic leukemia, are a group of syndromes characterized by abnormal proliferation of bone marrow cell lines, which all arise from a common pluripotential stem cell. These stem cells produce the progenitor erythroid, granulocytic, monocytic, and megakaryocytic cell lines. The myeloproliferative syndromes include polycythemia vera, primary myelofibrosis with myeloid metaplasia, essential thrombocythemia, and chronic myelogenous leukemia. All of these disorders result in new clones that have a proliferative advantage over the normal marrow cells, which they gradually replace, and all have genetic instability, which predisposes to the development of an acute leukemia. The probability of progression to acute leukemia is greatest in chronic myelogenous leukemia (*i.e.,* chronic myelogenous leukemia in blast crisis).[29]

The diagnostic features of chronic myelogenous leukemia are the Philadelphia chromosome marker (a translocation between chromosomes 9 and 22) and decreased leukocyte alkaline phosphatase activity in circulating granulocytes. Chronic myelogenous leukemia in blast crisis represents 20% of acute leukemias and usually occurs in the fourth decade of life. Histopathologically, the bone marrow shows granulocytic hyperplasia with marked hypercellularity, an increased myeloid to erythroid cell ratio, and variable fibrosis.[28,30] Splenomegaly, which is sometimes massive, is found in nearly all cases. Chemotherapy does not increase survival time in chronic myelogenous leukemia, and induction of remission is not possible without bone marrow transplantation.

Splenomegaly, a leukoerythroblastic peripheral smear, and fibrotic marrow with occasional osteosclerosis characterize agnogenic myeloid metaplasia with primary myelofibrosis.[31] The marrow fibrosis commonly results in a dry aspirate. Bone marrow biopsy demonstrates hypercellularity with an increased number of megakaryocytes, increased fibrosis, and decreased fat content (Fig. 12–19). The cause of the myelofibrosis appears to be related to growth factor and factor IV produced by abnormal megakaryocytes.[32] Vascular clumps of hematopoietic cells are found in distended marrow sinusoids. Increased hemosiderin may be present secondary to repeated blood transfusions to correct the associated anemia or to loss of iron uptake due to lack of effective erythropoiesis.

Secondary causes of myelofibrosis are numerous and include the following:

- metastatic carcinoma
- leukemia
- lymphomas
- tuberculosis
- Gaucher's disease
- Paget's disease
- irradiation
- toxin exposure.[29]

Magnetic Resonance Appearance. Most chronic leukemias tend not to involve yellow marrow areas, and, in adults, are characterized by a moderate to marked decrease in marrow signal in normal red marrow areas on T1-weighted images (Fig. 12–20). Since red to yellow marrow conversion is complete in adults, leukemic involvement is more likely to be identified in the axial skeleton, pelvis, and proximal femurs. In children, leukemic involvement is more likely to be identified in the more peripheral sites of red marrow stores, such as the metaphysis, with diaphysial or epiphysial extension. Marrow cellularity can also be noninvasively assessed with MR imaging.

In the acute phase of chronic leukemia, particularly in chronic myelogenous leukemia patients in blast crisis, there is almost complete replacement of both red and yellow marrow areas. The decreased signal on T1-weighted sequences represents replacement of marrow fat by tumor cells, which have a significantly longer T1 relaxation time. On STIR images, tumor cells appear as white within a black or gray background.

Severe anemias or other marrow invasive processes may have a similar appearance. Myeloma is rather variable, but is generally less symmetrical, more patchy, and irregular in distribution.

In primary myelofibrosis, T1-weighted images show patchy involvement with low signal intensity on T1- and T2-weighted images (Fig. 12–21). T2*-weighted images have been used to evaluate areas of susceptibility where fibrous tissue and hemosiderin have been identified. With STIR techniques, the imaging characteristics of areas of involvement are identical to those of normal hematopoietic marrow—intermediate to mild increased signal intensity. T2*-weighted images, however, do not display typical red marrow imaging characteristics—isointensity with surrounding fat marrow.

Hairy Cell Leukemia. Hairy cell leukemia, representing 2% of all leukemias, is a form of chronic leukemia which evolves from B lymphocytes.[28] It typically occurs in adult males, and classically presents as pancytopenia with splenomegaly. In hairy cell leukemia, the distribution of marrow involvement is irregular and patchy, with a propensity for focal marrow involvement. Focal or extensive involvement with reticulin limits productive marrow aspirations. Bone core biopsy is the definitive diagnostic procedure, and reveals mononuclear cells in clusters or sheets within a fine reticulin mesh in a patchy or diffuse pattern. The marrow may be hypercellular or hypocellular (Fig. 12–22).[33] Hairy cells are reactive to tartrate resistant acid phosphatase, which distinguishes hairy cell leukemia from other lymphoproliferative malignancies.[34] Magnetic resonance imaging demonstrates both a patchy, lymphomalike marrow pattern and a second pattern with a diffuse marrow infiltrate that resembles the distribution of chronic myelogenous leukemia (Fig. 12–23).[35]

Bone Marrow Transplantation

Over the past ten years, therapy for patients with hematologic malignancies has become progressively more

(text continues on page 983)

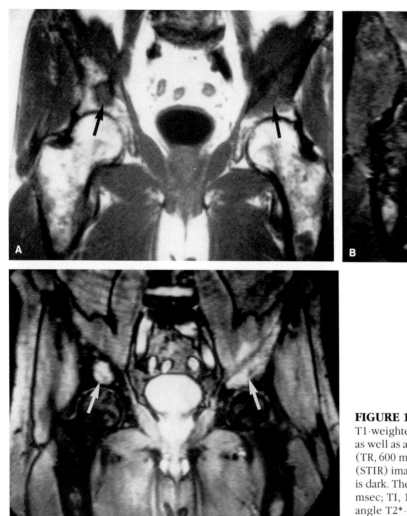

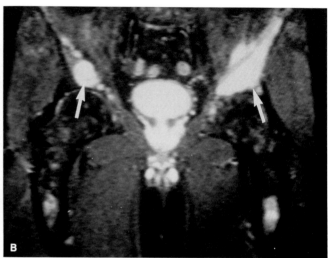

FIGURE 12–15. Recurrent acute myelocytic leukemia. (**A**) A T1-weighted spin-echo image shows a dark focal recurrent tumor as well as a dark, diffuse background of marrow fibrosis (*arrows*). (TR, 600 msec; TE, 30 msec.) (**B**) On a short TI inversion recovery (STIR) image, the tumor (*arrows*) is hyperintense, and the fibrosis is dark. Therefore, these sequences are complementary. (TR, 1400 msec; TI, 140 msec; TE, 40 msec.) (**C**) Although the limited flip angle T2*-weighted image appears similar to the STIR image, it has lower marrow and soft-tissue contrast (*arrows*). (TR, 400 msec; TE, 20 msec; flip angle, 25°.)

FIGURE 12–16. Extensive myelofibrosis occurred after chemotherapy for acute leukemia. The bone marrow exhibits extensive marrow fibrosis, which appears as spindled cells with an abundant collagen matrix (*solid straight arrow*) filling the marrow space between the trabecular bone (*curved arrow*). Osteoblastic activity can also be seen (*open arrows*). (H & E stain; original magnification ×100.)

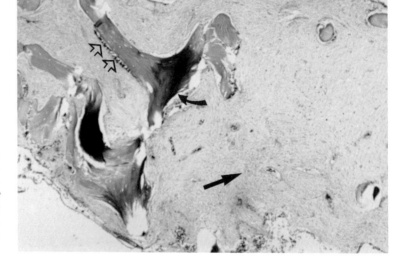

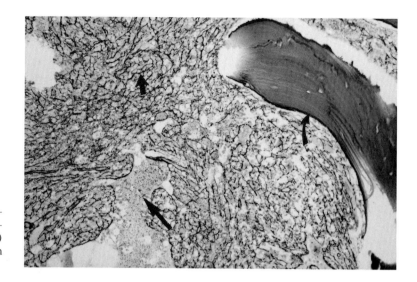

FIGURE 12–17. In myelofibrosis, bone marrow displays abundant reticulin fibers (*short arrow*). Vascular sinusoids (*long arrow*) and trabecular bone (*curved arrow*) can be seen. (Silver reticulin stain; original magnification ×150.)

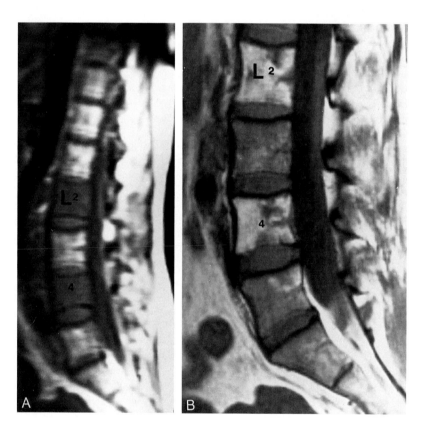

FIGURE 12–18. Marrow response to chemotherapy. T1-weighted images of the lumbar spine (**A**) prechemotherapy and (**B**) postchemotherapy for metastatic colonic carcinoma. Metastatic disease demonstrates low signal intensity on L2 and L4 prior to chemotherapy, and high signal intensity fatty replacement after chemotherapy. Adjacent uninvolved vertebral bodies also show a flip-flop in signal intensity as the red marrow is activated.

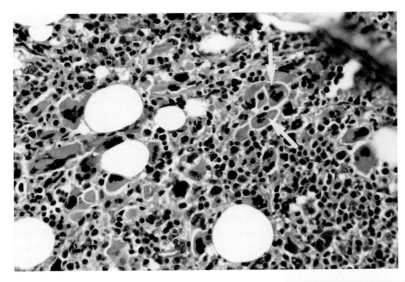

FIGURE 12–19. In myeloproliferative disorder (*i.e.,* the cellular phase of agnogenic myeloid metaplasia with primary myelofibrosis), the bone marrow is hypercellular, with an 85:15 cell-to-fat ratio. Abnormal megakaryocytes are increased in number and tend to cluster (*arrows*). Megakaryocytes secrete factors responsible for the extensive marrow fibrosis seen in late stages of the disease. (H & E stain; original magnification ×400.)

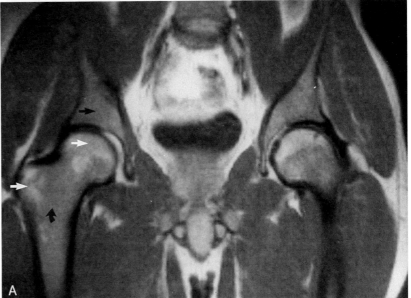

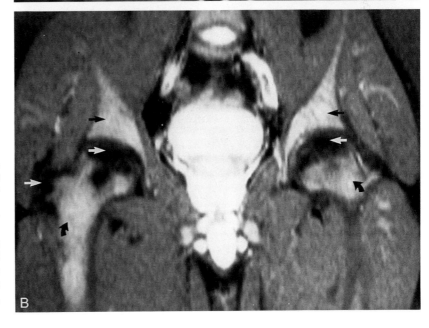

FIGURE 12–20. In chronic myelogenous leukemia, diffuse marrow involvement infiltrates regions of previous red marrow stores in the femurs (*curved arrows*) and acetabulum (*straight black arrows*) and demonstrates (**A**) low signal intensity on a T1-weighted image and (**B**) high signal intensity on a corresponding short TI inversion recovery (STIR) image. Spared sites of yellow marrow (*i.e.,* greater trochanter, femoral epiphysis) demonstrate high signal intensity on the T1-weighted image and low signal intensity (*i.e.,* nulled fat signal) on the STIR sequence (*white arrows*). (A: TR, 600 msec; TE, 20 msec; B: TR, 1400 msec; TI, 125 msec; TE, 40 msec.)

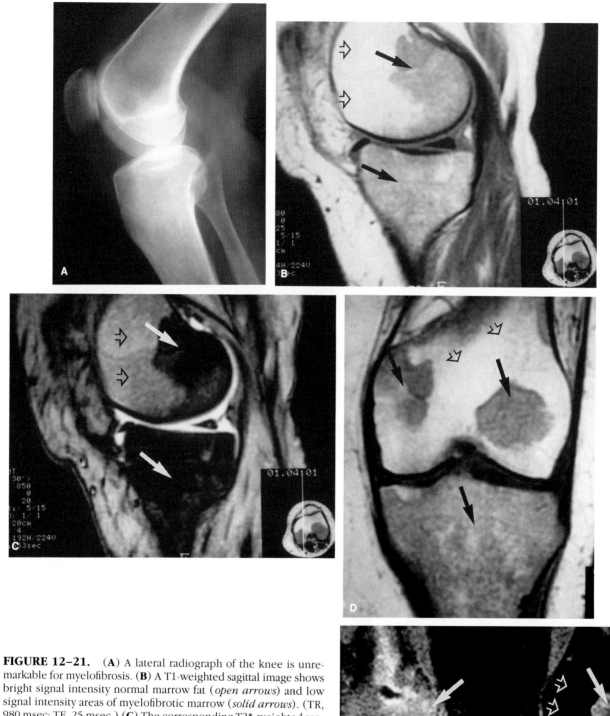

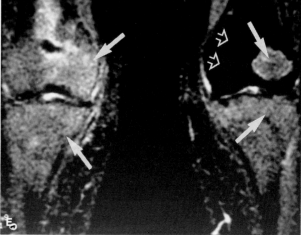

FIGURE 12–21. (**A**) A lateral radiograph of the knee is unremarkable for myelofibrosis. (**B**) A T1-weighted sagittal image shows bright signal intensity normal marrow fat (*open arrows*) and low signal intensity areas of myelofibrotic marrow (*solid arrows*). (TR, 980 msec; TE, 25 msec.) (**C**) The corresponding T2*-weighted sagittal image shows intermediate signal intensity normal marrow fat (*open arrows*) and dark signal intensity myelofibrosis (*solid arrows*). The susceptibility of fibrous tissue and hemosiderin contributes to the extreme dark marrow signal intensity. (TR, 850 msec; TE, 20 msec; flip angle, 30°.) Coronal (**D**) T1-weighted and (**E**) short TI inversion recovery (STIR) images characterize the patchy involvement of myelofibrosis (*solid arrows*) in contrast to normal marrow fat (*open arrows*). Marrow fat is black on the STIR image, whereas myelofibrosis displays intermediate signal intensity resembling red marrow. This may be secondary to compensatory hematopoiesis. (D: TR, 980 msec; TE, 25 msec; E: TR, 1500 msec; TI, 100 msec; TE, 40 msec.)

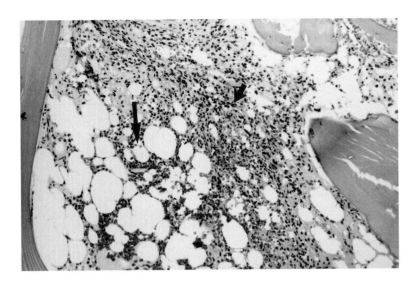

FIGURE 12–22. Bone marrow cellularity is low (*i.e.,* 40:60 cell-to-fat ratio) in hairy cell leukemia. Mononuclear cells (*short arrow*) enveloped in reticulin form solid areas and infiltrate between the remaining fat cells (*large arrow*). (H & E stain; original magnification ×100.)

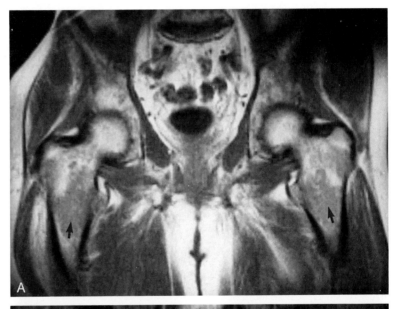

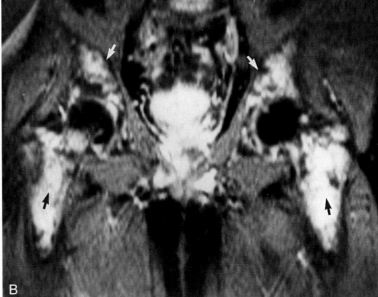

FIGURE 12–23. The patchy pattern of marrow involvement in hairy cell leukemia mimics the appearance of lymphoma. Leukemic infiltration demonstrates (**A**) low signal intensity (*black arrows*) on a T1-weighted image and (**B**) high signal intensity (*all arrows*) on a short TI inversion recovery sequence. (A: TR, 600 msec; TE, 20 msec; B: TR, 1400 msec; TI, 125 msec; TE, 40 msec.)

intensive. Such intensive therapy encompasses the use of maximum dosage chemotherapy and multiagent regimens. However, maximally intensive multiagent chemotherapeutic regimens result in significant side effects, notably lethal bone marrow cytotoxicity. Bone marrow transplantation is an attempt to circumvent this side effect by providing stem cells to repopulate normal marrow elements. Marrow available for transplantation is of three types, syngeneic (*i.e.,* from an identical twin), allogeneic (*i.e.,* from an HLA matched donor), and autologous (*i.e.,* from the patient).[36] In addition to leukemia treatment, autologous bone marrow transplantation has been implemented in therapy of ovarian tumors, testicular tumors, breast cancers, small cell carcinoma of the lung, Hodgkin's disease, and non-Hodgkin's lymphoma. Preliminary results have been encouraging, and increased use of bone marrow transplantation, in conjunction with aggressive chemotherapy, is anticipated.[37]

Procedure. Prior to bone marrow transplantation, the patient is treated with standard chemotherapy, which ideally induces a state of remission. To eradicate any residual neoplastic cells, the patient then undergoes intensive high-dose chemotherapy, either alone or in combination with total-body irradiation. This also eradicates the patient's immune system, preventing graft resistance in the case of an allogeneic transplantation. After ablation therapy, patients receive donor marrow by intravenous therapy. Histopathologic evidence of stem cell engraftment in the bone marrow is first seen one or two weeks after transplantation as small clusters of erythroid cells. Obvious engraftment is usually seen by three weeks. Blood counts start to rise between 4 and 8 weeks after transplantation. In the case of autologous bone marrow transplantation, the patient's own marrow is harvested after the induction of a remission state and cryopreserved for later infusion. Various ex vitro techniques are available, and the ability to purge autologous marrow of contaminating neoplastic cells prior to reinfusion is continuously being improved.[36]

Graft-*versus*-Host Disease. Graft-*versus*-host disease, one of the major complications of marrow transplantation, may occur with allogeneic HLA-matched marrow. It occurs when there is an immunologic reaction by the engrafted lymphoid cells against the tissues of the host, particularly the skin, gastrointestinal tract, and liver.[38] The possibility of graft-*versus*-host disease increases with patient age, which usually limits this form of marrow transplant to patients younger than 40 years of age.

Magnetic Resonance Appearance. Bone marrow transplantation produces characteristic changes on MR

studies of vertebral bone marrow.[39] Magnetic resonance changes in the spine have been identified as early as three weeks post-transplantation. On T1-weighted images, there is a peripheral zone of intermediate signal intensity that represents repopulated hematopoietic cells and a central zone of high signal intensity fatty marrow. Short TI inversion recovery images show a reciprocal change, with increased signal intensity in the peripheral zone of hematopoietic cells, and decreased signal intensity in the central zone, because signal from fat is nulled. The alternating zones form a characteristic band pattern. Loss of this band may signify relapse, as a homogeneous area of decreased signal intensity replaces the vertebral body. Repopulation of hematopoietic marrow follows vascular sinusoid pathways, which enter the periphery of the vertebral body; this produces the peripheral region of intermediate signal intensity. These sinusoids drain into the basivertebral vein located in the central portion of the vertebral body. On STIR images used to evaluate repopulated marrow in the spine and pelvis after ablation therapy and bone marrow transplant, it is possible to differentiate red marrow from recurrent tumor (Fig. 12–24).

In patients with chronic myelogenous leukemia, post-transplant increases in marrow signal intensity have been observed in the pelvis and proximal femur, as compared with pretreatment T1-weighted images.[15] The intensity of signal, however, is less than that seen in disease-free marrow. Hypoplastic fatty marrow may be seen prior to hematopoietic repopulation (Fig. 12–25).

Malignant Lymphoma

Lymphomas are neoplastic growths of lymphoid cells that normally reside in primary lymphoid tissue such as lymph nodes. The two major types of lymphomas are Hodgkin's disease and non-Hodgkin's lymphomas. Bone marrow examination is an important component of the staging process for patients with malignant lymphoma. Demonstration of marrow involvement may advance the stage of disease and contraindicate the use of nodal radiotherapy. After treatment, marrow study is crucial in following the patient for evidence of therapeutic response or lymphomatous relapse.

Hodgkin's Disease. In its most common presentation, Hodgkin's disease is localized to a single group of lymph nodes (*i.e.,* cervical, cervicoclavicular, mediastinal, paraaortic) and spreads to contiguous lymph nodes by way of lymphatic channels. Only when malignant cells enter the blood via a major lymphatic duct does the disease invade the bone marrow; this occurrence portends a potential fatal outcome. The disease is usually not generalized in the marrow, but presents focally in nodules (Fig. 12–26). On a microscopic level, Hodgkin's lesions in the bone marrow vary from primarily cellular to primarily fibrotic. The unifying histopathologic feature of Hodgkin's disease is the presence of Reed–Sternberg cells, which are large cells with a bilobed nucleus exhibiting prominent nucleoli set in the proper cellular and architectural background (Fig. 12–27). The exact cell of origin in Hodgkin's disease is still under debate.

Although four distinct histologic subtypes of Hodgkin's disease have been identified (*i.e.,* lymphocyte predominant, nodular sclerosis, mixed cellularity, lymphocyte depleted), the prognosis of Hodgkin's disease rests primarily in the clinical and pathologic stage of disease rather than histologic subtype.[40]

Non-Hodgkin's Lymphoma. Malignant lymphomas other than Hodgkin's disease are referred to as non-Hodgkin's lymphoma. Within this classification is a diverse group of diseases that span various morphologic and immunologic types. They range from low-grade indolent processes to highly aggressive lesions which, if left untreated, are rapidly fatal. The various types of non-Hodgkin's lymphoma differ in their response to therapy. In contrast to Hodgkin's disease, the prognosis of non-Hodgkin's lymphomas is more directly related to histologic subtype than to the clinical and pathologic stage.

Low-grade non-Hodgkin's lymphoma is compromised predominantly of small cells and may also be called small cleaved cell lymphoma or well-differentiated small lymphocytic cell lymphoma. When initially diagnosed, low-grade non-Hodgkin's lymphoma almost always involves widespread lymph nodes at multiple sites in an asymmetrical distribution above and below the diaphragm. In 50% of cases, the bone marrow is affected at the time of diagnosis. On a microscopic level, small cleaved cell lymphomas may be diffuse, or may tend to form nodules in a peritrabecular location. Involvement of the spleen is usually in the form of small miliary nodules centered in the white pulp zones.[41]

High-grade non-Hodgkin's lymphoma (*i.e.,* large cell lymphoma) may be formally designated as histiocytic or reticulum cell, immunoblastic, lymphoblastic, Burkitt's, or non-Burkitt's lymphoma. High-grade non-Hodgkin's lymphoma represents the most heterogeneous type of lymphoma morphologically and immunologically. It is the most common primary lymphoma arising in bone, and the type that occurs most often in acquired immunodeficiency syndrome (AIDS) (Fig. 12–28). In contrast to the low-grade (*i.e.,* small cleaved cell) lymphoma, microscopic marrow involvement in large cell lymphoma can be focal or widespread, but there is no peritrabecular bony preference.

A rapidly growing mass at a single nodal or extranodal site is the typical clinical presentation in large cell lymphoma (Fig. 12–29). Liver and spleen involvement, not common at the time of diagnosis, consists of large masses,

as opposed to the small miliary nodules typical of low-grade lymphomas. Large cell lymphomas are rapidly fatal if not treated. However, with current aggressive multi-agent chemotherapy, complete remission can be achieved in 60% to 80% of patients. In contrast, low-grade lymphoma is relatively resistant to chemotherapy, although it exhibits an indolent clinical course.[41]

Lymphoblastic Lymphoma. Lymphoblastic lymphoma, also a high-grade lymphoma, is usually diffuse in the bone marrow. It commonly occurs in adolescence and represents approximately one-third of childhood non-Hodgkin's lymphomas. It often progresses to extensive, diffuse bone marrow involvement and frank leukemia. The presentation is usually mediastinal.

Burkitt's Lymphoma. Burkitt's lymphoma is another diffuse, high-grade lymphoma (Fig. 12–30). In nonendemic areas such as the United States, it usually occurs in older children and presents as a rapidly growing abdominal mass with marrow involvement, malignant pleural effusions, and ascites.

Magnetic Resonance Findings. Unlike leukemia, lymphoma tends to form nodules or marrow tumors (Fig. 12–31),[42,43] although it may at times be diffuse and simulate leukemia on MR imaging (Fig. 12–32).[44] When diffuse, it can usually be detected by posterior crest marrow biopsy. Not infrequently, however, sampling error produces a negative marrow biopsy in lymphoma, especially with asymmetric involvement (Figs. 12–33 and 12–34). Bone scanning is also frequently negative, even in lymphoma patients with known marrow involvement.

With MR imaging, marrow involvement can be detected because of the ability to sample a large volume of marrow through imaging. Since detection of marrow tumor in patients with lymphoma affects both staging and treatment, this is potentially one of the more important areas for clinical MR imaging of the body. Staging is of particular importance in Hodgkin's disease, because bone marrow involvement portends a potentially fatal outcome and is therefore treated with more aggressive multiagent chemotherapy. Mediastinal tumor is common in the supradiaphragmatic presentation of Hodgkin's disease (Fig. 12–35), and MR can also identify bone marrow involvement not appreciated at the time of diagnosis. An additional benefit of MR imaging, particularly when STIR imaging is used, is that lymph node invasion can also be detected (Figs. 12–36 and 12–37). Although CT is highly accurate for lymph node detection, it is insensitive to marrow involvement in the absence of bone destruction. Focal marrow lymphoma may simulate metastatic disease (Fig. 12–38). In contrast to Hodgkin's disease, non-Hodgkin's lymphoma demonstrates early bone marrow involvement.

(text continues on page 994)

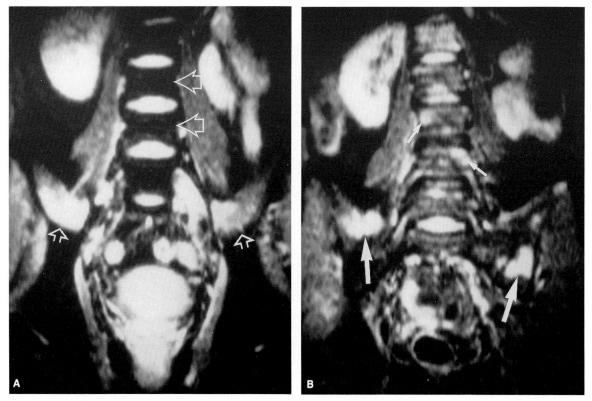

FIGURE 12-24. Recurrent tumor after bone marrow transplantation is seen on coronal short TI inversion recovery images. (**A**) After total body irradiation and bone marrow transplant, there is severe marrow hypoplasia (*i.e.,* dark fatty marrow; *large open arrows*) and biopsy edema (*small open arrows*). (**B**) Nine months later, the marrow has repopulated with hematopoietic cells which demonstrate intermediate signal intensity spotted with hyperintense recurrent tumor (*arrows*). (TR, 1400 msec; TI, 125 msec; TE, 40 msec.)

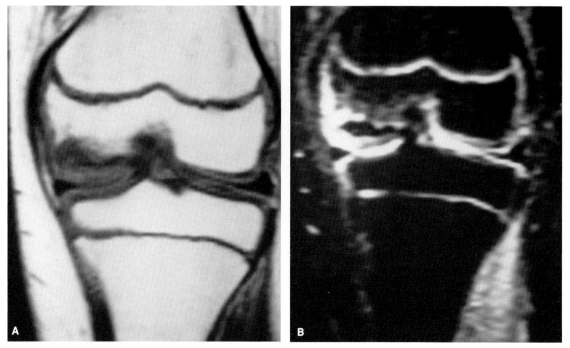

FIGURE 12-25. A 13-year-old girl presented with knee pain after a bone marrow transplant for chronic myelogenous leukemia. Hypoplastic marrow demonstrates (**A**) bright fat marrow signal intensity on coronal T1-weighted images and (**B**) dark fat marrow signal intensity on short TI inversion recovery images in the metaphyseal regions of the femur and tibia. A focus of symptomatic osteonecrosis can be identified in the medial femoral condyle (*arrow*). (A: TR, 600 msec; TE, 30 msec; B: TR, 1400 msec; TI, 125 msec; TE, 40 msec.)

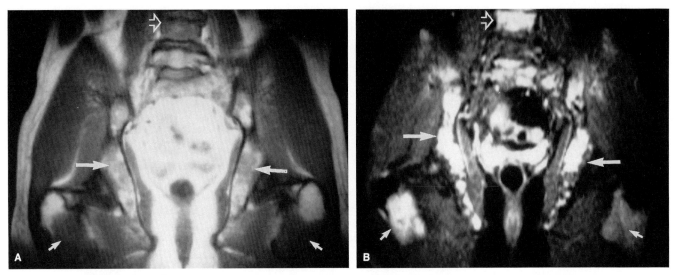

FIGURE 12–26. Severe patchy marrow involvement is present in the nodular presentation of Hodgkin's disease, which resembles hairy cell leukemia. Coronal (**A**) T1-weighted and (**B**) short TI inversion recovery images show vertebral body involvement (*open arrow*), iliac crest tumor (*large solid arrow*), and proximal femur tumor (*small solid arrow*). (A: TR, 600 msec; TE, 30 msec; B: TR, 1400 msec; TI, 140 msec; TE, 40 msec.)

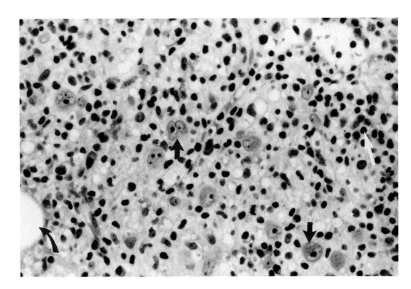

FIGURE 12–27. High magnification of bone marrow illustrates the Hodgkin's cells (*straight black arrows*) scattered among a fibrocellular background. The smaller cells consist of a polymorphous population of lymphocytes, plasma cells, and histiocytes (*white arrow*). Fat cells (*curved black arrow*) are decreased in the areas of Hodgkin's involvement. (H & E stain; original magnification ×400.)

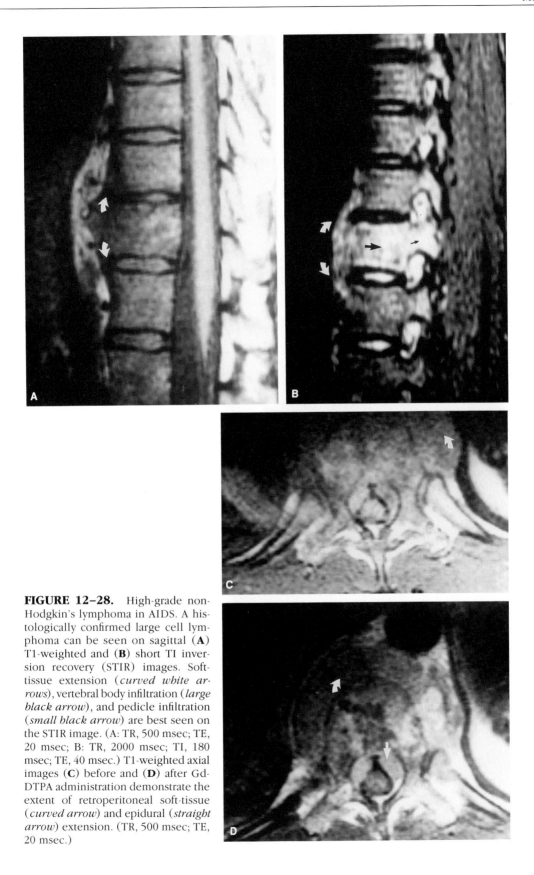

FIGURE 12–28. High-grade non-Hodgkin's lymphoma in AIDS. A histologically confirmed large cell lymphoma can be seen on sagittal (**A**) T1-weighted and (**B**) short TI inversion recovery (STIR) images. Soft-tissue extension (*curved white arrows*), vertebral body infiltration (*large black arrow*), and pedicle infiltration (*small black arrow*) are best seen on the STIR image. (A: TR, 500 msec; TE, 20 msec; B: TR, 2000 msec; TI, 180 msec; TE, 40 msec.) T1-weighted axial images (**C**) before and (**D**) after Gd-DTPA administration demonstrate the extent of retroperitoneal soft-tissue (*curved arrow*) and epidural (*straight arrow*) extension. (TR, 500 msec; TE, 20 msec.)

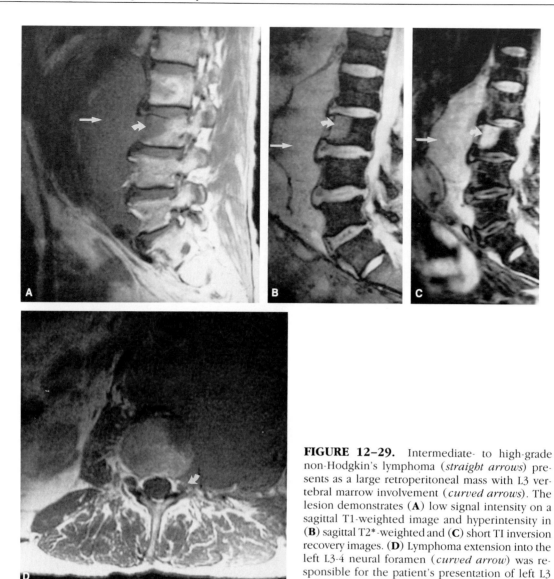

FIGURE 12–29. Intermediate- to high-grade non-Hodgkin's lymphoma (*straight arrows*) presents as a large retroperitoneal mass with L3 vertebral marrow involvement (*curved arrows*). The lesion demonstrates (**A**) low signal intensity on a sagittal T1-weighted image and hyperintensity in (**B**) sagittal T2*-weighted and (**C**) short TI inversion recovery images. (**D**) Lymphoma extension into the left L3-4 neural foramen (*curved arrow*) was responsible for the patient's presentation of left L3 radiculopathy.

FIGURE 12–30. High magnification of bone marrow that has been extensively replaced by a monotonous population of round immature cells displaying the cytologic features of Burkitt's high-grade lymphoma. There is granular individual cell necrosis (*arrow*) between the cells. (H & E stain; original magnification ×400.)

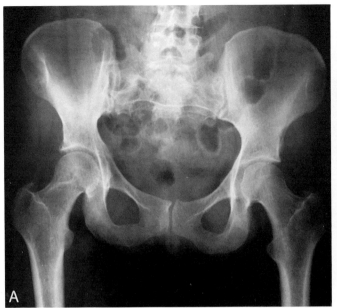

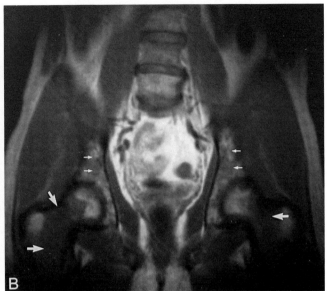

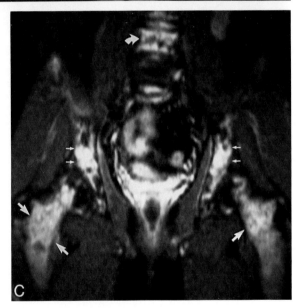

FIGURE 12–31. (**A**) An anteroposterior radiograph of the pelvis is negative for nodular pattern lymphoma. (**B**) A T1-weighted coronal image shows nonspecific low signal intensity proximal femurs (*large arrows*) and acetabuli (*small arrows*). The fatty marrow of the epiphysis and greater trochanter is spared. (TR, 600 msec; TE, 20 msec.) (**C**) A short TI inversion recovery image shows patchy nodularity of lymphomatous marrow involvement, which demonstrates high signal intensity in the proximal femurs (*large arrows*), acetabulum (*small arrows*), and L4 vertebral body (*curved arrow*). The spared yellow marrow of the greater trochanter and femoral epiphysis appears black. (TR, 1400 msec; TI, 125 msec; TE, 40 msec.)

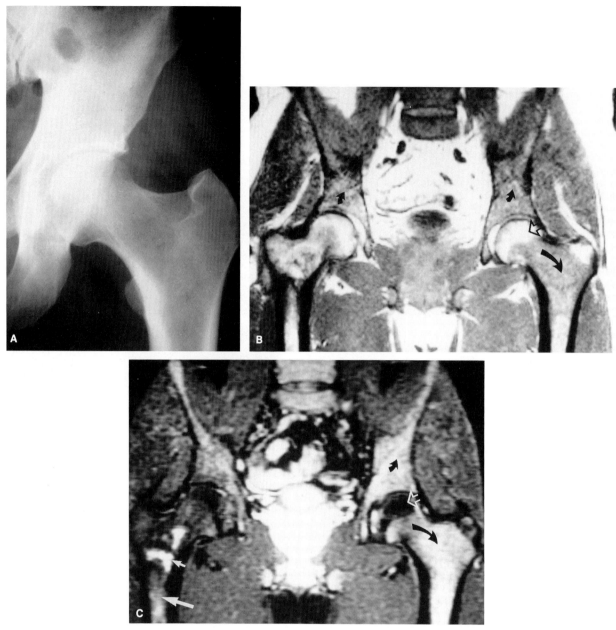

FIGURE 12–32. (**A**) An anteroposterior radiograph of the left femur and hip is negative for low-grade non-Hodgkin's lymphoma. (**B**) On a T1-weighted coronal image, diffuse distribution of low signal intensity infiltration, or replacement of normal marrow with histologically proven well-differentiated small lymphocytic cell lymphoma, can be seen. Acetabular (*small curved arrow*) and femoral (*large curved arrow*) sites are shown. Distribution of the tumor corresponds to adult sites of anatomic red marrow. Yellow marrow locations in the femoral head (*open arrow*) and greater trochanter are not involved. The status of the right femur is difficult to assess postradiation. (**C**) On a coronal short TI inversion recovery image, dark signal intensity postradiation fatty marrow is seen with recurrent tumor (*large solid white arrow*) and postbiopsy fluid (*small solid white arrow*) in the right femur. Hyperintense left acetabular (*small curved arrow*) and femoral (*large curved arrow*) infiltrations are shown on either side of normal femoral head fat marrow (*open arrow*).

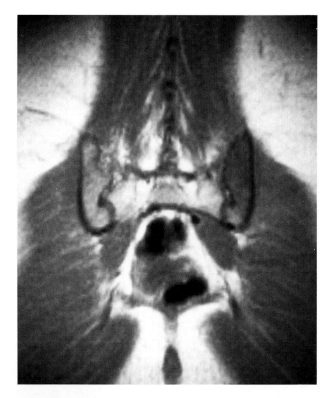

FIGURE 12–33. Characteristic asymmetric involvement of lymphoma is shown as a low signal intensity infiltration in the left posterior iliac bone on a T1-weighted coronal image. (TR, 600 msec; TE, 20 msec.)

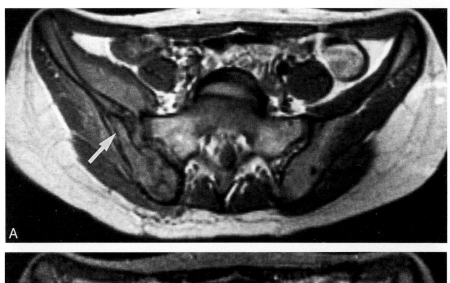

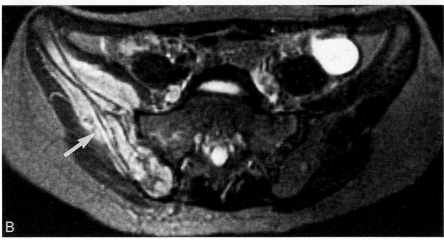

FIGURE 12–34. (**A**) An asymmetric pattern of low signal intensity lymphoma involving the right ilium (*arrow*) is seen on an intermediate-weighted image. (TR, 2000 msec; TE, 20 msec.) (**B**) On a T2-weighted image, the lesion demonstrates high signal intensity (*arrow*). (TR, 2000 msec; TE, 60 msec.)

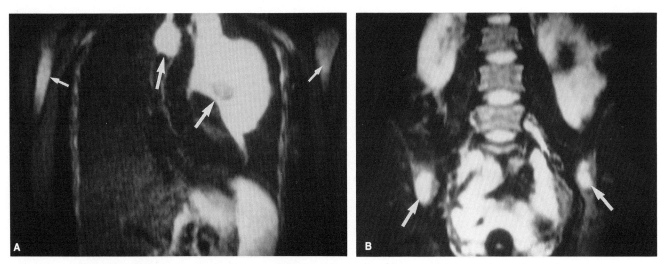

FIGURE 12–35. Coronal short TI inversion recovery images in Hodgkin's and Gaucher's disease show (**A**) a large mediastinal mass (*large arrows*) and Gaucher's marrow signal abnormality (*small arrows*) in the humeri and (**B**) focally hyperintense infiltration in nonsampled marrow with Hodgkin's disease. (TR, 400 msec; TI, 140 msec; TE, 40 msec.)

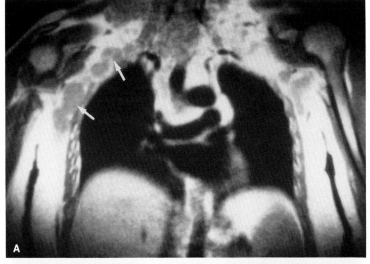

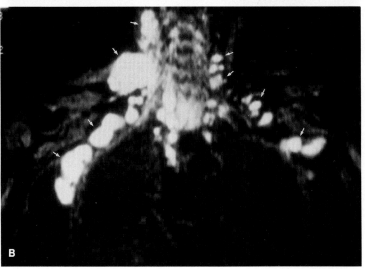

FIGURE 12–36. A 51-year-old woman with aggressive non-Hodgkin's lymphoma (*arrows*). Coronal (**A**) T1-weighted images are not as sensitive for detection as (**B**) short TI inversion recovery images. Nodes and marrow lesions as small as 4 mm can be detected due to their high signal intensity. This patient's marrow is uninvolved. (A: TR, 600 msec; TE, 30 msec; B: TR, 1400 msec; TI, 140 msec; TE, 40 msec.)

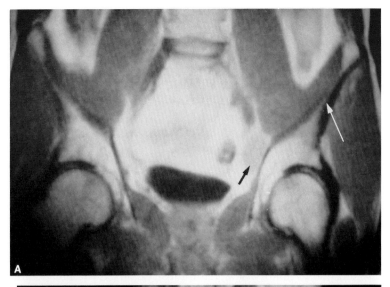

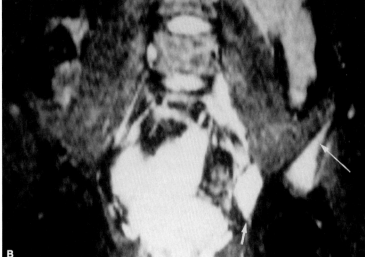

FIGURE 12–37. Nodular large cell lymphoma with negative posterior iliac crest biopsy shows left iliac marrow involvement (*long arrows*) and an enlarged node (*short arrows*) on (**A**) coronal T1-weighted and (**B**) short TI inversion recovery (STIR) images. The marrow tumor and node are hyperintense on the STIR image. The node and marrow lesions are resolved in follow-up MR after chemotherapy.

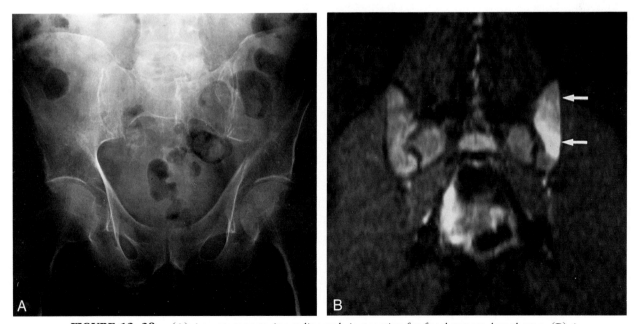

FIGURE 12–38. (**A**) An anteroposterior radiograph is negative for focal pattern lymphoma. (**B**) A short TI inversion recovery sequence shows a high signal intensity lymphoma with an asymmetric pattern of marrow involvement (*arrows*) in the posterior ilium. (TR, 1400 msec; TI, 125 msec; TE, 40 msec.)

The AIDS-related lymphomas, which are high-grade and of B-cell origin, frequently demonstrate both marrow dissemination and soft-tissue disease. Short TI inversion recovery contrast is most effective in characterizing these sites of tumor involvement (see Fig. 12–28). Magnetic resonance provides better detail than CT in imaging soft-tissue pathology (Fig. 12–39).

Changes in lumbar vertebral bone marrow have also been characterized in MR scans on patients receiving radiation therapy for Hodgkin's disease.[45,46] In response to treatment with 1500 to 5000 rads, increased signal intensity can be detected on STIR images within two weeks. Magnetic resonance changes are thought to reflect marrow edema and necrosis. On T1-weighted images, increased heterogeneity of signal intensity, caused by the predominance of high signal intensity fat, can be identified three to six weeks postradiation. Late marrow changes, including fatty marrow replacement, occur six weeks to fourteen months after radiation therapy. On MR scans, these changes are seen as either homogeneous fatty marrow replacement of the vertebral body or as peripheral hematopoietic intermediate signal intensity marrow adjacent to a central zone of fatty marrow (Fig. 12–40). The delineation between irradiated and nonirradiated areas can be sharply defined on STIR images, which show fat with dark or black signal intensity and adjacent hematopoietic marrow with intermediate signal intensity. On T1-weighted images, the postradiation identification of low signal intensity vertebral body marrow, especially in the presence of fat marrow signal intensity seen at other levels, is consistent with recurrent disease (Fig. 12–41). T1-weighted and STIR images are most sensitive in identifying recurrent disease in or adjacent to the field of radiation (Fig. 12–42). Coronal T1-weighted and STIR images are also useful in evaluating internal changes in tumor size and recurrent disease in Hodgkin's disease and non-Hodgkin's lymphoma after whole body irradiation and bone marrow transplantation (Fig. 12–43). Monoclonal antibodies tagged to a radioisotope or chemotherapeutic agent have also been used in lymphoma treatment (Fig. 12–44). On STIR images, red marrow stores can be differentiated from lymphoma by the significantly increased signal intensity in lymphomatous infiltration.

Histiocytic Proliferative Disorders

Histiocytosis X. Three related diseases, eosinophilic granuloma, Letterer-Siwe disease, and Hand-Schuller-Christian disease, are included under the designation histiocytosis X. The three differ with respect to the extent of organ involvement and the prognosis. These diseases currently represent neoplasia of a special form of histiocyte known as the Langerhans cell.

The unifocal bone lesion (*i.e.,* eosinophilic granuloma) is a benign disorder that typically occurs in children and young adults.[47] In some cases, spontaneous healing and fibrosis occur within a year or two of presentation. Other cases require curettage or local irradiation. Magnetic resonance findings in eosinophilic granuloma are characterized by nonaggressive lesions that demonstrate low signal intensity on T1-weighted images and increased signal intensity on T2-weighted images (Fig. 12–45). Long-bone involvement, typically diaphyseal, may involve the metaphysis or extension to the physeal plate. There may be localized bone expansion with a low signal intensity sclerotic peripheral border. The lesions may be associated with perilesional or peritumoral edema. In the vertebral body, eosinophilic granuloma may present as a vertebral plana with diffuse infiltration of the vertebral body. Typical characteristics on T1- and T2-weighted images, however, are nonspecific for the diagnosis of eosinophilic granuloma. Age, in addition to location and morphology of signal intensity, are important in determining a differential diagnosis.

The multifocal form of the disease is known as Hand-Schuller-Christian disease, and it usually presents in patients younger than 5 years of age. Systemic symptomatology is common; the classic triad of calvarial bone lesions, exophthalmos, and diabetes insipidus due to posterior pituitary or hypothalamic involvement are diagnostic for Hand-Schuller-Christian disease.

The most aggressive form of histiocytosis X is Letterer-Siwe disease, which classically affects infants and young children. It involves virtually all the organs of the body, including bone marrow. Current chemotherapy has improved the prognosis for this disease; a 40% to 50% 5-year survival rate has been attained.[48]

Myeloma

Multiple myeloma, the most common primary neoplasm of bone, is primarily a disease of the elderly and is caused by the uncontrolled proliferation of malignant plasma cells within the marrow.[49] The neoplastic plasma cells secrete nonfunctional monoclonal immunoglobulins; these immunoglobulins can be measured in the serum to aid in the diagnosis. The ability of myeloma to destroy the skeleton, resulting in punched-out osteolytic lesions or diffuse osteopenia, is attributed to the production of an osteoclastic stimulating factor by the neoplastic plasma cells.[49,50] Amyloidosis may occasionally complicate myeloma.

The two variants of myeloma are the solitary bone plasmocytoma and extramedullary plasmocytoma. Solitary lesions, or plasmacytomas, are more common in young or middle-aged adults, and may be accompanied by back pain and cord compression.

Nuclear scintigraphy using technetium is limited in

the detection of multiple myeloma. Plain film radiography requires significant medullary bone involvement before osteoporosis or lytic lesions can be detected.

Magnetic Resonance Appearance. Involvement of the marrow is characteristically multifocal; this is clearly demonstrated in MR scans (Fig. 12–46). The patchy asymmetric process of focal deposits is distinguishable from metastases by signal intensity characteristics and morphology. Multiple myeloma may also present as complete marrow replacement, simulating leukemia. Areas of involvement demonstrate low signal intensity on T1-weighted images and bright signal intensity on T2-weighted, STIR, and Gd-DTPA–enhanced images (Fig. 12–47). Short TI inversion recovery images demonstrate greater lesion contrast than that seen on corresponding conventional T2-weighted images.

Metastatic Disease of the Marrow

In adults, marrow metastases usually result from carcinoma of the prostate (Fig. 12–48), breast (Fig. 12–49), lung (Figs. 12–50 and 12–51), kidney (Fig. 12–52), gastrointestinal tract (Fig. 12–53), and melanoma of the skin (Fig. 12–54). In pediatric patients, the most common primary cancers for metastases to the marrow are neuroblastoma, rhabdomyosarcoma (Fig. 12–55), and Ewing's sarcoma (Fig. 12–56). Invasion of the marrow by metastatic cancer occurs by hematogenous dissemination. The high frequency of metastases to pelvic bones and vertebrae is attributed to the abundant vascular supply afforded by the vertebral venous plexus, which serves as a major venous pathway.[51] Metastatic tumor deposits in the marrow can be accompanied by necrosis, fibrosis, bone destruction (*i.e.,* osteolytic activity) or bone production (*i.e.,* osteoblastic activity; Fig. 12–57).[52]

Magnetic Resonance Appearance. The potential contrast between metastatic tumor and normal adult marrow is high, because almost all metastatic tumors are characterized by long T1 and variably long T2 relaxation times. T1-weighted SE sequences are very useful in this situation. Short TI inversion recovery images have even higher contrast between metastatic tumor and normal or irradiated marrow (Fig. 12–58). The latter has a characteristic appearance on MR scans. The T2 relaxation time of metastatic deposits is often unpredictably variable, and lesions may be difficult to separate from normal fatty marrow. Depending on the degree of T2 prolongation *versus* the amount of blastic bone, the net signal is often variable, heterogeneous, and may even be decreased due to decreased proton density.

Short TI inversion recovery and short TR/TE sequences have replaced the more time-consuming T2-weighted pulse sequences in most cases. If spinal cord or thecal sac impingement is suspected, however, T2-weighted scans are useful, because increased signal in the cerebrospinal fluid (CSF) improves the detection of sac compression. Although STIR sequences also result in bright CSF, spatial resolution is not as good; as the tumor is also of high signal intensity, it may be difficult to distinguish between the tumor and CSF.

Short TI inversion recovery scans are used to screen the axial skeleton for metastatic disease. If this sequence shows no focal area of high signal intensity, the likelihood of microscopic marrow tumor involvement is low. Symptomatic individuals, however, occasionally have an inhomogeneous distribution of red marrow that may simulate metastatic disease, particularly in the proximal femurs. Osteomyelitis or infection may have to be excluded on clinical grounds (Fig. 12–59). Adenopathy or extension across the disc space indicates infection.

Metastatic disease has been successfully detected on MR T1-weighted and STIR images, even when bone scans are negative or equivocal (Figs. 12–60 and 12–61). Magnetic resonance provides an excellent means of assessing soft-tissue involvement, including adenopathy (Fig. 12–62), and Gd-DTPA enhancement is useful in the assessment of pathologic fractures and epidural spread (Fig. 12–63). The morphology of the posterior vertebral body cortex should be evaluated for convexity, a sign associated with metastatic tumor extension. A chronic, benign compression fracture frequently demonstrates fat marrow signal intensity (*i.e.,* bright on T1-weighted images, dark on STIR images; Fig. 12–64). In more acute compression fractures, subchondral reaction often parallels the endplate without the more central or heterogeneous involvement seen in metastatic disease. Disease progression (Fig. 12–65) and peritumoral reaction (Fig. 12–66) can be monitored on baseline or serial MR studies.

Lipid Storage Diseases

Gaucher's Disease

Gaucher's disease is a metabolic storage disorder caused by deficient activity of glucocerebrosidase, a lysosomal enzyme. There are three phenotypic forms of Gaucher's disease. Type I, the common adult form, spares the central nervous system but progressively involves the osseous system and viscera. Types II and III are much rarer childhood forms that have neurological manifestations. The progressive histiocytic proliferation secondary to accumulation of undegraded glycolipids results in displacement of normal hematopoietic cells in the marrow, eventually resulting in peripheral blood cytopenia. Bone erosion may result and precipitate fractures. Rarely, necrosis of bone marrow (*i.e.,* osteonecrosis) is associated with this disorder.[53]

(text continues on page 1017)

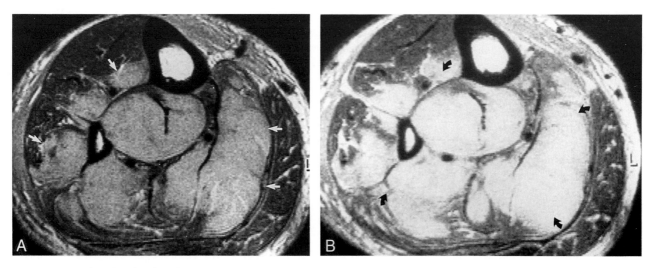

FIGURE 12–39. (**A**) On a T1-weighted axial image, the soft-tissue masses of histiocytic lymphoma (*arrows*) demonstrate intermediate signal intensity. (TR, 1000 msec; TE, 40 msec.) (**B**) On a T2-weighted sequence, the lesions demonstrate high signal intensity. (TR, 2000 msec; TE, 80 msec.)

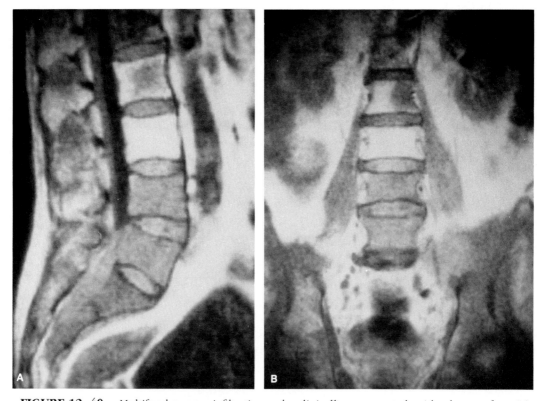

FIGURE 12–40. Multifocal marrow infiltration and a clinically unsuspected epidural tumor from L5 to S2 are detected with MR. Radiation induced marrow changes are imaged with vertebral fat marrow signal intensity on (**A**) T1-weighted sagittal and (**B**) coronal images, and with (**C**) bright signal intensity on a coronal short TI inversion recovery image.

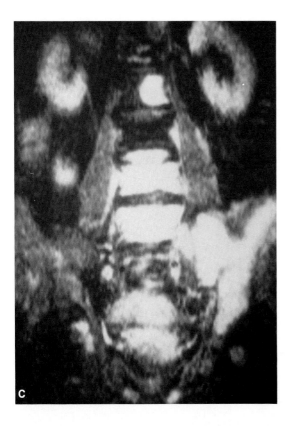

FIGURE 12–40. *(Continued)*

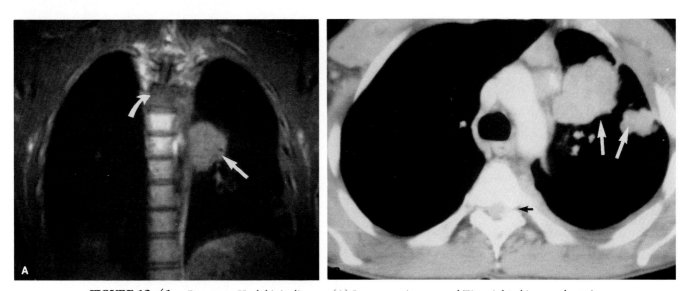

FIGURE 12–41. Recurrent Hodgkin's disease. (**A**) In a screening coronal T1-weighted image, thoracic vertebral marrow disease is identified in an area of previous irradiation (*curved arrow*). Left hilar adenopathy is also seen (*straight arrow*). (TR, 500 msec; TE, 30 msec.) (**B**) The corresponding CT scan shows hilar involvement (*white arrows*) with equivocal epidural tumor (*black arrow*). T1-weighted (**C**) sagittal and (**D**) axial images image marrow (*arrow*) and extensive epidural (*arrow*) tumor more accurately than the corresponding CT scans. (TR, 600 msec; TE, 30 msec.) *(continued)*

FIGURE 12–41. *(Continued)*

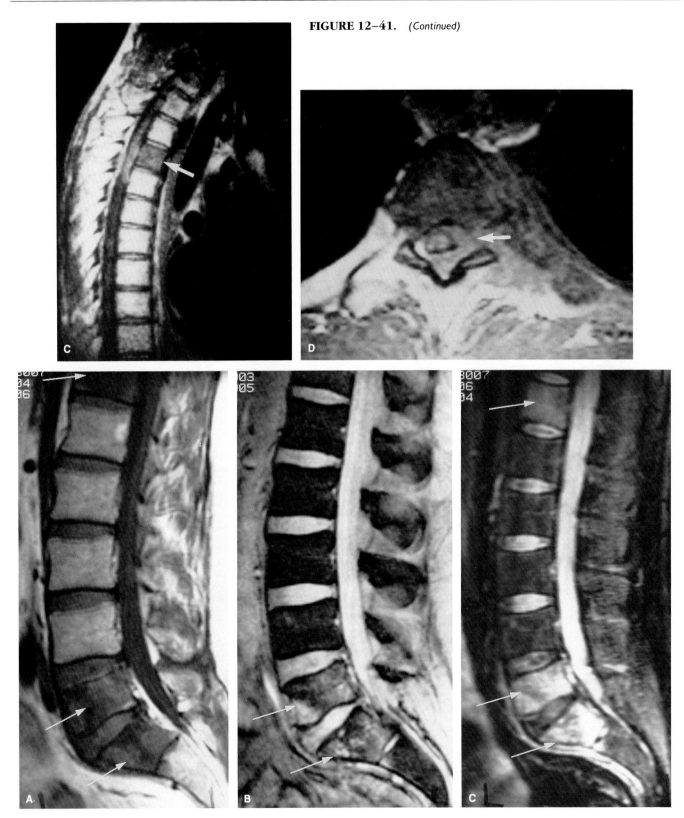

FIGURE 12–42. Hodgkin's disease. Vertebral body marrow infiltration (*arrows*) in the lumbar and lower thoracic spine is seen on (**A**) T1-weighted, (**B**) T2*-weighted and (**C**) short TI inversion recovery images. Marrow involvement was clinically unsuspected in this patient, whose status was post subtotal nodal radiation. Normally, the risk for marrow involvement is higher in patients with an advanced stage of disease than it is at the time of diagnosis. (A: TR, 600 msec; TE, 20 msec; B: TR, 400 msec; TE, 15 msec; flip angle, 20°; C: TR, 200 msec; TI, 160 msec; TE, 40 msec.)

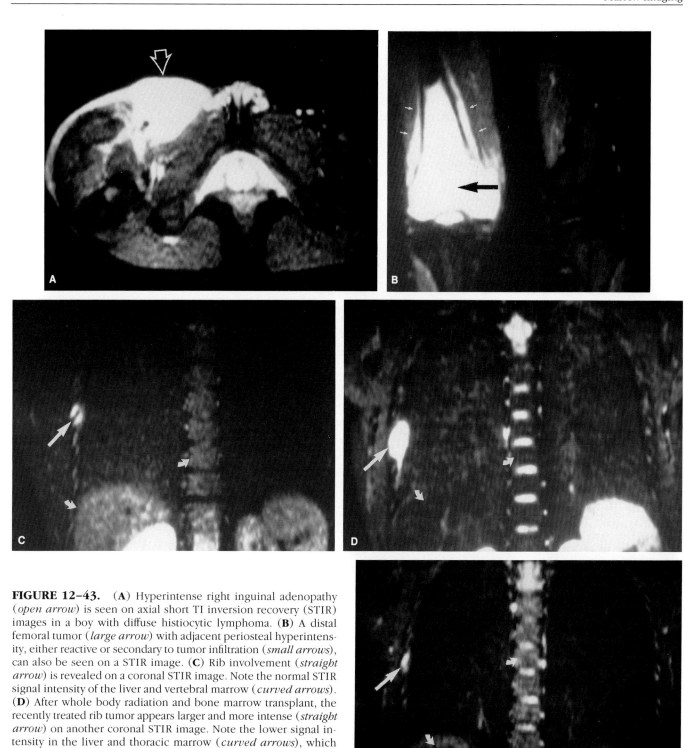

FIGURE 12–43. (**A**) Hyperintense right inguinal adenopathy (*open arrow*) is seen on axial short TI inversion recovery (STIR) images in a boy with diffuse histiocytic lymphoma. (**B**) A distal femoral tumor (*large arrow*) with adjacent periosteal hyperintensity, either reactive or secondary to tumor infiltration (*small arrows*), can also be seen on a STIR image. (**C**) Rib involvement (*straight arrow*) is revealed on a coronal STIR image. Note the normal STIR signal intensity of the liver and vertebral marrow (*curved arrows*). (**D**) After whole body radiation and bone marrow transplant, the recently treated rib tumor appears larger and more intense (*straight arrow*) on another coronal STIR image. Note the lower signal intensity in the liver and thoracic marrow (*curved arrows*), which indicates increased fat content. (**E**) Nine months after radiation and bone marrow transplant, residual rib signal intensity (*straight arrow*) is still seen on another coronal STIR image. Such lesions may take 12 months to resolve. Liver and marrow signal intensity have normalized (*curved arrows*).

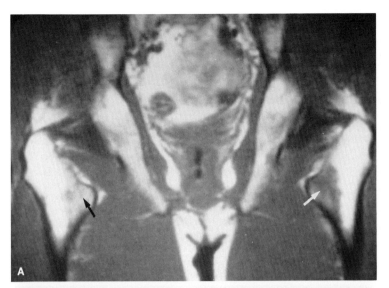

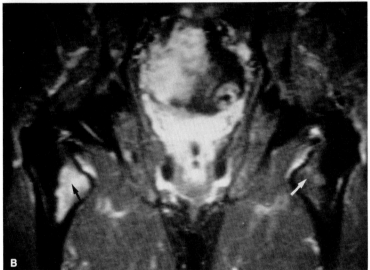

FIGURE 12–44. Non-Hodgkin's lymphoma in a 36-year-old man after monoclonal antibody therapy. (**A**) On a T1-weighted coronal image, a low signal intensity area within the left trochanter simulating tumor (*white arrow*) can be identified. A mild decrease in signal intensity in the right lesser trochanter (*black arrow*) appears less ominous. (**B**) On the corresponding coronal short TI inversion recovery image, a markedly hyperintense tumor is present in the right lesser trochanter (*black arrow*) and a mildly hyperintense normal red marrow signal intensity is seen in the left lesser trochanter (*white arrow*).

FIGURE 12–45. Solitary eosinophilic granuloma of histiocytosis X. (**A**) An anteroposterior radiograph shows thickened periosteal reaction (*arrow*) along the lateral femoral cortex. Bright signal intensity perilesional edema (*large white arrow*) and marrow involvement (*small white arrow*) and low signal intensity thickened medial femoral cortex (*black arrow*) are seen on (**B**) intermediate-weighted and (**C**) T2-weighted images. (TR, 2000 msec; TE, 20, 60 msec.) (**D**) A T1-weighted coronal image of eosinophilic granuloma of histiocytosis X involving the femoral diaphysis and metaphysis shows patchy areas of low signal intensity histiocytic infiltration (*arrows*). (TR, 600 msec; TE, 20 msec.)

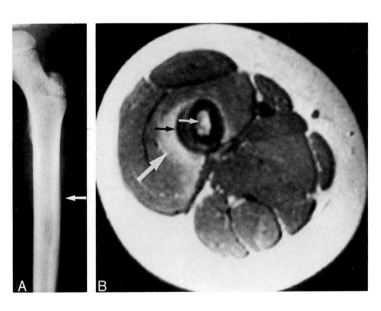

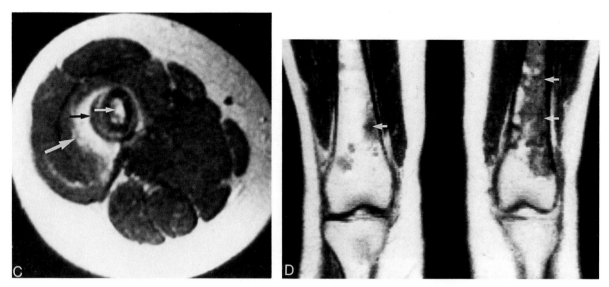

FIGURE 12–45. *(Continued)*

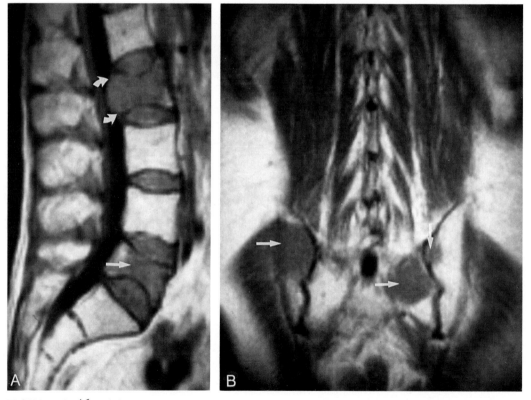

FIGURE 12–46. (**A**) A T1-weighted sagittal image shows multiple low signal intensity foci of myelomatous involvement in the lumbar spine. Collapse of L5 (*straight arrow*) and convexity to the posterior margin of L2 (*curved arrows*) are characteristic of metastatic disease. The corresponding (**B**) T1-weighted and (**C**) short TI inversion recovery (STIR) coronal images in the same patient show deposits of multiple myeloma (*arrows*), which generate increased signal intensity in STIR contrast. (**D**) On a T1-weighted image in a different patient, a diffuse pattern of multiple myeloma (*arrows*) demonstrates low signal intensity replacement of normally bright signal intensity marrow. *(continued)*

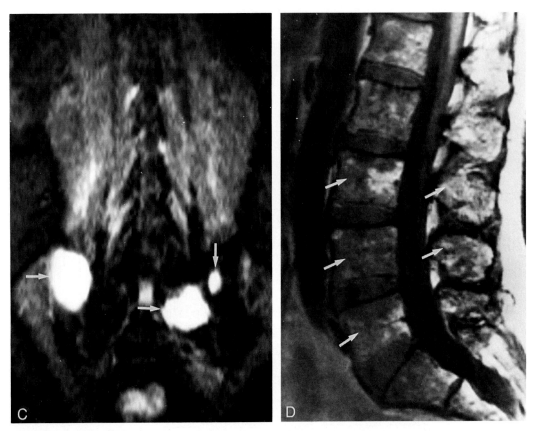

FIGURE 12–46. *(Continued)*

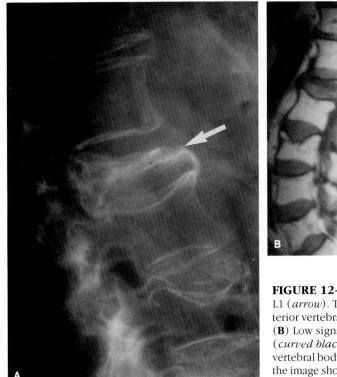

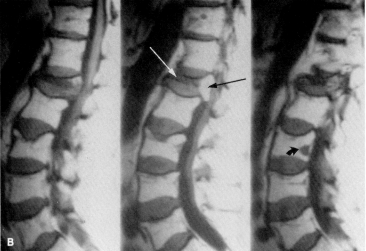

FIGURE 12–47. (**A**) Myeloma presenting as a pathologic fracture of L1 (*arrow*). The anterior osteophyte and relative preservation of the posterior vertebral body height could be misinterpreted as a benign process. (**B**) Low signal intensity myeloma is present in L1 (*white arrow*) and L3 (*curved black arrow*). Normal fat marrow is present in the posterior L1 vertebral body (*straight black arrow*). (**C**) After Gd-DTPA administration, the image shows myeloma enhancement in vertebral bodies of L1 (*straight white arrow*) and L3 (*curved black arrow*).

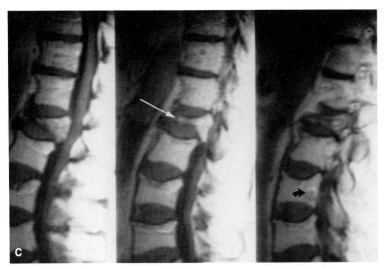

FIGURE 12–47. *(Continued)*

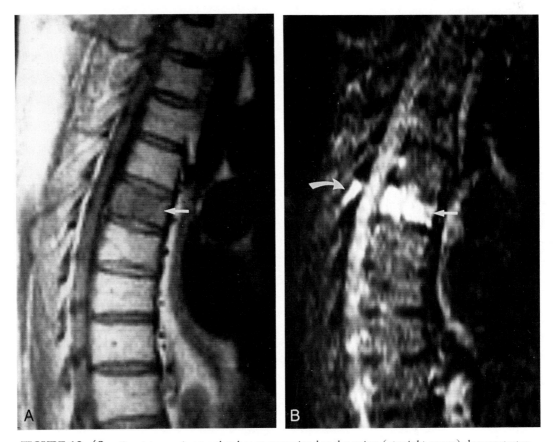

FIGURE 12–48. Prostate carcinoma that has metastasized to the spine (*straight arrow*) demonstrates (**A**) low signal intensity in a T1-weighted sagittal image and (**B**) high signal intensity on a short TI inversion recovery (STIR) sequence. In addition, posterior element involvement (*curved arrow*) is uniquely demonstrated on the STIR image. In a different patient, the affected L5 vertebral body demonstrates (**C**) low signal intensity on T1-weighted image, and (**D**) high signal intensity in Gd-DTPA–enhanced image. Gadolinium contrast enhancement allows enhancement of the tumor while the cerebrospinal fluid remains low in signal intensity. *(continued)*

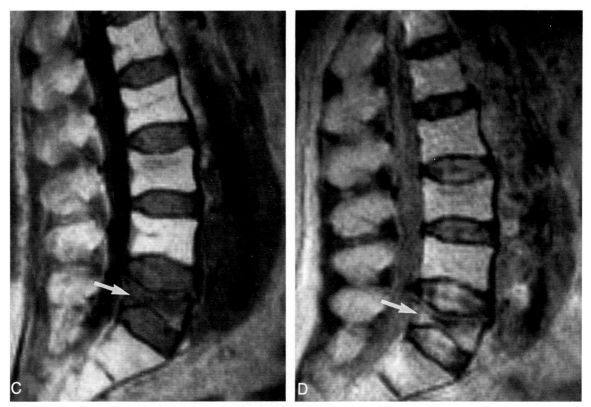

FIGURE 12–48. *(Continued)*

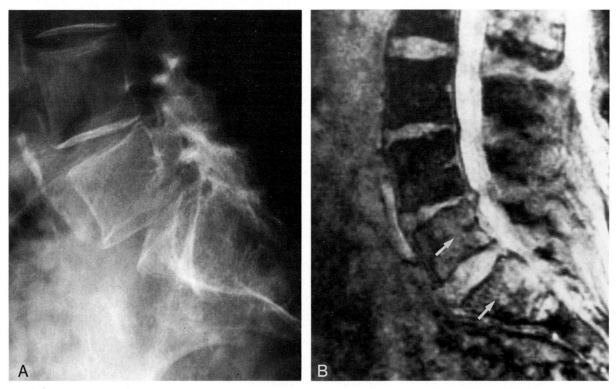

FIGURE 12–49. (**A**) A lateral radiograph is negative for metastatic breast carcinoma. (**B**) A T2*-weighted refocused sagittal image demonstrates high signal intensity metastatic infiltration of marrow in L5 and S1 vertebral bodies (*arrows*). (TR, 400 msec; TE, 15 msec; flip angle, 30°.)

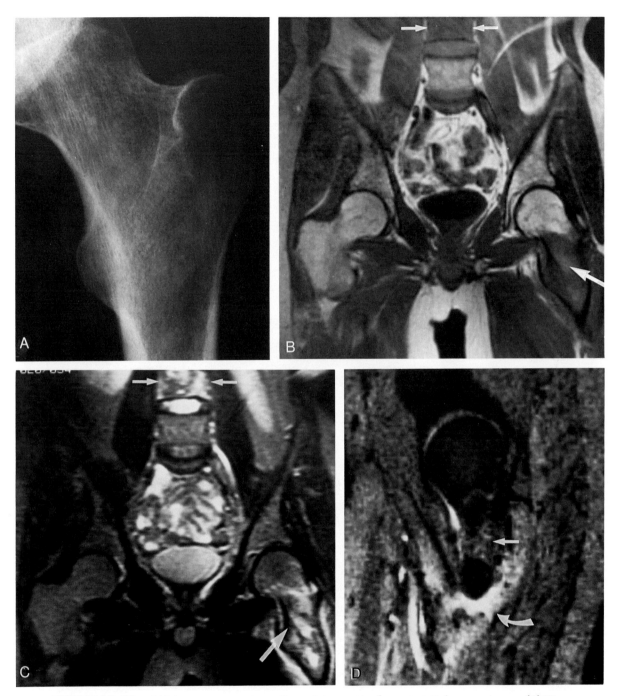

FIGURE 12–50. (**A**) An anteroposterior radiograph is negative for metastatic lung carcinoma. (**B**) T1-weighted and (**C**) T2-weighted images show low and high signal intensity, respectively, in L4 (*small arrows*) and the proximal femur (*large arrow*). (B: TR, 800 msec; TE, 20 msec; C: TR, 2000 msec; TE, 60 msec.) (**D**) A sagittal T2*-weighted image shows a high signal intensity metastatic deposit (*straight arrow*) and peritumoral edema (*curved arrow*). (TR, 400 msec; TE, 30 msec; flip angle, 30°.)

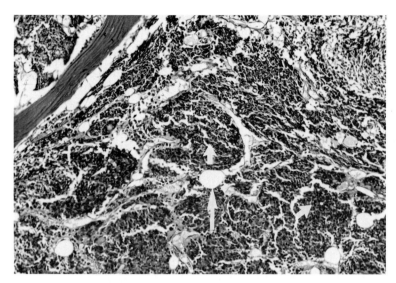

FIGURE 12–51. Extensive bone marrow replacement occurred secondary to metastatic small cell carcinoma of the lung. The marrow is hypercellular and composed of small hyperchromatic cells (*short arrow*) which have replaced the normal hematopoietic elements. Few fat cells (*long arrow*) are present. (H & E stain; original magnification ×120.)

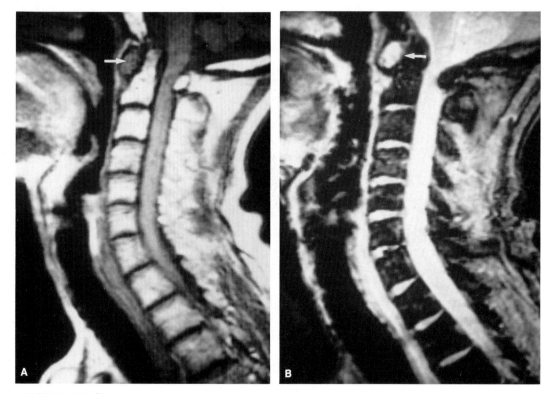

FIGURE 12–52. (**A**) A T1-weighted sagittal image of the cervical spine in a patient with metastatic renal cell carcinoma shows low signal intensity tumor replacement of fat marrow in the anterior arch of the atlas (*white arrow*). Subtle, mild signal intensity inhomogeneity of C3 through C7 is present. (TR, 500 msec; TE, 20 msec.) (**B**) A T2*-weighted image shows increased signal intensity in C1 (*white arrow*) with limited increase in metastatic tumor in C3 through C7. (TR, 400 msec; TE, 15 msec; flip angle, 20°.) (**C**) A STIR image shows hyperintense marrow tumor in C1 (*white arrow*) and C2 through C7 (*black arrows*). (TR, 2000 msec; TI, 160 msec; TE, 43 msec.)

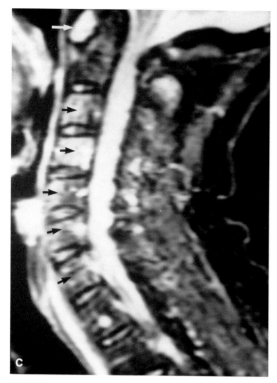

FIGURE 12–52. *(Continued)*

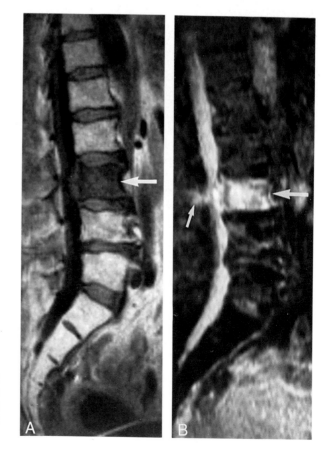

FIGURE 12–53. Metastatic colon carcinoma of L4 (*large arrows*) demonstrates (**A**) low signal intensity on a T1-weighted sagittal image and (**B**) high signal intensity on a short TI inversion recovery (STIR) sequence. The STIR image displays spinous process involvement as well (*small arrow*).

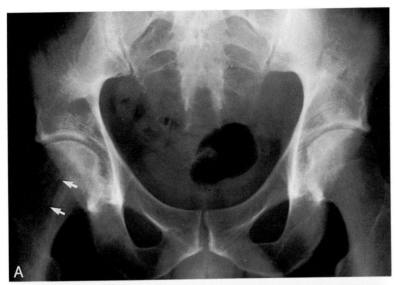

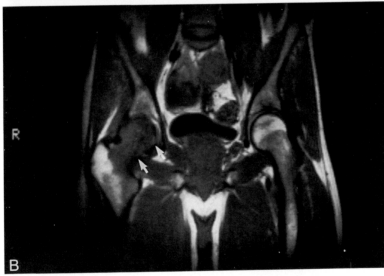

FIGURE 12–54. (**A**) On an anteroposterior radiograph, a metastatic melanoma lesion is seen as a lytic area in the lateral femoral neck (*arrows*). (**B**) On a T1-weighted coronal image, nonspecific low signal intensity marrow replacement (*arrows*) is evident. (TR, 500 msec; TE, 30 msec.)

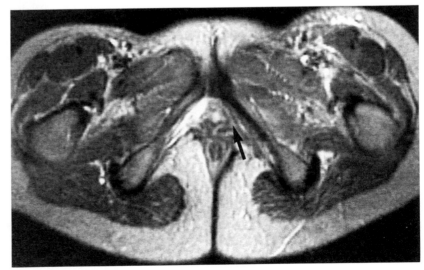

FIGURE 12–55. Postoperative rhabdomyosarcoma. A T2-weighted axial image of postoperative fibrous scarring of the pelvis (*arrow*), which demonstrates low to intermediate signal intensity. (TR, 2000 msec; TE, 60 msec.)

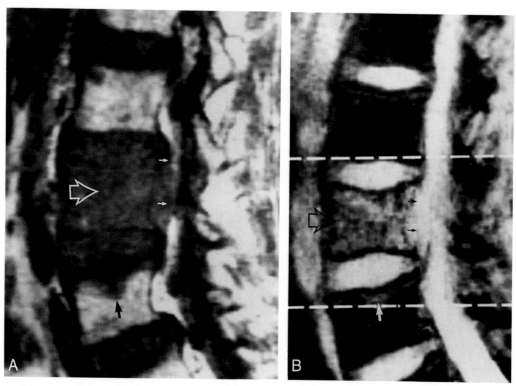

FIGURE 12–56. Ewing's sarcoma metastatic to L3 (*open arrows*) with epidural involvement (*small solid arrows*) demonstrates (**A**) low signal intensity on T1-weighted image and (**B**) high signal intensity in T2*-weighted image. Schmorl's node of the L5 endplate (*large solid arrows*) should not be mistaken for tumor. (A: TR, 600 msec; TE, 30 msec; B: TR, 400 msec; TE, 25 msec; flip angle, 30°.)

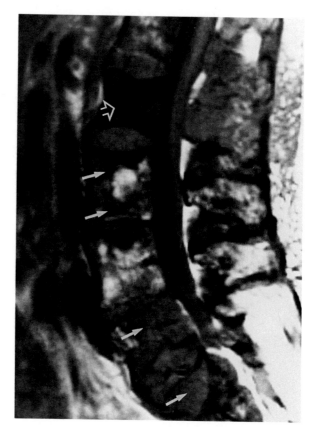

FIGURE 12–57. Lytic and blastic metastases. A T1-weighted sagittal image shows low signal intensity metastatic breast carcinoma (*solid arrows*) and diffuse low signal intensity isolated blastic vertebrae (*open arrow*). (TR, 600 msec; TE, 20 msec.)

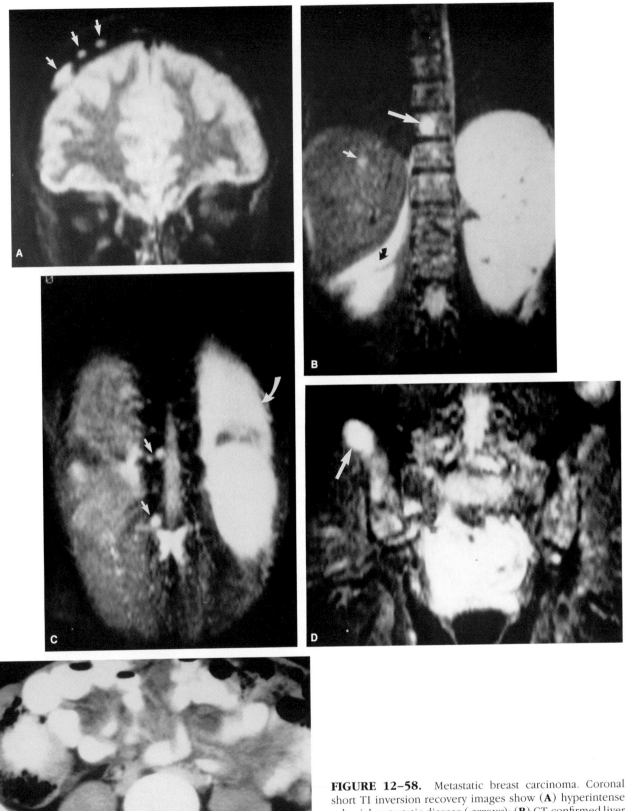

FIGURE 12–58. Metastatic breast carcinoma. Coronal short TI inversion recovery images show (**A**) hyperintense calvarial metastatic disease (*arrows*); (**B**) CT-confirmed liver metastasis (*small white arrow*) to the thoracic spine (*large white arrow*) and ascites (*curved black arrow*); (**C**) conspicuous (hyperintense) pedicle and laminar metastasis (*straight arrows*) and left pleural effusion (*curved arrow*); and (**D**) posterior iliac crest metastasis (*arrow*) with hyperintense inhomogeneity of marrow. (TR, 1400 msec; TI, 140 msec; TE, 40 msec.) (**E**) A CT image confirms lytic metastasis (*arrow*) in right ilium.

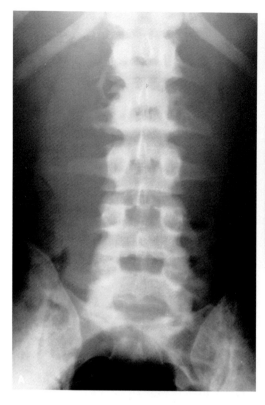

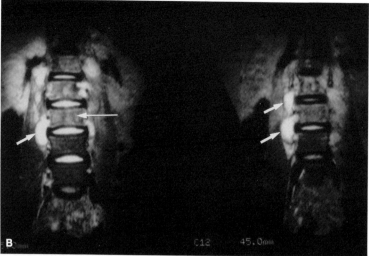

FIGURE 12–59. Coccidiomycosis. Biopsy-proven coccidiomycosis with marrow hyperemia and adenopathy. The findings (*i.e.,* vertebral body and pedicle erosion) simulate (**A**) lymphoma on a plain film radiograph and (**B**) adenopathy (*short arrows*) and marrow lesions (*long arrow*) in a coronal short TI inversion recovery image. (B: TR, 1400 msec; TI, 140 msec; TE, 40 msec.)

FIGURE 12–60. (**A**) A coronal short TI inversion recovery (STIR) image of the abdomen and pelvis, performed to evaluate possible lymphadenopathy, shows abnormal signal in S2 (*long arrow*). Muscle edema from a recent iliac biopsy is hyperintense (*short arrows*). (**B**) A bone scan made two days earlier was negative, even in retrospect. (**C**) A sagittal T1-weighted image shows abnormal marrow signal in S2 (*arrow*). (**D**) The corresponding STIR image shows marked hyperintensity (*arrow*) of this biopsy-confirmed metastasis from Ewing's sarcoma.

(continued)

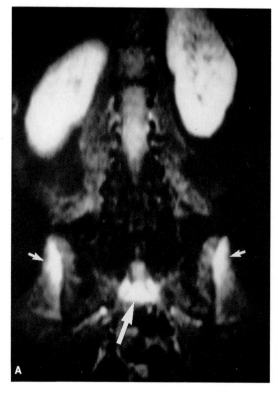

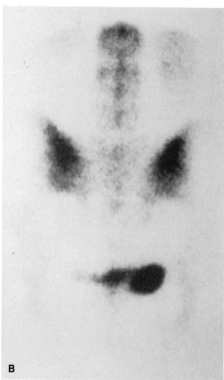

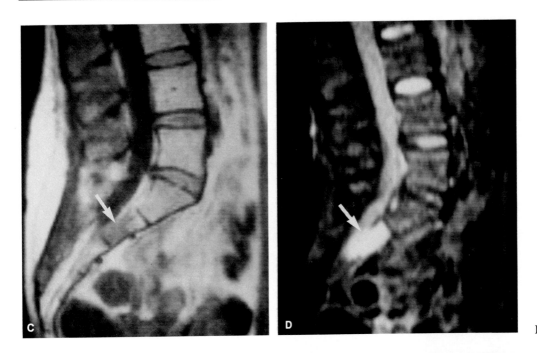

FIGURE 12–60. *(Continued)*

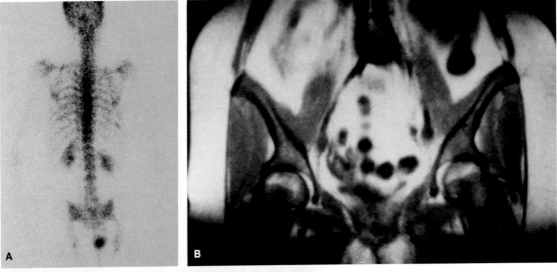

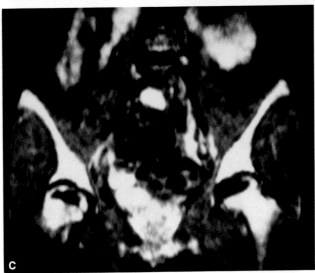

FIGURE 12–61. Metastatic breast cancer with a biopsy-proven tumor was clinically occult. (**A**) A bone scan is equivocal, with uptake in only two small rib lesions. (**B**) A T1-weighted coronal image of the pelvis and coronal short TI inversion recovery images of the (**C**) pelvis, (**D**) thoracic spine, and (**E**) humeri reveal nearly complete marrow replacement by metastatic tumor in this 45-year-old man, who had no bone pain at presentation. There was, however, splenic enlargement and an elevated carcinoembryonic antigen. Note that the humeral and femoral epiphyseal fat marrow stores were spared.

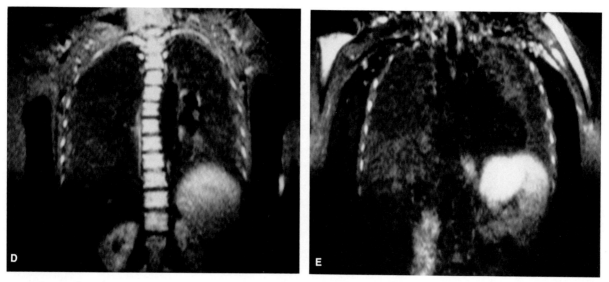

FIGURE 12–61. *(Continued)*

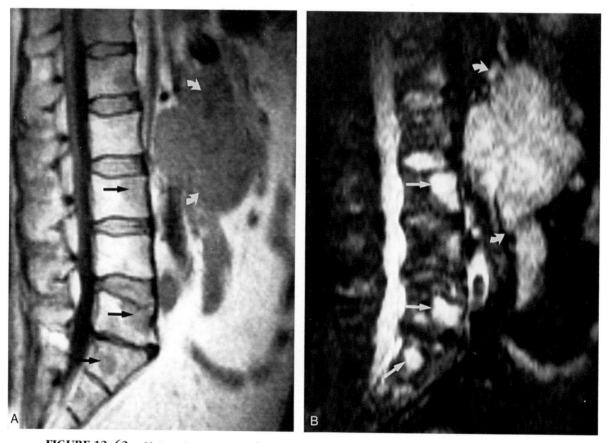

FIGURE 12–62. Metastatic carcinoma of the testis involving the lumbar spine (*straight arrows*) and periaortic lymph nodes (*curved arrows*) demonstrates (**A**) low signal intensity on a T1-weighted image and (**B**) high signal intensity on a short TI inversion recovery sequence.

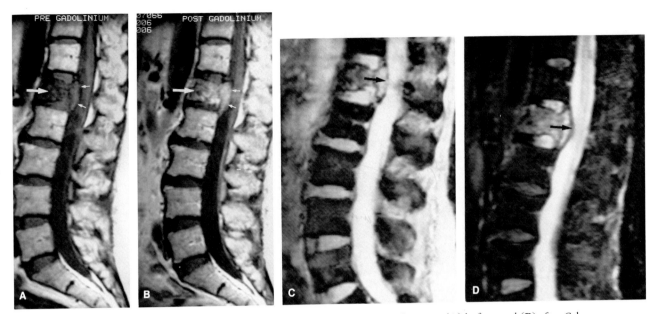

FIGURE 12–63. Metastatic lung carcinoma. T1-weighted sagittal images (**A**) before and (**B**) after Gd-DTPA administration show metastatic tumor infiltration (*large arrows*) and aggressive extension through the posterior vertebral cortex (*small arrows*). The tumor is enhanced on the post-Gd-DTPA image. (TR, 500 msec; TE, 20 msec.) A comparison of (**C**) sagittal T2*-weighted and (**D**) short TI inversion recovery images reveals posterior convexity of the L1 vertebral body, a sign characteristic of aggressive metastatic marrow replacement. (C: TR, 400 msec; TE, 15 msec; flip angle, 20°; D: TR, 2000 msec; TI, 140 msec; TE, 40 msec.)

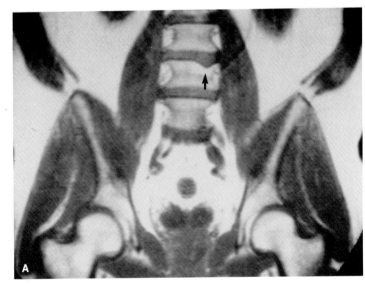

FIGURE 12–64. Benign marrow endplate changes. Fatty marrow endplate conversion in an area of benign endplate compression demonstrates (**A**) bright signal intensity (*arrow*) on a T1-weighted coronal image and (**B**) dark signal intensity (*small arrow*) on a coronal short TI inversion recovery (STIR) image. Normal hematopoietic marrow demonstrates intermediate signal intensity (*large arrow*) on the STIR image. The yellow marrow of the femoral heads and greater trochanter is also dark.

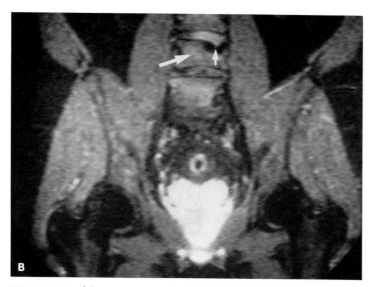

FIGURE 12–64. *(Continued)*

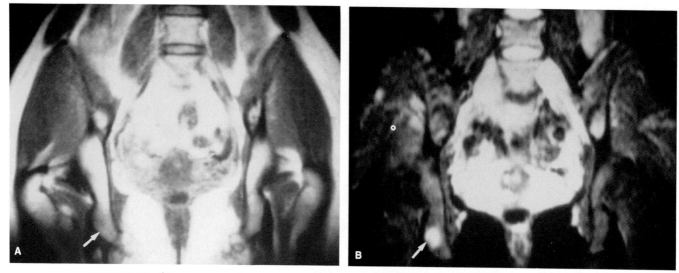

FIGURE 12–65. Metastatic breast cancer. (**A**) On a T1-weighted coronal image, the iliac crest marrow tumor (*arrow*) is poorly visualized. (**B**) On a coronal short TI inversion recovery (STIR) image, the focal metastatic tumor (*arrow*) is more clearly seen. A follow-up exam confirms disease progression (*arrows*) on (**C**) coronal T1-weighted and (**D**) STIR images. (C: TR, 600 msec; TE, 30 msec; D: TR, 1400 msec; TI, 140 msec; TE, 40 msec.)

(continued)

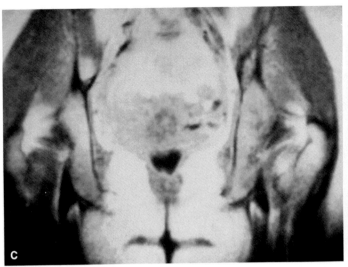

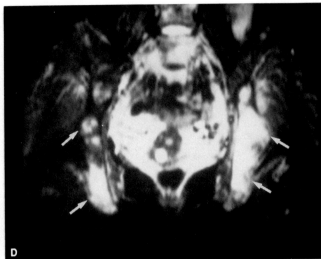

FIGURE 12–65. *(Continued)*

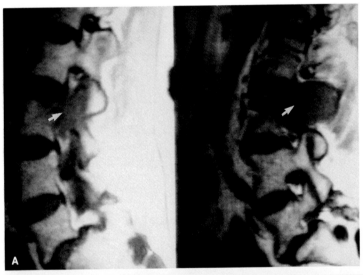

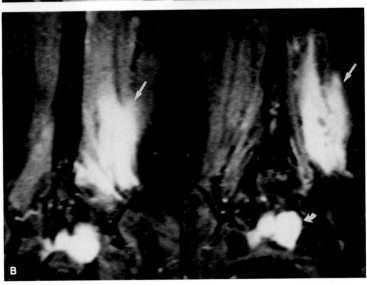

FIGURE 12–66. Metastatic lung carcinoma. (**A**) A T1-weighted sagittal image shows metastatic involvement of the left pedicle of L3 (*arrows*), which is expansile. Compression of the corresponding L2 and L3 nerve roots is present. (TR, 600 msec; TE, 30 msec.) (**B**) A coronal short TI inversion recovery image displays reactive peritumoral edema, which is poorly marginated and extends along the fibers of the spastic quadratus lumborum muscle (*straight arrows*). A benign sacral arachnoid cyst is also present (*curved arrow*). (TR, 1400 msec; TI, 140 msec; TE, 40 msec.)

Magnetic Resonance Appearance. Glucocerebroside-laden cells produce patchy, coarse, decreased signal intensity on T1- and T2-weighted images,[47,53] and increased signal intensity on STIR images (Fig. 12–67). There is a predilection for hematopoietic marrow stores in the axial skeleton, pelvis, and metaphyses of long bones (Fig. 12–68). Appendicular skeletal involvement proceeds from proximal to distal epiphyseal involvement, and in extensive marrow disease, there is generalized distal involvement. Preferential involvement of the distal femurs causes the characteristic Erlenmeyer flask deformity. The mucopolysaccharidoses, which are an unrelated group of hereditary disorders characterized by dwarfism and a specific enzyme deficiency, also demonstrate relative hyperintensity on STIR images (Fig. 12–69).

Marrow infarction, a complication of Gaucher's disease, is seen on T1-weighted images as sharply demarcated lesions of low signal intensity. The bright signal intensity described by Rosenthal and colleagues represents unaffected fatty marrow.[47] Short TI inversion recovery images depict increased signal intensity in more subacute or acute infarcts. Red marrow signal characteristics may be depicted in Gaucher's disease, but are less noticeable than in other marrow infiltrative disorders such as lymphoma.

Iron Storage Assessment

To assess iron stores directly, it is usually necessary to sample one of the two iron-storing organs, the liver or the bone marrow. Marrow iron stores are normal or mildly increased in anemias caused by chronic disease and thalassemia minor, and in homozygous hemoglobinopathies such as sickle-cell disease. Iron stores are greatly increased in chronic conditions requiring repeated blood transfusions, such as thalassemia major and myeloproliferative–myelodysplastic syndrome, as well as in long-standing aplastic anemia. In hemochromatosis, intestinal iron absorption and deposition is increased (Fig. 12–70). Errors of iron quantification are not uncommon due to the small amount of the biopsied sample and the chelation effect of the decalcified marrow biopsy specimen.[54]

Stored iron can also be assessed by evaluating urinary excretion of iron after the administration of a chelating agent, usually deferoxamine. This test is useful in detecting iron overload, but is less accurate in assessment of iron-deficiency states.[55]

Another method of estimating iron stores in rats, an *in vivo* method based on the magnetic susceptibility of ferritin in hemosiderin, was reported in 1967.[56]

Magnetic resonance imaging can also be used to assess iron stores (see Fig. 12–70). Iron stores of ferritin and hemosiderin cause decreased fatty marrow signal intensity on T1- and T2-weighted images. No studies of the correlation between the amount of iron deposition and the degree of decrease in marrow signal intensity have been performed.

Bone Marrow Changes in Females

Signal intensity changes representing reconversion of fatty marrow to hematopoietic marrow can be depicted on T1-weighted and STIR images. During pregnancy, accelerated erythropoiesis, representing an actual increase of approximately 25% in the red cell mass, takes place, as does an increase in circulating erythropoietin in the last two trimesters. Human placental lactogen has been shown to stimulate erythropoiesis in the mouse. Additionally, deficiencies of iron during pregnancy may result in anemia, making the finding of marrow reconversion during pregnancy not surprising.[57]

A common observation in the mature skeleton of females is red marrow inhomogeneity in metaphyseal and diaphyseal sites (Fig. 12–71). The cause has not been fully elucidated,[58] but one theory implicates a latent iron-deficient state as the stimulus for marrow reconversion. In latent iron deficiency, the patient may be asymptomatic, and the blood hemoglobin levels may be normal. More sophisticated testing, however, shows elevated erythrocyte protoporphyrin levels and absence of stainable iron in the marrow.[59] Delayed (*i.e.,* incomplete) conversion of red to yellow marrow also produces inhomogeneity. Red marrow stores, of low signal intensity on T1-weighted images, demonstrate isointensity on T2*-weighted images, minimal hyperintensity on T2-weighted images, and varying degrees of increased signal intensity on STIR images (Fig. 12–72).

Aplastic Anemia

In aplastic anemia, the marrow is extremely hypoplastic (*i.e.,* yellow) and exhibits less than 30% residual hematopoietic elements microscopically (Fig. 12–73). Aplastic anemia is believed to be caused by injury or failure of a common pluripotential stem cell affecting all hematopoietic cell lines. It may present as an acute disorder, or may have a more prolonged chronic course, with signs and symptoms related to the pancytopenia.[60]

The etiology is unknown in approximately 50% of patients; the anemia is diagnosed as idiopathic aplastic anemia in this case. The remainder of the cases are attributed to exposure to drugs, chemicals, toxins, radiation, and severe viral infections. Uncommonly, congenital disorders such as Fanconi's anemia may be accompanied by a genetic predisposition to aplastic anemia. Although a mild form of aplastic anemia may be successfully treated with marrow-stimulating drugs such as androgens, the mainstay of therapy is bone marrow transplantation.[61] Iatrogenically-induced aplastic marrows are encountered in the course of aggressive chemotherapy in the treatment of acute leukemia or in preparation for bone marrow transplantation. Radiotherapy may result in focal aplastic marrow.

Magnetic Resonance Appearance

Aplastic marrow is characterized by increased signal intensity on T1-weighted images and intermediate signal intensity on T2-weighted images. These signal intensity changes are attributed to replacement of hematopoietic marrow by fatty marrow.[62,63] On T1-weighted images, focal low signal intensity heterogeneity is seen during treatment for aplastic anemia. This heterogeneity may represent hematopoiesis recovery or fibrosis. Although MR imaging demonstrates primarily high signal intensity fatty marrow in aplastic anemia, islands of hematopoiesis may produce a patchy appearance of lower signal intensity areas surrounded by bright signal intensity fat on T1-weighted images. Aplastic anemia may be difficult to discriminate from normal bone marrow in adult patients because of the conversion to fatty marrow signal intensity. Diagnosis and monitoring of aplastic anemia may be improved with chemical-shift imaging techniques.

Hemoglobinopathies

Sickle-Cell Anemia

Approximately 0.15% of black children in the United States are homozygous for hemoglobin S (HbS) and have full-blown sickle-cell disease. This disorder is caused by a specific molecular lesion—the substitution of valine for glutamic acid at the beta chain of hemoglobin.[64] When oxygen tension is reduced, erythrocytes containing HbS become sickle-shaped. These rigid, nondeformable sickle cells cause occlusion of small vessels, and their abnormal shape subjects them to premature pitting by the spleen, resulting in accelerated red blood cell destruction (*i.e.,* hemolytic anemia). These two features, small vessel occlusion and hemolytic anemia, account for the various clinical manifestations in sickle-cell disease. Like other patients with congenital hemolytic anemia, sickle-cell patients demonstrate radiographic abnormalities due to expansion of the red marrow. Vascular occlusion leads to a development of bony infarctions.

Magnetic Resonance Appearance. Sickle-cell anemia is characterized by yellow to red marrow reconversion with low to intermediate signal intensity hema-

topoietic marrow identified on T1-weighted images and hematopoietic or red marrow characteristics on STIR images (Fig. 12–74). Marrow conversion can involve the diaphysis, metaphysis, and epiphysis.[65,66] Patients with marrow ischemia present with bone marrow infarction on MR images. Acute infarcts may demonstrate increased signal intensity on T2-weighted images.

Thalassemia

The thalassemias are a diverse group of congenital disorders in which there is a defect in the synthesis of one or more of the subunits of hemoglobin. As a result of the decreased production of hemoglobin, red blood cells are microcytic and hypochromic. Thalassemias are quantitative abnormalities of synthesis of either the beta or alpha hemoglobin subunit. As a result of the imbalance in the subunit synthesis, patients with the thalassemias exhibit varying degrees of ineffective erythropoiesis and hemolytic anemias. The severity of the resultant anemias is related to the number of the deficient subunit chains, which, in turn, is related to whether gene expression is homozygous, intermediate, or heterozygous.[67]

Magnetic Resonance Appearance. As in sickle-cell anemia, MR scans in thalassemia major demonstrate low to intermediate signal intensity within hematopoietic marrow, involving both fatty and red marrow stores (*i.e.,* epiphyseal extension). In thalassemia minor, MR imaging demonstrates increased red marrow stores and delayed development of ossification centers.[12]

Miscellaneous Marrow Lesions

Paget's Disease

Paget's disease is initially characterized by uncontrolled osteoclastic activity (*i.e.,* bone resorption), followed by vascular fibrous connective tissue production, and ends with osteoblastic activity (*i.e.,* bone production). In the final stages of this disease, bone is composed of dense trabecular bone organized in a haphazard fashion, resulting in irregular, mosaic cement lines. The composition of this altered bone is disorganized and, although dense, it is structurally weak and prone to fracture.

Paget's disease is most likely to affect individuals over 40 years of age, who are primarily of European extraction. Serum alkaline phosphatase levels are markedly increased in this disorder. Various electron-microscopic studies have implicated viral agents related to measles or respiratory syncytial viruses as possible etiologic agents. This disorder may involve a limited portion of the skeleton or may be more generalized. Pelvic bones

(text continues on page 1027)

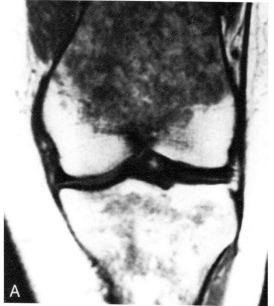

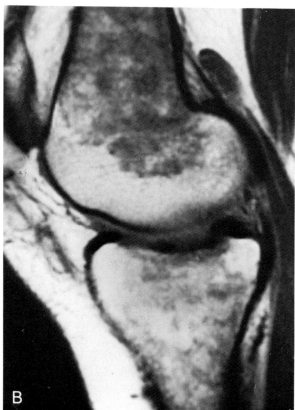

FIGURE 12–67. Low signal intensity marrow infiltration can be seen extending into the epiphysis on (**A**) T1-weighted coronal and (**B**) sagittal images. Gaucher's disease involves a defect of cerebroside metabolism in which lipid material accumulates in the reticuloendothelial cells. (TR, 800 msec; TE, 30 msec.)

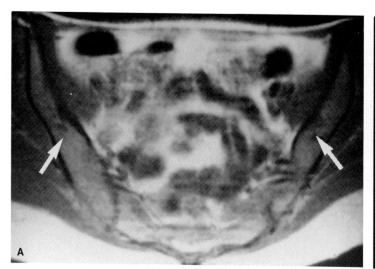

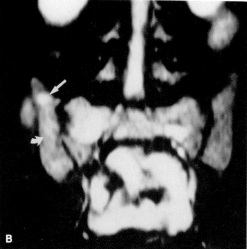

FIGURE 12–68. Hodgkin's disease and Gaucher's marrow. (**A**) On a T1-weighted axial image, diffuse low signal intensity iliac marrow (*arrows*) is present. (**B**) On a coronal short TI inversion recovery image, the Hodgkin's marrow involvement is hyperintense (*straight arrow*) relative to the heterogeneous high signal intensity Gaucher's marrow (*curved arrow*). (TR, 1400 msec; TI, 140 msec; TE, 40 msec.)

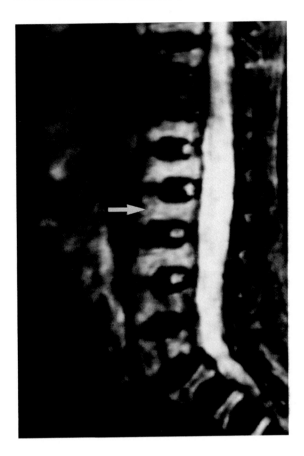

FIGURE 12–69. A sagittal short TI inversion recovery (STIR) image in a child with mucopolysaccharidosis type IV (*i.e.,* Morquio-Brailsford disease; Morquio's syndrome). The accumulation of mucopolysaccharides secondary to deficiency of galactosamine-6-sulfate sulfatase produces hyperintensity on STIR contrast (*arrow*). Note the platyspondyly (*i.e.,* flattening) and slight rounding of the vertebral bodies.

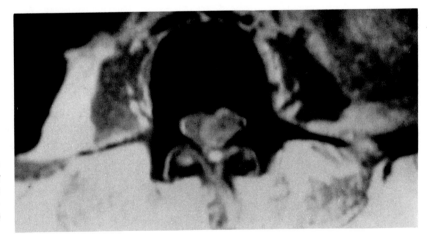

FIGURE 12–70. Iron deposition in hemochromatosis demonstrates diffuse low signal intensity on a T1-weighted axial image. This simulates the appearance of a gradient refocused or short TI inversion recovery sequence. (TR, 1000 msec; TE, 20 msec.)

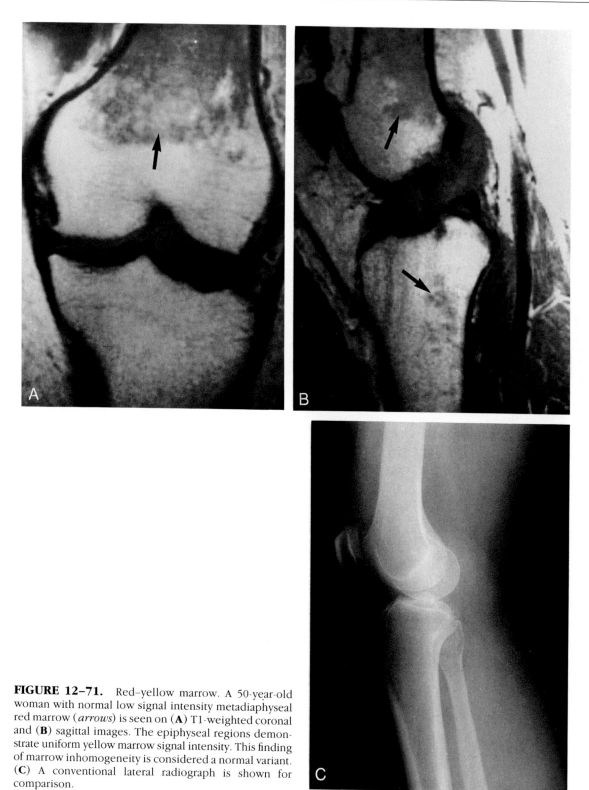

FIGURE 12–71. Red–yellow marrow. A 50-year-old woman with normal low signal intensity metadiaphyseal red marrow (*arrows*) is seen on (**A**) T1-weighted coronal and (**B**) sagittal images. The epiphyseal regions demonstrate uniform yellow marrow signal intensity. This finding of marrow inhomogeneity is considered a normal variant. (**C**) A conventional lateral radiograph is shown for comparison.

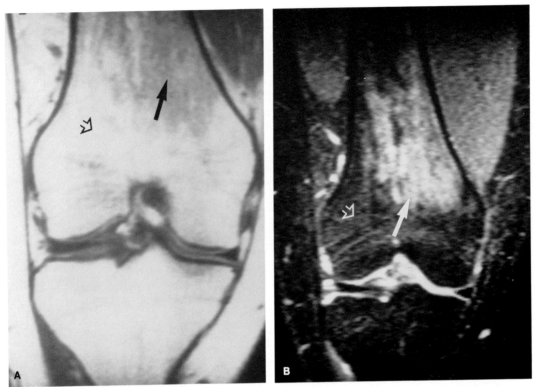

FIGURE 12–72. A normal 40-year-old woman shows normal red marrow and yellow marrow inhomogeneity in metaphyseal diaphyses. (**A**) A T1-weighted coronal image displays bright signal intensity fat marrow (*open arrow*) and hematopoietic or red marrow (*solid arrow*). (**B**) A corresponding coronal short TI inversion recovery image shows dark fat marrow (*open arrow*) and increased signal intensity red marrow (*solid arrow*).

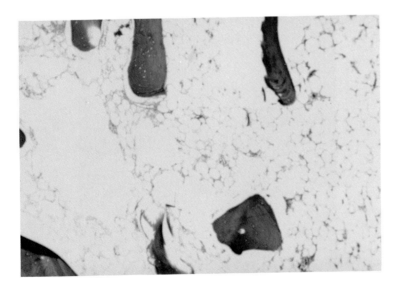

FIGURE 12–73. Bone marrow exhibits marked hypocellularity and is essentially 100% fat in aplastic anemia. (H & E stain; original magnification ×100.)

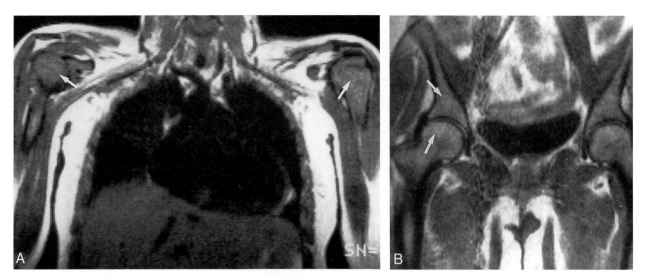

FIGURE 12–74. T1-weighted coronal images show diffuse low signal intensity (*arrows*) in (**A**) the humeri and (**B**) the pelvis in two patients with sickle cell anemia and persistent red marrow hypercellularity. (TR, 800 msec; TE, 20 msec.)

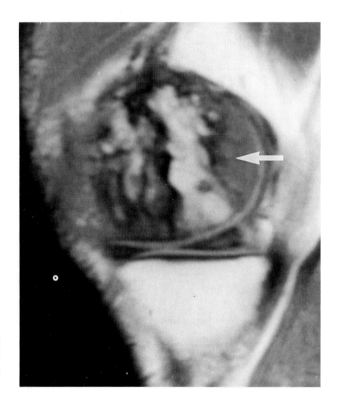

FIGURE 12–75. On a T1-weighted sagittal image, coarse-fibered bone in Paget's disease is seen as areas of low signal intensity intermixed with yellow marrow; this creates an inhomogeneous appearance in the medial femoral condyle (*arrow*). (TR, 800 msec; TE, 20 msec.)

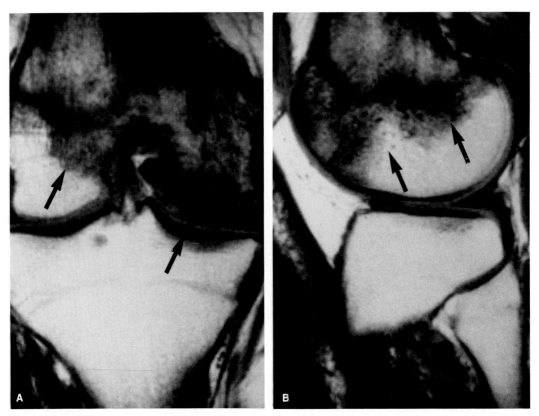

FIGURE 12–76. T1-weighted (**A**) coronal and (**B**) sagittal images in a patient with Paget's disease show geographically well-defined lysis and low signal intensity sclerosis (*arrows*) extending into the subarticular region of the distal femur. Initial tibial involvement is frequently diaphyseal. (TR, 600 msec; TE, 20 msec.)

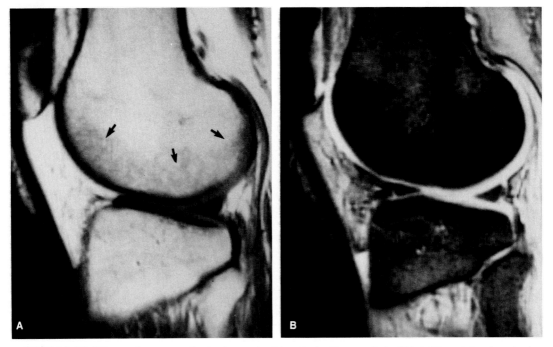

FIGURE 12–77. Reflex sympathetic dystrophy (*i.e.,* Sudeck's atrophy). (**A**) A T1-weighted sagittal image shows subarticular low signal intensity marrow (*arrows*). (TR, 600 msec; TE, 20 msec.) (**B**) The corresponding T2*-weighted sagittal image is unremarkable. (TR, 600 msec; TE, 15 msec; flip angle, 20°.) (**C**) An axial short TI inversion recovery image through the proximal tibia shows marrow hyperemia (*arrows*) with hyperintense signal intensity. (TR, 2000 msec; TI, 160 msec; TE, 43 msec.)

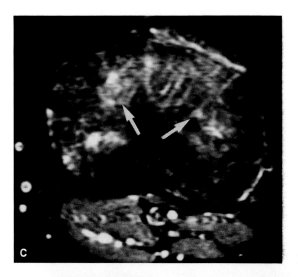

FIGURE 12–77. *(Continued)*

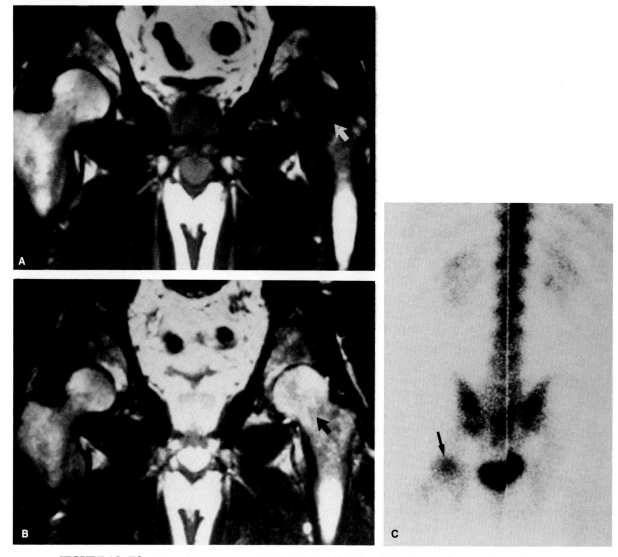

FIGURE 12–78. Transient osteoporosis of the hip. (**A**) A T-weighted coronal image shows low signal intensity in the left femoral head and neck (*arrow*) without an osteonecrotic focus. (TR, 600 msec; TE, 20 msec.) (**B**) On the corresponding T2-weighted coronal image, there is increased signal intensity in the left femoral head and neck (*arrow*). (TR, 2000 msec; TE, 80 msec.) (**C**) A technetium bone scan, posterior view, shows uptake in left femoral head (*arrow*).

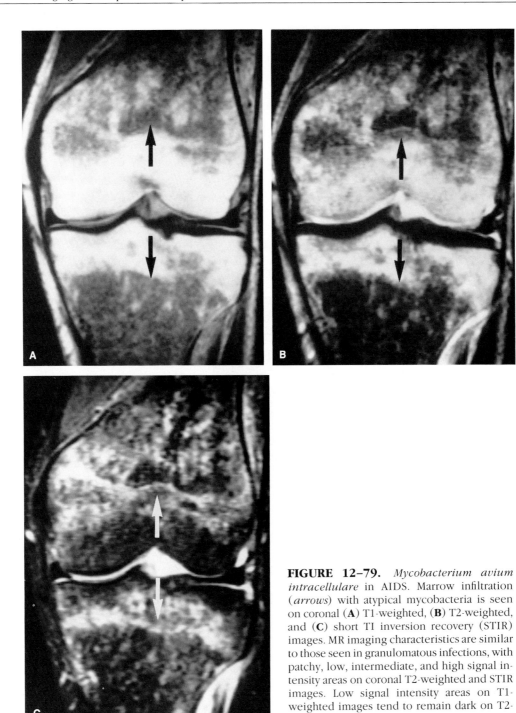

FIGURE 12–79. *Mycobacterium avium intracellulare* in AIDS. Marrow infiltration (*arrows*) with atypical mycobacteria is seen on coronal (**A**) T1-weighted, (**B**) T2-weighted, and (**C**) short TI inversion recovery (STIR) images. MR imaging characteristics are similar to those seen in granulomatous infections, with patchy, low, intermediate, and high signal intensity areas on coronal T2-weighted and STIR images. Low signal intensity areas on T1-weighted images tend to remain dark on T2-weighted and STIR images.

are most commonly involved, followed in incidence by the femur, skull, tibia, lumbosacral spine, dorsal spine, clavicles, and ribs. Secondary malignant sarcomatous transformation arises in preexisting Paget's disease in less than 1% of cases.[68]

Magnetic Resonance Appearance. In the lytic, mixed, and sclerotic presentation of Paget's disease, a coarsened appearance of the marrow is identified on T1-weighted images (Fig. 12–75).[69] Although no increase in signal intensity is observed on T2-weighted or T2*-weighted images, bright signal intensity may be identified on STIR images. The sclerotic pattern of Paget's may resemble diffuse osteonecrosis with diffuse low signal intensity marrow replacement on T1-, T2-, or T2*-weighted images (Fig. 12–76).

Localized Osteoporosis

Reflex sympathetic dystrophy, or Sudeck's atrophy, is a painful neurovascular disorder.[70] Dystrophic soft-tissue changes, swelling, distal extremity predilection, and periarticular as well as diffuse osteoporosis are characteristic. Reflex dystrophy syndrome is mediated by the sympathetic nervous system and may be initiated by minimal trauma or fracture. T1-weighted and STIR images are more sensitive than T2*- or conventional T2-weighted images in identifying hyperemic marrow (Fig. 12–77). Periarticular low signal intensity regions are displayed on T1-weighted images, whereas corresponding STIR images demonstrate a diffusely hyperintense signal intensity.

Transient regional osteoporosis is a self-limited condition characterized by localized osteoporosis and pain. The etiology is unknown. The joint space and articular cartilage are preserved, in contrast to septic arthritis. Transient regional osteoporosis is subdivided into regional migratory osteoporosis and transient osteoporosis of the hip (see Chapter 3). Regional migratory osteoporosis involves the joints of the lower extremity (*i.e.,* the knee, ankle, and foot), has a predilection for those in middle age, and is symptomatic for 6 months to 1 year. Unlike reflex sympathetic dystrophy, there is frequent clinical recurrence in other joints. Transient osteoporosis of the hip typically affects middle-aged men, although it was initially described in women in the third trimester of pregnancy. Either hip may be involved, with a self-limited course of demineralization and pain.

On T1-weighted images, femoral head and neck hyperemia demonstrates low signal intensity on T1-weighted images and increased signal intensity on T2-weighted and STIR images (Fig. 12–78). The acetabulum is not usually involved, although joint effusions are common. Early avascular necrosis may present with similar MR findings, and an osteonecrotic focus should be excluded on follow-up examination.

Acquired Immunodeficiency Syndrome

Patients with acquired immunodeficiency syndrome (AIDS) exhibit a multitude of disorders that may be reflected in various bone marrow changes. Infectious disorders, particularly disseminated mycobacterial (Fig. 12–79), cryptococcal, or histoplasma infection, may extensively involve the marrow. Histopathologically, discrete granulomas are not typically formed in immunodeficient patients. Instead, the causative organisms are detected within histiocytic aggregates and sheets. A diffuse histiocytic proliferation related to viral infection (*i.e.,* virus-associated hemophagocytic syndrome) has been observed in patients with AIDS.

High-grade lymphomas are frequently observed in AIDS and may involve bone marrow in a patchy or diffuse manner. Occasionally, this may present as extensive marrow necrosis associated with severe bone pain.

Some nonspecific changes reported in the bone marrow of AIDS patients include serous atrophy of fat with hypocellular marrow and accumulation of hyaluronic acid, hypocellularity, and decreased storage iron.[71,72]

REFERENCES

1. Kricun ME. Red-yellow marrow conversion: its effect on the location of some solitary bone lesions. Skeletal Radiol 1985;14:10-19.
2. Moore SG, Dawson KL. Magnetic resonance appearance of red and yellow marrow in the femur: spectrum with age. Radiology 1990;175:219.
3. Vogler JB III, Murphy WA. Bone marrow imaging. Radiology 1988;168:679.
4. Dooms GC, et al. Bone marrow imaging: magnetic resonance studies related to age and sex. Radiology 1985;155:429.
5. Weiss L. Histopathology of the bone marrow. In: Gordon AS, ed. Regulation of hematopoiesis. New York: Appleton-Century-Crofts, 1970.
6. Quesenberry P, Levitt L. Hematopoietic stem cells. N Engl J Med 1979;301:755.
7. Vogler JB, Murphy WA. Bone marrow imaging. Radiology 1988;168:679.
8. Custer RP, Ahlfeldt FE. Studies on the structure and function of the bone marrow. J Lab Clin Med 1932;17:960.
9. Le Bruyn PPH, Breen PC, Thomas TB. The microcirculation of the bone marrow. Anat Rec 1970;168:55.
10. Piney A. The anatomy of the bone marrow. Br Med J 1922;2:792.
11. Maniatus A, Vavassoli M, Crosby WH. Factors affecting the conversion of yellow to red marrow. Blood 1971;37:581.
12. Moore SG, Sebag GH. Primary disorders of bone marrow. In: Cohen MD, Edwards MK, eds. Magnetic resonance imaging of children. Philadelphia: Decker, 1990:765.

13. Wehrli FW, et al. Mechanisms of contrast in NMR imaging. J Comput Tomogr 1984;8:369.

14. Mitchell DG, et al. The biophysical basis of tissue contrast in extracranial MR imaging. AJR 1987;149:831.

15. Olson DL, et al. Magnetic resonance imaging of the bone marrow in patients with leukemia, aplastic marrow and lymphoma. Invest Radiol 1986;21:540.

16. Sebag GH, Moore SG. Effect of trabecular bone on the appearance of marrow in gradient echo imaging of the appendicular skeleton. Radiology 1990;174(3):855.

17. Brateman L. Chemical shift imaging: a review. AJR 1980;146:971. 1987

18. Foon KA, Casciato DA. Acute leukemia. In: Casciato DA, Lowitz BB, eds. Manual of clinical oncology. 2nd ed. Boston: Little, Brown and Company, 1990:386.

19. Foon KA, Todd RF. Immunologic classification of leukemia and lymphoma. Blood 1986;68:1.

20. Moore SG, et al. Bone marrow in children with acute lymphocytic leukemia: MR relaxation times. Radiology 1986;160:237.

21. Rosen BR, et al. Hematologic bone marrow disorders: quantitative chemical shift MRI imaging. Radiology 1988;169:799.

22. Thomsen C, et al. Prolonged bone marrow T1-relaxation in acute leukemia: in vivo tissue characterization by magnetic resonance imaging. Magn Reson Imaging 1987;5:251.

23. Sugmura K, et al. Bone marrow diseases of the spine: differentiation with T1 and T2 relaxation times in MR imaging. Radiology 1987;165:541.

24. Jensen KE, et al. Changes in T1 relaxation process in the bone marrow following treatment in children with acute lymphoblastic leukemia: a magnetic resonance imaging study. Pediatr Radiol 1990;20:464.

25. McKinstry CS, et al. Bone marrow in leukemia and aplastic anemia: MR imaging before, during and after treatment. Radiology 1987;162:701.

26. Wittels B. Bone marrow biopsy changes following chemotherapy for acute leukemia. Am J Surg Pathol 1980;4:135.

27. Islam A, Catovsky D, Galton DA. Histological study of bone marrow regeneration following chemotherapy for acute myeloid leukemia and chronic granulocytic leukemia in blast transformation. Br J Haematol 1980;45:535.

28. Foon KA, Casciato DA. Chronic leukemias. In: Casciato DA, Lowitz BB, eds. Manual of clinical oncology. 2nd ed. Boston: Little, Brown and Company, 1990:360.

29. Adamson JW, Fialkow PJ. Pathogenesis of the myeloproliferative syndromes. Br J Haematol 1978;38:299.

30. Wiernik PH. The chronic leukemias. In: Kelley WN, ed. Textbook of internal medicine. vol. 1. Philadelphia: JB Lippincott, 1989:1177.

31. Deisseroth AL, Wallerstein RO. Bone marrow failure. In: Kelley WN, ed. Textbook of internal medicine. vol. 1. Philadelphia: JB Lippincott, 1989:1202.

32. Moore MAS. Pathogenesis in myelofibrosis. In: Hoffman AV, ed. Recent advances in hematology. Edinburgh: Churchill-Livingstone 1982:132.

33. Burke JS. The value of the bone marrow biopsy in the diagnosis of hairy cell leukemia. Am J Clin Pathol 1978;70:876.

34. Golomb HM. Hairy cell leukemia. In: Williams WJ, et al, eds. Hematology. New York: McGraw-Hill, 1983:999.

35. Thompson JA, et al. MRI of bone marrow in hairy cell leukemia: correlation with clinical response to alpha-interferon. Leukemia 1987;1:315.

36. Gale RP, Champlin RE. Bone marrow transplantation in acute leukemia. Clin Haematol 1986;15:851.

37. Nadler BW. Malignant lymphoma. In: Harrison TR, ed. Principles of internal medicine. 12th ed. New York: McGraw-Hill, 1991:1608.

38. O'Reilly RG. Allogenic bone marrow transplantation: current state and future directions. Blood 1983;62:941.

39. Stevens SK, et al. Repopulation of marrow after transplantation: MR imaging with pathologic correlation. Radiology 1990;175:213.

40. O'Caroll DL, McKenna RW, Brunning RD. Bone marrow histology in Hodgkin's disease. Cancer 1976;38:1717.

41. Coller BS, Chabner BA, et al. Frequencies and patterns of bone marrow involvement in non-Hodgkin's lyphomas. Am J Hemat 1977;3:105.

42. Shields AF, et al. The detection of bone marrow involvement by lymphoma using magnetic resonance imaging. J Clin Oncol 1987;5(2):225.

43. Linden A, et al. Malignant lymphoma: bone marrow imaging versus biopsy. Radiology 1989;173(2):335.

44. Richard MA, et al. Low field strength magnetic resonance imaging of bone marrow in patients with malignant lymphoma. Br J Cancer 1988;57(4):412.

45. Stevens SK, et al. Early and late bone marrow changes after irradiation: MR evaluation. Am J Roentgenol 1990;154(4):745.

46. Casamassima F, et al. Hematopoietic bone marrow recovery after radiation therapy: MRI evaluation. Blood 1989;73(6):1677.

47. Rosenthal DI, et al. Evaluation of Gaucher disease using magnetic resonance imaging. J Bone Joint Surg [Am] 1986;68:802.

48. Murra JM. Histiocytoses in bone tumors: clinical, radiologic and pathologic correlations. Philadelphia: Lea & Febiger, 1989:1021.

49. Bergsagel DE. Plasma cell myeloma. In: Williams WJ, et al, eds. Hematology. New York: McGraw-Hill, 1983:1078.

50. Mundy, GR et al. Evidence for the accretion of an osteoclast stimulating factor in myeloma. N Eng J Med 1976;291:1041.

51. Jaffe HL. Tumors and tumorous conditions of the bones and joints. Philadelphia: Lea & Febiger, 1961:589.

52. Anner RM et al. Frequency and significance of bone marrow involvement by metastatic solid tumors. Cancer 1977;39:1337.

53. Lanir A, et al. Gaucher disease: assessment with MR imaging. Radiology 1986;161:239.

54. Fong TP, et al. Stainable iron in aspirated and needle biopsy specimens of marrow: a source of error. Am J Hemat 1977;2:47.

55. Harker LA. Evaluation of storage iron by chelates. Am J Med 1968;45:105.

56. Bauman JH. Estimation of hepatic iron stores by in vivo measurement of magnetic susceptibility. J Lab Clin Med 1967;70:246.

57. Jepson JH, et al. Erythropoietin in plasma of pregnant mice and rays. Com J Physiol Pharm 1968;45:573.

58. Deutsch AL, et al. Incidental detection of hematopoietic hyperplasia on routine knee MR imaging. AJR 1989;153(3):655.

59. Wintrobe M. Iron deficient and iron deficiency anemia. In: Wintrobe M, ed. Clinical hematology. 8th ed. Philadelphia: Lea & Febiger, 1981:618.

60. Gale RP, et al. Aplastic anemia: biology and treatment. Ann Intern Med 1981;95:477.

61. Camitta BM, et al. Aplastic anemia: pathogenesis, diagnosis, treatment and prognosis. N Eng J Med 1982;306:645.

62. McKinstry CS, Steiner TR, et al. Bone marrow in leukemia and aplastic anemia: MR imaging before, during, and after treatment. Radiology 1987;162:701.

63. Kaplan PA. Bone marrow patterns in aplastic anemia: observations with 1.5-T MR imaging. Radiology 1987;164:441.

64. Benz ED. The hemoglobinopathies. In: Kelley WN, ed. Textbook of internal medicine. Philadelphia: JB Lippincott, 1989:1423.

65. Sebes JI, et al. Diagnostic imaging of bone and joint abnormalities associated with sickle cell hemoglobinopathies. AJR 1989;152:1153.

66. Van Zanten TEG, et al. Imaging of bone marrow with magnetic resonance during a crisis and in chronic forms of sickle cell disease. Clin Radio 1989;40:486.

67. Henry J. Clinical diagnosis and management. Philadelphia: WB Saunders, 1984:679.

68. Cotran RS, Robbins SL. The musculoskeletal system. In: Pathologic basis of disease. 4th ed. Philadelphia: WB Saunders, 1989: 1328.

69. Roberts MC, et al. Paget disease: MR imaging findings. Radiology 1989;173:341.

70. Malkin LH. Reflex sympathetic dystrophy syndrome following trauma to the foot. Orthopaedics 1990;13(8):851.

71. Osborne BM, Guarda LA, Bertler JJ. Bone marrow biopsies in patients with the acquired immunodeficiency syndrome. Human Pathol 1984;15:1048.

72. Seaman JP, Kjeldsberg CR, Linhur A. Gelatinous transformation of the bone marrow. Human Pathol 1978;9:685.

Bone and Soft-Tissue Tumors

The superior contrast discrimination provided by magnetic resonance (MR) imaging has proved extremely valuable in the assessment of bone and soft-tissue tumors.[1-9] T1 and T2 relaxation times are prolonged in a variety of malignant tissue types; therefore, malignant change tends to demonstrate low to intermediate signal intensity on T1-weighted images, and bright signal intensity on T2-weighted images. Although computed tomography (CT) may provide superior cortical detail, MR imaging is much more sensitive to marrow involvement by edema or tumor and provides soft-tissue definition of the surrounding musculature, fascial planes, and neurovascular bundles without artifact from cortical bone.

IMAGING TECHNIQUES

In the evaluation of tumors, a combination of both T1 weighting (*i.e.,* inversion recovery) and T2 weighting (*i.e.,* spin-echo or gradient-echo) is essential. With short TI inversion recovery (STIR) imaging sequences, T1 and T2 contrast are additive.[10,11] T1-weighted images provide excellent contrast for identification of marrow, cortical, and soft-tissue involvement. In particular, T1-weighted images allow differentiation between fat and tumor as well as definition of muscular planes and separate anatomic compartments.

Gadolinium (Gd-DTPA) has been used to enhance contrast on T1-weighted images to better characterize osseous and soft-tissue tumor involvement.[12–14] On Gd-DTPA–enhanced images, regions of low signal intensity are thought to represent areas of nonviable tumor or necrosis (Fig. 13–1). Gadolinium-enhanced images may also be useful for differentiating peritumoral edema from underlying tumor and recurrent tumor from scar or fibrosis.

T2-weighted images are valuable in distinguishing muscle from tumor and can increase diagnostic specificity in evaluating marrow infiltration, seen as areas of low signal intensity on T1-weighted images.

Magnetic resonance may not be as sensitive as CT to cortical disruption, fine periosteal reactions, and small calcifications, although the sensitivity of MR *versus* CT needs further documentation. With proper imaging planes and resolution, we have been able to distinguish early endosteal and cortical erosions, as well as periosteal changes on MR images (Fig. 13–2).

Although each MR examination must be tailored to the patient and pathology in question, certain general guidelines can be followed. The longitudinal extent of tumors can be seen on T1-weighted coronal or sagittal images. If a lesion is difficult to differentiate from (*i.e.,* is isointense with) adjacent tissues, either a conventional spin-echo or a fast-scan T2*-weighted scan should be obtained. T1- and T2-weighted sequences in the axial plane provide the most important images in delineating the relationship of a tumor to adjacent neurovascular structures and compartments—essential information in preoperative limb salvage planning. In addition, the proximal and distal extent of tumor involvement can be assessed by evaluating multiple axial sections. The region of abnormality should be positioned as close to the center of the coil as possible. The patient's position—prone or supine—is determined by the area of abnormality. Prior to imaging the particular region of interest, a large field-of-view localizer using an increased diameter surface coil or body coil may be necessary to exclude skin lesions or to accurately determine the proximal and distal extension of a large mass.

GENERAL MAGNETIC RESONANCE APPEARANCE

Direct multiplanar imaging facilitates improved preoperative and pretherapy evaluation of the exact extent of a lesion. In addition, since there is minimal artifact from nonferromagnetic implants with MR imaging, it is often possible to identify postoperative and post-treatment fibrous tissues not seen on CT. A tumor bed with postoperative scarring demonstrates low signal intensity on both T1- and T2-weighted images. If, however, T1- and T2-weighted images show intermediate and high signal intensity, respectively, the possibility of recurrent tumor is more likely. This distinction often cannot be made on CT scans.

It is often not possible to distinguish benign from malignant lesions of bone and soft tissue on the basis of MR signal characteristics alone. Both benign and malignant lesions may demonstrate areas of low signal intensity on T1-weighted images and increased signal intensity on T2-weighted images. Malignant lesions tend to be more extensive, involving marrow, cortical bone, and soft tissues; but these criteria do not always distinguish benign from malignant lesions. No correlations have been shown matching T1 and T2 relaxation times with corresponding histopathology.[15] If the neurovascular bundle is involved, the lesion is likely to be malignant. A fluid–fluid level is a nonspecific finding in bone and soft-tissue lesions. Tumors with fluid–fluid levels include fibrous dysplasia, simple bone cysts, malignant fibrous histiocytoma (MFH), osteosarcoma, aneurysmal bone cysts, hemangioma, and synovial sarcoma.[16]

Infectious processes (*e.g.,* osteomyelitis) and benign neoplasms have been found to have a low signal intensity peripheral margin in 33% of patients studied.[17] This margin is rarely seen in malignant lesions because a well-defined sclerotic interface is not present. It is important to perform MR studies prior to biopsy, to avoid postsurgical inflammation and edema that may prolong T2 values of uninvolved tissues. Muscle edema is nonspecific and may be associated with trauma, infection, and vascular insults. On T1-weighted images, high signal intensity in the surrounding musculature can be seen in atrophy with fatty infiltration or neuromuscular disorders, and should not be mistaken for tumor. Venous varicosities may scallop subcutaneous tissue and demonstrate low signal intensity on T1-weighted images. This appearance is characteristic, and can be distinguished from neoplastic soft-tissue extension or tumor vascularity.

Red-to-yellow marrow conversion in middle-aged women is seen in metaphyseal or diaphyseal areas of low signal intensity (*i.e.,* red marrow) without extension into the epiphysis (Fig. 13–3). These lesions become isointense with adjacent marrow on heavily T2-weighted images and demonstrate increased signal intensity on STIR images. Inhomogeneity of metaphyseal red and yellow marrow may also be observed in the immature skeleton.

BONE TUMORS

Benign Lesions

Benign Osteoblastic Lesions

Osteoid Osteoma. Osteoid osteomas are small, benign, osteoblastic lesions characteristically seen in young patients between 7 and 25 years of age.[18] Osteoid osteomas are composed of osteoid and trabeculae of newly formed osseous tissue embedded in a substriated, highly vascularized osteogenic connective tissue with a surrounding peripheral zone of dense sclerotic bone. They rarely exceed 1 cm in diameter and are usually located in either the spongiosa or the cortex of the bone. Most commonly, they affect long tubular bones; the femur is the most common site of involvement. The clinical hallmark of this lesion is pain that is most prominently at night and can be relieved with salicylates (*i.e.,* aspirin).[18-20]

Magnetic Resonance Appearance. On T1-weighted images, the nidus of the lesion images with low to intermediate signal intensity (Figs. 13–4, 13–5, and 13–6). On T2-weighted images, the central nidus demonstrates moderate to increased signal intensity.[21,22] Intraarticular osteoid osteomas of the hip usually cause a synovial inflammatory response, and are associated with joint effusions.[23] Reactive sclerosis demonstrates low signal intensity on T1- and T2-weighted images. There may be extensive marrow edema associated with osteoid osteomas, and STIR images can be used to screen for this reactive edema. Thin section CT may be necessary to identify intracortical lesions, however.

Osteoblastoma. Initially known as giant osteoid osteoma, osteoblastoma commonly presents in patients between 10 and 20 years of age.[20,24] Local pain is inconsistently relieved with salicylates. Osteoblastoma most frequently involves the flat bones or posterior osseous elements of the vertebrae. Histologically, osteoblastomas present a more variable picture than osteoid osteomas. There is well-vascularized connective tissue containing osteoid and primitive woven bone rimmed by osteoblasts. In contrast to osteoid osteoma, trabecular maturation, degree of calcification, and overall architectural patterns vary greatly in osteoblastoma.[20] A diffuse inflammatory response involving bone and adjacent soft tissue was reported in one MR study of a case of vertebral osteoblastoma.[25] Heterogeneity or homogeneity of signal intensity

may be seen on T2-weighted images. Computed tomography may be more accurate in identifying small foci of matrix calcification.

Benign Chondroblastic Lesions

Enchondroma. Enchondromas are benign intramedullary lesions composed of circumscribed lobules of hyaline cartilage that occasionally exhibits flecks of calcification. Cellularity may be increased in tumors in children and adolescents, but these histologic features do not imply chondrosarcoma. Radiologic findings are critical for accurate diagnosis.[26] Approximately 40% to 65% of solitary enchondromas occur in the hands, and approximately 25% occur in the long tubular bones.[20,26] Multiple enchondromatosis (*i.e.,* Ollier's disease) was originally described in 1899. This rare, nonhereditary disorder is characterized by multiple asymmetric chondromatous lesions. In childhood, these lesions predispose the bone to fracture; in adulthood, there is an increased risk (about 30% to 50%) of malignant transformation.[27] Lesions that continue to grow after the cessation of normal body growth should raise the suspicion of malignant transformation.

Magnetic Resonance Appearance. Magnetic resonance imaging is useful in identifying enchondromas, which are well defined with low signal intensity on T1-weighted images. Satellite cartilaginous foci are often seen in association with enchondromas. Chondroid elements demonstrate hyperintensity on T2-weighted, T2*-weighted, or STIR images (Figs. 13–7 and 13–8). In the multiple enchondromas of Ollier's disease, the foci of cartilaginous tissue or matrix are seen as areas of low to intermediate signal intensity on T1-weighted images and high signal intensity on T2-weighted images (Figs. 13–9 and 13–10). This appearance is secondary to the long T1 and T2 relaxation times of chondroid tissue. Enchondromas in Ollier's disease may show aggressive features (*e.g.,* cortical irregularities) without malignant degeneration (see Fig. 13–9). Enchondromas are common in the tubular bones of the hands and feet (Fig. 13–11).

Enchondromas can be differentiated from bone infarcts by the following features:

The lack of central fat signal intensity on T1-weighted images
Peripheral borders that are not as serpiginous as those seen in infected tissue
Central areas of increased signal intensity on T2-weighted images.[28,29]

Central calcifications are best seen on T2*-weighted images (Fig. 13–12). However, it is difficult to differentiate enchondroma from low-grade chondrosarcoma on the basis of signal intensity alone. The presence of a positive bone scan in the absence of pain cannot be used as

(text continues on page 1042)

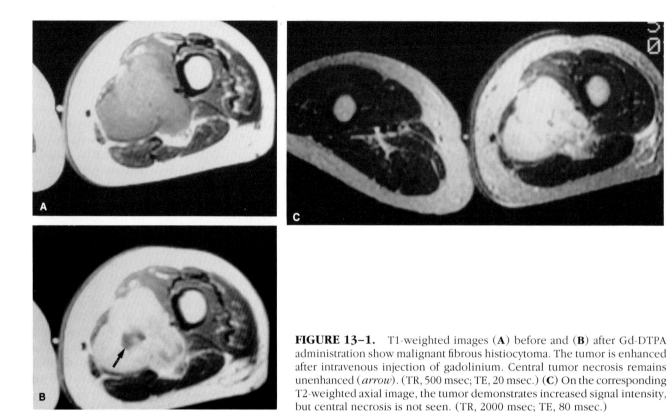

FIGURE 13–1. T1-weighted images (**A**) before and (**B**) after Gd-DTPA administration show malignant fibrous histiocytoma. The tumor is enhanced after intravenous injection of gadolinium. Central tumor necrosis remains unenhanced (*arrow*). (TR, 500 msec; TE, 20 msec.) (**C**) On the corresponding T2-weighted axial image, the tumor demonstrates increased signal intensity, but central necrosis is not seen. (TR, 2000 msec; TE, 80 msec.)

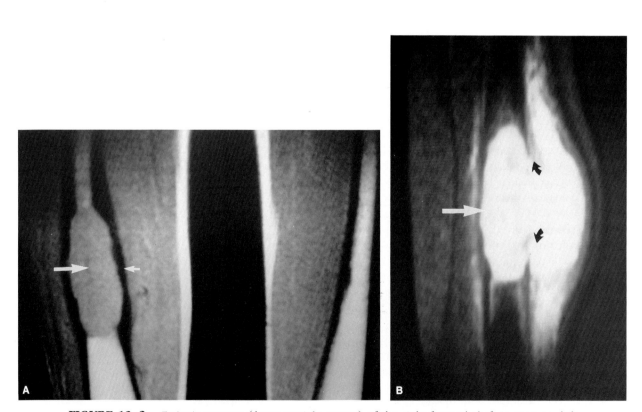

FIGURE 13–2. Ewing's sarcoma (*large straight arrows*) of the right femoral shaft is seen on (**A**) coronal T1-weighted and (**B**) sagittal short TI inversion recovery (STIR) images. Cortical thickening (*small straight arrow*) demonstrates low signal intensity on the coronal T1-weighted image. Histologically confirmed hyperintense subcortical tumor infiltration (*curved arrows*) is identified with STIR contrast. (**A:** TR, 600 msec; TE, 30 msec; **B:** TR, 1400 msec; TI = 100 msec; TE, 40 msec.)

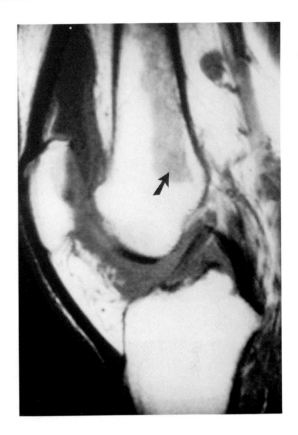

FIGURE 13–3. Red marrow inhomogeneity (*arrow*) without extension across the physeal scar can be seen in the diaphysis and metaphysis of the femur on a T1-weighted sagittal image. (TR, 600 msec, TE, 20 msec.)

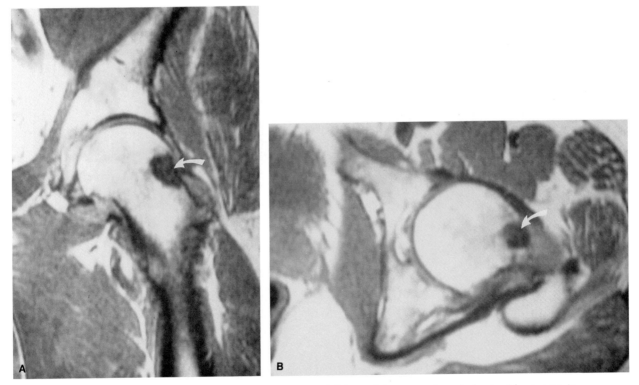

FIGURE 13–4. On T1-weighted (**A**) coronal and (**B**) axial images, subcortical osteoid osteoma is seen as a low signal intensity nidus (*curved arrows*) in the left femoral neck. (TR, 600 msec; TE, 20 msec.)

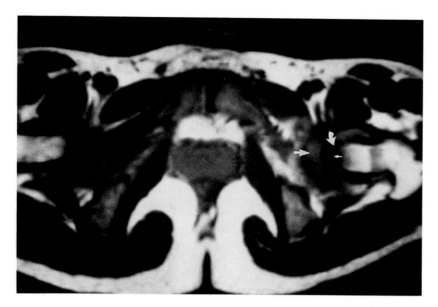

FIGURE 13–5. An intracortical osteoid osteoma of the left femoral neck with a circular nidus of intermediate signal intensity (*small straight arrow*), low signal intensity cortical thickening (*curved straight arrow*), and intermediate signal intensity effusion (*large arrow*) is seen on a T1-weighted axial image. (TR, 600 msec; TE, 20 msec.)

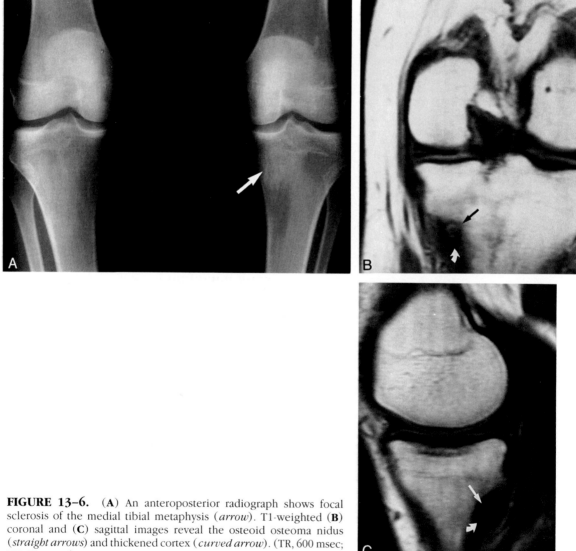

FIGURE 13–6. (**A**) An anteroposterior radiograph shows focal sclerosis of the medial tibial metaphysis (*arrow*). T1-weighted (**B**) coronal and (**C**) sagittal images reveal the osteoid osteoma nidus (*straight arrows*) and thickened cortex (*curved arrow*). (TR, 600 msec; TE, 20 msec.)

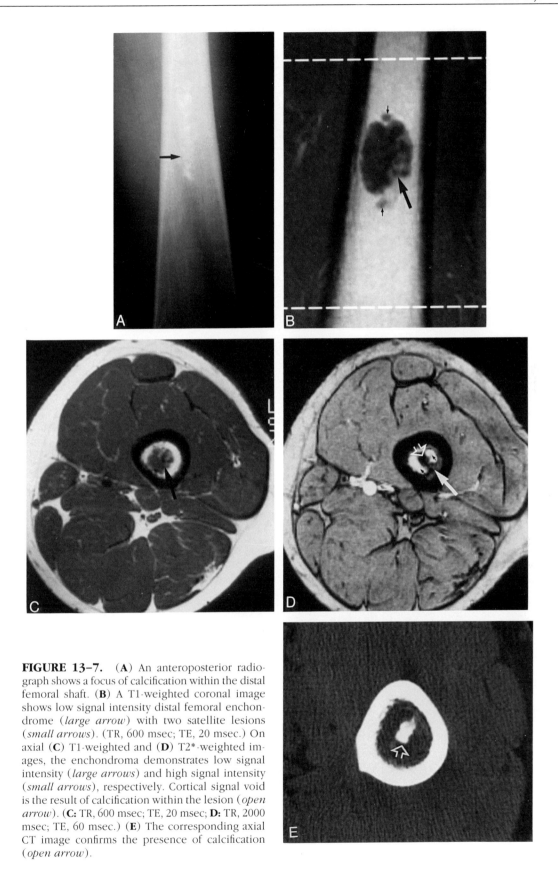

FIGURE 13–7. (**A**) An anteroposterior radiograph shows a focus of calcification within the distal femoral shaft. (**B**) A T1-weighted coronal image shows low signal intensity distal femoral enchondrome (*large arrow*) with two satellite lesions (*small arrows*). (TR, 600 msec; TE, 20 msec.) On axial (**C**) T1-weighted and (**D**) T2*-weighted images, the enchondroma demonstrates low signal intensity (*large arrows*) and high signal intensity (*small arrows*), respectively. Cortical signal void is the result of calcification within the lesion (*open arrow*). (**C:** TR, 600 msec; TE, 20 msec; **D:** TR, 2000 msec; TE, 60 msec.) (**E**) The corresponding axial CT image confirms the presence of calcification (*open arrow*).

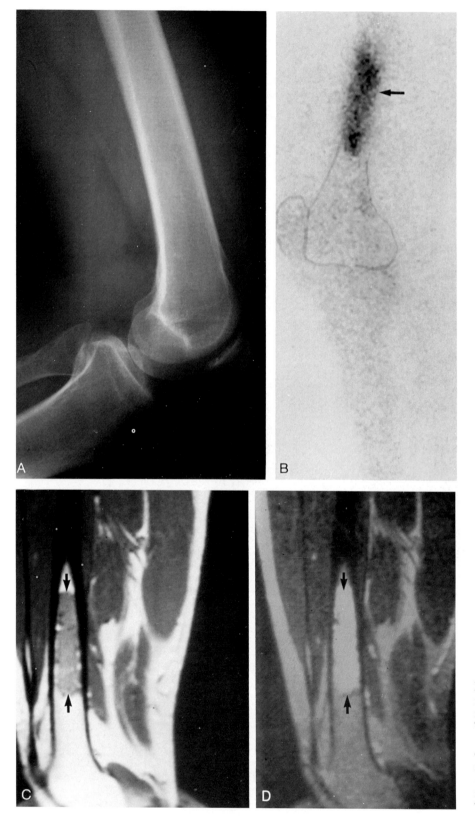

FIGURE 13–8. (**A**) A lateral radiograph is unremarkable for enchondroma. (**B**) On nuclear scintigraphy, there is uptake of ^{99m}TC-MDP bone tracer in the distal femur (*arrow*). On MR scans, benign enchondroma (*arrows*) demonstrates (**C**) low signal intensity on a T1-weighted image and (**D**) high signal intensity on a T2-weighted image. (**C:** TR, 1000 msec; TE, 20 msec; **D:** TR, 2000 msec; TE, 60 msec.)

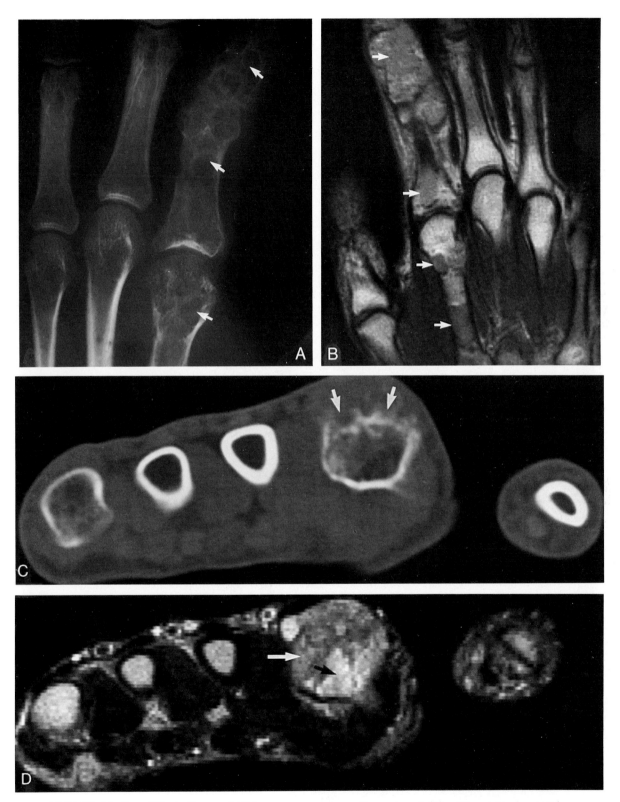

FIGURE 13–9. Ollier's disease. (**A**) An anteroposterior radiograph and (**B**) a T1-weighted coronal image show multiple enchondromatous foci (*arrows*) in the second ray. (**B:** TR, 1000 msec; TE, 40 msec.) (**C**) The corresponding axial CT image shows cortical irregularity (*arrows*). (**D**) On an axial spin-echo T2-weighted sequence, increased signal intensity is seen in cartilaginous foci (*black arrow*) within the affected digit (*white arrow*). (TR, 2000 msec; TE, 80 msec.)

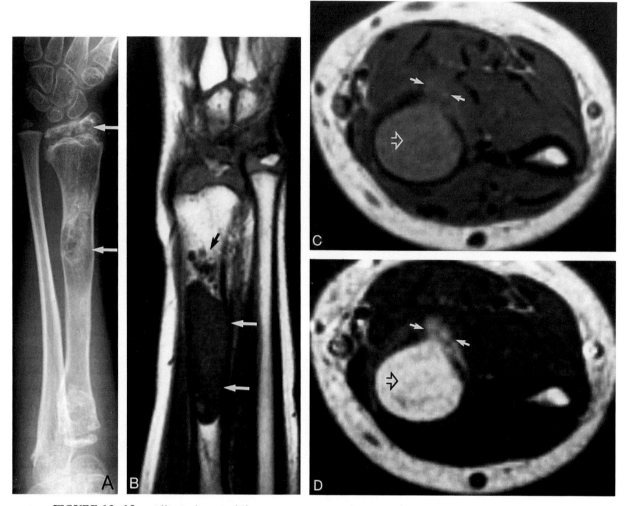

FIGURE 13–10. Ollier's disease. (**A**) An anteroposterior forearm radiograph demonstrates proximal and distal radius lesions (*arrows*). (**B**) A T1-weighted coronal image of distal radius lesions shows satellite enchondromas (*black arrow*) and a larger low signal intensity chondrosarcoma (*white arrows*). (TR, 600 msec; TE, 20 msec.) Chondrosarcoma (*open arrows*) on axial (**C**) T1-weighted and (**D**) T2-weighted images demonstrates low and high signal intensity, respectively, with disruption of cortical bone (*solid arrows*). (**C:** TR, 600 msec; TE, 20 msec; **D:** TR, 2000 msec; TE, 60 msec.)

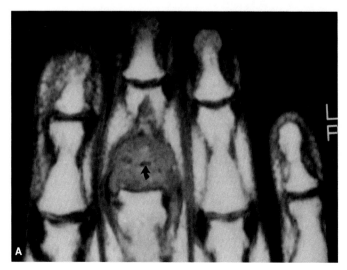

FIGURE 13–11. Expansile enchondroma of the base of the middle phalanx is seen on coronal (**A**) T1-weighted and (**B**) T2*-weighted images. Central calcification can be seen (*arrows*). (**C**) The corresponding CT image shows central stippled chondroid tumor calcification (*black arrow*) and cortical interruption (*white arrow*).

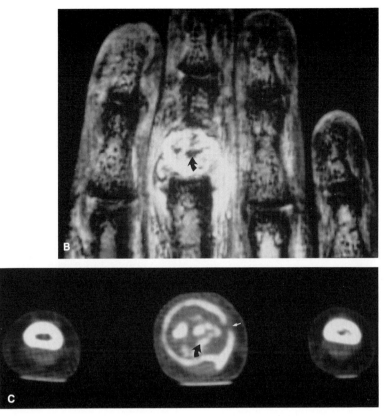

FIGURE 13–11. *(Continued)*

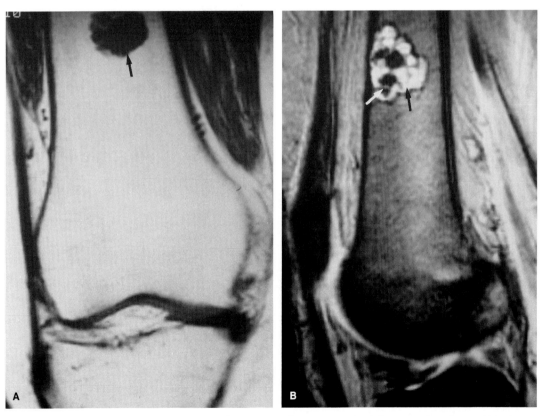

FIGURE 13–12. Central calcification (*white arrow*) occurs in distal femur enchondroma (*black arrows*). (**A**) Compared with a T1-weighted coronal image, the chondroid tissue is (**B**) hyperintense on a T2*-weighted sagittal image. (**A:** TR, 600 msec; TE, 20 msec; **B:** TR, 400 msec; TE, 15 msec; flip angle, 20°.)

a criteria for malignant conversion of enchondromas. Nonaggressive features include the absence of a soft-tissue mass and absence of interval growth on serial MR studies.

In juxtacortical or periosteal chondroma, soft-tissue calcification may mimic myositis ossificans (Fig. 13–13). Localized increases in signal intensity on T2-weighted images may occur without underlying involvement of the adjacent bone.

Osteochondroma. Osteocartilaginous exostosis (*i.e.,* osteochondroma) is one of the most common bone tumors in children. Solitary osteochondroma is a frequent lesion; opinions differ as to whether it represents a true neoplasm or a developmental physeal growth defect.[26] The vast majority of these lesions present in patients younger than 20 years of age. With the exception of a proliferative cartilage cap, the spongiosa and cortex in exostosis are continuous with the adjacent shaft. The thickness of the cartilaginous cap correlates with the age of the patient.[26] In children or adolescents, the cap may be as thick as 3 cm. In adults, however, the cap is thinner, presumably secondary to wear and tear. Findings of a cartilage cap thicker than 1 cm, an irregular cartilaginous cap, renewed growth with pain in an adult, or a combination of these raises the possibility of chondrosarcomatous transformation.[20,26,30,31] Such malignant transformation is rare in solitary osteochondroma, but has been reported with increased frequency in cases of multiple osteocartilaginous exostoses.

Magnetic Resonance Appearance. Osteochondromas are metaphyseal-based tumors that usually involve the long bones (Fig. 13–14). When the flat bones are involved, the lesion may present with a more cauliflower or expansile configuration (Figs. 13–15 and 13–16). On MR examination, benign osteochondromas are isointense with normal marrow. The intact cartilage cap demonstrates intermediate signal intensity on T1-weighted images and high signal intensity on T2-weighted images (see Fig. 13–14). With malignant degeneration, the signal intensity of the exostosis decreases on T1-weighted images and increases on T2-weighted images. Disruption of the high signal intensity cartilaginous cap may also be observed with aggressive tumor invasion. T2*-weighted sequences are useful in defining the thickness of high signal intensity cartilaginous cap, which may be as thick as 3 cm in adolescents and less than 1 cm in adults. Growth deformity is associated with multiple exostoses (Fig. 13–17).

Chondroblastoma. The benign chondroblastoma is an epiphyseal cartilage tumor that generally arises in a long tubular bone and occurs most frequently in the second decade of life.[32] Periarticular bone involvement can present with accompanying joint effusions. Histologic findings include a cellular proliferation of chondroblasts

with irregularly dispersed multinucleated osteoclast giant cells.[32] In 50% of cases, benign peripheral sclerosis, intralesional punctate, lacelike calcifications, and chondroid are present. Older lesions may exhibit necrosis, resorption, or reparative fibrosis with metaplastic osseous areas; this contributes to the variability seen in this lesion.

Magnetic Resonance Appearance. Benign chondroblastoma demonstrates a well-defined area of low signal intensity on T1-weighted images and heterogeneity with increased signal intensity in a noncalcified chondroid matrix on T2-weighted images (Figs. 13–18 and 13–19). Chondroblastoma characteristically involves the long-bone epiphyses of the humerus, tibia, and femur; MR imaging can be used to identify eccentric locations and the associated sclerotic border.[33] Epiphyseal and metaphyseal marrow edema associated with the diametaphyseal periosteal reaction is a frequent finding, seen in up to 57% of cases of long-bone involvement.[34] Magnetic resonance imaging is sensitive to this extensive reactive marrow edema, which demonstrates decreased signal intensity in T1-weighted images and increased signal intensity in T2-weighted or STIR images (Fig. 13–20).

Benign Fibrous and Related Lesions

Fibrous Cortical Defect. Fibrous cortical defects, histologically identical to large nonossifying fibromas (see Nonossifying Fibroma), demonstrate low to intermediate signal intensity on T1-weighted images and increased signal intensity on T2*-weighted images. The increased signal intensity observed on T2-weighted images is secondary to T2 prolongation in the varied cellular constituents (*e.g.,* fibrous stroma, multinucleated giant cells, foam cells, cholesterol crystals, stromal red blood cells in hemorrhage) (Fig. 13–21).[20]

Nonossifying Fibroma. Nonossifying fibromas are frequently found in the long bones of children and are thought to represent one end of the spectrum of benign cortical defects. Histologically, both nonossifying fibromas and fibrous cortical defects are composed of spindle-shaped fibroblasts arranged in interlacing patterns. On T1-weighted images, these lesions are low in signal intensity and have a lobulated contour with an eccentric epicenter (Figs. 13–22 and 13–23).

Gadolinium has been used to enhance the peripheral border in fibrous metaphyseal defects.[35] Benign fibrous histiocytomas, also histologically similar to nonossifying fibromas, present in an older population group and may be associated with symptoms of bone pain and local recurrence after treatment (Fig. 13–24).[33]

Ossifying Fibroma. Ossifying fibromas are benign fibro-osseous lesions that most commonly arise in the facial bones of young females.[20] These lesions, as opposed to fibrous dysplasia, are well demarcated and therefore amenable to surgical curettage and enucleation. The histologic features of this lesion consist of random trabecular woven bone or dystrophic calcification set in a fibrous stroma.

Fibrous and Osseous Fibrous Dysplasia. Fibrous and osseous fibrous dysplasias demonstrate low signal intensity on T1-weighted images and increased signal intensity on T2-weighted images (Fig. 13–25). The lesions are bordered by a thick, low signal intensity sclerotic border and may demonstrate homogeneous increased signal intensity that is less than that of fluid on T2-weighted images (Fig. 13–26). The intracortical cystic lesions of osseous fibrous dysplasia may mimic adamantinoma and demonstrate heterogeneity on T2-weighted images (Fig. 13–27). Fibrous dysplasia may exhibit monostotic or polyostotic involvement. The femoral neck is a common location for monostotic fibrous dysplasia.

Miscellaneous Benign Tumors and Non-neoplastic Lesions

Unicameral Bone Cyst. A solitary unicameral bone cyst enters into the differential diagnosis of benign bone lesions. In patients younger than 16 years of age, unicameral bone cysts may occur in the proximal humerus or femur, in close proximity to the cartilaginous growth plate, and they may recur following surgical removal. Malignancy in a solitary unicameral bone cyst has been reported, but it is extremely rare.

Magnetic Resonance Appearance. The unicameral bone cyst has a characteristic MR appearance. On T1-weighted images, it is well defined and demonstrates low signal intensity secondary to simple fluid within the cyst. On T2-weighted images, the fluid contents demonstrate uniformly increased signal intensity (Figs. 13–28 and 13–29). Internal hemorrhage may alter T1 and T2 signal characteristics. A low signal intensity peripheral border representing reactive sclerosis often demarcates this lesion.[33] Although fracture may occur as a complication, there should be no associated soft-tissue mass.

Aneurysmal Bone Cyst. The aneurysmal bone cyst is an expansile, blood-filled lesion that is osteolytic on conventional radiographs. In the hip or pelvis, aggressive cortical expansion and soft-tissue extension may simulate a malignant process or pseudotumor. Aneurysmal bone cysts, which occur in children and young adults (approximately 80% occur in patients younger than 20 years of age), are most commonly found in the posterior osseous elements of the vertebrae and the shafts of the long bones.[36] They are reported to involve the femur in 13% of cases and the innominate bone in 9% of cases. Aneurysmal bone cysts contain varying amounts of blood, fluid, and fibrous tissue. In many cases, they arise from preexisting bone lesions such as a giant cell tumor, osteoblastoma, chondroblastoma, fibrous dysplasia, or chondromyxoid fibroma.[36]

Histologic features include blood-filled channels supported by fibrous septa, which contains multinucleated giant cells and osteoid. Careful microscopic assessment is required to rule out the elusive telangiectatic variant of osteosarcoma, which may mimic an aneurysmal bone cyst both clinically and radiographically.[36-38] The favored theory regarding the pathogenesis of aneurysmal bone cysts suggests an altered vascular flow resulting in a local circulatory failure.[36]

Magnetic Resonance Appearance. On MR examination, aneurysmal bone cysts tend to be well circumscribed but heterogeneous, with areas of both low and high signal intensity.[39] The expansile lesion may have internal septations, a fluid level, and areas of bright signal intensity on both T1- and T2-weighted images, depending on the chronicity of the associated hemorrhage (Figs. 13–30 and 13–31).[40] Fluid–fluid levels have been identified in an expansile aneurysmal bone cyst of the distal tibia (Fig. 13–32). The fluid–fluid level probably represents layering of uncoagulated blood within the lesion.[41] On T1-weighted images, increased signal intensity in the gravity dependent layer represents methemoglobin. It may be difficult to exclude associated malignant tissue when severe inhomogeneity of signal intensity is observed. Cortical bowing and septation (*i.e.,* trabeculation) may be seen in a low signal intensity contour of cortical bone.

Hemangioma. Hemangiomas are benign bone lesions classified as capillary, cavernous, or venous vascular proliferations. Those hemangiomas that are highly cellular may be confused with a malignant vascular neoplasm.[42] Hemangiomas may occur in patients from 20 to 60 years of age, but the incidence increases after middle age. The spine and flat bones of the skull and mandible are most frequently involved. When there is vertebral involvement, standard radiographs demonstrate coarse vertical trabeculations with a corduroy-cloth appearance.

Magnetic Resonance Appearance. Hemangiomas are variable in appearance. On T1-weighted images, they can demonstrate low, intermediate, or high signal intensity (Fig. 13–33). There is usually some increase in signal intensity on T2-weighted or STIR images. Reinforced trabeculae are more difficult to appreciate on MR than CT scans.

Intraosseous Lipoma. Intraosseous lipomas are rare, constituting approximately 0.1% of bone tumors.[17] Approximately 10% of these are discovered within the calcaneus.[17] Both simple bone cysts and lipomas exhibit a pyramidal shape and are situated in the center of the trigonum calcis, which raises the question of some form

(text continues on page 1058)

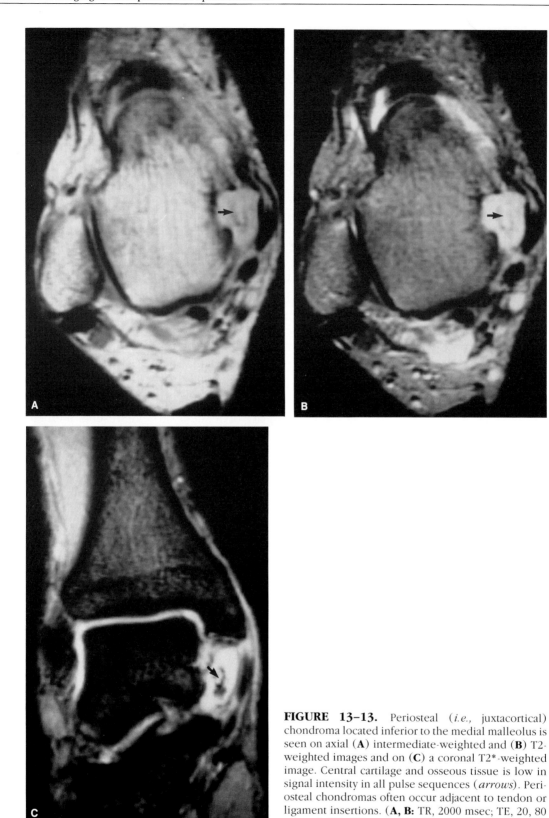

FIGURE 13–13. Periosteal (*i.e.,* juxtacortical) chondroma located inferior to the medial malleolus is seen on axial (**A**) intermediate-weighted and (**B**) T2-weighted images and on (**C**) a coronal T2*-weighted image. Central cartilage and osseous tissue is low in signal intensity in all pulse sequences (*arrows*). Periosteal chondromas often occur adjacent to tendon or ligament insertions. (**A, B:** TR, 2000 msec; TE, 20, 80 msec; **C:** TR, 400 msec; TE, 20 msec; flip angle, 25°.)

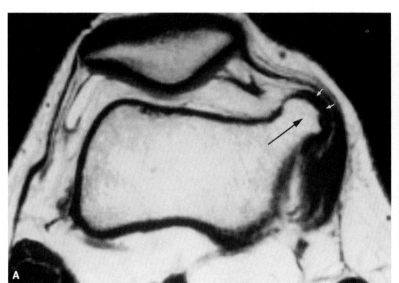

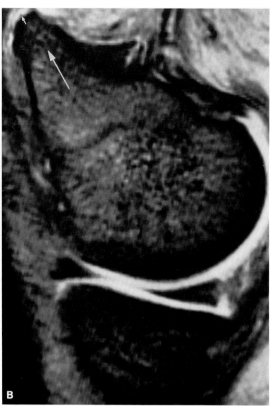

FIGURE 13–14. Osteochondroma. Metaphyseal exostosis with continuity of marrow and cortex (*long arrows*) is present. The cartilage cap (*short arrows*) demonstrates (**A**) low to intermediate signal intensity on a T1-weighted image and (**B**) high signal intensity on a T2*-weighted image. (**A:** TR, 600 msec; TE, 20 msec; **B:** TR, 400 msec; TE, 15 msec; flip angle, 20°.)

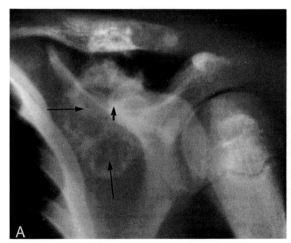

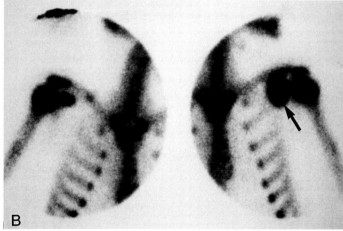

FIGURE 13–15. Benign osteochondroma. (**A**) An anteroposterior radiograph shows a cauliflowerlike bony excrescence (*long arrows*) arising from the coracoid process (*short arrow*). (**B**) Nuclear scintigraphy shows increased uptake of bone tracer in region of left coracoid. (**C**) On an axial CT image, the enlarged cartilage cap (*white arrows*) can be seen continuous with cortex and spongiosa of adjacent bone (*open arrow*). (**D**) On a T1-weighted coronal image, a low signal intensity mass can been seen emanating from the low spin density coracoid (*white arrow*). The cartilage cap is difficult to distinguish from the cortex without a T2-weighted pulse sequence. (TR, 600 msec; TE, 20 msec.) *(continued)*

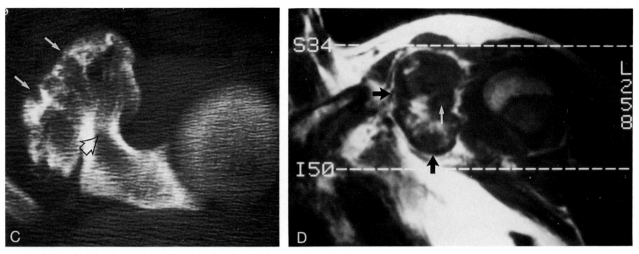

FIGURE 13–15. *(Continued)*

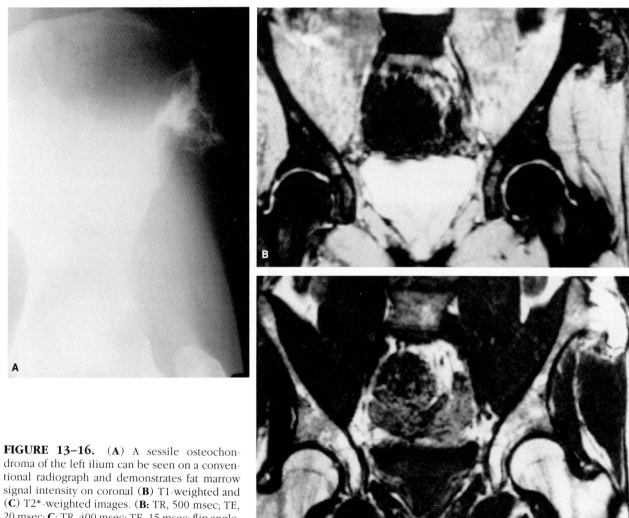

FIGURE 13–16. (**A**) A sessile osteochondroma of the left ilium can be seen on a conventional radiograph and demonstrates fat marrow signal intensity on coronal (**B**) T1-weighted and (**C**) T2*-weighted images. (**B:** TR, 500 msec; TE, 20 msec; **C:** TR, 400 msec; TE, 15 msec; flip angle, 20°.)

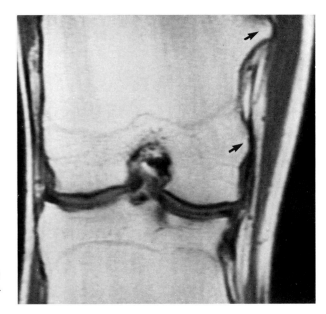

FIGURE 13–17. Undertubulation of the knee and exostosis (*arrows*) are seen on a T1-weighted coronal image of multiple hereditary exostosis. (TR, 600 msec; TE, 20 msec.)

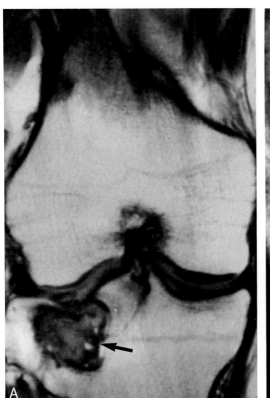

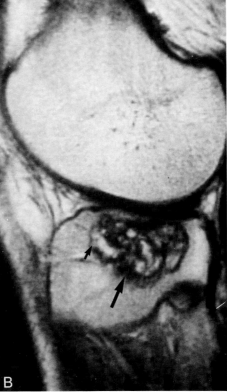

FIGURE 13–18. (**A**) On a T1-weighted image, chondroblastoma of the tibial epiphysis (*arrow*) demonstrates intermediate signal intensity. (TR, 600 msec; TE, 20 msec.) (**B**) On a T2-weighted sagittal image, the chondroblastoma (*large arrow*) demonstrates nonuniform increased signal intensity (*small arrow*). (TR, 2000 msec; TE, 60 msec.)

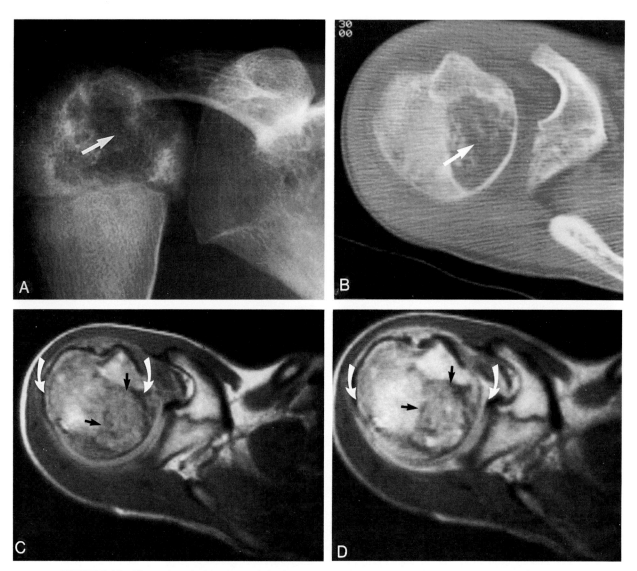

FIGURE 13–19. Chondroblastoma of the humeral epiphysis is identified as a lytic defect (*arrows*) on (**A**) an anteroposterior radiograph and (**B**) an axial CT scan. On a T2-weighted sequence, a cartilage tumor (*straight black arrows*) of the humeral head (*curved white arrows*) (**C**) demonstrates low to intermediate signal intensity on the first echo and (**D**) is an inhomogeneous area of mixed signal intensity on the second echo. (TR, 1500 msec; TE, 20, 60 msec.)

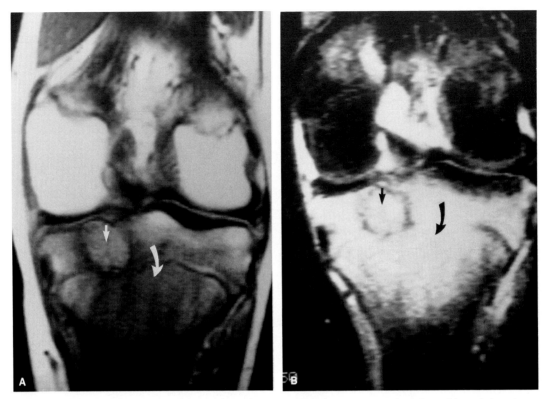

FIGURE 13–20. Extensive marrow edema (*curved arrows*) in reaction to epiphyseal-based chondroblastoma (*straight arrows*) demonstrates (**A**) low signal intensity on a T1-weighted image and (**B**) hyperintensity on a short TI inversion recovery image.

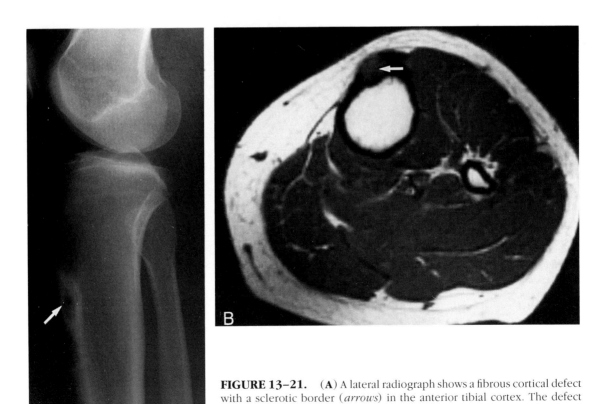

FIGURE 13–21. (**A**) A lateral radiograph shows a fibrous cortical defect with a sclerotic border (*arrows*) in the anterior tibial cortex. The defect demonstrates low and high signal intensity on axial (**B**) T1-weighted and (**C**) T2-weighted images, respectively.

(continued)

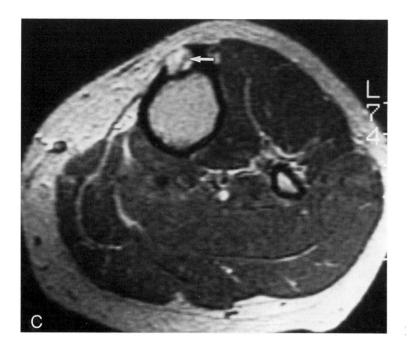

FIGURE 13-21. *(Continued)*

FIGURE 13-22. (**A**) An antero-posterior radiograph shows the scle-rotic border (*straight arrows*) of a nonossifying fibroma. An incidental biopsy site for Ewing's sarcoma can also be seen (*curved arrow*). (**B**) A T1-weighted image shows lobulated low signal intensity in the distal femoral metaphysis (*arrows*). (TR, 600 msec; TE, 20 msec.)

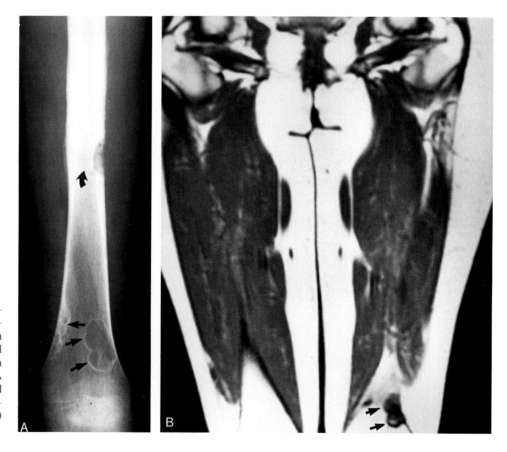

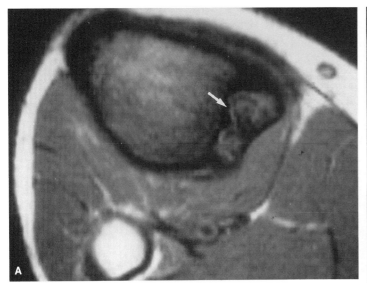

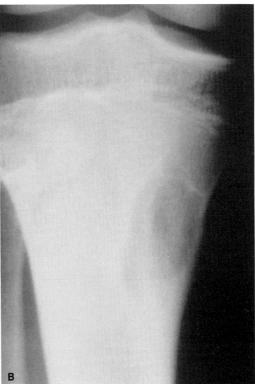

FIGURE 13–23. (**A**) A T1-weighted axial image shows nonossifying fibroma with a pathologic fracture. (TR, 500 msec; TE, 20 msec.) (**B**) The corresponding anteroposterior radiograph displays the eccentric location of the lesion.

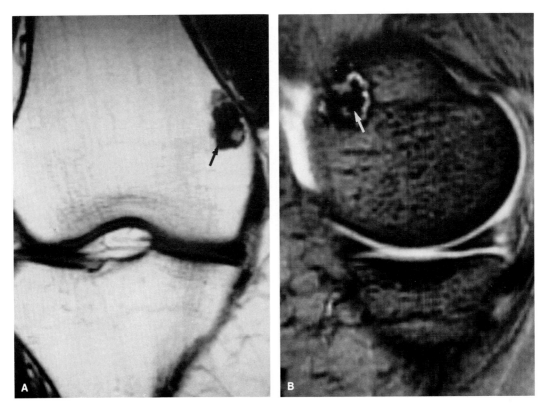

FIGURE 13–24. A clinically benign fibrous histiocytoma (*arrows*) may present with pain. MR characteristics are the same as those of a nonossifying fibroma: low signal intensity on (**A**) coronal T1-weighted and (**B**) sagittal T2* images. (**A:** TR, 500 msec; TE, 20 msec; **B:** TR, 400 msec; TE, 15 msec; flip angle, 20°.)

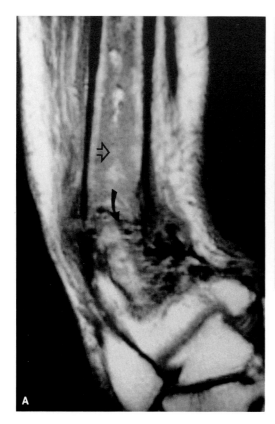

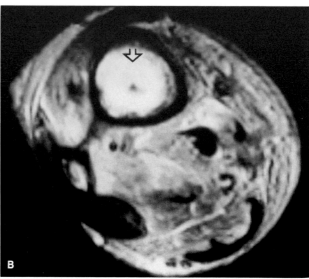

FIGURE 13–25. Fibrous dysplasia (*open arrows*) with pathologic fracture (*curved arrow*) involving the distal tibial diaphysis and metaphysis is present. Fibrous tissue expansion of the medullary cavity demonstrates (**A**) low to intermediate in signal intensity on a coronal T1-weighted image and (**B**) bright in signal intensity on an axial T2-weighted image.

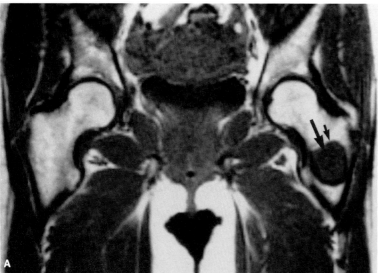

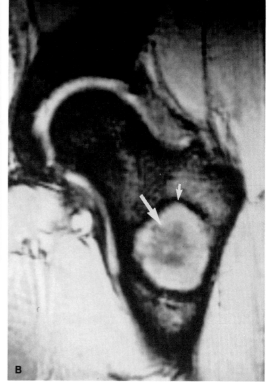

FIGURE 13–26. Monostotic fibrous dysplasia (*large arrows*) of the left femoral neck—a common location—demonstrates (**A**) low signal intensity on a coronal T1-weighted image and (**B**) increased signal intensity on a coronal T2*-weighted image. Note the central area of lower signal intensity on the T2*-weighted image and the thick cortical low signal intensity sclerotic rind (*small arrows*).

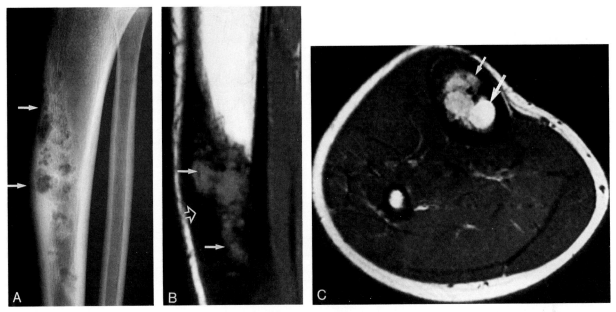

FIGURE 13–27. (**A**) A lateral radiograph shows a sclerotic, bubbly lesion in the anterior tibial shaft (*arrows*). (**B**) A T1-weighted sagittal image shows intermediate signal intensity osseous fibrous dysplasia (*solid arrows*) and low signal intensity thickened cortical tissue (*open arrow*). (TR, 600 msec; TE, 20 msec.) (**C**) A T2-weighted axial image shows increased signal intensity within fibrous dysplasia (*small arrow*), separate from the tibial shaft (*large arrow*). (TR, 2000 msec; TE, 60 msec.)

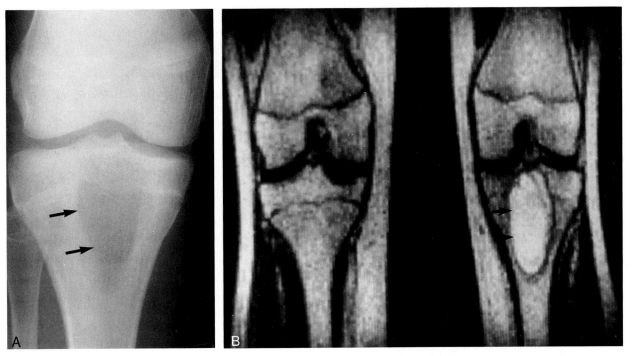

FIGURE 13–28. Unicameral bone cyst. (**A**) An anteroposterior radiograph shows a lytic lesion in tibial metaphysis (*arrows*). (**B**) A T2-weighted coronal image shows uniform increased signal intensity within the cyst fluid contents (*arrows*). (TR, 2000 msec; TE, 60 msec.)

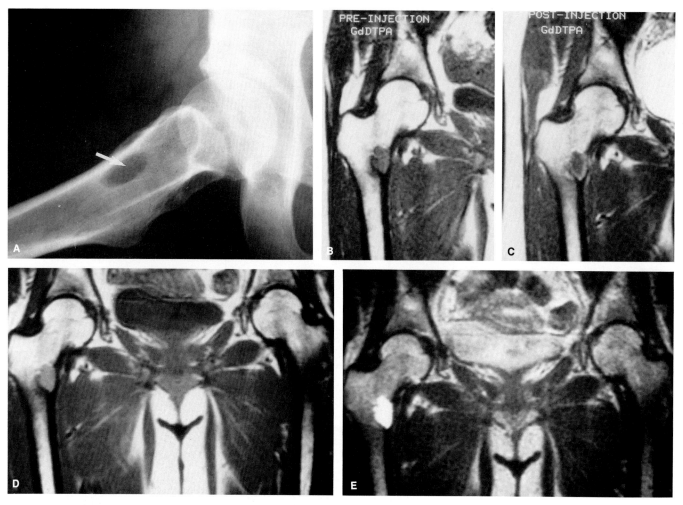

FIGURE 13–29. (**A**) A simple bone cyst (*arrow*) is oriented with the long axis of the femur. T1-weighted images (**B**) before and (**C**) after Gd-DTPA administration show no increased signal intensity in the medial epicentered cyst. (TR, 500 msec; TE, 20 msec.) Coronal (**D**) intermediate-weighted and (**E**) T2-weighted images display a progressive increase in signal intensity. (**D, E:** TR, 2000 msec; TE, 20, 80 msec.)

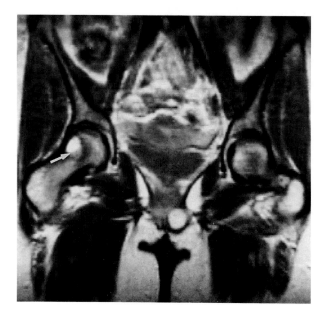

FIGURE 13–30. A T1-weighted coronal image shows an aneurysmal bone cyst. The hemorrhagic fluid–fluid level (*arrow*) is visualized with high and low signal intensity, as is characteristic of bone cysts. (TR, 1000 msec; TE, 40 msec.)

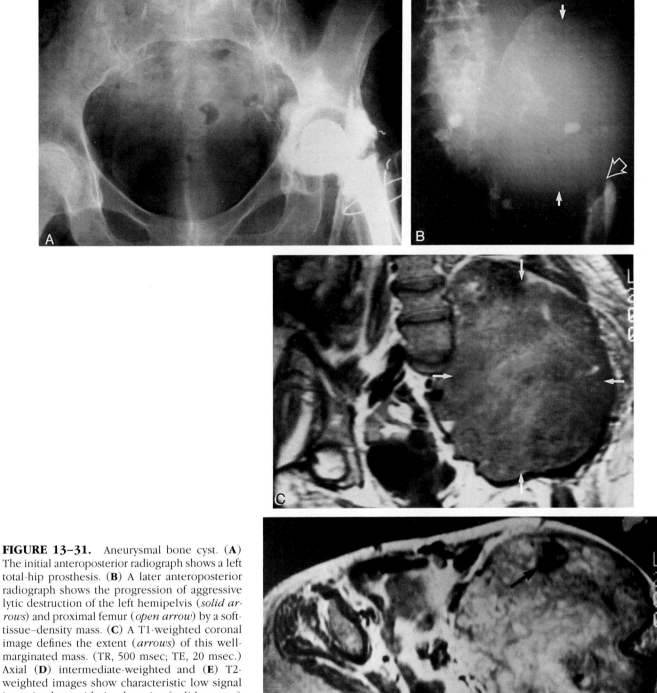

FIGURE 13–31. Aneurysmal bone cyst. (**A**) The initial anteroposterior radiograph shows a left total-hip prosthesis. (**B**) A later anteroposterior radiograph shows the progression of aggressive lytic destruction of the left hemipelvis (*solid arrows*) and proximal femur (*open arrow*) by a soft-tissue–density mass. (**C**) A T1-weighted coronal image defines the extent (*arrows*) of this well-marginated mass. (TR, 500 msec; TE, 20 msec.) Axial (**D**) intermediate-weighted and (**E**) T2-weighted images show characteristic low signal intensity hemosiderin deposits (*solid arrows*) mixed with high signal intensity hemorrhagic elements (*open arrow*). (**D, E:** TR, 2000 msec; TE, 20, 60 msec.) (**F**) The corresponding axial CT image of the lesion (*arrows*) is nonspecific for hemorrhagic constituents.   (*continued*)

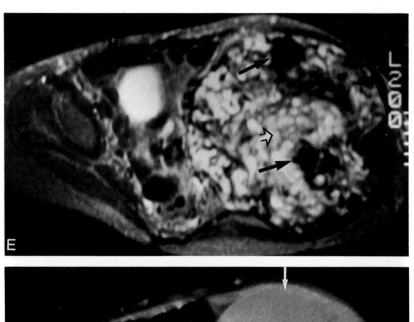

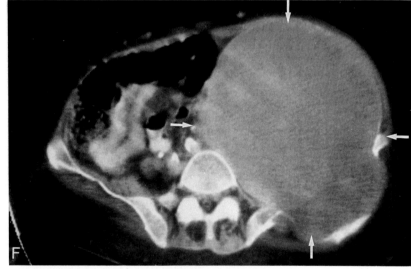

FIGURE 13–31. *(Continued)*

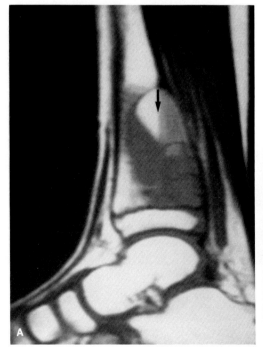

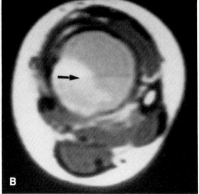

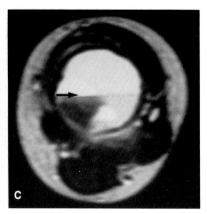

FIGURE 13–32.

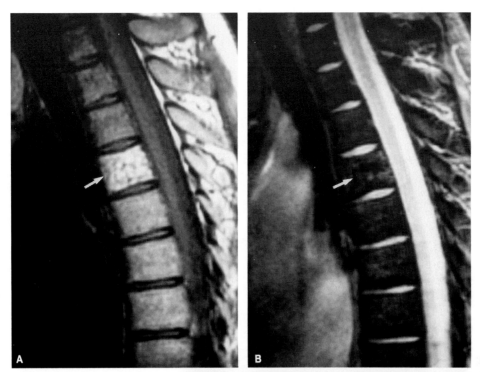

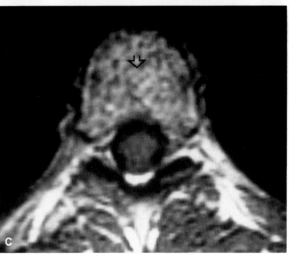

FIGURE 13–33. (**A**) A T1-weighted sagittal image shows thoracic vertebral body involvement with a bright signal intensity hemangioma (*arrow*). (TR, 600 msec; TE, 20 msec.) (**B**) The corresponding T2*-weighted sagittal image does not show significant increased signal intensity (*arrow*). Hemangiomas, however, frequently display increased signal intensity on T2-weighted or short TI inversion recovery images. (TR, 400 msec; TE, 15 msec; flip angle, 20°.) (**C**) The hemangioma (*arrow*) has a corduroy appearance on a T1-weighted axial image. (TR, 600 msec; TE, 20 msec.)

◄ **FIGURE 13–32.** A metaphyseal-based aneurysmal bone cyst is eccentric and expansile, with a hemorrhagic fluid–fluid level, (*arrows*) as seen on sagittal (**A**) T1-weighted and (**B**) intermediate-weighted images and (**C**) an axial T2-weighted image.

of relationship between the two entities. However, the precise explanation remains uncertain.[17]

The staging classification for intraosseous lipomas incorporates three categories based on the degree of histologic involvement.[17,43]

In stage 1 tumors, viable fat cells can be demonstrated.
In stage 2 tumors, there are both viable fat cells and mixed areas of fat necrosis and calcification.
In stage 3 tumors, necrotic fat, calcification, cyst formation, and reactive woven bone are present.

Magnetic Resonance Appearance. An intraosseous lipoma can be differentiated from a simple cyst in the calcaneus by diffuse fat signal intensity or a thick rind of adipose tissue. This tissue demonstrates bright signal intensity on T1-weighted images, and circumscribes a central hemorrhagic component, which demonstrates low signal intensity on T1-weighted images and bright signal intensity on T2-weighted images (Figs. 13–34 and 13–35). In addition to their appearance in the calcaneus, intraosseous lipomas are known to affect the long tubular bones, including the fibula, tibia, and femur (Fig. 13–36). Intraosseous lipomas demonstrate the same signal intensity as that of fat (*i.e.,* bright on T1-weighted images and intermediate on T2-weighted images), and therefore appear black on STIR images, for which fat signal intensity is nulled.

Bone Infarct. Bone infarcts, usually metaphyseal-based, are circumscribed by a serpiginous low-signal intensity border that corresponds to the rim of reactive sclerosis that is often detected in plain radiographs (Fig. 13–37).[44] In the acute and subacute stages, signal from the central island of the infarct is isointense with fatty marrow signal. T2 weighting may demonstrate linear bright signal parallel with the outline of the lesions. Except for location, the imaging characteristics of subarticular degeneration and sclerosis may be similar to those seen in bone infarcts.

Eosinophilic Granuloma. The solitary and diffuse lesions of eosinophilic granuloma may be confused with osteomyelitis or Ewing's sarcoma on MR images. Subperiosteal new bone and high signal intensity peritumoral edema have been identified on both T1- and T2-weighted images (Fig. 13–38).[45] The site for histiocytic proliferation demonstrates increased signal intensity on T2-weighted images.

Benign/Malignant Lesions

Giant Cell Tumor

Giant cell tumors exhibit unpredictable biologic behavior. They can be aggressive, and are usually treated by surgical removal. Forty percent recur locally, and approximately 10% to 20% have potential for malignant transformation.[46] Others exhibit local soft-tissue extension or systemic tumor implantation. The majority of these tumors are seen in patients 20 to 40 years of age.[46,47] The long tubular bones are most commonly affected. Giant cell tumors commonly present about the knee (*e.g.,* distal femur, proximal tibia) and abut the subchondral bone.[48] When spinal bones are involved, there is a predilection for anterior elements (*i.e.,* vertebral bodies). Giant cell tumors of bone originate in the distal metaphysis of the long bones and abut the physeal plate.[49] They do not occur in or cross the physis prior to fusion of the epiphysis and metaphysis, at which time the tumor occupies a subchondral position.

Histologically, these lesions exhibit a uniform distribution of giant cells against a cellular background of ovoid spindle stromal cells that exhibit mitotic activity. Osteoid foci can be seen within these lesions, and are usually associated with areas of hemorrhage or within a fracture callus.[46] The pathologic histologic grading system which was instituted at one time in an attempt to predict the biologic aggressiveness of these lesions, has fallen out of favor in light of unpredictable behavior in the presence of histologically benign features. Tumor implantation at distant sites, typically the lungs, in patients with histologically benign giant cell tumors occurs in approximately 1% to 3% of cases.[46] These are regarded as passive vascular transports related to surgical curettage. If these pulmonary lesions are identical histologically to the primary giant cell tumor, they generally do not lead to the demise of the patient.

Malignant transformation, which can occur in a previously benign-appearing giant cell tumor, usually occurs following irradiation of the original tumor.[11,13,15,16]

Magnetic Resonance Appearance. The MR appearance of giant cell tumors of the long bones is generally well defined. In MR images, giant cell tumors demonstrate low to intermediate signal intensity in T1-weighted images and high signal intensity in T2-weighted images (Figs. 13–39 and 13–40).[49] Heterogeneity in T2-weighted images may represent central areas of liquefaction, hemorrhage, or necrosis (Figs. 13–41 and 13–42).

Gradient refocused images may help to identify areas of tumor recurrence after excision and packing with methylmethacrylate (Fig. 13–43). In one case, a cystic giant cell tumor of the calcaneus demonstrated low to intermediate signal intensity on T1-weighted sequences and high signal intensity on T2-weighted sequences (Fig. 13–44). A fluid–fluid level was identified in this lesion on MR scans, but it was not revealed on corresponding CT sections.[50] Areas of necrosis (*i.e.,* signal inhomogeneity), cortical erosion, and associated effusions may be characterized in MR images. Intratumoral hemorrhage may produce bright signal intensity on T1- and T2-weighted images, although the tumor generally demonstrates low signal intensity on T1-weighted images and increased signal intensity on T2-weighted images.

Soft-tissue involvement and rare joint invasion can be evaluated with pretherapeutic MR staging.[51] A thin rim of sclerotic bone may be identified at the tumor interface with uninvolved fatty marrow in less aggressive lesions. Contrast inhomogeneity and multilobular configuration was seen in one case of giant cell tumor involving the flat pubic bone of the pelvis.

Malignant Lesions

Since the primary component of most malignant bone tumors has prolonged T1 and T2 tissue relaxation times, these tumors demonstrate low signal intensity on T1-weighted images and bright signal intensity on T2-weighted images.[1] Nonuniformity of signal intensity is most evident on T2-weighted images in the areas of necrosis or hemorrhage. Neurovascular bundle encasement, peritumoral edema, and irregular margins are secondary evidence of the malignant nature of these lesions. Except in cases of postradiation marrow edema, extensive marrow involvement by edema or tumor is highly suggestive of either a malignancy or an infection.

When there is marrow involvement in neoplastic or inflammatory disease, the MR signal characteristics depend on whether the marrow in the affected limb is yellow or red. On T1-weighted images, neoplastic or inflammatory involvement of yellow marrow demonstrates low signal intensity within or adjacent to bright marrow fat and increased signal intensity with progressive T2 weighting. When the affected limb is primarily red marrow, however, lesions often appear isointense with normal hematopoietic marrow on T1-weighted images and bright on T2-weighted images.

In the postoperative evaluation of malignant neoplasms, there may be some initial edema and inflammatory changes that demonstrate low signal intensity on T1-weighted images and bright signal intensity on T2-weighted images. This bright signal intensity on T2-weighted images is feathery, infiltrative, and conforms to the contour of the muscle. With increased time, the surgical field is replaced with fibrous tissue that demonstrates low to intermediate signal intensity on T1- and T2-weighted scans. Postoperative hematomas and seromas are well margined, confined to the region of surgery, and demonstrate uniform increased signal intensity with long TR and TE settings. Chronic hemorrhage with hemosiderin deposits remains dark on T1- and T2-weighted images because of the paramagnetic effect of iron.

Certain MR changes, including the following, strongly suggest tumor recurrence:

The reappearance of edema, characterized by low signal intensity on T1-weighted images and bright signal intensity on T2-weighted images

A new area of increased signal intensity on T2-weighted images with a corresponding area of intermediate signal intensity on T1-weighted images

A change in the contour of a muscle or postoperative surgical field, such that the margins are convex instead of concave.

Osteosarcoma

Osteosarcoma is the most common primary malignant bone tumor in childhood. Excluding multiple myeloma, osteosarcomas are the most common primary malignancy of bone and are considered one of the most aggressive and histologically varied neoplasms. The identifying feature of all osteosarcomas is the presence of malignant stromal cells that produce osteoid. From a clinical viewpoint, there are two main categories, primary (*i.e., de novo*) and secondary osteosarcomas.[27,52]

Primary Osteosarcoma. Primary (*i.e., de novo*) conventional osteosarcomas predominantly affect individuals younger than 20 years of age. There is a slight predominance in males. In 96% of cases, the tumor develops in the long bones and limbs. The lesion is usually metaphyseal, destroys trabecular and cortical bone, invades the soft tissues, and may extend into the epiphysis.[52]

The role of genetic factors in the pathogenesis of osteosarcoma is of interest, especially in children. Those patients with genetic retinoblastoma who show a point mutation at chromosome 13q14 band demonstrate a 500-fold increased risk of developing osteosarcoma.[31] Cytogenic and molecular genetics have uncovered the Rb gene, a tumor suppressor gene that plays a role in the pathogenesis of osteosarcoma.[31] Suppression of the p53 gene appears to be common in osteosarcoma.[53]

Secondary Osteosarcoma. Osteosarcoma that occurs in older individuals (*i.e.,* secondary osteosarcoma) arises in a setting of preexisting bone disease (*e.g.,* Paget's disease, bone infarcts) or after exposure to a mutagenic event such as irradiation (Fig. 13–45). In osteosarcoma associated with Paget's disease, bones other than the long bones (*e.g.,* the pelvis, skull, facial bones, scapula) are involved. Osteosarcomas arising in Paget's disease have a poorer prognosis than more conventional *de novo* osteosarcomas.[31]

Classification. Several histologic patterns of osteosarcomas have been identified. Histologic assessment of telangiectatic osteosarcomas is especially difficult, because the viable cells and anaplastic cells are obscured by hemorrhage and necrosis or camouflaged within benign reactive cells of the walls, which simulates an aneurysmal bone cyst.[36,37] According to some investigators, telangiectatic osteosarcomas have a more aggressive clinical course. On conventional radiographs, the telangiectatic variant appears lytic because of the lack of demonstrable bone production. Magnetic resonance scans show an aggressive, destructive lesion, usually accompanied by an associated soft-tissue mass. The inhomogeneity of signal intensity with both low and high signal intensity areas on T1- and T2-weighted images reflect the high degree of vascularity and large hemorrhagic cystic spaces present (Fig. 13–46).

Approximately 10% of primary osteosarcomas are tremendously rich in bone production (*i.e.,* sclerosing or osteoblastic osteosarcoma).[52] At times, the bone and osteoid are deposited in massive solid amounts. Frequently, the mineralization extends into the soft tissues.[54] Blastic components remain low in signal intensity on T1- and T2-weighted images. Associated peritumoral edema or nonsclerotic areas, however, generate increased signal intensity on heavily T2-weighted or STIR images.

Chondroblastic osteosarcoma is seen in approximately 5% of cases.[52] The generation of chondroid elements, whether benign or malignant, contributes to increased signal intensity on T2-weighted images.

Osteosarcomas that produce large amounts of spindly fibroblasts are classified as fibroblastic osteosarcoma, which is seen in approximately 4% of cases.[52] Studies have reported no convincing evidence that chondroblastic or fibroblastic subtypes of osteosarcoma have different prognoses.[52]

Central, low-grade osteosarcoma, a rare type of osteosarcoma arising in medullary bone, is so well differentiated that it is frequently mistaken for a benign condition both radiologically and histopathologically. The patients are usually young adults and may have symptoms for years. Much of the lesion appears well circumscribed, simulating fibrous dysplasia. A search for small foci of cortical destruction may be paramount for accurate diagnosis. The prognosis in low-grade osteosarcoma is excellent. Metastasis occurs late, if ever; but local recurrences may be a serious problem if surgery is inadequate.[52] On MR scans, the low-grade central osteosarcoma may be difficult to distinguish from a conventional osteosarcoma, which has an identical radiographic appearance.

There are three additional subtypes of osteosarcomas, referred to as juxtacortical osteosarcomas. They account for 7% of all osteosarcomas and arise on the surface of the bone rather than within the medulla. These juxtacortical subtypes are:

- periosteal osteosarcoma
- parosteal osteosarcoma
- high-grade surface osteosarcoma.

Periosteal osteosarcoma, which accounts for 0.3% of all osteosarcomas, favors the diaphyseal surface of long tubular bones and forms an irregular thickened cortex. Histologically, hyaline chondrosarcomatous elements are a prominent feature.[55] Parosteal osteosarcoma, another rare form of osteosarcoma (0.8%) occurs most frequently on the metaphyseal surface of long tubular bones within the parosteal soft tissue, and forms a lobulated mass. Histologically, these subtypes are characterized by a fibrous proliferation surrounding parallel lamellar bony spicules. The fibrous component can appear externally bland, mimicking a fibrous dysplasia. As opposed to periosteal osteosarcoma, chondrosarcomatous elements are minimal or absent.[56,57]

Treatment. Management of patients with conventional osteosarcoma has changed drastically in the last 20 years, which has resulted in a significant improvement in prognosis. Preoperative chemotherapy has contributed to this change by facilitating conservative surgical procedures. The effectiveness of preoperative chemotherapy is assessed by evaluating the sensitivity of the tumor to chemotherapy. Although this can be approximated on a clinical and radiological basis, histopathologic assessment of the amount of tumor necrosis in the postresection specimen remains the best way to evaluate response.[53] Direct coronal or sagittal MR images of the tumor are also helpful in planning pre- or postoperative therapeutic regimens.

Magnetic Resonance Appearance. Magnetic resonance imaging affords superior soft-tissue discrimination in the evaluation of osteosarcoma. Osteosarcoma, chondrosarcoma, giant cell tumors, and Ewing's sarcoma are statistically the primary bone neoplasms that are likely to involve the lower extremities. The distal femur, proximal tibia, and humerus are common sites of involvement in conventional osteosarcoma (Fig. 13–47). With MR imaging, intramedullary marrow involvement, soft-tissue extension, skip-lesion metastases, and postoperative recurrence can be accurately assessed (Figs. 13–48 and 13–49). Marrow infiltration can be mapped on MR scans, even when standard radiographs are negative. In addition to occurring as a primary extremity neoplasm, osteosarcoma is a known complication of osteogenesis imperfecta, and tumoral callus may mimic osteosarcoma (see Fig. 13–45). Magnetic resonance imaging can be used to differentiate exuberant bone, which is isointense with yellow marrow, from osteosarcoma, which causes both T1 and T2 prolongation. On MR scans of an aggressive, dedifferentiated osteosarcoma, a necrotic, hemorrhagic fluid–fluid level was imaged within the more distal marrow cavity, a unique feature not demonstrated by corresponding CT (Fig. 13–50).

In many cases, evidence of tumor crossing the physis, not evident on conventional radiographs, has been

(text continues on page 1072)

FIGURE 13–34. An intraosseous lipoma is typically located between the anterior and middle one-thirds of the calcaneus. The increased signal intensity on a T1-weighted image is secondary to fat composition (*arrow*). (TR, 500 msec; TE, 20 msec.)

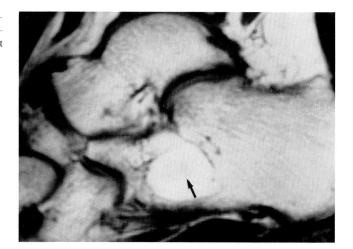

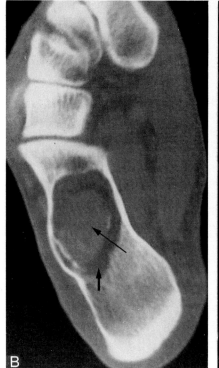

FIGURE 13–35. (**A**) A lateral radiograph shows intraosseous lipoma as a lytic area in the calcaneus (*arrow*). (**B**) The corresponding axial CT image delineates the low-attenuation periphery (*short arrow*) and higher-attenuation central component (*long arrow*). (**C**) On a T1-weighted image, the high signal intensity fat (*solid arrows*) surrounds the low signal intensity hemorrhagic fluid contents (*curved arrow*). (TR, 600 msec; TE, 20 msec.) (**D**) On a T2-weighted axial image, the fat periphery demonstrates decreased signal intensity (*solid arrow*), whereas central fluid contents (*curved arrow*) generate increased signal intensity. (TR, 2000 msec; TE, 60 msec.)

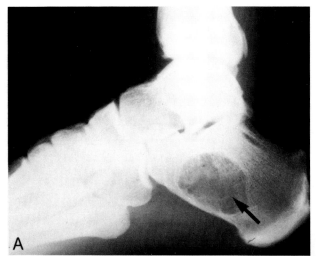

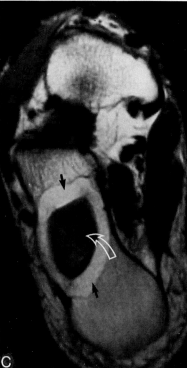

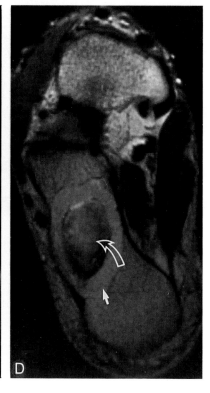

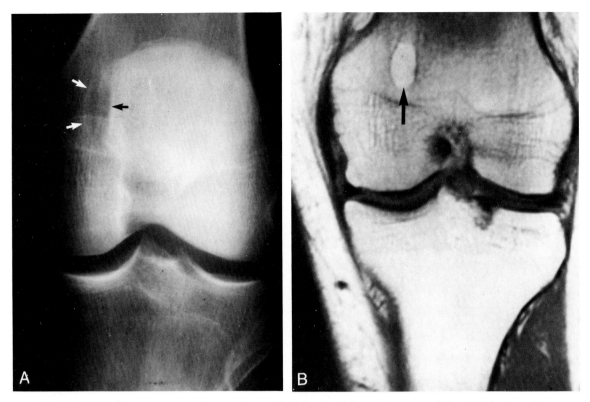

FIGURE 13–36. Intraosseous lipoma (*arrows*) of the distal femur is seen as (**A**) a lytic lesion with sclerotic borders on a conventional radiograph and as (**B**) a high signal intensity focus on a T1-weighted coronal image.

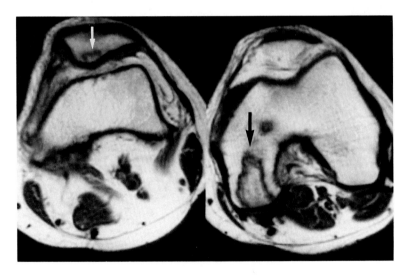

FIGURE 13–37. Low signal intensity circumscribed bone infarcts are present in the patella (*white arrow*) and medial femoral condyle (*black arrow*), as seen on a T1-weighted axial image. Central fat marrow signal intensity is characteristic of bone infarction. The location of an infarct in the medial femoral condyle should be viewed as having the same significance as osteochondritis or an osteonecrotic lesion and demonstrates diffuse low signal intensity. (TR, 500 msec; TE, 20 msec.)

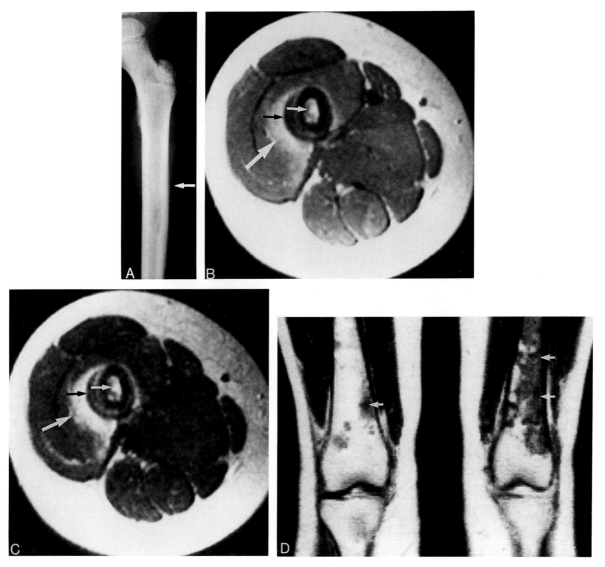

FIGURE 13–38. Solitary eosinophilic granuloma of histiocytosis X. (**A**) An anteroposterior radiograph shows thickened periosteal reaction (*arrow*) along the lateral femoral cortex. Bright signal intensity perilesional edema (*large white arrow*) and marrow involvement (*small white arrow*) and low signal intensity thickened medial femoral cortex (*black arrow*) are seen on (**B**) intermediate-weighted and (**C**) T2-weighted images. (TR, 2000 msec; TE, 20, 60 msec.) (**D**) A T1-weighted coronal image of eosinophilic granuloma of histiocytosis X involving the femoral diaphysis and metaphysis shows patchy areas of low signal intensity histiocytic infiltration (*arrows*). (TR, 600 msec; TE, 20 msec.)

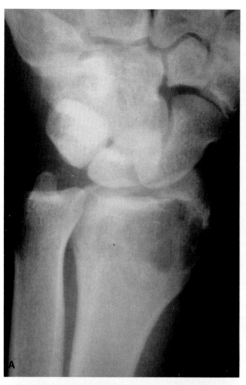

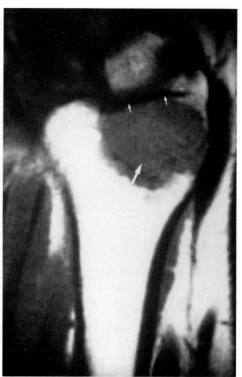

FIGURE 13–39. (**A**) An antero-posterior radiograph shows an eccentric osteolytic lesion involving the subchondral bone of the distal radius. Cortical thinning and expansion are seen. Coronal (**B**) T1-weighted and (**C**) T2*-weighted images show subchondral extension (*small arrows*) of the giant cell tumor (*large arrows*). Tumor contents demonstrate low signal intensity on the T1-weighted image and are hyperintense on the T2*-weighted image.

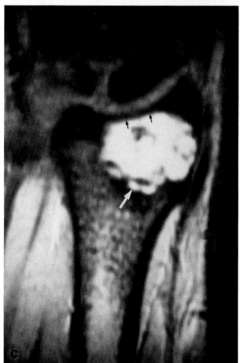

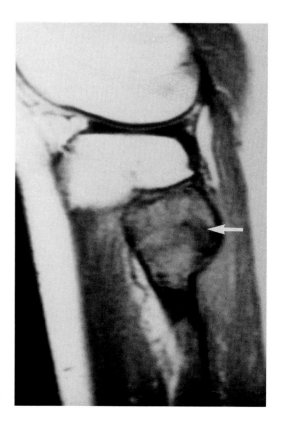

FIGURE 13–40. Expansile giant cell tumor (*arrow*) of the proximal fibula demonstrates low signal intensity on a T1-weighted sagittal image. (TR, 600 msec; TE, 20 msec.)

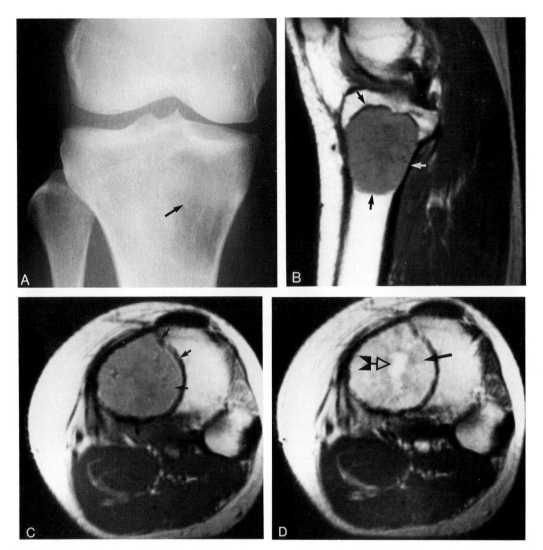

FIGURE 13–41. Giant cell tumor. (**A**) A lytic focus on the medial tibial metaphysis and epiphysis (*arrow*) is seen on a radiograph. T1-weighted (**B**) sagittal and (**C**) axial images demonstrate a well-circumscribed low signal intensity tumor (*black arrows*) with intact overlying cortex (*white arrow*). (TR, 600 msec; TE, 20 msec.)   (**D**) A T2-weighted image shows central necrosis (*flagged arrow*) within the high signal intensity lesion (*straight arrow*). (TR, 2000 msec; TE, 60 msec.)

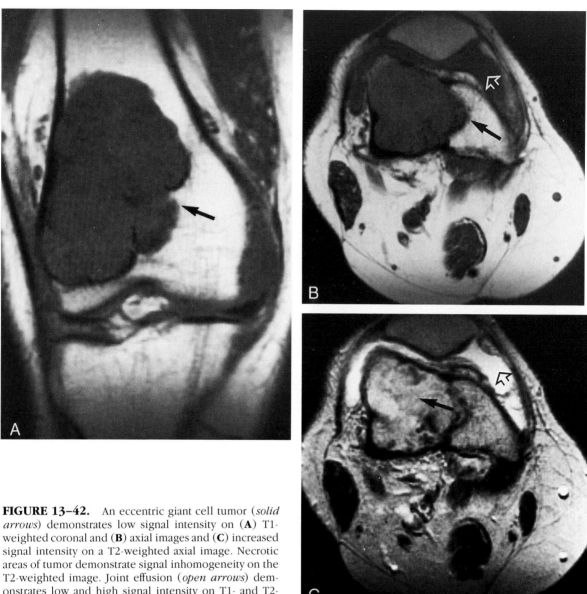

FIGURE 13–42. An eccentric giant cell tumor (*solid arrows*) demonstrates low signal intensity on (**A**) T1-weighted coronal and (**B**) axial images and (**C**) increased signal intensity on a T2-weighted axial image. Necrotic areas of tumor demonstrate signal inhomogeneity on the T2-weighted image. Joint effusion (*open arrows*) demonstrates low and high signal intensity on T1- and T2-weighted images, respectively.

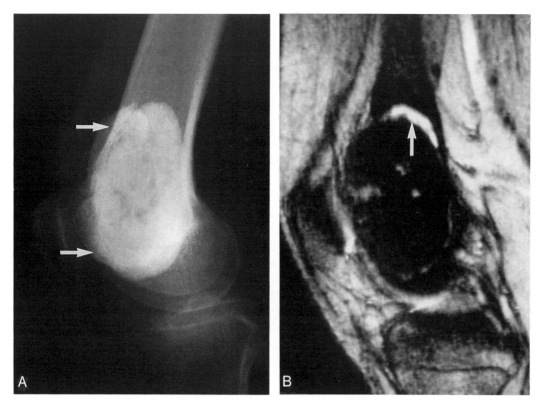

FIGURE 13–43. (**A**) A lateral radiograph shows a methylmethacrylate packed cavity after operative resection of giant cell tumor (*arrows*). (**B**) The corresponding T2*-weighted image reveals a recurrent giant cell tumor, which demonstrates bright signal intensity (*arrow*). Methylmethacrylate generates dark signal intensity. (TR, 400 msec; TE, 30 msec; flip angle, 30°.)

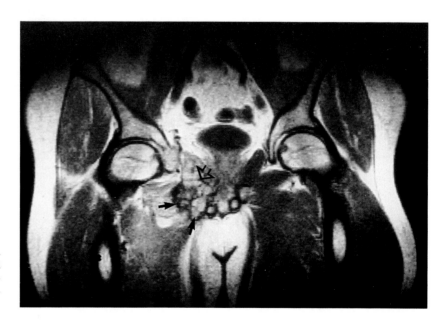

FIGURE 13–44. A multilobulated giant cell tumor (*solid arrows*), arising from the pubic rami (*open arrow*), demonstrates nonuniform intermediate signal intensity on an intermediate-weighted image. (TR, 1500 msec; TE, 28 msec.)

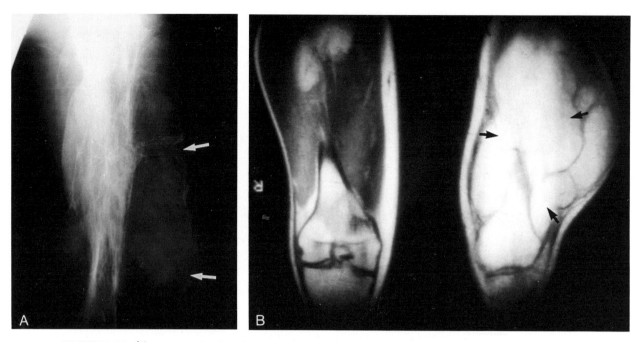

FIGURE 13–45. Tumoral callus (*all arrows*) in osteogenesis imperfecta of the femur is seen on (**A**) an anteroposterior radiograph and (**B**) a T1-weighted coronal image. Exuberant osteoid tissue demonstrates normal yellow marrow signal intensity. No malignant degeneration to osteosarcoma is seen.

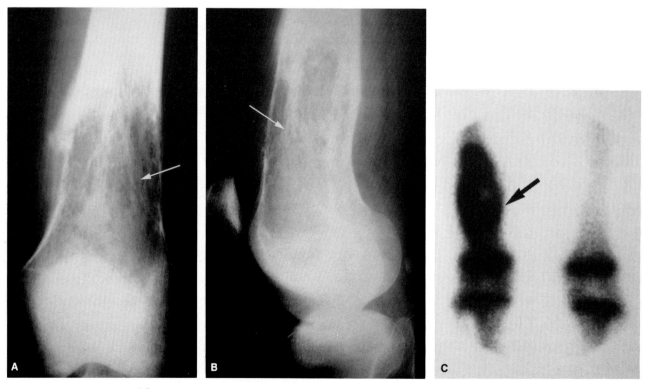

FIGURE 13–46. Telangiectatic osteosarcoma. (**A**) Anteroposterior and (**B**) lateral radiographs show an osteolytic tumor (*arrows*) with trabecular and cortical destruction. (**C**) Bone scintigraphy shows uptake of tracer in the distal femur (*arrow*). Uptake is present beyond the confines of the femur (*i.e.,* the convex margins). Coronal (**D**) T1-weighted and (**E**) T2-weighted images show intra- and extraosseous tumor extension with heterogeneous cystic hemorrhagic components. (**D:** TR, 500 msec; TE, 30 msec; **E:** TR, 2000 msec; TE, 120 msec.)

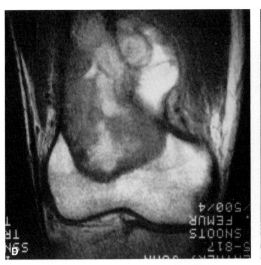
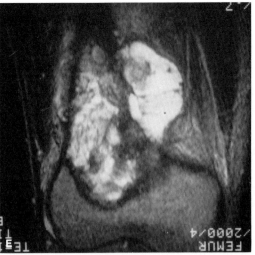

FIGURE 13-46. *(Continued)*

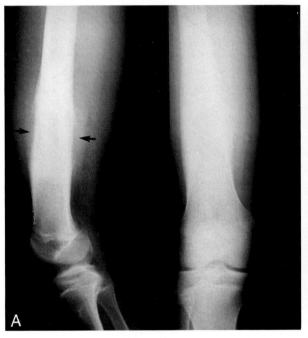

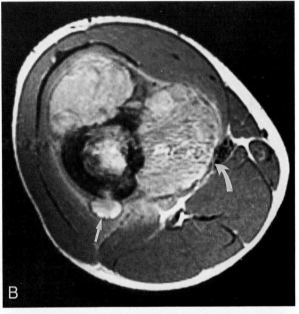

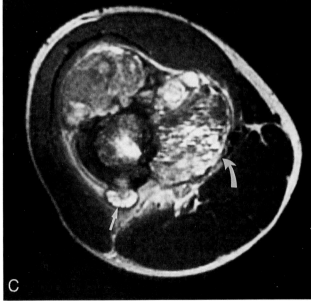

FIGURE 13-47. Osteosarcoma. (**A**) Anteroposterior (*left*) and lateral (*right*) radiographs show aggressive cortical destruction with periosteal reaction (*arrow*). Axial (**B**) intermediate-weighted and (**C**) T2-weighted images show a high signal intensity tumor with cortical transgression (*curved arrows*) and soft-tissue extension (*straight arrows*).

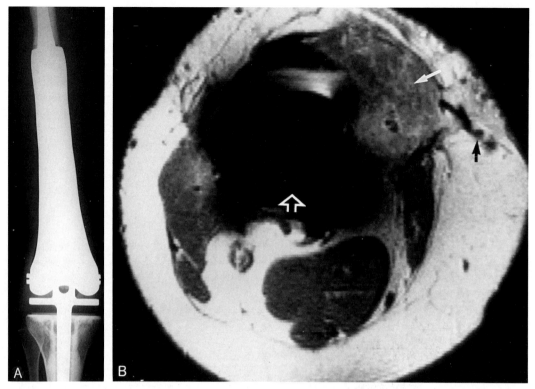

FIGURE 13–48. Postoperative osteosarcoma. (**A**) An anteroposterior radiograph shows limb salvage with a total knee prosthesis. (**B**) The corresponding intermediate-weighted axial image shows postoperative fibrous tissue (*solid white arrow*), the surgical incision site (*solid black arrow*), and a prosthesis signal artifact (*open arrow*). (TR, 1500 msec; TE, 40 msec.)

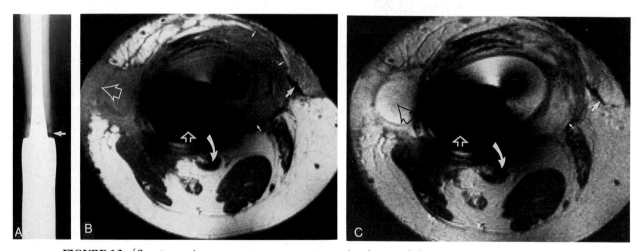

FIGURE 13–49. Interval postoperative osteosarcoma with infection. (**A**) An anteroposterior radiograph shows cortical irregularity at the prosthesis–bone interface (*arrow*). Abscess formation (*large open arrows*) in lateral soft tissues demonstrates (**B**) low signal intensity on an axial T1-weighted image and (**C**) high signal intensity on an axial T2-weighted image. A metallic artifact (*small open arrows*), fibrous tissue (*small solid arrows*), the surgical incision site (*large solid arrows*), and the popliteal vessels (*curved arrows*) are shown. (**B:** TR, 600 msec; TE, 20 msec; **C:** TR, 2000 msec; TE, 60 msec.)

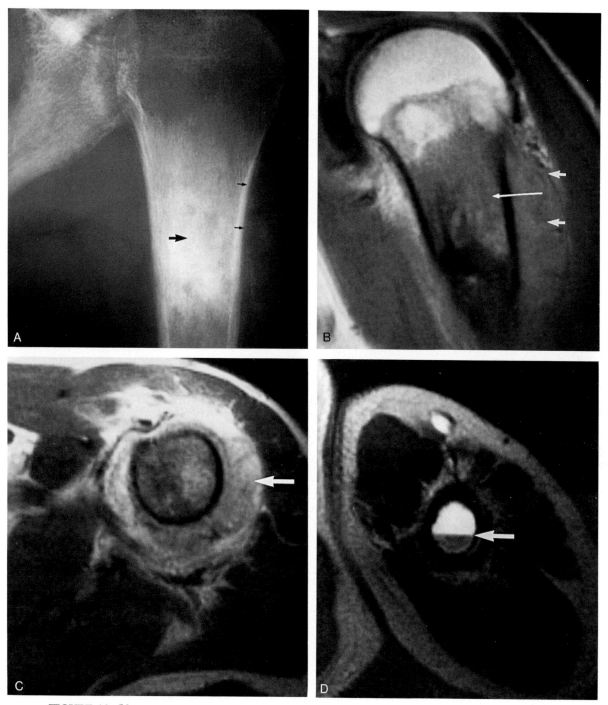

FIGURE 13–50. Differentiated osteosarcoma involving the proximal humerus. **(A)** An anteroposterior radiograph shows sclerosis (*large arrow*) and aggressive periosteal reaction (*small arrows*). **(B)** The corresponding T1-weighted coronal image demonstrates a soft-tissue mass (*short arrows*) and marrow involvement (*long arrow*). (TR, 600 msec; TE, 20 msec.) T2-weighted axial images display increased intensity in **(C)** the circumferential soft-tissue component (*arrow*) proximally and **(D)** the fluid–fluid level (*arrow*) in area of marrow necrosis distally. (**C, D:** TR, 2000 msec; TE, 60 msec.)

demonstrated with MR imaging (Fig. 13–51). Although osteosarcomas tend to image with low signal intensity on T1-weighted sequences and high signal intensity on T2-weighted sequences, specific cellular constituents (*e.g.,* fibrous, chondroid, blastic, or telangiectatic components) can modify signal characteristics.[54]

There is excellent correlation between the MR appearance of the extent of the marrow, cortical bone, and soft-tissue involvement and the gross pathologic specimen (Fig. 13–52).[58] Lesions that are primarily blastic and therefore sclerotic on plain film radiographs, demonstrate low signal intensity on both T1- and T2-weighted sequences (Fig. 13–53). Even in lesions with extensive sclerosis, areas of increased signal intensity may be identified on T2-weighted images. Hemorrhagic components within telangiectatic osteosarcoma demonstrate focal areas of high signal intensity on T1- and T2-weighted images (see Fig. 13–46). Skip lesions and multiple sites of involvement are common in multicentric osteosarcoma, which affects a younger age group (Fig. 13–54).[59]

In cases of parosteal osteosarcoma, the precise involvement of cortex and marrow can be assessed using sagittal plane images (Fig. 13–55). Both edema and tumor extension may encase vessels, and multiple axial images are usually necessary to distinguish edema that conforms and tracks along specific muscle groups.

Magnetic resonance imaging is superior to CT in determining the exact extent of marrow involvement by tumor and edema, particularly important in limb salvage procedures (Fig. 13–56). Interval response of tumor and edema to chemotherapy can be monitored by serial MR scans prior to surgery (Fig. 13–57).[60,61] Pan and colleagues reported on four MR patterns found in postchemotherapy osteosarcoma.[61]

1. A dark pattern of low to intermediate signal intensity areas on T1- and T2-weighted images corresponds to calcified osteoid or cartilage matrix, dense granulation tissue, and hemosiderin.

2. A mottled or speckled pattern of intermediate signal intensity on T1-weighted images and high signal intensity on T2-weighted images is best appreciated on T2-weighted images and corresponds to tumor matrix, edematous granulation tissue, and hemosiderin deposits.

3. A distinct multicystic or bubbly appearance in the cystic pattern, of intermediate to high signal intensity on T1-weighted images and high signal intensity on T2-weighted images, is thought to correspond to either blood-filled cysts with viable tumor cells or tumor matrix mixed with edematous granulation tissue. Foci of residual viable tumor could not be specifically diagnosed, however.

4. Skip metastases can also be accurately identified, as well as a reduction in peritumoral edema, the development of a dark rim of collagenous capsule continuous with the periosteum, bone infarcts, and intramedullary vascular channels.

Holscher and colleagues have reported a correlation between a positive response to chemotherapy and signal intensity changes on T2-weighted images of the extraosseous tumor component and in overall tumor volume.[60] No correlation was observed between chemotherapy and intraosseous tumor signal intensity or volume and histology. Sanchez and colleagues have studied patients receiving intraarterial chemotherapy and reported similar signal intensities in viable tumor, necrosis, edema, and hemorrhage, which demonstrated the limitations of unenhanced spin-echo images in the accurate assessment of the percentage of tumor necrosis.[62]

Chondrosarcoma

Chondrosarcomas occur about one-half as often as osteogenic sarcomas. They are malignant cartilage-producing neoplasms which arise primarily in adulthood and old age. The peak incidence is in the fourth, fifth, and sixth decades of life. Chondrosarcomas most commonly arise in the central skeleton (*i.e.,* pelvis and ribs) and within the metadiaphysis of the femur and humerus. More than in other primary bone malignancies, their clinical and biologic behavior depends on their histologic grade, which is proportional to the level of anaplasia. Grade 1 (*i.e.,* well-differentiated) chondrosarcomas consist of pure hyaline cartilage exhibiting mild anaplasia and mild increased cellularity. The cellularity and anaplasia is greatest in the poorly differentiated or grade 3 variant. The 5-year survival rates of patients with grades 1, 2, and 3 disease are approximately 90%, 81%, and 43%, respectively.[31] Grades 1 and 2 neoplasms (*i.e.,* the majority of chondrosarcomas) do not usually metastasize, whereas grade 3 neoplasms demonstrate a tendency to form hematogenous metastases. The majority (approximately 75%) of chondrosarcomas arise *de novo* (*i.e.,* are primary chondrosarcomas). The remainder (*i.e.,* secondary chondrosarcomas) arise by malignant transformation of preexisting cartilaginous lesions such as multiple enchondromatosis (*e.g.,* Ollier's disease, Maffucci's syndrome) and exostosis, especially multiple osteochondromatosis (Fig. 13–58).[31] These neoplasms, whether situated peripherally or centrally, are composed of characteristic lobules of gray–white translucent tissue with spotty calcification.[31] The adjacent cortex may be thickened or eroded, with extension of the neoplasm into the surrounding soft tissues (Fig. 13–59).

Magnetic Resonance Appearance. Magnetic resonance imaging can be used to characterize changes of marrow involvement prior to medullary expansion (Fig. 13–60). T2*-weighted images are sensitive to matrix calcifications and associated soft-tissue masses (Fig. 13–61). On T2- and T2*-weighted images, calcifications are identified as low signal intensity foci that contrast with the bright signal intensity tumor. On T2- or T2*-weighted images, low signal intensity fibrous septa may separate homogeneous high signal intensity lobules of hyaline cartilage.[41] Heterogeneity of signal intensity correlates with higher grade, more cellular lesions.[63]

Although extremely rare in childhood, chondrosarcoma has been known to arise from malignant transformation of an enchondroma in Ollier's disease (see Fig. 13–58). On T2-weighted images, these areas demonstrate greater signal intensity than adjacent enchondromas. Malignant degeneration or transformation can be inferred by the presence of frank cortical disruption, soft-tissue extension, periosteal reaction, and disproportionate size of lesion relative to satellite enchondromas. Although these findings have been confirmed by pathologic evaluation, reliable MR criteria have not been developed to characterize these aggressive cartilage lesions.

Ewing's Sarcoma

Ewing's sarcoma is seen primarily during the last part of the first decade and the first one-half of the second decade of life. It is the second most common malignant bone tumor in childhood, and although any bone in the body may be affected, the femur, ilium, humerus, and tibia are the most common sites. Ewing's sarcoma is one of the malignant round cell tumors involving bone. Although its histogenesis remains uncertain, evidence suggests a neuroectodermal origin.[64] Specific chromosomal translocation of the long arms of chromosomes 11 and 22 have been found in Ewing's sarcoma.[65]

Magnetic Resonance Appearance. Ewing's sarcoma demonstrates low signal intensity on T1-weighted sequences and bright signal intensity on T2-, T2*-weighted, and STIR sequences (Fig. 13–62).[66,67] Marrow involvement and peritumoral edema are clearly delineated (Fig. 13–63).

Magnetic resonance imaging is superior to CT or to plain film radiography in the evaluation of Ewing's sarcoma, because the soft-tissue component, which is usually substantial, is better evaluated with MR, especially in the distal extremities (Fig. 13–64). Since MR imaging provides excellent delineation of soft tissues, the extent of muscular and neurovascular involvement in extraosseous Ewing's sarcoma can also be assessed (Fig. 13–65). Ewing's sarcoma originating in bone marrow can be identified in the early stages, before cortical erosion and periostitis have developed (Fig. 13–66).

Plasmacytoma

Plasmacytoma is a solitary neoplasm of plasma cells that sometimes converts into multiple myeloma.[68] Solitary plasmacytomas affect the middle age group (50 years), and frequently target the spine and pelvis. A solitary lytic or expansile lesion is common, although an ivory vertebral pattern has been reported in the spine. Magnetic resonance characteristics of plasmacytoma are nonspe-

specific—low to intermediate signal intensity on T1-weighted images and high signal intensity on T2-weighted images (Fig. 13–67). Aggressive cortical disruption and infiltration into soft tissue and adjacent structures, with discontinuity of adjacent low signal intensity cortical bone, can be identified on MR examination.

Adamantinoma

Adamantinoma of bone is a rare neoplasm with an uncertain histogenesis. The tibia is the site of involvement in 90% of cases. Immune histochemical data indicate an epithelial nature. Histologically, there is a spectrum of patterns ranging from spindled to squamoid, with characteristic basaloid cells. The peak incidence is in the third to fourth decades of life. Although these tumors are slow growing and appear histologically bland, approximately 20% metastasize.[69]

The MR imaging characteristics of adamantinoma may be similar to lesions of osteofibrous dysplasia, with low signal intensity sclerosis identified on T1- and T2-weighted images (Fig. 13–68). Peritumoral edema or small focal areas of hyperintensity may be identified within the tibial cortex. These areas of increased signal intensity may correspond to osteolytic defects adjacent to sclerotic bone. Adamantinomas are characteristically located in the middle one-third of the tibia, and have a cortical or eccentric epicenter.

Metastatic Disease

Magnetic resonance is very sensitive in evaluating metastatic disease.[70–73] In general, metastatic bone disease appears as focal lesions that involve both cortical bone and marrow and demonstrate low signal intensity on T1-weighted sequences and bright signal intensity on T2-weighted sequences. T1-weighted and STIR images are more sensitive than T2*-weighted images in identifying increased signal intensity in metastatic deposits or surrounding edema (Figs. 13–69 and 13–70). Gadolinium has been used to enhance osseous and soft-tissue metastases on T1-weighted images (Figs. 13–71 and 13–72). Neuroblastoma has a high frequency of metastases in both bone and soft tissue (*e.g.,* paraspinal lesions; Fig. 13–73). Nuclear scintigraphy may produce false-positive scans or may be negative even with very aggressive lesions (Fig. 13–74). Metastatic deposits can be identified on MR scans in patients with negative conventional radiographs (Fig. 13–75). Vascularity may assist in determining the site of tumor origin (*e.g.,* renal cell carcinoma with low signal intensity vessels; Fig. 13–76). High bone detail in cortical or trabecular destruction may require correlation with corresponding CT scans (Fig. 13–77).

The MR appearance of metastatic lesions is nonspecific for the site of origin.[13] Peritumoral soft-tissue edema

(text continues on page 1092)

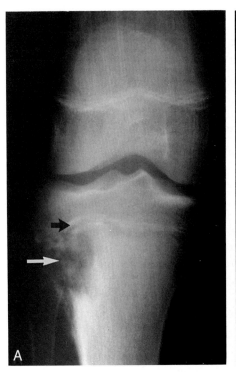
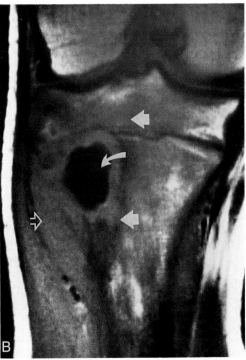

FIGURE 13–51. (**A**) An antero-posterior radiograph shows lytic metaphyseal-based osteosarcoma with aggressive cortical destruction (*white arrow*). No extension of tumor is seen proximal to the physeal line (*black arrow*). (**B**) The corresponding T1-weighted coronal image shows low signal intensity marrow infiltration involving the epiphysis, metaphysis, and proximal diaphysis (*solid straight arrow*). A soft-tissue mass with cortical breakthrough involves the medial tibial metaphysis (*open arrow*). The biopsy site, which is packed with gelfoam, is shown as a dark focus of low signal intensity (*curved arrow*). (TR, 800 msec; TE, 25 msec.)

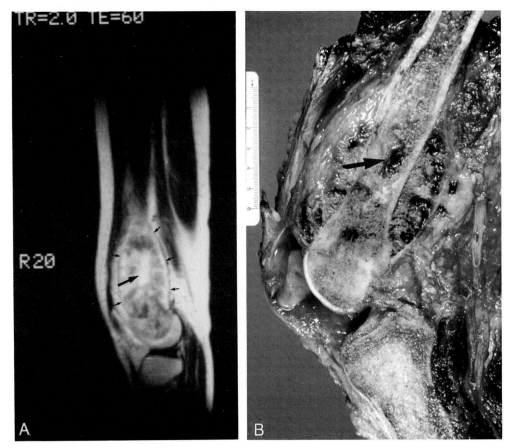

FIGURE 13–52. (**A**) A T2-weighted sagittal image shows osteosarcoma involving the femoral metaphysis (*small arrows*). Bright contrast portions of the high signal intensity tumor represent necrosis with hemorrhage (*large arrow*). (TR, 2000 msec; TE, 60 msec.) (**B**) The corresponding gross specimen shows central tumor necrosis (*arrow*).

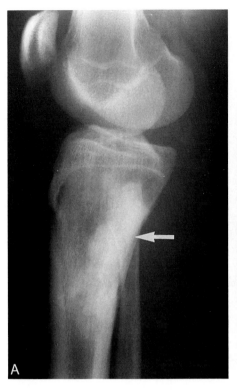

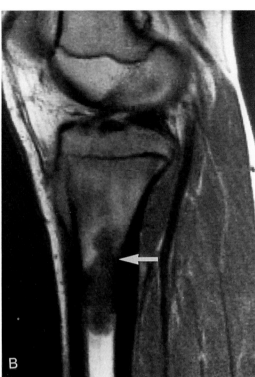

FIGURE 13–53. (**A**) A lateral radiograph shows a sclerotic response (*arrow*) to osteoblastic osteosarcoma. (**B**) The corresponding T1-weighted sagittal image shows a low signal intensity blastic tumor (*arrow*). (TR, 600 msec; TE, 20 msec.)

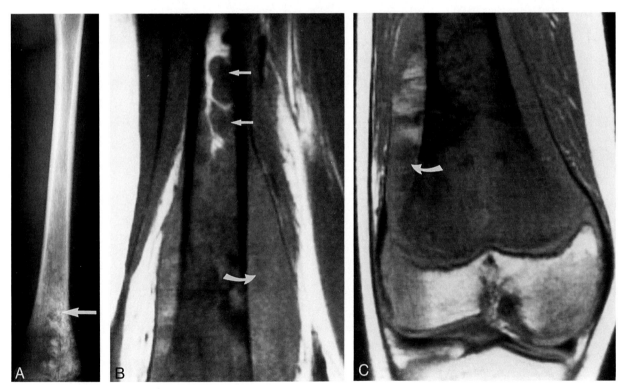

FIGURE 13–54. (**A**) An anteroposterior radiograph shows distal femoral lytic sclerotic reaction (*arrow*) to multicentric osteosarcoma. (**B**) Skip lesions (*straight arrows*) are seen on a T1-weighted sagittal image. (**C**) These lesions are located proximal to the primary tumor focus on T1-weighted coronal image. A soft-tissue mass is identified on both the sagittal and coronal views (*curved arrows*). (**B, C**: TR, 600 msec; TE, 20 msec.) (**D**) Intermediate-weighted and (**E**) T2-weighted axial images show increased signal intensity in the marrow and surrounding soft tissue. (**D, E**: TR, 2000 msec; TE, 20, 60 msec.) *(continued)*

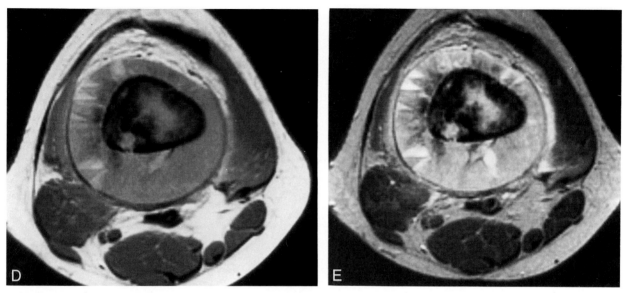

FIGURE 13–54. *(Continued)*

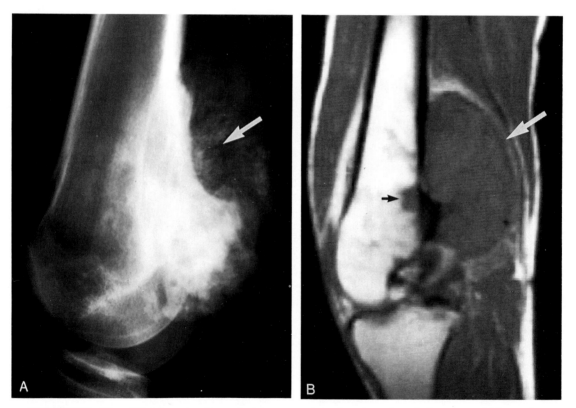

FIGURE 13–55. (**A**) A lateral radiograph shows posterior sclerosis and a soft-tissue osteoid (*arrow*). (**B**) On a T1-weighted sagittal image, soft-tissue parosteal osteosarcoma demonstrates low signal intensity (*white arrow*). The focus of marrow involvement (*black arrow*) was not revealed on plain film radiographs. (TR, 600 msec; TE, 20 msec.)

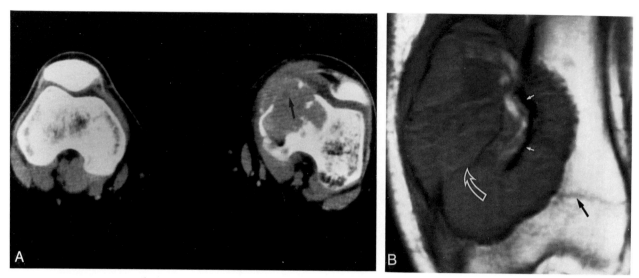

FIGURE 13–56. (**A**) An axial CT scan shows cortical breakthrough and a soft-tissue mass (*arrow*), which are characteristic of osteosarcoma. (**B**) A coronal T1-weighted image defines the proximal and distal extent of the tumor across the physis (*black arrow*), amount of soft-tissue involvement (*curved open arrow*), and amount of cortical destruction (*white arrows*) on a single section. (TR, 600 msec; TE, 20 msec.)

FIGURE 13–57. (**A**) On an anteroposterior radiograph, blastic osteosarcoma appears as a sclerotic metaphyseal focus. (**B**) On a T1-weighted coronal image, the lesion is seen as a low signal intensity area of marrow replacement (*arrows*). (TR, 1000 msec; TE, 40 msec.) The interval response to monthly chemotherapy in the (**C**) first, (**D**) second, and (**E**) third months of treatment is seen on T2-weighted images. Although the blastic foci of the tumor (*black arrows*) remain unchanged, popliteus muscle edema (*white arrows*) decreases with continued chemotherapy. The unfused tibial apophysis is demarcated (*open arrow*). (**F**) An anatomic gross section shows blastic tumor (*white arrows*) and tibial apophysis (*open arrow*). (**C–E:** TR, 2000 msec; TE, 60 msec.) *(continued)*

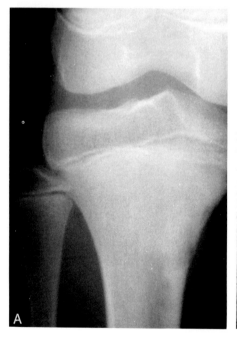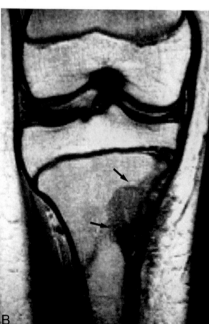

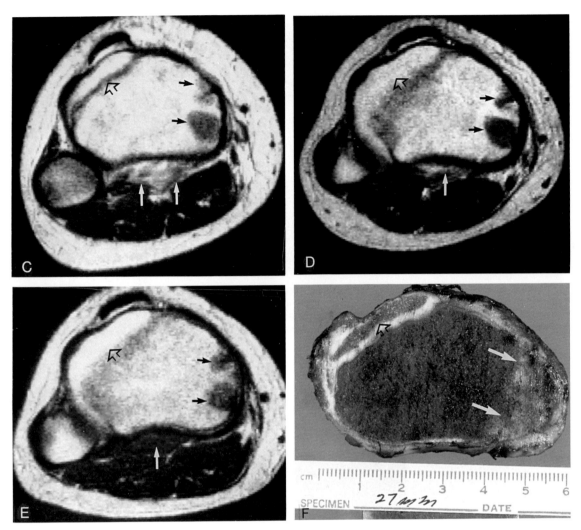

FIGURE 13–57. *(Continued)*

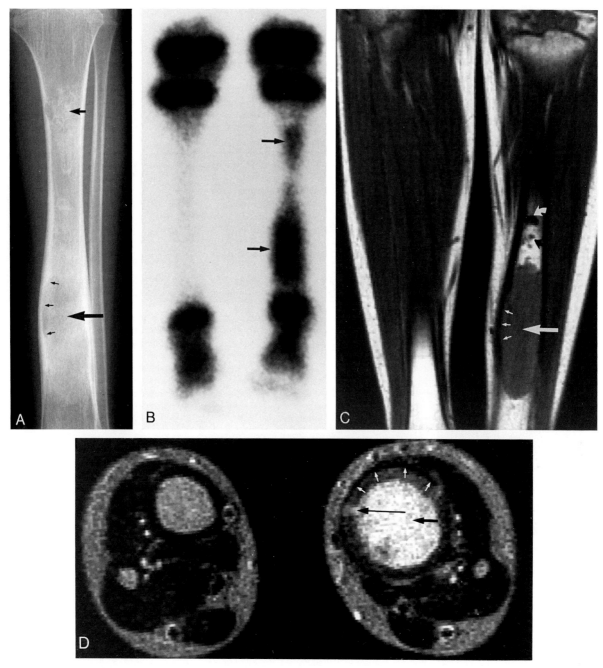

FIGURE 13–58. (**A**) An anteroposterior radiograph shows multiple enchondromas (*medium arrow*); a discrete lytic lesion in the distal femoral shaft represents transformation into a chondrosarcoma (*large arrow*). Endosteal scalloping is seen (*small arrows*). (**B**) Technetium bone scintigraphy shows increased uptake in the proximal femoral enchondromas and a larger distal lesion (*arrows*). (**C**) A T1-weighted coronal image shows a focus of malignant degeneration from an enchondroma to a chondrosarcoma (*large arrow*). Endosteal scalloping with bowing of low signal intensity cortical bone (*small arrows*) and satellite enchondromas (*curved arrow*) are shown also shown. (TR, 500 msec; TE, 40 msec.) (**D**) The corresponding T2-weighted axial image shows uniform increased signal intensity (*short black arrow*), cortical extension (*long black arrow*), and periosteal reaction (*small white arrows*). (TR, 2000 msec; TE, 80 msec.)

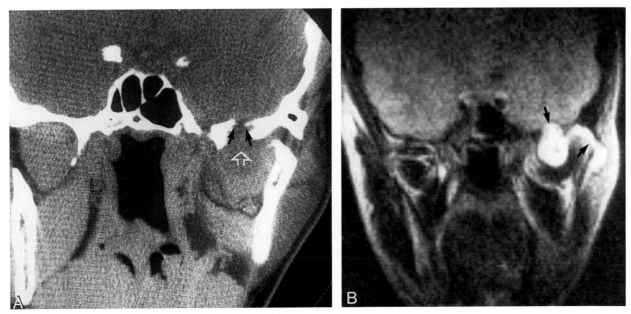

FIGURE 13–59. Chondrosarcoma of the temporomandibular joint. (**A**) Direct coronal CT shows a vague low attenuation mass (*open arrow*) and cortical destruction (*solid arrows*) extending to the middle cranial fossa. (**B**) The corresponding T2-weighted coronal image shows the exact location and boundaries of the bright signal intensity tumor (*arrows*).

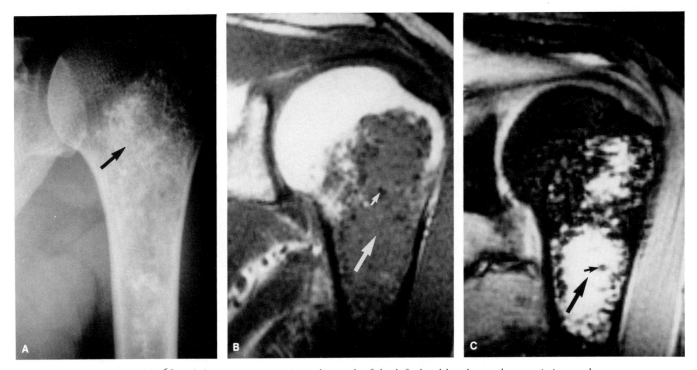

FIGURE 13–60. (**A**) An anteroposterior radiograph of the left shoulder shows characteristic annular and comma-shaped calcifications within central or medullary chondrosarcoma (*arrow*). Coronal (**B**) T1-weighted and (**C**) T2*-weighted images more accurately depict proximal marrow involvement (*large arrows*). Calcifications are seen as dark signal intensity foci (*small arrows*). The chondroid matrix is hyperintense on the T2*-weighted image.

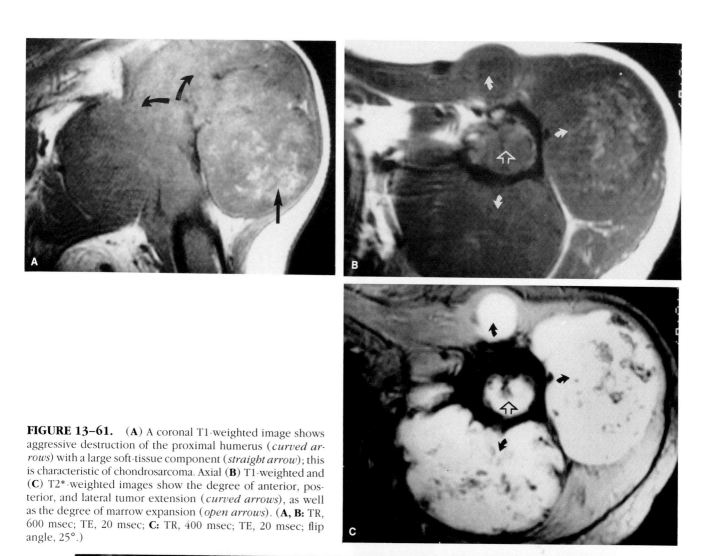

FIGURE 13-61. (**A**) A coronal T1-weighted image shows aggressive destruction of the proximal humerus (*curved arrows*) with a large soft-tissue component (*straight arrow*); this is characteristic of chondrosarcoma. Axial (**B**) T1-weighted and (**C**) T2*-weighted images show the degree of anterior, posterior, and lateral tumor extension (*curved arrows*), as well as the degree of marrow expansion (*open arrows*). (**A, B:** TR, 600 msec; TE, 20 msec; **C:** TR, 400 msec; TE, 20 msec; flip angle, 25°.)

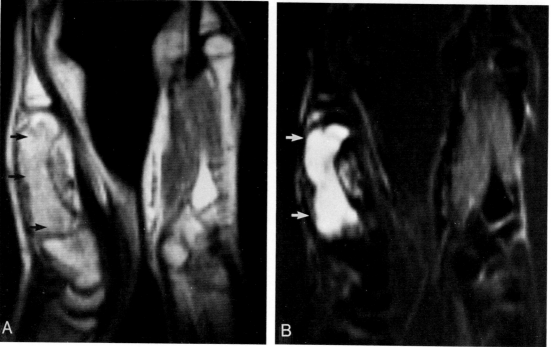

FIGURE 13-62. (**A**) Ewing's sarcoma (*arrows*) of the metacarpal in a patient undergoing radiation therapy is seen on a conventional T1-weighted sagittal image. (TR, 900 msec; TE, 40 msec.) (**B**) A short TI inversion recovery image shows high signal intensity contrast (*arrows*) in the infiltrated bone. The normal marrow appears black. (TR, 400 msec; TI, 125 msec; TE, 40 msec.)

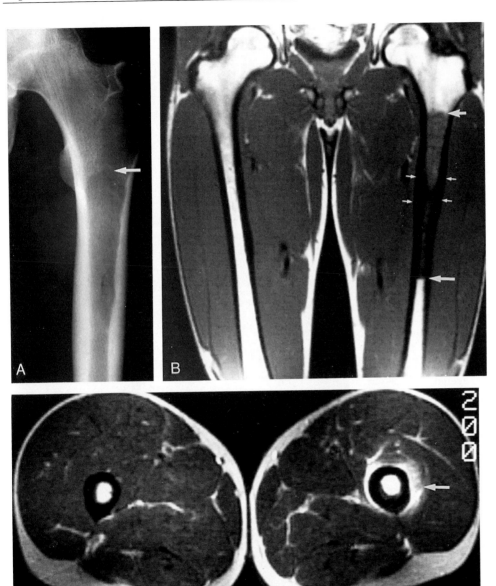

FIGURE 13–63. (**A**) An antero-posterior radiograph demarcates the proximal extent of medullary involvement (*arrow*) in Ewing's sarcoma. (**B**) The corresponding T1-weighted coronal MR image reveals both proximal (*medium arrow*) and distal (*large arrow*) marrow extension and periosteal thickening (*small arrows*). (TR, 500 msec; TE, 20 msec.) (**C**) A T2-weighted axial image shows high signal intensity peritumoral edema (*arrow*) without an associated soft-tissue mass. (TR, 2000 msec; TE, 60 msec.)

FIGURE 13–65. (**A**) On a balanced, weighted image, extraosseous Ewing's sarcoma demonstrates intermediate signal intensity (*arrow*). (TR, 1500 msec; TE, 40 msec.) (**B**) Signal intensity of the sarcoma (*arrows*) is low on a T1-weighted image and (**C**) high on a T2-weighted image. (**B:** TR, 600 msec; TE, 20 msec; **C:** TR, 2000 msec; TE, 60 msec.)

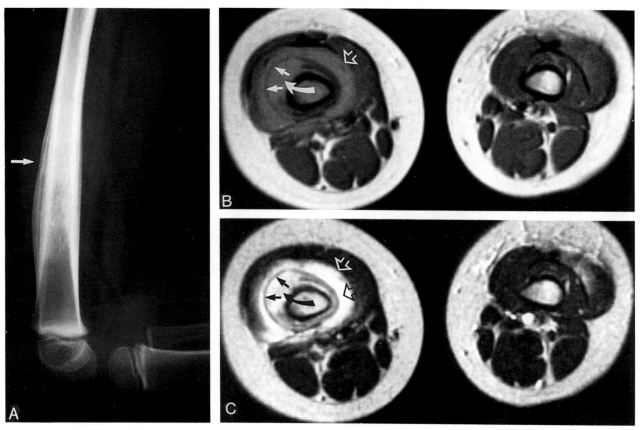

FIGURE 13–64. (**A**) A lateral radiograph shows an "onion skin" periosteal reaction in Ewing's sarcoma of the femur (*arrow*). Axial (**B**) T1-weighted and (**C**) T2-weighted images show a low signal intensity periosteal reaction (*solid arrows*), peritumoral edema (*open arrows*), and marrow and soft-tissue components (*curved arrows*). Edema, marrow, and soft-tissue components demonstrate low signal intensity on a T1-weighted image and bright signal intensity on a T2-weighted image. (**B:** TR, 600 msec; TE, 20 msec; **C:** TR, 2000 msec; TE, 60 msec.)

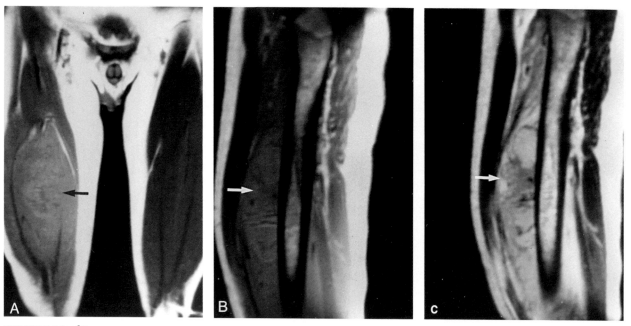

FIGURE 13–65.

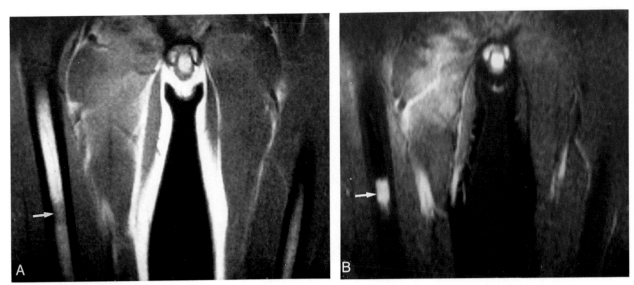

FIGURE 13–66. (**A**) On a T1-weighted image, early marrow involvement (*arrow*) of Ewing's sarcoma is seen as a focus of decreased signal intensity. (TR, 600 msec; TE, 20 msec.) (**B**) On a short TI inversion recovery image, the focus of involved marrow (*arrow*) shows increased signal intensity. (TR, 1400 msec; TI, 125 msec; TE, 40 msec.)

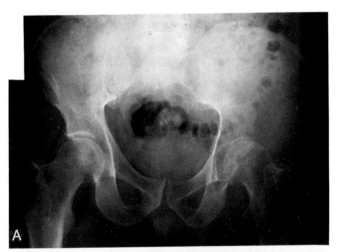

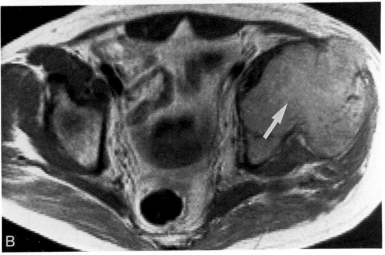

FIGURE 13–67. Plasmacytoma of the ilium. (**A**) An anteroposterior radiograph of the pelvis shows destruction of the left ilium. (**B**) A T1-weighted axial MR image reveals an intermediate signal intensity mass (*arrow*) with aggressive cortical transgression and soft-tissue extension. (TR, 600 msec; TE, 20 msec.) (**C**) An axial CT image shows disrupted cortical bone (*arrows*).

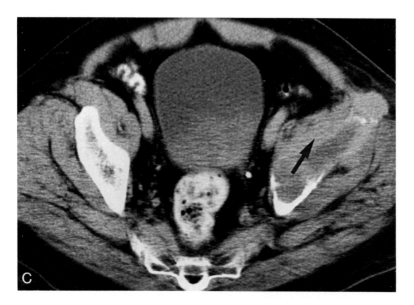

FIGURE 13–67. *(Continued)*

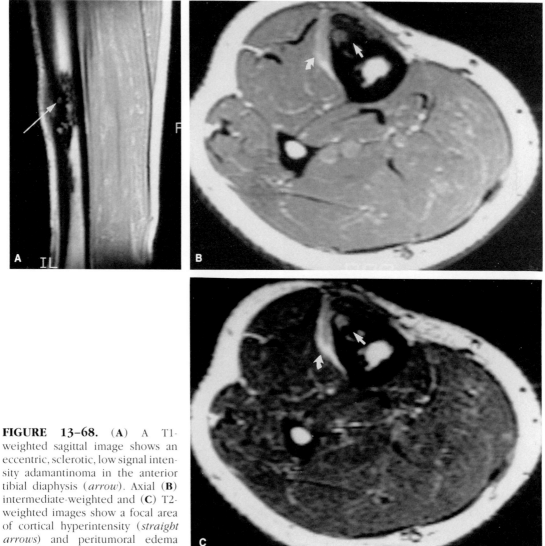

FIGURE 13–68. (**A**) A T1-weighted sagittal image shows an eccentric, sclerotic, low signal intensity adamantinoma in the anterior tibial diaphysis (*arrow*). Axial (**B**) intermediate-weighted and (**C**) T2-weighted images show a focal area of cortical hyperintensity (*straight arrows*) and peritumoral edema (*curved arrows*).

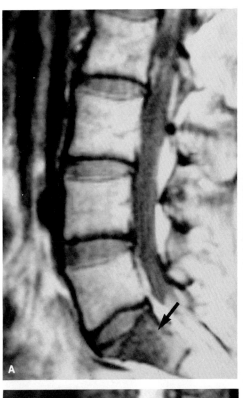

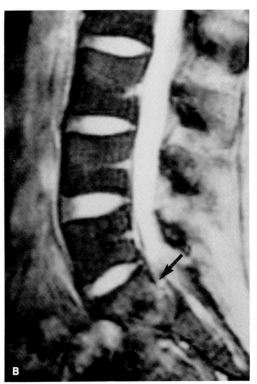

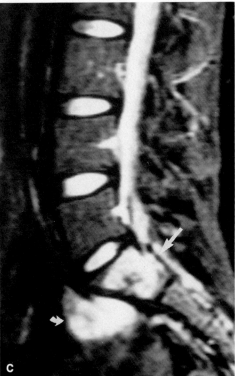

FIGURE 13–69. This metastatic tumor is of unknown primary origin. Metastatic fatty marrow replacement of the S1 vertebral body is present. The tumor (*straight arrows*) demonstrates (**A**) low signal intensity on a T1-weighted image and (**B**) is poorly delineated on the T2*-weighted image. (**C**) The greatest sensitivity for detection is seen on a short TI inversion recovery image. Normal bowel is identified anterior to S1 (*curved arrow*).

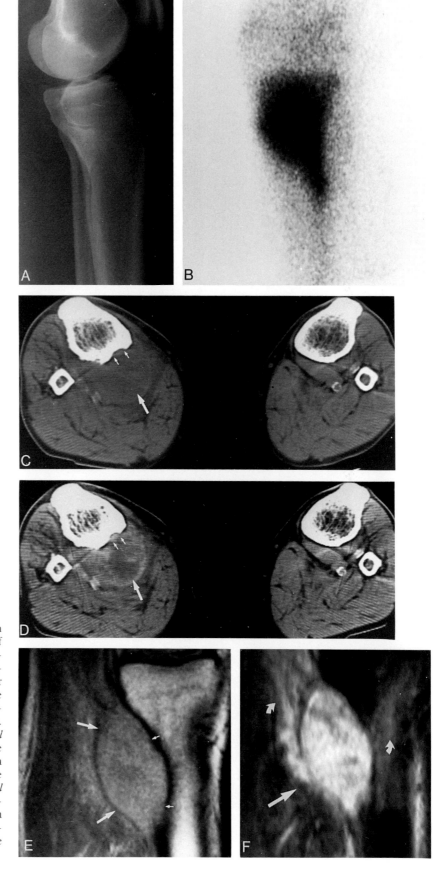

FIGURE 13–70. (**A**) A lateral radiograph shows subtle cortical irregularity, indicative of metastatic melanoma, along the proximal posterior tibial cortex. (**B**) Technetium bone scintigraphy reveals an uptake of tracer in the posterior tibia and soft tissues. Axial CT scans (**C**) before and (**D**) after contrast enhancement show hypervascularity of the soft-tissue mass (*large arrows*). Posteromedial cortical erosion is shown (*small arrows*). (**E**) On a T1-weighted sagittal image, the intermediate signal intensity metastatic melanoma is an elliptical mass (*large arrow*) invading the low signal intensity posterior tibial cortex (*small arrows*). (**F**) On the corresponding short TI inversion recovery image, the metastatic melanoma (*straight arrow*) demonstrates high signal intensity, as well as reactive marrow and soft-tissue edema (*curved arrows*).

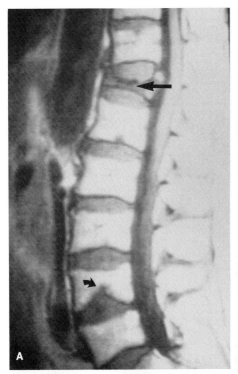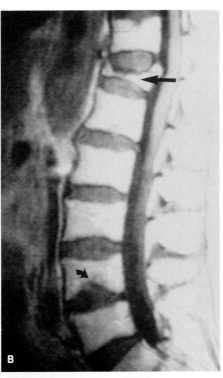

FIGURE 13–71. In metastatic lung cancer, T1-weighted sagittal images (**A**) before and (**B**) after Gd-DTPA enhancement show a pathologic fracture at T12 (*straight arrows*). A nonenhanced benign compression fracture at L4 is also indicated (*curved arrows*). (TR, 500 msec; TE, 30 msec.)

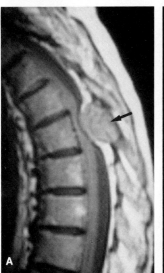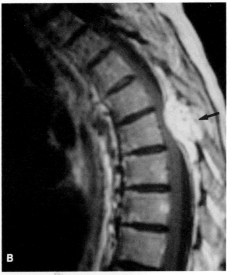

FIGURE 13–72. This metastatic adenocarcinoma (*arrows*) is from an unknown primary source. Sagittal T1-weighted images (**A**) before and (**B**) after Gd-DTPA enhancement show the tumor epicenter in the posterior elements of the thoracic spine, resulting in extradural cord compression. (TR, 500 msec; TE, 20 msec.)

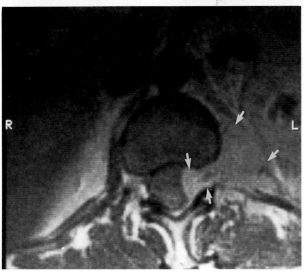

FIGURE 13–73. Metastatic neuroblastoma has infiltrated the left neural foramina (*arrows*) on this intermediate-weighted image. (TR, 2000 msec; TE, 28 msec.)

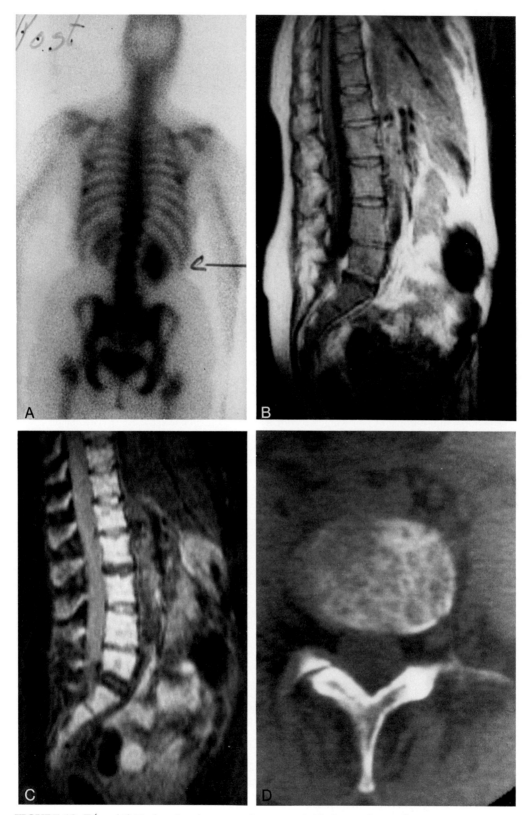

FIGURE 13–74. (**A**) Technetium bone scan is unremarkable in a patient with aggressive metastatic breast carcinoma. (**B**) T1-weighted and (**C**) short TI inversion recovery images show low and high signal intensity, respectively, in diffuse marrow involvement of the entire thoracic and lumbar spines. (**D**) The corresponding axial CT scan confirms lytic destruction of cancellous cortical bone.

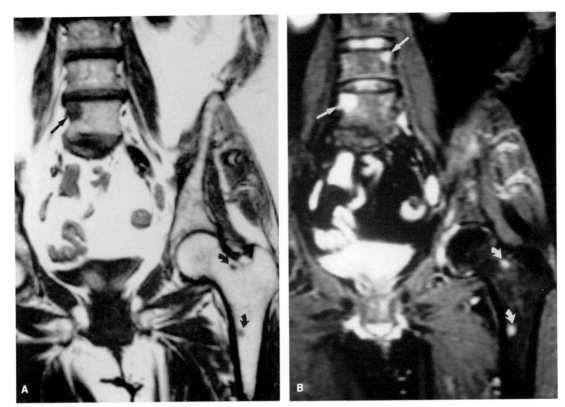

FIGURE 13–75. Unsuspected metastatic breast carcinoma was not detected on routine radiographs of the spine or hip. Coronal (**A**) T1-weighted and (**B**) short TI inversion recovery (STIR) images reveal metastatic foci in the L4 and L5 vertebral bodies (*straight arrows*) and left proximal femur (*curved arrows*). Note the greater sensitivity (*i.e.,* contrast) on the STIR image, which highlights the L4 metastatic tumor that is not seen on the T1-weighted image. (**A**: TR, 500 msec; TE, 20 msec; **B**: TR, 2000 msec; TI, 160 msec; TE, 40 msec.)

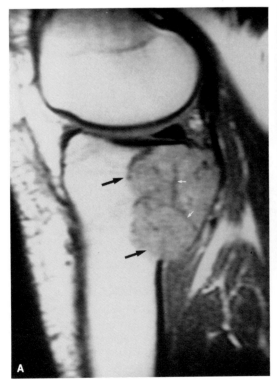

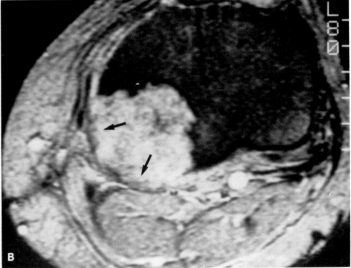

FIGURE 13–76. (**A**) A T1-weighted image shows expansile destruction of the posterior tibial cortex (*black arrows*) caused by metastatic renal cell carcinoma. Tumor vascularity is seen in low signal intensity linear segments (*white arrows*). (TR, 600 msec; TE, 200 msec.) (**B**) The corresponding axial T2*-weighted image shows hyperintense metastasis violating the posterior tibial cortex (*arrows*). (TR, 500 msec; TE, 20 msec; flip angle, 25°.)

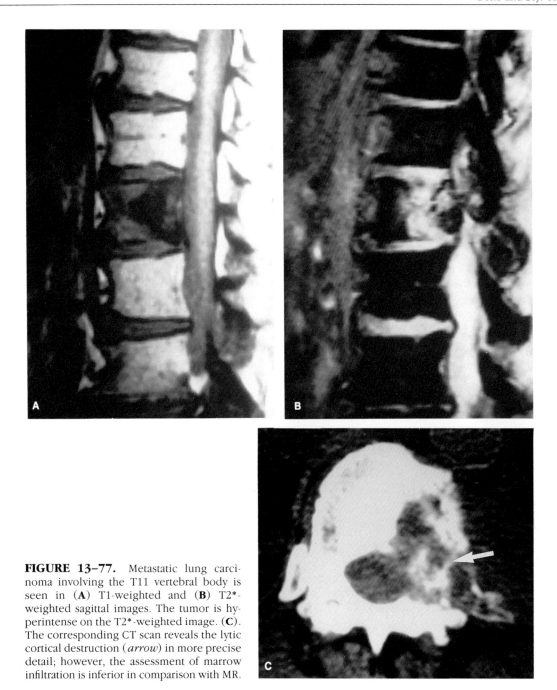

FIGURE 13–77. Metastatic lung carcinoma involving the T11 vertebral body is seen in (**A**) T1-weighted and (**B**) T2*-weighted sagittal images. The tumor is hyperintense on the T2*-weighted image. (**C**). The corresponding CT scan reveals the lytic cortical destruction (*arrow*) in more precise detail; however, the assessment of marrow infiltration is inferior in comparison with MR.

may be observed in the absence of a soft-tissue mass. Osteolytic metastatic lesions, commonly from carcinoma of the lung or breast, often demonstrate a more uniform signal intensity on T1- and T2-weighted images than do mixed sclerotic or osteoblastic deposits from carcinoma of the prostate or medulloblastoma (Fig. 13–78). Lesions of enostosis or osteopoikilosis may mimic blastic metastatic deposits; however, no aggressive features are associated with enostosis or osteopoikilosis (Figs. 13–79 and 13–80).

Primary Lymphoma of Bone

Originally designated "reticulum cell sarcoma of the bone"[74,75] by Parker and Jackson in 1989, this clinicopathologic disorder is now defined as a malignant lymphoma that arises within the medullary cavity of a single bone and occurs without concurrent regional lymph node or visceral involvement within a 6 month period (Fig. 13–81).[74,75] This rare disorder represents approximately 2% to 3% of malignant bone tumors and 5% of all extranodal lymphomas. Although all pathohistologic types of non-Hodgkin's lymphoma have been reported to occur in bone, large cell (*i.e.,* reticulum cell) lymphoma is the most common. Primary lymphoma of bone carries a better prognosis than disseminated non-Hodgkin's lymphoma with secondary involvement of bone.[76]

SOFT-TISSUE NEOPLASMS

In the evaluation of soft-tissue tumors, MR imaging offers the following advantages over CT:

- both cortical and marrow involvement can be evaluated
- improved depiction of the tissue planes surrounding the lesion
- neurovascular involvement can be assessed.[4,5,77–80]

Gadolinium enhancement may be used to further characterize the extent, degree of necrosis, and recurrence of soft-tissue tumors.[81,82]

Benign Soft-Tissue Neoplasms

Benign soft-tissue tumors are usually homogeneous and clearly marginated, and do not involve neurovascular structures. Malignant soft-tissue lesions tend to be inhomogeneous, with irregular margins and surrounding muscle edema. With long TR/TE sequences (TR, 2500 msec; TE, 80 msec), a tumor may demonstrate higher signal intensity than associated edema.

Fibromatosis

Axial and sagittal planar images may also be used to assess the fibrous lesions of plantar fibromatosis. These fibrous nodules, which involve the plantar aponeurosis, demonstrate low signal intensity on T1- and T2-weighted sequences. Xanthofibromas may also demonstrate low signal intensity on T1- and T2-weighted images (Fig. 13–82). In a series of 26 patients, the MR appearance of soft-tissue fibromatoses was variable, with hyperintense, isointense, hypointense, or mixed signal intensity relative to adjacent skeletal muscle.[83] Increased signal intensity on T1-weighted images was attributed to fat, protein, or both. Lesions of fibromatosis may show varying degrees of increased signal intensity on T2, T2*, and STIR protocols.

Lipoma

Soft-tissue lipomas are homogeneous and clearly marginated, with or without internal fibrous separations. Lipomas are the most frequent of the soft-tissue tumors, and they usually appear in the fifth or sixth decades of life. Most commonly, these soft-tissue neoplasms are found in the subcutaneous regions of the back and shoulder, but they can be found in any subcutaneous location. Less frequently, they occur in deeper locations such as within the thigh, anterior mediastinum, retroperitoneum, and gastrointestinal wall. Deep-seated intramuscular lipomas, especially in the paraspinal region, are rarely encapsulated; these frequently recur.[84]

Magnetic Resonance Appearance. Lipomas demonstrate bright signal intensity on T1-weighted images and do not increase in signal intensity on T2-weighted sequences (Figs. 13–83 and 13–84).[4] On STIR images, the fat signal in these lesions is nulled (Figs. 13–85 and 13–86). Low signal intensity septations may occur within these lesions on T1- and T2-weighted images.

Deep lipomas occurring in the extremities commonly involve either the shoulder or thigh. Although intramuscular lipomas are almost always well-defined lesions, on occasion they may have ill-defined borders and may demonstrate infiltration into adjacent muscle tissue (Fig. 13–87).

Hemangioma

Hemangiomas can occur in bone or soft tissues, and may vary widely in appearance. Histopathologically, they range from the cavernous type, with very large vascular spaces separated by fibrous tissue, to the capillary type, which is very cellular and lacks fibrous septa (Figs. 13–88, 13–89, and 13–90). Intramuscular hemangiomas are noncircumscribed tumors with a predilection for the thigh muscles of young adults (Fig. 13–91).[85] Pain is frequently the presenting symptom. The intramuscular type of hemangioma is associated with variable amounts of fat, smooth muscle, myxoid stroma, and hemosiderin. Although clearly benign histologically, these intramuscular hemangiomas may recur.[84]

Magnetic Resonance Appearance. Hemangiomas generate low to intermediate signal intensity on T1-weighted images and bright signal intensity on T2-weighted images (Fig. 13–92).[86] Paramagnetic effects cause central hemorrhage with hemosiderin deposits or peripheral hemosiderin-laden macrophages to demonstrate low signal intensity on T1- and T2-weighted images (Fig. 13–93). In selected cases, feeding vessels can be identified on STIR images (Fig. 13–94).

Hemangiopericytoma

Hemangiopericytomas are hypervascular soft-tissue tumors thought to originate from the capillary cell wall.[20] Pericytes (*i.e.,* cells present in the walls of capillaries and venules) can be demonstrated with electron microscopy and identified as the exact cell of origin. Most of these neoplasms are small, but, on rare occasions, they may achieve diameters of 8 cm or more. Although these tumors may exhibit a benign histopathologic pattern, they can recur, and as many as 50% metastasize to lungs, bone, and liver. Their biologic behavior, therefore, cannot be predicted from histology in all cases. Hemangiopericytomas usually present as a deep, soft-tissue mass of the thigh.[84]

Magnetic Resonance Appearance. The peripheral arterial branching seen in angiograms is depicted on T2-weighted MR images as an intricately packed network of vessels demonstrating signal void, in contrast to the adjacent tumor, which is bright (Fig. 13–95).

Ganglion Cyst

Ganglion cysts, thin-walled cysts filled with clear mucinous fluid, occur in soft tissues near joints. They are most commonly found around the hands and feet, especially the wrist, and are felt to represent either synovial herniations or mucinous degenerations of dense fibrous connective tissue, possibly related to trauma. Occasionally, these lesions may erode adjacent bone and become totally intraosseous.[87] The most common site of the intraosseous ganglion cyst is the medial malleolus of the tibia. Synovial ganglion cysts project into the soft tissues, are well defined, and demonstrate low signal intensity on T1-weighted images and high signal intensity on T2-weighted images (Fig. 13–96). Septations, when present, are best seen on T2-weighted images where they are outlined by the bright signal intensity of fluid.

Hemorrhage

Intramuscular hemorrhage and venous or arterial thrombosis may present with pain and can simulate a soft-tissue mass (Figs. 13–97 and 13–98).

Arteriovenous Malformation

Arteriovenous malformations of the soft tissues are seen as an irregular tangle of vessels that demonstrate low signal intensity on T1- and T2-weighted images in areas of rapidly flowing blood.

Desmoid Tumor

Desmoid tumors (*i.e.,* aggressive fibromatosis) exhibit biologic aggressiveness that lies somewhere between a reactive fibrous proliferation and a low-grade fibrosarcoma.[84] These lesions appear most frequently in the second to fourth decades, although they may occur at any age. They are usually large, infiltrative, poorly demarcated fibrous masses which tend to recur if incompletely surgically excised. They do not, however, exhibit the ability to metastasize. The desmoid tumor of soft tissue may present in the popliteal fossa and infiltrate surrounding musculature.[84,88]

Magnetic Resonance Appearance. Desmoid tumors are characterized by low signal intensity fibrous bands traversing the tumor, which demonstrates low to intermediate signal intensity on T1-weighted images and high signal intensity on T2- and T2*-weighted images (Fig. 13–99). In contrast, juvenile fibromatosis demonstrates uniformly low signal intensity on T1- and T2-weighted images.

Juvenile Fibromatosis

Juvenile fibromatosis is a locally invasive tumor that demonstrates low signal intensity on T1- and T2-weighted images (Fig. 13–100). It resembles fibrous desmoid tumors, and may recur after initial excision.

Cystic Hygroma

Cystic hygromas, usually found in the neck, exhibit the same signal intensity as fluid in T1- and T2-weighted images (Fig. 13–101).[89] In one case of cystic hygroma involving the axilla, recurrence, after initial resection, was identified in MR examination.

Neurofibromatosis

Neurofibromatosis is a hereditary, autosomal dominant, hamartomatous disorder that involves the neuroectoderm, mesoderm, and endoderm. Neurofibromas represent an unencapsulated nerve sheath lesion, which occurs in three forms:

1. Solitary localized nodules
2. Diffuse thickening of skin and subcutaneous tissues
3. "Plexiform" tumor representing wormlike multinodular growths that expand to contiguous major or minor nerves.

The "plexiform" pattern is characteristic of neuro-fibromatosis.[84]

Magnetic Resonance Appearance. In neurofibromatosis, MR imaging is used not only to evaluate the soft-tissue extent of disease, but also to assess spinal canal, adjacent cortical bone, and marrow involvement.[90] Neurofibromas demonstrate low to intermediate signal intensity on T1-weighted sequences and uniform bright signal intensity on T2-weighted images (Figs. 13–102 and 13–103). They also demonstrate increased signal intensity on T2*-weighted images and on Gd-DTPA–enhanced T1-weighted images.

Plexiform neurofibromas may be distinguished from nonplexiform types by the presence of longitudinal tracking along neural fascicles in a lobulated fashion (see Figs. 13–102 and 13–103; Fig 13–104). The nonplexiform lesions that do not involve multiple fascicles are more likely to infiltrate into adjacent tissue and are visualized with greater signal inhomogeneity (Fig. 13–105).

Malignant Soft-Tissue Neoplasms

Liposarcoma

Arising from primitive mesenchymal cells rather than adult fat cells, liposarcomas appear anywhere in the body without regard to adipose tissue. They are frequently found in the extremities, and the myxoid type commonly involves the thigh and popliteal region.[91] Peak incidence is in the fifth to seventh decades. These neoplasms arise in deep structures, and although they appear deceptively well circumscribed, they are commonly multilobular, with projections that creep between tissue planes. Areas of hemorrhage, necrosis, and cystic softening may be present. Four histopathologic variants have been characterized:

1. Well differentiated
2. Round cell
3. Myxoid
4. Pleomorphic.

Myxoid liposarcomas are the most commonly observed variant. Biologic aggressiveness and a tendency for distant metastases is expressed primarily in the round cell and pleomorphic variants.

Magnetic Resonance Appearance. Liposarcomas are more inhomogeneous than lipomas (Fig. 13–106).[84,92] On T1-weighted images, lesions with a greater cellular component may visualize with lower signal intensity relative to fatty elements. Focal areas of malignant change within a lipomatous matrix demonstrate low to intermediate signal intensity on T1-weighted sequences and high signal intensity on T2-weighted sequences.[93]

Gadolinium-enhanced MR imaging has been used to demonstrate central myxoid degeneration in a liposarcoma that was not seen on unenhanced T2-weighted images.

Leiomyosarcoma

In one case, a leiomyosarcoma of the posterolateral calf demonstrated isointensity with muscle tissue on T1-weighted images and a uniform increase in signal intensity on T2-weighted images (Fig. 13–107).

Neurofibrosarcoma

The development of neurofibrosarcoma may be characterized by irregular areas of necrosis. It demonstrates increased heterogeneity on T1- and T2-weighted images.

Synovial Sarcoma

The term synovial sarcoma is considered a misnomer, because studies do not support the synovial cell as the cell of origin. Instead, a multipotential mesenchymal cell has been identified as the likely source of these tumors.[84,94] Synovial sarcomas tend to occur in younger patients, 15 to 35 years of age, in close proximity to joints. They commonly involve the lower extremities in an extraarticular location. Less than 10% of these tumors arise within the joint cavity. In one patient with recurrent intraarticular synovial sarcoma, a nodule of malignant tissue was imaged adjacent to the anterior horn of the lateral meniscus.

Spotty calcification is present in 15% of cases, and the histopathologic pattern is biphasic with epithelial and spindled areas.[84] Synovial sarcomas have a propensity to metastasize to lymph nodes.

Magnetic Resonance Appearance. In a series of synovial sarcomas involving the ankle and foot, we used MR imaging to stage intra- and extraarticular involvement (Fig. 13–108). The propensity of synovial sarcoma to track along tendon sheaths and invade adjacent bone allowed prospective MR diagnosis in five of six cases studied. The lesions demonstrated low to intermediate signal intensity on T1-weighted images and were homogeneously bright on T2-weighted images. Small areas of central necrosis were demonstrated as regions of higher signal intensity. Focal calcifications, although detected on MR images, were better delineated on CT images. In a separate series of 12 cases of synovial sarcoma, a heterogeneous, multilocular mass with internal septation was the characteristic feature on MR images. Extensive loculations with multiple fluid–fluid levels secondary to hemorrhage were observed in three cases.[95] Infrapatellar fat-pad edema as well as recurrent tumor imaged with increased signal intensity in T2-weighted images (Fig. 13–109).

(text continues on page 1116)

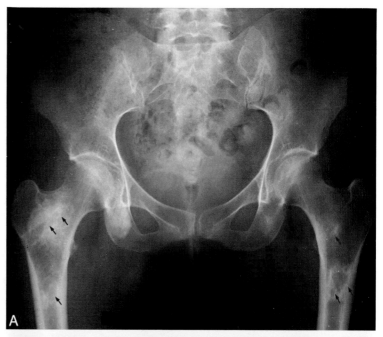

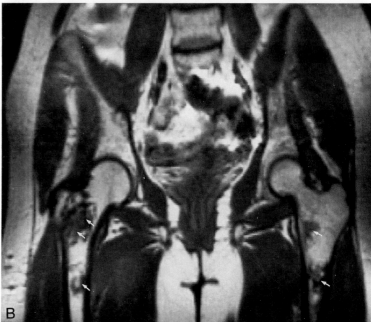

FIGURE 13-78. (A) An anteroposterior radiograph of the pelvis shows mixed lytic and sclerotic femoral lesions (*arrows*). (B) On the corresponding T1-weighted coronal image, metastatic deposits of medulloblastoma (*arrows*) demonstrate nonuniform low to intermediate signal intensity. (TR, 500 msec; TE, 40 msec.)

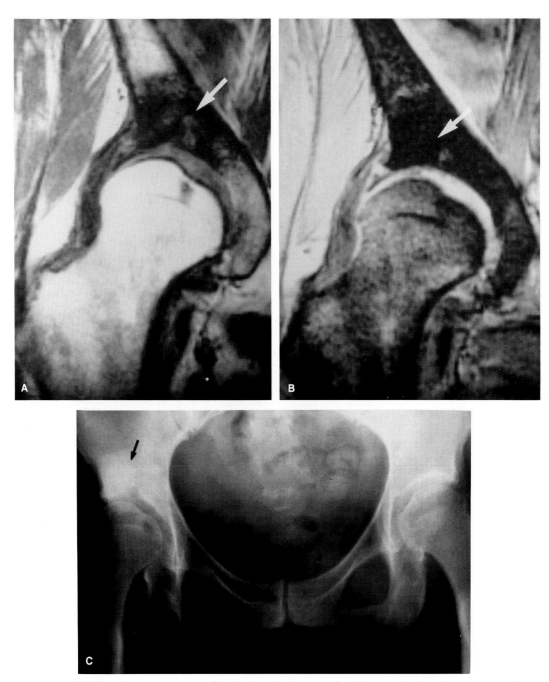

FIGURE 13–79. A large enostosis (*i.e.,* bone island; *arrows*) of the acetabulum demonstrates low signal intensity on coronal (**A**) T1-weighted and (**B**) T2*-weighted images. Without the aggressive features of soft-tissue mass or marrow hyperemia, this should not be diagnosed as a sclerotic metastasis. (**A**: TR, 500 msec; TE, 20 msec; **B**: TR, 400 msec; TE, 20 msec; flip angle, 25°.) (**C**) The corresponding antero-posterior radiograph shows a superior acetabular sclerotic focus (*arrow*).

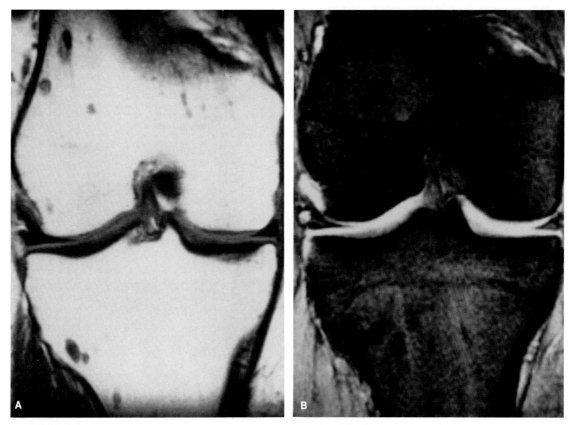

FIGURE 13–80. Asymptomatic low signal intensity multiple bone islands are seen on coronal (**A**) T1-weighted and (**B**) T2*-weighted knee images. The morphology and distribution of these islands are characteristic of osteopoikilosis. (**A**: TR, 600 msec; TE, 20 msec; **B**: TR, 400 msec; TE, 15 msec; flip angle, 20°.)

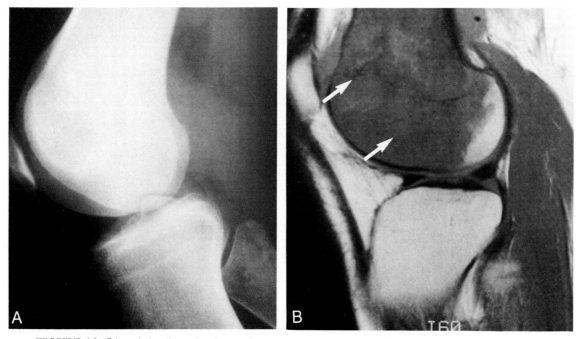

FIGURE 13–81. (**A**) A lateral radiograph is negative in a patient with osseous lymphoma. (**B**) On a T1-weighted sagittal image, low signal intensity lymphomatous marrow replacement is seen crossing the physeal scar and involving the subchondral bone (*arrows*). (TR, 800 msec; TE, 20 msec.)

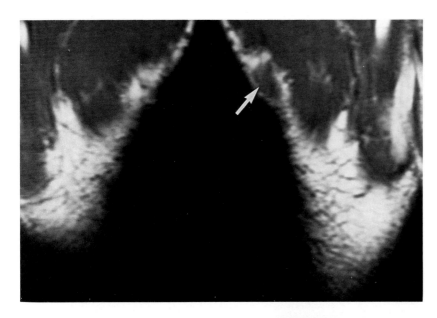

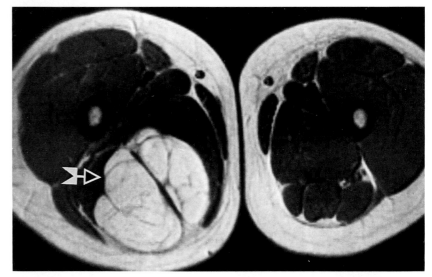

FIGURE 13–82. Low signal intensity xanthofibroma is seen scalloping the subcutaneous tissue on the medial plantar surface of the foot (*arrow*) on a T1-weighted axial image. (TR, 600 msec; TE, 20 msec.)

FIGURE 13–83. A lipoma (*arrow*) located between the semimembranosus and semitendinosus muscles demonstrates subcutaneous fat signal intensity on a T1-weighted axial image. (TR, 600 msec; TE, 20 msec.)

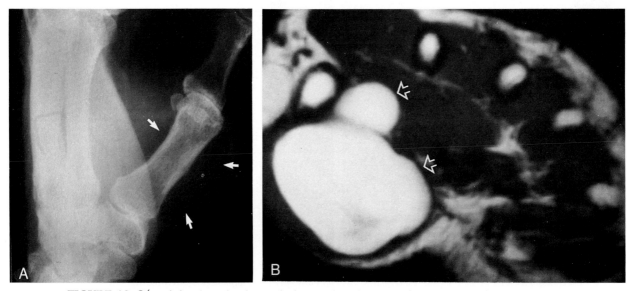

FIGURE 13–84. (**A**) A lateral radiograph shows a low-density, soft-tissue mass of thenar eminence (*arrows*). (**B**) The corresponding T1-weighted axial image shows multilobulated lipoma with subcutaneous and marrow signal intensity (*arrows*). (TR, 600 msec; TE, 20 msec.)

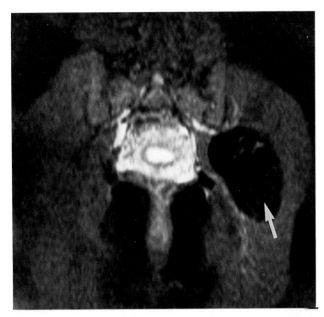

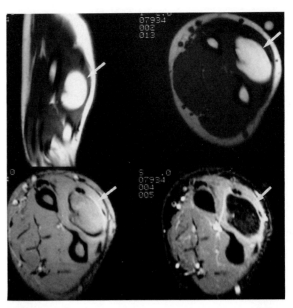

FIGURE 13–85. Lipoma of the left thigh (*arrow*) demonstrates nulled or dark fat signal intensity on a short TI inversion recovery image. (TR, 1400 msec; TI, 125 msec; TE, 40 msec.)

FIGURE 13–86. Lipoma (*arrows*) demonstrates bright fat signal intensity on T1-weighted sagittal (*top, left*) and axial (*top, right*) images. Lipomatous tissue is isointense with surrounding musculature and soft tissue on a T2*-weighted axial image (*bottom, left*); the tissue demonstrates dark signal intensity in an axial short TI inversion recovery image (*bottom, right*).

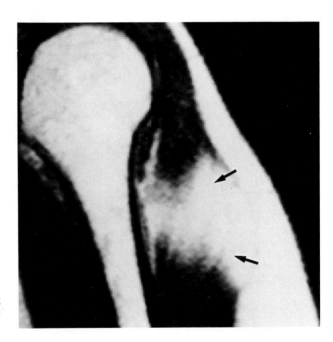

FIGURE 13–87. A high signal intensity lipoma (*arrows*) is infiltrating the deltoid muscle laterally on a T1-weighted coronal image. (TR, 500 msec; TE, 31 msec.)

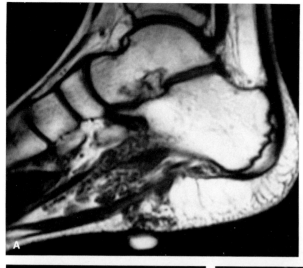

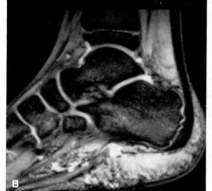

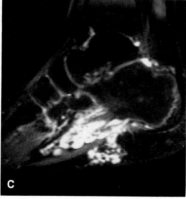

FIGURE 13–88. Hemangioma, with dilated, serpiginous vessels, in the plantar aspect of the foot demonstrates (**A**) low signal intensity on a T1-weighted sagittal image and bright signal intensity on (**B**) T2*-weighted and (**C**) short TI inversion recovery (STIR) images. Characteristic extension to the skin and subcutaneous tissues is most accurately defined on T1-weighted and STIR images. (**A**: TR, 600 msec; TE, 20 msec; **B**: TR, 400 msec; TE, 20 msec; flip angle, 25°; **C**: TR, 2000 msec; TI, 160 msec; TE, 43 msec.)

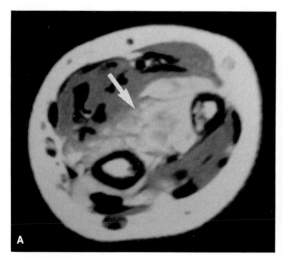

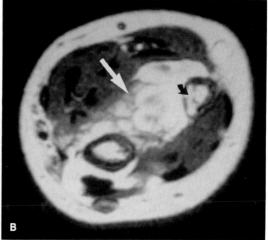

FIGURE 13–89. Axial (**A**) intermediate-weighted and (**B**) T2-weighted images show hyperintense hemangioma with lobulated, sinusoidal, blood-filled spaces (*straight arrows*). Marrow and cortex hemangiomatous tissue are shown (*curved arrow*).

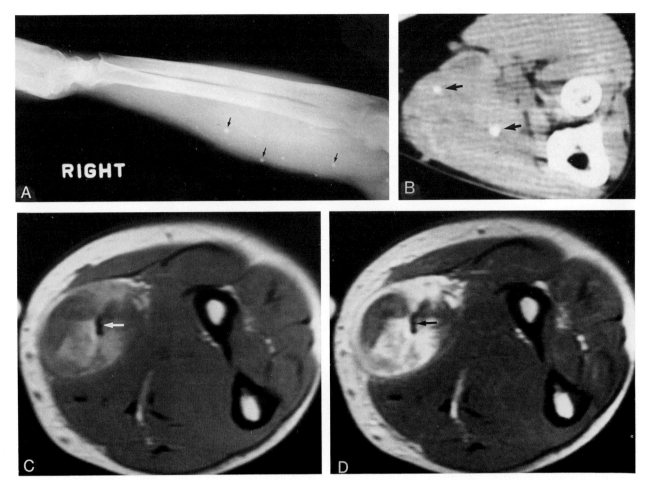

FIGURE 13–90. (**A**) A lateral radiograph shows a volar soft-tissue hemangioma with phleboliths (*arrows*) in the forearm. (**B**) An axial CT image demonstrates punctate calcifications and an indistinct soft-tissue mass within the pronator teres and flexor digitorum superficialis (*arrows*). Axial (**C**) intermediate-weighted and (**D**) T2-weighted images show a progressive increase in signal intensity. The central vessel, with signal void, is indicated (*arrows*). (**C, D**: TR, 2000 msec; TE, 20, 80 msec.)

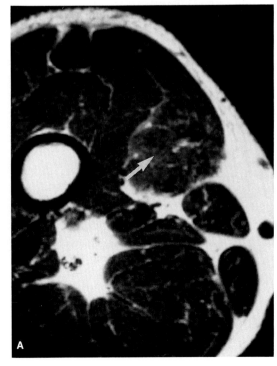

FIGURE 13–91. Soft-tissue hemangioma (*arrows*) involving the vastus medialis muscle is seen on axial (**A**) T1-weighted, (**B**) intermediate-weighted, and (**C**) T2-weighted images. Dilated vessels are isointense with muscle on the T1-weighted image and become hyperintense with progressive T2 weighting. (**A**: TR, 500 msec; TE, 20 msec; **B, C**: TR, 2000 msec; TE, 20, 80 msec.   *(continued)*

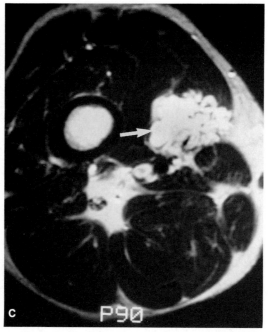

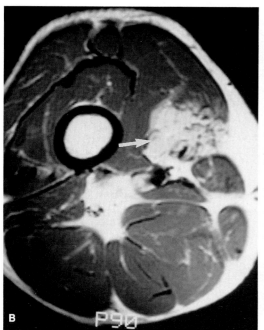

FIGURE 13–91. *(Continued)*

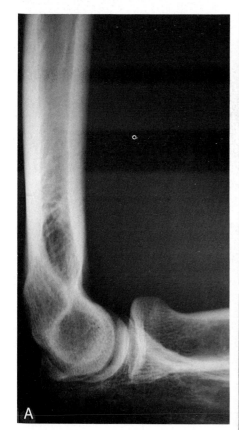

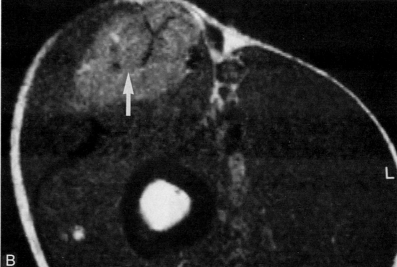

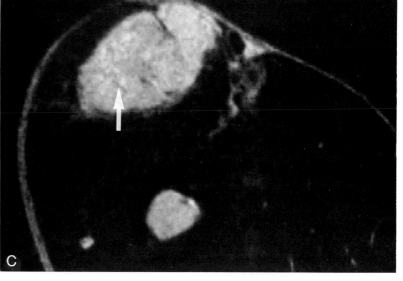

FIGURE 13–92. (**A**) A lateral radiograph of the distal humerus and elbow is normal. (**B**) On a T1-weighted image, an intermediate signal intensity soft-tissue hemangioma is revealed deep to the biceps brachii. (TR, 800 msec; TE, 20 msec.) (**C**) The hemangioma increases in signal intensity (*arrows*) on T2-weighted images. (TR, 2000 msec; TE, 80 msec.)

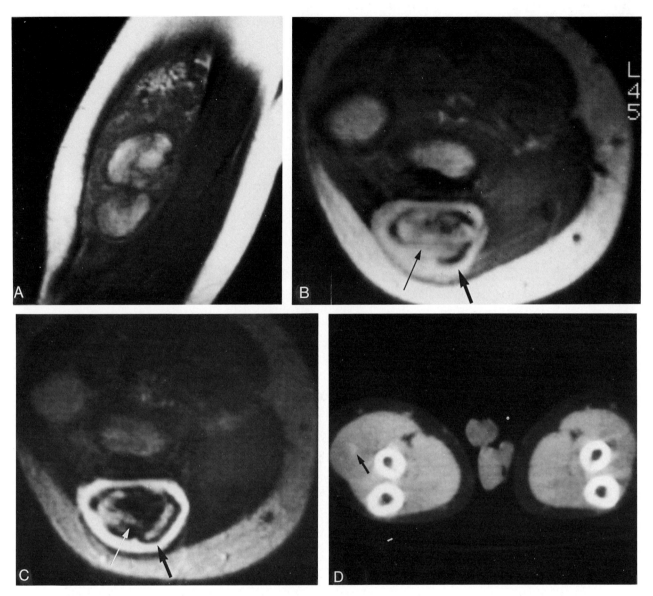

FIGURE 13–93. (**A**) On a T1-weighted coronal image of the forearm, hemorrhagic intramuscular hemangioma demonstrates high signal intensity elements. (TR, 800 msec; TE, 20 msec.) (**B**) On the corresponding T1-weighted axial image, a high signal intensity central portion (*thin arrow*) and a surrounding high signal intensity peripheral ring (*thick arrow*) can be seen. (TR, 800 msec; TE, 20 msec.) (**C**) With T2 weighting, the central hematoma (*white arrow*) becomes less intense due to the T2-shortening effect, whereas the outer core of more chronic blood and clot demonstrates bright signal intensity (*black arrow*). (TR, 2000 msec; TE, 80 msec.) (**D**) An axial CT scan shows a nonspecific soft-tissue mass with a focal area of high attenuation (*arrow*).

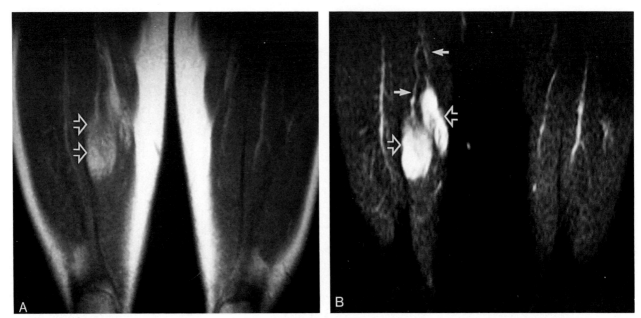

FIGURE 13–94. High signal intensity hemangioma (*open arrows*) of the vastus medialis muscle is seen on both (**A**) T1-weighted and (**B**) short TI inversion recovery (STIR) images. The supplying vessels demonstrate high signal intensity contrast in the STIR sequence (*solid arrows*). The symmetry of vessel size with adjacent vasculature excludes fistula from the differential diagnosis. (**A**: TR, 600 msec; TE, 20 msec; **B**: TR, 1400 msec; TI, 125 msec; TE, 40 msec.)

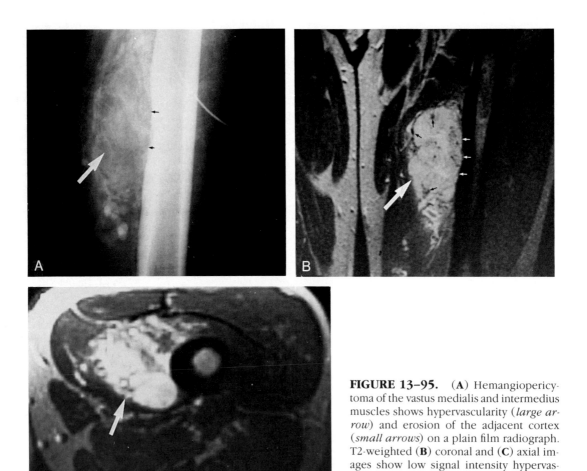

FIGURE 13–95. (**A**) Hemangiopericytoma of the vastus medialis and intermedius muscles shows hypervascularity (*large arrow*) and erosion of the adjacent cortex (*small arrows*) on a plain film radiograph. T2-weighted (**B**) coronal and (**C**) axial images show low signal intensity hypervascularity (*small black arrows*), cortical erosion (*small white arrows*), and bright signal intensity (*large arrow*). (**D**) The corresponding axial CT shows a vague soft-tissue mass. (**B**, **C**: TR, 2000 msec; TE, 60 msec.)

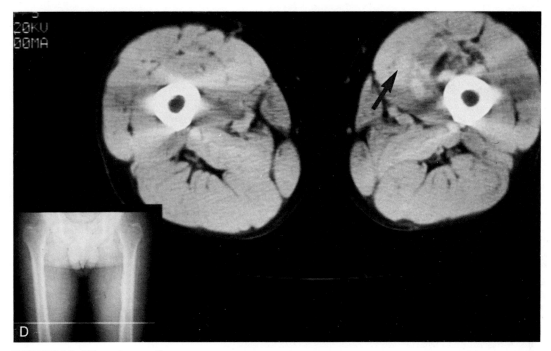

FIGURE 13–95. *(Continued)*

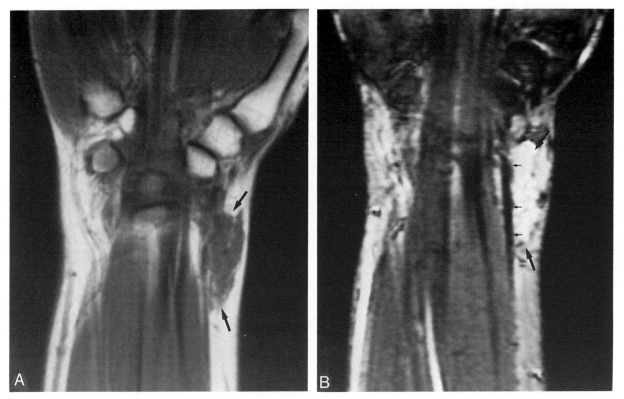

FIGURE 13–96. A synovial wrist ganglion (*large arrows*) associated with the flexor carpi radialis tendon (*small arrows*) is seen on coronal (**A**) T1-weighted and (**B**) T2*-weighted images, and on axial (**C**) T1-weighted and (**D**) T2-weighted images. The relationship of the cyst (*curved arrow*) to the flexor tendon (*medium arrow*) is evident on the axial image. Mucinous synovial contents demonstrate low signal intensity on T1-weighted images and high signal intensity on T2-weighted images. (**A, C**: TR, 600 msec; TE, 20 msec; **B**: TR, 400 msec; TE, 30 msec; flip angle, 30°; **D**: TR, 2000 msec; TE, 60 msec.)

(continued)

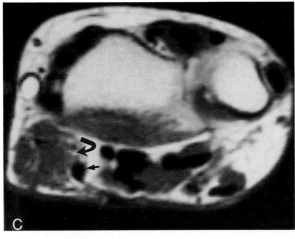

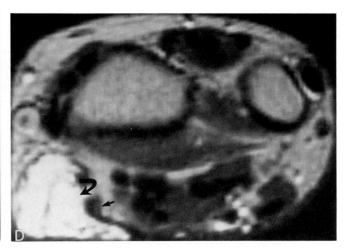

FIGURE 13–96. *(Continued)*

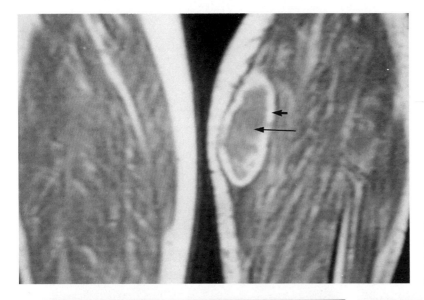

FIGURE 13–97. Soleus muscle hemorrhage (*long arrow*) with subacute blood demonstrates a high signal intensity periphery (*short arrow*) on T1-weighted coronal image. (TR, 800 msec; TE, 20 msec.)

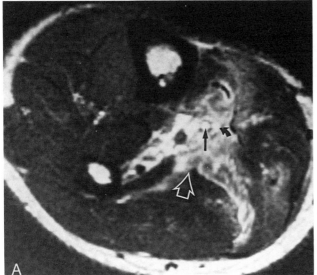

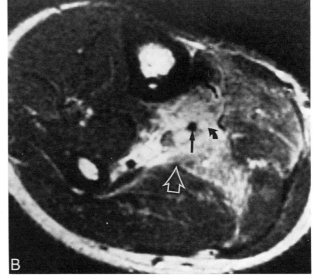

FIGURE 13–98. Arterial embolus. (**A**) Slow flow in the posterior tibial artery (*solid straight arrow*) and vein (*curved arrow*) demonstrates high signal intensity on T2-weighted axial image. Surrounding muscle edema (*open arrow*) demonstrates high signal intensity. (TR, 2000 msec; TE, 80 msec.) (**B**) Lack of flow in the posterior tibial artery on an inferior axial image is seen as signal void (*solid straight arrow*), whereas the adjacent vein maintains high signal intensity (*curved arrow*). Edema (*open arrow*) conforms to the regional arterial supply. (TR, 2000 msec; TE, 80 msec.)

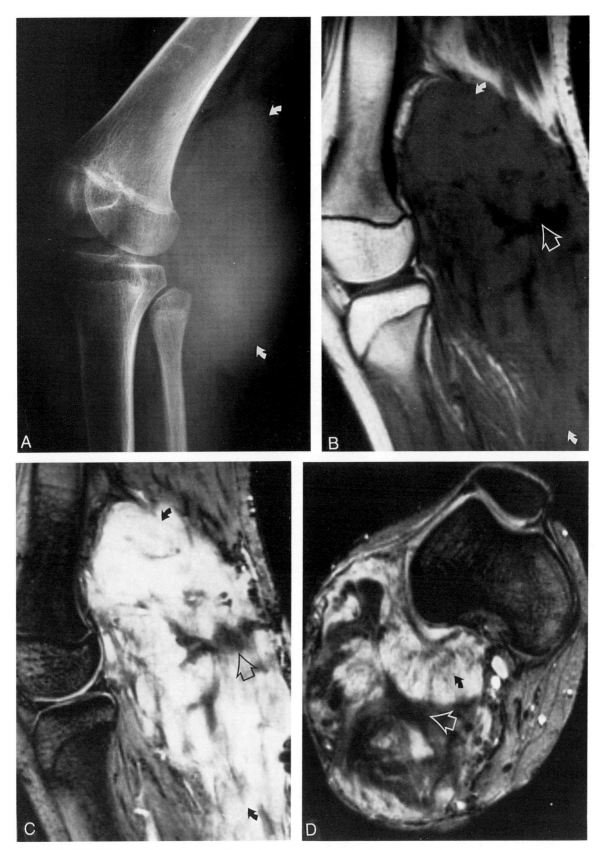

FIGURE 13–99. (**A**) A lateral radiograph shows a popliteal soft-tissue mass (*curved arrows*). (**B**) A T1-weighted sagittal image shows an intermediate signal intensity desmoid tumor (*curved arrows*) and dark signal intensity fibrous bands (*open arrow*). (TR, 600 msec; TE, 20 msec.) (**C**) Sagittal and (**D**) axial T2*-weighted images show a high signal intensity tumor (*curved arrows*) with low signal intensity fibrous stroma (*open arrows*). (TR, 400 msec; TE, 30 msec; flip angle, 30°.)

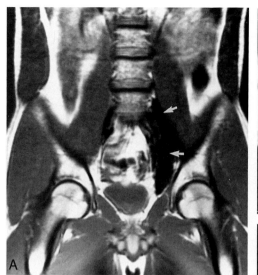

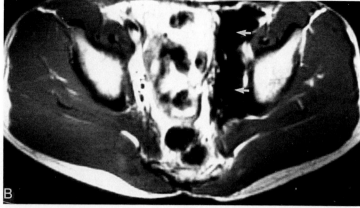

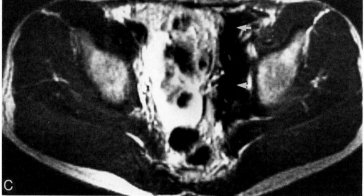

FIGURE 13–100. In juvenile fibromatosis, fibrous tissue demonstrates uniform low signal intensity (*arrows*) on T1-weighted (**A**) coronal and (**B**) axial images and on (**C**) a T2-weighted axial image. (**A, B**: TR, 800 msec; TE, 20 msec; **C**: TR, 2000 msec; TE, 80 msec.)

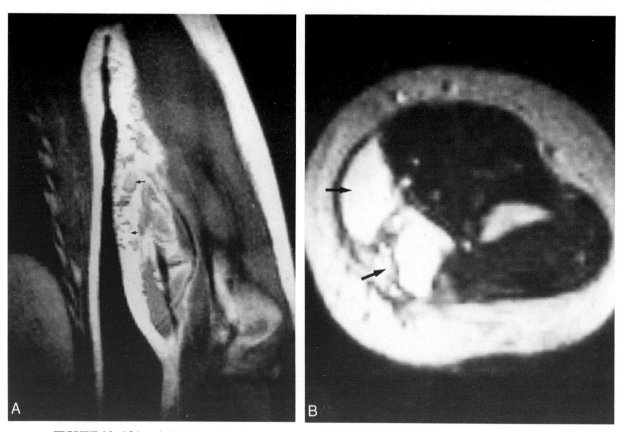

FIGURE 13–101. (**A**) A T1-weighted coronal image shows areas of inhomogeneous low signal intensity (*arrows*) in the axillary subcutaneous fat; these are indicative of cystic hygroma. (TR, 500 msec; TE, 40 msec.) (**B**) On a T2-weighted axial image through the upper arm, the fluid-filled cystic structures (*arrows*) demonstrate high signal intensity. (TR, 2000 msec; TE, 60 msec.)

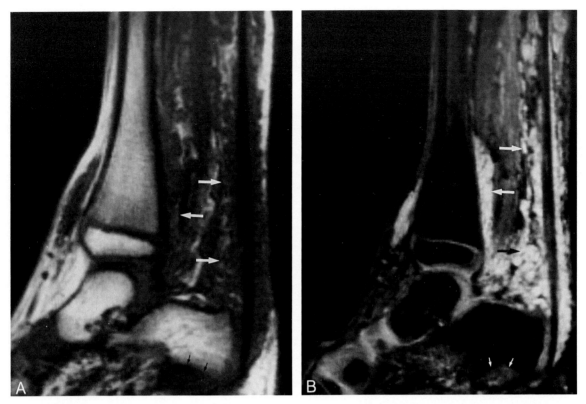

FIGURE 13–102. (**A**) T1-weighted and (**B**) T2*-weighted images of the ankle show low and high signal intensity, respectively, in a plexiform neurofibroma that courses longitudinally along the nerve bundles. Neurofibromas have a characteristic lobulated contour (*large arrows*). Undercutting or erosion of the inferior calcaneal surface is shown (*small arrows*). (**A**: TR, 600 msec; TE, 20 msec; **B**: TR, 400 msec; TE, 30 msec; flip angle, 30°.)

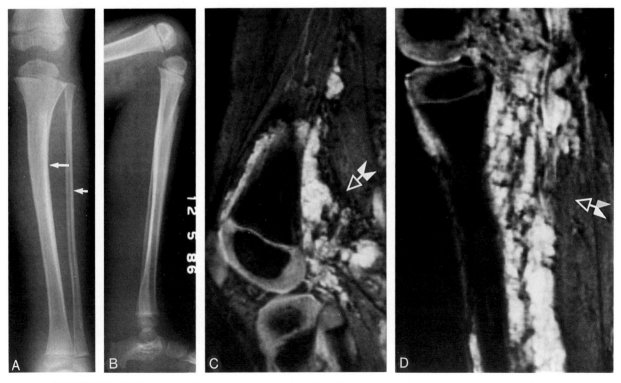

FIGURE 13–103. Neurofibromatosis in a 5-year-old child. Tibial dysplasia–bowing (*long arrow*) and a gracile fibula (*short arrow*) is seen on (**A**) anteroposterior and (**B**) lateral radiographs. On T2*-weighted images, high signal intensity plexiform neurofibromas (*flagged arrows*) can be seen from (**C**) the popliteal fossa to (**D**) the soft tissue posterior to the tibia. (**C, D**: TR, 400 msec; TE, 30 msec; flip angle, 30°.)

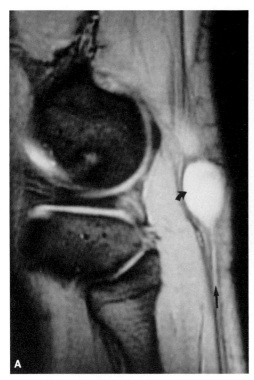

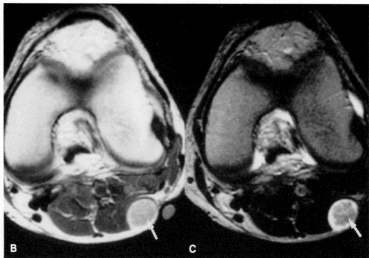

FIGURE 13–104. (**A**) On a sagittal T2*-weighted image, plexiform neurofibroma (*curved arrow*) of the common peroneal nerve (*straight arrow*). (TR, 600 msec; TE, 15 msec; flip angle, 20°.) On (**B**) intermediate-weighted and (**C**) T2-weighted images, individual distended fascicles (*arrows*) can be seen. (**B, C**: TR, 2000 msec; TE, 20, 80 msec.)

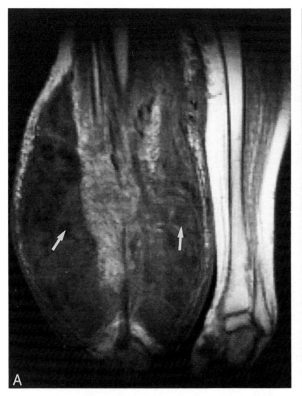

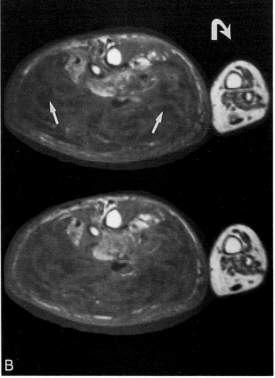

FIGURE 13–105. T1-weighted (**A**) coronal and (**B**) axial images show a large, infiltrating, nonplexiform neurofibroma invading and replacing soft-tissue elements in the leg. Lower signal intensity areas of inhomogeneity represent fibrous components (*straight arrows*). The opposite leg is shown for comparison (*curved arrow*). (TR, 500 msec; TE, 40 msec.)

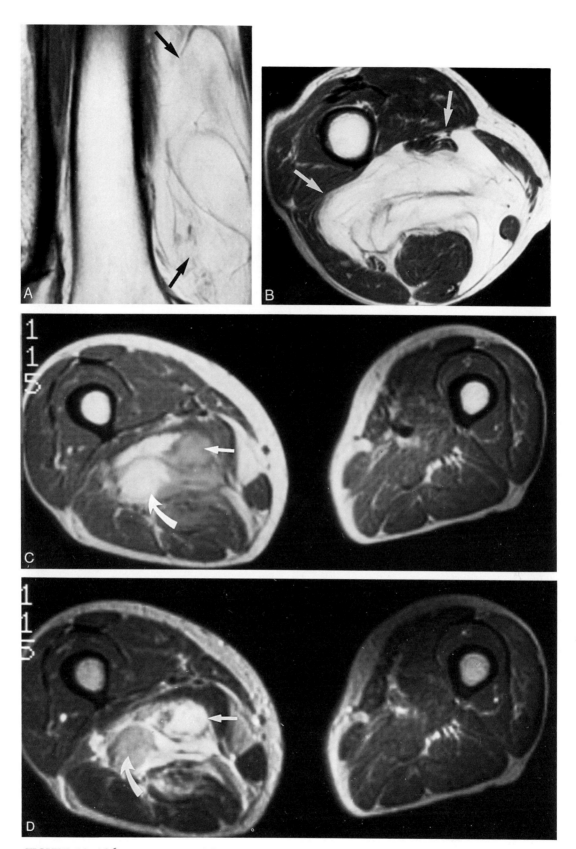

FIGURE 13–106.　T1-weighted (**A**) sagittal and (**B**) axial images through the distal femur display popliteal high signal intensity lipomatous tissue (*arrows*) in the popliteal fossa. (TR, 500 msec; TE, 20 msec.) (**C**) An intermediate-weighted axial image shows sarcomatous change at a lower signal intensity (*straight arrow*) than adjacent lipomatous tissue (*curved arrow*). (TR, 2000 msec; TE, 20 msec.) (**D**) Flip-flop of signal intensity occurs on a T2-weighted axial image—liposarcoma demonstrates high signal intensity (*straight arrow*), whereas the adjacent lipoma is isointense with subcutaneous fat (*curved arrow*). (TR, 2000 msec; TE, 60 msec.)

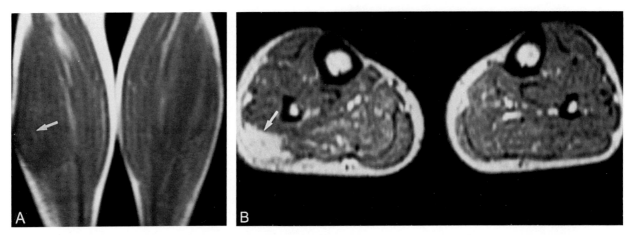

FIGURE 13–107. (**A**) A T1-weighted coronal image shows a posterolateral soft-tissue mass that is isointense with muscle (*arrow*). (TR, 600 msec; TE, 20 msec.) (**B**) The leiomyosarcoma (*arrow*) shows a uniform increase in signal intensity on the T2-weighted axial image. (TR, 2000 msec; TE, 60 msec.)

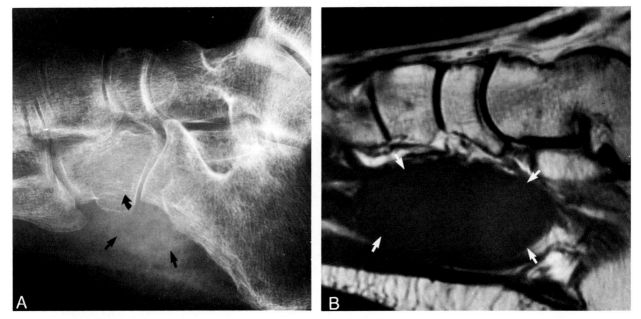

FIGURE 13–108. (**A**) A lateral radiograph shows a subtle plantar soft-tissue mass (*straight arrows*) of synovial sarcoma. Localized osteoporosis and distortion of normal trabecular lawn is seen in the adjacent cuboid (*curved arrow*). The corresponding sagittal (**B**) T1-weighted and (**C**) T2*-weighted images show a large, primary, soft-tissue synovial sarcoma (*arrows*) that demonstrates low and high signal intensity, respectively. (**B**: TR, 600 msec; TE, 20 msec; **C**: TR, 400 msec; TE, 30 msec; flip angle, 30°.) (**D**) An axial T2-weighted image shows cuboid bone invasion (*solid arrows*) and the proximity of the sarcoma to the flexor and peroneal tendons (*open arrows*). (TR, 2000 msec; TE, 60 msec.)

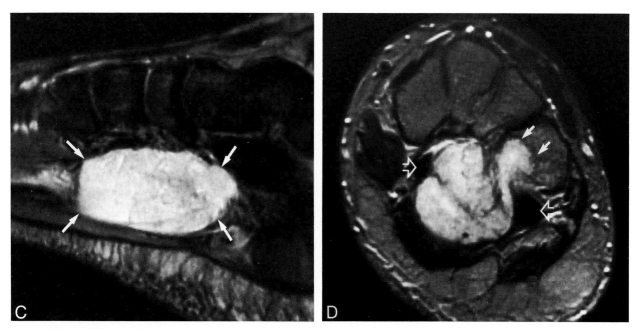

FIGURE 13–108. *(Continued)*

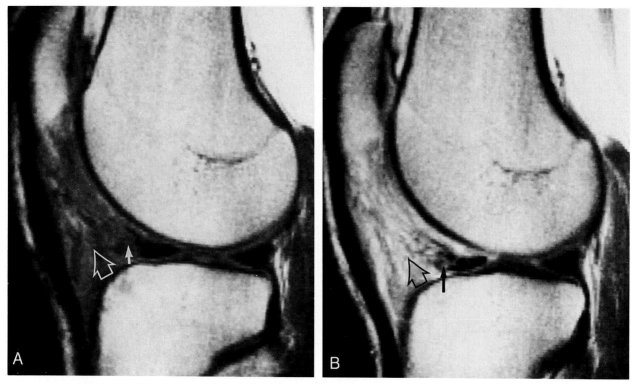

FIGURE 13–109. A recurrent intraarticular synovial sarcoma nodule is seen adjacent to the anterior horn of the lateral meniscus on sagittal (**A**) T1-weighted and (**B**) T2-weighted images. Infrapatellar fat-pad edema (*open arrows*) and sarcoma (*solid arrows*) demonstrate low signal intensity on the T1-weighted image and high signal intensity on the T2-weighted image.

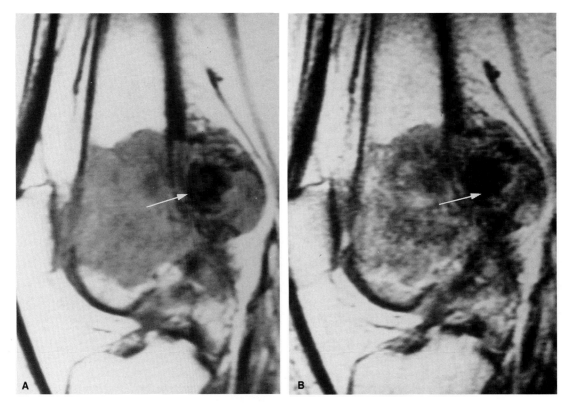

FIGURE 13–110.   Malignant fibrous histiocytoma is manifest as a destructive lesion of the distal femur with subchondral extension and an extraosseous soft-tissue component (*arrows*). The lesion demonstrates (**A**) intermediate signal intensity on the T1-weighted sagittal image and (**B**) signal heterogeneity on the T2-weighted sagittal image.

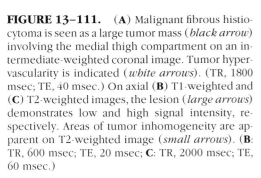

FIGURE 13–111.   (**A**) Malignant fibrous histio-cytoma is seen as a large tumor mass (*black arrow*) involving the medial thigh compartment on an in-termediate-weighted coronal image. Tumor hyper-vascularity is indicated (*white arrows*). (TR, 1800 msec; TE, 40 msec.) On axial (**B**) T1-weighted and (**C**) T2-weighted images, the lesion (*large arrows*) demonstrates low and high signal intensity, re-spectively. Areas of tumor inhomogeneity are ap-parent on T2-weighted image (*small arrows*). (**B**: TR, 600 msec; TE, 20 msec; **C**: TR, 2000 msec; TE, 60 msec.)

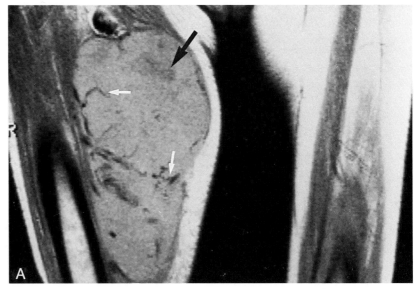

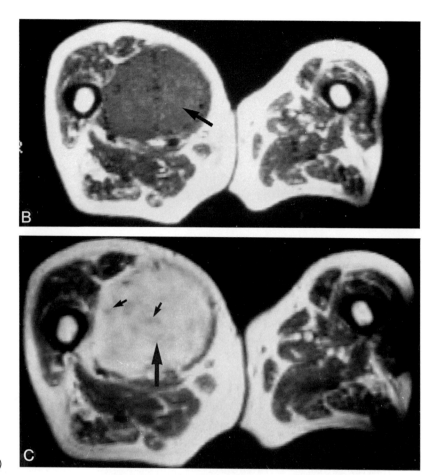

FIGURE 13–111. *(Continued)*

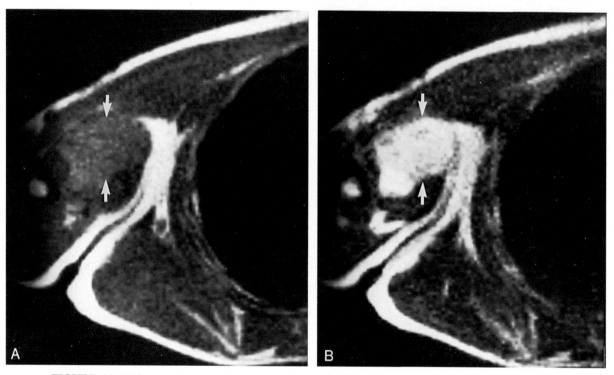

FIGURE 13–112. A soft-tissue fibrosarcoma (*arrows*) of the upper arm involves the biceps brachii muscle group medially. The tumor demonstrates (**A**) low signal intensity on a T1-weighted axial image and (**B**) high signal intensity on a T2-weighted axial image. (**A**: TR, 500 msec; TE, 28 msec; **B**: TR, 1500 msec; TE, 56 msec.)

Malignant Fibrous Histiocytoma

Malignant fibrous histiocytoma of both bone and soft tissue has been characterized on MR images (Figs. 13–110 and 13–111).[96] Malignant fibrous histiocytoma is a soft-tissue sarcoma that occurs most frequently in patients 50 to 70 years of age. Areas of hemorrhage and necrosis are common within this often large, multinodular, hypervascular tumor. Magnetic resonance features of MFH are nonspecific. Signal inhomogeneity with low to intermediate intensity on T1-weighted images and high intensity on T2-weighted images reflect the distribution of hemorrhage, necrosis, and calcification. Low signal intensity vessels correspond to hypervascular regions of the tumor.

Fibrosarcoma

Fibrosarcoma is a rare malignant tumor with a fibrous, proliferative matrix devoid of any cartilage, osteoid, or bone. Fibrosarcoma of bone has a poorer prognosis than primary soft-tissue fibrosarcoma.[96] Magnetic resonance characteristics of fibrosarcoma include low signal intensity on T1-weighted images, reflecting histologic differentiation, and uniform high signal intensity on T2-weighted images (Fig. 13–112).[97] In one case of soft-tissue fibrosarcoma involving the upper arm, the lesion was identified without evidence of cortical transgression. Fibrosarcomas that occur in children are different from those seen in adults. In children, the tumor usually occurs within the first 2 years of life, and the prognosis is more favorable than in adults.

REFERENCES

1. Zimmer WD, et al. Magnetic resonance imaging of bone tumors: comparison with CT. Radiology 1985;155:709.
2. Bloem JL, et al. Magnetic resonance imaging of primary malignant bone tumors. RadioGraphics 1987;7:425.
3. Wetzel LH, et al. A comparison of MR imaging and CT in the evaluation of musculoskeletal masses. RadioGraphics 1987;7:851.
4. Petasnick JP, et al. Soft-tissue masses of the locomotor system: comparison of MR imaging with CT. Radiology 1986;160:125.
5. Totty WG, et al. Soft tissue tumors: MR imaging. Radiology 1986;160:135.
6. Tehranzadeh J, et al. Comparison of CT and MR imaging in musculoskeletal neoplasms. J Comput Assist Tomogr 1989;13:466.
7. Dalinka NK, et al. Use of magnetic resonance imaging in the evaluation of bone and soft-tissue tumors. Radiol Clin North Am 1990;28:461.
8. Lenkinski RE, et al. Combined MR imaging and spectroscopy of bone and soft tissue tumors. J Comput Assist Tomogr 1990;14:1.
9. Sundaram M, et al. MR imaging of tumor and tumorlike lesions of bone and soft tissue. AJR 1990;155:817.
10. Porter B, et al. Magnetic resonance imaging of bone marrow disorders. Radiol Clin North Am 1986;24:269.
11. Golfieri R, et al. Role of the STIR sequence in magnetic resonance imaging examination of bone tumours. Br J Radiol 1990;63:251.
12. Erlemann R. Musculoskeletal neoplasms: dynamic Gd-DTPA-enhanced MR imaging: reply. Radiology 1990;177:288.
13. Erlemann R, et al. Musculoskeletal neoplasms: fast low-angle shot MR imaging with and without Gd-DTPA. Radiology 1990;176:489.
14. Erlemann R, et al. Musculoskeletal neoplasms: static and dynamic Gd-DTPA-enhanced MR imaging. Radiology 1989;171:767.
15. Pettersson H, et al. Musculoskeletal tumors: T1 and T2 relaxation times. Radiology 1988;167:783.
16. Tsai JC, et al. Fluid-fluid level: a nonspecific finding in tumors of bone and soft tissue. Radiology 1990;175:779.
17. Mirra JM, Picci P. Tumors of fat. In: Mirra J, ed. Bone tumors—clinical, radiologic, and pathologic correlations. Philadelphia: Lea & Febiger, 1989:1480.
18. Lichentenstein L. Osteoid osteoma. In: Lichentenstein L, ed. Bone tumors. 5th ed. St. Louis: CV Mosby, 1977:89.
19. Cohen MD, Herrington TM, et al. Osteoid osteoma: 95 cases and a review of the literature. Semin Arthritis Rheum 1983;12:265.
20. Resnick D, Kyriakos M, Greenway G. Tumors and tumorlike lesions of bone: imaging and pathology of specific lesions. In: Resnick D, Niwayama G, eds. Diagnosis of bone and joint disorders. 2nd ed. Philadelphia: WB Saunders, 1988:3621.
21. Harms SE, et al. MRI of the musculoskeletal system. In: Scott WW, et al, eds. CT of the musculoskeletal system. New York: Churchill-Livingstone, 1987:171.
22. Glass RBG, et al. MR imaging of osteoid osteoma. J Comput Assist Tomogr 1986;10:1065.
23. Schlesinger AE, et al. Intracapsular osteoid osteoma of the proximal femur: findings on plain films and CT. AJR 1990;154:1241.
24. Kroon HM, et al. Osteoblastoma: clinical and radiologic findings in 98 new cases. Radiology 1990;175:783.
25. Crim JR, et al. Widespread inflammatory response to osteoblastoma: the flare phenomenon. Radiology 1990;177:835.
26. Milgram JW. The origin of osteochondromas and enchondromas: a histopathologic study. Clin Orthop 1983;174:264.
27. Liu J, et al. Bone sarcomas associated with Ollier's disease. Cancer 1987;59:1376.
28. Crim JR, et al. Enchondroma protuberans: report of a case and its distinction from chondrosarcoma and osteochondroma adjacent to an enchondroma. Skeletal Radiol 1980;19:431.
29. Unger EC, et al. MR imaging of Maffucci syndrome. AJR 1988;150:351.
30. Evans HL, et al. Prognostic factors in chondrosarcoma of bone. A clinicopathologic analysis with emphasis on histologic grading. Cancer 1977;40:818.
31. Cotran R, et al. The musculoskeletal system. In: Cotran R, et al, eds. Robbins' pathologic basis of disease. Philadelphia: WB Saunders, 1989;1336.
32. Springfield DS, et al. Chondroblastoma: a review of 70 cases. J Bone Joint Surg [Am] 1985;67:748.
33. Greenspan A. Orthopaedic radiology: a practical approach. Gower, 1988:15.2.
34. Brower AC, et al. Frequency and diagnostic significance of periostitis in chondroblastoma. AJR 1990;154:309.
35. Fletcher BD, et al. Musculoskeletal neoplasms: dynamic Gd-DTPA-enhanced MR imaging. Radiology 1990;177:287.
36. Ruiter DJ, von Rijssel TG, VanderVelde EA. Aneurysmal bone cysts: a clinicopathological study of 105 cases. Cancer 1977;39:2231.
37. Kaufman RA, Towbin RB. Telangiectatic osteosarcoma simulating the appearance of an aneurysmal bone cyst. Pediatr Radiol 1982;11:102.
38. Huvos AG, Rosen G, Bretsky SS, Butler A. Telangiectatic osteogenic sarcoma: a clinicopathologic study of 124 patients. Cancer 1982;49:1679.
39. Munk PL, et al. MR imaging of aneurysmal bone cysts. AJR 1989;153:99.
40. Beltran J, et al. Aneurysmal bone cysts: MR imaging at 1.5T. Radiology 1985;158:689.

41. Moore SG. Tumors of the musculoskeletal system. In: Cohen MD, ed. Magnetic resonance imaging of children. Philadelphia: BC Decker, 1990.

42. Mirra JM. Vascular tumors. In: Mirra J, ed. Bone tumors—clinical, radiologic, and pathologic correlations. Philadelphia: Lea & Febiger, 1989:1335.

43. Milgram JW. Intraosseous lipomas: radiologic and pathologic manifestations. Radiology 1988;167:155.

44. Munk PL, et al. Immature bone infarcts: findings on plain radiographs and MR scans. AJR 1989;152:547.

45. Haggstrom JA, et al. Eosinophilic granuloma of the spine: MR demonstration. J Comput Assist Tomogr 1988;12:344.

46. Mirra J. Giant cell tumors. In: Mirra J, ed. Bone tumors—clinical, radiologic, and pathologic correlations. Philadelphia: Lea & Febiger, 1989:941.

47. Eckardt JJ, Grogan TJ. Giant cell tumors of bone. Clin Orthop 1986;204:45.

48. Brandy TJ, et al. NMR imaging of forearms in healthy volunteers and patients with giant-cell tumors of bone. Radiology 1982;144:549.

49. Mosrer RP, et al. Giant cell tumor of the upper extremity. Radiographics 1990;10:83.

50. Stark DD, Bradley WG, eds. Magnetic resonance imaging. St Louis: CV Mosby, 1988:1323.

51. Herman SD, et al. The role of magnetic resonance imaging in giant cell tumor of bone. Skeletal Radiol 1987;16:635.

52. Mirra J, Gold R, Picci P. Osseous tumors of intramedullary origin. In: Mirra J, ed. Bone tumors—clinical, radiologic, and pathologic correlations. Philadelphia: Lea & Febiger, 1989:303.

53. Picci P, Bacci G, Companacci M, et al. Histologic evaluation of necrosis in osteosarcoma induced by chemotherapy. Regional mapping of viable and nonviable tumor. Cancer 1985;56:1515.

54. Seeger LL, et al. Cross-sectional imaging in the evaluation of osteogenic sarcoma. Semin Roentgenol 1989;24:174.

55. Farr G, Huvos A. Juxtacortical osteogenic sarcoma. An analysis of fourteen cases. J Bone Joint Surg [Am] 1972;54:1205.

56. Companacci M, Picci P, et al. Parosteal osteosarcoma. J Bone Joint Surg [Am] 1984;66:313.

57. Mirra J, ed. Bone tumors—clinical, radiologic, and pathologic correlations. Philadelphia: Lea & Febiger, 1989:1743.

58. Gillespy T III, et al. Staging of intraosseous extent of osteosarcoma: correlation of preoperative CT and MR imaging with pathologic macroslides. Radiology 1988;167:765.

59. Hopper KD, et al. Osteosarcomatosis. Radiology 1990;175:233.

60. Holscher HC, et al. Value of MR imaging in monitoring the effect of chemotherapy in bone sarcomas. AJR 1990;154:763.

61. Pan G, et al. Osteosarcoma: MR imaging after preoperative chemotherapy. Radiology 1990;174:517.

62. Sanchez RB, et al. Musculoskeletal neoplasms after intraarterial chemotherapy: correlation of MR images with pathologic specimens. Radiology 1990;175:237.

63. Cohen EK, et al. Hyaline cartilage-origin bone and soft tissue neoplasms: MR appearance and histologic correlation. Radiology 1988;167:477.

64. Yunis EJ. Ewing's sarcoma and related small round cell neoplasms in children. Am J Surg Pathol 1986;10(Suppl):54.

65. Turc-Carel C, Phillip T, Berger MP, et al. Chromosome study of Ewing's sarcoma (ES) cell lines. Consistency of a reciprocal translocation (11:22) (q24:q12). Cancer Genet Cytogenet 1984;12:1.

66. Boyko OB, et al. MR imaging of osteogenic and Ewing's sarcoma. AJR 1987;148:317.

67. Frouge C, et al. Role of magnetic resonance imaging in the evaluation of Ewing's sarcoma: a report of 27 cases. Skeletal Radiol 1988;17:387.

68. Frassica DA, et al. Solitary plasmacytoma of bone: Mayo Clinic experience. Int J Radiat Oncol Biol Phys 1989;16:43.

69. Huvos AG. Adamantinoma of long bones. A clinicopathologic study of fourteen cases with vascular origin suggested. J Bone Joint Surg [Am] 1975;57:148.

70. Gold RH, et al. Integrated approach to the evaluation of metastatic bone disease. Radiol Clin North Am 1990;28:471.

71. Avrahami E, et al. Early MR demonstration of spinal metastases in patients with normal radiographs and CT and radionuclide bone scans. J Comput Assist Tomogr 1989;13:598.

72. Colman LK, et al. Early diagnosis of spinal metastases by CT and MR studies. J Comput Assist Tomogr 1988;12:423.

73. Smoker WRK, et al. The role of MR imaging in evaluating metastatic spinal disease. AJR 1987;149:1241.

74. Boston H, et al. Malignant lymphoma (so-called reticulum cell sarcoma) of bone. Cancer 1974;34:1131.

75. Ostrowski M, et al. Malignant lymphoma of bone. Cancer 1986;12:2646.

76. Demas BE, et al. Soft-tissue sarcomas of the extremities: comparison of MR and CT in determining the extent of disease. AJR 1988;150:615.

77. Kransdorf MJ, et al. Soft-tissue masses: diagnosis using MR imaging. AJR 1989;153:541.

78. Sundaram M, et al. Magnetic resonance imaging of soft tissue masses: an evaluation of 53 histologically proven tumors. Magn Res Imag 1988;6:237.

79. Berquist TH, et al. Value of MR imaging in differentiating benign from malignant soft-tissue masses: study of 95 lesions. AJR 1990;155:1251.

80. Sundaram M, et al. Soft-tissue masses: histologic basis for decreased signal (short T2) on T2-weighted MR images. AJR 1987;148:1247.

81. Herrlin K, et al. Gadolinium-DTPA enhancement of soft tissue tumors in magnetic resonance imaging. Acta Radiol 1990;31:233.

82. Fletcher BD, et al. Musculoskeletal neoplasms: dynamic Gd-DTPA-enhanced MR imaging. Radiology 1990;177:287.

83. Quinn SF, et al. MR imaging in fibromatosis: results in 26 patients with pathologic correlation. AJR 1991;156:539.

84. Braaks J. Disorders of soft tissue. In: Sternberg S, ed. Diagnostic surgical pathology. vol. 1. New York: Raven, 1989:161.

85. Buetow, PC, et al. Radiologic appearance of intramuscular hemangioma with emphasis on MR imaging. AJR 1990;154:563.

86. Hawnaur JM, et al. Musculoskeletal hemangiomas: comparison of MRI with CT. Skeletal Radiol 1990;19:251.

87. Bullough P. Joint diseases. In: Sternberg S, ed. Diagnostic surgical pathology. vol. 1. New York: Raven, 1989:214.

88. Sundaram M, et al. Synchronous multicentric desmoid tumors (aggressive fibromatosis) of the extremities. Skeletal Radiol 1988;17:16.

89. McCarthy SM, et al. Magnetic resonance imaging of fetal anomalies in utero: early experience. AJR 1985;145:677.

90. Levine E, et al. Malignant nerve-sheath neoplasms in neurofibromatosis: distinction from benign tumors by using imaging techniques. AJR 1987;149:1059.

91. Sundaram M, et al. Myxoid liposarcoma: magnetic resonance imaging appearances with clinical and histological correlation. Skeletal Radiol 1990;19:359.

92. Dooms GC, et al. Lipomatous tumors and tumors with fatty component: MR imaging potential and comparison of MR and CT results. Radiology 1985;157:479.

93. London J, et al. MR imaging of liposarcomas: correlation of MR features and histology. J Comput Assist Tomogr 1989;13:832.

94. Tsumyoshi M. Synovial sarcoma: a clinicopathologic and ultrastructural study of 42 cases. Acta Pathol 1983;33:23.

95. Morton MJ, et al. MR imaging of synovial sarcoma. AJR 1991;156:337.

96. Petasnick JP, et al. Soft-tissue masses of the locomotor system: comparison of MR imaging with CT. Radiology 1986;160:125.

97. Beltran J, et al. Gadopentetate dimeglumine-enhanced MR imaging of the musculoskeletal system. AJR 1991;156:457.

Index

Page numbers followed by *f* indicate figures; those followed by *t* indicate tables.

ISBN 0-397-51144-2

9 780397 511440